Essentials of
HUMAN DISEASES *and* CONDITIONS

7TH EDITION

Essentials of

HUMAN DISEASES and CONDITIONS

7TH EDITION

MARGARET SCHELL FRAZIER

RN, CMA (AAMA), BS

Retired

Former Chair, Health and Human Services
   Division
Program Chair, Medical Assisting Program
Ivy Tech State College, Northeast
Fort Wayne, Indiana
Clinical Director
Faith Community Health Clinic
Angola, Indiana

Presently

President/Consultant/Author, M & M Consulting
Hudson, Indiana

TRACIE FUQUA

BS, CMA (AAMA)

Program Director and Instructor
Medical Assisting Program
Wallace State Community College
Hanceville, Alabama

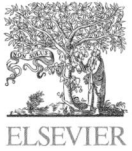

ELSEVIER

Elsevier
3251 Riverport Lane
St. Louis, Missouri 63043

ESSENTIALS OF HUMAN DISEASES
AND CONDITIONS, SEVENTH EDITION

ISBN: 978-0-323-71267-5

Notice

Practitioners and researchers must always rely on their own experience and knowledge in evaluating
and using any information, methods, compounds or experiments described herein. Because of rapid
advances in the medical sciences, in particular, independent verification of diagnoses and drug dosages
should be made. To the fullest extent of the law, no responsibility is assumed by Elsevier, authors,
editors or contributors for any injury and/or damage to persons or property as a matter of products
liability, negligence or otherwise, or from any use or operation of any methods, products, instructions,
or ideas contained in the material herein.

Previous editions copyrighted 2016, 2013, 2009, 2004, 2000, and 1996.

Library of Congress Control Number: 2020942171

Director, Private Sector Education Content: Kristin Wilhelm
Director, Content Development: Laurie Gower
Senior Content Development Specialist: Rebecca Leenhouts
Publishing Services Manager: Julie Eddy
Senior Project Manager: Abigail Bradberry
Design Direction: Brian Salisbury

Printed in China

Last digit is the print number: 9 8 7 6 5 4 3 2 1

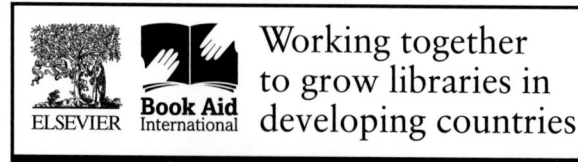

Contributors and Reviewers

CONTRIBUTORS

Brandon Brooks, BS, CPhT
Program Director–Pharmacy Technology
Wallace State Community College
Hanceville, Alabama

Cindy Pavel, MPA, CMA (AAMA)
Program Director
Medical Assistant Program
North Idaho College
Coeur d'Alene, Idaho

REVIEWERS

Tonya Alleshouse RN, IBCLC
Obstetrics Nurse
Parkview Noble Hospital
Kendallville, Indiana

Brandon Brooks, BS, CPhT
Program Director–Pharmacy Technology
Wallace State Community College
Hanceville, Alabama

Patricia A. Brubaker BSN, RN
Retired
Cameron Memorial Community Hospital
Angola, Indiana

Louise L. Crago, BGS, CMA (AAMA), CPhT, HIT
Health Education Coordinator, Apprenticeship Program
    Coordinator
Alaska Primary Care Association
Anchorage, Alaska

Diane Howe, MSN, RN, FNP-C
Family Nurse Practitioner
Cameron Memorial Community Hospital
Angola, Indiana

Cindy Pavel, MPA, CMA (AAMA)
Program Director
Medical Assistant Program
North Idaho College
Coeur d'Alene, Idaho

Acknowledgments

Special thanks go to the Elsevier experts involved in the publication of this text. We gratefully acknowledge Kristin Wilhelm, Director, Private Sector Education, for her guidance and suggestions during the rewriting of this book. We also thank Rebecca Leenhouts, Senior Content Development Specialist, for her patience while interpreting our files and arranging them all in an acceptable form. It was a pleasure working with her. We are grateful to Abigail Bradberry, Senior Project Manager, for her expert diligence as she prepared our words and illustrations as final pages for print.

Recognition goes to our contributing authors and many professional reviewers: Brandon Brooks, BS; K. Minchella; Cindy Pavel, MPA, CMA(AAMA); Diane Howe, FPN; Patricia Brubaker, BSN; Tonya Alleshouse, RN, IBCLC; Louise Crago, CMA(AAMA).

Appreciation goes to Mischelle R Quegan, RN; Mary Adomaitis, MSEd; Margaret (Pegi) Boswell MS, LFMT; and Aggie Osterholt-Poulston, MSW-LCSW for being there to kindly answer my many questions about their experiences with children dealing with mass shootings, with PANDAS, with their experiences with individuals and the opioid crisis and with suicidal individuals and grieving. They provided me with observations about pet therapy and assistance animals.

A special acknowledgment goes to Brandon Brooks who answered our many questions regarding pharmaceutical products and medications. We are grateful to Brandon for sharing his knowledge of pharmaceuticals with us.

Special recognition and gratitude goes to Jeanette Drzymkowski, RN, BS for the many years that we worked together as authors to produce previous editions.

To my family that was patient with and understanding of me through the past 25 years I have been working on these books, a huge thank you is expressed.

Finally, to Tracie Fuqua, it has been a long friendship through AAMA and writing years. Tracie you stepped in when I was injured and have been of great assistance to me and the rest of the development and production team. Thanks.

Thanks and hugs to all. Margie

To Dave, my forever soulmate and the love of my life.
Our love for each other has sustained me as you traveled into the sunset.
To my parents, Alfred O. and Emma M. Schell, thank you for believing in me.

Hugs and Love, Margie

To my husband of 24 years Michael David, and our children Ethan and Kaitlynn,
for always showing me their love and support. To my parents John and Ann Griffin,
for teaching me to work hard and be thankful for my blessings. To my sister Lisa Pipes
who is my rock as we both care for our aged parents.
And to Margie for showing her faith in me as her co-author for this edition.

Love you always, Tracie

Preface

Essentials of Human Diseases and Conditions, Seventh Edition, is a user-friendly reference intended to serve as a stimulating and practical textbook for students and an invaluable tool as a handbook for health care providers in any type of health care setting. Instructors of anatomy and physiology, disease conditions, medical insurance coding, pharmacology, massage therapy, and medical transcription may appreciate the value of this edition as a required text. This encyclopedic, but simplified, handbook includes comprehensive information on hundreds of diseases and conditions. Students in the field of medical assisting, medical transcription, medical insurance coding, pharmacy technology, massage therapy, or other allied health programs with prior introduction to basic anatomy and physiology of the human body and medical terminology will find the text format orderly, concise, and easy to comprehend.

Because the *International Statistical Classification of Diseases and Related Health Problems*, 10th edition (ICD-10) is the preferred resource for diagnostic codes, references to ICD-9 have been removed from this edition.

Distinctive Features of Our Approach

Content and topics new to this edition include the following:
- In Chapter 2, two updated illustrations of premature infants have been added. Another new illustration of 2.6-oz premature infant has been added. Discussion on a drug recently approved by the U.S. Food and Drug Administration (FDA) for the treatment of Duchenne muscular dystrophy is included. New approaches to drug therapy for cystic fibrosis have evolved and are now included. An Alert box regarding the importance of vaccines has been added.
- Chapter 3 includes new findings relevant to the statistics on human immunodeficiency virus (HIV) infection and on home testing kits for the disease. A new drug approved for the treatment of rheumatoid arthritis (RA) has been added. Signs and symptoms of juvenile idiopathic arthritis have been updated. Diagnosis for ankylosing spondylitis has been revised. New drug treatment for multiple sclerosis is discussed.
- Chapter 4 includes information regarding continual glucose-monitoring systems. Illustrations on the signs of hypocalcemia and a newer image for Cushing syndrome have been added.
- In Chapter 5, dry eye syndrome has been added. New illustrations of subconjunctival hemorrhage, conjunctivitis, and vernal conjunctivitis have been added.

- Chapter 6 presents recent information on the treatment of atopic dermatitis. New treatment options for psoriasis are discussed. Information concerning the vaccine, Shingrix, which was introduced in 2017 and is now the preferred vaccine for the prevention of shingles, is also included. Illustrations of seborrheic dermatitis, urticaria, and rosacea have been added.
- New illustrations of scoliosis, ganglion cyst on wrist, and gouty arthritis have been added to Chapter 7.
- In Chapter 8, more details on fatty liver disease have been added as an Enrichment box on the subject. New or updated illustrations include those of leukoplakia, esophageal varices, esophagitis, esophageal adenocarcinoma, Barrett esophagus, ulcers, Crohn disease, ulcerative colitis, diverticulosis, colorectal cancer, chronic pancreatitis, and carcinoma of the pancreas. Additionally, recent approaches to the treatment of hepatitis C are discussed.
- In Chapter 9, updated illustrations of deviated septum and nasal polyps are included. Potential complications of peritonsillar abscess are discussed. Recent recommendations for replacing warfarin after treatment of pulmonary embolism are added. There is a suggestion for a recently introduced medication to treat influenza. Another important patient teaching point is to report any abdominal pain immediately to the health care provider. Although rare, spontaneous splenic rupture is a medical emergency. There is an Enrichment box on vaping and electronic cigarettes.
- Chapter 10 includes a new disorder, broken heart syndrome. The topic of PANDAS is introduced. An additional discussion about the possible cause of non-Hodgkin lymphoma has been included. Updated or recent illustrations that have been added include pericarditis, effects of pericardial effusion, bacterial endocarditis, causative factors of endocarditis, artificial valves, and a mitral valve replacement.
- In Chapter 11, warnings regarding patients with kidney disease not taking NSAIDs have been included. New or updated images include uremic frost, the nephron, polycystic kidney, chronic pyelonephritis, end-stage glomerulopathy/chronic glomerulonephritis, urinary calculi, acute cystitis, chronic cystitis, and renal cell carcinoma.
- In Chapter 12, an update on symptoms of gonorrhea has been provided. A discussion on contraception has been added, along with chancroid of the testes, nodular prostatic hyperplasia, and adenocarcinoma of the prostate. Illustrations of ovarian serous tumors, mature cystic teratoma (dermoid cyst) of the ovary, uterine leiomyomas, pelvic inflammatory disease, and bilateral and asymmetric cervical

os with surrounding, invasive, exophytic cervical carcinoma have been added. Information regarding new therapies for postmenopausal breast cancer has been included.

- In Chapter 13, two new Enrichment boxes on the Wounded Warrior Project and Chiari malformation have been added. Information on use of the spinal cord stimulator for degenerative disk disease has been added. A new class of migraine medications approved by the FDA in 2018, called calcitonin gene-related peptide (CGRP) inhibitors, is discussed. Information on treatment options for epilepsy has been updated and includes implanted vagus nerve stimulator (VNS).

- Chapter 14 includes discussions on mass shootings and PANDAS. Illustrations of subdural and epidural hematomas and a new photo of the nasal continuous positive airway pressure (CPAP) mask have been added.

- In Chapter 15, a discussion on suicide has been included.

A logical and orderly approach to exploring pathophysiologic conditions flows from a discussion of diseases as they progress from general concepts to the beginning of life and to diseases and conditions of childhood.

General concepts of diseases are presented in Chapter 1 as a basis for the discussion of conditions. Chapter 1 introduces the reader to the general principles of pathophysiology. In conjunction with a breakdown of the mechanisms of disease, the subject matter flows through integrant aspects important for the student to consider in the study of human diseases, such as genetics, immune disorders, preventive health care, nontraditional medicine, and patient teaching. Additionally, the topic of cancer is introduced in Chapter 1 with foundational information about the pathology, pathogenesis, and prognostic indicators of the disease (*staging* and *grading* of malignant tumors). Specific sites and types of cancers are then comprehensively addressed in subsequent chapters. This is followed by a discussion of pediatric situations in Chapter 2. After these general discussions, the text progresses through body systems from Chapters 3 to 12. Chapter 3 introduces the student to the immune system, including discussions of immunodeficiency disorders and autoimmune disorders. In Chapter 4, the endocrine system, its disorders resulting from both deficiency and overactivity, is dealt with. This is followed by the special senses of sight and hearing in Chapter 5. Chapter 6 progresses to the largest sensory organ, the skin, or the integumentary system, and its disorders. Chapter 7 describes the upright structure of the human body, its movement, and the disorders that disrupt the normal functioning of the musculoskeletal system. Chapter 8 addresses the body's nourishment system: the gastrointestinal system and its accessory organs. Chapter 9 presents discussions on the oxygen–carbon dioxide exchange, the respiratory system. The cardiovascular system (including the heart, blood, and blood vessels) is the topic of Chapter 10. Chapter 11 follows with a discussion of the urinary system, which maintains homeostasis and is a major factor in excretion of urinary waste products. Chapter 12 discusses both male and reproductive systems, pregnancy, and disorders of the breast. Chapter 13 covers the diseases and conditions of the neurologic system. Chapter 14

provides a discussion of mental disorders, including phobias, grief response, posttraumatic stress disorders, alcohol abuse, sleep disorders, and other conditions covered by the *Diagnostic and Statistical Manual of Mental Disorders*, fifth edition (DSM-V). This chapter also includes a comprehensive chart on drugs of abuse, their street names, and their effects on the abuser. Chapter 15 includes information to help health care providers with practical knowledge to deal with a variety of traumatic injuries. This material includes lightning injuries; insect, animal, and snake bites; child abuse; psychological abuse; elder abuse; sexual abuse; intimate partner violence; rape; and suicide.

Organization of Material

Each chapter is introduced with a brief review of the normal function of the specific body system discussed in the chapter, and this review is reinforced with clear illustrations. Important pathologic mechanisms are explained and illustrated as well. A disease entity is presented with a description and discussion of the symptoms experienced by the patient and the signs detected by the physician. The chapter continues with sections devoted to etiologic factors, diagnosis, treatment options, prognosis, prevention, and patient teaching related to the disease entity. A diagnostic code is assigned to each disease entity. (See important notes at the end of the preface.) **ICD-10-CM codes are included to aid in locating appropriate insurance codes.** This format also follows the inherent progression of a patient's experience: (1) The individual reports symptoms to a health care provider, usually in a clinical setting; (2) abnormal signs of a clinical disorder may be elicited during the physical examination and/or subsequent diagnostic testing; (3) an appropriate treatment option is initiated and monitored for results; (4) the patient is given appropriate teaching to encourage compliance and thus to ensure an optimal outcome. The usual prognosis for the condition and the possible preventive measures are discussed.

Italicized words found in the chapters are defined in the Glossary for purposes of review or clarification of meaning. The advantages to the student and health care worker in better understanding clinical terminology include (1) great professional gain when one comprehends the effects that a disease has on a person, (2) increased communication skills with the entire health care team, and (3) personal education that has many practical applications.

We believe it is important to define the role of *patient screening* in each discussion. Therefore, the discussion of each disease entity begins with a feature called Patient Screening; the remarks therein usually are tailored to the disease entity being discussed. Because the vast majority of patients first seek access to health care services over the telephone, many health care facilities have a written, standardized protocol for medical personnel who take incoming calls. The comments offered in the *Patient Screening* feature of this text are not intended to help diagnose the caller's medical condition or give curative advice. The feature typically offers *general clues* to recognizing the urgency for an appointment, identifying emergencies, and discerning the kind of calls that require referral to the physician for action. This feature is not to be confused with the skill of medical triage, which state practice acts generally reserve for certain licensed professionals. Careful listening to the patient who is calling often identifies information that helps the telephone screener select the appropriate action required by the caller. Ideally the outcome of telephone communication between the caller and the screener will benefit the patient and avoid potential medical-legal problems. Maintaining sensitivity to human suffering, keeping strict confidentiality, and upholding the priority of meeting the needs of patients cannot be overemphasized as skills necessary in a medical telephone screener.

In this regard, we also would like to add a list of serious and life-threatening conditions that require immediate assessment and intervention. These include, but are not limited to:

- Sudden onset of unexplained shortness of breath
- Crushing pain across the center of the chest
- Difficult breathing occurring suddenly and rapidly worsening, often in the middle of the night
- Vomiting of blood that is bright red or has a very dark "coffee grounds" appearance
- Sudden onset of weakness and unsteadiness or severe dizziness
- Sudden loss of consciousness or paralysis
- Flashes of light in field of vision
- Sudden and progressively worsening abdominal, flank, or pelvic pain

- Sudden onset of blurred vision accompanied by severe throbbing in the eye

A report of any of these symptoms must be immediately relayed to the physician. The physician will then offer additional instructions to give to the individual calling for help.

The appendices offer valuable information about diagnostic testing, pharmacology, and resource agencies. The appendix Common Laboratory and Diagnostic Tests discusses tests often ordered by the physician. Reference values for laboratory tests are listed, followed by possible causes of each variation above normal or below normal. Reference values or expected normal results are discussed for imaging and other studies. Again, causes of variations from normal are provided. It is imperative that the reader using this information recognize that reference values may vary, depending on the laboratory in which the test is performed and reported. Another appendix contains pharmacology information, which has been updated and revised. Representative drugs are listed by group and include the name of the drug, the usual intended therapeutic objective, possible side effects, and general comments. The presentation of this appendix follows the chapters in the text. Once again, the reader must recognize that drugs and drug substances may be continually changing and that any specific material must be confirmed by referencing a current drug reference or pharmacology reference source.

Chapter Features

Key features of each chapter include:

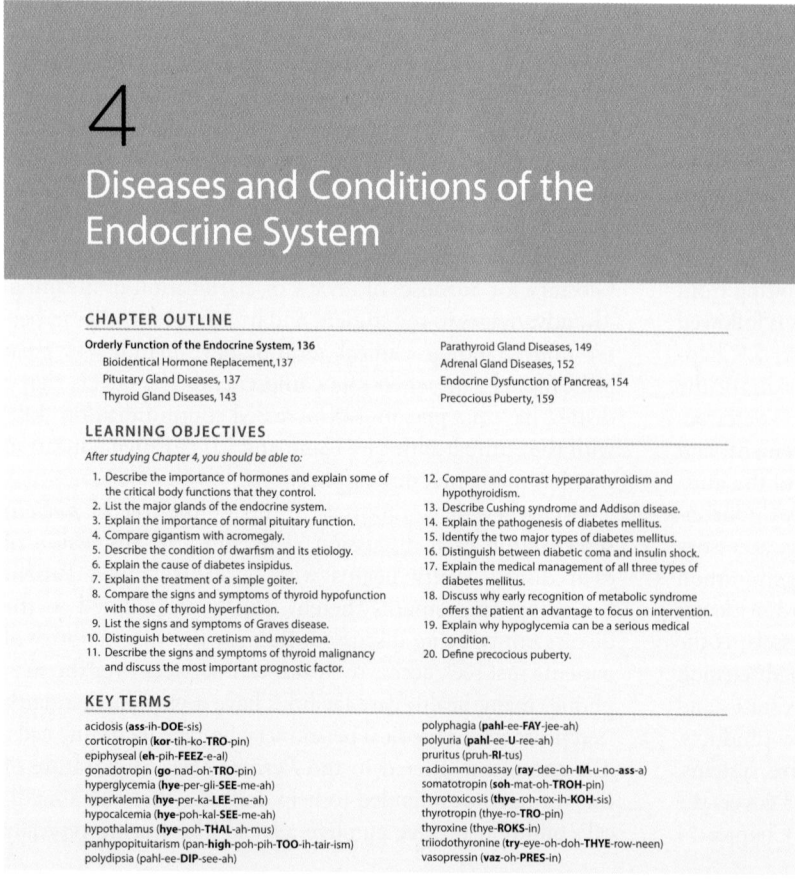

4

Diseases and Conditions of the Endocrine System

CHAPTER OUTLINE

Orderly Function of the Endocrine System, 136
  Bioidentical Hormone Replacement, 137
Pituitary Gland Diseases, 137
Thyroid Gland Diseases, 143

Parathyroid Gland Diseases, 149
Adrenal Gland Diseases, 152
Endocrine Dysfunction of Pancreas, 154
Precocious Puberty, 159

LEARNING OBJECTIVES

After studying Chapter 4, you should be able to:

1. Describe the importance of hormones and explain some of the critical body functions that they control.
2. List the major glands of the endocrine system.
3. Explain the importance of normal pituitary function.
4. Compare gigantism with acromegaly.
5. Describe the condition of dwarfism and its etiology.
6. Explain the cause of diabetes insipidus.
7. Explain the treatment of a simple goiter.
8. Compare the signs and symptoms of thyroid hypofunction with those of thyroid hyperfunction.
9. List the signs and symptoms of Graves disease.
10. Distinguish between cretinism and myxedema.
11. Describe the signs and symptoms of thyroid malignancy and discuss the most important prognostic factor.
12. Compare and contrast hyperparathyroidism and hypothyroidism.
13. Describe Cushing syndrome and Addison disease.
14. Explain the pathogenesis of diabetes mellitus.
15. Identify the two major types of diabetes mellitus.
16. Distinguish between diabetic coma and insulin shock.
17. Explain the medical management of all three types of diabetes mellitus.
18. Discuss why early recognition of metabolic syndrome offers the patient an advantage to focus on intervention.
19. Explain why hypoglycemia can be a serious medical condition.
20. Define precocious puberty.

KEY TERMS

acidosis (**ass**-ih-**DOE**-sis)
corticotropin (**kor**-tih-ko-**TRO**-pin)
epiphyseal (**eh**-pih-**FEEZ**-e-al)
gonadotropin (**go**-nad-oh-**TRO**-pin)
hyperglycemia (**hye**-per-gli-**SEE**-me-ah)
hyperkalemia (**hye**-per-ka-**LEE**-me-ah)
hypocalcemia (**hye**-poh-kal-**SEE**-me-ah)
hypothalamus (**hye**-poh-**THAL**-ah-mus)
panhypopituitarism (pan-**high**-poh-pih-**TOO**-ih-tair-ism)
polydipsia (pahl-ee-**DIP**-see-ah)

polyphagia (**pahl**-ee-**FAY**-jee-ah)
polyuria (**pahl**-ee-**U**-ree-ah)
pruritus (pruh-**RI**-tus)
radioimmunoassay (**ray**-dee-oh-**IM**-u-no-**ass**-a)
somatotropin (**soh**-mat-oh-**TROH**-pin)
thyrotoxicosis (**thye**-roh-tox-ih-**KOH**-sis)
thyrotropin (thye-ro-**TRO**-pin)
thyroxine (thye-**ROKS**-in)
triiodothyronine (**try**-eye-oh-doh-**THYE**-row-neen)
vasopressin (**vaz**-oh-**PRES**-in)

Each chapter begins with a set of **Learning Objectives** that list important actions the student will be able to perform after reading the chapter content.

The **Key Terms** list provides pronunciations for important words related to chapter content. Boldfaced words found in the text are listed in the Key Terms at the beginning of each chapter and in the Glossary unless the term has been adequately defined within the text of the chapter.

Enrichment boxes give the reader pertinent or relevant information that enhances knowledge of a discussion topic in the text.

36 CHAPTER 2 Developmental, Congenital, and Childhood Diseases and Disorders

◆ ENRICHMENT

Conjoined Twins

During the conception process, the fertilized egg (the embryo) may divide, creating identical twins. Conjoined twins result when the separation process of identical twins fails to complete before the 13th day after fertilization. As with identical twins, the embryo originates from a single fertilized ovum and occupies one placenta. For an unidentifiable reason, however, the normal separation of the embryo into twins stops before completion, resulting in a partially separated embryo that continues to mature into conjoined fetuses. Conjoined twins occur more often in female embryos than in male embryos and result in two fetuses that are joined at some point on their bodies. More of these children are being born alive as a result of specific prenatal diagnosis and surgical intervention to facilitate the delivery.

These children may be joined at different locations of the body and may share various organs. The attachment to each other may involve a small portion of tissue or may be as extensive as fusion at the head or sharing of an organ or body part. Common types or variations usually are categorized by the location and involvement of the junction through the term *pagus,* meaning fastened, included in the classification terminology.

Twins with a cranial union are called *craniopagus twins.* Those with anterior junction at the chest, often sharing the heart and vital portions of the chest wall and internal organs, are called *thoracopagus conjoined twins.* Thoracopagus is the most common form of conjoined twins. The term *pygopagus twins* describes those joined posteriorly at the rump. Another posterior junction occurring at the sacrum and coccyx is termed *ischiopagus.* When the connection proceeds from the breastbone to the waist, the term *omphalopagus* describes the junction. A very rare form, *dicephalus,* is the condition in which the individual has one body and two separate heads and necks.

Modern technology and medical advances have recently helped physicians and surgical teams to successfully separate some of these twins. In some separation procedures, one or both of the children have died during or shortly after the surgery. The children and their families require emotional support and education about the possible outcomes of the condition (Fig. 2.3).

652 CHAPTER 15 Disorders and Conditions Resulting from Trauma

Victimization of individuals has become so prevalent that health care providers are now trained to identify people who have been victimized, to treat their physical and emotional trauma, and to report incidents or suspicion of abuse, as required by law.

Violence occurs in all areas of society, affecting both sexes, occurring at all socioeconomic levels, and including the entire age spectrum. The number of occurrences continues to increase, even though societal and cultural values typically expressed in the United States do not condone such behavior. Health care providers are encouraged to provide unconditional support to victims and to direct them to support groups or counseling for appropriate therapy.

Violence has taken on a new dimension in the past few years in the form of terrorist attacks and bioterrorism. (Refer to the Alert box about Bioterrorism for additional information.)

❶ ALERT!

Bioterrorism

Bioterrorism is a source of great public concern. Anthrax, smallpox, plague, botulism, and radiation exposure are possible sources of danger. Government agencies and health care providers are researching these conditions and exploring treatment options. Silent and deliberate attacks can seriously threaten life and cause social disruption. Awareness of the likelihood of the threats and knowledge of these conditions and possible intervention measures may prevent a potentially catastrophic final outcome. Updates about these conditions will be provided by the health care communities and government agencies.

The following are thumbnail sketches of bioterrorism agents that a terrorist group would be likely to choose:

Anthrax

Anthrax is a bacterial infection caused by *Bacillus anthracis;* it can affect the skin, intestinal tract, or respiratory system. Anthrax traditionally has affected mainly agricultural animals and their handlers. However, pulmonary anthrax has recently been reported in the United States and has been suspected to be the result of terrorist activity.

Pulmonary anthrax begins when a sufficient amount of spores suspended in the air are inhaled into the lungs. Once infected, victims complain of fever, fatigue, muscle aches, chest pain, cough, and severe respiratory distress; without very early medical intervention, most will die. As soon as exposure to the disease is confirmed, administration of vaccine and antibiotic therapy is begun. Diagnosis is confirmed by examination of blood, skin lesions, or respiratory secretions. Presence of the anthrax bacterium or elevated antibodies causes increased amounts of the protein to be produced directly as a response to the infection. Every effort is made to find the source of the infection. This form of anthrax is not considered contagious.

Skin anthrax starts as a raised, itching lesion; within a day or two, the lesion resembles a blister that ulcerates and develops a coal black center.

Caregivers must wear gloves because the skin lesions may be infectious with direct skin contact. This disease is usually not fatal if treated promptly with antibiotics.

Plague

A bioterrorism outbreak of plague would most likely be brought about by the inhalation of the causative bacteria, causing a severe life-threatening lung disease within a few days of exposure. The onset is sudden and includes very severe respiratory symptoms. Prompt antibiotic treatment is required to save the infected person. Precautions are necessary to prevent the spread of the disease via face-to-face contact.

Smallpox

Smallpox is a highly contagious viral infection caused by the variola virus (a member of the poxvirus family) that can be spread in aerosol form as a biologic weapon. It was once eradicated worldwide through vaccination, but now there is growing concern because people younger than 30 years of age have never been vaccinated, and some adults vaccinated as children may no longer be immune.

Early symptoms resemble a mild viral infection. After a variable incubation (7 to 17 days), symptoms worsen and include high fever, malaise, headache, delirium, and a rash that begins over the face and spreads to the extremities. The rash turns into pustules that leave pitted scars. No cure has been developed, and the only treatment is supportive. Immediate isolation of the infected individual is required, and every case must be reported to health authorities. Vaccine is once again available and is being given or has been given to the military, certain public safety providers, and some health care providers. Provisions are in progress to accomplish mass citizen vaccination should there be an endemic occurrence.

Botulism

Botulism toxin, a powerful poison, is easy to make and store, and can be easily aerosolized. Although other forms of botulism exist, it is the inhalation form that could possibly be used in a bioterrorist attack.

Within a day or two after exposure to the toxin, the infected person experiences a cluster of flulike symptoms. Shortly thereafter, rapid progression of neurologic symptoms begins and can result in complete respiratory failure. Early intervention with an antitoxin may be helpful in cases in which the toxin is attached to nerve endings. Additionally treatment with human botulism immune globulin may be used. No other drugs are available to treat botulism toxin or poisoning at this time.

Alert boxes provide essential warnings (cautions and precautions) that require discussion or may require special treatment.

Refractive Errors

Refractive errors are the most common cause for diminished visual acuity. Refractive errors that result in the eye being unable to focus light effectively on the retina are identified as hyperopia, myopia, astigmatism, and presbyopia.

Hyperopia (Farsightedness)

Description
Hyperopia (farsightedness) occurs when light that enters the eye is focused behind the retina rather than on the retina, requiring refocusing by the internal lens or the use of an external corrective lens to reposition the viewed object on the retina to sharpen the image. With this condition, near vision is particularly impaired. Hyperopia occurs when the eyeball is abnormally short, as measured from front to back (Fig. 5.2).

ICD-10-CM Code   H52.03 *(Hypermetropia, bilateral)*
(H52.00-H52.03 = 4 codes of specificity)

Myopia (Nearsightedness)

Description
Myopia (nearsightedness) is the result of light rays entering the eye being focused in front of the retina, causing blurred vision. Near objects can be seen clearly, but distant objects are blurry, and the image being viewed cannot be sharpened by the internal lens of the eye. Myopia occurs when the eyeball is abnormally long, as measured from front to back (Fig. 5.3).

ICD-10-CM Code   H52.13 *(Myopia, bilateral)*
(H52.10-H52.13 = 4 codes of specificity)

Astigmatism

Description
Astigmatism is an irregular focusing of the light rays entering the eye. It usually is caused by the cornea not being spherical. The front of the cornea may be more egg-shaped than spherical, thereby causing light rays to be unevenly or diffusely focused across the retina. This causes some images to appear clearly defined, whereas others appear blurred.

ICD-10-CM Code   H52.209 *(Unspecified astigmatism, unspecified eye)*
(H52.20-H52.229 = 12 codes of specificity)
Refer to the physician's diagnosis and then to the current edition of the ICD-10-CM coding manual to ensure the greatest specificity of pathology.

Presbyopia

Description
Presbyopia is the inability of the internal lens of the eye to focus on near objects due to the loss of elasticity of the lens. This condition is related to aging and usually starts in people in their mid-40s.

ICD-10-CM Code   H52.4 *(Presbyopia)*

Symptoms and Signs
The primary symptoms of a refractive error are blurred vision and eye fatigue, which can lead to squinting, frequent rubbing of the eyes, and headaches.

Patient Screening
Schedule a comprehensive refractive examination for a patient complaining of changes in visual acuity or clearness or sharpness of visual perception.

A **diagnostic code** used in the health care setting has been assigned to each disease entity in this publication to help students and workers in the health care setting understand the ICD-10-CM coding process when reporting clinical information.

Extensive Supplemental Resources

Student Workbook

The workbook features comprehensive additional review exercises and practice activities in a variety of formats to reinforce chapter topics. The workbook has been updated to include information added to this edition.

- **Word Definitions** and **Glossary Terms** review important key terms covered in each chapter.
- **Short Answer** and **Fill-in-the-Blank** questions review key chapter concepts.
- An **Anatomical Structures** section in select chapters presents diagrams representing key body structures to be labeled by the student.
- A **Patient Screening** section guides students in the practice of appointment scheduling or specialist referral based on a patient's described signs and symptoms.
- A **Patient Teaching** section guides students in the practice of providing patient education regarding various diseases and disorders.
- **Essay** questions invite students to further investigate key chapter topics.
- A **Certification Exam Review** helps students prepare for the certification exam with questions focused on chapter content in multiple-choice format.

Evolve

The specially designed complementary Evolve website provides important assets to students and instructors. For students, critical thinking case study exercises linked to each chapter can be found on the Evolve website, available at http://evolve.elsevier.com/Frazier/essentials/.

Test Bank

The Test Bank located on the Evolve site in the ExamView format gives instructors the option of evaluating students' retained knowledge by chapter in a comprehensive format. This tool is capable of assessing retention of essential information necessary for excellence in functioning in the workplace. The seventh edition's Test Bank has been updated and revised to now include answer rationales. Also, the questions have been updated to include more stem-type questions as seen on credentialing examinations, rather than statement questions which conclude with the answer options.

TEACH Instructor Resources

The TEACH lesson plans help instructors prepare for class and make full use of the rich array of ancillaries and resources that come with the textbook. The content covered in each textbook chapter is divided across one or more lesson plans, each designed to occupy 50 minutes of class time. Lesson plans are organized into easily understandable sections that are each tied to the chapter learning objectives:

- Instructor Preparation—This section provides a checklist of all the things you need to do to prepare for class, including a list of all the items that you need to bring to class to perform any activity or demonstration included in the lesson plan, and all pertinent key terms covered in that lesson.

- Student Preparation—Textbook readings, study guide exercises, online activities, and other applicable homework assignments for each lesson are provided here, along with the overall estimated completion time.
- The 50-Minute Lesson Plan—A lecture outline that reflects the chapter lecture slides that come as part of TEACH is included, as well as classroom activities and online activities, one or more critical thinking questions, and time estimates for the classroom lecture and activities. Corresponding PowerPoint slides are provided to help the instructor save valuable preparation time and create a learning environment that fully engages the student.
- Assessment Plan—To ensure that your students have mastered all the objectives, the new TEACH includes a separate "Assessment Plan" section. An easy-to-use table maps each assessment tool to the lesson plans and chapter objectives so that you can see all your assessment options—by chapter, by lesson, and by objective—and choose accordingly.
- Answer Keys to the text and the workbook

All the above features are available to the instructor for easy download from the Evolve site, allowing the instructor to apply his or her creativity; all of these features may be revised to accommodate any instructor's lesson plan.

Important Information

The information presented in this book represents research into the mainstream of medical knowledge and its application in clinical practice. In the actual practice of the dynamic art and science of medicine, great variations and opposing views result in either more conservative or more aggressive concepts. The material presented in this text should not take the place of individualized consultation with medical experts.

Regarding the *diagnostic codes* included in this publication, it is imperative to consider the following: Medical coding is an intricate and intense process requiring study and understanding to ensure maximum reimbursement from insurance companies, for participation in Medicare and Medicaid programs, and for statistical tabulation. Diagnostic codes are subject to changes, revisions, and additions; therefore it is imperative that you always refer to the *current*

listing of ICD-10-CM codes. We have kept in mind that financial reimbursement directly correlates with the reporting of current, valid codes, which may require modification to ensure greatest specificity found in the most current coding manual and guidelines. Therefore we recommend that you refer to the current edition of a coding manual or to digital coding tools.

With regard to *patient teaching*, we are mindful of the legal parameters addressed in state acts governing the practice of medical assistants. *Readers, please consult your state code for licensing with regard to the rules and regulations applying to medical assistant practice.* State practice laws vary; they identify the tasks the properly prepared medical assistant can perform. With regard to the responsibility issue, the medical assistant in a medical office must know who his or her supervisor is; it may be the physician. Medical assistants should ask about a written office policy regarding delegation of tasks by the health care providers they work for, whether it be a physician, physician assistant, or nurse practitioner.

We consider it important, and in the patient's best interests, that all health care workers, as members of a clinical team, understand the principles, goals, and specifics of patient teaching. *Licensing regulations and state practice acts generally permit only nurses, nurse practitioners, physician assistants, and physicians to perform patient teaching and make triage judgments. Medical assistants in some states do perform some patient teaching if directed by the health care provider.*

Students completing education in medical assisting will find this book an invaluable tool as they move into the professional arena. The text has been designed to provide information relevant in the medical office environment and will remain a handy reference during employment. The website updates will offer a resource that covers current changes in the health care field to help keep the graduate current.

The established health care provider, whether a medical assistant, nurse, transcriber, coder, respiratory therapist, massage therapist, receptionist, emergency medical technician, paramedic, pharmacy technician, or other, will find this reference material a valuable resource in his or her work with the patient. Knowledge of diseases and related factors is essential in the provision of quality care.

Margaret Schell Frazier, RN, CMA (AAMA), BS
Tracie Fuqua, BS, CMA (AAMA)

Contents

1   Mechanisms of Disease, Diagnosis, and Treatment, 1

2   Developmental, Congenital, and Childhood Diseases and Disorders, 31

3   Immunologic Diseases and Conditions, 100

4   Diseases and Conditions of the Endocrine System, 135

5   Diseases and Disorders of the Eye and Ear, 162

6   Diseases and Conditions of the Integumentary System, 204

7   Diseases and Conditions of the Musculoskeletal System, 243

8   Diseases and Conditions of the Digestive System, 280

9   Diseases and Conditions of the Respiratory System, 342

10   Diseases and Conditions of the Circulatory System, 381

11   Diseases and Conditions of the Urinary System, 449

12   Diseases and Conditions of the Reproductive System, 477

13   Neurologic Diseases and Conditions, 533

14   Mental Disorders, 574

15   Disorders and Conditions Resulting from Trauma, 620

Appendix I   Common Laboratory and Diagnostic Tests, 664

Appendix II   Pharmacology, 685

Glossary, 703

Index, 711

Mechanisms of Disease, Diagnosis, and Treatment

CHAPTER OUTLINE

Pathology at First Glance, 2

Mechanisms of Disease, 2

    Predisposing Factors, 2

    Inflammation and Repair, 3

    Infection, 3

    Genetic Diseases, 6

    Genetic Counseling, 7

    Cancer, 7

    Immune Disorders, 14

    Physical Trauma and Chemical Agents, 15

    Malnutrition, 15

    Aging, 15

    Psychological Factors, 16

    Mental Disorders, 16

    Diagnosis of Disease, 16

    Treatment of Disease, 19

    Cultural Diversity, 20

    Gene Therapy, 20

    Stem Cell Research, 20

    Pain, 21

    Preventive Health Care, 24

    Nontraditional Medicine, 25

Patient Teaching, 27

    General Principles of Patient Teaching, 27

    Goals of Patient Teaching, 28

    Reasons for Patient Teaching, 28

    The Specifics of Patient Teaching: Addressing the Patient's Concerns, 28

    Special Considerations for the Patient with Cancer or Life-Threatening Disease, 29

Conclusion, 29

LEARNING OBJECTIVES

After studying Chapter 1, you should be able to:

1. Explain how a pathologic condition affects the homeostasis of the body.
2. Describe the difference between:
   - Signs and symptoms of disease
   - Acute and chronic diseases
3. Identify the predisposing factors of disease.
4. Explain the body's natural defense system against infection.
5. Explain the terms *superbugs* and *super strains* as they relate to infection.
6. Describe the ways in which pathogens may cause disease.
7. Describe the difference between benign and malignant neoplasms.
8. Explain the relationship between mutations in the genetic code in cancer and other diseases.
9. List the prevention guidelines for cancer.
10. Recall the two systems used to stage and grade cancer tumor cells.
11. Describe how chemotherapy treatment fights cancer.
12. Describe the hospice concept of care.
13. Recall three classes of immune disorders that result in the breakdown of the body's defense system.
14. Explain how mild to very severe symptoms of an allergic response can be triggered in the body.
15. Explain the inappropriate response of the body in an autoimmune disease.
16. Track the essential steps in diagnosis of disease.
17. Define *holistic approach to medical care.*
18. Explain why recognition of cultural diversity is important in clinical practice.
19. Describe (1) the physiology of pain, (2) how pain may be treated, and (3) what is meant by *referred pain.*
20. Name two ways an individual can practice positive health behavior.
21. Describe examples of nontraditional medical therapies.
22. Define *integrative medicine.*
23. Discuss the principles and goals of patient teaching.

KEY TERMS

allergen (**AL**-ler-jen)
anaphylaxis (**an**-ah-fih-**LAK**-sis)
antigen (**AN**-tih-jen)
asymptomatic (a-sim-toh-**MAH**-tik)
auscultation (**aws**-kel-**TAY**-shun)
cachexia (kah-**KEX**-e-ah)
carcinogenic (**kar**-sih-no-**JEN**-ik)
chromosome (**KRO**-mo-sohm)
genotype (**JEN**-o-type)
homeostasis (**ho**-me-o-**STA**-sis)
hospice (**HAUS**-pis)

ischemia (is-**KEY**-me-ah)
karyotype (**KARE**-ee-o-type)
metastasis (meh-**TAS**-tah-sis)
mutation (meu-**TAY**-shun)
nociceptor (**no**-see-**SEHP**-tor)
oncogene (**AHN**-ko-jeen)
pathogenesis (**path**-o-**JEN**-eh-sis)
phagocytic (**fag**-o-**SIT**-ik)
probiotic (pro-bi-ah-**TIC**)
somatoform (so-**MAT**-o-form)

Pathology at First Glance

Pathology, the scientific study of disease, is the objective description of the traits, causes, and effects of abnormal conditions. Pathologic conditions involve measurable changes in normal structure and function that threaten the internal stability, or homeostasis, of the body.

In human disease, the negative characteristics, or departures from normal status, are described subjectively by patients as symptoms. Signs, or abnormal objective findings, are the evidence of disease found by physical examination and diagnostic testing. Signs of disease often correlate with the symptoms. In other instances, the signs of disease may be noted in an asymptomatic patient, as in the discovery of a painless tumor or the finding of an abnormal blood pressure reading in a person with undiagnosed essential hypertension. A defined collection of signs and symptoms that characterize a disorder or condition is termed a *syndrome.*

The development of disease occurs in stages, described as the pathogenesis. In the course of infection, for instance, the pathogenesis may include an incubation period, a period of full-blown symptoms, and then remission or convalescence. The pathogenesis of a disease varies with the individual patient, the causative factors, and the medical intervention.

Diseases often are described as acute or chronic. *Acute* refers to an abrupt onset of more or less severe symptoms that run a brief course (usually < 6 months) and then resolve or, in some cases, result in death. When a disease develops slowly, is intermittent, or lasts longer than 6 months, it is described as *chronic.* Persons who have continuous pain as part of chronic syndromes often experience depression.

Mechanisms of Disease

Human disease, a universal occurrence, has varied manifestations, any of which threatens a person's ability to adapt to internal and external stressors and to maintain a state of well-being. Systemic health, or internal equilibrium, is preserved by numerous body organs and structures that work in concert to meet specific cellular needs. Any disruption of the body's equilibrium produces degenerative changes at the cellular level that may produce signs and symptoms of disease. Major disruptions in the body's cellular equilibrium that threaten homeostasis include fluid and electrolyte imbalance and excessive acidity (acidosis) or alkalinity (alkalosis).

Elements involved either directly or indirectly in pathogenesis include predisposing factors, access to preventive health care, genetic diseases, infection, inflammation and repair, neoplasms, physical trauma, chemical agents, malnutrition, immune disorders, aging, psychological factors, and mental disorders.

Predisposing Factors

Predisposing factors, also called *risk factors,* make a person or group more vulnerable to disease. Although the recognition of risk factors may be significant in prevention, diagnosis, and prognosis, it does not precisely predict the occurrence of disease, nor does the absence of predisposing factors necessarily protect against the development of disease. A person may be susceptible, to a greater or lesser degree, as a result of one or more risk factors that overlap or occur in combination. Predisposing factors include age, gender, lifestyle, environment, heredity, and *immunodeficiency.*

- Age: From complications during pregnancy and the postpartum period to maladies associated with aging, some increased risks of diseases are simply intrinsic to one's stage in the human life cycle.
- Gender: Certain diseases are more common in women (e.g., multiple sclerosis and osteoporosis), and other disorders are more common in men (e.g., gout and Parkinson disease).
- Lifestyle: Occupation, habits, or one's usual manner of living can have negative cumulative effects that can threaten a person's health. It is possible to alter some known risk factors associated with lifestyle, thereby promoting health instead of predisposing one to disease; examples include smoking, excessive drinking of alcohol,

risky sexual behavior, poor nutrition, lack of exercise, and certain psychological stressors.

- Environment: Air pollution and water pollution are considered major risk factors for illnesses, such as cancer and pulmonary disease. Poor living conditions, excessive noise, chronic psychological stress, and a geographic location conducive to disease proliferation also are environmental risk factors.
- Heredity: Genetic predisposition (inheritance) currently is considered a major risk factor. Family histories of coronary disease, cancer, certain arthritic conditions, and renal disease are known hereditary risk factors. Many other genetic links to diseases are rapidly being discovered. Hereditary factors in disease that appear regularly in successive generations are likely to affect males and females equally. Hereditary or genetic diseases often develop as a result of the combined effects of inheritance and environmental factors. Examples are mental illness, cancer, hypertension, heart disease, and diabetes. Some evidence shows that smoking, a sedentary lifestyle, and a diet high in saturated fat, combined with a positive family history, compound a person's risk for heart disease and cancer. Schizophrenia may result from a combination of genetic predisposition and numerous psychological and sociocultural causes.
- Immunodeficiency: An inadequate or absent immune system makes an individual susceptible to infections, diseases, and harmful substances. The degree of risk depends on which components of the immune system are inadequate or absent and are the cause of the immunodeficiency. In cases of autoimmune disease, the immune response is misdirected at one's own body tissue, potentially causing damage.

Inflammation and Repair

Injury and disease impose stress on the body's equilibrium and disrupt or destroy cellular function. Acute inflammation, a normal protective physiologic response to tissue injury and disease, is accompanied by redness, heat, swelling, pain, and loss of function. Widespread inflammation is marked by systemic symptoms, such as fever, malaise, and loss of appetite. Blood testing may reveal an elevated white blood cell (WBC) count or an elevated erythrocyte sedimentation rate (ESR). Cross-reactive protein (CRP) is a blood test marker used to detect inflammatory disorders, among other pathologies. The intensity of inflammation depends on the cause, the area of the body involved, and the physical condition of the person. An inflammatory response is considered a nonspecific immune response. Infection with pathogens, the effects of toxins, physical trauma, ischemia, and necrosis are some conditions that induce the inflammatory response.

Acute inflammation, an exudative response, attempts to wall off, destroy, and digest bacteria and dead or foreign tissue. Vascular changes allow fluid to leak into the site; this fluid contains chemicals that permit phagocytic activity by WBCs. The process prevents the spread of infection through antibody action and other chemicals released by cells with more specific immune activity. After the mechanisms of inflammation have contained the insult and "cleaned up" the damaged area, repair and replacement of tissue can begin (Fig. 1.1). A normal inflammatory response can be inhibited by immune disorders, chronic illnesses, or the use of certain medications, especially long-term steroid therapy.

When an inflammatory response is chronic or too intense, damage to the affected tissue can result, thereby inhibiting the healing process. Diseases with a chronic inflammation component include arthritis, asthma, and eczema.

Infection

Infectious diseases are caused by pathogens. The cardinal signs of local infection are redness, swelling, heat, pain, fever, pus, enlarged lymph glands, and red streaks. Symptoms of widespread infection are fever, headache, body aches, weakness, fatigue, loss of appetite, and delirium.

When disease-causing organisms find ideal conditions in which to grow and multiply in the body, they cause disease by (1) invasion and local destruction of living tissue and (2) intoxication or production of substances that are poisonous to the body. The result is tissue damage that has the potential for producing systemic involvement.

The sources of infection can be endogenous (originating within the body) or exogenous (originating outside the body). Modes of transmission of pathogenic organisms are direct or indirect physical contact, inhalation or droplet nuclei, ingestion of contaminated food or water, or inoculation by an insect or animal. Pathogenic agents include bacteria, viruses, fungi, and protozoa (Table 1.1).

A communicable or contagious disease can be transmitted directly from one person to another. Carriers are asymptomatic persons or animals that harbor in their bodies pathogens that can be transferred to others.

The body's natural defense systems against infection include (1) natural mechanical and chemical barriers, such as the skin, the cilia, body pH, and normal body flora; (2) the inflammatory response; and (3) the immune response. When these mechanisms of defense fail to contain or eliminate infection, appropriate and prompt medical intervention is required to treat the host and to control transmission of the infectious disease. This is accomplished by first isolating and identifying the organism through laboratory testing. Subsequently, appropriate antimicrobial therapy using antibiotic (antibacterial), antifungal, antiparasitic, or antiviral agents can begin. Analgesics for pain and antipyretic agents for fever, as well as other comfort measures, are dispensed. Adequate fluid intake, infection control measures, and rest are important for management.

Fundamental to preventing the spread of certain infections are isolation of the infected individual, when necessary, implementation of immunization programs, and rudimentary public health teaching. To facilitate early intervention and infection control measures, many infectious diseases (e.g., encephalitis, syphilis, and tuberculosis)

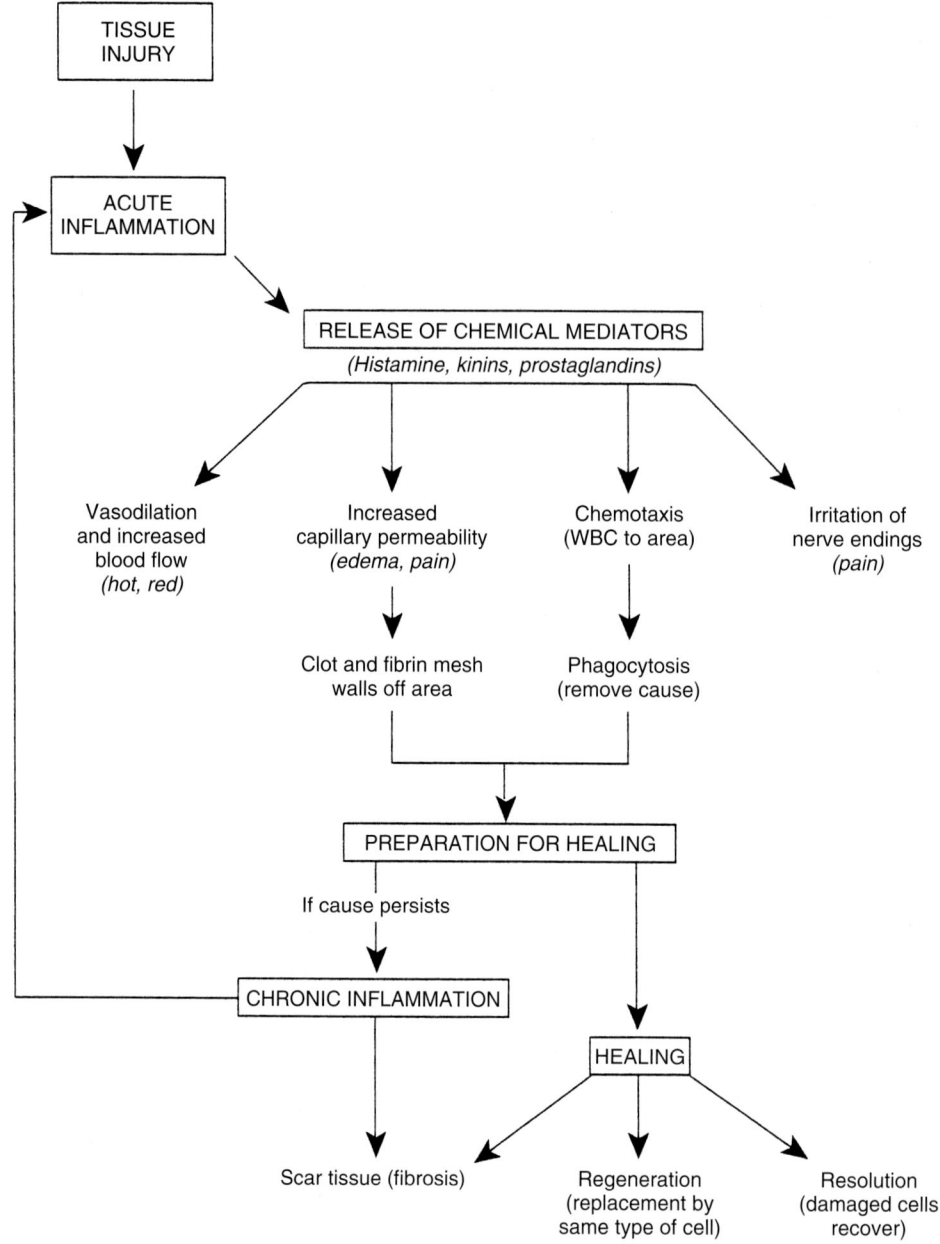

• **Fig. 1.1** The course of inflammation and healing. *WBC,* White blood cell. (From Gould BE: *Pathophysiology for the health professions,* ed 4, St Louis, 2011, Saunders.)

must be reported to the local health department. The Centers for Disease Control and Prevention (CDC) publishes notifiable diseases in the United States. In hospitals, the control of postsurgical bacterial wound infections relies on breaking the chain of transmission by killing the pathogen, isolating infected persons, and using precautions, such as hand washing and sterilization, to prevent cross-contamination.

Of special concern is the emergence of new, virulent antibiotic-resistant strains of bacteria (commonly referred to as *superbugs* or *super strains*), which present a danger even to the young and healthy. Methicillin-resistant strains of *Staphylococcus aureus* (MRSA) began showing up in hospitals, jails,

crowded living quarters, and other community environments. MRSA is to blame for aggressive skin and soft tissue infections, sometimes mistaken for spider bites; these lesions quickly develop into abscesses and cellulitis. In addition to skin infections, MRSA can cause fatal pneumonia, bone infections, and septicemia. Many MRSA strains of bacteria are currently resistant to several different antibiotics. Occasionally toxic and resistant strains of MRSA have been termed *flesh eating bacteria* because of the rapid spread of infection resulting in destruction of human skin. MRSA continues to be a leading cause of surgical wound infections in hospitals. The pathogen is easily transmitted from person to person and can survive for a long time nearly anywhere in

TABLE 1.1 Common Pathogens and Some Infections or Diseases That They Produce

Organism	Reservoir	Infection or Disease
Bacteria		
Escherichia coli (E. coli)	Colon, manure	Enteritis, mild to severe
Staphylococcus aureus Note: See section on Infection for discussion on methicillin-resistant strains of *S. aureus* ("superbugs")	Skin, hair, anterior nares	Wound infection, pneumonia, food poisoning, cellulitis
Streptococcus (β-hemolytic group A) organisms	Oropharynx, skin, perianal area	"Strep throat," rheumatic fever, scarlet fever, impetigo
Streptococcus (β-hemolytic group B) organisms	Adult genitalia	Urinary tract infection, wound infection, endometritis
Clostridium difficile (C. difficile)	Contaminated surfaces or spores transferred on unclean hands of others	Serious intestinal conditions such as colitis
Mycobacterium tuberculosis	Lungs	Tuberculosis
Neisseria gonorrhoeae	Genitourinary tract, rectum, mouth, eye	Gonorrhea, pelvic inflammatory disease, infectious arthritis, conjunctivitis
Rickettsia rickettsii	Wood tick	Rocky Mountain spotted fever
Staphylococcus epidermidis	Skin	Wound infection, bacteremia
Pseudomonas aeruginosa	Skin, water, soil	Pneumonia, urinary tract infection, meningitis
Viruses		
Hepatitis A virus	Feces, blood, urine	Hepatitis A (infectious hepatitis)
Hepatitis B virus	Feces, blood, all body fluids and excretions	Hepatitis B (serum hepatitis)
Hepatitis C virus	Blood and body fluids	Liver disease may become chronic
Herpes simplex virus	Lesions of mouth, skin, blood, excretions	Cold sores, aseptic meningitis, sexually transmitted disease
Human immunodeficiency virus (HIV)	Blood, semen, vaginal secretions (also isolated in saliva, tears, urine, breast milk, but not proven to be sources of transmission)	Acquired immunodeficiency syndrome (AIDS)
Hantavirus	Deer mouse urine, feces, saliva	Upper respiratory infection (URI) to lower respiratory infection (LRI) to adult respiratory distress syndrome (ARDS)
Ebola hemorrhagic fever (HF)	Contaminated blood or body fluid, fruit bat	Hemorrhagic fever, vascular permeability, shock, and death; potential bioterrorism threat
West Nile virus	Mosquito-borne	Fever, rash, hepatitis, encephalitis
Fungi		
Aspergillus organisms	Soil, dust	Aspergillosis, allergic bronchopulmonary
Candida albicans	Mouth, skin, colon, genital tract	Thrush, dermatitis
Protozoa		
Plasmodium falciparum	Mosquito	Malaria

Modified from Potter P, Perry A: *Fundamentals of nursing: concepts, process, and practice,* ed 6, St Louis, 2006, Mosby.

the environment. About 1 in 100 persons in the United States has the organisms in his or her body without showing signs of infection; however, the person may transmit MRSA bacteria to others. Healthy persons are at lower risk for infection. Because of the constant threat of infection, everyone must be considered a risk for MRSA, particularly hospitalized patients. Fortunately, a few antibiotics that are effective against strains of MRSA are available, but they are used judiciously to prevent the emergence of new antibiotic-resistant strains. Excellent hygiene practices help prevent the spread of MRSA. Stricter infection control measures throughout U.S. health care systems have reduced MRSA infections significantly. Participating medical facilities have implemented active surveillance testing, such as nasal swab tests on patient admission. Individuals with history of MRSA may be placed in isolation. Public education stresses thorough and frequent hand washing across the board as an effective practice of infection control in the community as well. Vancomycin-resistant *Enterococcus* (VRE) is a growing problem in chronic care facilities and hospitals because there are only a few antibiotics that can be used to treat VRE. This resistant bacterial infection is spread from person to person and can cause many types of infection.

Another family of germs, termed *carbapenem-resistant Enterobacteriaceae (CRE)*, has caused special concern in the health care setting. Recently, the CDC has sounded an alarm about the incidence of CRE infections that are difficult to treat because they have high levels of resistance to even the "last resort" antibiotics. Infections with CRE more commonly occur among patients who are receiving treatment for other infections, and CRE can be deadly. As of this writing, there are no new antibiotics in development to combat this super strain lying in wait.

Yet another multidrug-resistant bacterium, *Acinetobacter baumannii*, is capable of causing infection and death, especially in those with compromised immune systems, the frail elderly, and chronically hospitalized. It was introduced to North America by troops returning to Canada from the Middle East.

Genetic Diseases

Genetics, the study of genes and their heredity, will continue to occupy center stage in the practice of medicine. Genetic factors can guide treatment decisions and preventive strategies. Application of genetics may influence genetic counseling, newborn screening, and carrier screening. At this point, several thousand human genetic disorders have been described and cataloged.

Every cell in the body is coded with genetic information arranged on 23 pairs of chromosomes; one chromosome from each pair is inherited from the father and the other from the mother. The X and Y chromosomes are known as the *sex chromosomes,* whereas the remaining 22 pairs are called *autosomes.* Each cell in an individual's body contains the same chromosomes and genetic code (genotype). A karyotype is an ordered arrangement of photographs of a full chromosome set (Fig. 1.2). Genes, the basic units of heredity, are small stretches of a deoxyribonucleic acid (DNA) molecule, situated at a particular site on a chromosome.

Genetic diseases are (1) produced by an abnormality in, or a mutation of, the genetic code in a single gene; (2) caused by several abnormal genes (producing the so-called *polygenic diseases*); (3) caused by the abnormal presence or absence of an entire chromosome; or (4) caused by alteration in the structure of chromosomes. Harmful genetic mutations, or changes in the genetic code, passed from one generation to the next may occur spontaneously or be caused by agents known to disrupt the normal sequence of DNA units. Agents (called *mutagens*) that can damage DNA include certain chemicals, radiation, and viruses.

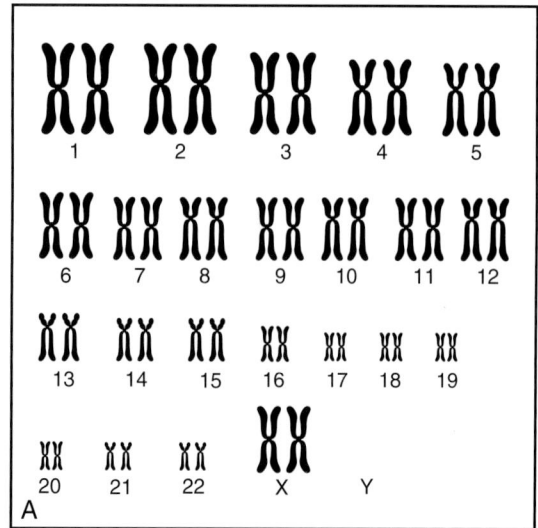 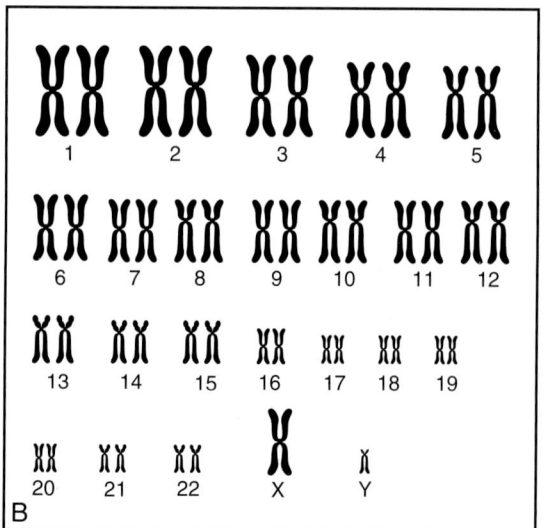

• **Fig. 1.2** Examples of Karyotypes. (A) Normal female (46,XX). (B) Normal male (46,XY). (From Damjanov I: *Pathology for the health professions,* ed 4, St Louis, 2011, Saunders.)

The main modes of inheritance for genetic diseases are as follows:
- Autosomal dominant: The gene in question is located on an autosome, and the mutant *phenotype* is seen even if a normal gene is present on the other chromosome in the pair. Examples include Marfan syndrome and Huntington disease.
- Autosomal recessive: The gene is located on an autosome but is insufficient to produce the mutant phenotype in the presence of a normal gene on the paired chromosome. Both genes must be mutated for disease to occur. Examples include cystic fibrosis and phenylketonuria.
- X-linked (sex-linked) recessive: The gene is located only on the X chromosome. Males are much more commonly affected by these diseases than are females. Examples include Duchenne muscular dystrophy and hemophilia A.

Individuals who have only one copy of a recessive gene and appear outwardly normal are known as *carriers* of the defective gene. The mutant gene may produce an abnormal protein that causes a disease, or it may fail to produce its normal cellular function. Hereditary diseases often are noted at birth, but they may not appear until later in life. Many genetic mutations are compatible with life, but some are not.

The following examples of genetic abnormalities are discussed in this book:
- Huntington chorea
- Down syndrome
- Robinow syndrome (dwarfism)
- hypertrophic cardiomyopathy
- hemophilia
- Klinefelter syndrome
- polycystic kidney
- albinism
- hyperopia
- hemolytic anemia
- cystic fibrosis
- epilepsy
- Hirschsprung disease
- phenylketonuria
- Turner syndrome
- hemolytic disease of newborn
- cleft palate
- myopia

Genetic Counseling

For many genetic diseases, the responsible gene or chromosomal abnormality has been identified, and it is possible to test for the presence of the mutation in an individual. The discovery of a genetic disease in a family member often raises questions as to whether other family members are affected, whether others are carriers of the disease, and whether future offspring will be affected by it. Genetic counseling is a communication process that is centered on the occurrence or risk of occurrence of a genetic disorder in a family. Such counseling should be offered to all families affected by the diagnosis of a genetic disease in one or more members.

Genetic counseling is more than simply reproductive counseling concerning inherited disorders; it helps bridge the gap between complicated medical and scientific concepts and the emotional aspects of being diagnosed with a certain condition. Attending physicians and other counselors help the family understand the diagnosis, course of the disease, and available treatment options. They talk about heredity and risk of occurrence in other family members and future offspring. If genetic testing is available for the disorder, the counselors first explain the test and the benefits of taking or not taking the test. They help prepare the family for any outcome of the genetic test. Common feelings experienced after receiving a diagnosis of a genetic disorder are a sense of being "labeled," guilt that other family members may be affected, worry about insurance discrimination, or a sense of hopelessness if the disease has no cure. Even if the patient receives the "good" news that he or she is not affected, there may be a feeling of "survivor guilt." With the increase in availability of genetic testing for many conditions, genetic counselors are usually available at most major hospitals.

Cancer

> **NOTE**
> What follows is a general introduction to the pathology and pathogenesis of cancer, including prognosis, as demonstrated by *staging* and *grading* of tumors. Broad measures of prevention, diagnosis, and treatment are also discussed. Current statistics are included. Specific sites and types of cancers are addressed in subsequent chapters.

Cancer, a leading cause of death in the United States, refers to a group of diseases characterized by uncontrolled cell proliferation. This abnormal growth leads to the development of tumors or *neoplasms*, a relentlessly growing mass of abnormal cells that proliferate at the expense of the healthy organism. Tumors are characterized as malignant or benign and according to the cell type and tissue of origin (Tables 1.2 and 1.3). Some of the main general types of cancer are carcinoma, cancer of the epithelial cells; sarcoma, cancer of the supportive tissues of the body, such as bone and muscle; lymphoma, cancer arising in the lymph nodes and tissues of the immune system; leukemia, cancer of blood cell precursors; and melanoma, cancer of the melanin-producing cells of the body.

Benign tumors usually develop slowly and can arise from any tissue. They tend to remain encapsulated and do not infiltrate surrounding tissue. When examined microscopically, benign tumor cells are well differentiated; they resemble the tissue of origin. Because these tumors take up space, complications can result from compression of tissue by the lesion or obstruction of organs. Benign tumors rarely recur after surgical removal.

Malignant tumors can represent a serious threat to the health and life and well-being of a person. Cancer cells are variable in appearance and disorderly (anaplastic) with irreversible changes in structure. Malignant tumors have the

TABLE 1.2 Comparison of Benign and Malignant Tumors

Characteristics	Benign Tumors	Malignant Tumors
Mode of growth	Relatively slow growth by expansion; encapsulated; cells adhere to each other	Rapid growth; invade surrounding tissue by infiltration
Cells under microscopic examination	Resemble tissue of origin; well differentiated; appear normal	Do not resemble tissue of origin; vary in size and shape; abnormal appearance and function
Spread	Remain localized	Metastasis; cancer cells carried by blood and lymphatics to one or more other locations; secondary tumors occur
Other properties	No tissue destruction; not prone to hemorrhage; may be smooth and freely movable	Ulceration and/or necrosis; prone to hemorrhage; irregular and less movable
Recurrence	Rare after excision	A common characteristic
Pathogenesis	Symptoms related to location with obstruction and/or compression of surrounding tissue or organs; usually not life-threatening unless inaccessible	Cachexia; pain; fatal if not controlled

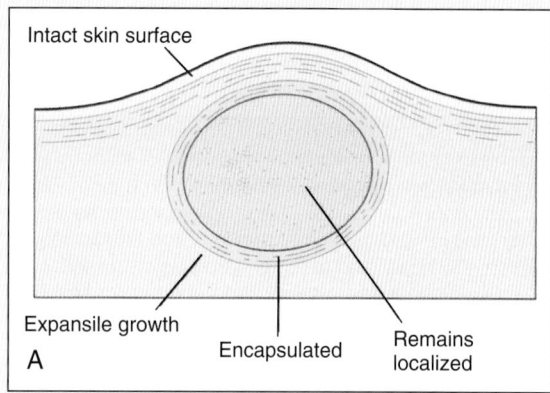 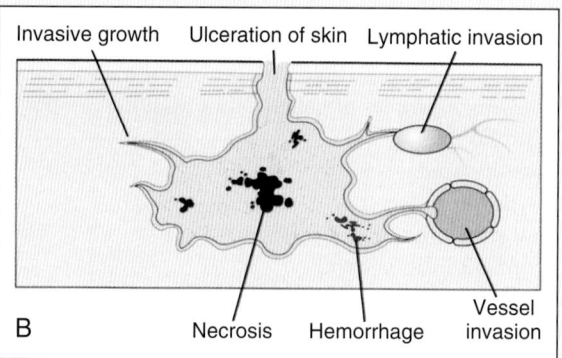

Gross appearance of benign (A) and malignant (B) tumors.

TABLE 1.3 Classification of Neoplasms by Tissue of Origin

Tissue of Origin	Benign	Malignant
Connective tissue		Sarcoma
Embryonic fibrous tissue	Myxoma	Myxosarcoma
Fibrous tissue	Fibroma	Fibrosarcoma
Adipose tissue	Lipoma	Liposarcoma
Cartilage	Chondroma	Chondrosarcoma
Bone	Osteoma	Osteogenic sarcoma
Epithelium		Carcinoma
Skin and mucous membrane	Papilloma	Squamous cell carcinoma
Glands		Basal cell carcinoma Transitional cell carcinoma
	Adenoma	Adenocarcinoma
	Cystadenoma	Cystadenocarcinoma

TABLE 1.3	Classification of Neoplasms by Tissue of Origin—cont'd	
Tissue of Origin	**Benign**	**Malignant**
Pigmented cells (melanocytes)	Nevus	Malignant melanoma
Endothelium		Endothelioma
Blood vessels	Hemangioma	Hemangioendothelioma Hemangiosarcoma Kaposi sarcoma
Lymph vessels	Lymphangioma	Lymphangiosarcoma Lymphangioendothelioma
Bone marrow		Multiple myeloma Ewing sarcoma Leukemia
Lymphoid tissue		Malignant lymphoma Lymphosarcoma Reticulum cell sarcoma
Muscle Tissue		
Smooth muscle	Leiomyoma	Leiomyosarcoma
Striated muscle	Rhabdomyoma	Rhabdomyosarcoma
Nerve Tissue		
Nerve fibers and sheaths	Neuroma Neurinoma Neurilemmoma	Neurogenic sarcoma
	Neurofibroma	Neurofibrosarcoma
Ganglion cells	Ganglioneuroma	Neuroblastoma
Glial cells	Glioma	Glioblastoma
Meninges	Meningioma	Malignant meningioma
Gonads	Dermoid cyst	Embryonal carcinoma Embryonal sarcoma Teratocarcinoma

(From Black JM, Matassarin-Jacobs E: *Medical-surgical nursing,* ed 6, Philadelphia, 2001, Saunders.)

ability to invade the surrounding tissue. Often malignant cells enter the bloodstream or the lymphatic vessels and lead to tumor growth in other areas of the body. These secondary tumors are known as *metastases.* Metastasis makes the neoplasm more difficult to eradicate from the body.

Cancer is actually many different diseases with numerous causes. Cancer may be caused by both external exposure to *carcinogens* (chemicals, radiation, and viruses) and internal factors (hormones, immune conditions, and inherited mutations). Many years may pass between exposures or mutations and the onset of detectable cancer. Cancer can develop in anyone, but the frequency increases with age. Fig. 1.3 shows the leading sites of cancer incidence and death.

Recommendations for decreasing the risk of cancer encompass guidelines and appropriate screening tests for early detection and treatment. Primary prevention guidelines include the following:
- Consume a diet rich in fruits, vegetables, and whole grains. Limit consumption of processed and red meats.
- Eliminate active and passive exposure to cigarette smoke.
- Limit skin exposure to sunlight.
- Limit use of alcohol.
- Avoid excessive exposure to radiation and radon.
- Avoid chemical agents known to be carcinogenic.
- Increase physical activity.
- Maintain a healthy weight.
- Protect against sexually transmitted infections, including getting the human papillomavirus (HPV) vaccine.

Cancer is very prevalent in the United States. According to statistics from the American Cancer Society, nearly 1.6 million Americans are diagnosed with invasive cancer, and greater than 500,000 die of cancer every year. One out of every four deaths in the United States is cancer related.

Early cancer detection employs physical examination, medical history taking, and laboratory screening tests. Screening examinations can detect cancers of the breast, rectum, colon, prostate, cervix, testis, oral cavity, and skin early, which is when treatment is more likely to succeed. These

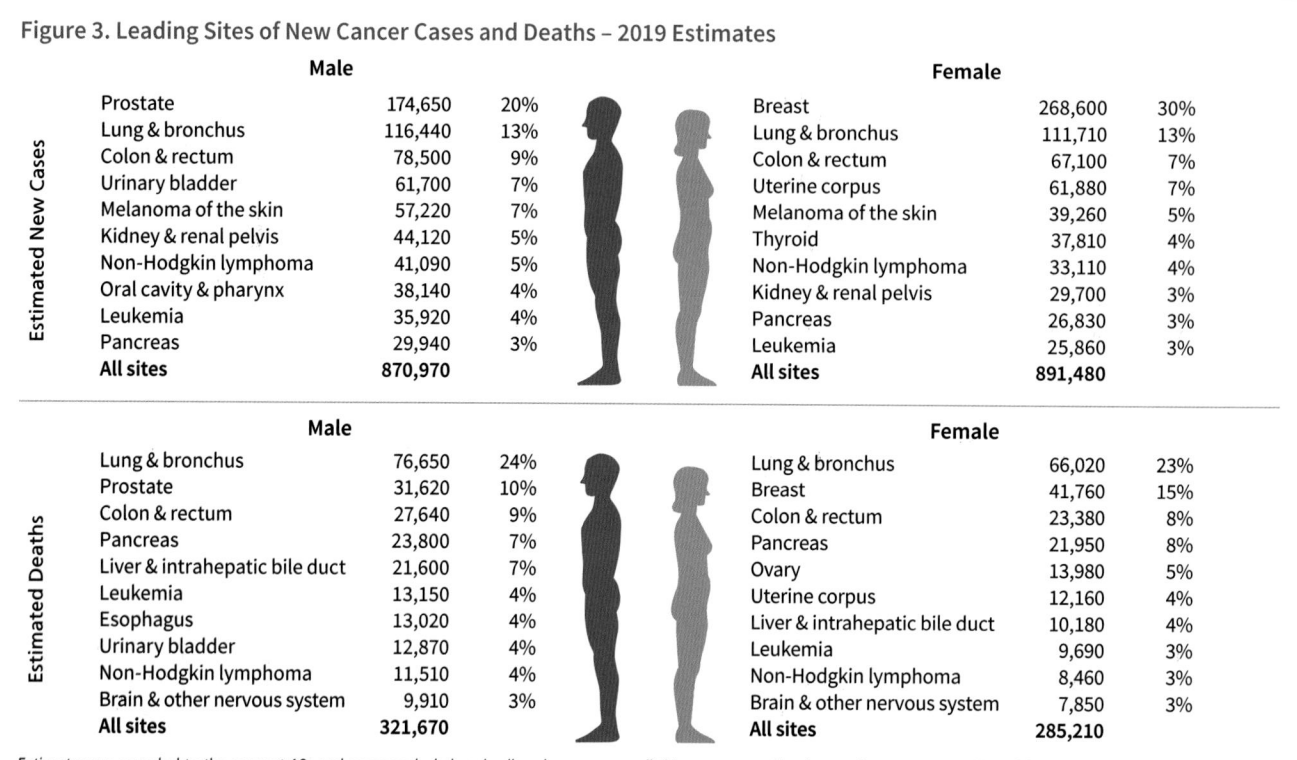

Figure 3. Leading Sites of New Cancer Cases and Deaths – 2019 Estimates

Estimated New Cases

Male				Female		
Prostate	174,650	20%		Breast	268,600	30%
Lung & bronchus	116,440	13%		Lung & bronchus	111,710	13%
Colon & rectum	78,500	9%		Colon & rectum	67,100	7%
Urinary bladder	61,700	7%		Uterine corpus	61,880	7%
Melanoma of the skin	57,220	7%		Melanoma of the skin	39,260	5%
Kidney & renal pelvis	44,120	5%		Thyroid	37,810	4%
Non-Hodgkin lymphoma	41,090	5%		Non-Hodgkin lymphoma	33,110	4%
Oral cavity & pharynx	38,140	4%		Kidney & renal pelvis	29,700	3%
Leukemia	35,920	4%		Pancreas	26,830	3%
Pancreas	29,940	3%		Leukemia	25,860	3%
All sites	**870,970**			**All sites**	**891,480**	

Estimated Deaths

Male				Female		
Lung & bronchus	76,650	24%		Lung & bronchus	66,020	23%
Prostate	31,620	10%		Breast	41,760	15%
Colon & rectum	27,640	9%		Colon & rectum	23,380	8%
Pancreas	23,800	7%		Pancreas	21,950	8%
Liver & intrahepatic bile duct	21,600	7%		Ovary	13,980	5%
Leukemia	13,150	4%		Uterine corpus	12,160	4%
Esophagus	13,020	4%		Liver & intrahepatic bile duct	10,180	4%
Urinary bladder	12,870	4%		Leukemia	9,690	3%
Non-Hodgkin lymphoma	11,510	4%		Non-Hodgkin lymphoma	8,460	3%
Brain & other nervous system	9,910	3%		Brain & other nervous system	7,850	3%
All sites	**321,670**			**All sites**	**285,210**	

Estimates are rounded to the nearest 10, and cases exclude basal cell and squamous cell skin cancers and in situ carcinoma except urinary bladder. Estimates do not include Puerto Rico or other US territories. Ranking is based on modeled projections and may differ from the most recent observed data.

©2019, American Cancer Society, Inc., Surveillance Research

• **Fig. 1.3** Leading sites of new cancer cases and deaths, 2019 estimates. (American Cancer Society. *Cancer Facts and Figures 2019.* Atlanta, 2019, American Cancer Society, Inc.)

cancers account for approximately half of all new cancer cases.

Some tumor cells produce and secrete substances called *tumor markers.* Screening tests for elevation of blood serum levels of tumor markers, when considered with other diagnostic data, are shown to have clinical value in (1) helping determine the diagnosis of cancer, (2) evaluating response to therapy, and (3) screening for disease recurrence. For example, in primary and metastatic prostate cancer, elevated prostate-specific antigen (PSA) may be found.

If cancer is suspected, additional diagnostic investigation is achieved by using high-technology imaging techniques and, most decisively, by performing *biopsy* of the lesion.

After a cancer diagnosis has been confirmed, the patient undergoes an evaluation to determine the stage of the neoplasm. The *stage* reflects tumor size and the extent of tumor spread. It has important implications for prognosis and in the determination of treatment choice. Staging is a terminology that institutions can use to communicate patient information, so the procedures and staging systems used for staging must be standardized worldwide. Types of cancer that are more prevalent in less developed countries, such as cervical cancer, are often staged clinically and without use of technologies, such as magnetic resonance imaging (MRI) and computed tomography (CT). For some types of cancer, such as endometrial neoplasms, complete staging requires surgical removal of the affected organ and examination of the specimen by an experienced pathologist.

Although a number of different staging systems exist, the majority of cancers use the tumor–node–metastasis (TNM) system. TNM staging assesses the neoplasm in three different areas: (1) the size or extent of the primary tumor (T); (2) the extent of regional lymph node involvement by the tumor (N); and (3) the number of distant metastases (M). Once all three parameters are defined, they are combined to assign a stage number: I, II, III, or IV to the cancer. Stage I is an early stage tumor and carries the best prognosis, whereas stage IV is the most advanced stage. Within each stage, subcategories are defined (Ia, Ib, and so on) to further aid in treatment planning and facilitation of communication among institutions and physicians. See Table 1.4 for an example of staging.

The stage usually offers the best indicator of prognosis. The prognosis reflects the estimation of the likelihood of cancer recurrence and death, independent of the treatment given. In general, the diagnosis of cancer in an early stage offers a greater chance for cure. The prognosis is usually reported statistically as the percentage of patients with that cancer who are still alive after a certain period. The patient may be cured of the disease, in remission, or still undergoing treatment. The most frequently reported survival period is

TABLE 1.4	Melanoma Staging System of the American Joint Committee on Cancer		
Primary Tumor (pT)			
TX	Primary tumor cannot be assessed		
T0	No evidence of primary tumor		
Tis	Melanoma in situ (atypical melanotic hyperplasia, severe melanotic dysplasia)		
T1	Tumor ≤ 1 mm in thickness, a = without ulceration and mitosis < 1/mm²; b = with ulceration and mitoses ≥ 1/mm2		
T2	Tumor > 1 mm but not > 2 mm in thickness, a = without ulceration; b = with ulceration		
T3	Tumor > 2 mm but not > 4 mm in thickness, a = without ulceration; b = with ulceration		
p4	Tumor > 4 mm in thickness, a = without ulceration; b = with ulceration		
Lymph Node (N)			
NX	Regional lymph nodes cannot be assessed		
N0	No regional lymph node metastasis		
N1	One positive lymph node, a = intralymphatic micrometastasis; b = macrometastases		
N2	Two to three positive lymph nodes, a = micrometastasis; b = macrometastases; c = in transit metastasis without metastatic nodes		
N3	≥ 4 metastatic nodes or matted nodes or in transit metastasis with metastatic nodes		
Distant Metastasis (M)			
MX	Presence of distant metastasis cannot be assessed		
M0	No distant metastasis		
M1a	Metastases to skin, subcutaneous tissue, or distant lymph nodes; normal lactate dehydrogenase (LDH)		
M1b	Metastases to lung, normal LDH		
M1c	All other visceral metastases with normal LDH, any distant metastasis with elevated LDH		
Clinical Stage Grouping			
Stage 0	Tis	N0	M0
Stage IA	T1a,	N0	M0
Stage IB	T1b, T2a	N0	M0
Stage IIA	T2b,T3a	N0	M0
Stage IIB	T3b, T4a	N0	M0
Stage IIC	T4b	N0	M0
Stage III	Any T	N1, N2, or N3	M0
Stage IV	Any T	Any N	M1

5 years. It can be reported as "overall 5-year survival," which takes into account all the people, regardless of stage, with that cancer who are still alive; or it can be reported to reflect the 5-year survival rate for people in the various stages of cancer. For example, the overall 5-year survival rate for all types of cancer combined is 68% (i.e., for every 100 people diagnosed with cancer, 68 will be alive 5 years later), but the 5-year survival rate for stage IV colon cancer is 6%. It is important to note, however, that the current 5-year survival rate actually represents data from patients diagnosed with cancer at least 8 years ago and does not reflect more recent advances in treatment.

Depending on the type of neoplasm, other factors can impact prognosis. Examples include age of the patient, serum concentration of any tumor markers, time between diagnosis and treatment, and grade of the tumor. Tumor grade is determined through microscopic evaluation of the tumor or a biopsy specimen. Grade is assigned on the basis of the degree of differentiation of the tumor cells. *Well-differentiated,* low-grade tumor cells still retain features of the tissue cells from which they are derived. *Poorly differentiated,* high-grade tumor cells are more abnormal in appearance and do not resemble the tissue from which they are derived. High-grade tumor cells usually have a greater number of mitoses (divide more rapidly) and are associated with poorer survival.

One type of cancer in which grade is a very important indicator of prognosis is prostate cancer. The grading system is known as the *Gleason grade,* and this system was designed with the knowledge that prostate cancer has different patterns of growth and that multiple patterns coexist in the prostate. Analysis of prostate tumor histology is performed, and the two predominant patterns are recorded and scored from 1 to 5 (1 represents a well-differentiated histology; 5 is the most poorly differentiated). Both scores are summed to give a Gleason score from 2 to 10. The Gleason grade correlates with extent of disease throughout the body and with prognosis.

The goal of cancer treatment is to eradicate every cancer cell in the body. Treatment options involve localized therapy (e.g., surgery and radiation) along with systemic modalities (e.g., chemotherapy, hormonal therapy, and immunotherapy). Surgery alone is curative only for some early-stage tumors. Usually, more than one treatment option is employed. *Neoadjuvant therapy* may be administered preoperatively to shrink the tumor to facilitate surgical removal.

Surgery is important for the treatment of solid cancers and is often used in the staging evaluation as well. As a treatment modality, the goal is either cure or palliative symptom control. When surgery is employed as a curative measure, surgeons try to achieve negative margins around the tumor—that is, the surgeon will remove a certain amount of normal tissue along with the tumor to ensure that the entire tumor has been removed. If negative margins are not achieved, surgery must be performed again or another type of treatment must be tried. At the time of surgery, the regional lymph nodes may be evaluated to determine whether the cancer cells have entered the lymphatic system and invaded the nodes. Affected nodes are generally removed. Palliative surgery is performed to relieve troublesome symptoms, such as an obstruction. Relief can be achieved by tumor resection, bypass, stenting, or laser *ablation.*

Chemotherapy involves the use of medicines to destroy cancer cells. Most of the drugs affect cell replication, so chemotherapy is most effective against rapidly dividing cells, such as cancer cells. Normal cells in other parts of the body that are known to divide rapidly also are destroyed, and this accounts for many of the classic side effects of chemotherapy. These cell populations (and the related side effects) include hair cells (alopecia); gastrointestinal (GI) mucosal cells (anorexia, vomiting, and diarrhea); hematopoietic cells (anemia and bruising); and reproductive organs (infertility). Often drugs that affect different steps in cell replication are administered at the same time (combination chemotherapy). Chemotherapy usually is given in cycles that include a treatment period followed by a recovery period and is often performed in the outpatient setting. Although cancer cells may be initially responsive to the drugs, cells tend to develop resistance to the drugs over time, and new drugs or different treatment modalities must then be employed.

The use of hormone therapy and immunotherapy in the treatment of cancer is continually evolving. Hormone therapy can be effective in hormone-dependent cancers, such as breast cancer and prostate cancer. It may involve the administration of drugs that suppress hormone synthesis, such as luteinizing hormone-releasing hormone (LHRH) antagonists or aromatase inhibitors that are used to treat prostate cancer; drugs that block the action of hormones, such as the estrogen receptor modulator tamoxifen used to treat breast cancer; or surgical removal of hormone-producing glands, such as an *oophorectomy* and *orchiectomy.*

Immunotherapy stimulates the body's own immune system to fight cancer. It can involve the use of cancer vaccines (see the Enrichment box on Cancer Vaccines), infusion of cellular products, such as T cells or natural killer (NK) cells, which may or may not have been modified prior to administration, or *monoclonal antibodies* designed to target certain products of cancer cells that are not found in normal cells. These antibodies may generate an anticancer effect in one of three ways: (1) they can trigger an immune response against the tumor cell, (2) deliver a lethal dose of radiation to the cell, or (3) release a deadly chemical inside the cell. Several antibodies are currently approved for use by the U.S. Food and Drug Administration (FDA). They include trastuzumab (Herceptin), approved for use in breast cancers that overexpress the human epidermal growth factor receptor 2 (HER2/neu) protein; rituximab (Rituxan) for use in non-Hodgkin lymphoma; alemtuzumab (Campath) for use in chronic lymphocytic leukemia; and ipilimumab (Yervoy) for metastatic melanoma. Newer-generation medications to treat breast cancer include three newer drugs, which are CDK4 and CDK6 inhibitors (cyclin-dependent kinases). Abemaciclib (Verzenio), palbociclib (IBRANCE), and ribociclib (Kisqali) all belong to this class of drugs.

◆ ENRICHMENT

Cancer Vaccines

Although there are currently some vaccines that may be given to prevent cancer (e.g., the human papillomavirus (HPV) vaccine that protects against cervical cancer and the hepatitis B vaccine that helps protect against liver cancer), research is currently underway to produce vaccines that may treat cancer in patients who already have the disease. Researchers are trying to isolate proteins from cancer cells, which, when injected into a patient with cancer, can trigger an immune response in the patient to attack and destroy the cancer cells. Others are attempting to inject a substance that will cause a more generalized immune response within tumor tissue to destroy it. Many cancer vaccines are in clinical trials, and one that has received the U.S. Food and Drug Administration (FDA) approval for use in patients with metastatic hormone refractory–prostate cancer who are minimally symptomatic is sipuleucel-T (Provenge). This novel approach to cancer therapy could be a way to enhance the body's natural defense mechanisms to combat this disease.

For patients with metastatic disease, a cure may not be possible, but these same treatment modalities may be useful in prolonging life or improving the quality of life for the patient. Even after the patient has achieved remission, he or she must be followed up closely for several years. Micrometastases may exist at the time of diagnosis that can lead to eventual recurrence of the cancer if they are not eradicated by systemic therapy.

Advances in radiation and chemotherapy have diminished the need for radical surgery. However, these modalities have significant side effects that require constant surveillance and management. Pain management both during and after treatment is a major concern in patients and includes generous use of various analgesics and noninvasive techniques that promote relaxation and distraction. Terminally ill persons can be referred to hospice care for compassionate, holistic case management (see the Enrichment box on Hospice Care).

◆◆ ENRICHMENT

Hospice Care

The word *hospice* describes a unique concept of care developed to help patients and their families deal with life-threatening illness. The hospice philosophy of care includes compassionate staff pledged to respect the patient's choice for care and to provide comfort, dignity, and privacy. The focus is on comfort and supportive care for the family unit during the illness and the bereavement period. Hospice care is covered by health insurance if a patient has a terminal illness and a physician certifies that the patient likely has less than 6 months of life remaining, although the amount covered may vary by insurer.

The philosophy of hospice affirms life and neither hastens nor postpones death. Dying is recognized as a normal process, even when it is the result of disease. Through appropriate care and the promotion of a caring community sensitive to their needs, patients and families may be free to attain a degree of mental and spiritual preparation for death that is satisfactory to them. The hospice team may include a physician, a registered nurse available day and night, a social worker, a home health aide as needed, a chaplain as needed, volunteers, therapists, and a pharmacist. Hospice provides a full range of care in a variety of settings, such as a residential hospice care center, a skilled nursing facility, or the patient's home.

The field of palliative medicine has grown out of the need to incorporate the philosophy of hospice into the acute medical care setting. Many hospitals now have palliative care teams that concentrate on the psychosocial care of the patient and family and on the management of advanced disease. Involving a palliative care team early on in the course of a terminal illness can provide much-needed support even before the patient qualifies for hospice care.

One aspect of cancer treatment that is becoming more important as a greater number of patients are being cured of their cancer is the consequence of therapy. Chemotherapy and radiation therapy are very toxic, not only to cancer cells but also to the body in general. Some of the effects of this toxicity are not seen until many years after therapy. Patients are predisposed to the development of other malignancies,

especially lymphomas and leukemias. The late effects of cancer therapy are even more dramatic in children. Delayed growth and cognitive impairment are not uncommon. Still, cancer therapies are constantly evolving and methods are being developed that may not have such drastic long-term side effects, as seen in the physical state of cachexia (e.g., see the Enrichment box on Stereotactic Radiosurgery).

◆◆ ENRICHMENT

Stereotactic Radiosurgery

Stereotactic radiosurgery (SRS) has been available for several years as an alternative to conventional radiation therapy (RT) for cancer tumors. Traditional RT involves giving small doses of radiation with a single beam for many cycles (25–30), whereas SRS involves many beams of low-dose radiation coming in at different angles to converge on one point so that the target tumor (or lesion) will get intense radiation, but the normal tissue each single beam passes through only gets a small amount. An analogy might be many people in a circle shining flashlights onto the same point. That one point will be very bright, but the individual beams themselves give off very little light. The advantages of SRS over RT are that normal tissues experience much less toxicity. Usually only one or few treatments are required with a short or no recovery time. Generally fatigue is the most common side effect. Other possible side effects are specific to the area of external beam radiation and are monitored and treated by a radiation oncologist. SRS offers hope in the treatment of cancer in sites considered inoperable by conventional surgery.

CyberKnife is a sophisticated precise system of radiation treatment considered a major advance in SRS technology. It is now available at many hospitals on an outpatient basis for the noninvasive and extremely precise treatment of many types of malignant tumors. The system provides increased access to tumors particularly in the brain, the base of the skull, or the spine; however, it may be used anywhere in the body and provides a more relaxed treatment experience. Real-time imaging is combined with intelligent robotics; so when the patient moves slightly, the robot immediately adjusts the beams so the target tumor (or lesion) remains at the center of the beam. CyberKnife does not require the invasive external fixation used with traditional radiosurgery (Gamma Knife and LINAC) to stabilize patient movement. CyberKnife has been used to investigate the pancreas, prostate, and lungs.

RT is still preferred in some cases, such as for a large tumor or when the tumor is near a cranial nerve or a speech/language center of the brain.

Research continually provides useful information about new, promising approaches to cancer treatment. Certain forms of cancer are inherited; thus much of the current research is focused on cancer at its genetic roots. Scientists are investigating genetic switches that cause healthy cells to become disorderly. It has been observed that broken genes can send cells into spirals of cancerous growth. Such oncogenes and tumor suppressor genes are proposed targets for therapy. One drug currently targeting an oncogene is imatinib (Gleevec), which inhibits the *BCR-ABL* tyrosine kinase (an abnormal enzyme) in chronic myelogenous leukemia.

Specific types of cancer are discussed in subsequent chapters of this book.

Immune Disorders

The immune system is a complex network of specialized cells and organs that has evolved to defend the body against attacks by foreign organisms. Immune disorders are the result of a breakdown in the body's defense system that may generate (1) hypersensitivity (allergy), (2) autoimmune diseases, or (3) immunodeficiency disorders.

Allergic disease is a hypersensitivity of the body to a substance (**allergen**) ordinarily considered harmless. Common allergens include inhalants (dust, molds, and fungi), food, animal dander, drugs, insect venom, chemicals, and physical agents (heat, cold, and radiation). Initial exposure to an allergen, which acts as an **antigen** (a substance that causes the allergic response), stimulates the production of immunoglobulin E (IgE) antibodies, and the person thus is sensitized. Subsequent exposures trigger the allergic response, which is an antigen–antibody reaction causing the release of histamine and other chemicals (Fig. 1.4). The chemicals cause a variety of persistent and bothersome symptoms, including nasal congestion, sneezing, coughing, wheezing, itching, burning, swelling, and diarrhea. Common allergic conditions include seasonal allergic rhinitis (hay fever), allergic sinusitis, bronchial asthma, urticaria (hives), and eczema. These conditions may range from mild and self-limiting ones to severe and life-threatening ones.

Although allergies cannot be cured, they can usually be controlled with proper diagnosis and treatment. Diagnosis includes allergy blood testing and/or allergy skin testing. When the offending allergens can be identified, they are eliminated from the diet or the environment. Symptomatic treatment includes the use of antihistamines, bronchial dilators, and corticosteroids. Desensitization with a series of injections may be recommended to build immunity to some antigens.

Severe systemic manifestations of allergic responses include **anaphylaxis**, serum sickness, arthralgia, and status asthmaticus. For example, anaphylaxis (anaphylactic shock), the result of a severe systemic allergic reaction, calls for emergency life-saving intervention. Common causes of anaphylaxis include insect stings, food, latex, and medications.

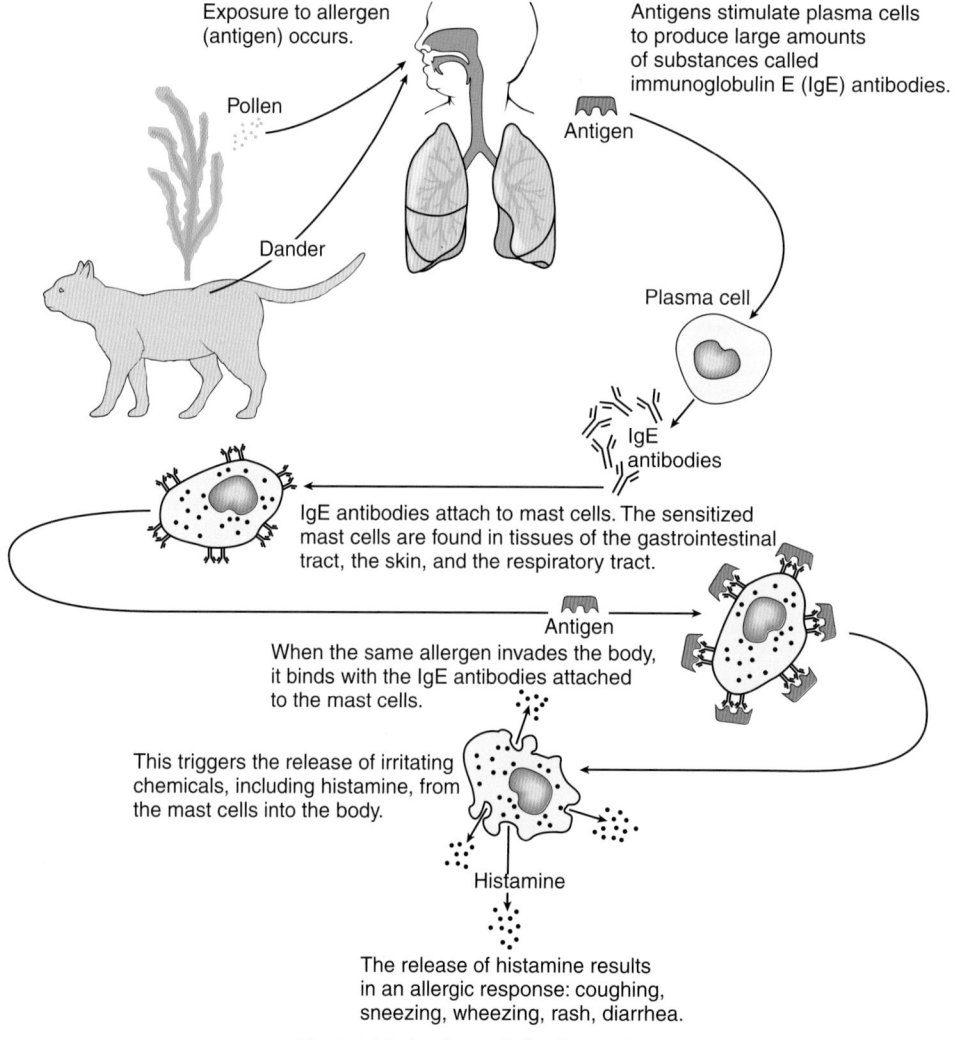

Exposure to allergen (antigen) occurs.

Pollen

Dander

Antigens stimulate plasma cells to produce large amounts of substances called immunoglobulin E (IgE) antibodies.

Antigen

Plasma cell

IgE antibodies

IgE antibodies attach to mast cells. The sensitized mast cells are found in tissues of the gastrointestinal tract, the skin, and the respiratory tract.

Antigen

When the same allergen invades the body, it binds with the IgE antibodies attached to the mast cells.

This triggers the release of irritating chemicals, including histamine, from the mast cells into the body.

Histamine

The release of histamine results in an allergic response: coughing, sneezing, wheezing, rash, diarrhea.

• **Fig. 1.4** Mechanisms of allergic reaction.

Individuals who are prone to systemic allergic reaction often carry prescribed epinephrine kits for self-administration until they can reach an emergency facility.

Autoimmune diseases represent a large group of disorders marked by an inappropriate or excessive response of the body's defense system that allows the immune system to become self-destructive. Normally the immune system is able to distinguish self-antigens, which are harmless, from foreign antigens, which present a threat to the body. In autoimmune diseases, antibodies are formed against self-antigens mistakenly identified as foreign. Why the body becomes confused or what triggers an autoimmune response remains a mystery. Many serious diseases appear to have a strong autoimmune component. Examples are glomerulonephritis (see Chapter 11), Hashimoto disease (see Chapter 4), and rheumatoid arthritis (see Chapter 3).

Immunodeficiency disorders result from a depressed or absent immune response. Causative factors can be primary, manifested by a characteristic decrease in the number of T cells and B cells, leaving the body unable to adequately defend itself against infection and tumors. Immunodeficiency also may be secondary to disease, infection, and aging or may be the result of damage to the immune system caused by drugs, radiation, or surgery. Acquired immunodeficiency syndrome (AIDS), a prominent example of an immunodeficiency state, is caused by infection by human immunodeficiency virus (HIV).

Chapter 3 discusses specific diseases of the immune system.

Physical Trauma and Chemical Agents

Physical trauma is the major cause of death in children and young adults. Common mechanisms of acute injury are falls; motor vehicle accidents, including those involving pedestrians; physical abuse; physical injury from incidents of domestic violence; penetrating injuries; multiple types of injuries sustained in military combat; drowning; and burns. Emergency management begins with triage to determine the priorities of care. Persons who sustain trauma require precise assessment and management to prevent infection, to minimize the insult to the body's tissues, to combat shock and hemorrhage, and to restore homeostasis.

Chemical agents or irritants that are potentially injurious include pollutants, poisons, drugs, preservatives, cosmetics, and dyes. There are known bioterrorism infectious agents that can cause severe toxic trauma to humans in a bioterrorism attack (see Alert box in Chapter 15). Extreme heat or cold, radiation, electrical shock, and insect and snake bites are other instruments of injury to the body.

See Chapter 15 for a discussion of specific types of trauma.

Malnutrition

Disorders of nutrition, as discussed in Chapter 8, may be the result of a deficient diet or of disease conditions that do not allow the body to break down, absorb, or use food. An example of a severe deficiency disease is protein-calorie malnutrition (kwashiorkor), the starvation associated with famine. Other nutritional disorders include eating disorders, iron deficiency, anemia, obesity, and hypervitaminoses.

Aging

Because of the gradual diminishment of body functions, the aging process, although not considered a disease in itself, is a risk factor for the onset of many health problems. With aging comes *immunosenescence,* which is a gradual deterioration of the functions of the immune system. As a result, older adults are at higher risk for infections and less able to achieve full protection from vaccinations. This along with other age-related risk factors explains why bacterial community-acquired pneumonia is responsible for a high incidence of death in older adults. A yearly physical examination with specific screening tests is recommended after age 50 years. Screening examinations include determination of blood cholesterol levels for hyperlipidemia, electrocardiography (ECG) for heart disease, rectal examination for bowel cancer and prostate enlargement, PSA serum blood test to determine prostate health, blood pressure check for hypertension, Papanicolaou (Pap) smear for cervical cancer, mammography for breast cancer, and urinalysis for possible diabetes and renal disease.

The nature of geriatrics is changing as the life span in the United States has reached an all-time high (78.7 years) because of preventative health care and innovations in medical management. Knowing the special needs of older persons is becoming a more critical component of health care because the percentage of Americans over age 65 years is growing dramatically. Currently, 14.9% of the population is older than age 65 years of age, and they account for greater than one-third of all health expenditures. It is predicted that this percentage will double over the next 20 years as the "baby boomers" approach late adulthood. Attention must be paid to the functional status and to the health issues of older patients. Common concerns are substance abuse, overmedication, loss of mental acuity, depression, and nutritional problems. Regular exercise three to five times a week, proper nutrition, and creating a hazard-free environment to prevent falls should all be emphasized. Each year, 1 in 3 adults age 65 years and older falls, causing moderate to severe injuries.

Older adults can have many significant life stresses, such as financial hardship, relocation, loss of normal roles in life, and death of loved ones and friends. Skyrocketing health care costs and medical insurance premiums are troubling to seniors living on fixed incomes. Such added stress in a person's life may be a contributing factor in disease development or progression. Drug therapy is another major issue, because many older adults take a number of different prescribed medications, in addition to nonprescription drugs that the health care professionals providing care might not know about. These older persons are at high risk for adverse drug reactions and may have to be hospitalized for such problems. Older adults are often given daily doses of intestinal probiotics to ward off antibiotic-associated diarrhea and infection with *Clostridioides difficile* which can cause life-threatening bowel inflammation. A recent study has cast doubt on the effectiveness of routine prescription of probiotics along with antibiotics for older patients.

Older adults also may not be able to tolerate the standard dose of medications because of metabolic and other changes in body composition (increased adipose tissue, decreased total body water, and so on) that occur with aging. Severe cognitive impairment from any one of several forms of dementia may present substantial hardship to the older person and to family members and caregivers. Other conditions frequently associated with aging include urinary incontinence and sensory isolation because of visual and/or hearing impairment. Generally the state of frailty makes older people more vulnerable to infection, injury, and inability to tolerate invasive therapies.

Psychological Factors

The constant interaction between mind and body can potentially affect a person's state of wellness or illness. When a person seeks medical attention, assessment of mental status is intertwined with physical evaluation. Psychological evaluation encompasses the observation of behavior, appearance, mood, communication, judgment, and thought processes. Because people react differently to disease or the threat of illness, treatment plans must be tailored to meet their psychological needs as well. Preservation of self-esteem is of great importance.

Illness can disrupt daily activities; it can significantly change a patient's life and also the lives of involved family members. In the face of disease, the person experiences an altered body image and emotional and social changes that are best understood in terms of past personal experience and perception. For example, when the patient was a child, did illness elicit empathy and a "chicken soup" approach, or was illness met with aversion and a "tough it out" attitude?

Chronic disease is a stressor that can affect a person's self-esteem and behavior. Fear, helplessness, and lack of control are typical feelings. Patients pass through stages of anxiety, shock, denial, anger, withdrawal, and depression as they adjust to the presence of disease. If these stages are sustained and the person fails to accept the reality of the disease, the patient may develop psychological disturbances in addition to physical alterations.

Mental Disorders

Generally mental disorders are described as clinically significant behavioral or psychological syndromes that are associated with psychic pain or distress or impairment of function. Although sometimes cloaked in mystery, the common occurrence of mental disorders and their potential for causing disability dictate the need for the same careful handling as for any other sickness. Chapter 14 discusses mental disorders in more detail, including grief response, dementia, mood disorders, and somatoform disorders.

Diagnosis of Disease

When a person seeks medical attention and describes symptoms and/or exhibits signs of disease, the clinician begins an orderly series of steps to investigate the cause and make a diagnosis (Fig. 1.5). Establishing a diagnosis is a decision-making process in which data collected from the medical history, physical examination, and diagnostic tests are analyzed, integrated, and interpreted. A diagnosis provides a logical basis for determining treatment and prognosis.

The importance of the patient's medical history cannot be overstated; as the primary source of data, it provides vital clues and background information that help direct the remainder of the assessment. During the patient interview, medical information (e.g., family history, predisposing factors or preexisting conditions, drug allergies, and current therapies) is carefully noted. This can provide the foundation for an individualized treatment plan. And, finally, the clinician focuses questions on the onset and nature of the present illness.

Next, a methodical physical examination of the patient from head to toe (a systems review) is performed to detect the physical signs of disease. Assessment skills used to evaluate health status are inspection (observation and measurement, including vital signs), auscultation (trained listening), palpation (investigation by sense of touch), and percussion (tapping that produces vibration and sound). The information gathered is then measured against norms or standards.

The final source of assessment data is that which can be obtained by conducting a wide variety of appropriate diagnostic studies and laboratory tests. These include microscopic examination of cells and tissues and chemical analysis. Although diagnostic testing is considered an important scientific measure of function, these laboratory data are not interpreted apart from other clinical data gathered from the history and physical examination. In the process of deciding or confirming the identification of a disease, the results of diagnostic studies are integrated with the medical history and physical examination findings. In fact, physicians now have computerized systems that can analyze large numbers of patient records to quantify probabilities and to devise an orderly approach to diagnosis (a decision tree). As a result, the physician is reminded of a full range of possible diagnoses for a given set of symptoms and signs; in other words, the physician is aided in making a *differential diagnosis,* especially when two or more diseases resemble one another in respect to signs and symptoms.

Laboratory tests, particularly biochemical profiles obtained by testing blood and urine, are used routinely to screen for imbalances or to detect early signs of disease. They also are used to monitor the effectiveness of therapeutic medications and other medical treatment (Box 1.1).

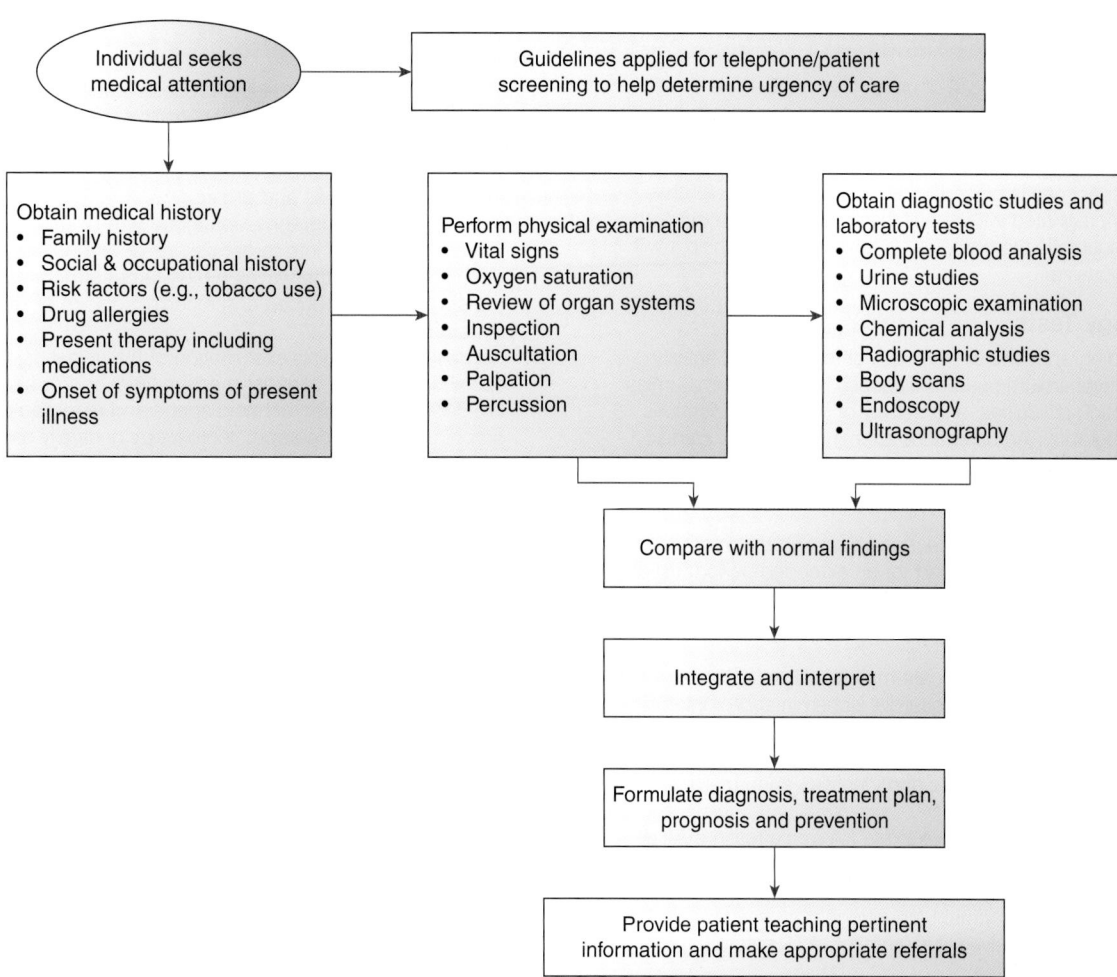

• **Fig. 1.5** Essential steps in diagnosis.

<table>
<tr><td>• BOX 1.1</td><td>Common Laboratory and Diagnostic Tests</td></tr>
</table>

Blood Analysis

Complete blood count (CBC): Evaluation of cellular components of the blood; includes red blood cell (RBC) count, RBC indices, white blood cell (WBC) count, WBC differential, hemoglobin (Hgb), hematocrit (HCT), and platelet count; sometimes referred to as *hemogram;* often the differential must be ordered specifically as CBC with differential

Hgb: Measurement of the oxygen-carrying pigment of the RBCs

HCT: Measurement of the percentage of RBCs in a volume of whole blood

Glycosylated hemoglobin: Measurement of Hgb to which glucose is bound; also known as *HgbA1c*

Chemistries: Normal chemistry profiles may contain blood serum levels for albumin, alkaline phosphatase, aspartate aminotransferase (AST), bilirubin, calcium, creatinine, lactate dehydrogenase (LD), phosphorus, total protein, urea nitrogen, and uric acid

Thyroid function tests: Thyroid thyroxine (T_4), triiodothyronine (T_3), and thyroid-stimulating hormone (TSH)

Lipid profile: Total cholesterol, triglycerides, high-density lipoprotein (HDL) cholesterol, and low-density lipoprotein (LDL) cholesterol

Electrolytes (lytes): Blood serum test for chloride, potassium, sodium, and carbon dioxide

Clotting and coagulation studies: Partial thromboplastin time (PTT), prothrombin time (PT), platelet (thrombocyte) count, and bleeding times

Erythrocyte sedimentation rate (ESR): The rate at which RBCs (erythrocytes) fall out of well-mixed whole blood to the bottom of the test tube

Glucose tolerance test (GTT): Fasting blood glucose (FBG) levels

Toxicology studies: Drug screens

Drug levels: Digoxin, digitoxin, theophylline, lidocaine, lithium, and various drugs for therapeutic and/or toxic levels

Arterial blood gas (ABG) analysis: Measurement of dissolved oxygen (O_2) and carbon dioxide in arterial blood. Also measures pH and O_2 saturation of arterial blood

Cardiac enzymes: Creatine kinase (CK), CK isoenzymes, LD, LD isoenzymes, AST (serum glutamic oxaloacetic transaminase [SGOT]), and alanine aminotransferase (ALT; serum glutamic pyruvate transaminase [SGPT])

Cross-reactive protein (CRP): A blood test used to detect bacterial infection and inflammatory disorders; an indicator of possible acute myocardial infarction

Urine Studies

Urinalysis (UA): A screening test using a urine specimen that gives a picture of the patient's overall state of health and the state of the urinary tract. Measurements include pH and specific gravity of the urine, presence of ketones, protein, sugars, bilirubin, and urobilinogen. Color and odor are noted, as is the presence of abnormal blood cells, casts, bacteria, other cells, and crystals.

Continued

• **BOX 1.1** **Common Laboratory and Diagnostic Tests—cont'd**

Culture and sensitivity (C&S) of urine: *Culture:* Sample of urine specimen is placed in/on culture medium to see whether microbial growth occurs. If growth occurs, identification of the pathogenic microbe is determined. *Sensitivity:* A portion of the specimen is placed on a sensitivity disk (which has been impregnated with specific antibiotics) to determine to which antibiotic the pathogen is resistant or to which it will be responsive.

Cardiology Tests

Electrocardiography (ECG): A record of the electrical activity of the myocardium used to diagnose ischemia, arrhythmias, conduction difficulties, and activity of cardiac medications

Echocardiography: An ultrasound examination of the cardiac structure to define the size, shape, thickness, position, and movements of the cardiac structures, including valves, walls, and chambers

Holter monitor: A miniature electrocardiograph that records the electrical activity of the heart for an extended period, usually 24 to 48 hours; patient records all activities during the time period for the examiner to correlate activity with cardiac abnormalities

Thallium scan: A scan to indicate myocardial profusion and the location and extent of myocardial ischemia and/or infarction and to predict the possible prognosis of the cardiac condition

Multigated acquisition (MUGA) scan: A scan that assesses the function of the left ventricle and identifies abnormalities of the myocardial walls

Stress testing, treadmill, and exercise tolerance testing: An assessment of cardiac function during moderate exercise after 12-lead ECG

Pulse oximeter: An instrument (spectrophotometer) that provides a noninvasive measurement of O_2 saturation of arterial blood

Cardiac catheterization: Fluoroscopic visualization of right or left side of heart by passing a catheter into right or left chamber and injecting dye. Angiography consists of the catheter being passed into the coronary vessels where the dye is injected and fluoroscopic images are recorded.

Imaging Studies

Radiography: Visualization of internal organs and structures by electromagnetic radiation. Radiographs of bone; the abdomen; the chest; paranasal sinuses; kidneys, ureters, and bladder (KUB); and mammograms that do not require contrast medium; contrast medium used to distinguish soft tissue and some organs, such as the gallbladder, esophagus, stomach, and small and large intestines

Magnetic resonance imaging (MRI): Uses a magnetic field instead of radiation to visualize internal tissues; it is possible to view tissue and organs in a three-dimensional manner with MRI. Helpful in determining blood flow to tissues and organs, in studying condition of blood vessels, in detecting tumors, in differentiating healthy and diseased tissues, and in detecting sites of infection; patient not exposed to ionizing radiation during MRI

Computed tomography (CT): A radiographic technique using a scanner system that can provide images of the internal structure of tissue and organs both geographically and characteristically

Positron emission tomography (PET): A highly specialized imaging technique that uses a small amount of radioactive material to produce three-dimensional colored images that reveal how body tissues and organs are functioning by providing information about the body's chemistry

Fluoroscopy: A real-time imaging process that provides continuous visualization of the area undergoing radiography; still films and video recordings are made of the process for more extensive examination; used in procedures and to study the functioning of tissues and organs

Sonography, ultrasonography, echography: A beam of sound waves is projected into target tissues or organs, resulting in a bouncing back of the waves off the target structure; outline of the structure is produced and recorded on film or videotape for examination

Myelography: An imaging examination of the spinal cord and spinal nerve roots; contrast medium (dye) and/or air are injected into the subarachnoid space and recorded on radiographic film and videotape; fluoroscopy generally used in this procedure

Stool Analysis

Guaiac tests: For occult blood
Ova and parasite tests

Sputum Analysis

Sputum studies: Microscopic studies of sputum, including C&S, acid-fast bacteria culture and stain, Gram staining, and cytology studies

Endoscopy Tests

Endoscopy: Visual inspection of internal organs and/or cavities of the body using appropriate scope; procedures named after the body area or organ to be visualized or treated

Gastroscopy: Visualization of the stomach by a gastroscope

Colonoscopy: Visualization of the colon with a colonoscope

Sigmoidoscopy: Visualization of the sigmoid portion of the colon and the rectum with a sigmoidoscope

Proctoscopy: Visualization of the rectum with a proctoscope

Cystoscopy: Visualization of the structures of the urinary tract with a cystoscope

Colposcopy: Visualization of the cervical epithelium, vagina, and vulvar epithelium with a colposcope

Bronchoscopy: Visualization of the trachea and bronchi with a bronchoscope

Pulmonary Function Studies

Peak flow: The patient blows into a flowmeter to determine the volume of an expiratory effort

Spirometry: A measurement of lung capacity, volume, and flow rates by a spirometer

Methacholine challenge: A test for asthma in which measurement of lung volumes is taken before and after the inhalation of methacholine, a bronchial constrictor

Pulmonary function: Tidal volume, expiratory reserve volume, residual volume, and inspiratory reserve volume

Miscellaneous Tests

C&S: *Culture:* Sample of specimen is placed in/on culture medium to see whether microbial growth occurs; if growth occurs, identification of the pathogenic microbe is determined; *Sensitivity:* A portion of the specimen is placed on a sensitivity disk (which has been impregnated with specific antibiotics) to determine which antibiotic the pathogen is resistant to or to which it will be responsive; the specimen could be blood, stool, urine, sputum, any discharge fluid, or from a wound

Genetic testing has varied applications, such as forensic DNA testing in certain courtroom cases, or paternity genetic testing for proving or disproving paternity

• **BOX 1.1** Common Laboratory and Diagnostic Tests—cont'd

Bone marrow studies: Aspiration of bone marrow by needle from the sternum, posterior or superior iliac spine, or the anterior iliac crest for diagnosis of neoplasms, metastasis, and blood disorders

Immune and immunoglobulin studies: Studies of the functioning or nonfunctioning of the patient's immune system

Serologic testing: Analysis of blood specimens for antigen-antibody reactions. Used to detect bacterial infections, including syphilis, Lyme disease, chlamydia, and streptococcal infections; antibodies from viral sources, including infectious mononucleosis, rubella, hepatitis, rabies, human immunodeficiency virus (HIV), herpes, and cytomegalovirus; antibodies from fungal sources, such as histoplasmosis and *Candida;* and antibodies from the parasitic source, toxoplasmosis

Biopsy: The excision of tissue from the living body, followed by microscopic examination, for purpose of exact diagnosis

Lumbar puncture (LP): A surgical procedure to withdraw spinal fluid for analysis

Electroencephalography (EEG): A recording of the electrical activity of the cerebral cortex of the brain

Electromyelography (EMG): An electrodiagnostic assessment and recording of the activity of the skeletal muscles

Gastric analysis: Used in the diagnosis of pernicious anemia and peptic ulcers

Pregnancy tests: All pregnancy tests are based on the detection of human chorionic gonadotropin (hCG). Used in diagnosis of pregnancy, abortion, ectopic pregnancy, and uterine pathology

Gram staining: Used to identify gram-positive or gram-negative microorganism of infectious process

Polysomnography (PSG): Sleep studies indicated in excessive snoring, excessive daytime sleeping or drowsiness, insomnia or sleep time cardiac rhythm disturbances

Screening

Hepatic screening: Liver function tests, liver profile; usually includes ALT, alkaline phosphatase, AST, bilirubin, and gamma-glutamyl transpeptidase.

Tuberculosis (TB) screening: Mantoux test: An intradermal injection of tuberculin is done usually on the inner aspect of the lower arm; localized thickening of the skin in the area, along with redness, indicates the presence of active or dormant TB; positive reaction requires further investigation, usually including chest radiograph

Prostate-specific antigen (PSA): A serum blood test to determine the level of PSA; increased levels may indicate benign prostatic hypertrophy, prostate cancer, or inflammatory conditions of the prostate; should be followed by a digital rectal examination of the prostate gland to determine any abnormalities; often additional diagnostic studies indicated

Papanicolaou (Pap) smear: A cytologic examination of cells that have been scraped or aspirated from the cervix and cervical os; screen test done annually, especially before any female hormones are prescribed

Mammogram: A radiographic examination of the breast tissue; screen test done on an annual basis for women older than 40 years of age to detect the presence of breast disease; should be accompanied by a manual examination of the breast tissue by a physician; monthly breast self-examinations recommended

These are many of the common diagnostic procedures that may be ordered and performed. Many more diagnostic procedures may be used in the process of arriving at the patient's diagnosis and prognosis. More diagnostic tests and procedures are discussed, along with the corresponding disease or condition, in subsequent chapters. Refer to Appendix I for additional information regarding normal and abnormal values and indications for tests.

Treatment of Disease

After the initial assessment is completed and a diagnosis is established, appropriate medical intervention is implemented. The plan of treatment is directly related to an identified expected outcome. The goal may be specifically to cure, to control symptoms, or to be supportive, or it may be a combination of these. Therapeutic elements of a conventional medical care plan may be used conservatively or aggressively and include one or more of the following: preventive measures, therapeutic procedures, administration of medications, measures for relief of pain, surgery, physical therapy, diet modification, psychotherapy, patient education, and follow-up care.

After a medical treatment plan is implemented, it is evaluated and modified, as needed. The current trend is to involve patients directly in the choices of treatment and to emphasize their responsibility to make choices that promote their recovery. The physician is the expert advisor who must inform and empower the patient. A team approach to medical treatment, involving the patient, medical personnel, family, and community support systems, is optimal for complicated cases.

Encouraging the patient's active participation in the recovery process is essential to this system of care. Feelings of love, humor, hope, and enthusiasm are part of the healing process, whereas feelings of hostility, fear, anger, grief, rage, shame, and greed fuel the illness process.

The concept of holistic medicine is comprehensive care that focuses on the needs of the whole person (Fig. 1.6). The physical and psychological well-being of the individual are dependent on each other. It is this established mind–body interaction that compels the holistic health care provider to consider the patient as a whole person. Rather than narrowly defining a disease *only* in terms of physical pathologic changes, the clinician also considers the patient's social, emotional, intellectual, and spiritual components. Individualizing care is important; the personality, environment, and lifestyle of the patient all need to be factored into the care plan. The holistic practitioner acknowledges the uniqueness of the patient with regard to his or her needs, aspirations, perception, comprehension, and insight. The illness or health-altering event is considered to be a dysfunction of the entire, or whole, person and not just an isolated dimension.

The absence of illness does not necessarily indicate optimal health. Holistic care encourages the patient to consciously pursue the highest possible expressions of being, including those of spirit, mind, emotion, environment, socialization, and physical being. Although integrating all the needs of a patient is compatible with the comprehensive

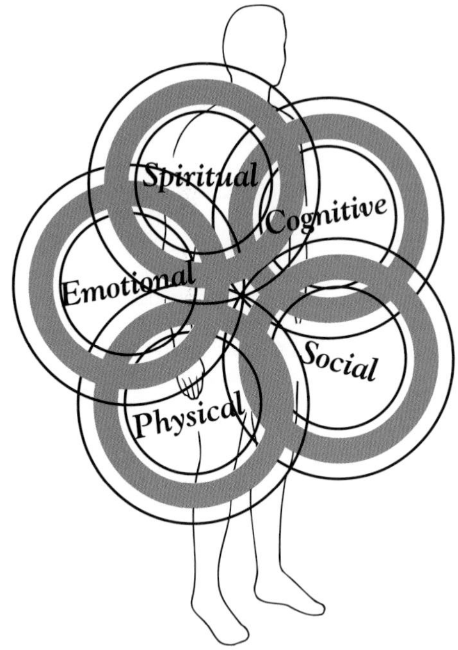

• **Fig. 1.6** Human beings from a holistic viewpoint. The expanding and receding circles represent the dynamic interaction of the physical, social, emotional, spiritual, and cognitive needs that constitute humanness. (From Luckmann J, Sorensen K: *Medical-surgical nursing: a pathophysiologic approach,* Philadelphia, 1987, Saunders.)

treatment plans of traditional medicine, holistic medicine may also incorporate a variety of nontraditional methods of treatment, which may be empirical or experimental. A discussion on nontraditional methods of treatment can be found later in this chapter.

Cultural Diversity

One important aspect of holistic medicine is recognition of the cultural diversity of patients. The United States continues to grow more culturally diverse. According to the U.S. Census Bureau, the number of foreign-born U.S. residents increased from 19 million to about 40 million between 1990 and 2010. Health care providers must be aware of the challenges of caring for such a diverse population, such challenges as differences in language, religious beliefs, views about health issues, and life experiences. Stereotyping can be misleading in caring for a patient. Some hospitals use a cultural pocket guide, noting such traditions as birth and death rituals and dietary preferences.

Overcoming the challenges that cultural diversity presents begins with a willingness on the part of the health care provider to learn about cultural issues, to overcome language barriers, and to take the time necessary to understand what the patient is trying to convey. Many hospitals and clinics have interpreters available to facilitate communication with more prominent minority groups in their communities. Assistance with a Navigation Program can help steer patients through the treatment process. Even so, it

takes time, patience, and flexibility to acquire knowledge of different cultures and their ways of explaining, understanding, and treating health problems.

Gene Therapy

Gene therapy refers to the experimental intervention of adding, repairing, or blocking the expression of specific genes to treat a disease. A therapeutic gene is delivered by using a vector (a chaperone molecule that accompanies and aids in the safe delivery of DNA). Most of the vectors used for DNA delivery, to date, involve viruses (most commonly *adenovirus* or adeno-associated virus), but nonviral vectors, such as liposomes (small, spherical, artificial particles consisting of a lipid bilayer that encloses, in this case, the gene to be delivered), are being investigated as well. Protocols may be done ex vivo (outside the body) or in vivo (inside the body). In ex vivo protocols, the cells to be modified are removed from the body, modified, and returned to the patient. In vivo therapies treat the patient with a gene delivery vehicle that will target the desired cells for the gene modification. Gene therapy aims to treat autosomal or X-linked recessive diseases by addition of a functional copy of the defective gene. The goal for autosomal dominant disease is to inhibit or repair the defective gene. Experimental gene therapy protocols have been designed to treat diseases, such as cystic fibrosis, sickle cell anemia, hemophilia B, and various forms of cancer. Recently, trials in hemophilia B have begun to show significant benefit for some patients. Still, much research needs to be done before this type of treatment can become the standard of care. Because of the recent promising results, researchers believe that they will soon be able to surmount the technical difficulties that currently prohibit the use of gene therapy in the treatment of a wide variety of illnesses.

Stem Cell Research

Scientists study stem cells to investigate their potential to repair damaged tissue in a field called *regenerative medicine.*

A stem cell is an unspecialized cell that has the potential to give rise to cells specialized for any tissue in the body. When the stem cell divides, the daughter cell has the potential to become another stem cell or to differentiate into liver, lung, heart, or other specific types of cells. In the human embryo, stem cells give rise to the specialized cells that make up the lungs, heart, brain, and other tissues. Stem cells still exist in many adult tissues, such as bone marrow, skin, and liver, to replace cells lost through disease, injury, or normal use. As long as a person is alive, his or her stem cells are able to divide, differentiate, and replenish the various cells in the body. Specialized cells, in contrast, can only give rise to other specialized cells.

Stem cell research has already resulted in an important advance in medicine, that is, bone marrow transplantation. Stem cells from the bone marrow are used in this procedure to treat several types of cancer, aplastic anemia, sickle cell anemia, immunodeficiencies, and other diseases. Other uses of stem cell-generated tissues include burn therapy (skin grafts), bone grafts, and tissue for corneal transplants. These stem cell successes continue to spur on researchers who hope to one day use stem cells to treat humans suffering from Parkinson disease, cancer, organ failure, and other diseases. Important questions stem cell research hopes to answer include:

- What are the signals involved in getting a stem cell to differentiate?
- Can stem cell lines be used to test the efficacy and safety of new drugs?
- Can stem cells be used to generate new human tissue that can be used to treat disease?

If scientists can reliably direct the differentiation of stem cells into specific cell types, the resulting cells could be used to treat diabetes, spinal cord injury, muscular dystrophy, heart disease, and many other conditions. The use of stem cells and regenerative medicine holds exciting promise of novel therapies, but much research still needs to be done before these ideas become reality.

Pain

All of us experience pain at some time in our lives. What is pain? How do we describe pain? How do we interpret pain? What are the types of pain? Why are tolerance levels different for different people? Why do we have pain at all? Knowing the answers to these questions is a necessary component of developing an understanding of pain and how the health care provider can facilitate relief of pain for patients. In addition to established medical options for pain management, there are doctors who specialize in pain management. Certain nonsurgical interventions and focused physical therapy offer new approaches for those who suffer with chronic discomfort, such as back pain.

Describing Pain

Pain is subjective, individualized, and perceived only by the individual experiencing it. It can be physiologic or psychological. The vocabulary people use to express their sensations of pain varies widely; pain may be described as an uncomfortable sensation, an unpleasant experience, distress, strong discomfort, suffering, agony, or, simply, hurting. *Dull* and *aching* are words used often to describe pain resulting from overuse of the musculoskeletal system. Pain along a nerve route that is described as "burning" is often an indication of peripheral nerve insult. Patients use the term *cramping* to characterize an abdominal–visceral type of pain. Head pain or pain felt along a blood vessel commonly is described as *throbbing*. Other descriptive terms include *shooting, stabbing,* and *stinging*. In reference to thermal injury, pain may be described as a burning sensation. When expressing concern about how pain is affecting them, patients may use such terms as *frightening, sickening, tiring, discomforting, intense, unbearable, mild, excruciating,* and *vicious* to categorize the pain.

Because pain interpretation is subjective, the intensity with which it is felt depends on many factors. An individual's perception of pain and response to pain may be based on cultural values, past experiences, religious beliefs, emotional support or lack thereof, anxiety, level of education, and the specific situation in which pain is being felt. Pain perception may be absent when a person is in the middle of a life-threatening situation and returns only when the person has escaped the danger. A variety of pain rating scales, using numbers and figures, are sometimes used to help measure an individual's perception of pain intensity and quality (Fig. 1.7). Often the patient may be asked to use a numerical scale from 0 to 10 to classify the intensity of pain: 1 to 3 as mild, 4 to 5 as moderate, or 6 to 10 as severe or "as bad as you can imagine." The way a patient describes their pain is taken seriously. In the clinical setting, assessment of a patient's pain is noted when vital signs are taken. This information is helpful in tracking the patient's response to treatment.

Physiology of Pain

Pain is a necessary entity in life. The physiology of pain involves the stimulation of specialized nerve endings called nociceptors. These pain receptors are found on free sensory nerve endings in the superficial portions of skin, in some tissues of internal or visceral organs, in joint capsules, in the periosteum of bones, surrounding the walls of blood vessels, and in certain deep tissues. Pain often is a signal of injury or tissue damage and, as such, is a protective mechanism that makes people aware of tissue insult.

Pain is the result of tissue insult from noxious (harmful) stimuli, including heat and cold, pressure, chemicals, electrical shock, and trauma. Pain receptors respond to three types of stimuli: (1) temperature extremes; (2) mechanical damage; and (3) dissolved chemicals, including potassium, acids, histamines, acetylcholine, bradykinin, and prostaglandins. A very strong stimulus may excite all three types, creating a burning-type sensation. Additional causes of painful stimuli include hypoxia and ischemia to the tissue and muscle spasms.

Pain impulses travel from the nerve ending through the spinal cord to the thalamus and then proceed to the sensory cortex in the parietal lobe of the brain. Adaptation to painful stimuli does not occur because the receptors continue to respond as long as the stimulus remains, stopping only when the tissue damage has ended.

Pain is a signal that helps locate and eliminate or reduce the source of tissue damage. Pain may be a part of the normal healing process, too, as a reaction to the inflammatory process. It is also possible for pain to occur in the absence of physical injury; this is referred to as *psychological pain*. Psychological or emotional pain is as real as pain with a physical cause to the person experiencing it. This type of pain also can be acute, chronic, transient, or *intractable*.

Pain is not always reported accurately. Stress can alter both perception and response to pain. The cerebral cortex is responsible for the interpretation of pain and therefore must

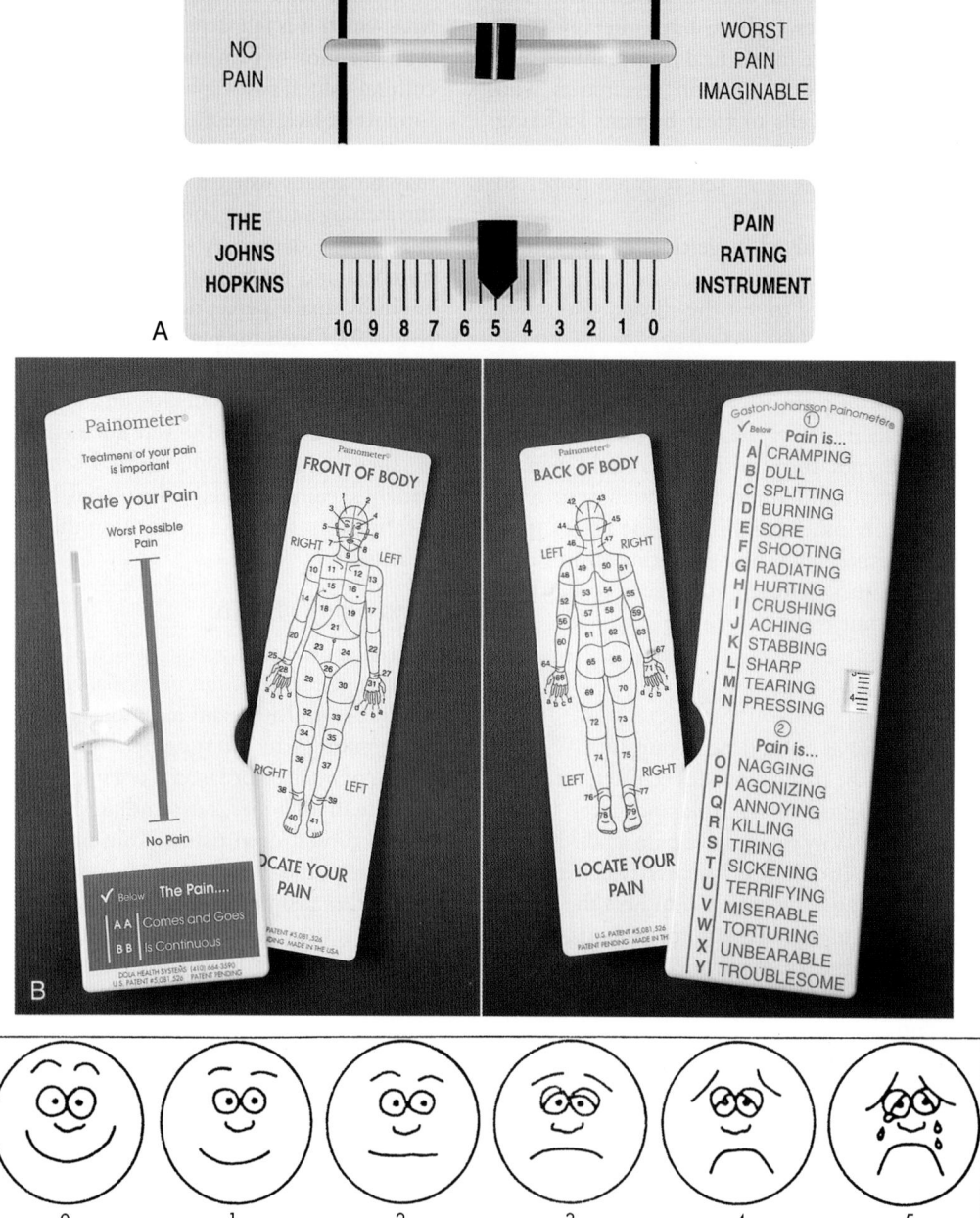

• **Fig. 1.7** Pain Rating Scales and Instruments. (A) Self-contained, portable, pain-rating instrument that can provide an immediate assessment of pain. (B) Painometer. (C) The Wong-Baker FACES Rating Scale. (A, From Grossman SA, Sheidler VR, McGuire DB, et al: A comparison of the Hopkins Pain Rating Instrument with standard visual analogue and verbal descriptor scales in patients with cancer pain, *J Pain Symptom Manage* 7(4):196–203, 1992. B, Courtesy Dr. Fannie Gaston-Johansson, School of Nursing, Johns Hopkins University. C, From Hockenberry MJ, Wilson D: *Wong's essentials of pediatric nursing*, ed 8, St Louis, 2009, Mosby.)

be functioning at normal capacity for interpretation to occur. Many of the internal organs are poorly supplied with nociceptors, and therefore the tissue insults in these organs are not always reported as such. The free nerve endings have large receptive fields, consequently making it difficult to determine the true source of the pain stimuli. Additionally, neurons from certain organs may travel a parallel pathway along the spinal cord to the brain, resulting in *referred pain*. Generally referred pain follows a *dermatome* that is supplied by the same spinal nerve as the nerve that has been stimulated by the insult, causing the pain to be projected to the body surface. For example, the patient experiencing myocardial ischemia or angina describes the pain as chest pain radiating to the left arm. Likewise, the nervous tissue of the

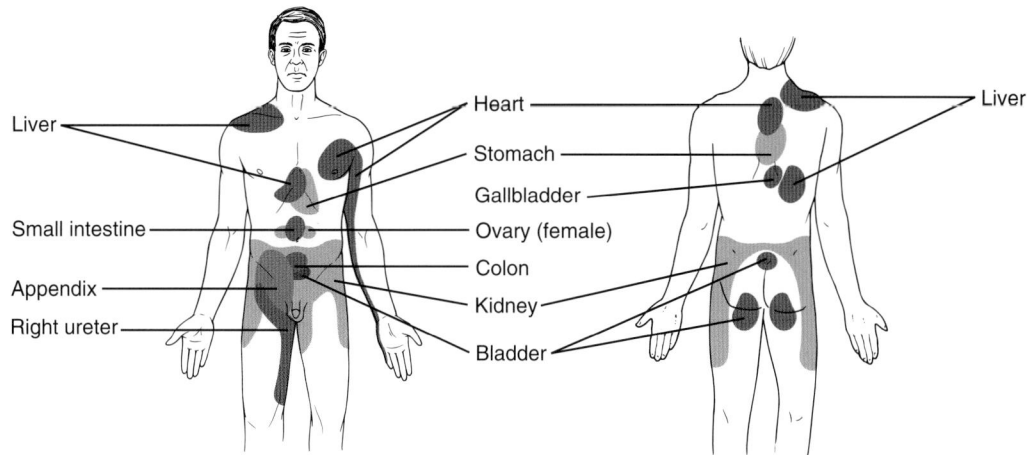

• **Fig. 1.8** Referred pain, anterior and posterior views. (From Miller-Keane BF: *Encyclopedia and dictionary of medicine, nursing, & allied health,* ed 7, Philadelphia, 2003, Saunders.)

brain has no pain receptors; nevertheless, headaches are commonly reported. Often the pain is caused by pressure on the blood vessel walls or the meninges. Tissue insult or inflammation of the gallbladder often results in pain referred to the right scapular region (Fig. 1.8).

Pain Classification

Pain may be classified as acute, chronic, transient, or intractable. Acute pain usually has a sudden onset and is severe in intensity. It also usually is of short duration. Individuals with acute pain have a tendency to guard the painful area; may exhibit distractive behavior, such as crying or moaning; are restless, anxious, or listless; and may have altered thought processes. Blood pressure and pulse often increase, whereas respiratory rates may increase or decrease. Occasionally sudden onset of very severe pain may cause vascular collapse and a resulting state of shock. Facial movements may indicate a grimace, and the skin may become *diaphoretic.* Chronic pain is usually less severe, with a duration of greater than 6 months. Pain from inflammatory conditions, such as arthritis and bursitis, is considered chronic. Patients with chronic pain often exhibit weight loss or gain, insomnia or altered sleep patterns, anorexia, inability to continue normal activities, and guarded movements. Psychosocial relationships may be altered. Chronic intractable pain, usually generated by nerve damage or cancer, is debilitating and can cause depression. Transient pain comes and goes, usually has a brief duration, and often is not significant.

Pain also can be classified as superficial, deep, or visceral. Superficial pain is described as being located on the body surface. Deep pain usually is correlated with muscles, joints, or tendons. Visceral pain is attributed to internal organs.

Pain Relief

Acute pain, such as the pain experienced as a result of myocardial infarction, postoperative pain after surgical intervention, pain resulting from severe trauma, and pain felt during terminal illness, can be treated with narcotics or opioid-related drugs. A device called a *patient-controlled analgesia (PCA) pump* allows a prescribed dose of an analgesic to be dispensed intravenously at safe intervals for effective control of acute pain. Aspirin is the most widely used analgesic in the world. Cannabis and cannabidiol (CBD) oils and preparations are also used to treat pain.

Chronic pain often is treated with acetaminophen, steroids, or antiinflammatory agents, such as nonsteroidal antiinflammatory drugs (NSAIDs). More recently, evidence-based guidelines for the treatment of chronic pain have suggested that antidepressants and anticonvulsants can be used for chronic neuropathic pain. Transcutaneous electrical nerve stimulation (TENS) sends types of electrical impulses to the nerve endings with the intention of blocking nerve transmission to the brain and may be of benefit to persons experiencing acute or chronic pain. In some cases, surgical intervention is necessary to remove the source of pain or block the transmission of pain.

Complementary and alternative methods of pain control include physical therapy and massage of the painful area to increase the blood flow to and from the area and to increase the flow of lymph from the area. Acupuncture, an ancient therapeutic treatment, is thought to elicit pain relief by way of the needles used to stimulate nerves deep in the tissue, thus arousing the pituitary gland and other parts of the brain to cause release of *endorphins,* the brain's own natural opioids. Endorphins reduce the perception of pain while the stimulus remains. A more extensive discussion of nontraditional medicine can be found later in this chapter.

> **NOTE**
>
> See Appendix II, Pharmacology, under the section for Chapter 1, for more information on drugs for pain.

Preventive Health Care

Preventive health care places emphasis on strategies for preventing disease and injury. Included is the trend to be proactive in one's own health care. Current statistical evidence indicates that positive personal health behavior, in conjunction with prophylactic medical services, may reduce the mortality rate associated with certain diseases, such as cardiovascular disease. Identifying risk factors and employing specific screening tests to detect alterations give individuals information they can use to modify their lifestyles. Using available medical measures can help prevent the onset of disease or at least minimize complications. Of particular concern is scientific evidence that smoking tobacco and exposure to secondhand smoke is the *single greatest avoidable cause of death and disease.* Public education in this regard has led to laws that prohibit smoking in many restaurants and other public arenas (see Alert box on Health Effects of Exposure to Tobacco Smoke).

! ALERT!

Health Effects of Exposure to Tobacco Smoke

There is supporting scientific evidence that even *passive exposure* to tobacco smoke has negative consequences for children and adults. Here are some facts that demonstrate ways smoking has immediate and long-term health consequences:

- Secondhand smoke contains hundreds of chemicals known to be toxic or carcinogenic (cancer causing), including formaldehyde, benzene, vinyl chloride, arsenic, ammonia, and hydrogen cyanide.
- Children who are exposed to secondhand smoke are at an increased risk for sudden infant death syndrome (SIDS), acute respiratory infections, ear problems, and more severe asthma.
- Breathing secondhand smoke (which is more toxic than what is inhaled by the smoker) has immediate adverse effects on the cardiovascular system.
- Short exposures to secondhand smoke can irritate and damage the lining of the airways even in healthy people.
- Separating smokers from nonsmokers and cleaning the ventilating and air-conditioning systems of buildings cannot eliminate exposures of nonsmokers to secondhand smoke.
- Smoking is the single greatest avoidable cause of death and disease.
- Research confirms that smoking can increase the risk for coronary artery disease.

(From U.S. Department of Health and Human Services: *The health consequences of involuntary exposure to tobacco smoke: a report of the Surgeon General,* U.S. Department of Health and Human Services, Centers for Disease Control and Prevention, National Center for Chronic Disease Prevention and Health Promotion, Office on Smoking and Health, 2006.)

Health care institutions are challenged daily to uphold infection control measures that protect patients against hospital-acquired infections (known as *nosocomial infections*). Continuing education requirements fulfilled by physicians and other health care providers give them the skills that help diminish occasions of *iatrogenic* disorders, that is, those diseases or conditions that are a result of medical procedures or

treatment. Another example is that some hospital emergency rooms have awareness programs that monitor alcohol abuse in teenagers to promote early intervention.

Some U.S. companies are embracing wellness program initiatives that motivate employees to lose weight, quit smoking, and learn how to manage chronic conditions. These onsite programs provide the worker with tools and incentives to improve health and thereby boost worker productivity.

Many injuries may be prevented by implementing (1) improved safety measures involving the operation of machinery and automobiles; (2) protective labeling and packaging of food, drugs, and toxic products; and (3) general public safety education. Family violence, another possible threat to an individual's health, is a serious and growing epidemic in the United States, resulting in both psychological stress and physical trauma. In many cases, early intervention may prevent such abuse. Involving legal, social, and medical authorities early on can serve to identify and protect those caught up in the cycle of domestic violence before serious medical consequences result. Currently, medical literature shines a light on how chronic stress can affect certain functions within the brain and adversely impact health. Interventions to help reduce and manage stress include meditation and ways to increase confidence in one's ability to self-regulate emotion and mood. Exercise that involves a structured program to improve physical fitness has proven to be health enhancing to the body and mind as well (Box 1.2).

Vaccines are important for adults, adolescents, and children for protection against many communicable diseases. Vaccine recommendations for adolescents and adults are

---

• BOX 1.2 Key Physical Guidelines for Adults

All adults should avoid inactivity. Some physical activity is better than none, and adults who participate in any amount of physical activity gain some health benefits.

For substantial health benefits, adults should do at least 150 minutes (2.5 hours) a week of moderate-intensity aerobic activity or 75 minutes (1.25 hours) a week of vigorous-intensity aerobic activity, or an equivalent combination of moderate- and vigorous-intensity aerobic activities.

Aerobic activity should be performed in episodes lasting at least 10 minutes and should be spread throughout the week.

For additional and more extensive health benefits, adults should increase their aerobic physical activity to 300 minutes (5 hours) a week of moderate-intensity or 150 minutes (2.5 hours) a week of vigorous-intensity aerobic physical activity, or an equivalent combination of moderate- and vigorous-intensity activity. Additional health benefits are gained by engaging in physical activity beyond this amount.

Adults should also do muscle strengthening activities that are moderate or high intensity and involve all major muscle groups 2 or more days a week because these activities provide additional health benefits.

(From U.S. Department of Health and Human Services: 2008 physical activity guidelines for Americans, *health.gov* [website]: www.health.gov/paguidelines. Accessed February 3, 2015.)

based on a variety of factors including age, overall health status, and medical history. Contraindications and precautions associated with each specific vaccine are factored in for the individual before immunization is begun. In general, vaccines for adults include:

- tetanus-diphtheria vaccine (all adults, every 10 years)
- seasonal influenza (flu) vaccine (adults age 50 years and older)

> **NOTE**
>
> The composition of the 2013–2014 influenza vaccine, in most cases, includes the H1N1 H1N2, and other viral components.

- pneumococcal vaccine (adults age 65 years and older)
- hepatitis B vaccine (adults at risk), three doses
- hepatitis A (two doses)
- measles-mumps-rubella (MMR) vaccine (susceptible adults) contraindicated in HIV infection and pregnancy
- varicella (chickenpox) vaccine (susceptible adults but contraindicated in pregnancy)
- meningococcal vaccine (college freshmen living in dormitories)
- HPV vaccine (all previously unvaccinated females and males through age 26 years)
- Gardasil (HPV) vaccine (can be given for young men)
- Shingrix vaccine to help prevent shingles (herpes zoster) in adults 60 years of age or older except when contraindicated (pregnancy and HIV infection)
- tetanus toxoid, reduced diphtheria toxoid, and acellular pertussis (Tdap) vaccine is recommended for adults 19 to 64 years of age and for certain adults 65 years of age and older (specific recommendations for Tdap vaccine exist for persons 11 to 18 years of age)
- vaccines for travelers (specific recommendations are found on the CDC website)
- special recommendations for polio vaccine

No vaccine is completely risk free or completely effective. Side effects can occur. The national program that monitors the safety of vaccines, after they are licensed, is called the *Vaccine Adverse Event Reporting System (VAERS).* Although unexpected reactions are rare, anyone can report a possible problem to VAERS, where the information is monitored by the FDA and the CDC.

Nontraditional Medicine

Many patients and practitioners now accept safe complementary and alternative medicine (CAM) as an adjunct to conventional medicine.* Patient demand for integrative medicine (integrating mainstream medicine with CAM) is evident by the big gain in percentage of hospitals offering one or more types of CAM services. The National Center for Complementary and Alternative Medicine (NCCAM), a component of the National Institutes of Health (NIH), is the government's lead agency for classification and scientific research of CAM. The agency states that although some scientific evidence exists regarding some CAM therapies, for *most,* there are key questions that are yet to be answered through well-designed scientific studies, questions as to whether these therapies are safe and whether they work for the diseases or medical conditions for which they are used.

By definition, *complementary* medicine is used *together with* conventional medicine. An example of a complementary therapy is using aromatherapy to help lessen a patient's discomfort following surgery. *Alternative* medicine is used *in place of* conventional medicine. An example of an alternative therapy is using a special diet to treat cancer instead of undergoing surgery, radiation, or chemotherapy that has been recommended by a conventional doctor.

Osteopathy is probably the most widely accepted form of alternative medicine. In the United States, osteopathic physicians (doctors of osteopathy [DOs]) are trained medical doctors who emphasize stimulation of the body's natural processes as a means to promote healing and well-being. In addition to traditional medical and surgical concepts, osteopathic physicians use manipulation techniques to realign body structure, thereby restoring balance and promoting healing.

Chiropractic medicine is based on the concept that the body's nervous system is the foundation of health and that undue pressure on or an insult to the nervous system may result in pain and disease. Correct alignment of the spinal vertebrae is emphasized; therefore, many chiropractic adjustments involve manipulation of the spine.

Massage, although not a new concept, is just now being recognized by the U.S. medical community as a valid alternative therapy or type of medicine. According to Eastern philosophy and also Swedish concepts, massage encourages drainage of the lymphatic system and increases circulation to the tissue.

Reflexology, a form of massage, directs its efforts primarily toward massage of the feet and sometimes of the hands. The theory is that the body is divided into zones and that these zones are reflected in specific areas of the feet or hands. Manipulation of these areas is expected to cause a therapeutic effect on the organ or system represented in that zone.

Aromatherapy uses essential oils to promote wellness and healing and to relieve stress. Although this therapy mainly involves inhalation and the olfactory system (Fig. 1.9), the oils used are absorbed through the skin and transported to the various body tissues and systems by the circulatory system as well. The essential oils are diluted and then massaged into the skin or placed in a steam inhaler for inspiration. Some of the more common essential oils used in aromatherapy are chamomile, clary sage, clove, eucalyptus, geranium, ginger, lavender, orange, peppermint, rosemary, sage, tea tree, evening primrose, and ylang ylang. Often aromatherapists mix the oils to meet the specific needs of their patients.

Herbs have been used as medicines for many centuries, with ancient Egyptians being the first known to record lists of herbs. Sometimes called *natural medicines,* herbs now are being substituted for pharmaceutical products by some.

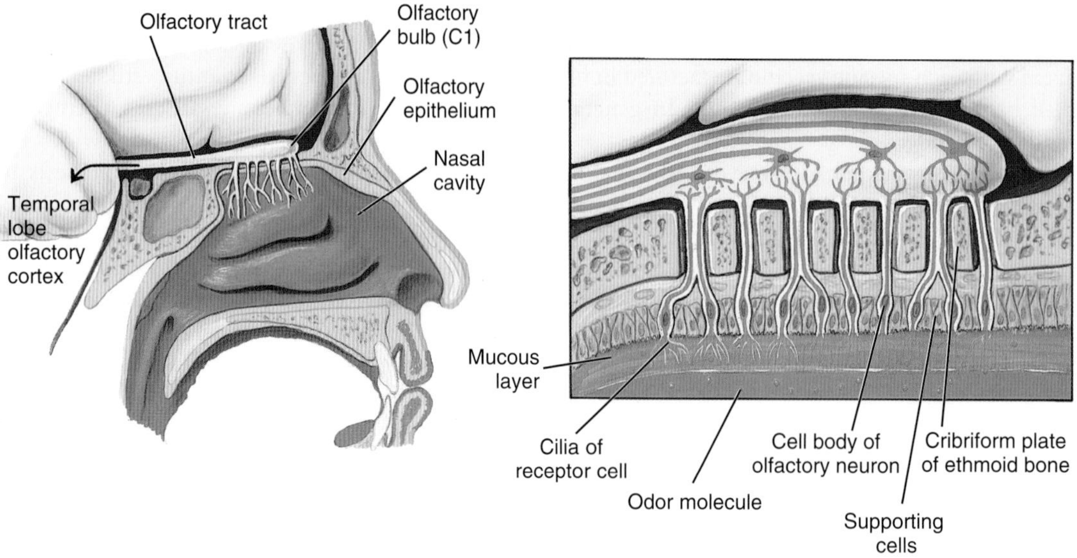

Olfactory tract

Olfactory bulb (C1)

Olfactory epithelium

Nasal cavity

Temporal lobe olfactory cortex

Mucous layer

Cilia of receptor cell

Odor molecule

Cell body of olfactory neuron

Cribriform plate of ethmoid bone

Supporting cells

• **Fig. 1.9** Structure of the olfactory receptors. (From Applegate EJ: *The anatomy and physiology learning system,* ed 4, St. Louis, 2011, Saunders.)

Common herbal products include ginkgo biloba, garlic, saw palmetto, ginseng, passion flower, angelica, chamomile, fennel, lavender, peppermint, rosemary, sage, St. John's wort, valerian, and yarrow. Herbs may be purchased in a pharmacy, in a herbal drug store, or by mail. Herbal remedies are professed to treat allergies, arthritis, gastrointestinal (GI) problems, headaches, hypertension or hypotension, insomnia, urinary problems, menstrual or menopausal symptoms, and skin diseases. Many of these products do not have FDA approval and may damage health if taken unwarily or in conjunction with prescription drugs. For example, the most used dietary supplement, ginkgo biloba, was recently studied for evidence of positive effects on memory and other clinical uses. Results were mixed and inconclusive, resulting in narrowed indications for its use and a list of contraindications and cautions. Lack of FDA regulation also means that the ingredients stated on the outside of the bottle may not necessarily be inside the bottle or may not be present in the amounts indicated.

Diet and nutrition therapy certainly is not a new concept; however, many are following special diets and addressing nutritional needs, hoping to eliminate toxins from the body and allow it to function at the optimal level. Diet therapy may include fat-free, low-saturated-fat, low-sugar, high-protein, low-carbohydrate, vegetarian, no- or low-caffeine, and seafood diets. Vitamin and mineral supplements often are added to the daily routine but this should be done with caution because megadoses may be toxic. Patients should check with a physician or pharmacist before starting any nutritional supplement regimen.

Acupuncture, an Asian therapy that uses meridians, attempts to adjust the body's energy (*chi* [chee]) flow by inserting needles into acupuncture points (Fig. 1.10). After insertion, the needles are manipulated by twirling or by a gentle pumping action. Recent advances in techniques use electrical or laser stimulation. Only professionals trained in

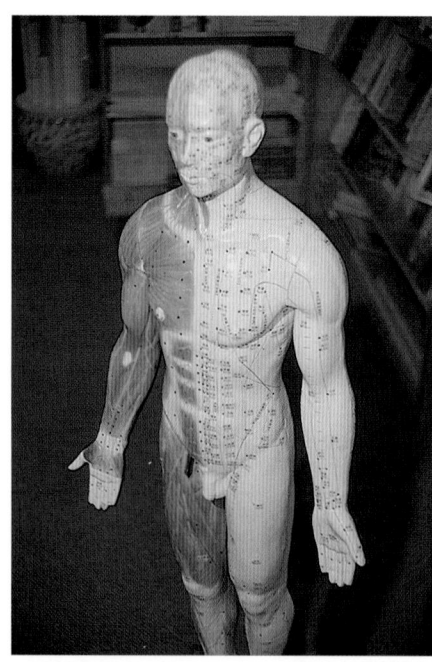

• **Fig. 1.10** Acupuncture sites on a male model. (From *Mosby's dictionary of medicine, nursing & health professions,* ed 9, St Louis, 2013, Elsevier/Mosby.)

it should attempt acupuncture. Patients with cardiac pacemakers and other electronic devices are advised to talk with their doctor before beginning acupuncture.

Acupressure, similar to acupuncture, involves the manipulation of acupoints by means of finger pressure. The intent is to balance the flow of energy along the meridians to promote healthy functioning of internal organs. Acupressure often is incorporated into massage as a method of muscle relaxation and stress reduction.

Therapeutic touch is derived from an ancient technique called *laying-on of hands.* It is based on the premise that it is the healing force of the therapist that affects the patient's recovery; healing is promoted when the body's energies are in balance; and, by passing their hands over the patient, healers can attempt to identify energy imbalances.

Shiatsu (she-AT-sue), a form of therapy from Japan that is similar to acupressure, usually is performed on a mat on the floor. The patient remains clothed, and the therapist applies pressure to the acupoints and along the meridians using the fingertips, knuckles, elbows, knees, or even the feet.

Magnetic therapy, a relatively new concept in the United States, has not been approved by the FDA. However, it is being used extensively in veterinary medicine, especially in equine veterinary medicine. In Europe and the United Kingdom, magnetic therapy has been accepted for use in humans as well. Although the theory has not been proved according to FDA standards, it is believed that magnets increase circulation to the area being treated, thereby increasing the available amount of oxygen (O_2) and nutrients, at the same time transporting away the waste products of metabolism and the inflammatory process. It also is postulated that the magnetic field interferes with the conduction of the sensory nerves by preventing movement of the sodium (Na1) and potassium (K1) ions in and out of the nerve cell; this reduces the conduction capability of the sensory nerve. Advocates of this therapy state that magnets are useful in relieving muscle and nerve pain, reducing inflammation, and mitigating migraines.

Hypnosis and hypnotherapy have been accepted means of psychological therapy only for approximately the past 40 years. The therapist places the patient in a trancelike state, often resembling sleep. While in this trance, the subject follows acceptable suggestions. Often relaxation and pain relief can be achieved by using this therapy. Only a qualified practitioner who is trained specifically in the performance of hypnosis should attempt this therapy.

Relaxation can be thought of as a form of self-hypnosis. Many techniques for achieving relaxation are available to the individual. Physical relaxation usually is the starting point for the subject, with psychological relaxation often being the next step. Relaxation is used to treat stress-related physical and emotional problems, pain, anxiety, asthma, arthritis, depression, panic attacks, and hypertension. Many forms of relaxation include repetition of an action, images, or sounds that then passively erase everyday thoughts from the mind. Some meditation techniques can be used to establish a relaxation response and are used in stress reduction programs. However, meditation is contraindicated for patients with certain personality disorders or active psychosis.

Prayer is considered a mind–body therapy and is used by many as a source of healing and comfort. Some recent studies link positive patient outcomes to prayer; other studies report uncertain scientific evidence of a relationship between prayer and recovery. Nevertheless, some schools are including the value of spirituality in holistic models of care.

Reiki (ray-KEE) claims to transfer healing energy from the practitioner to the patient. Usually the practitioner starts the ritual at the patient's head and either touches the head or moves the hands close to the head within the patient's aura. The practitioner's hands then touch other parts of the patient's body, or the hands move into the aura space outlining the body. Healing energy then is transferred to the patient. The intention of this therapy is the promotion of physical, emotional, and spiritual well-being.

Music therapy recognizes the involvement of vibrations, rhythms, and sound in the well-being of individuals. Listening to music by composers of the Baroque period, such as Mozart, can help achieve relaxation. Music along with anesthesia or pain medication is used to elevate mood, to create a calming effect, to lessen muscle tension, and to alleviate feelings of fear and anxiety by manifesting a state of relaxation. Patients undergoing chemotherapy for cancer can benefit from music that induces relaxation. Trained and qualified music therapists design the therapy to fit the particular patient's needs.

Homeopathy, polarity therapy, Rolfing, *tai chi* (tie-CHEE), iridology, naturopathy, hydrotherapy, and Ayurveda are some additional forms of alternative medicine. Although any of these therapies may be considered a form of alternative medicine, the patient and practitioner should check with the physician before attempting to include these therapies in the course of treatment. When used, they should be considered as adjunct treatment and not necessarily proven medical treatment. Health care providers should inquire routinely about a patient's use of alternative therapies because a large percentage of the population does use them, and many do not think to report this use to their physicians.

Patient Teaching

> ### ✕ NOTE
>
> Please consult your state code regarding licensing regulations for an explanation of the rules and regulations governing medical assistant practice in your location. Practice laws address what tasks the properly prepared medical assistant can perform; these laws differ from state to state. It is important that medical assistants know who their legally responsible supervisor is in a medical office; it may be the physician. Medical assistants should ask to see the written office policy regarding any delegation of tasks by the physician or nurse.

We consider it important, and in the patient's best interests, that all health care workers, as members of a clinical team, understand the principles, goals, and specifics of patient teaching. *Licensing regulations and state practice acts generally permit only nurses and physicians to actually do patient teaching and make triage judgments.*

Under these regulations, medical assistants often contribute significantly to patient education according to the discretion of the supervising physician or licensed professional.

General Principles of Patient Teaching

- The concept of patient teaching is based on patient-centered care, with the patient being a partner in the process of learning skills, solving problems, and preventing complications.

- Effective patient teaching requires skillful listening as patients express their understanding of their situations, their worries, and their hopes. The education process is ongoing, interactive, and directed toward achieving the patient's plan of care.
- Patient teaching is a course of action that involves assessment, critical thinking, and compromise directed toward successful compliance.
- Effective patient teaching policies indicate who has primary legal responsibility for patient teaching and documentation (outlined in nurse state practice acts).

Goals of Patient Teaching

- Encourage the patient to comply with the personalized medical treatment plan to assure recovery.*
- Offer guidance, support, and clear instruction both to the patient who requires medical attention and to the family or the caregiver.
- Develop a trusting relationship with patients through empathy, effective communication, and knowledge about the subject matter being taught.
- Help patients learn how to effectively deal with their conditions by making healthy lifestyle choices.
- Give the individual the confidence needed to take responsibility for his or her health or recovery.

Reasons for Patient Teaching

- Ease anxiety.
- Answer questions.
- Instill confidence through individualized education.
- Evaluate the patient's perception of the treatment plan, and make any necessary adjustments.
- Reinforce the physician's instructions.
- Highlight reasonable goals for recovery.
- Encourage the individual to take responsibility for his or her health care.
- Help build the esteem that creates a sense of self-sufficiency and control.
- Educate the primary caregiver or family about specific aspects of the care plan.
- Improve patient/family coping.
- Provide an opportunity to practice skills associated with care.
- Reduce clinic visits and hospitalization.
- Supply the patient and caregiver with educational materials (booklets, websites, and community resources).
- Suggest participation in appropriate social support groups.
- Supply a list of phone numbers to call for answers to questions or medical concerns during recovery.
- Stress the importance of keeping future appointments for follow-up care.

> **NOTE**
>
> Modern information technology is an essential component of all health care and a powerful tool for patient education. Electronically generated materials can be customized according to almost any patient's need for knowledge and practical application of the prescribed treatment plan. Electronic learning (e-learning) teaching methods include videos or educational websites that demonstrate activities for rehabilitation or using home equipment, such as an oxygen support system or a glucose monitoring system. It is wise to integrate e-learning with face-to-face or telephone contact for reinforcement of patient education to help ensure a safe and positive outcome.

The Specifics of Patient Teaching: Addressing the Patient's Concerns

"What's wrong with me?"

Answering this question provides an opportunity to reinforce or explain *only what has been expressed to the patient by the medical professional with primary responsibility for care.* It is not appropriate to "second guess" or give false or unsubstantiated information to a patient.

"What are these tests for?"

Again, your response will depend on guidelines given by the medical professional ordering the tests.

- Explain any special preparation and the purpose for the test.
- In plain words, explain the procedure and what to expect during and after the procedure.
- Make sure the patient understands warning signs of complications that may occur, if any.
- Tell the patient when to expect the test results and advise when to call or wait to be called for those results.
- Be prepared to discuss the cost to the patient or insurance company, if asked.

"What is this disease?"

You should review and explain the diagnosis made by the physician. When possible, use illustrations and plain language to explain the pathophysiology of the disease. Try to point to the history of symptoms that may relate to the disease. This will help the patient monitor changes in symptoms during recovery.

"What causes this disease?"

Review the physician's explanation of the cause(s) and contributing factors. This could include the source of infection, genetic influences, lifestyle, age, diet, trauma, or epidemic factors. Understanding prevention measures is helpful in some cases.

"Why do I need this medication?"

Explain the purpose and expected results. Review the dosage schedule and route of administration. Discuss the common side effects and what side effects to report to the physician. Give special instructions such as how to handle skipped doses, and explain why some medications must not be stopped abruptly without the advice of the doctor. Be sure to mention over-the-counter drugs to avoid.

"When should I call the doctor?"

Review warning signs of possible complications from the disease or any medical intervention that require notification of the nurse or physician: sudden increase in pain, signs of infection or bleeding, neurologic changes, muscle pain or weakness, and so on. Advise the patient on how to obtain refills for medications.

"How long do I have to undergo this therapy?"

Explain the goal(s) of treatment or therapy: physical therapy, therapeutic topical applications of heat or ice, eye drops, wound care, extra rest, or avoidance of certain activity. Demonstrate and give the patient time to practice a prescribed treatment or evaluation, such as glucose monitoring or the use of an inhaler.

"Would you explain this diet?"

Instruct the patient on the relationship between diet and his or her recovery and health. Warn the patient about the possible interactions between specific herbs and certain medications. List the signs of dehydration. Refer to a dietitian, as needed.

"The doctor says I need an operation."

Preoperative Care

- Offer reasonable assurance, because preoperative anxiety is universal.
- Review the preoperative instructions given by the physician.
- Ask the patient if he or she understands what to expect from the operation and offer as much information as possible to the family or caregiver. Determine whether the patient needs further clarification about the benefits and risks of the operation.
- Arrange for any preoperative blood work, radiology, or scans. Answer related questions. Give laboratory phone numbers and hours of service.
- Give the patient complete directions and parking instructions.

Postoperative Care

- After surgery, make sure the patient understands the medical plan: wound care, how to take medications, and when to resume activity and return to work.
- The patient needs reassurance about pain control and what to expect during the recovery process.
- Explain warning signs of complications: fever, bleeding, infection, shock, dehydration, and emotional depression.
- The patient and caregiver should be given written instructions and the phone numbers of the nurse or physician to call for answers to questions.
- Make appropriate referrals to support groups.

"When do I have to be seen again?"

Make a follow-up appointment for the patient. Explain the importance of ongoing care during the recovery process. Encourage the patient to ask questions about any aspect of his or her medical care. Long-term treatment and medical concerns are addressed on an ongoing basis.

Special Considerations for the Patient with Cancer or Life-Threatening Disease

When the clinician interrelates with patients and families faced with life-shortening illness, he or she has many opportunities to offer important responses and guidance. Seriously ill patients benefit from an interdisciplinary approach to the clinical management of their diseases. Clinicians can expect to address many special needs of the person diagnosed with the disease itself and also with side effects of therapeutic interventions. The issues to be addressed are many and varied:

- Keep patients and families from feeling abandoned by providing support based on their personal needs and goals.
- Give verbal and written instructions.
- Welcome feedback on all aspects of the care plan.
- Encourage discussion about side effects of medications, especially chemotherapy, radiation, or any therapeutic procedures.
- Review warning signs to report to the physician (i.e., weight loss, dehydration, or pain that is not controlled by prescription medication).
- Address the physical, psychological, social, and spiritual aspects of care.
- Bear in mind the two main fears of those with life-threatening illness: being in pain and becoming a burden to others.
- Make appropriate and timely referrals to support groups or comprehensive programs of end-of-life care, such as hospice.
- Reinforce the concept of palliative care being prescribed when curative treatment offers no hope; the goal is to prevent and ease suffering and can be delivered at any time in the course of an illness.
- If spiritual distress is identified, offer a referral to a hospital chaplain.
- Address the caregiver's concerns, including adjusting to role changes, providing physical care, and ethical issues and dilemmas.

Conclusion

Human pathologic processes involve complex mechanisms that can be weighed separately as elements of the disease process but that ultimately converge into the total picture of how and why an individual is sick and what is required as a remedy.

It is worth the effort to strive to understand the nature and impact of human disease on the person and on humankind. One can expect to find great personal and professional satisfaction in knowing the nature, signs, symptoms, causes, and treatment of the pathologic conditions that alter or seriously threaten health. This knowledge also fosters insight into the scenario imposed by diseases and fosters compassion for the people affected by them.

Review Challenge

Answer the following questions:

1. How may the following predisposing factors make a person more vulnerable to disease?
   a. Age
   b. Gender
   c. Lifestyle
   d. Environment
   e. Heredity
2. Describe three ways that genetic diseases are caused.
3. Name three of the body's natural defense mechanisms.
4. How does acute inflammation protect against infection?
5. Discuss the behavioral characteristics of malignant neoplasms.
6. What is the goal of cancer treatment, and what therapeutic measures may be used?
7. What is allergic disease? What are the symptoms, and how may they be treated?
8. List the normal sequence of steps in formulating diagnosis.
9. What is the difference between benign and malignant tumors?
10. What is the emphasis in preventive health care?
11. Explain the importance of knowing the types of pain, the possible causes, and how it may be described by the patient.
12. List some of the stresses and special needs of older persons.
13. What are the components of the holistic concept of medical care?
14. Discuss osteopathy as a form of alternative medicine.
15. How does genetic counseling help families?
16. How does good patient teaching affect the positive outcome of disease?
17. What are some of the harmful health effects of exposure to tobacco smoke?
18. What does MRSA stand for? Why is MRSA considered a threat to public health?

Internet Assignments

1. Explore the plethora of information available for information and research from the National Cancer Institute (www.cancer.gov). Report on your personal points of interest on this subject.
2. Navigate the website for the Centers for Disease Control and Prevention (CDC; www.cdc.gov), available in English or Spanish, and explore the available materials, such as the Health Topics A–Z page.
3. Explore the Genetic Alliance website (www.geneticalliance.org) for available resources regarding any particular genetic disease.
4. Access the American Academy of Allergy and Immunology website (www.aaaai.org), and explore the pages, such as the National Allergy Bureau (NAB) report on pollen and mold.

Critical Thinking

1. Explain this statement: "The absence of illness does not necessarily indicate optimal health."
2. It is said that *cancer* refers to a group of diseases with numerous causes. Explain.
3. Describe some challenges a health care worker might encounter caring for a person from a foreign culture.
4. Suggest ways in which chronic and/or severe stress can adversely affect health.
5. Generally speaking, what are the reasons good communication in patient teaching is an essential component of all health care?
6. What is implied in the statement: "The physician is the expert advisor who must inform and empower the patient?"
7. Choose one of the goals of patient teaching as listed in the textbook. Explain how you or someone you know has benefited from such patient teaching.

2

Developmental, Congenital, and Childhood Diseases and Disorders

CHAPTER OUTLINE

Developmental and Congenital Disorders, 32

Developmental Characteristics and Congenital Anomalies, 32

Congenital Anomalies, 32

Genetic Disorders and Syndromes, 33

Methods of Prenatal Diagnosis, 34

Prematurity, 35

Genetic Syndromes and Conditions, 43

Diseases of the Nervous System, 47

Congenital Cardiac Defects, 55

Musculoskeletal Conditions, 60

Genitourinary Conditions, 63

Diseases of the Digestive System, 65

Metabolic Disorders, 67

Endocrine Syndromes, 69

Childhood Diseases, 72

Infectious Diseases, 72

Respiratory Diseases/Disorders, 80

Gastrointestinal Disorders, 86

Blood Disorders, 90

Miscellaneous Diseases, Syndromes, and Disorders, 95

LEARNING OBJECTIVES

After studying Chapter 2, you should be able to:

1. List the possible causes of congenital anomalies.
2. Discuss genetic disorders and syndromes.
3. Discuss the purpose and procedure of amniocentesis.
4. Describe the condition of prematurity and associated disorders: the causes and treatments.
5. List possible risk factors of retinopathy of prematurity (ROP).
6. List symptoms and signs of Down syndrome.
7. List and discuss diseases of the pediatric nervous system.
8. Distinguish between muscular dystrophy (MD) and cerebral palsy (CP).
9. Describe patent ductus arteriosus (PDA).
10. Name and describe the most common congenital cyanotic cardiac defect.
11. List and discuss musculoskeletal conditions of newborns and young children.
12. List and discuss pediatric genitourinary conditions.
13. List and discuss pediatric diseases of the digestive system.
14. List and discuss pediatric metabolic disorders.
15. List the major clinical manifestations of cystic fibrosis (CF).
16. Distinguish between Klinefelter syndrome and Turner syndrome.
17. List and discuss contagious diseases of children.
18. Describe the clinical condition of congenital rubella syndrome.
19. Discuss possible causes and prevention of sudden infant death syndrome (SIDS).
20. Distinguish between croup and epiglottitis.
21. Describe the symptoms, signs, and treatment for tonsillitis and adenoid hyperplasia.
22. Discuss the treatment of asthma.
23. Discuss causes and treatment of bronchiolitis.
24. List the types of worms that may infest the gastrointestinal (GI) tract.
25. List the symptoms and signs of anemia; describe the pathology of leukemia.
26. Explain the etiology of erythroblastosis fetalis.
27. Name some warning signs of lead poisoning.
28. Describe the infant born with fetal alcohol syndrome (FAS).

KEY TERMS

acetabulum (**ass**-eh-**TAB**-u-lum)
acyanotic (a-**sigh**-ah-**NOT**-ik)
adenosarcoma (**ad**-eh-no-sar-**KO**-mah)
amniocentesis (**am**-nee-o-sen-**TEE**-sis)
anencephalic (**an**-en-seh-**FAL**-ik)
ataxic (ah-**TACH**-sik)
azoospermia (azo-**SPIR**-me-a)
bicornuate (bye-**KOR**-nate)
contracture (kon-**TRACK**-chur)
dysplasia (dis-**PLAY**-zee-ah)
dystrophy (**DIS**-troe-fee)

electromyography (e-**LECK**-tro-my-**og**-ra-fee)
foramen ovale (for-**A**-men o-**VAL**-a)
meconium (meh-**KOH**-nee-um)
meninges (men-**IN**-jeez)
neonates (**NEE**-o-nates)
pylorus (pye-**LOR**-us)
stenosis (ste-**NO**-sis)
syncope (**SIN**-koh-pee)
tachypnea (**tack**-ip-**NEE**-ah)
trisomy (**TRY**-so-me)

Developmental and Congenital Disorders

Developmental Characteristics and Congenital Anomalies

The developmental process begins with conception (Fig. 2.1A) and progresses as a gradual modification of the structure and characteristics of the individual (see Fig. 2.1B). The first 2 months of the gestational period is considered the embryonic period, after which the developing human being is considered a fetus. At any point in this prenatal development, during the birth process (perinatal period), or during the neonatal and postnatal periods, development may diverge from normal, generating a developmental dilemma. Causes of these dilemmas can be many or even unknown.

Pregnant women are encouraged to abstain from smoking, consuming alcohol, and taking any form of medication or drugs without their physician's knowledge and consent and to prevent any situation that may expose the developing fetus to toxic substances. Table 2.1 describes the specific stages of development during this important period of life.

Congenital Anomalies

Congenital anomalies can be mental or physical and can vary widely in severity, from trivial to fatal. They are present at birth but might not be detected until later in infancy or childhood. The limbs or organs may be malformed, duplicated, or entirely absent. Organs sometimes fail to move to their proper location or fail to open or close at the right

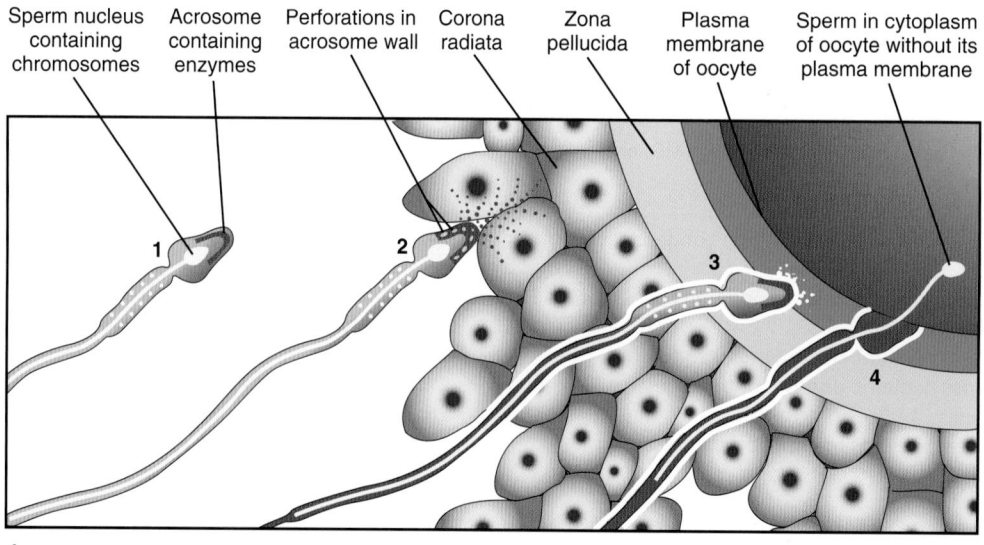

A

• **Fig. 2.1** (A) Acrosome reaction and sperm penetration of an oocyte. *1,* Sperm during capacitation. *2,* Sperm undergoing the acrosome reaction. *3,* Sperm forming a path through the zona pellucida. *4,* Sperm entering the cytoplasm of the oocyte.

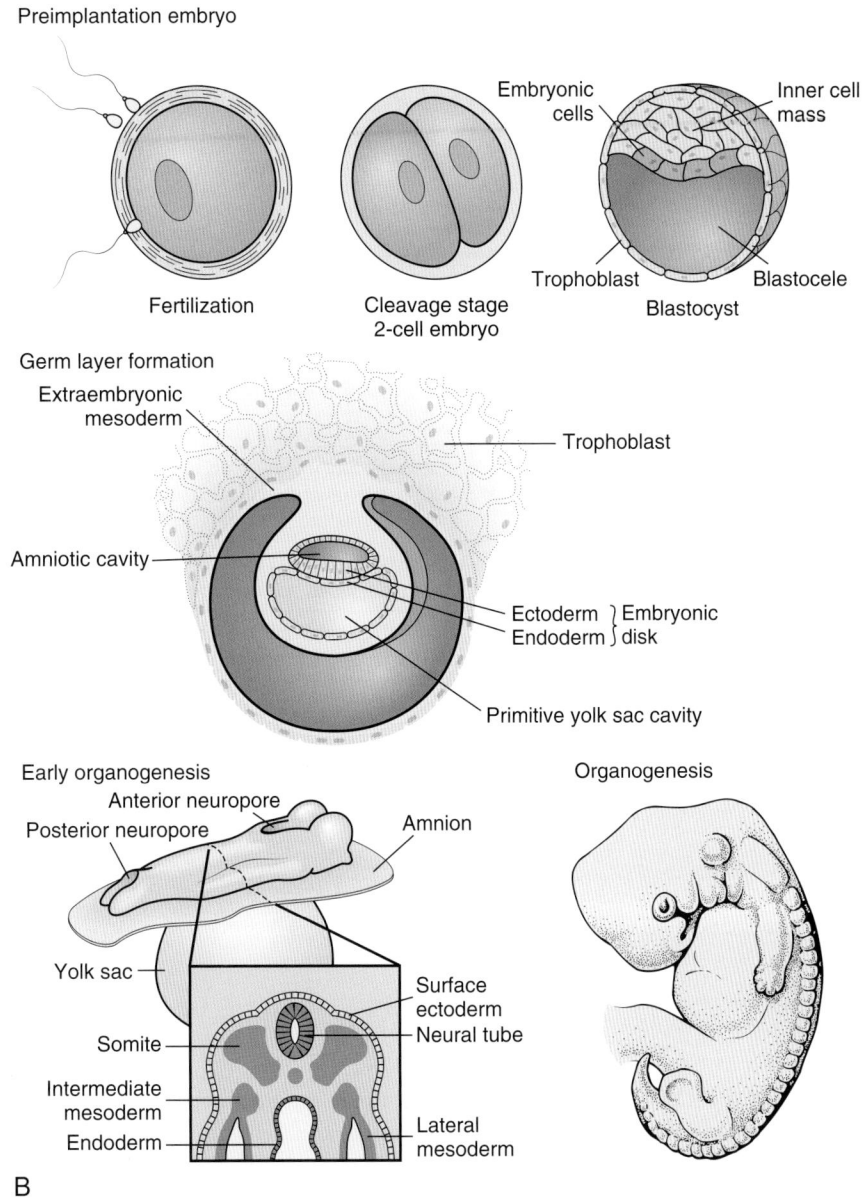

• **Fig. 2.1, cont'd** (B) Normal prenatal development can be divided into several stages. (A, From Moore KL, Persaud TVN, Torchia MG: *Before we are born: essentials of embryology and birth defects,* ed 8, St Louis, 2013, Saunders. B, From Damjanov I: *Pathology for the health professions,* ed 4, St Louis, 2011, Saunders.)

time. Anomalies are seldom isolated and are likely to occur in multiple forms and/or organs or organ tissues.

The cause of congenital defects may be genetic, nongenetic, or a combination of both. Nongenetic causes include infection in the mother, drugs taken by the mother, the age of the mother, radiographic examination made early in pregnancy, or injury to the pregnant woman or the fetus. The cause often is unknown. However, prenatal care and advanced surgical techniques have greatly improved the management of anomalies that are compatible with life. Parents of a special-needs child face emotional and physical challenges and deserve medical attention. A team approach is ideal, including medical assessment by physicians and appropriate therapy for the child, as well as family involvement and participation in a support group for the parents.

Genetic Disorders and Syndromes

Genetic syndromes are a form of congenital anomaly. Genetic information is contained in microscopic thread-like structures in the nucleus of human body cells. The genetic material contained within the genes is responsible for inheritance traits. Each cell within the human body contains 46 chromosomes arranged in 23 pairs. Twenty-two pairs of the chromosomes are termed *homologous pairs,* and the remaining pair comprises the sex chromosomes.

Genetic disorders and syndromes are the result of an abnormal gene taking up residence on one of the 22 pairs of nonsex chromosomes. The 22 pairs of homologous pairs are also identified as autosomes. When the abnormal gene that

TABLE 2.1	Monthly Changes During Prenatal Development	
End of Month[a]	Size of Embryo or Fetus	Developments During the Month
1	6 mm	Arm and leg buds form; heart forms and starts beating; body systems begin to form.
2	23–30 mm, 1 g	Head nearly as large as body; major brain regions present; ossification begins; arms and legs distinct; blood vessels form and cardiovascular system fully functional; liver enlarges.
3	75 mm, 10–45 g	Facial features present; nails develop on fingers and toes; can swallow and digest amniotic fluid; urine starts to form; fetus starts to move; heartbeat detected; external genitalia develop.
4	140 mm, 60–200 g	Facial features well formed; hair appears on head; joints begin to form.
5	190 mm, 250–450 g	Mother feels fetal movement; fetus covered with fine hair called *lanugo hair;* eyebrows visible; skin coated with vernix caseosa, a cheesy mixture of sebum and dead epidermal cells.
6	220 mm, 500–800 g	Skin reddish because blood in the capillaries is visible; skin wrinkled because it lacks adipose in the subcutaneous tissue.
7	260 mm, 900–1300 g	Eyes open; capable of survival but high mortality rate; scrotum develops; testes begin their descent.
8	280–300 mm, 1400–2100 g	Testes descend into the scrotum; sense of taste is present.
9	310–340 mm, 2200–2900 g	Reddish skin fades to pink; nails reach tips of fingers and toes or beyond.
10	350–360 mm, 3000–3400 g	Skin smooth and plump because of adipose in subcutaneous tissue; lanugo hair shed; fetus usually turns to a head-down position; full-term.

[a]These are 4-week (28-day) months.
(From Applegate EJ: *The anatomy and physiology learning system,* ed 4, St. Louis, 2011, Saunders.)

causes the condition is on one of the 22 pairs of autosomes, the condition is termed an *autosomal inherited condition.*

Some of the autosomal inherited conditions have a dominant pattern of inheritance; other conditions may be the result of autosomal recessive traits. Dominant inheritance occurs when only one gene of the pair has the ability to produce symptoms, thus making it dominant over the normal gene. The parent who carries the abnormal gene has a 50% chance of transmitting the defective gene to each of his or her offspring. When the condition is considered as autosomal recessive inheritance, the parent's abnormal genetic makeup must have genetic errors on both of the genes of the pair, resulting in the carrier usually having no symptoms of the disorder. The autosomal recessive disorder has a 25% chance of surfacing when two carrier parents conceive a child. The child could be affected by the autosomal inherited condition when the pair of affected genes is present.

Methods of Prenatal Diagnosis

Congenital anomalies in a fetus can be diagnosed by taking a fluid sample from the amniotic sac between the 15th and 18th weeks of pregnancy. This procedure, known as **amniocentesis**, allows amniotic fluid to be tested and cells to be microscopically examined for abnormal substances or chromosomal abnormalities. An example of an abnormal substance is an elevated alpha-fetoprotein (AFP) level. Amniocentesis is not without risk to the mother and the baby.

Abnormalities of the spine, skull, and many organs, such as the heart and kidneys, may be discovered during ultrasound studies of the fetus. An alternative procedure called *chorionic villus biopsy* (CVB) can be performed in the second month of pregnancy. The gynecologist, guided by ultrasonography, directs an instrument toward the placenta in the womb and obtains a tissue sample. The safety of this procedure has not been proven, and some data link this test to limb abnormalities.

Many, but not all, congenital disorders can be detected through prenatal diagnosis (Fig. 2.2). The diagnosis of potential genetic or neural tube deficit disorders may provide future parents with time to obtain counseling and to prepare for the many health needs of the infant before the child's birth. When the testing indicates a potential abnormality, the delivery and nursery staff is provided with the opportunity to prepare for the delivery.

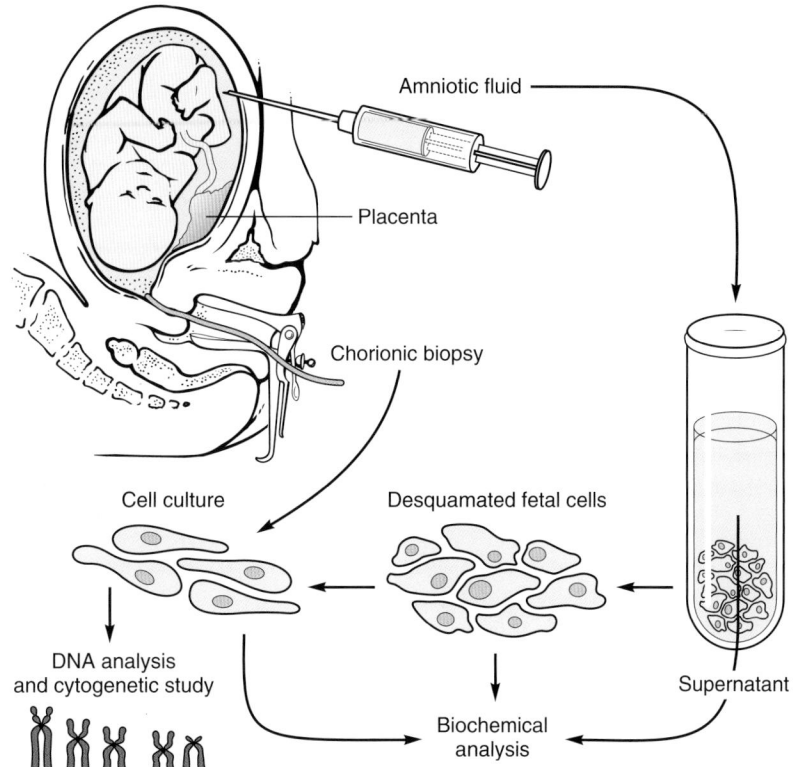

• **Fig. 2.2** Methods of prenatal diagnosis. (From Damjanov I: *Pathology for the health professions,* ed 4, St Louis, 2011, Saunders.)

Prematurity

Preterm Birth or Prematurity

Description

Preterm birth, or prematurity, is the result of birth before the 37th gestational week. The condition of prematurity describes the birth of a low-weight, underdeveloped, and short-gestation infant and is considered the leading cause of death during the neonatal period. These high-risk infants are born with incomplete development of organ systems. Compared with full-term infants, these infants are at a greater risk for developing serious health problems, including cerebral palsy (CP), intellectual developmental disorder, chronic lung disease, gastrointestinal (GI) problems, vision and hearing loss, and multisystem developmental delays.

ICD-10-CM Code   P07.00 *(Extremely low birth weight newborn, unspecified weight)*
(P07.00-P07.03 = 4 codes of specificity)
P07.10 *(Other low birth weight newborn, unspecified weight)*
(P07.10-P07.18 = 6 codes of specificity)

Usually implies a birth weight of less than 1000 grams. This code requires the additional code for weeks of gestation (765.20–765.29).

ICD-10-CM Code   P07.00 *(Extremely low birth weight newborn, unspecified weight)*
(P07.00-P07.03 = 4 codes of specificity)
P07.10 *(Other low birth weight newborn, unspecified weight)*
(P07.10-P07.18 = 6 codes of specificity)

Usually implies birth weight of 1000–2499 grams. This code requires the additional code for weeks of gestation (765.20–765.29).

Weeks of Gestation

ICD-10-CM Code   P07.20 *(Extreme immaturity of newborn, unspecified weeks)*
(P07.20-P07.26 = 7 codes of specificity)
P07.30 *(Other preterm newborn, unspecified weeks)*
(P07.31-P07.39 = 9 codes of specificity)
P07.21 *(Extreme immaturity of newborn, gestational age less than 23 completed weeks)*
P07.22 *(Extreme immaturity of newborn, gestational age 23 completed weeks)*

Conjoined Twins

During the conception process, the fertilized egg (the embryo) may divide, creating identical twins. Conjoined twins result when the separation process of identical twins fails to complete before the 13th day after fertilization. As with identical twins, the embryo originates from a single fertilized ovum and occupies one placenta. For an unidentifiable reason, however, the normal separation of the embryo into twins stops before completion, resulting in a partially separated embryo that continues to mature into conjoined fetuses. Conjoined twins occur more often in female embryos than in male embryos and result in two fetuses that are joined at some point on their bodies. More of these children are being born alive as a result of specific prenatal diagnosis and surgical intervention to facilitate the delivery.

These children may be joined at different locations of the body and may share various organs. The attachment to each other may involve a small portion of tissue or may be as extensive as fusion at the head or sharing of an organ or body part. Common types or variations usually are categorized by the location and involvement of the junction through the term *pagus,* meaning fastened, included in the classification terminology.

Twins with a cranial union are called *craniopagus twins.* Those with anterior junction at the chest, often sharing the heart and vital portions of the chest wall and internal organs, are called *thoracopagus conjoined twins.* Thoracopagus is the most common form of conjoined twins. The term *pygopagus twins* describes those joined posteriorly at the rump. Another posterior junction occurring at the sacrum and coccyx is termed *ischiopagus.* When the connection proceeds from the breastbone to the waist, the term *omphalopagus* describes the junction. A very rare form, *dicephalus,* is the condition in which the individual has one body and two separate heads and necks.

Modern technology and medical advances have recently helped physicians and surgical teams to successfully separate some of these twins. In some separation procedures, one or both of the children have died during or shortly after the surgery. The children and their families require emotional support and education about the possible outcomes of the condition (Fig. 2.3).

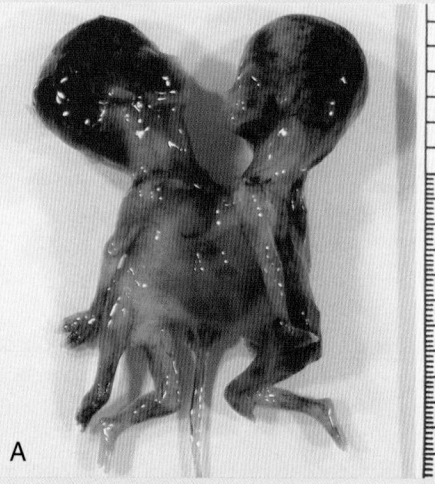
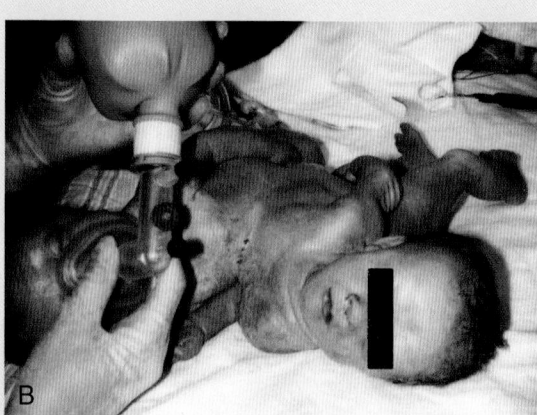

• **Fig. 2.3** (A) Conjoined twins at 12 weeks of development. (B) Conjoined twins after birth. (A, From Moore KL, Persaud TVN, Shiota K: *Color atlas of clinical embryology,* ed 2, Philadelphia, 2000, Saunders; Courtesy Dr. D.K. Kalousek, Department of Pathology, University of British Columbia, Children's Hospital, Vancouver, British Columbia, Canada. B, From Callen P: *Ultrasonography in obstetrics and gynecology,* ed 5, Philadelphia, 2008, Saunders.)

Weeks of Gestation

P07.23 *(Extreme immaturity of newborn, gestational age 24 completed weeks)*

P07.24 *(Extreme immaturity of newborn, gestational age 25 completed weeks)*

P07.25 *(Extreme immaturity of newborn, gestational age 26 completed weeks)*

P07.26 *(Extreme immaturity of newborn, gestational age 27 completed weeks)*

P07.31 *(Preterm newborn, gestational age 28 completed weeks)*

P07.32 *(Preterm newborn, gestational age 29 completed weeks)*

P07.33 *(Preterm newborn, gestational age 30 completed weeks)*

P07.34 *(Preterm newborn, gestational age 31 completed weeks)*

P07.35 *(Preterm newborn, gestational age 32 completed weeks)*

P07.36 *(Preterm newborn, gestational age 33 completed weeks)*

P07.37 *(Preterm newborn, gestational age 34 completed weeks)*

P07.38 *(Preterm newborn, gestational age 35 completed weeks)*

P07.39 *(Preterm newborn, gestational age 36 completed weeks)*

P07.30 *(Preterm newborn, unspecified weeks)*

Symptoms and Signs

Premature babies may weigh as low as 12 ounces or less at the time of birth. Their physical development is at various stages, depending on the length of gestational time. The smaller of these infants have little subcutaneous fat, palms and soles with few creases, possible undescended testes in males, and a prominent clitoris in females. Many of these very tiny and immature babies lack the ability to suck or swallow or have weakened sucking or swallowing reflexes. The lungs are often underdeveloped, leading to respiratory dangers. The immature neurologic system can lead to some difficulties in maintenance of body temperature, problems in controlling cardiac function, and spontaneous episodes of apnea or may result in seizure activity. An immature immune system makes the risk of infection high.

Patient Screening

Pregnant patients who contact the physician to say they may be in labor require prompt attention. When the pregnant patient thinks she is in labor more than 3 weeks before her due date, she must be assessed as quickly as possible. Many physicians prefer that these patients go directly to the hospital where the delivery is planned to take place. Others prefer to see the patient in the office as soon as possible. When the patient arrives at the office, she should be placed in the examination room and the physician promptly notified that she is in the office.

Etiology

There are many reasons that premature infants enter the world before reaching the traditionally accepted gestational age of 40 weeks and thus have very low birth weights. Causes of premature labor resulting in a premature infant are an incompetent cervix; bicornuate uterus; toxic conditions; maternal infection; trauma; premature rupture of the amniotic membranes; history of previous miscarriages; multiple gestations; intrauterine fetal delayed growth; and other physical conditions of the mother, such as pregnancy-induced or chronic hypertension. Diabetes, heart disease, kidney disease, poor nutrition, substance abuse, and lack of prenatal care also contribute to the incidence of the mother giving birth to a preterm infant. In some cases, the etiology is never identified. Attempts may be made to halt premature labor by having the mother on complete bed rest or using drug therapy to slow or halt contractions. The mother is often given a short course of steroids to aid fetal lung maturation. Many times, efforts to allow the fetus more time to grow and mature in the mother's uterus are unsuccessful.

Diagnosis

Diagnostic criteria include a gestational age of less than 37 weeks. Neonates diagnosed as small for gestational age (SGA) are low-weight infants (< 5 lb 8 oz) that may or may not be premature.

Treatment

Treatment varies, depending on the gestational age, weight, present or subsequent conditions, anomalies, and nutritional status. Intravenous (IV) fluids and hyperalimentation are necessary to encourage the growth and development of the premature infant. Airway management and pulmonary functioning are monitored very closely. Many of the smallest babies are intubated endotracheally, and respiration is maintained by mechanical ventilation. Recent advances in respiratory care for tiny premature infants permit extubation of the infant and maintenance of the airway by continuous positive airway pressure (CPAP) through the nose. Pulse oximeters constantly monitor oxygen (O_2) saturation levels and heart rate. Body temperature is monitored closely and maintained at normal levels (Fig. 2.4). When infection is a risk caused by maternal prenatal infection or extended time of ruptured amniotic sac, vigilance is required for the onset of any symptoms of infection, and antibiotics are

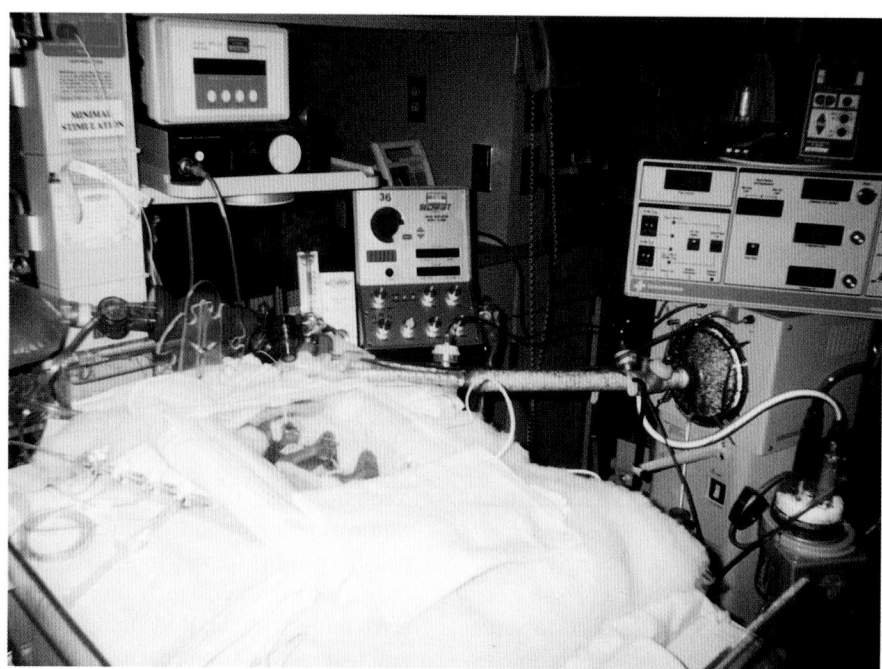

• **Fig. 2.4** Infant in neonatal intensive care unit (NICU) born at 28 weeks, weighing 2 lb 6 oz. (Photo Courtesy Kim and LilliAnna Kervin.)

often started presumptively. When early signs of infection occur, aggressive treatment is introduced. Monitoring of blood glucose, blood pressure, and body temperature is performed on a frequent and regular basis, and any treatment necessary is instituted to maintain optimal levels.

Comfort measures include placing an article with the mother's scent in the isolette or crib with the infant. These tiny babies are swaddled to simulate the closeness and feeling of the womb. Lights are kept at a dim level, and harsh auditory stimuli are kept at a minimum.

Prognosis

Advances in technology have made survival of low weight and short gestation infants possible. The prognosis for these

children varies, depending on gestational age, weight, and the occurrence of anomalies and developmental deficits. There are documented cases of 12-ounce and/or 22-gestational-week babies surviving. They fall into the 1% of premature babies born at that weight and gestational age. Because they are born before the normal prenatal development is complete, these children often have many problems to overcome (Fig. 2.5).

One of the primary risks is cerebral bleeding, which may occur during the labor and delivery process or may result from handling after delivery. The cerebral bleeding may cause the development of CP, mental functioning deficiencies, or other neurologic conditions.

Another major concern is underdevelopment of the pulmonary system, including the lung tissue and the airway. Some pulmonary conditions these infants experience are infant respiratory distress syndrome (IRDS), bronchopulmonary **dysplasia** (BPD), laryngomalacia, tracheomalacia, and bronchomalacia. Lack of body fat can affect the maintenance of body temperature. Any stress or increased or high supplemental O_2 flow may be responsible for retinopathy of prematurity (ROP) and possible blindness. Necrotizing enterocolitis (NEC) is a danger in the digestive system because of the reduced tolerance of the alimentary tract. Atrial septal defect (ASD) and patent ductus arteriosus (PDA) often are present because the fetal circulatory system has failed to mature.

The generally accepted gestational age for 50% of infants to survive the birth process and perinatal period is 24 weeks, with a greater percentage of infants surviving as gestational age increases. Improvements in technology are making it possible for more and more of these tiniest infants to survive (Fig. 2.6).

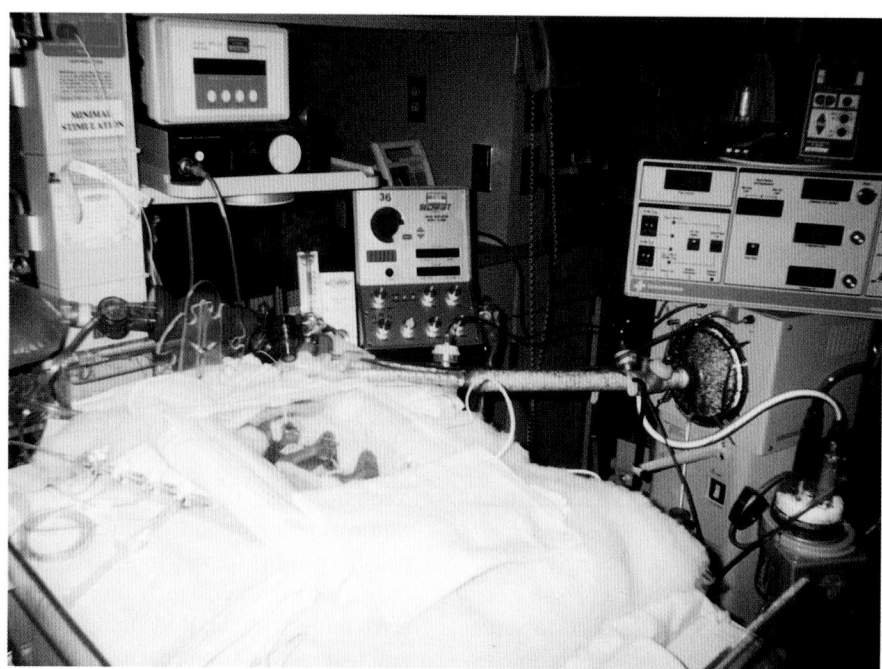

• **Fig. 2.5** Four-day-old premature infant. Weight is 14.6 oz and gestational age is 22 weeks. (Courtesy David L. Frazier, 1999.)

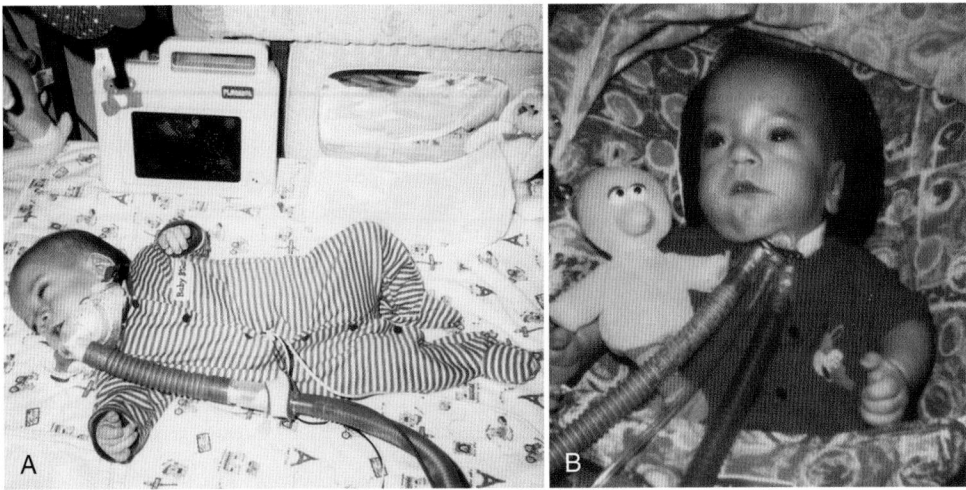

• **Fig. 2.6** (A) Same premature infant from Fig. 2.5 at age 9 months; weight 11 lb 8 oz. (B) Same infant at age 10 months, weight 13 lb. (Courtesy David L. Frazier, 1999.)

Prevention

Preventing prematurity requires good prenatal care, adequate nutrition, and assessment of the pregnant patient's risk factors for premature labor. Abstaining from consuming alcohol and smoking cigarettes helps reduce the risk of premature birth and/or low birth weight. Additionally, bed rest of the expectant mother may delay the onset of premature labor and create more time for the fetus to develop. Drug therapy may be used in an attempt to stop premature labor that results in premature birth (see Chapter 12).

Patient Teaching

Encouraging pregnant women to obtain prenatal care and to follow guidelines is important. Pregnant women should be instructed to contact their physicians at the first sign of labor, especially labor before the 37th week of gestation. Parents of premature infants need emotional support and should be educated in the possibility of complications resulting from prematurity.

Infant Respiratory Distress Syndrome

Description

IRDS, or hyaline membrane disease, is similar to adult respiratory distress syndrome in that the patient suffers acute hypoxemia caused by infiltrates within the alveoli.

ICD-10-CM Code	P22.0 *(Respiratory distress syndrome of newborn)* (P22.0-P22.9 = 4 codes of specificity)

Symptoms and Signs

Shortly after birth, the neonate exhibits signs of respiratory distress, including nasal flaring, grunting respirations, and sternal retractions. Blood gas studies indicate reduced oxygen tension and ineffective gas exchange. The infant becomes cyanotic with mottled skin.

Patient Screening

The infant is hospitalized, usually in a neonatal intensive care unit (NICU). The NICU staff observes the infant for signs of respiratory distress, and immediate intervention is instituted at the first signs of distress.

Etiology

The lungs of the neonate lack the surfactant needed to allow the alveoli to expand. The surfactant normally is produced relatively late in fetal life; consequently, premature infants are at risk. The outcome of this inability of the lungs to expand is inadequate surface area for proper gas exchange and a potentially fatal lack of oxygen in blood.

Diagnosis

The first indications of IRDS are increased respiratory efforts of the newborn and a history of prematurity. Blood gas studies demonstrate the reduced potential for adequate gas exchange. Radiographic chest films indicate the presence of the infiltrate or hyaline membrane.

Treatment

Treatment consists of the administration of carefully titrated supplemental oxygen, usually administered by mechanical ventilation and positive end-expiratory pressure (PEEP), and is of primary importance. Drug therapy, including the aerosol infusion of an exogenous surfactant, such as beractant (Survanta) or poractant alfa (Curosurf), into the pulmonary tree via an endotracheal tube as soon as possible after birth helps provide an artificial surfactant, allowing the alveoli to expand. This treatment should begin within the first 8 hours of life and be repeated once or twice, if needed, until the alveoli are expanded.

Prognosis

The prognosis for these infants' survival has improved greatly because of a better understanding of their condition and advanced technology in drug and respiratory therapies.

Prevention

Prevention is the best treatment; therefore, if time permits, the mother is injected with a corticosteroid (betamethasone [Celestone Soluspan]) 24 hours before delivery in an attempt to mature the surfactant-synthesizing system.

Patient Teaching

Give the parents printed information about the condition. Parents need emotional support and understanding. They should be referred to community support groups. Allow the parents to verbalize their anxieties and fears to a compassionate and understanding individual to provide validation of their feelings regarding the situation.

Unfortunately, the occurrence of IRDS, along with its treatment modalities, often predisposes premature infants to the development of BPD.

◆ ENRICHMENT

Laryngomalacia, Tracheomalacia, and Bronchomalacia

Laryngomalacia, tracheomalacia, and bronchomalacia all are forms of obstructive airway conditions. They can evolve as separate entities or can develop in a combination of two or even all three conditions. Although most often observed in the infant or young child, these conditions may be found in adults as well. The primary cause in all conditions is softened or underdeveloped cartilage (malacia), allowing the airway structure or structures to partially or completely collapse and compromise the airway.

The infant with laryngomalacia exhibits respiratory stridor that is louder on inspiration. The infant with tracheomalacia also exhibits respiratory stridor; however, the stridor is more pronounced on expiration. All these congenital conditions cause the infants to experience dyspnea and possibly episodes of cyanosis. Oxygen saturation levels decrease, and the infants may experience bradycardia. These infants occasionally experience feeding difficulties. Diagnostic studies include chest radiography, computed tomography (CT), flexible fiberoptic laryngoscopy, and bronchoscopy. Treatment is based on the underlying cause once it has been determined. Most of these children outgrow the disorders.

Bronchopulmonary Dysplasia

Description

BPD, a serious, chronic lung disease, results after an insult to the neonate's lungs. This may be a sequela to IRDS, a lung infection, or extreme prematurity. The lungs are stiff, obstructed, and hard to ventilate.

ICD-10-CM Code	P27.0 (Wilson-Mikity syndrome)
	(P27.0-P27.9 = 4 codes of specificity)
	P27.1 (Bronchopulmonary dysplasia originating in the perinatal period)
	P27.8 (Other chronic respiratory diseases originating in the perinatal period)

Symptoms and Signs

The infant experiences periods of dyspnea, including tachypnea, wheezing, cyanosis, nasal flaring, and sternal retractions. O_2 saturation decreases, as does heart rate. The infant may experience coughing and difficulty feeding. These babies appear to be working very hard to breathe, and they exhibit poor posture of the neck, shoulders, and upper body. Wet or crackling sounds are heard on auscultation of the lungs with a stethoscope.

Patient Screening

The infant is hospitalized, usually in an NICU. The NICU staff observes the infant for signs of respiratory distress, and immediate intervention is instituted at the first signs of distress.

Etiology

BPD occurs in many premature infants after IRDS, mechanical ventilation with supplemental oxygen, and infection or pneumonia. The pressure and oxygen needed to maintain life-sustaining oxygen levels can damage soft and fragile lung tissue, causing overinflation or scarring.

Diagnosis

Observation of the infant reveals early respiratory distress. Radiographs of the chest are abnormal, indicating alveolar damage, either scarring or overinflation, sometimes described as a "ground glass" appearance. Arterial blood gas (ABG) levels indicate a problem. Oxygen levels in the lungs may be low and carbon dioxide (CO_2) levels high.

Treatment

The goal of treatment is replacement of the damaged alveoli. Children grow new alveoli until about 8 years of age. Infants who have BPD need to grow new alveoli to replace those damaged by scarring. As this replacement occurs, the severity of the condition lessens. Supportive treatment includes supplemental oxygen and adequate nutritional support. The types of medications used include diuretics and bronchodilators, including beta$_2$-agonists, anticholinergic drugs, and theophylline. Antiinflammatory drugs, such as steroids, also may help.

Supplemental O_2 therapy may be needed for several weeks, occasionally for greater than 1 year. This therapy usually is given via a nasal cannula; however, if the infant has a tracheostomy, it may be delivered via the tracheostomy collar or via CPAP. O_2 saturation levels must be monitored with a pulse oximeter so that they can be maintained at 90% or greater. The pulse oximeter also monitors heart rate. As the infant grows and matures, blood oxygen saturation levels may be maintained on room air, usually by age 1 year.

Diuretics help reduce fluid accumulation in the lungs and reduce the incidence of pulmonary hypertension and right-sided heart failure. Bronchodilators are administered to reverse the narrowing of the bronchi resulting from inflammation or bronchospasm, thus allowing more oxygen to reach the lung tissue. These drugs may be administered orally as syrups or via aerosol inhalation. The antiinflammatory drugs help prevent the inflammatory process from becoming severe.

Adequate nutrition is needed for the infant's growth and to meet the increased caloric demand resulting from difficult breathing. High-calorie formulas are used. The infant must be held with the head raised slightly and the formula given frequently in small amounts to prevent gastroesophageal reflux disease (GERD). Some infants are given medications to prevent GERD and other medications, such as antacids or histamine-2 blockers, to reduce gastric acid.

Prognosis

Prognosis is good with early and aggressive intervention, prudent monitoring, and maintenance of adequate O_2 saturation levels and heart rate. Resolution of the condition is slow, and improvement is gradual. Complications include pulmonary edema and hypertension, right-sided heart failure (cor pulmonale), respiratory infections, apnea, tracheomalacia, asthma, GI reflux, and aspiration. These children are particularly susceptible to respiratory infections, such as bronchiolitis caused by respiratory syncytial virus (RSV). They may experience poor growth or delayed development. Many of these children outgrow the condition, but others may be susceptible to respiratory distress for life. Apneic periods and low oxygen saturation levels for an extended period may cause hypoxia of the brain, which may result in developmental deficits. Some infants may not survive.

Prevention

There is currently no way to prevent BPD; however, early weaning from mechanical respiratory support may reduce its incidence. Early and aggressive intervention and treatment may prevent complications and permanent conditions, even death.

Patient Teaching

Help parents find community support groups and agencies to help deal with emotional and financial stressors. The parents should receive emotional support because this condition in their child usually requires prolonged or frequent hospitalizations. Parents should be encouraged to become as involved as possible in the care of their infant, helping them become familiar with the infant's health care needs and promoting bonding with the infant.

Retinopathy of Prematurity

Description

ROP, or retrolental fibroplasia, is abnormal growth of blood vessels in the retinas of the infant's eyes. The condition occurs in the eyes of premature infants.

ICD-10-CM Code	H35.179 *(Retrolental fibroplasia, unspecified eye)*
	(H35.171-H35.179 = 4 codes of specificity)

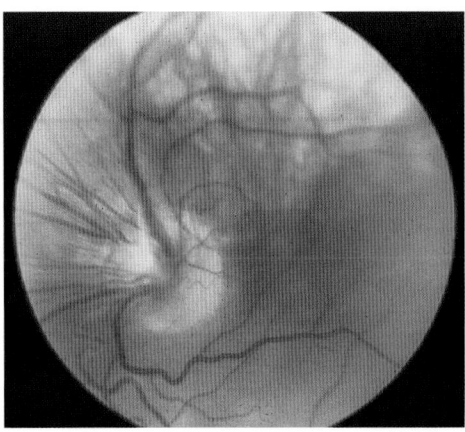

• **Fig. 2.7** Retrolental fibroplasia. (From Zitelli BJ, Davis HW: *Atlas of pediatric physical diagnosis,* ed 6, Philadelphia, 2012, Mosby.)

Symptoms and Signs

ROP occurs most often in infants born before 28 weeks of gestation. There are no visible symptoms. Screening examinations are performed routinely on premature infants weighing less than 1500 g or at a gestational age of less than 30 weeks. The entire retina is visualized to determine the stages of development of the blood vessels supplying it. These examinations are first performed when the infant is 4 to 6 weeks old (Fig. 2.7).

Patient Screening

The infant is hospitalized, usually in an NICU. An ophthalmologist performs routine examinations of the retina. If the infant has been dismissed from the hospital and later exhibits signs of complications, an immediate appointment or examination should be arranged.

Etiology

The vascularization of the retina begins at the back central part of the eye, as vessels grow out toward the edges. The blood vessels to the retina do not begin development until about the 28th week of gestation. In premature infants, this vascularization is incomplete. Regardless of gestational age at birth, most ROP originates 34 to 40 weeks after conception.

No specific risk factors for the development of ROP have been identified. Therefore, there is a group of risk factors that contribute to it. The more premature and the lower the birth weight of the infant, the greater is the risk of ROP. High supplemental oxygen concentrations are responsible for many incidents of ROP. Therefore, close monitoring of oxygen saturation levels and appropriate adjustment and titration of oxygen concentration levels to the infant reduce the risk. Certain drugs, such as surfactant and indomethacin administered to the neonate for treatment of immature lungs, as well as PDA, may increase the risk for the premature infant. Recently intense artificial lighting in the nursery or crib has been considered a risk factor. Other risk factors cited include seizures, mechanical ventilation, anemia, blood transfusions, and multiple spells of apnea and bradycardia.

Diagnosis

Diagnosis is made by an ophthalmologist using an indirect ophthalmoscope and scleral depression to visualize the retina. The lens and iris also are examined at this time.

Treatment

Most mild forms of ROP resolve without treatment. Laser treatment to the area anterior to the vascular shunt eliminates abnormal vessels before they deposit enough scar tissue to cause retinal detachment. Severe cases may require other procedures.

Prognosis

As previously mentioned, mild forms of this condition may resolve spontaneously. Laser surgery may be required in more serious cases. Blindness may result from serious damage. ROP that has resolved can have later complications. These include crossed or wandering eyes (strabismus), "lazy eye" (amblyopia), nearsightedness (myopia), glaucoma, and late-onset retinal detachment. Many of these children may require corrective glasses. Children who have been diagnosed with some retinal damage in the neonatal period require follow-up monitoring up to the toddler years, or even later if problems are detected. A partially or completely detached retina may occur in the most serious cases. Prompt intervention may result in repair of the detachment and prevention of blindness.

Prevention

There is no way to prevent ROP in the premature infant. Close monitoring and titration of oxygen concentrations have reduced the incidence of the condition. NICUs now protect premature infants' eyes from excessive exposure to artificial lighting. Attempts are made to avoid exposing premature infants to stress factors. Screening examinations, staging (determining extent of vascular damage), and appropriate intervention help reduce the severity of the condition and prevent blindness.

Patient Teaching

Parents should be told of the risk for this condition in the premature infant. Give them printed material about the condition, and help them contact support groups in the community. Encourage follow-up eye examinations for infants as prescribed by the ophthalmologist.

Necrotizing Enterocolitis

Description

NEC is an acute inflammatory process caused by ischemic necrosis of the mucosal lining of the small intestine, the large intestine, or both. It is a condition of premature infants or sick neonates that develops after birth, when the fragile intestinal tract of the premature or compromised newborn becomes active.

ICD-10-CM Code	P77.9 *(Necrotizing enterocolitis in newborn, unspecified)* (P77.1, Stage 1; P77.2, Stage 2; P77.3, Stage 3 = 4 codes of specificity)

Symptoms and Signs

Feeding intolerance, abdominal distention, bile-colored emesis, diarrhea, blood in the stool, decreased or absent bowel sounds, lethargy, and body temperature instability a few days after birth are some of the initial symptoms exhibited by the preterm or low birth weight infant. The state of well-being degrades as these infants experience respiratory problems related to brief apneic periods, reduced urine output, hyperbilirubinemia, and erythema. The abdomen is tender to palpation.

Patient Screening

The infant is hospitalized, usually in an NICU. The NICU staff observes the infant for signs of NEC, and the neonatologist is notified of any signs of distress so that immediate intervention can be instituted.

Etiology

The etiology of NEC is unknown; however, it is thought to be a breakdown in the normal defense systems of the GI tract, allowing the *normal flora* of the GI tract to invade the intestinal mucosa. This can happen when blood is shunted away from the GI tract, resulting in convulsive vasoconstriction of the mesenteric vessels and diminished blood supply, interfering with the normal production of protective mucus.

In addition to prematurity, factors that may predispose infants to NEC include hypovolemia, sepsis, umbilical catheters, exchange transfusions, and IRDS. Another factor is oral feeding of high-calorie concentrated formula.

Diagnosis

Observation of changes in the infant's feeding patterns or activity level, impaired body temperature maintenance, and respiratory difficulties, along with abdominal distention and tenderness, call for further investigation. Complete blood count (CBC) indicates an elevated white blood cell (WBC) count, and guaiac test results of stool specimens for occult blood are positive. Blood and stool cultures are performed and may confirm the presence of bacteria. Radiography of the intestine confirms the condition.

Treatment

Aggressive and immediate intervention is necessary if the infant is to survive. Feedings are stopped, making the infant's status NPO (nothing by mouth). A small tube is inserted into the stomach by way of the nose or the mouth for decompression. Fluids are administered intravenously, as are antibiotics. Respiratory status and pH are monitored by measuring ABGs. The infant's weight and intake and output (I&O) are monitored closely, and fluid and electrolyte balance is maintained. Abdominal distention is monitored through frequent measurements of the abdomen by a tape measure. Radiographic monitoring of the intestinal tract also is performed. Complications of intestinal perforation or peritonitis require surgical intervention with removal of the necrotic tissue. When necrosis is extensive, ileostomy or colostomy may be necessary until the infant grows, and closure with anastomosis can be performed.

Prognosis

Without immediate and aggressive intervention, many of these babies will die. NEC is a serious complication of prematurity, and some babies die even with aggressive treatment. Resection of a portion of the bowel can lead to an obstruction of the bowel or to malabsorption syndrome. Perforation can lead to sepsis and death.

Prevention

Most of these babies are still in the hospital when NEC develops. Prudent nursing observations and reporting of any symptoms of NEC are essential. Because the infection can be spread from infant to infant, meticulous hand washing must be followed. Breast milk appears to offer some protection from this condition. An awareness of the high-risk infant is fundamental in the prevention and early intervention of this disease.

Patient Teaching

Parents require emotional support along with information about the condition. Meticulous hand washing should be emphasized, and the dangers of infection should be explained to the parents.

Genetic Syndromes and Conditions

Robinow Syndrome

Description

Robinow syndrome is a condition of small stature and related incidence of interorbital distance, bulging (bossing) forehead, depressed nasal bridge, malaligned teeth, and short limbs. Other manifestations of the syndrome may be present.

Symptoms and Signs

Robinow syndrome may present in dominant or recessive forms. Characteristics of both types of the syndrome are typically present in both forms and are usually minor or moderate in nature. Box 2.1 lists typical manifestations of Robinow syndrome. Two types of this syndrome have been described (dominant and recessive), and the information presented in the box refers to both of them. The patients usually have most of these signs in a minor to moderate scale. Individuals with Robinow syndrome have been found to be of normal intelligence; however, they may experience medical issues throughout childhood and the developmental stages (Fig. 2.8A–B).

Patient Screening

Parents calling to arrange an appointment possibly are referred by the dentist or school nurse. The anxiety level will be high because the parents may not have any idea why they are being referred, usually because the child is small or because the dentist has encountered a small mouth with misaligned teeth. Children or adults with this syndrome usually are born after normal gestation and generally have a normal birth weight. Schedule an appointment as early as convenient for all.

Etiology

Robinow syndrome, an inherited condition, is a genetic syndrome. The gene responsible for the dominant form has not yet been established. The recessive form results from a mutation of a specific gene that has been identified as being located in chromosome 9q22. This gene deals with bone and cartilage formation. Typically, both parents are carriers of the recessive gene and are not affected.

• BOX 2.1   Medical Manifestations of Robinow Syndrome

Skeletal System

- Mild to moderate short stature (dwarfism)
- Short lower arms (mesomelic brachymelia)
- Small hands with clinodactyly usually of the fifth finger (abnormal lateral or medial bending of one or more fingers or toes) and brachydactyly (abnormally short fingers or toes)
- Small feet

Spinal Malformations

- Vertebral segmentation defects
- Dominant—at most a single butterfly vertebra
- Recessive—multiple vertebral segmentation defects (always multiple rib anomalies, fusions)
- Hemivertebrae, vertebral fusions, narrow interpediculate distances most common in the recessive form

Abnormalities of the Head and Facial Area (Craniofacial, Fetal Face)

- Flat facial profile with larger head (macrocephaly not necessarily associated with hydrocephaly)

- Prominent or bulging forehead with widely spaced eyes
- Short, upturned nose with anteverted nostrils and flat nasal bridge
- Wide triangular mouth; long philtrum with broad horizontal upper lip in the dominant form, short philtrum with an inverted V-shaped or tented upper lip in the recessive form
- Crowded, misaligned teeth and gum hypertrophy

Eyes and Ears

- Hypertelorism/hypoplastic, or shortened, S-shaped lower eyelids giving the impression of prominent eyes
- Ears are sometimes cup shaped, flapped, and/or low set

Genital Hypoplasia

- Males often have an underdeveloped penis, sometimes only visible when the surrounding skin is retracted
- Undescended testicles
- In females, the clitoris and labia minora (sometimes labia majora) are underdeveloped (hypoplastic)

Used with permission of Robinow Syndrome Foundation, Anoka, MN.

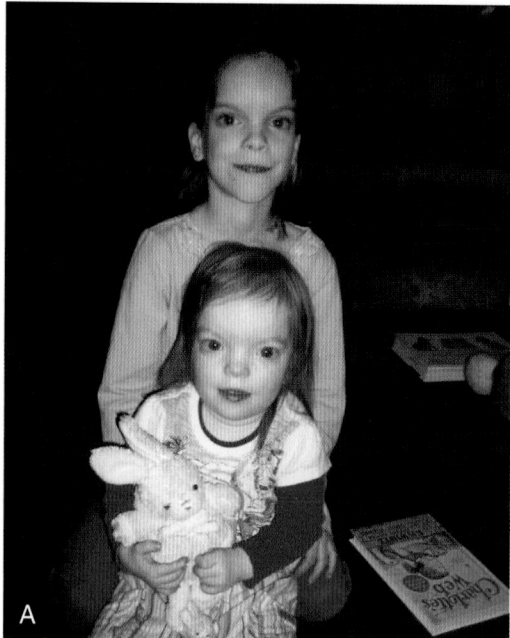
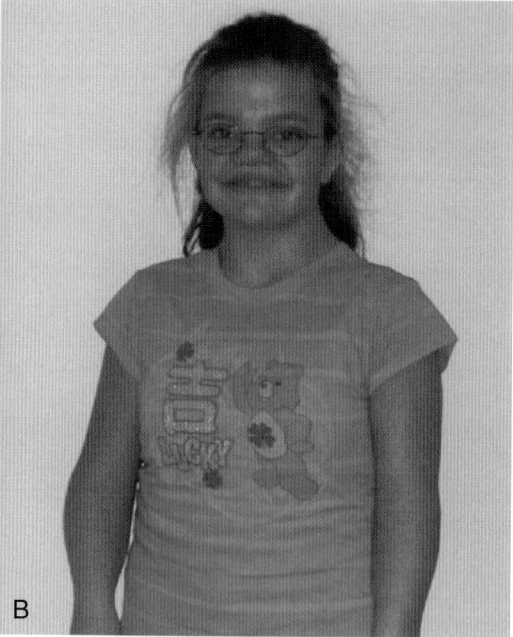

• **Fig. 2.8** (A) Sisters with autosomal dominant form of Robinow syndrome. (B) Teenage girl with autosomal recessive form of Robinow syndrome. (A, Courtesy David Frazier, 2007. B, Courtesy Karla Kruger, 2006.)

Diagnosis

The clinical picture of short stature and presence of some of the characteristic symptoms and signs help the physician make the diagnosis. The diagnosis is confirmed by a genetic study indicating the chromosomal defect. Additional genetic studies will confirm the presence of the syndrome.

In early life, the condition of many of these children is misdiagnosed as failure to thrive. The smallness of the body, along with eating and swallowing difficulties, tends to lead to the misdiagnosis. This diagnosis may place a social stigma on the parents and create problems for them with social services in the home community.

Treatment

This genetic condition has no cure. Treatment involves addressing any treatable conditions, such as dental abnormalities, cleft palate, and orthopedic conditions, including scoliosis. Genetic counseling may be recommended. For those with problems of self-image because of short stature and other typical abnormalities, psychosocial counseling could be recommended.

Prognosis

There is no cure for this condition. With supportive treatment, individuals with Robinow syndrome generally have a normal life span.

Prevention

There is no prevention for this hereditary condition. Genetic counseling is advised.

Patient Teaching

Encourage patients and parents to contact resource agencies for emotional and medical support.

◆ ENRICHMENT

Cri-du-Chat Syndrome (Cat's Cry Syndrome)

The deletion of genetic material from chromosome 5 results in the condition called *cri-du-chat*. This rare disorder, "cat's cry" syndrome, usually results in stillborn children or those who die shortly after birth. Those who survive the perinatal and neonatal periods may progress to maturity. These individuals may have various medical and mental problems.

Infants with cri-du-chat syndrome have an abnormally small head (microcephaly), with deficiency of cerebral brain tissue, and usually experience some level of intellectual developmental disorder. Those who are born alive have a weak, mewing, catlike cry. The orbits of the eyes are spaced far apart. Surviving children usually experience slow growth patterns, a small head, and poor muscle tone. Motor and language skills development may be delayed. Mental development may be slow, and behavioral problems may develop. Cri-du-chat syndrome is a hereditary condition and the result of a chromosomal aberration caused by deletion of part of the short arm of chromosome 5 of the B group. A genetic study indicating the chromosomal defect confirms the diagnosis.

Parents' awareness of the condition usually occurs when the child is born. Generally parents are anxious to discuss why the syndrome is present in the child and the possibility of subsequent children also having the same syndrome. Discussions should take place as soon as possible. Should the child survive and be in the home environment, the child should be seen immediately for any problem that arises.

Because there is no cure, treatment supports body functions as long as the infant survives. Many fetuses with this chromosomal aberration die in utero. Those infants who survive and progress into childhood need special schooling and supportive care. These individuals can possibly experience a normal life span.

There is no prevention for this hereditary condition. Parents are encouraged to contact community support groups.

Hypertrophic Cardiomyopathy

Description

Hypertrophic cardiomyopathy (HCM), a congenital disorder, occurs when a portion of the heart muscle thickens without any apparent cause. This condition is a major cause of sudden cardiac death in young athletes who have appeared to be completely healthy.

ICD-10-CM Code	I42.2 *(Other hypertrophic cardiomyopathy)*
	(I42.0-I42.9 = 10 codes of specificity for cardiomyopathy)
	I42.5 *(Other restrictive cardiomyopathy)*
	I42.8 *(Other cardiomyopathies)*

Symptoms and Signs

Tragically, the first sign is the collapse of a seemingly healthy young athlete during a strenuous sporting event or other period of stressful exercise. This collapse can be followed by cardiac arrest caused by cardiac arrhythmia. Many have no symptoms until the collapse. It is possible that some individuals experience no symptoms. Signs may be discovered during a physical examination. Symptoms, often ignored by young people, may include chest pain, syncope, hypertension, palpitations, or shortness of breath. Some report experiencing fatigue, shortness of breath when lying down, or reduced tolerance of activity.

Etiology

A portion of the myocardium becomes thickened without any obvious cause. The normal alignment of the myocardial cells is disturbed (myocardial disarray), resulting in disruption of cardiac electrical impulses.

This genetic disease is an inherited autosomal dominant trait.

Diagnosis

Diagnosis of young people who have collapsed during a strenuous exercise or sporting event and had a sudden cardiac arrest is made on autopsy. Before a collapse, the condition may be diagnosed with an investigation of a report involving any of the following symptoms: A drop in blood pressure may be noted during exercise; the person has a family history of cardiac arrest or sudden death at a young age along with a history of the individual experiencing palpitations or unexplained syncope; and the presence of life-threatening arrhythmias, which is recorded on a Holter monitor and is investigated.

Electrocardiography may indicate the presence of the hypertrophy. Echocardiography, radiography, or cardiac magnetic resonance imaging (MRI) may also indicate the thickness of areas of the myocardium (Fig. 2.9). A genetic test can be done to look for any of the known mutations leading to HCM.

Treatment

When arrhythmias are present, medications, including beta-blockers and calcium channel blockers, may be prescribed.

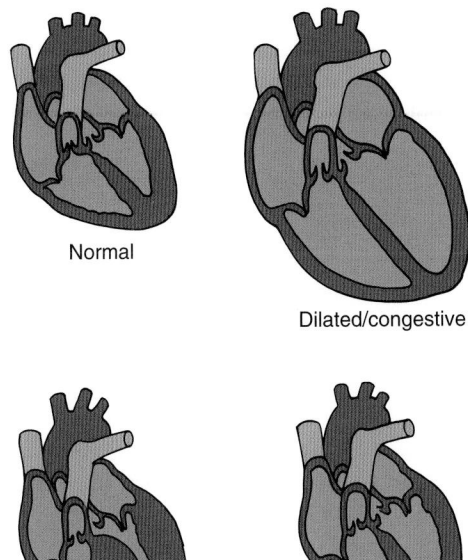

Normal

Dilated/congestive

Hypertrophic

Restrictive

• **Fig. 2.9** Drawing of heart with cardiomyopathy. (From Black JM, Hawks JH: *Medical-surgical nursing: Clinical management for positive outcomes,* ed 8, St Louis, 2009, Saunders.)

Some patients may require implantation of a pacemaker or implantable cardioverter-defibrillator (ICD). Should the thickening obstruct the flow of blood, a surgical myectomy may be performed. Patients should avoid strenuous exercise and stressful situations.

Prognosis

Young people with HCM are at a high risk for sudden cardiac death. Prognosis of the young person who has collapsed is very guarded because most do not respond to immediate cardiac resuscitation. Those who are diagnosed before a catastrophic event and who can follow medical guidelines, such as avoiding strenuous exercise, have a fair outlook. Some may not experience symptoms and may live a normal life span.

Prevention

There is no prevention for this genetic disorder. Genetic counseling is advised for the individual and his or her relatives. Electrocardiography performed during a sports physical can help identify those who are at risk for HCM.

Patient Teaching

Patients who have been diagnosed with HCM should be encouraged to follow their physician's advice about avoiding strenuous exercise. They should continue follow-up care with their physician and be compliant regarding medications that have been prescribed.

Down Syndrome

Description

Down syndrome (formerly called *mongolism*) is a genetic syndrome in which the individual has 47 chromosomes instead of the usual 46, resulting in a congenital form of mild to severe intellectual developmental disorder that is accompanied by characteristic facial features and distinctive physical abnormalities.

ICD-10-CM Code   R00.0 *(Tachycardia, unspecified)*

Symptoms and Signs

Down syndrome, in addition to mild to severe intellectual developmental disorder, is associated with heart defects and other congenital abnormalities. Typically, the infant has a small head with a flat back skull, a characteristic slant to the eyes, a flat nasal bridge, small low-set ears, a small mouth with a protruding tongue, and small, weak muscles (Figs. 2.10 and 2.11). The hands are short, with stubby fingers and a deep horizontal crease across the palm (simian line). There is an exaggerated space between the big and little toes.

Patient Screening

Down syndrome usually is diagnosed prenatally via ultrasonography, blood tests, and/or amniocentesis or during the neonatal period. Patients are monitored closely through normal infant and childhood office visits. When the parent of a child with Down syndrome calls requesting an appointment, assessment should be made depending on the complaint. Consider the anxiety level of the parent, and schedule an appointment for the next available time.

Etiology

Infants with Down syndrome have an extra chromosome number 21 (**trisomy** 21). It occurs in 1 in 700 live births

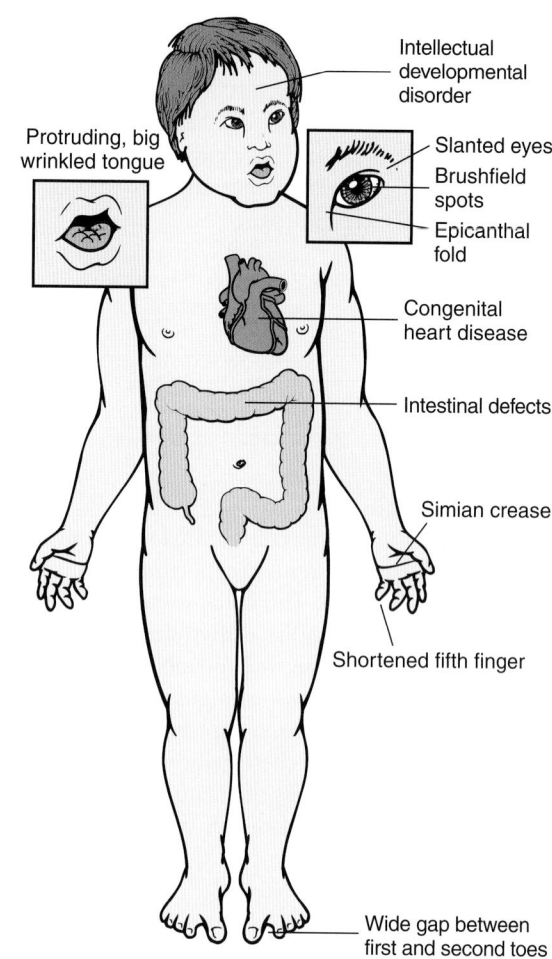

• **Fig. 2.11** Typical features of Down syndrome. (From Damjanov I: *Pathology for the health professions,* ed 4, St Louis, 2011, Saunders.)

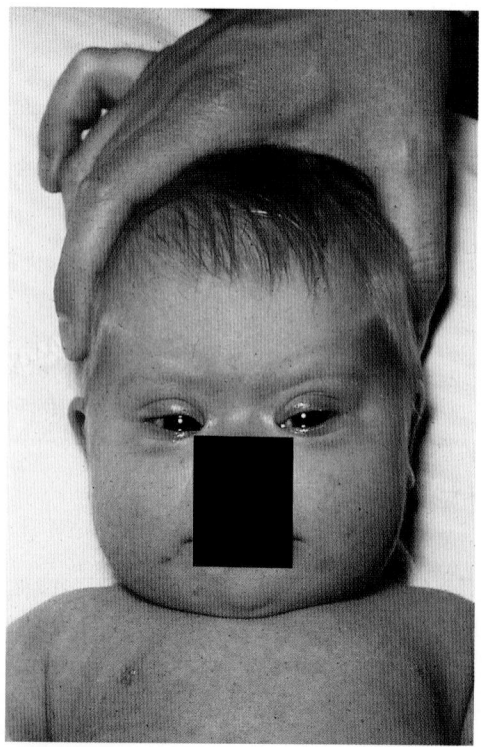

• **Fig. 2.10** Typical face seen in a child with Down syndrome. (From Zitelli BJ, Davis HW: *Atlas of pediatric physical diagnosis,* ed 6, Philadelphia, 2012, Mosby.)

and more often in infants born to women older than 35 years of age (Fig. 2.12).

Diagnosis

Infants with severe Down syndrome usually are identified at or before birth; milder forms are diagnosed later. The physical characteristics may be blatantly obvious. Findings on examination of the eyes may include the presence of small white dots on the iris. A karyotype showing the chromosomal abnormality can confirm the diagnosis.

Treatment

Care of the child with Down syndrome depends on the severity of the physical defects and the degree of mental impairment. There is no known cure. The treatment plan is individualized and includes a multidimensional approach to maximize the development of motor and mental skills. Life expectancy has been improved through surgical correction of cardiac defects and antibiotic therapy for susceptibility to pulmonary disease. Some individuals may receive care in their homes; others require residency at long-term care centers. Those who live longer are known for their affectionate and placid personalities.

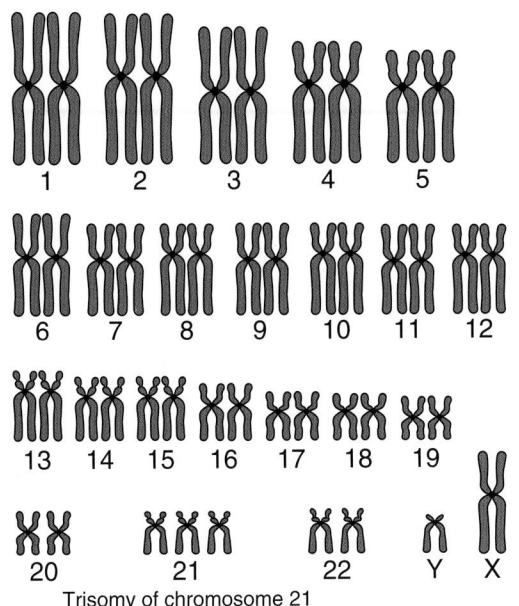

1 2 3 4 5

6 7 8 9 10 11 12

13 14 15 16 17 18 19

20 21 22 Y X

Trisomy of chromosome 21

• **Fig. 2.12** Karyotype of Down syndrome. (From Damjanov I: *Pathology for the health professions,* ed 4, St Louis, 2011, Saunders.)

Prognosis

There is no known cure for Down syndrome; however, some of these individuals may be educable and may be able to live independently in assisted or supervised living facilities.

Prevention

There is no prevention for this condition.

Patient Teaching

Help parents find and contact local support groups. Be available to answer parents' questions.

Diseases of the Nervous System

Cerebral Palsy

Description

CP, the most common crippling condition in children, consists of a group of disorders possibly involving cerebral and nervous system functions that deal with movement, learning, hearing, sight, and thinking. This disorder may be congenital or acquired and may be bilateral or unilateral in the form of a nonprogressive paralysis that results from damage to the central nervous system (CNS).

ICD-10-CM Code	G80.9 *(Cerebral palsy, unspecified)* (G80.0-G80.9 = 7 codes of specificity)

Infantile CP is coded by type. Refer to the physician's diagnosis and then to the current editions of the ICD-9-CM and ICD-10-CM coding manuals to ensure the greatest specificity of pathology.

Symptoms and Signs

This syndrome affects primarily motor performance and might be noticed shortly after birth, when the infant has difficulty with sucking or swallowing. The muscles may be floppy (like a rag doll) or stiff, with reduced voluntary movement. When the infant is lifted from behind, the legs may be difficult to separate and the infant may cross his or her legs. There are three major types of CP:

- Spastic CP is characterized by hyperactive reflexes or rapid muscle contractions. The older child manifests the scissor gait by walking on the toes and crossing one foot over the other. Approximately 70% of patients with CP fall into this category.
- Athetoid CP is characterized by involuntary muscle movements, especially during times of stress, and reduced muscle tone. The child has difficulty with speech. About 20% of cases of CP fall into this category.
- Ataxic CP is characterized by lack of control over voluntary movements, poor balance, and a wide gait.

A patient may exhibit signs of all three types in varying degrees from mild to severe. The symptoms tend to be more exaggerated as the child grows; however, they may be static (i.e., they neither get worse nor improve). Some patients have other related complications, including visual and auditory deficits, seizure activity, and intellectual developmental disorder.

Patient Screening

Most times, CP is suspected during routine well-baby or well-child visits. However, when a parent calls the office about previously mentioned symptoms, the child should be scheduled for an evaluation as soon as possible. The condition usually is not a life-threatening one; nevertheless, the parents' anxiety is high, and the condition may appear as an emergency to them.

Etiology

CP usually stems from inadequate blood or oxygen supply to the brain during fetal development, during the birth process, or in early childhood until about age 9 years. The syndrome is more common in premature infants and in male babies. Most insults to the brain result from an interruption in the circulation of blood to the brain during labor and delivery or from infection or head trauma during the first month of life. It often is impossible to determine the exact cause of CP.

Diagnosis

Diagnosis is made from the clinical picture and neurologic examination findings. The child is examined to determine the degree of physical and mental impairment.

Treatment

There is no cure for CP. Early treatment helps the child reach optimal accomplishments. In mild or severe cases, the goal of treatment is to minimize the handicap by providing every possible therapeutic measure to help the child reach his or her potential. This takes a team effort involving the family or the caregiver and various medical specialists. Physical therapy, speech therapy, and special education may be required. Orthopedic intervention with casts, braces, and traction or surgery may be indicated. If the child experiences seizure activity, anticonvulsant agents are prescribed. Muscle relaxants help reduce spastic muscle activity.

Prognosis

The brain damage cannot be reversed; therefore there is no cure for CP. Supportive treatment is important and is intended to provide the child with the best obtainable quality of life.

Prevention

Measures to prevent oxygen deprivation in the developing brain are essential during the prenatal, perinatal, and neonatal periods. Additional steps are important to prevent head injury or brain infection during these periods of cerebral development.

Patient Teaching

Encourage and help parents to contact community support groups. Reinforce the fact that there is no cure for CP and that parents should take advantage of support services available in the community. When possible, assist parents by giving them the names of agencies that provide services to children with CP and their families.

Muscular Dystrophy

Description

Muscular **dystrophy** (MD) is a progressive degeneration and weakening of the skeletal muscles where muscle fibers are abnormally vulnerable to injury. There are several types of the disease, but all are rare. The most common and best-known type is Duchenne MD, which is diagnosed soon after birth or during early childhood, usually before age 5 years.

ICD-10-CM Code	G71.0 *(Muscular dystrophy)*

MD is coded by type. Refer to the physician's diagnosis and then to the current editions of the ICD-9-CM and ICD-10-CM coding manuals to ensure the greatest specificity of pathology.

Symptoms and Signs

MD initially affects the muscles of the shoulders, hips, thighs, and calves of the legs, causing the characteristic waddling gait and toe walking. Affected muscles sometimes look larger than normal because fat replaces atrophied muscle. The child also may have lordosis or other spinal deformities. In addition, the child has difficulty climbing stairs and running, tends to fall easily, and has difficulty getting up. As the disease progresses, it involves all the muscles, causing crippling and immobility (Fig. 2.13). Contractures typically develop, and the child becomes increasingly susceptible to serious pulmonary infections, such as pneumonia. Also children with Duchenne MD often are impaired mentally.

Patient Screening

MD usually is first suspected during routine well-baby or well-child visits. However, when a parent calls the office about previously mentioned symptoms, the child should be scheduled for an evaluation as soon as possible. The condition usually is not a life-threatening one; nevertheless, the parents' anxiety is high, and the condition may appear as an emergency to them.

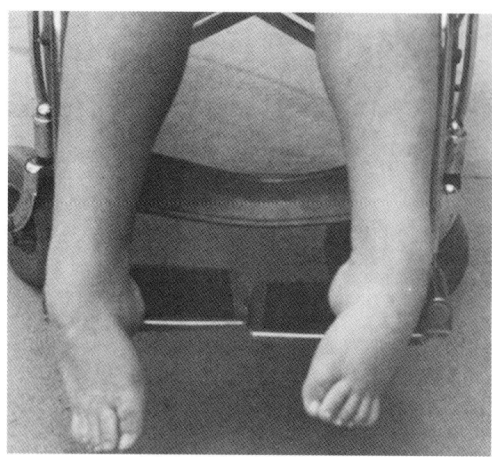

• **Fig. 2.13** Contracture of the feet in a patient with muscular dystrophy (MD). (From Jahss MH: *Disorders of the foot and ankle,* vol 1, ed 2, Philadelphia, 1991, Saunders.)

Etiology

Duchenne MD is the result of a genetic defect. It is caused by the absence of dystrophin, a protein involved in maintaining the integrity of muscle. As is the case for hemophilia and color blindness, the disease affects only males and generally is inherited through female carriers. In one-third to one-half of cases, there is no family history of MD. This means that the disease may be caused by a newly acquired mutation.

Diagnosis

Characteristic symptoms along with family history of MD suggest the diagnosis. Muscle biopsy and **electromyography** (EMG) confirm the diagnosis. Also, an elevated serum creatine kinase (CK) level is evident in the blood. Another diagnostic test is the deoxyribonucleic acid (DNA) blood test, which can indicate the presence of an abnormality of the protein dystrophin.

Treatment

In 2017, the U.S. Food and Drug Administration (FDA) approved the drug deflazacort (Emflaza) for the treatment of Duchenne MD. Experimental drugs based on genetic mutation are also being developed, so genetic research will play a role in future treatment options. Physical therapy, exercise, surgery, and the use of orthopedic appliances in some cases minimize deformities and preserve mobility. Metal rods may be implanted into the spine to assist the patient with staying upright, which assists with breathing. When swallowing becomes difficult, some patients require a feeding tube to prevent asphyxiation. Corticosteroids may be prescribed to slow muscle degeneration. Seizures and some muscle activity may be controlled with anticonvulsants. Delaying some damage to dying muscle cells may occur with use of immunosuppressants, and respiratory infections can be warded off with the use of antibiotics.

Prognosis

There is no cure for Duchenne MD, but the average life span has increased with advances in technology and treatment.

Some patients with Duchenne MD live into adulthood, and historically death usually results from cardiac or respiratory complications within 10 to 15 years of the onset of the disease. Mild cases have been known to progress slowly, allowing the child to attain early adulthood with only a mild disability.

Prevention
MD is genetic and therefore not preventable.

Patient Teaching
With no cure for MD available at present, parents and family members need emotional support. Help them contact support groups and services for patients with MD and for their families. Offer families educational material on the supportive treatment and care of the child with MD. As the child gets older, he or she will need wheelchair access vehicles for physician office visits. The patient may also need other assistive devices and walk-in shower access for rolling a bath wheelchair in for bathing.

Spina bifida

Description
Spina bifida is a group of malformations of the spine in which the posterior portion of the bony canal containing the spinal cord (usually in the lumbar region) is completely or partially absent (Fig. 2.14A). Also called *neural tube defects,* the three different levels of the condition originate during early weeks of gestation as the spinal cord and bony canal develop. During this developmental stage, there is failure of the posterior spinal processes to close, usually in the lumbar region. This failure of complete closure allows the meninges and, in severe cases, the spinal cord to herniate. Depending on the extent of the herniation and the amount of the neural tube that has herniated, various degrees of neural deficits or impairment occur. The three types of spina bifida are spinal bifida occulta, meningocele, and myelomeningocele.

Spina Bifida Occulta
Description. In the defect called *spina bifida occulta,* the posterior arches of the vertebrae, commonly in the lumbosacral area, fail to fuse, but there is no herniation of meninges or spinal cord. Usually there is no spinal cord or spinal nerve involvement.

ICD-10-CM Code	Q76.0 *(Spina bifida occulta)*
	Q05.8 *(Sacral spina bifida without hydrocephalus)*
	(Q05.0-Q05.9 = 10 codes of specificity) (codes for Cervical, Thoracic, Lumbar, and Sacral)

Spina bifida is coded according to involvement of hydrocephalus and region affected. Refer to the physician's diagnosis and then to the current editions of the ICD-9-CM and ICD-10-CM coding manuals to ensure the greatest specificity of pathology.

Symptoms and Signs. When this malformation occurs without displacement of the cord or the meninges, spina bifida occulta is asymptomatic. At other times, the only evidence of the neural tube defect is a dimpling, a tuft of hair, or a hemangioma over the site where the vertebrae have not completely fused.

Patient Screening. Most cases are discovered during the newborn examination. Parents requesting an appointment to discuss the condition should be scheduled as soon as possible. It is important to remember the amount of anxiety the parents may experience.

Etiology. The etiology of this congenital anomaly is unknown, but it has been associated with exposure to ionizing radiation during early uterine life. Reduced levels of vitamin A and folic acid consumed during pregnancy may contribute to the incidence of spina bifida. The condition occurs when the neural tube fails to close in the early stages of fetal development, possibly as a result of a metabolic imbalance leading to lack of these nutrients.

Diagnosis. Maternal blood levels of AFP may be measured to detect possible neural tube defects. Diagnosis is made by using prenatal ultrasonography or with postnatal physical examination, detection of neurologic symptoms, visual inspection of the spine, and spinal ultrasonography. If the infant is asymptomatic, the condition may not be discovered unless medical attention is sought.

Treatment. Spina bifida occulta usually requires no intervention other than prudent observation throughout the child's growth and development. Treatment depends on the degree of neurologic involvement. If the child becomes symptomatic with neurologic problems, surgical intervention to repair the defect is necessary.

Prognosis. The prognosis is good for children with spina bifida occulta.

Prevention. Because the etiology of this condition is unknown, methods of prevention are also unknown. However, avoiding exposure to ionizing radiation during pregnancy is a wise precaution and significant in the prevention of this disorder. Increased intake of folic acid is encouraged in females planning to become pregnant and during the early stages of pregnancy. Because many pregnancies are unplanned, all females of child-bearing age capable of becoming pregnant are encouraged to take the recommended amount of folic acid each day.

Patient Teaching. The value of regular observation during the growth and development period should be emphasized to both the child and the parents. In addition, the parents and the child should be urged to watch for and report any neurologic symptoms.

Meningocele
Description. The second level of failure of the spinal column to fuse during the developmental stage is called *meningocele.* The meninges protrude through an opening in the spinal column, thus forming a sac that becomes filled with cerebrospinal fluid (CSF) (see Fig. 2.14B).

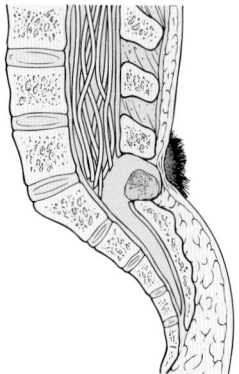

SPINA BIFIDA
Posterior vertebral arches
have not fused; there is no
herniation of the spinal cord
or meninges

A

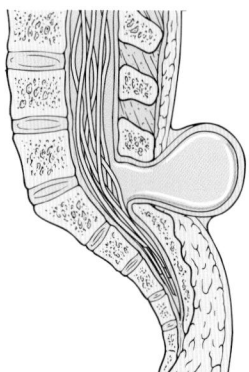

MENINGOCELE
External protruding sac
contains meninges and CSF

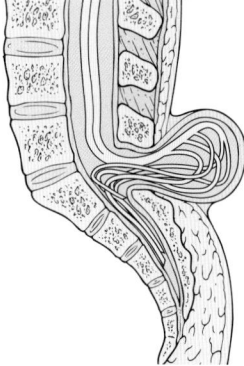

MYELOMENINGOCELE
External sac contains
meninges, CSF, and the
spinal cord

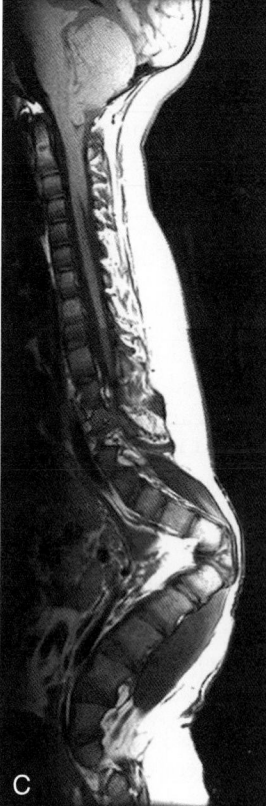

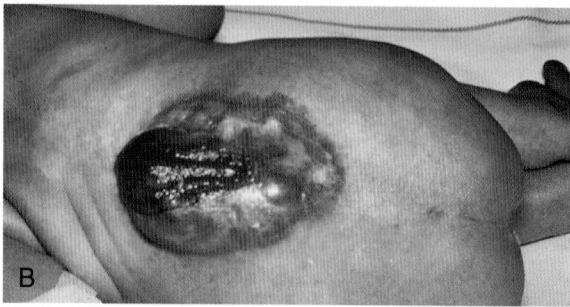

B

C

• **Fig. 2.14** (A) Congenital spinal cord defects. (B) Myelomeningocele. (C) Radiograph of myelomeningocele. *CSF,* Cerebrospinal fluid. (B, From Shiland B: *Mastering healthcare terminology,* ed 6, St Louis, 2019, Mosby. C, From Frank ED, Long BW, Smith BJ: *Merrill's atlas of radiographic positioning and procedures,* ed 12, St Louis, 2012, Mosby.)

ICD-10-CM Code   Q05.8 *(Sacral spina bifida*
without hydrocephalus)
Meningocele is coded according to the region affected.
Refer to the physician's diagnosis and then to the cur-
rent editions of the ICD-9-CM and ICD-10-CM coding
manuals to ensure the greatest specificity of pathology.

Symptoms and Signs. There is no nerve involvement; therefore the infant usually has no neurologic problems. The sac formed over the defect permits the passage of light during transillumination, indicating no spinal cord or neurologic involvement. The skin over the area may be fragile, and rupture of the sac is a potential problem.

Patient Screening. Most cases are discovered during the newborn examination. When parents request an appointment to discuss the condition, it should be scheduled as soon as possible. It is important to remember the anxiety parents may be experiencing. As the child grows and matures, the parents may detect the onset of neurologic symptoms. When this happens, the child requires immediate assessment.

Etiology. As in spina bifida occulta, the posterior portion of the neural tube fails to close. The exact cause is not known. However, genetic and environmental factors may play a role. It is possible that a metabolic abnormality in which there are reduced levels of vitamin A and folic acid may contribute to the incidence of spina bifida.

Diagnosis. Diagnosis is made by visual examination of the spinal area and verification of the presence of a sac. Radiographic studies of the spine confirm the clinical findings. The infant is assessed for hydrocephalus, which often is associated with neural tube defects.

Treatment. Treatment usually consists of surgical intervention to correct the defect in the first 24 to 48 hours of life. Because the spinal cord is not involved, paralysis usually does not occur. These children require prudent follow-up and usually develop normally.

Prognosis. With early surgical intervention, the outlook for these children is good.

Prevention. Because the etiology of this condition is unknown, methods of prevention are also unknown. However, avoiding exposure to ionizing radiation during pregnancy is a wise precaution and significant in the prevention of this disorder. Increased intake of folic acid is encouraged for females planning to become pregnant and during the early stages of pregnancy. Because many pregnancies are unplanned, all females of child-bearing age capable of becoming pregnant are encouraged to take the recommended amount of folic acid each day.

Patient Teaching. The value of regular observation during the growth and development period should be emphasized to both the child and the parents. In addition, the parents and child should be urged to watch for any neurologic symptoms and report them.

Myelomeningocele

Description. Myelomeningocele (also known as *spina bifida cystica*) is a protrusion of a portion of the spinal cord and the meninges through a defect in the spinal column, usually in the lumbar region (see Fig. 2.14A–B).

ICD-10-CM Code   Q05.8 *(Sacral spina bifida without hydrocephalus)*
Myelomeningocele is coded according to the region affected. Refer to the physician's diagnosis and then to the current editions of the ICD-9-CM and ICD-10-CM coding manuals to ensure the greatest specificity of pathology and any appropriate modifiers.

Symptoms and Signs. Myelomeningocele is the most severe form of spina bifida. Because spinal nerves or the spinal cord are present in this herniation, the infant exhibits neurologic symptoms. The infant may have musculoskeletal malformation, immobile joints, or paralysis of the lower extremities. Depending on the level of the anomaly, bowel or bladder control may be affected.

Patient Screening. This condition is apparent during the newborn examination. Parents requesting an appointment to discuss the condition should be scheduled as soon as possible. It is important to remember the amount of anxiety the parents may be experiencing. As the child grows and matures, the parents may detect the onset of increased neurologic symptoms. When this happens, the child requires immediate assessment.

Etiology. As in spina bifida occulta and meningocele, the neural tube fails to close during fetal development. This allows the meninges, spinal nerves, and spinal cord to herniate through the opening of the posterior aspect of the spinal column. The etiology may include genetic factors; spinal cord defects are more common when prior offspring of the mother have had a similar defect.

According to the Agent Orange Benefits Act, Public Law 104-204, which became law in 1996, the federal government and the U.S. Department of Veterans Affairs recognized the possibility that exposure of a parent before conception to Agent Orange could result in the child being born with a form of spina bifida.

Diagnosis. Diagnosis is made on the basis of physical examination and imaging findings. EMG is used to determine the extent of neurologic involvement. Surgical exploration verifies the severity of the disorder (see Fig. 2.14C).

Treatment. Treatment is surgical intervention, usually within the first 24 hours of life, to prevent further deterioration of the involved nerves, infection, and rupture of the herniation. As the child grows, additional procedures may be required to correct evolving problems. Children with myelomeningocele may have other anomalies, including hydrocephalus. Many of these children have no bowel or bladder control and may never be able to walk. A large number of these children die before age 2 years.

Prognosis. Nerve damage is irreversible. Surgical intervention in early life may halt the progression of any paralysis. Physical therapy, including leg braces, crutches, and ambulation training, helps increase the child's mobility. Bladder and bowel problems will not improve, and the child and family must be educated to provide care.

Prevention. As with other spina bifida conditions, the etiology of this condition is unknown, as are methods of prevention. However, avoiding exposure to ionizing radiation during pregnancy is a wise precaution and significant in the possible prevention of this disorder. Increased intake of folic acid is encouraged for females planning to become pregnant and during the early stages of pregnancy. Because many pregnancies are unplanned, all females of child-bearing age capable of becoming pregnant are encouraged to take the recommended amount of folic acid each day.

Patient Teaching. Parents are told that nerve damage is irreversible. Parents should be given information about spina bifida, along with help in locating and contacting support groups.

The value of regular observation during the growth and development period should be emphasized to both the child and the parents. In addition, the parents and child should be urged to watch for and report any neurologic symptoms.

Hydrocephalus

Description

In hydrocephalus, the amount of CSF is increased greatly or its circulation is blocked, resulting in an abnormal enlargement of the head and characteristic pressure changes in the brain. Hydrocephalus affects both pediatric and adult patients.

ICD-10-CM Code   Q05.4 *(Unspecified spina bifida with hydrocephalus)*
Q07.01 *(Arnold-Chiari syndrome with spina bifida)*
Q07.02 *(Arnold-Chiari syndrome with hydrocephalus)*
Q07.03 *(Arnold-Chiari syndrome with spina bifida and hydrocephalus)*
G91.0 *(Communicating hydrocephalus)*
(G91.0-G91.9 = 7 codes of specificity)
G91.1 *(Obstructive hydrocephalus)*

Symptoms and Signs

The fontanels begin to bulge, the sutures of the skull separate, and scalp veins become distended. Head circumference increases at a faster rate than expected for normal growth. The infant has a high-pitched cry, is irritable, and may have episodes of projectile vomiting. Eventually there is downward displacement of the eyes. Neurologic signs include abnormal muscle tone of the legs.

Patient Screening

Many cases of hydrocephalus are apparent during the newborn examination, and others may be detected during well-baby examinations. The head circumference should be measured and plotted on a growth chart at each office visit. Parents requesting an appointment to discuss the condition will have great anxiety, so the appointment should be scheduled as soon as possible. When a parent contacts the office with concern about the child's head appearing to be unusually large, the child requires prompt assessment. The same policy should apply to parents contacting the office with concerns about possible neurologic signs. When a parent or a patient with a shunt in place calls about possible problems with the shunt, an immediate appointment is required, or the patient should be sent to the nearest emergency facility for evaluation.

Etiology

In hydrocephalus, a large amount of CSF accumulates in the skull, causing increased intracranial pressure. An impairment of the circulation of the CSF in the ventricular circulation (obstructive hydrocephalus) may be caused by a lesion within the system or by a congenital structural defect. Impairment of the flow of CSF in the subarachnoid space (communicating hydrocephalus) prevents CSF from reaching the areas where it normally would be reabsorbed by the arachnoid villi. This may be the result of intracranial hemorrhage resulting from head trauma, a blood clot, prematurity, or infection (meningitis) (Figs. 2.15 and 2.16).

Diagnosis

Diagnosis is made on the basis of the clinical picture, physical examination, and radiographic skull studies. CT and MRI scans demonstrate the condition.

Treatment

Treatment consists of surgical intervention to place a shunt in the ventricular or subarachnoid spaces to drain off excessive CSF. Some catheters empty into the peritoneal cavity,

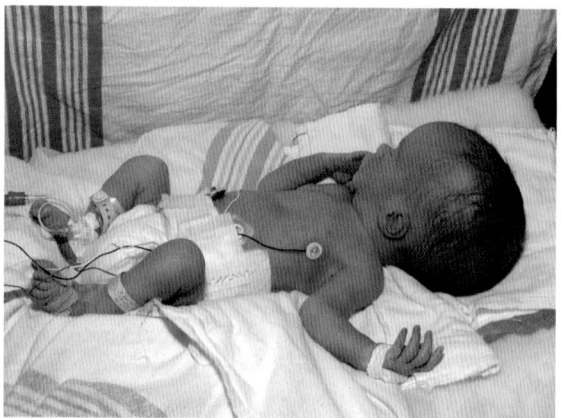

• **Fig. 2.15** Hydrocephalus. (From Kliegman R, Stanton BF, St. Geme JW, et al: *Nelson textbook of pediatrics,* ed 19, St Louis, 2011, Saunders/Elsevier.)

and other shunt catheters empty into the right atrium of the heart (Fig. 2.17). One-way valves help shunt the excessive CSF away from the cerebrospinal canal and to maintain a normal pressure. If left untreated, the increasing intracranial pressure of hydrocephalus causes intellectual developmental disorder and eventually death (see Fig. 2.15).

Prognosis

The prognosis for these children varies, depending on the extent of the condition and the success of corrective interventions. Most children can function normally in society. Parents and the child must watch for the onset of neurologic symptoms and seek medical assessment and treatment.

Prevention

There is no known prevention for the congenital form of this disorder. Good prenatal care, along with prudent observation and assistance during labor and delivery, helps prevent damage to the brain. Preventing infections and injury to the head during childhood, although challenging, may prevent some incidences.

Patient Teaching

Parents and the child should be taught to recognize signs of malfunctioning shunts. In addition, they should be told the importance of promptly reporting any neurologic signs or symptoms to the physician.

Anencephaly

Description

This most severe form of neural tube defect occurs early in gestation with failure of the cephalic aspect of the neural tube to close.

ICD-10-CM Code	Q00.0 *(Anencephaly)*

Symptoms and Signs

The anencephalic fetus or neonate has no cranial vault and little cerebral tissue. Bones of the base of the skull and the orbits are present (Fig. 2.18). The microcephalic fetus or neonate has very small amounts of cerebral tissue and may survive a few hours or days. Although most of these infants die before birth or during the birth process, a few survive for a short time.

Patient Screening

This anomaly may be found during prenatal ultrasonography. The mother or both parents should be scheduled for an office visit, at which the physician should discuss the ultrasonographic findings. When the anomaly is not apparent until birth, the infant usually is stillborn or dies shortly after birth. This event produces great anxiety, and parents may request an appointment for additional information. An appointment should be scheduled promptly.

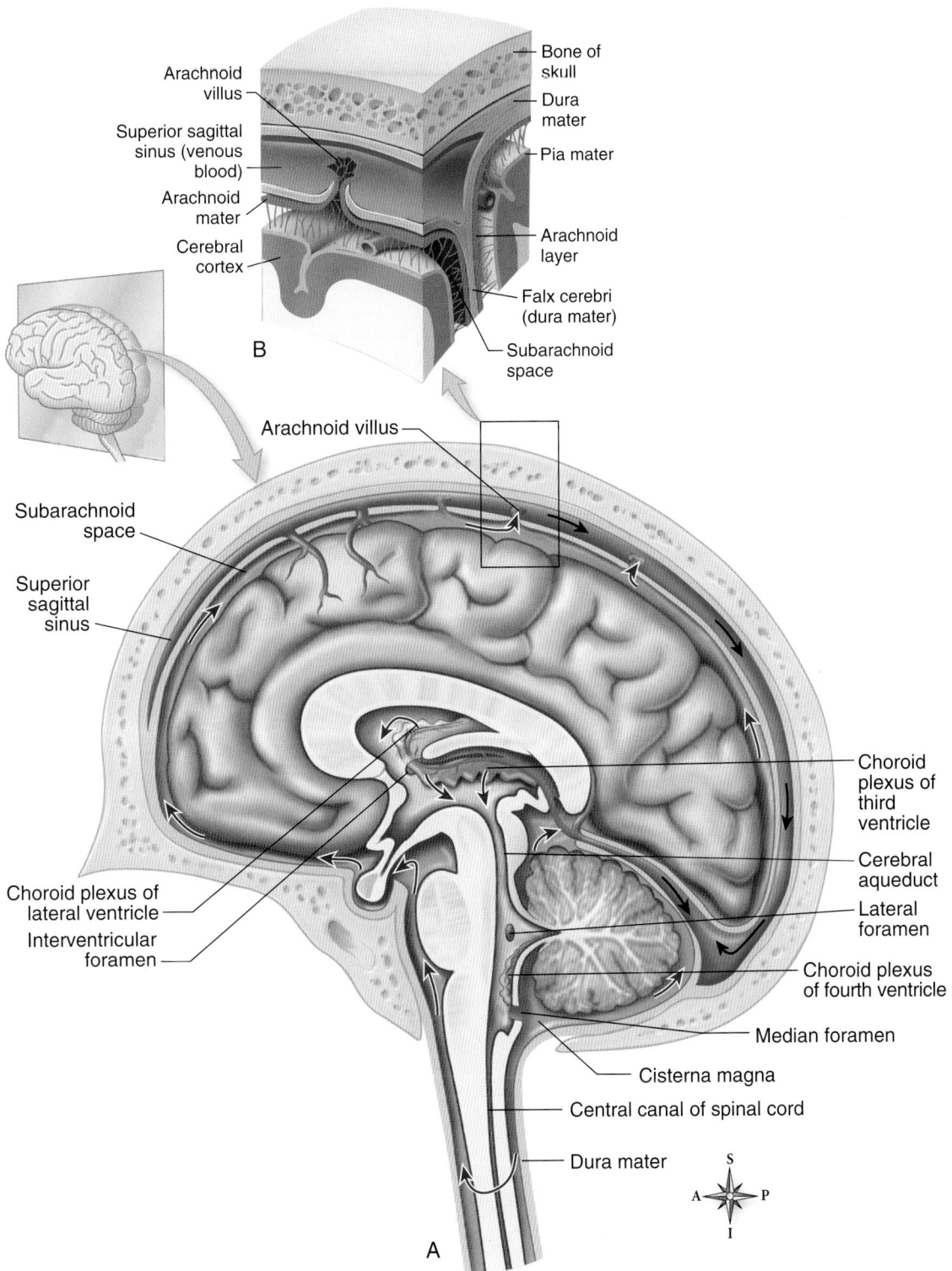

Arachnoid villus

Superior sagittal sinus (venous blood)

Arachnoid mater

Cerebral cortex

Bone of skull

Dura mater

Pia mater

Arachnoid layer

Falx cerebri (dura mater)

Subarachnoid space

B

Arachnoid villus

Subarachnoid space

Superior sagittal sinus

Choroid plexus of third ventricle

Cerebral aqueduct

Lateral foramen

Choroid plexus of lateral ventricle

Interventricular foramen

Choroid plexus of fourth ventricle

Median foramen

Cisterna magna

Central canal of spinal cord

Dura mater

A

S
A P
I

• **Fig. 2.16** Flow of cerebrospinal fluid (CSF). (From Patton KT, Thibodeau GA: *Anatomy and physiology,* ed 9, St Louis, 2016, Mosby.)

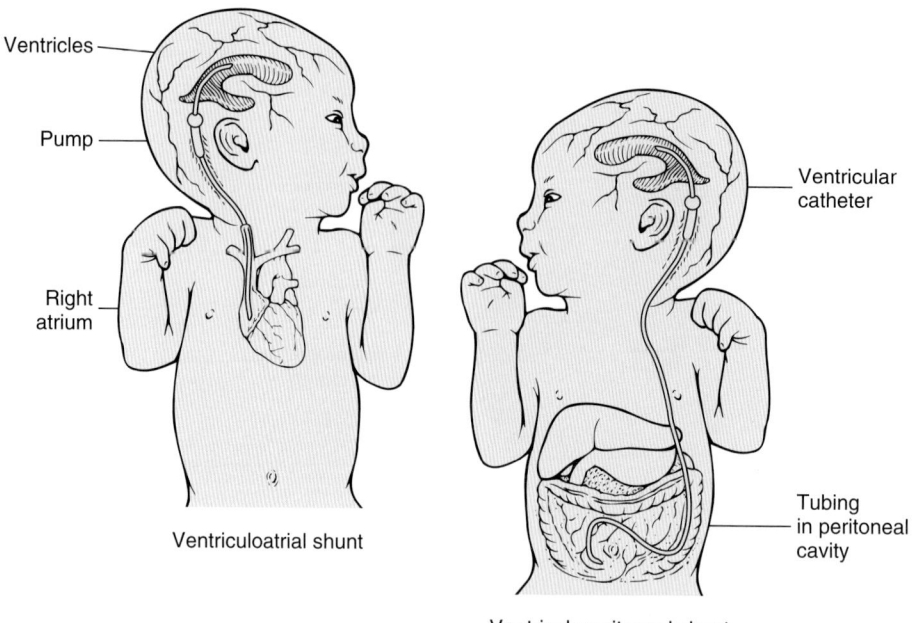

• **Fig. 2.17** Shunting procedures for hydrocephalus. Ventriculoperitoneal shunt is the preferred procedure.

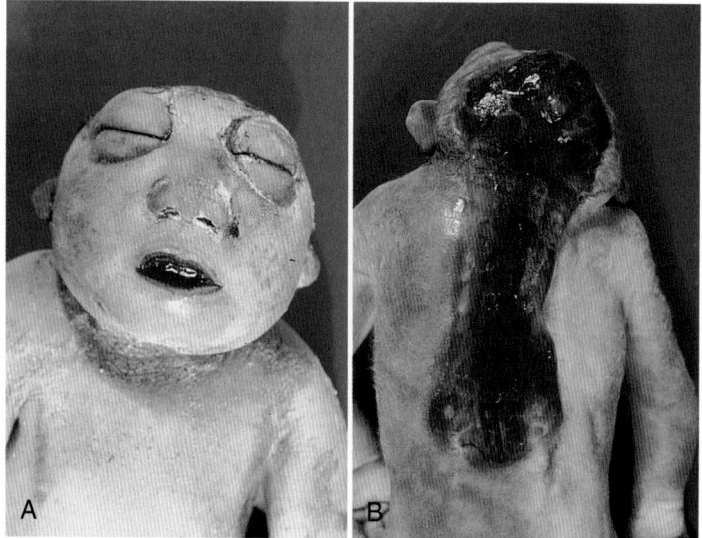

• **Fig. 2.18** Anencephaly. (From Damjanov I: *Pathology for the health professions,* ed 4, St Louis, 2011, Saunders.)

Etiology

The etiology is essentially unknown, but this anomaly is characterized by failure of the neural tube at the cephalic (cranial) end to close completely during the second or third week of gestation. The occurrence of this defect tends to be familial; females are affected more often compared with males. It is possible that the mother's diet and vitamin intake may be involved; therefore women of child-bearing age are encouraged to take folic acid supplements regularly to prevent neural tube deficits in their offspring.

Diagnosis

Diagnosis is made by ultrasonographic examination of the fetal head when blood tests of the mother indicate an

elevated AFP level. The ultrasonogram shows symmetric absence of normal cranial bone structure and brain tissue.

Treatment

There is no effective treatment of this anomaly. Infants who survive the birth process die shortly afterward because many have several other neural tube anomalies incompatible with life.

Prognosis

These fetuses or neonates lack sufficient cerebral tissue to sustain life.

Prevention

As with other neural tube defects, the etiology is unclear. All females of child-bearing age and capability are urged to avoid radiation exposure and take the recommended amount of folic acid daily.

Patient Teaching

Patient teaching includes answering the parents' questions. Encourage and help parents learn about appropriate community resources.

Congenital Cardiac Defects

Fetal Circulation

Oxygen and nutrients are supplied by the mother's blood to the developing fetus. The maternal blood supply also carries away waste products. The exchange takes place in the placental tissue. The umbilical vessels, two arteries and one vein, transport the blood between the placenta and the fetus (Fig. 2.19).

The umbilical vein transports oxygen-rich blood and nutrients to the fetus. The umbilical vein enters the fetal body by passing through the umbilical ring and then goes on to the liver. Fifty percent of this blood passes into the liver, and the other 50% bypasses the liver by way of the ductus venosus. The ductus venosus soon joins the inferior vena cava, allowing the oxygenated placental blood to mix with the deoxygenated blood coming from the lower fetal body. This blood then travels to the right atrium through the vena cava.

Because the fetal lungs are not functioning, this blood mostly bypasses the lungs. Most of the blood entering the right atrium by the inferior vena cava is shunted directly into the left atrium through the foramen ovale. On the left side of the atrial septum, there is a small valve called the *septum primum.* This valve keeps blood from going back into the right atrium. The remaining fetal blood that has entered the right atrium contains a large amount of oxygen-poor blood from the superior vena cava and travels to the right ventricle and into the pulmonary trunk. The pulmonary blood vessels have a high resistance to blood flow because of the collapsed state of the lungs; thus they only allow a small amount of blood to enter the pulmonary circulation. This small amount is enough to nourish the pulmonary tissue.

The blood that has been shunted away from the pulmonary circulation bypasses the lungs through the fetal vessel, the ductus arteriosus. This vessel connects the pulmonary trunk to the descending area of the aortic arch. The ductus arteriosus allows the blood with low oxygen concentration to bypass the lungs and also prevents it from entering the arteries leading to the brain.

The blood that has a high oxygen concentration and has been shunted to the left atrium by way of the foramen ovale mixes with the small amount of blood returning from the pulmonary circulation by way of the pulmonary veins. This blood flows into the left ventricle and then into the aorta. From the aorta, some blood travels to the coronary and the carotid arteries. A portion travels on through the descending aorta to other parts of the fetal tissue. The remaining blood travels into the umbilical arteries and back to the placenta for exchange of gases, nutrients, and waste.

After the birth process, the infant's respiratory effort, and the initial inflation of the lungs, the circulatory system undergoes important changes. The resistance to blood flow through the lungs is reduced by the inflation of the tissue, allowing an increased blood flow from the pulmonary arteries. An increased volume of blood now flows from the right atrium into the right ventricle and the pulmonary arteries. In addition, the volume of blood flowing through the foramen ovale into the left atrium is reduced. The volume of blood returning by way of the pulmonary veins from the

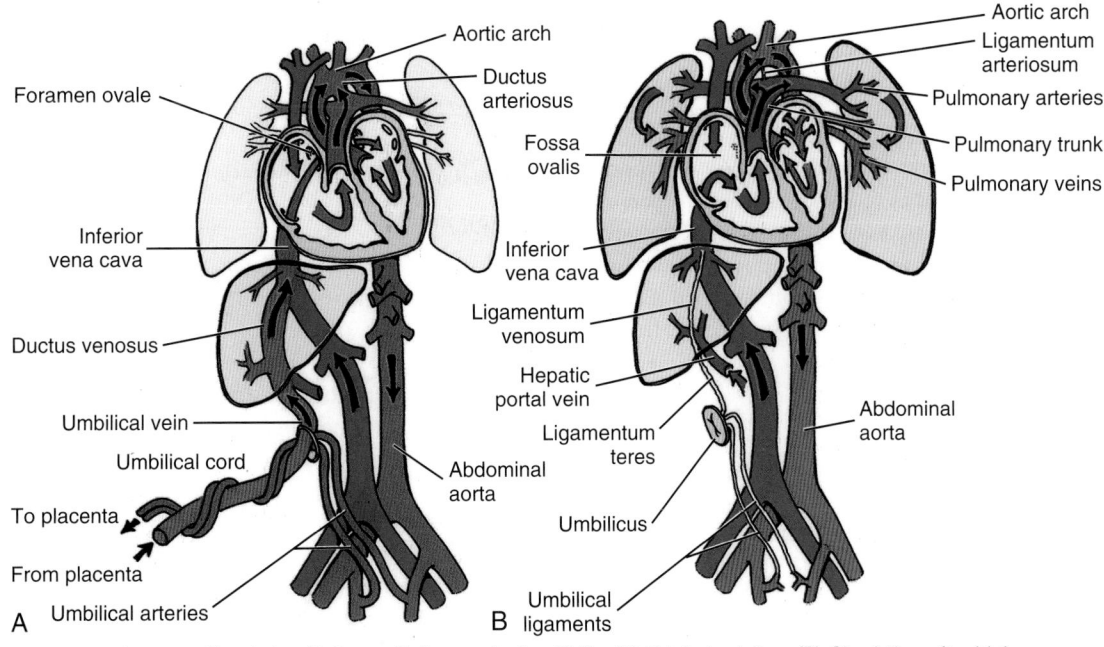

• **Fig. 2.19** Circulation Patterns Before and after Birth. (A) Fetal circulation. (B) Circulation after birth. (From Applegate EJ: *The anatomy and physiology learning system,* ed 4, Philadelphia, 2011, Saunders.)

lungs to the left atrium is increased, causing an increase in the pressure in the left atrium. Blood is forced against the septum primum by decreased right atrial pressure and increased left atrial pressure, and the foramen ovale closes. If this does not occur, the infant has an ASD (discussed subsequently under congenital anomalies). In most cases, however, the heart now is a two-sided pump.

With the lungs expanded and taking over the function of gas exchange, the infant no longer needs the ductus arteriosus to shunt blood from the pulmonary trunk to the descending aorta. Normally the ductus arteriosus closes in the first few days after birth. If it does not close, it is termed *patent*. PDA is a congenital birth defect (discussed subsequently).

Symptoms and Signs

Congenital cardiac defects are developmental anomalies of the heart or the great vessels of the heart. They are present at birth, and the defects cause mild to fatal stress of the cardiac muscle. Signs and symptoms vary, depending on the nature of the anomaly, the severity of the defect, and its effect on the heart and the circulatory system. One defect can be present, or a combination of defects can complicate the case. The common defects generally are categorized as follows: acyanotic, in which deoxygenated and oxygenated blood do not mix, and cyanotic, in which oxygenated and deoxygenated blood mix. The greatest medical concern for infants with acyanotic cardiac defects is congestive heart failure. The greatest concern for infants with cyanotic cardiac defects is hypoxia. Occasionally when the defects are minor, they may not be discovered until adulthood (Fig. 2.20).

Acyanotic Defects

Description

In this condition, oxygenated blood does not mix with deoxygenated blood, and the infant usually maintains a fairly normal pink skin color. Cyanosis is not prevalent.

Patient Screening

Most cases are discovered during the newborn examination. When parents request an appointment to discuss the condition, it should be scheduled as soon as possible. The parents may be experiencing great anxiety. Those cases not detected during the neonatal period of hospitalization may develop symptoms after discharge from the hospital. When parents contact the office to relay concerns and symptoms, the infant requires prompt assessment.

Ventricular Septal Defect

ICD-10-CM Code	Q21.0 *(Ventricular septal defect)* (Q21.0-Q21.9 = 7 codes of specificity)

The most common congenital cardiac disorder, VSD, is an abnormal opening between the right and the left ventricles (Fig. 2.21). When the defect is small, there is little functional disease; when it is large, the results are serious. In this condition, blood is shunted from the left to the right side of the heart as a result of higher pressure in the left ventricle. The characteristic murmur of VSD is described as harsh and holosystolic. The murmur is loudest when the defect is small, because a relatively large amount of blood is passing through a tiny opening. Clinical features include failure to gain weight, restlessness, irritability, sweating when feeding, and increased heart rate and respirations. This condition may go undetected until later in childhood, adolescence, or adulthood.

Patent Ductus Arteriosus

ICD-10-CM Code	Q25.0 *(Patent ductus arteriosus)* (Q25.0-Q25.9 = 10 codes of specificity)

PDA results when the ductus fails to functionally close. During normal fetal circulation, the patent ductus short circuits, shunting the circulation from the lungs, and instead directs blood from the pulmonary trunk to the aorta. If PDA continues after birth, circulation of oxygen is compromised because this abnormal opening is a shunt that allows oxygenated blood to recirculate through the lungs (Fig. 2.22). PDA is detected during a physical examination when a classic "machinery" murmur is heard on auscultation and palpitation reveals a thrill. The infant's growth and development may be slowed, and various signs of heart failure may be present. Closure may be attempted by drug therapy using an antiprostaglandin or ibuprofen. The other option is surgical closure of the ductus.

This condition is fairly common in premature infants and often is accompanied by ASD with failure of the foramen ovale to close.

The prognosis for these infants depends on the presence of other anomalies. Closure by using either drug therapy or surgical intervention establishes a normal postnatal circulation path and gives the infant the opportunity to grow and thrive. Currently no prevention is known.

Coarctation of the Aorta

ICD-10-CM Code	Q25.1 *(Coarctation of aorta)*

This defect is characterized by a narrowed aortic lumen, causing a partial obstruction of the flow of blood through the aorta (Fig. 2.23). The result is increased left ventricular pressure and workload, with decreased blood pressure distal to the narrowing. Signs and symptoms can be evident shortly after birth or may not surface until adolescence. They include signs of left ventricular failure with pulmonary edema. The patient is pale and cyanotic with weakness, dyspnea, and tachycardia. Systemic blood pressure is elevated when measured in the arms but decreased in the lower extremities. This defect is often associated with Turner syndrome.

MAJOR CYANOTIC DEFECTS

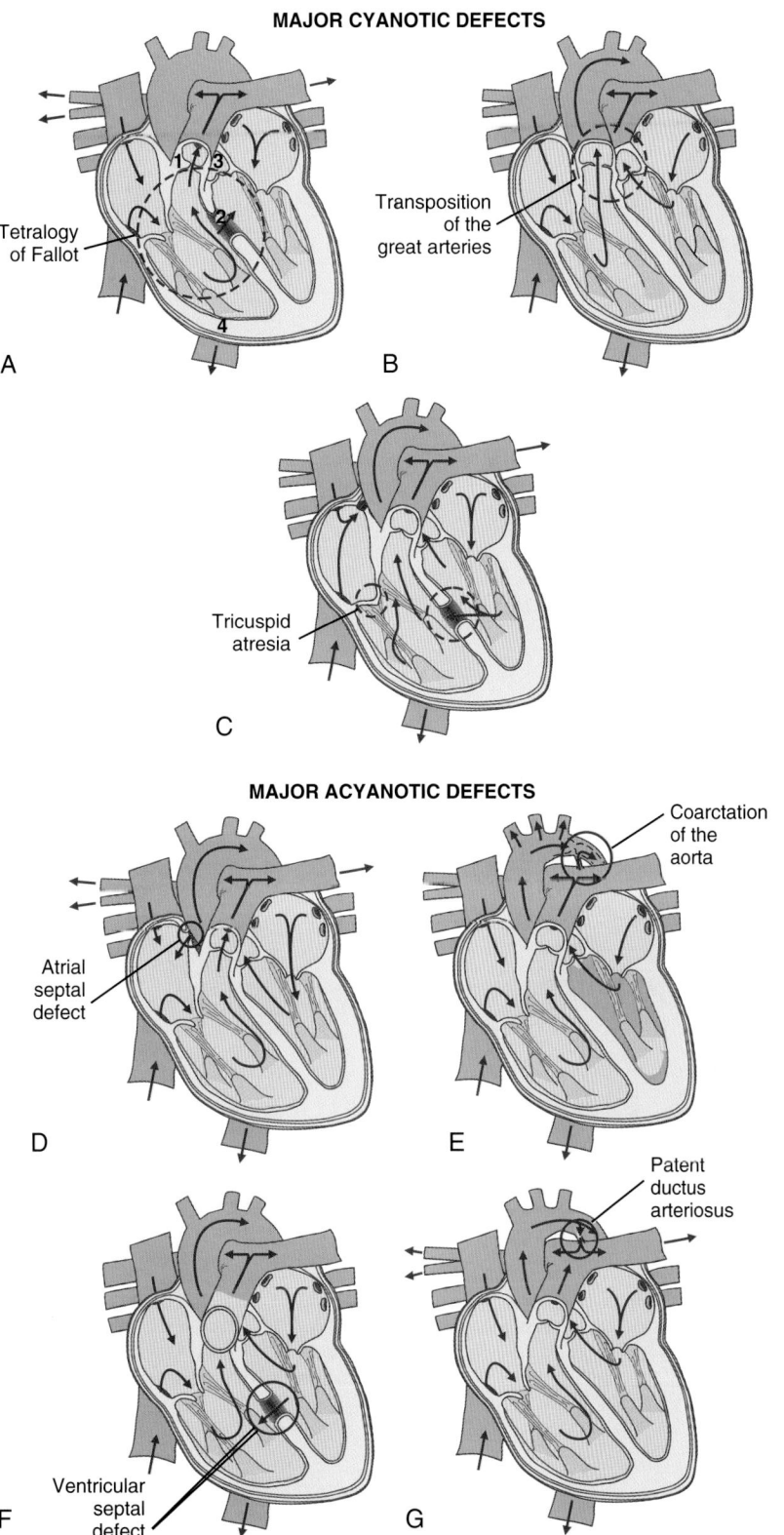

• **Fig. 2.20** Chart comparing acyanotic and cyanotic heart defects in newborn. (From Goodman CC, Fuller KS: *Pathology for the physical therapist assistant,* ed 1, St Louis, 2012, Saunders.)

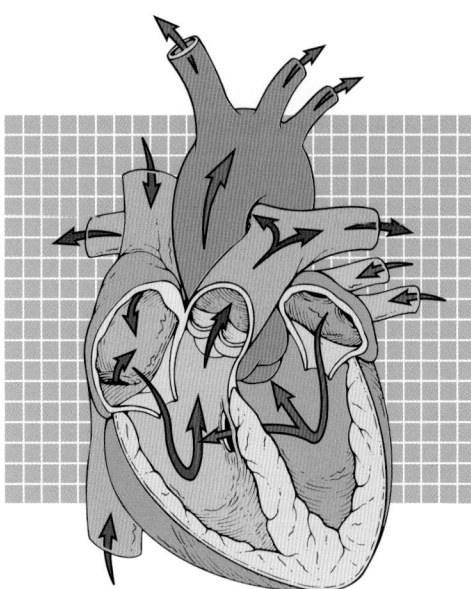

• **Fig. 2.21** Ventricular septal defect (VSD). (Used with permission of Ross Products Division, Abbott Laboratories, from Congenital heart abnormalities [Clinical Education Aid No. 7], 1992.)

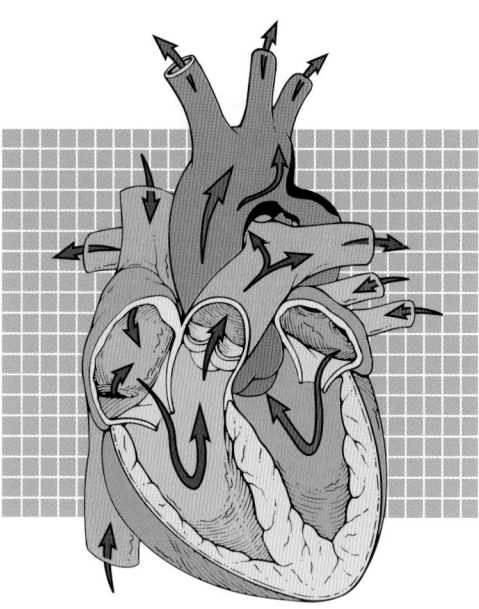

• **Fig. 2.23** Coarctation of the aorta. (Used with permission of Ross Products Division, Abbott Laboratories, from Congenital heart abnormalities [Clinical Education Aid No. 7], 1992.)

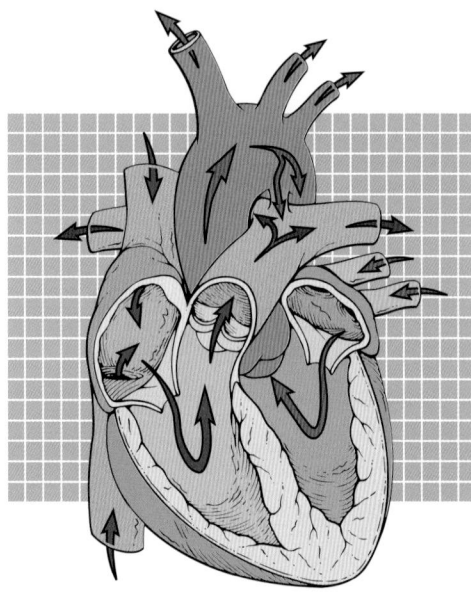

• **Fig. 2.22** Patent ductus arteriosus (PDA). (Used with permission of Ross Products Division, Abbott Laboratories, from Congenital heart abnormalities [Clinical Education Aid No. 7], 1992.)

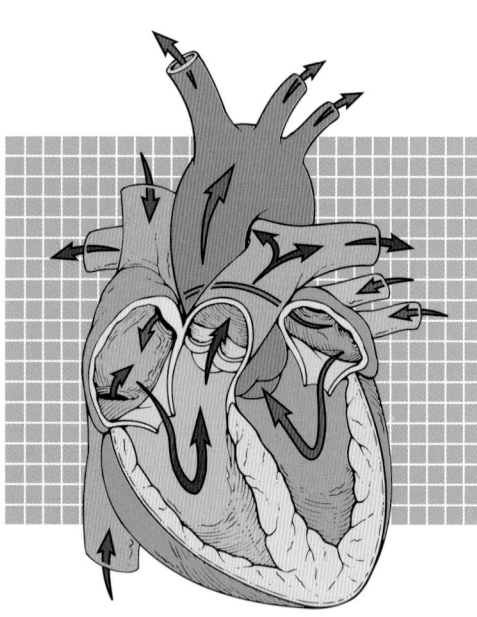

• **Fig. 2.24** Atrial septal defect (ASD). (Used with permission of Ross Products Division, Abbott Laboratories, from Congenital heart abnormalities [Clinical Education Aid No. 7], 1992.)

Atrial Septal Defect

ICD-10-CM Code   Q21.1 *(Atrial septal defect)*

ASD is an abnormal opening between the right and left atria (Fig. 2.24). Although the defect can vary in size and location, blood generally shunts from left to right in all ASDs. Small defects may be undetected or cause symptoms such as fatigue, shortness of breath, and frequent respiratory tract infections. A large defect causes pronounced cyanosis, dyspnea, and syncope. A classic systolic cardiac murmur can be heard with a stethoscope. This condition often is associated with prematurity and PDA, and closure is achieved with surgical repair.

Cyanotic Defects

Description

Central cyanosis is a sign that the atrial blood is not fully oxygenated. The infant appears cyanotic, with a blue tinge to the lips, tongue, and nail beds. The five main cardiac causes of central cyanosis are tetralogy of Fallot, transposition of the great arteries, truncus arteriosus, tricuspid atresia, and total anomalous pulmonary venous return. The two most common defects are discussed here.

Patient Screening

Some defects can be detected on prenatal ultrasonography. Most cases are discovered during the newborn examination. Appointments for parents seeking to discuss the condition should be scheduled as soon as possible. One must consider the great anxiety in the parents. Those cases not detected during the neonatal period of hospitalization may develop symptoms after discharge from the hospital. When parents contact the office to relay concerns and symptoms, the infant requires prompt assessment.

Tetralogy of Fallot

ICD-10-CM Code	Q21.3 *(Tetralogy of Fallot)*

The most common cyanotic cardiac defect is a combination of four congenital heart defects: (1) VSD, an abnormal opening in the ventricular septum; (2) pulmonary **stenosis**, a tightening of the pulmonary valve or vessel; (3) dextroposition (displacement to the right) of the aorta, which overrides (receiving circulation from both ventricles) the VSD; and (4) right ventricular hypertrophy, caused by increased pressure in the ventricle (Fig. 2.25).

Affected infants with severe obstruction are "blue babies" at birth. Deoxygenated blood enters the aorta, causing the symptoms of hypoxia: tachycardia, tachypnea, dyspnea, and seizures. Bone marrow hypoxia causes polycythemia, increased total red blood cell (RBC) mass. Physical examination may reveal delayed physical growth and development along with clubbing of the fingers and toes. Cardiac murmurs can

be heard. Older children assume a squatting position after exercise to relieve breathlessness caused by hypoxia.

Transposition of the Great Arteries

ICD-10-CM Code	Q20.3 *(Discordant ventriculoarterial connection)*

In this defect, the aorta and the pulmonary artery are reversed: the aorta originates from the right ventricle, and the pulmonary artery originates from the left ventricle. The result is two closed-loop circulatory systems: one between the heart and the lungs and the other between the heart and systemic circulation (Fig. 2.26). Within a few hours of birth, neonates with this defect exhibit cyanosis and tachypnea, followed by signs of heart failure.

Immediate surgical intervention is indicated. Prostaglandins are administered to the infant in an effort to keep the ductus arteriosus patent and the foramen ovale from closing. As soon as surgery is possible, the blood flow is redirected by correction of the defect.

The prognosis for these infants is poor unless a pediatric surgical unit is readily available and transportation to it is swift. Another factor in the survival of the infant with this condition is the infant's response to the drug therapy to maintain the fetal circulation and prevent the change to the normal postbirth circulatory system.

Methods of preventing this condition are unknown.

Etiology. The cause of congenital cardiac defects remains unknown. They may result from several factors, including chromosomal abnormalities and environmental conditions, such as maternal infections and the mother's use of certain drugs during gestation. Several congenital disorders result

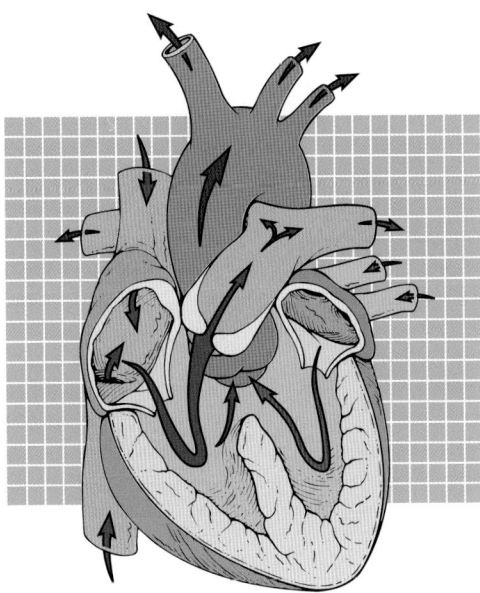

• **Fig. 2.25** Tetralogy of Fallot. (Used with permission of Ross Products Division, Abbott Laboratories, from Congenital heart abnormalities [Clinical Education Aid No. 7], 1992.)

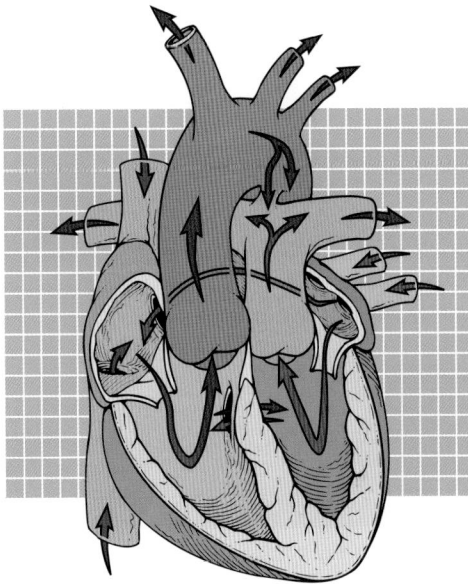

• **Fig. 2.26** Transposition of the great arteries. (Used with permission of Ross Products Division, Abbott Laboratories, from Congenital heart abnormalities [Clinical Education Aid No. 7], 1992.)

from the failure of the circulatory system to shift from the fetal route of blood flow at the time of birth.

Diagnosis. Physical examination and patient history are essential. The physician palpates the neck vessels and auscultates for blood pressure and murmurs. Diagnostic procedures depend on the initial findings and may include chest radiography, blood tests, cardiac catheterization, echocardiography, and electrocardiography. Many defects can be detected on a prenatal ultrasonography. The diagnostic investigation determines the presence and severity of any structural or functional abnormality or defect.

Treatment. The medical management of congenital cardiac defects is determined by the type of defect, the degree of symptoms and signs, and the presence of life-threatening complications. Advances in surgical techniques enable surgeons to close septal defects, to reconstruct or replace a valve, and to repair or join blood vessels. These procedures make it possible to save, improve, and extend the lives of individuals born with congenital cardiac defects. Medications are available to strengthen and regulate the heartbeat. Supportive measures include prophylactic antibiotic administration before dental procedures in some cases to ward off infection.

Prognosis. Prognosis varies and depends on the severity, the number of defects, and the gestational age of the infant or the child. Most defects can be surgically repaired.

Prevention. There is no known prevention for these defects. Good prenatal care accompanied by good nutrition is always wise during any pregnancy.

Patient Teaching. Parents and caregivers need understanding, encouragement, and teaching to cope with changes in individual and family lifestyle imposed by these conditions. Help and encourage parents to find and contact support groups in the community. It is recommended that individuals who have had surgical repair of cardiac defects maintain regular follow-up care with a cardiologist.

Musculoskeletal Conditions

Clubfoot (Talipes Equinovarus)

Description

Clubfoot is an obvious, nontraumatic deformity of the foot of the newborn in which the anterior half of the foot is adducted and inverted.

ICD-10-CM Code	Q66.0 *(Congenital talipes equinovarus)*

Symptoms and Signs

Besides the previously mentioned description, the heel is drawn up, with the lateral side of the foot being convex and the medial aspect being concave (Fig. 2.27A). A true clubfoot cannot be manipulated to the proper position, whereas distortions that are caused by intrauterine position usually can be.

Patient Screening

Most cases are discovered during the newborn examination. Appointments for parents seeking to discuss the condition should be scheduled as soon as possible. Remember the great anxiety the parents may be feeling. As treatment progresses, routine examinations are scheduled.

Etiology

Some sources suggest that fetal position is the cause, and other studies implicate genetic factors because of an abnormal development of the germ plasma during the embryonic stage.

Diagnosis

The deformity is obvious at birth, with a resistance of the foot to return to a neutral position during manipulation. In addition, the Achilles tendon is shortened.

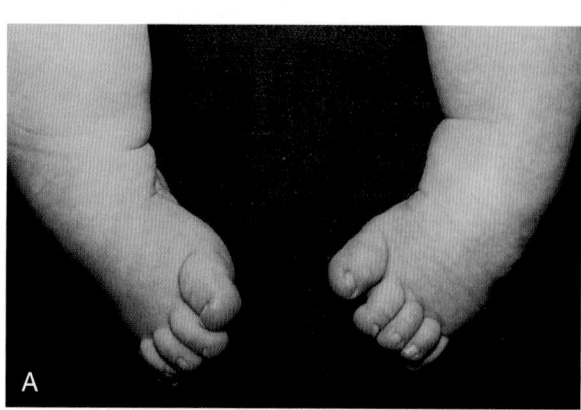
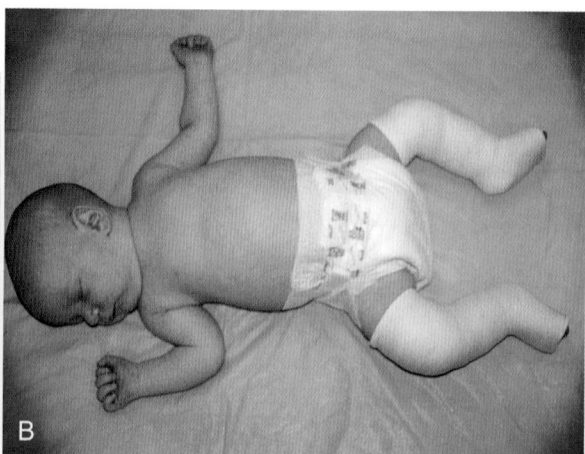

• **Fig. 2.27** (A–E) Congenital musculoskeletal diseases. (A, From Zitelli BJ, McIntire SC, Davis HW: *Zitelli and Davis' atlas of pediatric physical diagnosis,* ed 6, St. Louis, 2012, Saunders. B, From Perry S, Hockenberry M, Lowdermilk D, et al: *Maternal-child nursing care,* ed 3, St Louis, 2007, Mosby. C and E, From Behrman RE, Kliegman RM, Arvin AM: *Slide set for Nelson textbook of pediatrics,* ed 15, Philadelphia, 1996, Saunders. D, Courtesy Texas Scottish Rite Hospital for Children, Dallas, TX.)

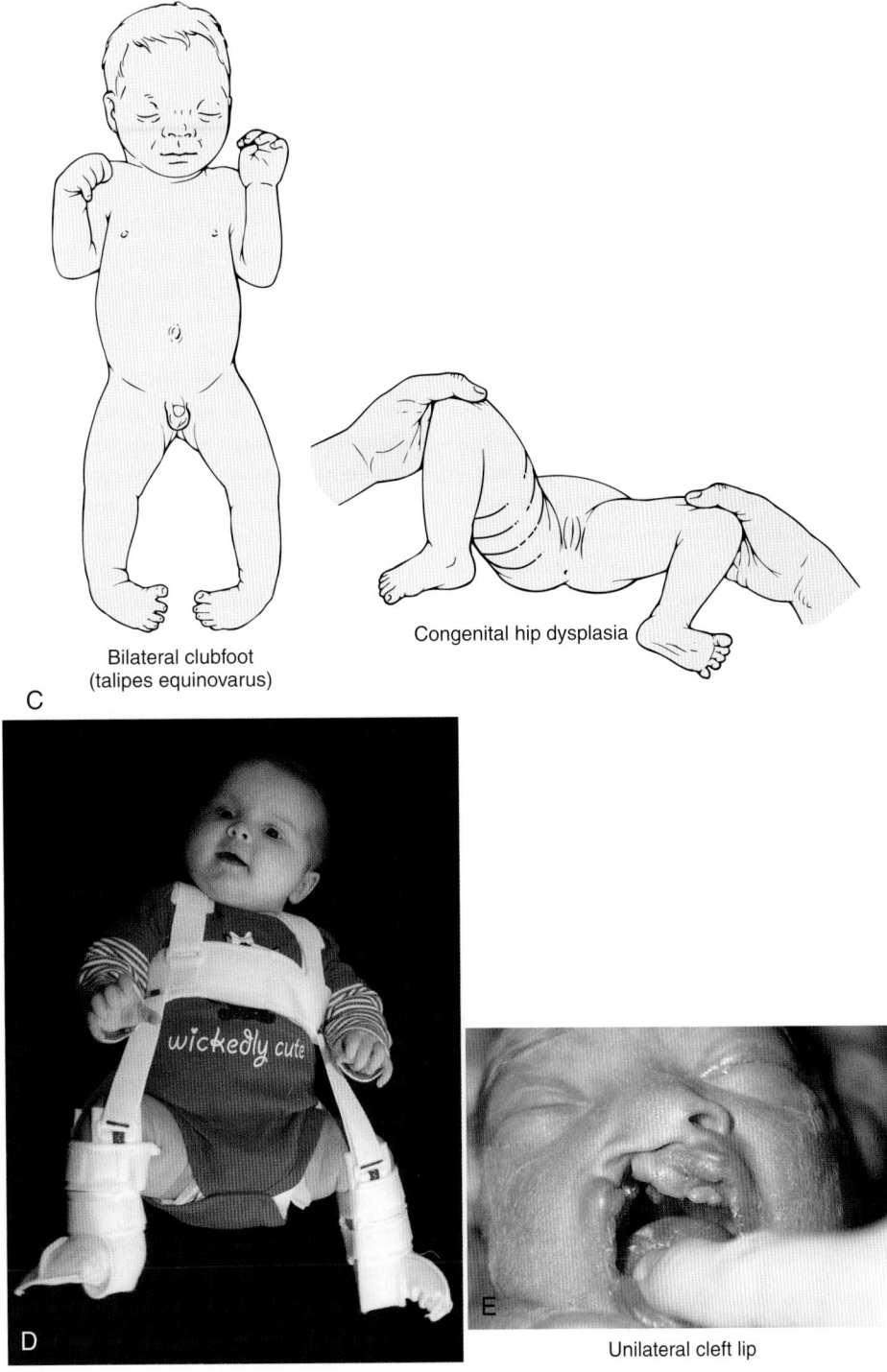

Bilateral clubfoot
(talipes equinovarus)

Congenital hip dysplasia

C

D

wickedly cute

E

Unilateral cleft lip

• **Fig. 2.27, con'd**

Treatment

Treatment consists of either cast application or the use of splints. Treatment must start early in the neonatal period. Casts are reapplied at frequent intervals as the correction increases and the infant grows (see Fig. 2.27B). Splints include a bar affixed to shoes; the infant is placed in the shoes, which hold the feet and legs in position. Many physicians employ a combination of manipulative methods, with cast application

followed by the use of splints as the child matures. The child must be observed throughout childhood for reversal of the improvement. If casting and splinting are unsuccessful, surgery may be indicated to correct the condition.

Prognosis

Prognosis is good for these children when casting is performed or splints can be used early in life. When these modes of treatment do not completely resolve the condition, surgical intervention usually corrects the deformity.

Prevention
No prevention of this deformity is known.

Patient Teaching
Parents will be extremely anxious and need information about this condition. Instruction on cast care and skin care is important. The importance of observing continuously for any reversal of correction is stressed.

Developmental Dysplasia of the Hip
Description
Developmental dysplasia of the hip (DDH), previously known as *congenital hip dysplasia* (CHD), is an abnormal development of the hip joint, ranging from an unstable joint to dislocation of the femoral head from the acetabulum.

ICD-10-CM Code	Q65.8 *(Other congenital deformities of hip)*
	(Q65.0-Q65.9 = 15 codes of specificity)
	Q65.2 *(Congenital dislocation of hip, unspecified)*

Refer to the physician's diagnosis and then to the current edition ICD-10-CM coding manual to ensure the greatest specificity of pathology.

Symptoms and Signs
Physical examination reveals asymmetric folds of the thigh of the newborn, with limited abduction of the affected hip. A shortening of the femur is noted when the knees and hips are flexed at right angles (see Figs. 2.27C and D).

Patient Screening
This dysplasia is apparent during the newborn examination. When parents request an appointment to discuss the condition, it should be scheduled as soon as possible. Remember the great anxiety the parents may be feeling. As treatment progresses, routine examinations are scheduled.

Etiology
The exact cause is unknown. Typical DDH occurs shortly before, during, or shortly after birth, possibly as a result of softening of the ligaments caused by the maternal hormone relaxin. DDH may result from a breech presentation and is more common in female infants.

Diagnosis
Abnormal signs, including positive Ortolani and Barlow maneuvers, may be detected at birth. Diagnosis is made during the physical examination and is confirmed with ultrasonography of the hip.

Treatment
Treatment includes the use of various devices to reduce the hip dislocation. After the femoral head is returned to its proper position in the acetabulum, the legs are held in place by a Pavlik harness, a splint, or a cast, allowing stable maintenance of the hip in a position of flexion and abduction. Early treatment offers the best results and may help avoid surgical intervention.

Prognosis
The prognosis for this deformity is good when therapy is instituted early in the neonatal period. If this therapy is unsuccessful, surgical intervention may be required.

Prevention
No prevention for this condition is known.

Patient Teaching
Parents should be taught to care for the skin and the correctional device. In addition, the need for compliance with the treatment should be stressed. After the condition appears to have been corrected, parents should be told of the importance of follow-up assessments of the child.

Cleft Lip and Palate
Description
Cleft lip (harelip) is a congenital birth defect consisting of one or more clefts in the upper lip (see Fig. 2.27E). Cleft palate is a birth defect in which there is a hole in the middle of the roof of the mouth (palate).

ICD-10-CM Code	Q37.9 *(Unspecified cleft palate with unilateral cleft lip)*
	(Q37.0-Q37.9 = 8 codes of specificity)

Cleft palate and lip are coded by type. Refer to the physician's diagnosis and then to the current editions of the ICD-9-CM and ICD-10-CM coding manuals to ensure the greatest specificity of pathology and any appropriate modifiers.

Symptoms and Signs
The cleft may extend completely through the hard and soft palates into the nasal area. The defects appear singularly or may be linked and vary in severity. Some infants have difficulty with nasal regurgitation and feeding because of air leaks around the cleft. A major problem is the infant's appearance.

Patient Screening
These birth defects are apparent during newborn examination. Parents may want an appointment to discuss the condition and treatment with the physician. Because of the great anxiety that the parents may be feeling, a prompt appointment should be scheduled. As the repair and correction of conditions progress, the parents may contact the office about problems the child is having, especially with feeding. Prompt response to their requests is required.

Etiology

The cause is a failure in the embryonic development of the fetus. It is considered a multifactorial genetic disorder and occurs in about 1 in 10,000 births (see the Genetic Disorders and Syndrome section).

Diagnosis

Cleft abnormalities are obvious during clinical examination at birth.

Treatment

Cleft deformities usually are repaired surgically as soon as possible. Extensive deformities require a second repair. Special feeding devices can be tried. The child often requires speech therapy.

Prognosis

Prognosis for this disorder is good with surgical repair. Advances in plastic surgery have made the repair look as natural as possible.

Prevention

No prevention of this disorder is known.

Patient Teaching

Parents need instruction on care of the surgical repair and feeding of the infant. Help and encourage them to find and contact support groups in the community. There are devices that are specifically made to enable the infant to nurse and keep food and liquid from entering an open palate. Encourage parents to seek out organizations with medical care specializing in care, treatment and financial assistance in infants and children with cranial–facial defects, primarily cleft deformations.

Genitourinary Conditions

Cryptorchidism (Undescended Testes)

Description

Cryptorchidism is failure of one or both of the testicles to descend from the abdominal cavity into the scrotum.

ICD-10-CM Code	Q53.9 *(Undescended testicle, unspecified)*
	(Q53.0-Q53.9 = 10 codes of specificity)

Symptoms and Signs

Cryptorchidism, or failure of the testicles to descend from the abdominal cavity into the scrotum, is detected at birth or shortly thereafter (Fig. 2.28). The condition may be unilateral or bilateral. During infancy and early childhood, there are no symptoms besides the absence of the testes. The condition is more common in premature infants.

Patient Screening

This condition is palpable and observed during the newborn examination. Parents may request an appointment to discuss the condition and possible treatment. The anxiety of the parents calls for an appointment at the earliest convenience of the parents and the physician.

Etiology

The cause of failure of the testes to descend during the final fetal development is not clearly understood. Some experts suspect that hormones play a role.

Diagnosis

Diagnosis is by visual inspection and by palpation, starting above the inguinal ring and pushing downward on the inguinal canal toward the scrotum. The examination reveals no evidence of one or both testes in the scrotal sac. When the condition is bilateral, the scrotum appears underdeveloped.

Treatment

The testes often descend spontaneously during the first year of life. If this does not happen by age 4 years, the treatment is to place the undescended testes into the scrotum by either surgical manipulation (orchiopexy) or hormonal drug therapy (beta-human chorionic gonadotropin [β-hCG] or testosterone). Treatment is important because

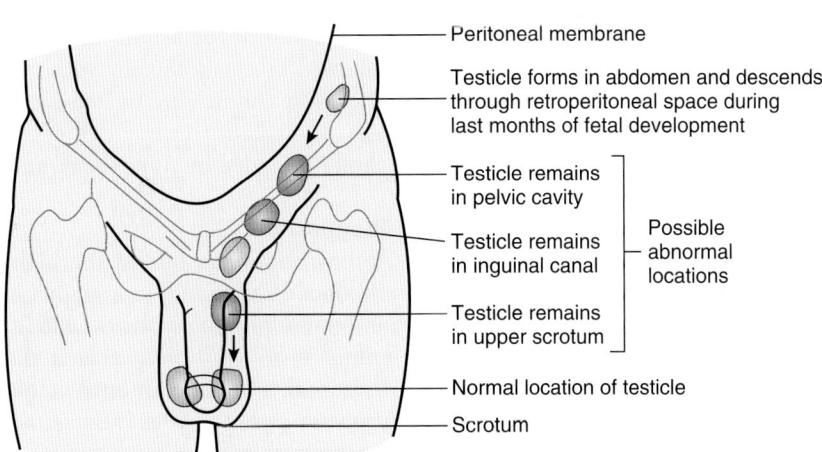

• **Fig. 2.28** Cryptorchidism and possible positions of the undescended testis. (From Gould BE: *Pathophysiology for the health professions*, ed 4, St Louis, 2011, Saunders.)

untreated cryptorchidism may lead to sterility in the adult male. There is an increased risk of testicular cancer in untreated cryptorchidism.

Prognosis

Prognosis is good when surgical intervention can move the testicles down into the scrotum and secure them. This procedure is necessary in early childhood to prevent sterility and possible cancer later in life.

Prevention

There is no accepted method of prevention.

Patient Teaching

Parents need to be told about the dangers of not utilizing the suggested surgical intervention. After the procedure, they need instructions in caring for the incisions.

Wilms Tumor

Description

Wilms tumor, or nephroblastoma, is a highly malignant neoplasm of the kidney that affects children younger than 10 years of age. It is the most common kidney tumor of childhood and the fourth most common childhood cancer.

ICD-10-CM Code	C64.9 *(Malignant neoplasm of unspecified kidney, except renal pelvis)* (C64.1-C64.9 = 3 codes of specificity)

Symptoms and Signs

The most common presentation is a mass in the kidney region, which is often discovered by a parent or an examining physician. The mass is firm, nontender, and usually confined to one side of the body. The patient may experience other symptoms resulting from compression caused by the tumor mass, metabolic alterations resulting from the tumor, or metastasis. These include hematuria, pain in the abdomen or chest, hypertension, anemia, vomiting, intestinal obstruction, constipation, weight loss, and fever.

Patient Screening

A child who is experiencing hematuria, pain, and vomiting and has a noticeable mass in the kidney region requires prompt assessment.

Etiology

Wilms tumor is an adenosarcoma arising from abnormal fetal kidney tissue that is left behind during early embryonic life (Fig. 2.29). Unrestrained cancerous growth of tissue begins after the child is born. About 20% of cases of Wilms tumor are hereditary; however, there is no method to identify gene carriers. Wilms tumor is associated with several congenital anomalies, such as aniridia (absence of the iris) and genitourinary anomalies (e.g., cryptorchidism and ambiguous genitalia), and is a part of some familial

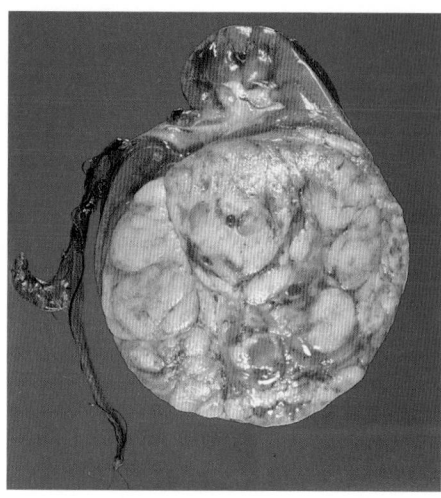

• **Fig. 2.29** Wilms tumor in the lower pole of the kidney with the characteristic tan-to-gray color and well-circumscribed margins. (From Kumar V, Cotran R, Robbins S: *Robbins basic pathology,* ed 8, Philadelphia, 2008, Saunders.)

cancer syndromes. Most tumors are unilateral, but 10% are bilateral or multicentric.

Diagnosis

A child suspected of having Wilms tumor often undergoes a physical examination to palpate the kidney mass, to seek associated congenital anomalies, and to look for signs of malignancy (e.g., increased size of liver and spleen and lymphadenopathy). Blood tests are done to assess for anemia and kidney and liver function. Specific tests that help determine the extent of disease include abdominal ultrasonography, CT, and urinalysis. Surgery is necessary for complete staging of the tumor. Staging is based on the degree the tumor extends beyond the kidney capsule, the presence of metastasis, and whether there is bilateral kidney involvement.

Treatment

Prompt recognition and treatment are imperative because the tumor is locally invasive and tends to metastasize. Surgical removal of the tumor and accessible metastatic sites is followed by chemotherapy with or without radiation therapy. Most children are treated according to research protocols at pediatric cancer centers. The specific treatment choice is guided by tumor stage and histology.

Prognosis

Wilms tumor has one of the highest survival rates of all childhood cancers. The prognosis is largely based on stage and tumor histology. Patients with a low stage and favorable tumor histology have a greater than 90% cure rate. For those with a late stage or unfavorable histology, the cure rate drops to close to 50%. Patients may suffer from renal impairment, hepatotoxicity, cardiotoxicity, or second malignancies as a result of their cancer therapy. Children should be followed up regularly after completion of therapy to assess for recurrence of primary tumor and development of late effects of treatment.

Prevention
No prevention is known.

Patient Teaching
Help and encourage parents to find and contact support groups in the community and resources that provide services to the child and the family.

Phimosis
Description
Phimosis is stenosis, or narrowing, of the opening of the foreskin in the male that leads to inability to retract the foreskin. It is rare for the foreskin to be retractable in the neonatal period. This is normal and, in some cases, can persist into adolescence. Phimosis can be problematic if acquired after the neonatal period.

ICD-10-CM Code	N47.0 *(Adherent prepuce, newborn)*
	N47.1 *(Phimosis)*
	N47.2 *(Paraphimosis)*
	(N47.0-N47.8 = 9 codes of specificity)

Symptoms and Signs
The child may experience difficulty with urination, or the parents may have difficulty with cleaning the area under the prepuce of the glans penis, resulting in accumulation of secretions. These symptoms may develop later in uncircumcised males, even into adulthood.

Etiology
Many male infants are born with phimosis; the cause is unknown.

Diagnosis
Diagnosis is made by visual examination and the inability to slide the prepuce back over the glans penis (Fig. 2.30).

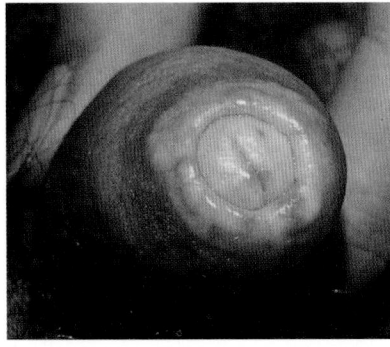

• **Fig. 2.30** Photo showing phimosis. (From Lewis SL, Dirksen SR, Heitkemper MM, Bucher L: *Medical-surgical nursing: Assessment and management of clinical problems,* ed 8, St Louis, 2011, Mosby.)

Treatment
Definitive treatment is circumcision, the surgical removal of the prepuce. This procedure, which used to be routine for male newborns, is usually performed in the first few days of life. An alternative treatment, when parents decide not to have the surgery performed on the male infant, is for the parents to gently wash the glans and prepuce with soap and water and gently slide the prepuce back over the glans. This procedure is done on a regular schedule, and the prepuce is never forced over the glans. Topical steroid cream may also be useful.

Prognosis
The prognosis is good.

Prevention
Newborn circumcision prevents this condition.

Patient Teaching
Parents require instruction in caring for the incised area. When the parents decide to attempt manual manipulation of the prepuce, instruction is provided, with emphasis on never forcing the prepuce over the glans. Parents must also be encouraged to cleanse and dry the area daily.

Diseases of the Digestive System
Congenital Pyloric Stenosis
Description
Pyloric stenosis (Fig. 2.31A), a congenital disorder, is a gastric obstruction associated with narrowing of the pyloric sphincter at the exit of the stomach. This condition may also be called *congenital hypertrophic pyloric stenosis.*

ICD-10-CM Code	Q40.0 *(Congenital hypertrophic pyloric stenosis)*

Symptoms and Signs
The infant has episodes of projectile vomiting after feedings (see Fig. 2.31B) and fails to gain weight. Symptoms usually begin when the infant is 2 to 3 weeks of age. The infant appears hungry, continues to feed, and yet fails to gain weight. If left untreated, the infant becomes dehydrated and experiences electrolyte imbalances. A small olive-shaped hard mass may be palpated in the region of the pyloric sphincter, and left to right peristalsis may be noted, followed by reverse peristalsis. The emesis contains no bile.

Patient Screening
The infant with sudden onset of projectile vomiting requires prompt assessment.

Etiology
There is a slight hereditary tendency, but the exact cause is unknown. It occurs four times more often in male than in female infants.

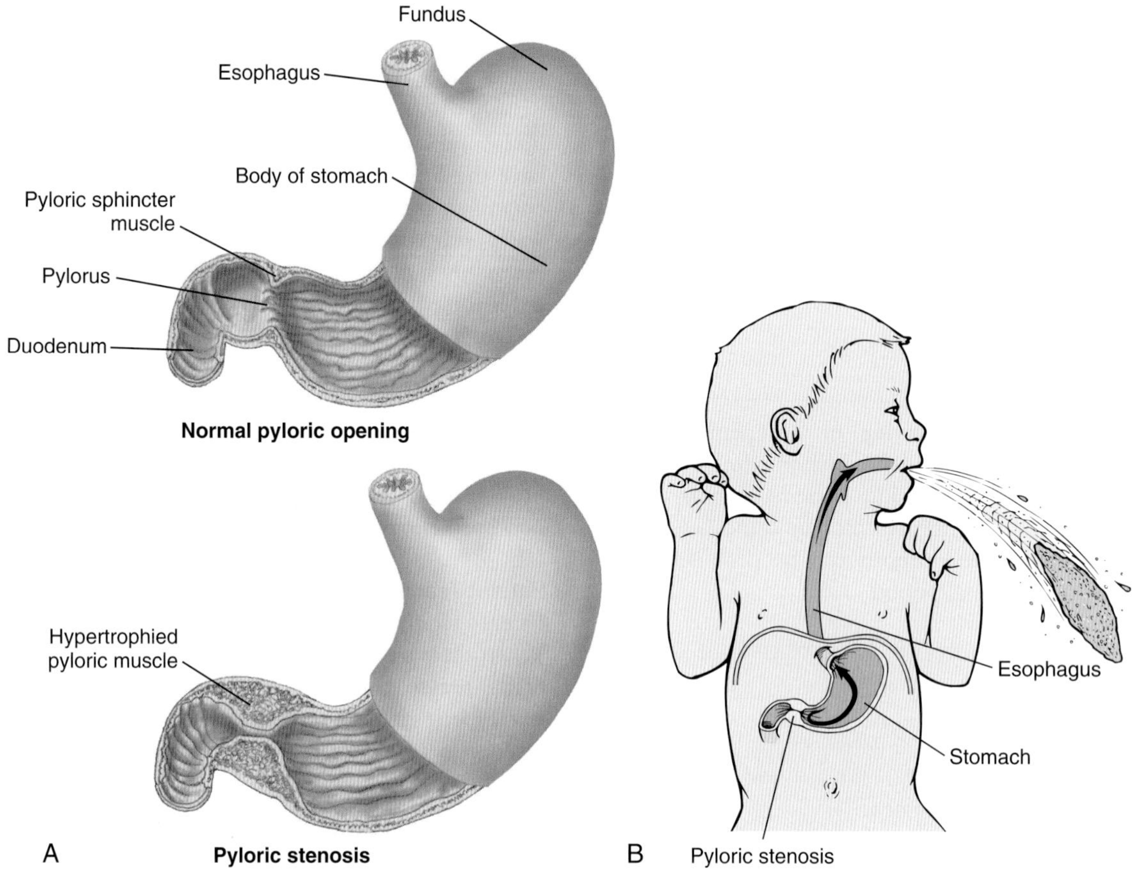

• **Fig. 2.31** (A) Congenital pyloric stenosis. (B) The abnormal narrowing of the opening of the pylorus causes episodes of projectile vomiting. (A, From Ashwill JW, Droske SC: *Nursing care of children: principles and practice,* ed 3, Philadelphia, 2007, Saunders.)

Diagnosis

The condition is diagnosed from the history and the patient's physical condition. Diagnostic studies include upper GI radiographic studies and ultrasonography of the **pylorus**.

Treatment

Treatment consists of surgical intervention, in which the constricted pylorus is incised (pyloromyotomy) and sutured to relieve the obstruction.

Prognosis

The prognosis is good with prompt surgical intervention.

Prevention

No prevention is known.

Patient Teaching

Parents need instruction in care of the incision. Reinforce the importance of postoperative visits.

Hirschsprung Disease (Congenital Aganglionic Megacolon)

Description

Hirschsprung disease, a congenital condition, is impairment of intestinal motility that causes obstruction of the distal colon (Fig. 2.32).

| ICD-10-CM Code | Q43.1 *(Hirschsprung's disease)* |

Symptoms and Signs

The symptoms and signs vary slightly, depending on the age of the child experiencing an exacerbation of the condition. In the neonatal period, the newborn fails to pass **meconium** within 48 hours after birth. The infant may have bile-stained or fecal vomitus and does not want to feed. The abdomen becomes distended.

After the neonatal period, the symptoms and signs include a failure to thrive, with obstinate constipation, vomiting, and abdominal distention. When the condition worsens, the infant may become feverish and may have explosive, watery diarrhea.

The older child exhibits more chronic symptoms, such as constipation, abdominal distention, ribbonlike stools that are foul smelling, easily palpable fecal masses, and visible peristalsis. The child appears malnourished and anemic.

Patient Screening

Infants or children with GI symptoms of bile-stained or fecal vomitus require prompt assessment, as do those children with obstinate constipation, especially when combined with vomiting and abdominal distention. Any child experiencing ribbonlike stools also should have prompt assessment.

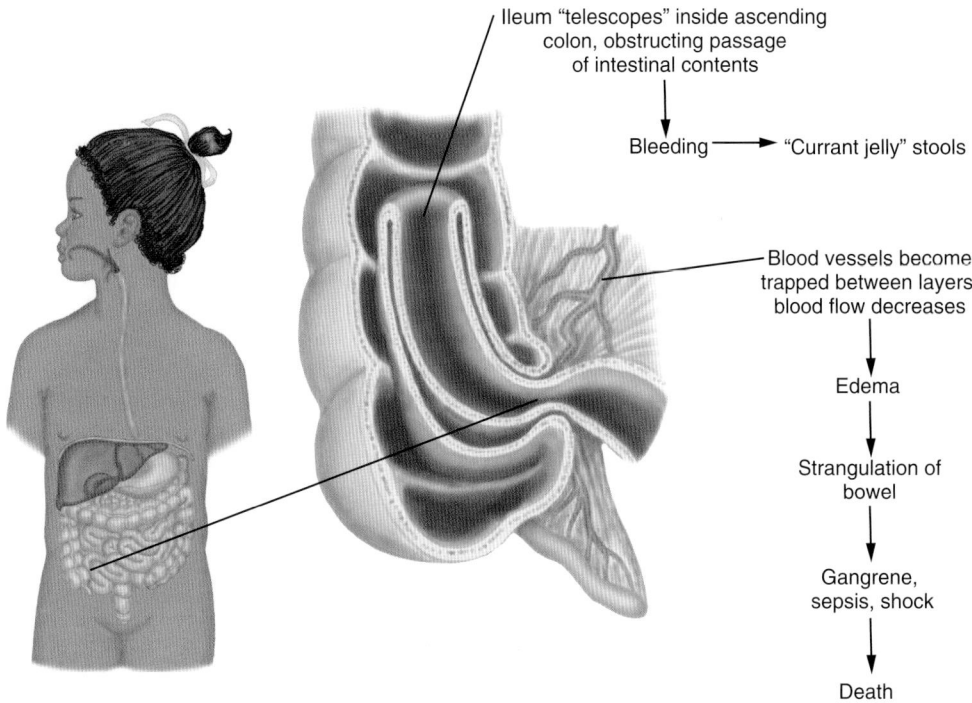

Ileum "telescopes" inside ascending colon, obstructing passage of intestinal contents

Bleeding ——→ "Currant jelly" stools

Blood vessels become trapped between layers; blood flow decreases

↓

Edema

↓

Strangulation of bowel

↓

Gangrene, sepsis, shock

↓

Death

• **Fig. 2.32** Hirschsprung disease. (From James K, et al.: *Nursing care of children,* ed 4, St Louis, 2013, Saunders.)

Etiology

The defect lies in the abnormal innervation of the intrinsic musculature of the bowel wall. In Hirschsprung disease, the parasympathetic nerve ganglion cells are absent in a segment of the colon, usually in the rectosigmoid area. This deficiency of innervation results in lack of peristalsis in the affected portion of the colon and the succeeding backup of fecal material. The proximal portion of the colon becomes grossly distended, and intestinal obstruction results.

Statistics indicate that males are more likely than females to have a megacolon and that the risk is increased in children with Down syndrome. It is believed to be a familial congenital disease.

Diagnosis

Diagnosis is based on family history, the clinical picture, radiographic studies of the bowel, and, finally, biopsy to confirm the absence of the ganglionic cells.

Treatment

Treatment consists of relief of the obstruction by surgical intervention; the affected bowel is excised, and the normal colon is joined to the anus. A temporary colostomy is performed proximal to the aganglionic section of the colon. Electrolyte and fluid balance must be maintained. After the colon recovers function (6 months to 1 year), the colostomy is closed.

Prognosis

The prognosis varies, depending on the extent of colon involvement and the success of surgical intervention. Ideally the colon will heal and the colostomy can be closed within a year.

Prevention

No prevention is known for this apparently familial congenital disease.

Patient Teaching

The parents and the child require training on caring for the stoma, as well as dealing with the colostomy bags and drainage. Help and encourage families to find and contact support groups and other community resources. The parents, the family, and the child may require counseling. Provide nutritional and dietary information.

Metabolic Disorders

Cystic Fibrosis

Description

Cystic fibrosis (CF), an autosomal recessive inherited disorder, is a chronic dysfunction of a gene called *cystic fibrosis transmembrane conductance regulator (CFTR)* that affects multiple body systems. It is the most common fatal genetic disease.

ICD-10-CM Code   E84.9 *(Cystic, fibrosis, unspecified)*
                       (E84.0-E84.9 = 5 codes of specificity)

Cystic fibrosis is coded according to the region involved. Refer to the physician's diagnosis and then to the current edition of the ICD-10-CM coding manual to ensure the greatest specificity of pathology.

Symptoms and Signs

Symptoms may become apparent soon after birth or may develop in childhood. The disease primarily attacks the lungs and the digestive system, producing copious thick and sticky mucus that accumulates and blocks glandular ducts. The clinical effects of CF can be immense and include dry paroxysmal cough, exercise intolerance, pneumonia, bulky diarrhea, vomiting, and bowel obstruction. Pancreatic changes occur, with fat and fiber replacing normal tissue. Involvement of sweat glands causes increased concentrations of salt in sweat. Normal growth and ability to thrive are reduced (Fig. 2.33). Sinus infections and diarrhea often accompany the other symptoms. Infertility is common.

Patient Screening

In many of these children, the disease is suspected during the neonatal period while they are still in the newborn nursery. The condition may become apparent during routine well-baby examinations. When parents report that the child has developed a cough producing thick, sticky mucus, or failure to thrive despite adequate intake, prompt assessment of the child is indicated.

Etiology

CF is an inherited disorder and is transmitted as an autosomal recessive trait (see the Genetic Disorders and Syndromes section).

Diagnosis

Genetic testing can be done prenatally if parents are known to be carriers of a genetic mutation for this disorder. The diagnostic workup includes family history, pulmonary function test, chest radiography, and stool studies. The sweat test reveals elevated levels of sodium and chloride and confirms the diagnosis.

Treatment

CF is considered a fatal disease. However, early diagnosis and treatment have greatly increased life expectancy

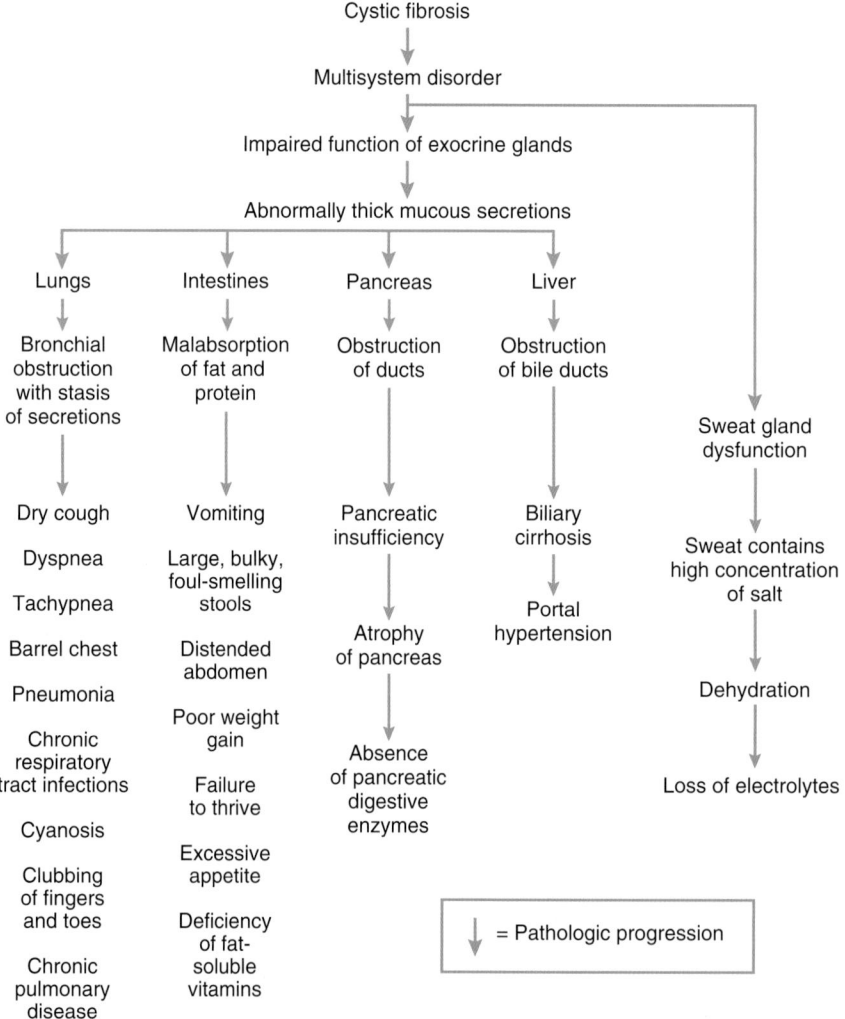

• **Fig. 2.33** Major clinical manifestations of cystic fibrosis (CF) in a child.

in the past few decades. Treatment includes supportive measures that help the child lead as normal a life as possible and that prevent pulmonary infections. These measures include the use of a high-calorie, high–sodium chloride diet; chest physiotherapy; supplementation of vitamins A, D, E, and K; increased fluid intake; and pancreatic enzyme supplementation to aid in digestion. Patients may require insulin to treat CF-associated diabetes. Broad-spectrum antibiotics are used aggressively to treat infection, and drugs that thin the mucus are given. Percussive therapy to dislodge mucus is helpful. Breathing treatments with aerosols using nebulizers is also helpful. Oxygen therapy may be required. Some patients with CF may be candidates for lung transplantation. Patients with CF are encouraged to avoid exposure to dust, dirt, household chemicals, smoke, fumes, fireplace smoke, mold, and mildew.

Prognosis

Because CF is considered a fatal disease, the long-term prognosis is not favorable. Early diagnosis and compliance with treatment have improved the chances for these children to have as near normal a life as possible and an increased life expectancy. At the present time, life expectancy of a patient with CF in the United States has extended into the 30s. Many have graduated from high school, and some have completed a college degree.

Prevention

CF is genetic, and no prevention is known.

Patient Teaching

The family needs emotional support and teaching about the disease; referral to genetic counseling is helpful. Help and encourage the family to find and contact support groups and other resources in the community.

Phenylketonuria

Description

Phenylketonuria (PKU) is an inborn error in the metabolism of amino acids and, when not corrected, causes brain damage and intellectual developmental disorder.

ICD-10-CM Code	E70.0 (Classical phenylketonuria)

Symptoms and Signs

In this defect, an enzyme needed to change an amino acid (phenylalanine) in the body into another substance (tyrosine) is lacking. As a result, phenylalanine accumulates in blood and urine and is toxic to the brain. Symptoms may not begin until the infant is 4 months old, when a characteristic musty odor of the child's perspiration and urine is noted. Other signs include rashes, irritability, hyperactivity, personality disorders, and evidence of arrested brain development.

Patient Screening

Screening of all newborns is mandatory in all the states, and a positive result on screening indicates immediate dietary intervention. Prompt assessment is indicated when a parent or a caregiver reports that the infant emanates a musty smell, especially in urine.

Etiology

PKU is inherited as an autosomal recessive trait and causes defective enzymatic conversion in protein metabolism, resulting in the accumulation of phenylalanine in blood (see the Genetic Disorders and Syndromes section).

Diagnosis

PKU is detected by mandatory screening of blood in the newborn. A positive Guthrie test result indicates the presence of phenylalanine in blood. Urine is tested for phenylalanine derivatives.

Treatment

The treatment is to place the infant on a phenylalanine-free diet, which allows the infant to grow with normal brain development. Individuals with PKU must eat a diet low in phenylalanine for the rest of their lives. Because natural proteins contain phenylalanine, the patient must remain on a protein-restricted diet. Restrictions or elimination of the following foods is required: meat, chicken, fish, cheese, nuts, and dairy products. The newborn cannot have breast milk because of its high levels of phenylalanine. Intake of some starchy foods, including potatoes, corn, pasta, and bread, requires close monitoring. The sweetener aspartame used in diet soda and diet food is metabolized into substances including phenylalanine.

Prognosis

The prognosis is excellent when the infant is placed on a phenylalanine-free diet soon after birth. Late dietary intervention does not reverse the brain damage.

Prevention

No prevention is known.

Patient Teaching

Close follow-up with testing for phenylalanine levels in blood may allow for some modification of the difficult dietary restrictions. Emotional support is important for the child and the parents. Genetic counseling is recommended. Help parents to find the essential dietary information listing foods and substances high in phenylalanine.

Endocrine Syndromes

Klinefelter syndrome and Turner syndrome are examples of genetic, chromosomal diseases that are not inherited. They result from nondisjunction, or the failure of a chromosome pair to separate, during *gamete* production (Fig. 2.34).

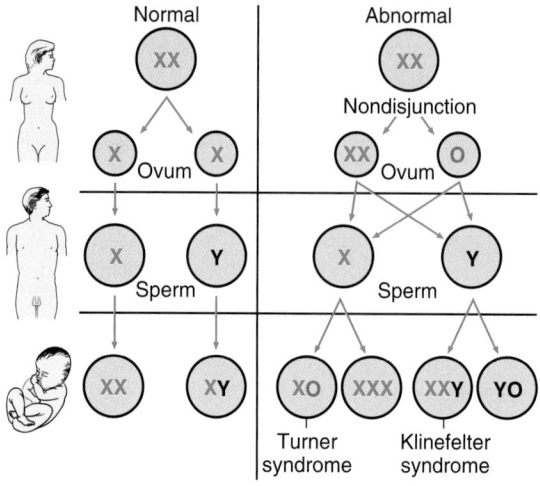

• **Fig. 2.34** Pathogenesis of sex chromosome abnormalities (Turner and Klinefelter). (From Damjanov I: *Pathology for the health professions*, ed 4, St Louis, 2011, Saunders.)

Humans normally have 46 chromosomes: 22 pairs of autosomes and two sex chromosomes. The technical notation for a human female is 46,XX and for a male, 46,XY. In a fertilized ovum, one chromosome from each pair of autosomes originates from the mother's ovum and the other from the father's sperm. Each ovum normally contains a single X chromosome. Sperm cells may contain either an X or a Y chromosome. If a sperm bearing the X chromosome fertilizes the ovum, the fetus develops into a female. A sperm carrying the Y chromosome produces a male fetus. Sometimes, through what may be described as an accident of nature, extra chromosomes or the absence of chromosomes in the fertilized ovum cause congenital syndromes with a variety of physical and mental developmental effects (Fig. 2.35).

Klinefelter Syndrome

Description

Klinefelter syndrome (XXY condition) is male hypogonadism, appearing in males after puberty with at least two X chromosomes and one or more Y chromosomes (typically the 47,XXY pattern).

ICD-10-CM Code	Q98.4 *(Klinefelter syndrome, unspecified)*
	(Q98.0-Q98.9 = 9 codes of specificity)

Symptoms and Signs

The presence of two X chromosomes in affected males causes abnormal development of the testes and reduced levels of the male hormone testosterone. Puberty begins at the usual time and usually results in a normal-size penis, but the testes are small, and body hair is scant. In general, the person appears normal, except for exceptionally long legs, above-average height, and reduced muscle development. The most significant problem associated with Klinefelter syndrome is infertility resulting from azoospermia. Only rarely are these patients fertile; they have the mosaic form that carries the extra X chromosome in only one cell line. Other alterations include a mild delay in language acquisition

and increased risk of behavioral and learning disabilities. Some affected individuals have mild to more significant intellectual impairment. The mammary glands may be enlarged in about half the cases. Possible complications include osteoporosis and chronic pulmonary diseases. Other complications may include autoimmune disorders, venous disease, osteoporosis, breast cancer, or tooth decay.

Patient Screening

The male infant appears normal at birth, and symptoms are usually not noted until puberty. The condition may be discovered during a routine sports or pre-camp physical. In other situations, parents may call to discuss the delay in sexual maturation of the young male. Considering the anxiety that the family may be experiencing, an assessment should be performed promptly.

Etiology

Klinefelter syndrome results from the presence of at least two X chromosomes, typically the 47,XXY pattern. The extra X chromosome may be of either maternal or paternal origin. Other variants include XXYY, XXXY, and XXXXY. The disease is not inherited but results from a nondisjunction during gamete formation. This disorder affects an estimated 1 in 500 to 600 liveborn males.

Diagnosis

The diagnostic workup includes a physical examination, serum and urine gonadotropin level determination, and semen analysis. A chromosomal smear analysis confirms the diagnosis and differentiates between the mosaic and true forms of Klinefelter syndrome.

Treatment

At the time of normal puberty, long-term hormone replacement with testosterone is given by injection or a transdermal patch, usually under the supervision of an endocrinologist. Testosterone is necessary for the maintenance of normal sexual function and normal muscle and bone mass. However, fertility cannot be restored. Many patients report an improvement in energy and emotional stability with hormone therapy. Supplemental calcium intake is prescribed to help prevent osteoporosis.

Prognosis

There is no cure for the syndrome, and natural fatherhood probably will never be achieved. Alteration of intelligence correlates with the number of extra X chromosomes. Many of these males achieve their goals in their chosen professions and are productive members of society.

Prevention

Because Klinefelter syndrome is a chromosomal disorder, no prevention is known.

Patient Teaching

Inform the patient and the family of the importance of follow-up appointments to monitor hormone replace-

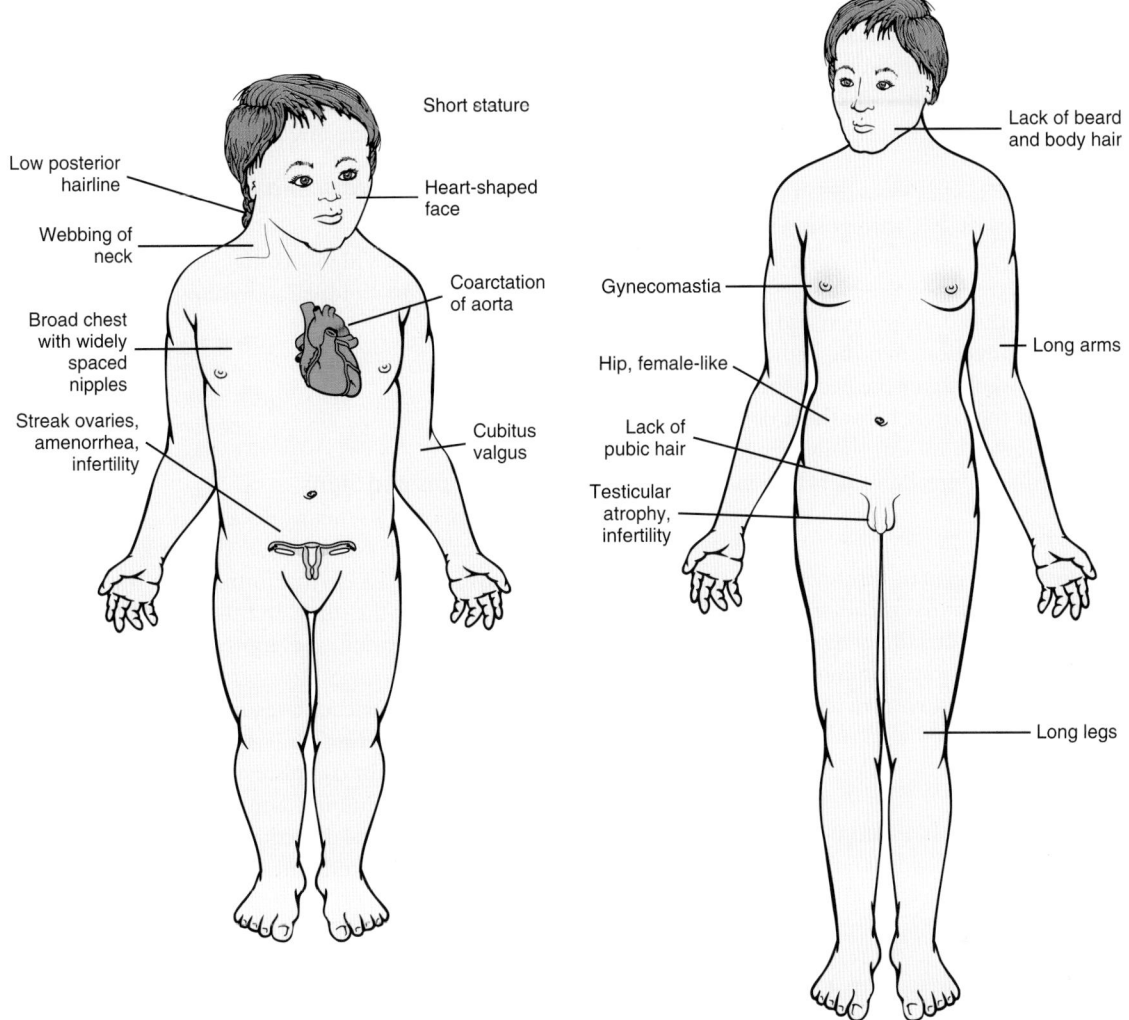

Short stature

Low posterior
hairline

Heart-shaped
face

Webbing of
neck

Coarctation
of aorta

Broad chest
with widely
spaced
nipples

Streak ovaries,
amenorrhea,
infertility

Cubitus
valgus

Lack of beard
and body hair

Gynecomastia

Long arms

Hip, female-like

Lack of
pubic hair

Testicular
atrophy,
infertility

Long legs

• **Fig. 2.35** Line art comparing features of individuals with Klinefelter syndrome and Turner syndrome. (From Damjanov I: *Pathology for the health professions,* ed 4, St Louis, 2012, Saunders.)

ment and identify the target dosage. Explain the importance of adhering to the prescribed dosage schedule of medication to maintain proper blood levels. Describe the possible adverse effects of testosterone therapy, such as insomnia, anxiety, tremors, and dizziness; tell the patient to report these or other symptoms to the attending physician. Refer the patient and the family to Klinefelter Syndrome and Associates for support, meetings, and conventions.

Turner Syndrome

Description

Turner syndrome is a chromosomal disease that occurs in females with a single sex chromosome, 45,XO.

ICD-10-CM Code	Q55.4 *(Other congenital malformations of vas deferens, epididymis, seminal vesicles, and prostate)*
	Q96.9 *(Turner's syndrome, unspecified)*
	(Q96.0-Q96.9 = 7 codes of specificity)

Symptoms and Signs

Turner syndrome is the most common disorder of gonadal dysgenesis in females. At birth, the ovaries are immature or absent, and the female infant appears short, with low-set ears, swollen hands and feet, and webbing of the neck. As these children grow, there is absence of sexual maturation, along with amenorrhea, sterility, dwarfism, and cardiac and kidney defects. Cardiac defects may include coarctation of the aorta in the infant and, in adulthood, aortic dissection caused by cardiovascular disease. If ovaries were present at birth, they slowly begin to disappear, leaving only small amounts of tissue. If the ovaries do not disappear, they typically contain no eggs, eliminating the possibility of pregnancy. Most of these female children may experience delayed speech and ambulation; however, they usually are of normal intelligence.

Patient Screening

Well-baby examinations may reveal signs of the disorder. The baby is referred for chromosome studies to confirm the diagnosis. As the child matures, appointments may be needed to assess possible cardiac or renal disorders.

Etiology

Turner syndrome results from loss of the second X chromosome caused by nondisjunction during gamete formation. The anomaly is seen in about 1 in 2500 live female births.

Diagnosis

Chromosomal smear studies show only one X chromosome instead of the normal 46,XX chromosomal pattern.

Treatment

Symptoms can be reduced by estrogen and growth hormone therapy. Surgical correction may be indicated for certain anomalies, such as webbing of the neck. Emotional support for the patient and the family helps them develop strategies for coping with low self-esteem, body image disturbance, and potential cardiac or renal disorders that may develop.

Prognosis

There is no cure for this genetic disorder; however, the prognosis is good if the patient has no other complicating conditions, including cardiac or kidney disorders. Moderate degrees of learning disorders are common. These females will never be able to conceive their own child because they have no ovaries to produce eggs.

Prevention

Because Turner syndrome is a chromosomal disorder, there is no prevention. These individuals are sterile; therefore they will have no offspring who could inherit the disorder.

Patient Teaching

Help the child and the parents find and contact support groups and community resources. Encourage the family to help the girl build self-esteem and confidence. Make referrals for genetic counseling, if requested.

Childhood Diseases

Nothing causes more anxiety than a seriously ill child. Pathologic processes in children pose special threats because children are constantly changing physically and functionally. The journey through childhood normally results in maturation and expansion of the body's natural immune defense mechanisms. In addition, rapid advances in treatment and preventive medicine have enabled us to control many infectious diseases that formerly caused serious illness, disabling complications, and even death. However, many infections and disease syndromes can interrupt the normal growth and development of any child. The following section describes common diseases that affect children.

Infectious Diseases

Although the infant acquires limited natural immunity from the mother, the growing child is vulnerable to many infectious diseases and the disabilities that they cause. Many of these communicable diseases can be prevented. Dramatic results have been achieved in pediatric medicine through routine prophylactic immunization with vaccines that build specific and prolonged protection. To prevent epidemics of contagious diseases, all states in the United States require that children receive vaccinations before entering school (Fig. 2.36) (see the discussion of immunity in Chapter 3).

Chickenpox (Varicella Zoster)
Description

Chickenpox is a highly contagious, acute viral infection that is common in children and young adults.

ICD-10-CM Code	B01.9 *(Varicella without complication)*
	(B01.0-B01.9 = 7 codes of specificity)

Symptoms and Signs

Chickenpox is a systemic disease with superficial cutaneous lesions that begin as red macules that progress to *papules* and then finally become *vesicles* that form crusts. The lesions first are seen on the face or the trunk and then spread over the extremities; they can be distributed everywhere on the body and even have been found internally. A day or two before the rash appears, the patient may experience fever, malaise, and anorexia. The lesions can continue to erupt for 3 to 4 days and cause intense itching. Recovery is usually complete within 2 weeks, leaving the person with lifetime immunity. Some possible complications include secondary bacterial infection, viral pneumonia, conjunctival ulcers, and Reye syndrome (Fig. 2.37).

Patient Screening

Contagious diseases present a challenge in the patient-screening process. Many physicians prefer not to have the contagious patient in the regular reception area. Many pediatricians have a sick child waiting room and a regular waiting room. At offices that have no sick child waiting area, the child is immediately placed in an examination room and the physician notified. Some physicians prefer to have a staff person make a telephone call to the parents ahead of the clinic appointment to obtain information on symptoms, body temperature, and so on, as well as the telephone number where the parent can be reached. The physician reviews the information and calls the parent back to discuss the situation.

Etiology

The causative organism is varicella-zoster virus (VZV), also known as *human herpes virus 3* (HHV-3), a member of the herpes virus group. The virus is transmitted via direct or indirect spread of droplet nuclei from the respiratory tract of the infected person or a carrier. Fluid from cutaneous lesions is also infectious, but dried crusty lesions are not contagious. The patient is considered contagious for 1 to 2 days before the eruptions until about 6 days after the eruptions. The incubation period is 2 to 3 weeks.

Diagnosis

Chickenpox usually is diagnosed on the basis of the history of exposure and the presence of characteristic cutaneous eruptions. Although laboratory testing is not usually necessary, VZV can

Table 1   Recommended Child and Adolescent Immunization Schedule for ages 18 years or younger United States, 2019

These recommendations must be read with the Notes that follow. For those who fall behind or start late, provide catch-up vaccination at the earliest opportunity as indicated by the green bars in Table 1. To determine minimum intervals between doses, see the catch-up schedule (Table 2). School entry and adolescent vaccine age groups are shaded in gray.

Vaccine	Birth	1 mo	2 mos	4 mos	6 mos	9 mos	12 mos	15 mos	18 mos	19-23 mos	2-3 yrs	4-6 yrs	7-10 yrs	11-12 yrs	13-15 yrs	16 yrs	17-18 yrs
Hepatitis B (HepB)	1st dose	←── 2nd dose ──→		←─────────────── 3rd dose ───────────────→													
Rotavirus (RV) RV1 (2-dose series); RV5 (3-dose series)			1st dose	2nd dose	See Notes												
Diphtheria, tetanus, & acellular pertussis (DTaP: <7 yrs)			1st dose	2nd dose	3rd dose		←──────── 4th dose ────────→					5th dose					
Haemophilus influenzae type b (Hib)			1st dose	2nd dose	See Notes		←─ 3rd or 4th dose, See Notes ─→										
Pneumococcal conjugate (PCV13)			1st dose	2nd dose	3rd dose		←──── 4th dose ────→										
Inactivated poliovirus (IPV: <18 yrs)			1st dose	2nd dose	←────────────── 3rd dose ──────────────→							4th dose					
Influenza (IIV)						Annual vaccination 1 or 2 doses					Annual vaccination 1 dose only						
or Influenza (LAIV)										Annual vaccination 1 or 2 doses		Annual vaccination 1 dose only					
Measles, mumps, rubella (MMR)					See Notes		←─ 1st dose ─→					2nd dose					
Varicella (VAR)							←─ 1st dose ─→					2nd dose					
Hepatitis A (HepA)					See Notes		2-dose series, See Notes										
Meningococcal (MenACWY-D ≥9 mos; MenACWY-CRM ≥2 mos)													See Notes	1st dose		2nd dose	
Tetanus, diphtheria, & acellular pertussis (Tdap: ≥7 yrs)														Tdap			
Human papillomavirus (HPV)														See Notes			
Meningococcal B														See Notes			
Pneumococcal polysaccharide (PPSV23)														See Notes			

Range of recommended ages for all children
Range of recommended ages for catch-up immunization
Range of recommended ages for certain high-risk groups
Range of recommended ages for non-high-risk groups that may receive vaccine, subject to individual clinical decision-making
No recommendation

Centers for Disease Control and Prevention | Recommended Child and Adolescent Immunization Schedule, United States, 2019 | Page 2

02/22/19

• **Fig. 2.36** Centers for Disease Control and Prevention (CDC) Schedule of Recommended Childhood and Adolescent Immunization.

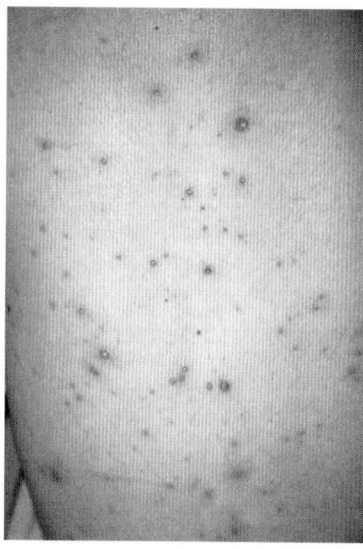

• **Fig. 2.37** Chickenpox (varicella). (From Hill MJ: *Skin disorders—Mosby's clinical nursing series,* St Louis, 1994, Mosby.)

be visualized when a culture of vesicular fluid is examined microscopically. After the infection, antibodies are found in serum.

Treatment

Palliative treatment to alleviate pruritus includes cool bicarbonate of soda baths, followed by cornstarch dusting or the application of calamine lotion. This helps control scratching that can lead to secondary infection and scarring. Other comfort measures include administration of acetaminophen for fever and pain. *Caution:* Aspirin is *not* given to children with chickenpox because of the risk of Reye syndrome. In some cases, treatment with antiviral drugs (e.g., acyclovir) may be prescribed. The patient must be isolated until all lesions have crusted.

Prognosis

Prognosis for recovery from chickenpox is good. The patient may have scarring resulting from the eruptions. Individuals who have had chickenpox are at risk of developing herpes zoster (shingles) later in life.

Prevention

A varicella virus vaccine (varicella virus vaccine [Varivax]) is available for protection against chickenpox. For children, an injection of the vaccine at age 12 to 18 months is recommended, with a second dose after age 24 months. For adolescents and adults, a second dose is administered 4 to 8 weeks after the first dose.

Patients who are immunocompromised or otherwise at high risk can be given the varicella-zoster immune globulin within 4 days of exposure.

Patient Teaching

Reinforce the need for thorough hand washing, use of tissues during coughing or sneezing episodes, and proper handling and disposal of soiled tissues. Encourage parents to minimize contact between these children and others during the contagious period, which is 1 to 2 days before the eruptions until about 6 days after the eruptions.

 ENRICHMENT

Recording Causes of Absenteeism in Schools

Some schools or school corporations are now requesting that parents calling in that their child is ill and unable to attend school to report symptoms. Records are kept concerning presence of elevated temperature, coughing, sneezing, upset stomach with nausea and vomiting, diarrhea, or any rash. This allows the tracking of trends of illnesses to be reported to the Centers for Disease Control and Prevention (CDC).

 ENRICHMENT

Prevention of Disease Spread During Athletic Events

Precautions to be taken during athletic events or participation help prevent the spread of bacteria and viruses. Observe ball handlers to see if they have a tendency to put their saliva on their hands to have a better grip on the ball (in football or basketball). Encourage individuals to wash hands with soap and water and to shower after athletic activities. Wrestling or any contact sport where a mat is used creates an area that holds body perspiration and saliva. After each contact set, it is important that the mat be washed down with a 10% bleach solution. Any uniform or piece of equipment that has blood on it must be cleansed with the 10% bleach solution. Athletes should shower after contact sports, such as wrestling.

 ENRICHMENT

Vaccines

A vaccine is a suspension of dead or attenuated organisms given to stimulate an active immune response that produces more or less permanent resistance to pathogenic organisms and viruses. Booster doses are smaller amounts of the original vaccine given at specified intervals to maintain serum antibody levels. Vaccines are controlled for potency and stability and are tested for safety and effectiveness. Some vaccines are grown in bird eggs or in animal organs or are weakened with chemicals. The patient is screened for certain allergies or previous reactions to vaccines. Local responses of soreness, redness, and swelling at the site of injection are common. Untoward responses include high fever, generalized swelling, difficulty breathing, severe headache, arthralgia, and seizures. Any of these symptoms should be reported immediately to the physician. It should be noted that there is no link between any vaccine and the development of autism spectrum disorders. Initial reports indicating a putative link have been retracted as falsified data, and in 2009, the U.S. vaccine court ruled that there is no evidence of any link between the measles–mumps–rubella (MMR) vaccine and autism. Parents expressing concerns should be counseled as to the true risks and benefits of vaccines.

Toxoids contain altered forms of bacterial toxins to stimulate antibody production and thereby impart protection against toxins.

Individuals with autoimmune diseases must not be given vaccines containing live microorganisms.

Diphtheria

Description

Diphtheria is an acute communicable disease that causes necrosis of the mucous membrane in the respiratory tract.

> ICD-10-CM Code   A36.9 *(Diphtheria, unspecified)*
> (A36.0-A36.9 = 12 codes of specificity)
> *Refer to the physician's diagnosis and then to the current edition ICD-10-CM coding manual to ensure the greatest specificity of pathology.*

Symptoms and Signs

The patient, most often a child, has sore throat, dysphagia, a cough, hoarseness, and chills. Fever, swollen regional lymph nodes, foul breath, and, in some cases, cyanosis can be noted. As the bacteria invade the nasopharynx, they multiply and produce a powerful exotoxin that travels in blood throughout the body. Locally, the infection and inflammation cause grayish patches of thick mucous membrane, known as *pseudomembrane* or *false membrane,* to appear along the respiratory tract. The membrane, which can be extensive, is composed of bacteria, inflammatory cells, dead tissue, and fibrin; it is surrounded by inflammation and swelling that can interfere with airway function, impairing swallowing and speech. As the toxin is absorbed, it affects other vital organ systems, with many possible complications, including otitis media, pneumonia, myocarditis, and paralysis.

Carriers, although infected, remain asymptomatic and do not experience active infection themselves.

Patient Screening

Children with fever, chills, and respiratory difficulties require prompt assessment. When a parent reports a child with respiratory difficulties, most protocols recommend that the child be seen in an emergency facility.

Etiology

The causative organism, *Corynebacterium diphtheriae,* is present in the nasopharynx of infected individuals or carriers and is transmitted via airborne respiratory droplets. The incubation period is 2 to 5 days. The patient is contagious for 2 to 4 weeks if untreated or for 1 to 2 days after initiation of antibiotic treatment. Carriers of the disease remain asymptomatic but can infect the inadequately immunized individual.

Diagnosis

The presence of the characteristic membrane adhering to the throat is diagnostic. Culture of the throat and staining is positive for *C. diphtheriae,* and antibodies are found in serum. Immunity or susceptibility can be determined by the Schick test.

Treatment

Diphtheria antitoxin is given as soon as possible. The administration of antibiotics, such as penicillin and erythromycin, is indicated to kill the organism. The patient is isolated, restricted to bed rest, and given a diet as tolerated. The patient is observed for the possible complications related to systemic involvement. Carriers are given antibiotics to eliminate the organisms from the respiratory tract.

Prognosis

With prompt intervention and completion of antibiotic drug therapy, the prognosis is good.

Prevention

Diphtheria, once common in North America and Europe, can be prevented by the administration of diphtheria toxoid to produce active immunity. Vaccination begins at 2 to 3 months in the form of the diphtheria–tetanus–pertussis (DTaP) vaccine, with booster doses given at appropriate intervals during childhood. Adults should receive booster vaccination to ensure that immunity is maintained. Therefore, when an injection to prevent tetanus is administered to adults, the inoculation tetanus–diphtheria–pertussis (TDaP) should be administered. This is also helpful in preventing outbreaks of whooping cough.

Patient Teaching

Reinforce the need for good hand washing and the use of tissues during coughing or sneezing episodes. Instruct on the handling and disposal of soiled tissues. Encourage parents to minimize contact between these children and others during the contagious period, which continues for 1 to 2 days after starting antibiotic therapy. Emphasize the importance of routine immunizations for children.

Mumps (Epidemic Parotitis)

Description

Mumps is an acute communicable viral disease causing inflammation and swelling of one or both parotid glands.

> ICD-10-CM Code   B26.9 *(Mumps without complication)*
> (B26.0-B26.9 = 11 codes of specificity)
> *Refer to the physician's diagnosis and then to the current edition of the ICD-10-CM coding manual to ensure the greatest specificity of pathology.*

Symptoms and Signs

The patient, usually a child, has tenderness in the neck in front of and below the ears in the region of the parotid glands and pain on swallowing (Fig. 2.38). Patients also may experience a rash, headache, muscle aches, and a low-grade fever, with loss of appetite and an earache that is aggravated by chewing. A common complication of the disease in the adult male is mumps orchitis, which may lead to sterility. Often the infection is subclinical, without noticeable symptoms.

Patient Screening

Contagious diseases present a challenge in the patient-screening process. Many physicians prefer not to have the

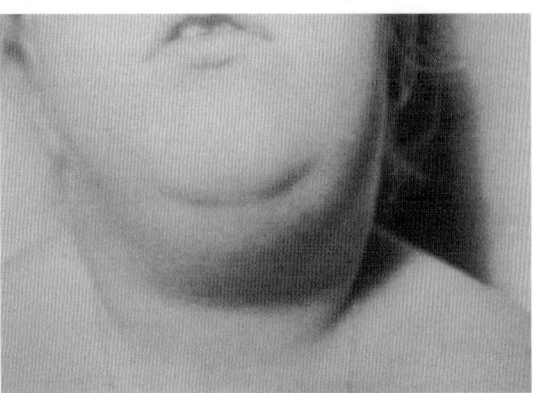

• **Fig. 2.38** Submaxillary mumps in an infant. (From Grimes D: *Infectious diseases—Mosby's clinical nursing series*, St Louis, 1994, Mosby.)

contagious patient in the reception area. When the parents feel an office visit is warranted, the child is immediately placed in an examination room and the physician notified. Some physicians prefer to have a staff person telephone the parents to obtain information on symptoms, body temperature, and so on, along with the telephone number where the parents can be reached. The physician reviews the information and either calls the parents back or has the staff member call them with instructions for care.

Etiology

The causative agent of mumps is an airborne virus that is spread by droplet nuclei from the respiratory tract. The incubation period is long, usually 14 to 21 days. The patient is contagious for 1 to 7 days before onset of the swelling of the parotid glands and up to 9 days thereafter. Lifelong immunity develops after a clinical or subclinical infection; active immunization with the mumps vaccine also affords prolonged immunity.

Diagnosis

Diagnosis is made from a history of exposure and a clinical picture that includes swelling of the parotid glands. The male patient is assessed for tenderness of the testes. Serum amylase is often elevated. A new polymerase chain reaction (PCR) test has been developed for diagnostic confirmation, when needed.

Treatment

Acetaminophen is given, and warm or cold compresses are applied for pain. A soft or liquid diet can help minimize discomfort when eating. The male patient who is experiencing testicular tenderness and swelling may need scrotal support. Isolation of the patient is helpful in preventing the spread of the disease.

Prognosis

Most children recover from mumps; however, orchitis, meningitis, and encephalitis are possible complications of mumps.

Prevention

Childhood immunization is the best prevention. Children should receive the first MMR immunization at age 12 months. The second dose should be given before the child enters school and can be given within 1 month of the initial immunization. An unimmunized person should be referred to a physician for active immunization within 48 hours of contact to prevent or alter the severity of the disease. Good hand washing and proper handling of soiled tissues helps prevent the spread of the disease among family members and other contacts.

Patient Teaching

Reinforce the need for good hand washing and proper handling and disposal of soiled tissues. Discuss the airborne viruses responsible for mumps and the means of preventing the spread of the disease. Emphasize the importance of routine immunizations for children.

Pertussis (Whooping Cough)

Description

Whooping cough is a highly contagious bacterial infection of the respiratory tract.

ICD-10-CM Code	A37.90 *(Whooping cough, unspecified species without pneumonia)* (A37.0–A37.91 = 8 codes of specificity)

Symptoms and Signs

The disease has three stages: (1) the highly contagious catarrhal stage, when the child seems to have a common cold; (2) the paroxysmal stage, when the cough becomes violent, ending in a high-pitched inspiratory whoop, often followed by vomiting of thick mucus; and (3) the convalescent stage, when the cough gradually diminishes.

Patient Screening

A child exhibiting symptoms of violent coughing with high-pitched inspiratory whoop and vomiting of thick mucus requires prompt attention.

Etiology

The pertussis bacillus *Bordetella pertussis* reproduces in the respiratory tract, where it releases a toxin that leads to necrosis of the mucosa, producing a thick exudate. It is transmitted by droplet nuclei spread via direct or indirect contact with the nasopharyngeal secretions of the contagious patient.

Diagnosis

Bacterial studies of nasopharyngeal mucus are positive for the pertussis bacillus. A PCR test can also be performed. The patient's WBC count usually is elevated.

Treatment

Erythromycin is the antibiotic of choice for treatment. Fluid intake is encouraged to prevent dehydration. A nutritious diet is important to prevent weight loss. Quiet and rest are required because the episodes of prolonged coughing cause exhaustion and weakness. The patient should be observed closely for respiratory distress. Bronchopneumonia, convulsions, or hemorrhages are possible complications of severe disease.

Prognosis

With prompt intervention, hydration monitoring and maintenance, and antibiotic therapy, the prognosis is good. However, if untreated, pertussis can be fatal.

Prevention

Pertussis can be prevented by immunization with the pertussis vaccine. Childhood immunization is the best prevention, and a booster is recommended in early adolescence. Good hand washing and proper handling of soiled tissues help prevent the spread of the disease among family members and other contacts. Emphasize the importance of routine immunizations for children. The newly developed acellular vaccine has been shown to be safer with fewer side effects. An increase in the incidence of whooping cough in adults has been noted. It is recommended that all adults receive TDaP immunization every 10 years to reduce the incidence of whooping cough.

Patient Teaching

Reinforce the need for good hand washing and proper handling and disposal of soiled tissues. Discuss the airborne microbe responsible for pertussis and the methods of preventing airborne spread of the disease. Emphasize the importance of routine immunizations.

Measles (Rubeola)

Description

Measles is an acute, highly contagious viral disease.

ICD-10-CM Code	B05.9 *(Measles without complication)* (B05.0-B05.9 = 7 codes of specificity)

Symptoms and Signs

Early symptoms include cough, coryza, conjunctivitis, and photophobia. The child has a fever, followed, in 3 to 7 days, by a red, blotchy rash. The rash starts behind the ears, hairline, and forehead and then progresses down the body (Fig. 2.39). Before the eruption of the rash, Koplik spots can be detected on the oral mucosa as tiny white spots on a red background (Fig. 2.40).

Patient Screening

Contagious diseases present a challenge in the patient-screening process. Many physicians prefer not to have the contagious patient in the reception area. When the parents feel an office visit is warranted, the child is immediately placed in an examination room and the physician notified. Some physicians prefer to have a staff person telephone the

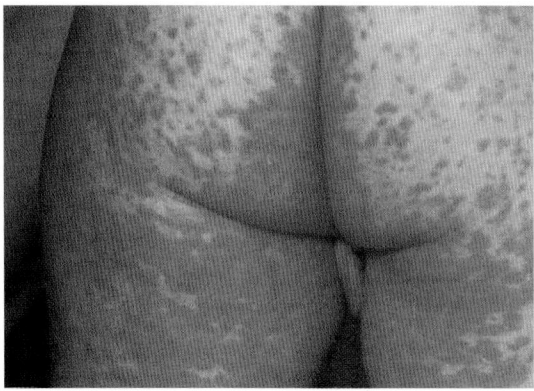

• **Fig. 2.39** Rubeola (measles) rash on the third day. (From Grimes D: *Infectious diseases—Mosby's clinical nursing series,* St Louis, 1994, Mosby.)

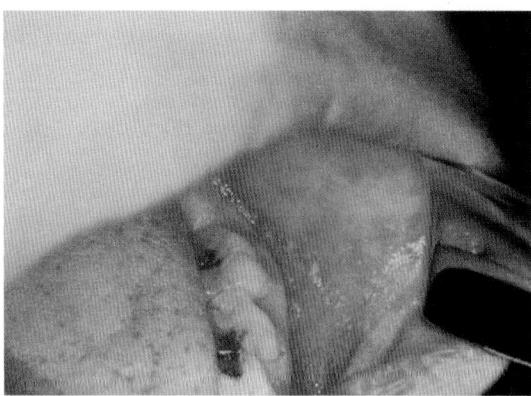

• **Fig. 2.40** Koplik spots on the buccal mucosa 3 days before eruption of rubeola (measles) rash. (From Grimes D: *Infectious diseases—Mosby's clinical nursing series,* St Louis, 1994, Mosby.)

parents to obtain information on symptoms, body temperature, and so on, as well as a contact telephone number. The physician reviews the information and either calls the parent back or has the staff person call the parents back with instructions for care.

Etiology

The causative agent of measles is the measles virus, specifically a *paramyxovirus* of the genus *Morbillivirus.* The infection is airborne, spread by direct contact with secretions from the nose or throat of the infected person. The patient is contagious from about 4 days before the onset of the rash until about 4 days after the onset. The incubation period is 8 to 12 days after exposure.

Diagnosis

Diagnosis is based on a history of exposure and the clinical picture, which includes a rash and the presence of Koplik spots on the oral mucosa.

Treatment

Uncomplicated measles runs its course in 7 to 10 days. Acetaminophen is given to treat the fever. If the fever is persistently high, tepid sponge baths may be given. The patient's eyes may be protected from bright light as a comfort measure. If secondary infection occurs, antibiotics are prescribed to treat the infection.

Prognosis

The prognosis for uncomplicated measles is good. The complications of measles include pneumonia, otitis media, conjunctivitis, and encephalitis. Refer to the Alert box about Subacute Sclerosing Panencephalitis regarding the delayed complications of the disease.

Prevention

Inoculation with the live measles vaccine is given during childhood to protect the individual and prevent epidemics of the disease. The first combination MMR vaccine is given at age 12 to 18 months, with a booster vaccine given when the child starts school. Measles immune globulin given 5 days after exposure to the disease creates passive immunity in unimmunized individuals at high risk. An attack of the disease usually creates immunity for life.

Patient Teaching

Reinforce the necessity of good hand washing and proper handling and disposal of soiled tissues. Discuss the airborne microbe responsible for measles, and discuss methods of preventing airborne spread of the disease. Emphasize the importance of routine immunizations for children.

 ALERT!

Recent outbreaks of measles, as well as mumps, have occurred in communities where parents have refused immunizations for their children.

Rubella (German Measles, 3-Day Measles)
Description

Rubella, a highly contagious viral disease, resembles measles clinically, but it has a shorter course and fewer complications.

ICD-10-CM Code	B06.9 *(Rubella without complication)* (B06.0-B06.9 = 8 codes of specificity)

Symptoms and Signs

In this viral disease, the child has a rose-colored, slightly elevated rash that appears first on the face and head and then progresses downward on the body (Fig. 2.41). In addition, the child has a low-grade fever and can have tenderness and enlargement of the lymph nodes. Complications include transient arthritis, myocarditis, and hemorrhagic manifestations.

Rubella causes great danger to the fetuses of pregnant women who contract the disease.

Patient Screening

Contagious diseases present a challenge in the patient-screening process. Many physicians prefer not to have the contagious patient in the reception area. When the parents feel an office visit is warranted, the child is immediately placed in an examination room and the physician notified.

Etiology

The causative agent is the rubella virus, which is spread by direct contact with nasal or oral secretions. The incubation period after exposure is 14 to 21 days. The patient is contagious from 1 week before eruption of the rash until 1 week

ALERT!

Subacute Sclerosing Panencephalitis

Parents are encouraged to have their children immunized against measles.

Subacute sclerosing panencephalitis (SSPE), an infectious condition of the CNS, is considered a rare disorder and is listed as such in the National Organization for Rare Disorders (NORD). SSPE, one of three forms of encephalitis occurring secondary to the measles virus, evolves after reactivation of the dormant measles virus. The reactivation of the latent measles virus causes a cerebral infection. This infectious process causes atrophy of the cortical areas of the brain, demyelination of the nerves, or ventricular dilation. The brain tissue is diffusely inflamed. Symptoms of this progressive neurologic disorder emerge with an insidious onset and are identified by progressive motor and mental or intellectual deterioration, including personality changes, and neurologic deterioration subsequently resulting in severe dementia. Seizures, blindness, and fever are additional symptoms. Motor involvement leads to periodic involuntary movements and eventual decerebrate rigidity. The patient usually is 5 to 20 years of age and has experienced an

attack of measles in the prior 2 to 10 years. Very rarely, onset of this inappropriate immune response follows measles immunization.

SSPE is diagnosed on the basis of symptoms and a history of previous occurrence of the measles or recent measles immunization. Cerebrospinal fluid (CSF) shows elevated gamma globulin levels. The antibody titer is elevated, indicating the presence of measles virus antibodies.

There is no effective therapy or cure for SSPE. The treatment includes supportive measures, including drug therapy for seizure control. The duration of this disorder is several years, with progressive deterioration of the CNS. The patient usually is nonresponsive and unable to care for himself or herself for some time before ultimate death.

The mother of a young English singer who was afflicted by this rare disorder at age 18 years urges all parents to have their children immunized against measles in the hope of preventing the condition that left her daughter blind and unable to speak. The daughter died 14 years after the onset of SSPE.

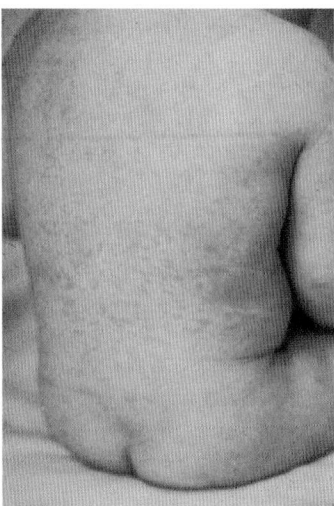

• **Fig. 2.41** Acquired rubella (German measles) in 11-month-old infant. (From Grimes D: *Infectious diseases—Mosby's clinical nursing series,* St Louis, 1994, Mosby.)

after the onset of the rash. Although rubella is preventable through immunization, sporadic epidemics still arise, often on college campuses.

Diagnosis

Diagnosis is made on the basis of a history of exposure and the clinical picture, including the rash. Because rubella resembles other diseases, a definitive diagnosis includes throat culture for the rubella virus and serologic studies to detect antibodies.

Treatment

Treatment consists of supportive measures, including the administration of a mild analgesic for fever and joint pain. The patient is isolated until the rash disappears.

Prognosis

The prognosis is good. (Refer to the Enrichment box about Congenital Rubella Syndrome.)

Prevention

Active immunity conferred by the rubella vaccine in a patient older than 12 months of age prevents the disease. (Refer to Fig. 2.36 for CDC guidelines for childhood immunizations.)

Patient Teaching

Reinforce the need for good hand washing and proper handling and disposal of soiled tissues. Discuss the microbe responsible for rubella and the methods of preventing the spread of the disease via the nasal and mucous routes. Emphasize the importance of routine immunizations for children.

Tetanus

Description

Tetanus is an acute, potentially deadly, systemic infection characterized by painful involuntary contraction of skeletal muscles.

ICD-10-CM Code   A35 *(Other tetanus)*

Symptoms and Signs

The patient is extremely febrile (temperature > 101°F), is irritable, and sweats profusely. He or she has a stiff neck, a tight jaw ("lockjaw"), spasms of the facial muscles, and difficulty swallowing. As the infection progresses, the muscles of the back and abdomen become rigid with generalized convulsive muscle spasm (opisthotonos). These tonic spasms may cause death caused by asphyxiation.

Patient Screening

Patients who have experienced a soft tissue wound, including animal bites and punctures from nails, burns, and abrasions, should be assessed for tetanus prophylaxis and instructed about the importance of receiving the tetanus shot. Patients experiencing high fever, irritability, and profuse perspiration accompanied by stiff neck, tight jaw (lockjaw), spasms of the facial muscles, and difficulty swallowing require immediate assessment and intervention.

Etiology

The bacillus *Clostridium tetani* is found in contaminated soil and animal excreta and enters the skin through a puncture wound, laceration, abrasion, burn, or other injury. Puncture wounds are excellent breeding grounds for the bacillus because they lack a good oxygen supply and the bacillus thrives in dead tissue, producing a powerful exotoxin that attacks the nervous system. The incubation period is 3 to 21 days, with the onset commonly occurring at about 8 days. Tetanus antitoxin immunizations followed by booster doses every 10 years create immunity.

Diagnosis

The patient's history may indicate inadequate immunization. The patient is acutely ill, as described previously. Laboratory test results do not always produce conclusive data for diagnosis.

Treatment

The medical management is chiefly supportive, with the administration of sedatives and muscle relaxants to relieve spasms and seizures; a quiet, dark environment promotes rest. If the patient suffers convulsions, respiratory integrity must be preserved.

The unimmunized patient at risk is given human tetanus immune globulin (TIG) within 72 hours of injury for temporary immunity. A booster injection of tetanus toxoid is needed if the injured person has not had tetanus immunization within 5 years.

Prognosis

Tetanus carries a 35% mortality rate, so prevention is important.

Prevention

The best course is childhood immunizations, timely booster doses, and prompt cleaning of wounds with hydrogen peroxide.

Patient Teaching

Encourage and stress the importance of tetanus booster immunizations. Cleansing of soft tissue injuries also should be stressed.

Influenza

Influenza is an acute, highly contagious viral infection of the respiratory tract. Its highest incidence is in school children, and it is more severe in young children. Influenza occurs sporadically or as an epidemic and is transmitted by droplet nuclei or direct contact with moist secretions. Children tend to have high fevers with influenza and are susceptible to pulmonary complications and Reye syndrome. Because of the latter, acetaminophen, and *not* aspirin, is given to children and adolescents for fever and pain. A full description of influenza can be found in Chapter 9.

Common Cold

Young children have several colds each year, and most colds are self-limiting and run their course in 4 to 5 days. In infants, the nasal congestion can cause difficulty with eating and breathing. Supportive treatment consists of rest, increased fluid intake, and diet as tolerated. The possibility of

secondary bacterial infection or extension of the infection into the lower respiratory tract or into the middle ear is potentially dangerous for the child. These complications warrant antibiotic therapy. For a complete discussion of the common cold, see Chapter 9.

Respiratory Diseases/Disorders

Sudden Infant Death Syndrome

Description

Sudden infant death syndrome (SIDS) is the sudden and unpredicted death of an infant younger than 1 year of age.

ICD-10-CM Code	R99 (Ill-defined and unknown cause of mortality)

Symptoms and Signs

SIDS, formerly called *crib death*, is defined officially as the sudden death of an infant younger than 1 year of age, for which a cause cannot be established. It is the number one cause of death among infants 1 to 12 months of age; 1 in 2000 infants dies mysteriously during the first year of life. Death occurs within seconds during sleep without sound or struggle, and the baby does not suffer. Most infants with SIDS appear healthy before death. When found, the dead infant may have a mottled complexion and cyanotic lips and fingertips.

Known causes and contributing factors for the sudden death of an infant are ruled out. These may include an immature respiratory control system, a susceptibility to deadly arrhythmias, congenital heart disease, and myocarditis.

Patient Screening

Any call regarding an infant not breathing is an emergency, and 911 emergency services should be called to the scene. When an infant dies, the situation usually becomes a coroner's case, and an autopsy is ordered. The parent desiring an appointment for an infant with near-miss SIDS should be seen as soon as possible. Adequate information should be obtained to determine whether the situation is an emergency and whether the child needs to be entered into the emergency care system or can be seen in the office. If the parent of a child who has died of diagnosed SIDS calls for an appointment, remember the magnitude of the situation, and schedule an appointment as soon as possible. During the entire process, remaining nonjudgmental is important.

Etiology

Although there are many theories and much misinformation about SIDS, the exact cause remains uncertain. Research studies and autopsies point to certain pathologic findings and have suggested more than one cause. Many maternal and infant risk factors are known: mother's age less than 20 years, poor prenatal care, smoking and drug abuse during pregnancy, exposure of the infant to second-hand smoke, prematurity, recent upper respiratory tract infection in the infant, sleeping in the prone position, and a sibling with apnea. The incidence is higher in males and during the winter months, likely as a result of over-bundling of the infant during sleep.

Diagnosis

When a complete postmortem investigation, including autopsy, a review of the child's medical history, and examination of the scene of death, has failed to identify the cause of death, it is diagnosed as SIDS.

Treatment

Resuscitation attempts fail. Currently, SIDS is not predictable or preventable. The American Academy of Pediatrics (AAP) has added sleeping in the prone position or on the side to the list of risk factors. To reduce that risk, the AAP recommends placing babies in bed on their backs instead of on their stomachs or sides.

Prognosis

Infants with near-miss SIDS are at risk for additional episodes and should be placed on their backs to sleep. Parents who have had an infant die as a result of SIDS are at higher risk of having another infant with SIDS.

Prevention

Recent studies have isolated the risk factors for SIDS. Although these risk factors may play a role in SIDS, parents must understand that of themselves, these factors do not cause SIDS.

As previously mentioned, the supine sleeping position carries the lowest risk for SIDS. Infants should not be placed in the prone position unless they are actively monitored by an adult. Exposure to cigarette smoke should be prevented. Use of firm bedding materials in a safety-approved crib is prudent. All blankets and pillows should be removed from the crib. Research shows that overheating an infant by dressing in excessive clothing, especially during illness, is to be avoided. Other important factors include good prenatal care and breastfeeding. Breastfeeding is a source of immunity to the newborn infant. An additional prevention is to avoid any contact of the infant with anyone with an upper respiratory illness or a GI upset, even if it is considered a minor episode. All individuals touching or handling the infant should wash their hands before any encounter with the infant. Infants who are high risk may be placed on apnea monitors during the first year of life.

Pregnant women should be advised to not smoke during their pregnancy.

Patient Teaching

Survivors of SIDS should be offered sensitive interventions to help them to deal with the grief and possible feelings of guilt and anger. The Sudden Infant Death Syndrome Alliance is a national voluntary organization in the United States dedicated to eliminating SIDS through medical research. Help families find and contact SIDS support groups.

Croup

Description

Croup is an acute, severe inflammation and obstruction of the respiratory tract.

ICD-10-CM Code	J05.0 (Acute obstructive laryngitis [croup])

Symptoms and Signs

It usually is preceded by an upper respiratory tract infection. The symptoms include hoarseness, fever, a harsh, high-pitched cough, and stridor during inspiration caused by narrowing of the upper airways. The child may experience dyspnea (fast and difficult respirations) that may be accompanied by a grunting noise or wheezing. When the child is not receiving enough oxygen, the skin becomes pale with circumoral cyanosis (slight blue tinge around the mouth). It is possible for the bronchi and lungs to become involved. The child may be anxious and frightened by the respiratory distress.

Patient Screening

Children experiencing signs and symptoms of respiratory distress, including hoarseness, fever, a harsh, high-pitched cough, and stridor during inspiration, require prompt, if not immediate, assessment and intervention.

Etiology

Croup is usually a viral disease that involves the larynx, trachea, and bronchi. Clinical manifestations are caused by edema and spasm of the vocal cords, creating varying degrees of obstruction (Fig. 2.42A).

Diagnosis

Croup must be distinguished from epiglottitis. If necessary, blood or throat cultures may be performed to identify certain bacterial causes. Laryngoscopy may be performed. Radiographs of the airway may show a characteristic "steeple sign" or be necessary to rule out an obstruction by a foreign body.

Treatment

The patient is treated symptomatically, with the administration of antipyretic agents, rest, increased fluid intake, cool humidification of air, and, if the cause is bacterial, antibiotic therapy. The steam from a warm shower may be beneficial. A dose of steroids may decrease airway edema. In severe cases, the patient is hospitalized for endotracheal intubation and oxygen therapy until the respiratory crisis passes. In most instances, the illness subsides in 3 to 4 days.

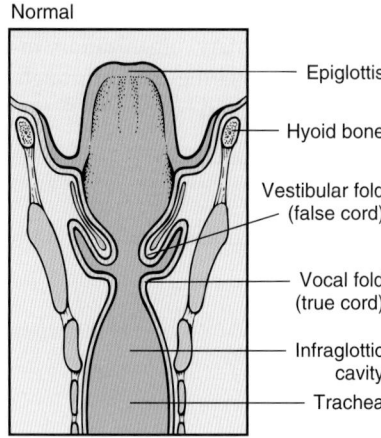

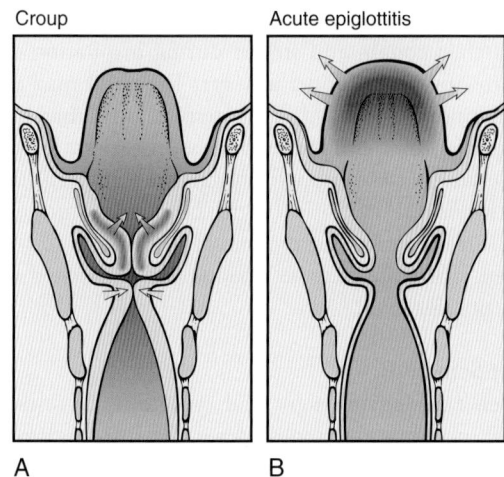

• **Fig. 2.42** Acute Inflammation of the Larynx. (A) Inflammation of the entire larynx, causing diffuse laryngeal swelling and laryngospasm (croup). (B) Inflammation localized to the epiglottis (so-called *acute epiglottitis*). (From Damjanov I: *Pathology for the health professions,* ed 4, St Louis, 2011, Saunders.)

Prognosis

The prognosis is good with prompt intervention. The child is likely to experience recurrences of the condition.

Prevention

Because croup is a viral disease, the only prevention is through avoidance of contact with respiratory viruses. Replace toothbrushes regularly and after any infectious process.

Patient Teaching

Instruct the parents *not* to place anything in the child's mouth until the child is assessed by a health care professional and epiglottitis is ruled out. Additional teaching includes instruction on handling and disposal of soiled tissues and the importance of good hand washing.

Epiglottitis

Description

Epiglottitis is inflammation of the epiglottis, the thin, leaf-shaped structure that covers the entrance of the larynx during swallowing.

ICD-10-CM Code   J05.10 *(Acute epiglottitis without obstruction)*
    J05.11 *(Acute epiglottitis with obstruction)*
    J37.0 *(Chronic laryngitis)*

Symptoms and Signs

Epiglottitis typically strikes children between ages 3 and 7 years. The symptoms include a sore throat, croupy cough, fever, and respiratory distress caused by laryngeal obstruction. Visual inspection reveals a red and swollen epiglottis. Rapidly increasing dyspnea and drooling are the most significant signs of this critical respiratory emergency (see Fig. 2.42B).

Patient Screening

Children experiencing any form of respiratory distress require immediate assessment and intervention. Instruct the parents *not* to place anything in the child's mouth until the child is assessed by a health care professional because airway spasm may result.

Etiology

Epiglottitis may follow an upper respiratory tract infection. The most common cause is *Haemophilus influenzae* type B (Hib). Other organisms that may be responsible for epiglottitis include *Streptococcus pneumoniae,* VZV, *Haemophilus parainfluenzae, Staphylococcus aureus,* and herpes simplex virus type 1 (HSV-1). Another form of epiglottitis, thermal epiglottitis, may be caused by heat damage to the epiglottis from ingestion of very hot liquids or food.

Diagnosis

Radiography of the neck may reveal an enlarged epiglottis. If the obstruction is not significant, the throat is examined to inspect the epiglottis. Nothing is placed in the child's mouth without the presence of a health care professional with the capability, equipment, and supplies needed to perform endotracheal intubation and tracheostomy.

Treatment

If the airway is obstructed, the child is hospitalized and given intensive care. The airway is established with tracheostomy or endotracheal intubation. Antibiotics, usually ampicillin, are given parenterally, and the patient is closely monitored.

Prognosis

Although this condition can be fatal if not treated, prompt treatment affords a good prognosis.

Prevention

The incidence of this potentially life-threatening condition has dramatically decreased following the introduction of the Hib conjugate vaccine. The AAP recommends that all children receive the Hib vaccine. Replace toothbrushes regularly and after any infectious process.

Patient Teaching

Instruct the parents *not* to place anything in the child's mouth until the child is assessed by a health care professional. Additional teaching includes instruction in the handling and disposal of soiled tissues and the importance of good hand washing. Reinforce the recommendation for immunization with the Hib conjugate vaccine.

Acute Tonsillitis

Description

Acute tonsillitis is a painful inflammatory and infectious process affecting the tonsils.

ICD-10-CM Code	J03.90 *(Acute tonsillitis, unspecified)*
	(J03.0-J03.91 = 9 codes for specificity)

Symptoms and Signs

Tonsillitis, or inflammation of the tonsils, usually has a sudden onset. The patient has a mild to severe sore throat, chills, fever, headache, malaise, anorexia, and muscle and joint pain. The tonsils appear inflamed and swollen, with yellowish exudate projecting from crypts. Lymph glands in the submandibular area are tender and enlarged (Fig. 2.43).

Patient Screening

An individual with pain, fever, and sore throat of sudden onset requires prompt assessment, with a culture and sensitivity test of the exudate obtained to determine the causative agent.

Etiology

Tonsillitis is caused by many organisms, with group A beta-hemolytic streptococci being the most common cause.

Diagnosis

The throat is examined, and a throat culture is performed to identify the causative organism. The WBC count may be elevated in response to the infection.

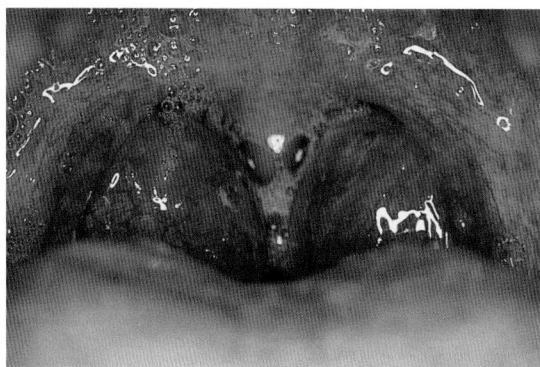

• **Fig. 2.43** Acute Tonsillitis. The tonsils are swollen and acutely inflamed, almost meeting in the middle. (From Stevens A, et al: *Core pathology*, ed 3, London, 2010, Mosby.)

Treatment

When the throat culture result is positive for group A streptococci ("strep throat"), a full 10-day course of penicillin is given. This strict regimen is necessary to prevent rheumatic fever, rheumatic heart disease, and renal complications. The child may need a liquid diet or saline throat irrigations if the pain is debilitating. Tonsillectomy may be recommended for chronic tonsillitis.

Prognosis

The prognosis is good with drug therapy. Surgery may be the option for chronic tonsillitis. Recovery from the surgical procedure usually is uneventful, although significant postoperative bleeding may occur. The patient should be evaluated in the emergency department should this occur.

Prevention

As with any infectious process, good hand washing and proper handling and disposal of soiled tissues helps prevent exposure to microbes. Toothbrushes should be replaced at least every 3 months or after any infectious process.

Patient Teaching

Teach the patient and family about the importance of hydration during illness. In addition, emphasize the importance of completing the entire recommended regimen of antibiotic therapy. Sharing of drinking glasses and eating utensils should be discouraged, and old toothbrushes should be replaced.

Adenoid Hyperplasia

Description

Adenoid hyperplasia is an abnormal enlargement of the lymphoid tissue located in the space above the soft palate of the mouth, causing a partial breathing blockage, especially in children.

ICD-10-CM Code	J35.2 *(Hypertrophy of adenoids)*
	(J32.0 J35.9 = 8 codes of specificity)

Refer to the physician's diagnosis and then to the current edition of the ICD-10-CM coding manual to ensure the greatest specificity of pathology.

Symptoms and Signs

Adenoids (and tonsils) are present at birth and play a role in the formation of immunoglobulins. After puberty, they normally atrophy.

Adenoid hyperplasia can contribute to recurrent otitis media and conductive hearing loss, resulting from obstruction of the eustachian tube. The child is usually a mouth breather and snores during sleep. In extreme cases, the obstruction may cause the child to experience episodes of sleep apnea. The child's speech has a nasal quality.

Patient Screening

Mouth-breathing children who snore should be evaluated for adenoid enlargement. Schedule the child for an assessment of adenoids, tonsils, nasopharynx, and oropharynx.

Etiology

The cause of adenoid hyperplasia is unknown. Contributing factors include repeated infections, chronic allergies, and heredity.

Diagnosis

The abnormal enlargement may be visualized on lateral pharyngeal radiographs or with a nasopharyngoscopic examination.

Treatment

Adenoidectomy is indicated for obstructive adenoids with recurrent otitis media or chronic serous otitis media with conductive hearing loss. It may also be indicated if the child is experiencing obstructive sleep apnea.

Prognosis

Surgical removal of the adenoids usually corrects the condition.

Prevention

No prevention is known.

Patient Teaching

Instruct the patient and the family about the importance of hydration during illness. Teach comfort measures and routine postoperative care when the adenoids have been removed.

Asthma

Description

Asthma is a chronic reversible obstructive disease caused by increased reactivity of the tracheobronchial tree to various stimuli. There are two major processes at work: constriction of the bronchioles and inflammation of the airway. It is a leading cause of chronic illness and school absenteeism in children.

ICD-10-CM Code	J45.909 *(Unspecified asthma, uncomplicated)*
	(J45-J45.998 = 18 codes of specificity)
	J45.998 *(Other asthma)*

Refer to the physician's diagnosis and then to the current edition of the ICD-10-CM coding manual to ensure the greatest specificity of pathology. Coding is done by extent of inflammation and type.

Symptoms and Signs

The child has an incessant productive or nonproductive cough, a pronounced expiratory wheeze, and rapid shallow respirations. The labored breathing results in a rapid pulse, pallor, profuse perspiration, and an inability to speak more than a few words without halting to breathe. The child often has nasal flaring and intercostal or sternal retractions. The patient often is anxious, is exhausted, and reports a "tight chest." The examining physician hears diminished breath sounds, with wheezes and rhonchi in the lungs. The bronchial spasms trap air and thick mucus in the lungs. An asthma exacerbation (Fig. 2.44) can be mild to severe, can last minutes or days, and may become a medical emergency. The attack may or may not have been preceded by a respiratory infection (Fig. 2.45) or exposure to a known trigger.

Patient Screening

Patients with asthma present an alarming clinical situation. A possible respiratory compromise requires prompt assessment and intervention.

Etiology

A hereditary factor is strongly associated with the disease. Asthma is the result of hyperactive and hypersensitive bronchial tubes. The bronchial spasms of asthma can be triggered by many extrinsic (allergic) or intrinsic (nonallergic) factors, including stress, heavy exercise, infection, and inhalation of allergens or other substances. Allergens may include pollen, cockroaches and their excrement, molds, household dust mites, and pet dander. Additional "triggers" include air pollutants and irritants (perfumes, colognes, and aftershaves), smoke and secondhand smoke, cold air, emotional upset, and exercise.

Diagnosis

The best tool available to reveal the degree of airway obstruction is the pulmonary function test. However, this test may show normal results between attacks. Chest radiography may show hyperinflation and changes in the lungs associated with mucous plugging. Specialists may order intradermal skin testing to identify inhalant and food allergies. Blood tests include a CBC with a differential leukocyte count, which may show an increased eosinophil count and elevated serum immunoglobulin E (IgE) levels (Fig. 2.46).

Treatment

Many individuals with chronic asthma require medical management under the care of an expert. Strict compliance with a regimen of medications to relax and widen the bronchi and to release excessive mucus is important. Some of the drugs used are cromolyn sodium, albuterol, theophylline, and aerosol corticosteroids. Allergy evaluation and skin testing may indicate immunotherapy by desensitization injections, commonly called *allergy shots*. Avoiding infection, known allergens, and other triggers is strongly advised. Individuals with asthma are encouraged to avoid smoking and exposure to secondhand smoke.

Severe acute asthma attacks are treated with injections of steroids and inhalation therapy. Steroids can reduce the airway inflammation, whereas inhaled albuterol decreases bronchoconstriction. The patient may require supplemental oxygen. In a severe attack that is refractory to drug therapy, a condition called *status asthmaticus* may lead to fatal respiratory failure and thus the need for endotracheal intubation. The patient requires hospitalization for aggressive medical treatment and follow-up. Occasionally some children may develop pneumonia concurrent with the asthma attack.

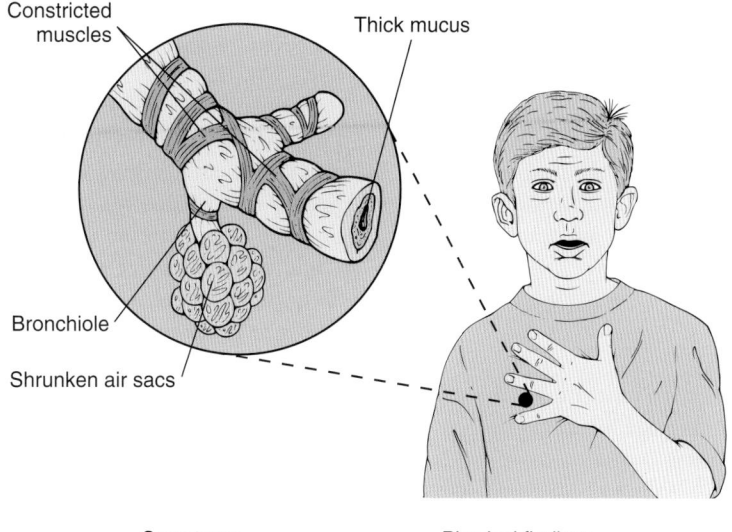

Symptoms	Physical findings
• Shortness of breath	• Rapid, shallow respirations
• Wheezing	• Rapid pulse
• Difficult breathing	• Pallor or cyanosis
• Cough	• Diminished breath sounds
• Anxiety	• Generalized retractions
	• Frequent pausing to catch the breath when talking
	• Hyperexpansion of the chest

• **Fig. 2.44** An asthma attack with respiratory distress.

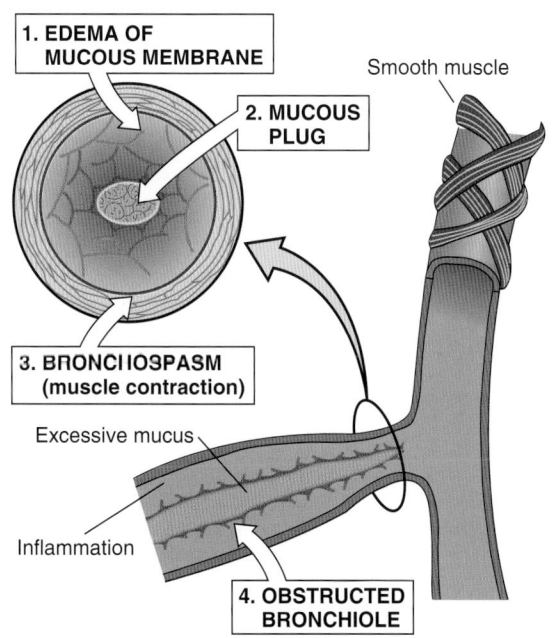

• **Fig. 2.45** Asthma—acute episode. (From Gould BE: *Pathophysiology for the health professions,* ed 4, St Louis, 2011, Saunders.)

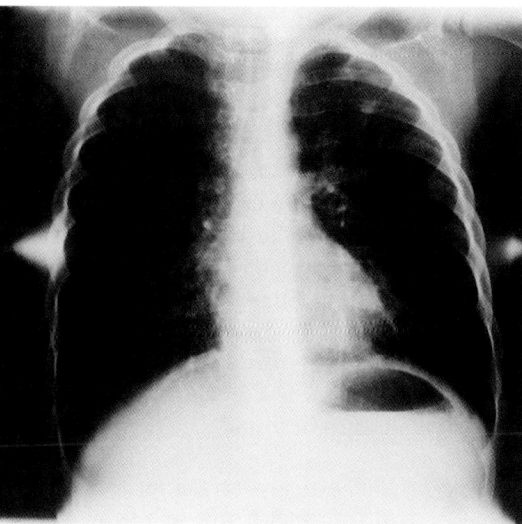

• **Fig. 2.46** Radiograph of lungs of child with asthma attack. (From Des Jardins T, Burton GC: *Clinical manifestations and assessment of respiratory disease,* ed 6, St Louis, 2011, Mosby.)

Prognosis

The prognosis varies, depending on the extent of the asthmatic attack and the causative factor. The use of prophylactic medications helps. Medication inhalers should be kept readily available at all times. Allergy testing may reveal the irritant, and allergy serum injections may help alleviate or reduce the severity of the attack. As previously mentioned, unresponsive asthma (status asthmaticus) may result in death.

Prompt medical intervention is necessary when an attack cannot be resolved by usual and available methods.

Prevention

The patient should take all controller medications as prescribed. Use of a daily controller medication helps to reduce the incidence and severity of the attacks. Avoiding any stimulating allergens and environments containing cigarette smoke is suggested. Injections of appropriate serum also may help prevent attacks.

Patient Teaching
Encourage patients to use prophylactic medications and to avoid known triggering allergens. Teach caregivers the importance of seeking medical help when an attack does not resolve quickly with normal intervention.

Bronchiolitis
Description
Bronchiolitis is inflammation of the bronchioles, the smallest air passages of the lungs, and is usually caused by viruses. It is a common disease in infancy.

ICD-10-CM Code	J21.8 (Acute bronchiolitis due to other specified organisms) (J21.0-J21.9 = 4 codes of specificity)

Symptoms and Signs
The infant or small child has a cough and nasal congestion that evolve into wheeze, tachypnea, and respiratory distress. Fever and posttussive emesis may be present. The patient may be breathing too fast to feed properly and can become dehydrated. In very young infants, especially in those who were premature, apnea may occur.

Patient Screening
Any infant with wheeze or respiratory distress must be evaluated immediately.

Etiology
Bronchiolitis is most commonly caused by infection with RSV. Many other viruses can cause this disease, including parainfluenza virus and adenovirus. Bronchiolitis is most common during the winter months (October through April). Infants in day care or who have school-age siblings are at highest risk. The natural progression of the infection is that symptoms worsen over the first few days of infection, peaking in severity around day 4 or 5, and then slowly improve.

Diagnosis
The diagnosis is made on the basis of patient history and physical examination. A chest radiograph may be obtained to rule out pneumonia. Rapid RSV testing is available in most emergency room settings to help with grouping of patients, but it does not affect management of the disease. Viral culture from the nasopharynx may also be obtained to determine etiology.

Treatment
Treatment is supportive care. Albuterol, racemic epinephrine, or hypertonic saline given via a nebulizer may improve respiratory symptoms. Supplemental oxygen may be required. If the patient is unable to feed, administration of IV fluids is necessary. In extreme cases, the patient experiences respiratory failure and must be intubated and mechanically ventilated until the infection runs its course.

Even after the acute infection, the airways may be sensitive for several weeks, leading to recurrent wheeze and cough.

Prognosis
Prognosis depends on the severity of the infection and early evaluation and initiation of supportive measures when needed. Premature infants and those with cardiac disorders or lung disease are at the greatest risk for complications. Children who receive prompt and appropriate care usually do quite well. There is a possible link between bronchiolitis and later development of asthma.

Prevention
Measures that reduce the spread of viruses, such as hand washing and avoidance of individuals symptomatic with respiratory infections, are the best ways of prevention. Infants who meet certain qualifications, such as prematurity, lung disease, and exposure to school-age siblings, may be able to receive vaccination with palivizumab, a monoclonal antibody against RSV. This immunization must be given monthly during the winter months when RSV infection is most prevalent. The qualification criteria are quite stringent because of the high cost of the vaccine.

Patient Teaching
Give the parents printed information about the disease. Parents need emotional support and understanding, especially when the child is hospitalized for treatment. Allow the parents to verbalize their anxieties and fears to a compassionate and understanding individual, thus providing a validation of their feelings in the situation.

Gastrointestinal Disorders
Infantile Colic
Description
Colic is intermittent distress in the newborn or during early infancy and has an unclear etiology.

ICD-10-CM Code	R10.9 (Unspecified abdominal pain) (R10.0-R10.9 = 29 codes of specificity)

Refer to the physician's diagnosis and then to the current edition of the ICD-10-CM coding manual to ensure the greatest specificity of pathology.

Symptoms and Signs
The infant intermittently draws up the legs, clenches the fists, and cries as if in pain. During the episode, the infant may pass gas via the mouth and the rectum. The episodes of colic are likely to occur in the late afternoon and evening. These babies usually thrive, gain weight, and appear to tolerate formula or mother's milk.

Patient Screening
Although not life-threatening, infantile colic is a very disruptive state in the life of the family with an infant with the

condition. This child requires prompt assessment, and an appointment should be scheduled as soon as convenient for all.

Etiology

The etiology of colic is unknown, although several theories have been advanced. One hypothesis suggests that improper feeding techniques may be responsible, and another theory blames overfeeding or swallowing of excessive air. Sensitivity to cow's milk may be the causative factor, even for the nursing infant. In this case, the nursing mother is urged to eliminate cow's milk from her own diet. Regardless of the cause, the infant is extremely uncomfortable and cries a great deal, with sleep pattern disturbance.

Diagnosis

Diagnosis is made by the symptoms and a physical examination to rule out other causes of the infant's fussiness.

Treatment

Investigation into possible causes is the first step in treatment. Eliminating any of the possible causative factors may help lessen the symptoms. The infant usually outgrows the condition at about age 3 months. Probiotics or simethicone can provide relief in some cases.

Prognosis

The prognosis for the child outgrowing colic type of symptoms is good. Parents can become exhausted both physically and emotionally with the colicky, constantly crying baby. Intervention by another family member or support person may be advised to prevent abuse of the baby.

Prevention

Because the etiology is unknown, prevention is also undetermined.

Patient Teaching

Encourage the use of support persons so that parents can get the needed rest. Many theories of treatment have been proposed; encourage parents to discuss these with the physician.

Helminth (Worm) Infestation

Description

Roundworms, pinworms, hookworms, and tapeworms all can take up residence in the GI tract. All of these worms are classified as helminths, and the term *helminth infestation* describes the presence of these parasites in the intestinal tract.

> ICD-10-CM Code B83.9 (Helminthiasis, unspecified)
> (B83.0-B83.9 = 7 codes for specificity)

Symptoms and Signs

Worm infestations in children occur as the eggs of parasites are introduced into their mouths from contaminated hands. After the pinworm *(Enterobius vermicularis)* eggs are swallowed, they hatch in the intestine. The female worms migrate to the perianal area at night, where they lay their eggs.

This process causes mild to intense itching and irritation in the area. The itching and scratching contaminates the fingers with the eggs and allows reingestion by the host.

Patient Screening

Children exhibiting behaviors that suggest the presence of intestinal worms require prompt assessment and intervention.

Etiology

E. vermicularis (pinworm) is one of many possible parasitic worms. It is the most common cause of helminth infestation in the United States, and most patients are preschool or school-age children and the mothers of infected children. Pinworms are transmitted directly or indirectly from human to human (Figs. 2.47 and 2.48).

Diagnosis

The diagnosis is made by detection of eggs or worms in the anal opening on transparent adhesive tape placed in the

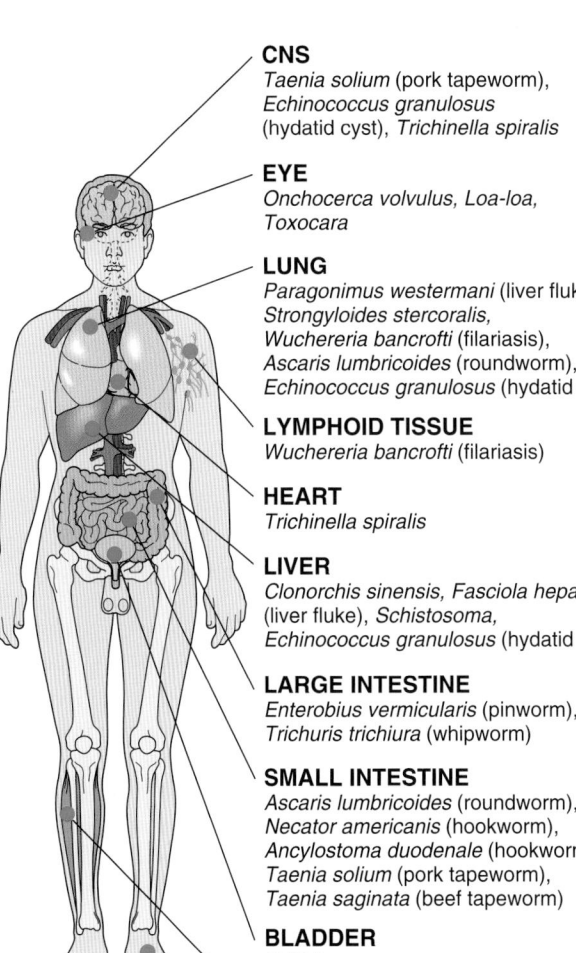

CNS
Taenia solium (pork tapeworm), *Echinococcus granulosus* (hydatid cyst), *Trichinella spiralis*

EYE
Onchocerca volvulus, Loa-loa, Toxocara

LUNG
Paragonimus westermani (liver fluke), *Strongyloides stercoralis, Wuchereria bancrofti* (filariasis), *Ascaris lumbricoides* (roundworm), *Echinococcus granulosus* (hydatid cyst)

LYMPHOID TISSUE
Wuchereria bancrofti (filariasis)

HEART
Trichinella spiralis

LIVER
Clonorchis sinensis, Fasciola hepatica (liver fluke), *Schistosoma, Echinococcus granulosus* (hydatid cyst)

LARGE INTESTINE
Enterobius vermicularis (pinworm), *Trichuris trichiura* (whipworm)

SMALL INTESTINE
Ascaris lumbricoides (roundworm), *Necator americanis* (hookworm), *Ancylostoma duodenale* (hookworm), *Taenia solium* (pork tapeworm), *Taenia saginata* (beef tapeworm)

BLADDER
Schistosoma

SKELETAL MUSCLE
Trichinella spiralis, Taenia solium (pork tapeworm)

SKIN
Onchocerca volvulus, Loa-loa, Toxocara

• **Fig. 2.47** Helminthic infestations. *CNS,* Central nervous system. (From Stevens A, et al.: *Core pathology,* ed 3, London, 2010, Mosby.)

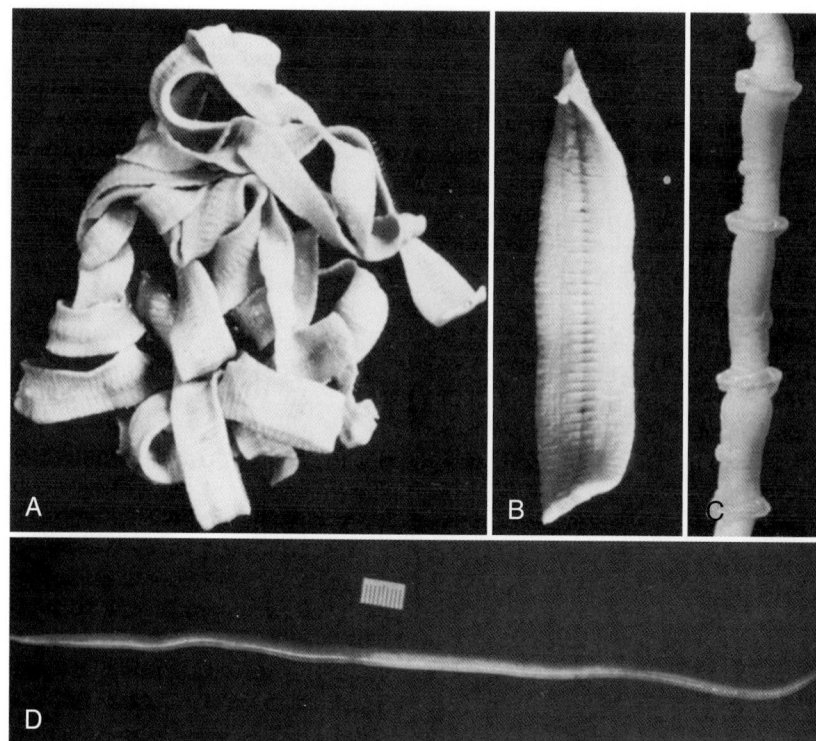

• **Fig. 2.48** Intestinal Worms. (A) Tapeworms. Part of the tapeworm *Diphyllobothrium latum*. The total length of the worm is greater than 30 feet. The head is about 1 mm in diameter, and the immature segments (proglottids) are much smaller than are the segments shown (×1.5). (B) Part of the worm shown in A. It is made up of many segments, each of which is wider than it is long. (C) Part of the tapeworm *Taenia saginata*. Each segment is longer than it is wide. (D) *Ascaris lumbricoides*. This worm is the largest roundworm parasite of humans and superficially resembles an earthworm (from the Latin lumbricus, an "earthworm"). It ranges in length from 15 to 35 cm. The specimen was approximately 20 cm (8 inches) in length. Other common roundworms are considerably smaller: *Trichuris trichiura*, 3 to 5 cm; *Enterobius vermicularis*, 8 to 13 mm; and *Ancylostoma duodenale*, up to 1 cm. (The scale above the roundworm shown is 1 cm.) (From Walter JB: *An introduction to the principles of disease*, ed 3, Philadelphia, 1992, Saunders.)

perianal area. A stool specimen examined microscopically may be positive.

Treatment

A complete course of anthelmintic agents is given; some physicians treat the entire family. Frequent showering and hand washing are advised. The worms and eggs also can be destroyed by the process of laundering clothing and linens in hot water with bleach.

Prognosis

The prognosis is good when the entire family is treated.

Prevention

Good hand washing and frequent showering help prevent infestation. Children should be encouraged not to touch or scratch the anus and not to put their hands in their mouths.

Patient Teaching

Stress the importance of good hand washing and other cleanliness measures. Point out to parents the importance of teaching children good hygiene habits, especially in the toileting process.

Diarrhea

Description

Diarrhea is rapid passage of stool through the intestinal tract, with a noticeable change in frequency, fluid content, appearance, and consistency.

ICD-10-CM Code   K52.2 *(Allergic and dietetic gastroenteritis and colitis)*

(K52.0-K52.9 = 7 codes of specificity)
K52.89 *(Other specified noninfective gastroenteritis and colitis)*
R19.7 *(Diarrhea, unspecified)*
Refer to the physician's diagnosis and then to the current edition of the ICD-10-CM coding manual to ensure the greatest specificity of pathology.

Symptoms and Signs

Diarrhea may be mild or severe, acute or chronic. In the infant or child, diarrhea can rapidly cause dehydration and electrolyte imbalance when fluid loss is profuse. Severe or prolonged diarrhea can produce metabolic acidosis; the patient may be lethargic and may hyperventilate. Depending on the cause, the symptoms could include intestinal cramping, weakness, nausea, irritability, and fever. Stool passage may become painful as a result of excoriation of the anus or skin in the diaper area.

Patient Screening

Children with diarrhea can become dehydrated rapidly. Prompt assessment is indicated.

Etiology

Diarrhea has multiple causes: infection (viral, bacterial, or parasitic), medications, allergic reactions, emotions, anatomic abnormalities, malabsorption syndromes, mechanical or chemical irritation resulting from the diet, and toxicity. The cause may be unknown.

Diagnosis

The clinician attempts to determine the degree of diarrheal disease, the underlying cause, and the fluid and electrolyte status of the patient. This requires a specific history of the onset and severity of symptoms, laboratory blood testing, stool cultures, and analysis of the stools.

Treatment

The treatment of diarrhea is directed at the cause, if known. Blood components are monitored for fluid and electrolyte balances. The frequency, color, consistency, and general composition of the stools are observed. Oral intake may be restricted to rest the intestinal tract and to reduce intestinal irritability. When infection is the cause, appropriate antibiotics may be given. Ignoring prolonged diarrhea in the infant or small child is dangerous. The patient may require hospitalization for IV fluid and electrolyte therapy.

Prognosis

The prognosis is good with prompt intervention. Dehydration and electrolyte imbalance are factors in the outcome of the condition. Hospitalization may be necessary to maintain hydration, stable electrolytes, and nutrition.

Prevention

Prevention is multifaceted because of the cause. Good hand washing is important in preventing microbial infections. Avoiding known allergens, certain medications, and dietary factors helps. Mechanical and chemical irritations in the diet may be eliminated. When the cause is anatomic abnormalities or malabsorption syndromes, preventive steps probably are few.

Patient Teaching

Emphasize the importance of hydration to the parents. Care of the anal area may be required as a result of the irritation caused by the loose and irritating stools. Good hand washing is necessary after handling soiled diapers or any other clothing that may contain stool. Teach the parents to observe urinary output for volume and color. When the child is in diapers, have the parents count the number of soiled or wet diapers within a set time and report this to the physician's office.

! ALERT!

Childhood Obesity

Childhood obesity has become a major health concern in the United States. Children with weights significantly beyond the average weight for age or height are often identified as having this serious health condition. As children become more and more obese, they are beginning a pattern that may plague them for the rest of their lives. Additionally, this condition may lead to health problems, such as diabetes, hypertension, hypercholesterolemia, respiratory ailments, and orthopedic problems. Another concern is that poor self-esteem and depression may occur in these children. They also may become targets for teasing and bullying by their peers.

The most common cause for childhood obesity is the combination of the eating too much food and not getting enough exercise. Types of food also play an important role in weight gain. Fast food restaurant type of food often has a content that is high in sugar and fat. Snacks, such as cookies, crackers, candy, and sodas, are high in calories and low in nutritional value. Many families consume prepared meals that are high in sodium and calories. Children today spend several hours a day sitting in front of a television screen or computer, communicating with peers or others on a cell phone or tablet, limiting quality exercise and the burning of calories.

Because parents usually make decisions regarding food and activity, they are encouraged to provide nutritious food for their children, as well as limiting the time the child spends watching TV, playing computer games, and sitting at a computer. Schools are being encouraged to provide nutritious meals containing fruits and vegetables and less fat and sugar. The schools also are urged to increase student physical activity with quality exercise. In addition to burning calories, exercise is essential for building strong bones and muscles.

During a well-child examination, the health care provider compares the child's weight and height with the Centers for Disease Control and Prevention (CDC) standard growth charts, and the child's body mass index (BMI) is measured as well. A child who has a BMI-for-age between the 85th and 94th percentiles is considered overweight. When a child has a BMI-for-age that is in the 95th percentile or above, he or she is considered obese. The health care provider takes into consideration the child's growth and development, family weight-for-height history, and skeletal and muscular structure of the body before making a diagnosis of obesity.

Five or more daily servings of fruit and vegetables are recommended. Many children consume fried potatoes as their five daily servings. Drinking sodas high in sugar content has increased steadily, whereas intake of milk has declined. Missed breakfasts, eating dinners outside the home, and increased snacking also contribute to the increasing incidence of obesity. Another factor in the increased incidence of obesity is a change in lifestyle. Many children ride buses or are driven to school rather than walking. Numerous children have no safe place to be physically active because of lack of outdoor lighting or a protected place to play or because of high rates of crime or unrestrained dogs in the neighborhood. Several neighborhoods do not have sidewalks where children can walk safely.

There is no simple answer to dealing with childhood obesity. It is a complex situation that involves lifestyle, intake of too much food, consumption of high-calorie foods and beverages, economic status, environmental circumstances, home location, transportation versus walking, decreased or restricted exercise activities, and increased TV, computer, or electronic game time. Family history, body structure, ethnic background, social factors, and genetics all play a role, along with diet and exercise, in the incidence of childhood obesity.

Vomiting

Description

Vomiting, or ejection of stomach contents through the mouth, is a common symptom in infants and children.

ICD-10-CM Code	R11.10 *(Vomiting, unspecified)*
	(R11.0-R11.2 = 6 codes of specificity)
	R11.11 *(Vomiting without nausea)*
	R11.12 *(Projectile vomiting)*

Symptoms and Signs

Vomiting can range from a mild regurgitation to projectile expulsion. The infant has a distended abdomen, is irritable, and often has a fever. Aspiration of vomitus into the lungs can result in pneumonia.

Patient Screening

Chronic or severe vomiting deserves special attention as a warning sign of disease or possible dehydration. Assessment is essential. Projectile vomiting requires prompt assessment.

Etiology

Vomiting, which is more common in infants than in children, usually results from trivial or temporary factors. However, it has a host of possible causes, including overfeeding, food allergy, gastric irritation, infection, drug poisoning, elevated intracranial pressure, defects (e.g., pyloric stenosis), and habitual voluntary vomiting.

Diagnosis

Vomiting in the infant or child always must be evaluated in the context of the child's total state of health. One assesses causative factors by performing a physical examination, taking the history, and monitoring the patient's vital signs, weight, nutritional status, and fluid and electrolyte balance. Radiographic studies of the intestinal tract may be indicated.

Treatment

Most vomiting can be expected to abate spontaneously. Food may be withheld for a time to rest the upper GI tract and to reduce gastric irritation. When treatment is indicated, it depends on the cause, severity, and nature of the vomiting. Infant feeding problems require changes in technique or intake. Other more serious causes, such as infection, poisoning, and congenital anomalies of the GI tract, may require direct medical or surgical intervention.

Prognosis

The prognosis varies, depending on the cause. Most vomiting subsides in a few hours. Longer periods of vomiting requiring medical or surgical intervention may or may not be corrected. Hydration, nutrition, and electrolyte balance are important factors in the resolution of the condition.

Prevention

Prevention varies depending on causative factors. Avoiding overfeeding, known food allergens, and substances that cause gastric irritation often is all that is necessary to prevent recurrence. Infection, drug poisoning, elevated intracranial pressure, defects (e.g., pyloric stenosis), and habitual voluntary vomiting may not be preventable.

Patient Teaching

Emphasize the importance of hydration and nutrition along with thorough hand washing after handling emesis.

Blood Disorders

Anemia

Description

Anemia is abnormal reduction in the concentration of RBCs or in the hemoglobin content of circulating blood. It is not a disease, but a symptom of various diseases. Anemia can lead to tissue hypoxia. See Chapter 10 for additional information on anemias.

ICD-10-CM Code	D64.9 *(Anemia, unspecified)*
	(D64.0-D64.9 = 9 codes of specificity)

Refer to the physician's diagnosis and then to the current edition of the ICD-10-CM coding manual to ensure the greatest specificity of pathology.

Symptoms and Signs

Pallor, weakness, fatigability, and listlessness are noted initially in the child or infant with anemia. Palpitations, tachycardia, cardiac enlargement, jaundice, and mental sluggishness are symptoms of severe anemia.

Laboratory studies show reduced hematocrit and hemoglobin concentration. Other laboratory results vary, depending on the underlying cause or type of anemia.

Patient Screening

When parents report that their child appears pale, weak, easily fatigued, and listless, prompt assessment is required.

Etiology

Iron deficiency is the most common cause of anemia in children. Other causes include acute or chronic blood loss, decreased blood formation, nutritional deficiency disorders, hemolytic diseases, inhibition or loss of bone marrow, and sickle cell disease.

Diagnosis

Diagnosis is based on findings from physical examination and laboratory testing for signs and symptoms of anemia. Diagnostic tests include determination of hemoglobin concentration, hematocrit levels, serum iron levels, RBC count, mean corpuscular hemoglobin levels, and bone marrow studies. It is often helpful to view a blood smear under a microscope.

Treatment

The first priority of treatment is to determine the cause of anemia. For iron deficiency anemia, iron-rich foods and oral preparations of ferrous sulfate are administered. When blood loss is the cause, blood volume is restored by transfusion. Replacement therapy is indicated in deficiency states (e.g., vitamin B_{12}, folic acid, and ascorbic acid deficiency). Specific hemolytic blood disorders are treated when the anemia is caused by excessive blood cell destruction. A planned program of activity balanced with rest is recommended during treatment.

Prognosis

The prognosis varies, depending on the cause. When diet modification can be recommended and followed, the prognosis is good. When the problem is bleeding and the source of the bleed can be determined and corrected, the prognosis is good with blood replacement and dietary supplement. Hemolytic disorders have a fair prognosis with aggressive treatment once the hemolytic disorder is identified.

Prevention

Diets meeting the daily requirement of iron and other vitamins and minerals help prevent iron deficiency anemia. Prompt exploration of any unexplained type of bleeding helps reveal underlying conditions and allows for prompt treatment.

Patient Teaching

Encourage parents to provide children with nutritious diets and the recommended nutritional supplements and pediatric vitamins and minerals. Emphasize the importance of follow-up appointments for these children.

Leukemia

Description

Leukemia, a cancer of blood-forming tissues, is the most common childhood malignancy. It is characterized by an abnormal increase in the number of immature WBCs or undifferentiated blastocytes.

ICD-10-CM Code	C95.9 (Leukemia, unspecified)
	(C90.1-C95.92 = 105 codes of specificity)

Refer to the physician's diagnosis and then to the current edition of the ICD-10-CM coding manual to ensure the greatest specificity of pathology.

Symptoms and Signs

Bone marrow infiltration by leukemic cells leads to anemia, susceptibility to infection resulting from neutropenia, and prolonged bleeding time resulting from the reduction in the amount of platelets. Common signs and symptoms include fever, easy bruising, pallor, weakness, weight loss, and bone and joint pain. The abnormal cells can invade various organs of the body, causing pressure symptoms in those areas. Lymph nodes and the spleen may become enlarged.

Patient Screening

When the parents report that their child has a fever, frequent infections, easy bruising, pallor, and weakness, prompt assessment is required.

Etiology

Two general types of leukemia are found in children, acute lymphoid leukemia (ALL) and acute myelogenous leukemia (AML). These main types are further divided into subtypes based on the specific aberrations of the WBCs. About 80% of childhood leukemias are ALLs. The etiology is unknown. Predisposing factors include congenital disorders, such as Down syndrome and radiation exposure. The peak age of incidence is between 2 years and 6 years. See Chapter 10 for additional discussion of leukemia.

Diagnosis

A peripheral blood smear shows immature forms of WBCs. Leukocytosis, neutropenia, anemia, and thrombocytopenia are often present. Laboratory studies also include measurement of uric acid levels, electrolytes, kidney and liver function, and coagulation studies. A specimen from bone marrow aspiration is examined. Chromosome analysis of the leukemic cells is performed for diagnosis and because the presence of different characteristic abnormalities has prognostic value. A lumbar puncture is performed to determine whether the CNS is involved because this determination can guide therapy.

Treatment

The disease is treated through systemic chemotherapy to eradicate leukemic cells and to induce remission. Chemotherapy is administered intrathecally to treat or as a prophylaxis against CNS invasion. The patient must be followed up closely for signs of tumor lysis syndrome, a group of metabolic complications that develop because of the destruction of leukemic cells when chemotherapy is initiated. Bone marrow transplantation (BMT) is a possible treatment for children with a poor prognosis or relapsed ALL or for children with AML (because AML carries a poorer prognosis than ALL when treated solely with chemotherapy). Psychological support for the child and the family must be provided.

Prognosis

The best prognostic indicators in determining long-term survival are the patient's age at diagnosis, WBC count at diagnosis, cytogenetics, and immunophenotype (T cell or B cell). For ALL, having a WBC count greater than 50,000/μL, age greater than 10 years or less than 1 year, and having certain cytogenic abnormalities, such as Philadelphia chromosome (a translocation between chromosomes 9 and 22), are associated with a poorer prognosis. For AML, a WBC count greater than 100,000/μL and certain chromosomal abnormalities, such as monosomy of chromosome 7, carry a poorer prognosis. In addition, failure to achieve remission by day 28 of therapy is associated with a poor prognosis.

Still, most children with leukemia survive the disease. Of those treated solely with chemotherapy, 80% achieve long-term, disease-free survival. Long-term survival for those undergoing BMT ranges from 25% to 50%. However, these long-term survivors can experience late adverse effects from the treatment, including CNS impairment, delayed growth, infertility, and even secondary cancers. Because of this, these children should be closely followed up after treatment.

Prevention
There is no known prevention.

Patient Teaching
Work with parents to contact support groups.

Erythroblastosis Fetalis (Hemolytic Disease of the Newborn)

Description
Erythroblastosis fetalis stems from the incompatibility of fetal and maternal blood, resulting in excessive rates of RBC destruction.

ICD-10-CM Code	P55.8 (Other hemolytic diseases of newborn)
	(P55.0-P55.9 = 4 codes of specificity)
	P55.9 (Hemolytic disease of newborn, unspecified)

Symptoms and Signs
Erythroblastosis fetalis is characterized by anemia, jaundice, kernicterus, and enlargement of the liver and the spleen. In the most severe form, called *hydrops fetalis,* the fetus or infant is in great jeopardy because of extreme hemolysis. If the infant survives, the condition is marked by heart failure, edema, pulmonary congestion, lethargy, seizures, and intellectual developmental disorder.

Patient Screening
Physicians caring for expectant mothers who have had prenatal care should understand the possibility of Rh incompatibility. New patients aware of possible Rh incompatibility because they know their Rh factor is negative should be scheduled to discuss the matter with the physician as soon as convenient for all parties. Newborn infants with hemolytic disease of the newborn are identified during the newborn examination if not before birth, and treatment will be instituted as soon as possible.

Etiology
The cause is Rh factor incompatibility. Rh factor is the antigen found on the RBCs of the Rh-positive individual. The mother, through a prior pregnancy, has become sensitized to the Rh factor (Rh isoimmunization) of the fetal RBCs. When sensitized maternal blood finds its way into fetal circulation, particularly during delivery, the antibodies in the mother's blood destroy the RBCs of the fetus (Figs. 2.49 and 2.50).

With an Rh-negative woman and an Rh-positive man, some or all of the infants will be Rh positive. During pregnancy, blood from the Rh-positive fetus may move from fetal circulation into the mother's bloodstream, where it stimulates the mother's body to form antibodies against the Rh factor. When sufficient quantities of the antibodies pass back into the infant's circulation, the antibodies can clump and destroy Rh-positive cells, causing the symptoms of erythroblastosis fetalis.

Diagnosis
Blood typing of the mother and the father is essential. The maternal history includes pregnancy, elective and spontaneous abortions, and blood transfusions. The direct Coombs test of the umbilical cord blood measures Rh-positive antibodies in the newborn; the bilirubin test for bilirubinemia and hematocrit determination also are performed on the infant's blood. The amniotic fluid may be analyzed for hemolysis.

Treatment
The treatment is dictated by the degree of erythroblastosis fetalis and its effect on the fetus or the newborn. Intrauterine transfusions may be indicated when the fetus shows signs of distress. When necessary, the delivery of the infant is planned 2 to 4 weeks before term. Through exchange transfusion, the infant is given fresh group-O, Rh-negative blood. Phototherapy and albumin infusion are used to reduce the amount of circulating bilirubin in the newborn.

Prognosis
The prognosis is good when the disease is discovered early in pregnancy and closely monitored. Early delivery with immediate transfusion usually treats this condition successfully. Mothers with Rh-negative blood factor need to continue Rho-GAM injections for protection in subsequent pregnancies, including any spontaneous or induced abortions.

Prevention
Protection is now available for Rh-negative mothers who have never been sensitized, preventing the possibility of harm to an Rh-positive baby. Rho(D) immune globulin is given at 28 weeks in the Rh-positive identified pregnancy and as soon as possible to the woman at risk after each exposure to Rh-positive blood (most often by giving birth to an Rh-positive infant) to prevent maternal Rh isoimmunization and complications in subsequent pregnancies.

Patient Teaching
Emphasize the importance of Rh screening to all pregnant females. Those who are Rh negative require information about Rh-negative mothers with Rh-positive babies. Provide help with finding and contacting community support groups.

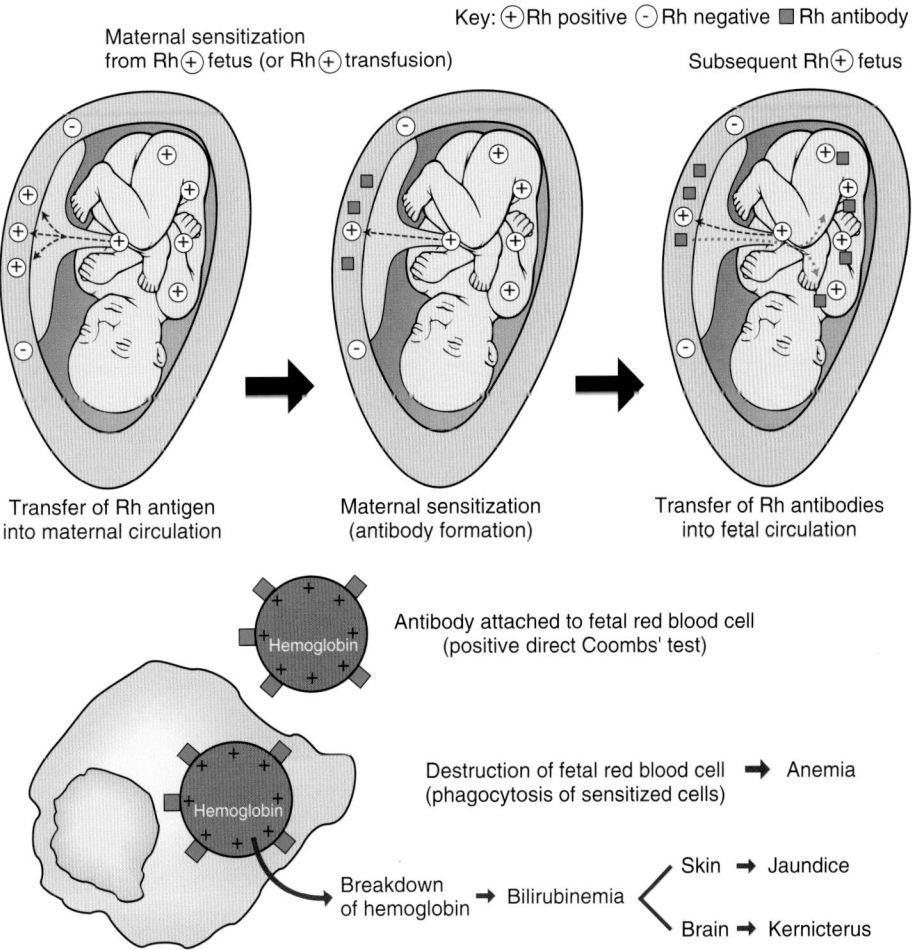

Key: ⊕ Rh positive ⊖ Rh negative ■ Rh antibody

Maternal sensitization from Rh⊕ fetus (or Rh⊕ transfusion)

Subsequent Rh⊕ fetus

Transfer of Rh antigen into maternal circulation

Maternal sensitization (antibody formation)

Transfer of Rh antibodies into fetal circulation

Antibody attached to fetal red blood cell (positive direct Coombs' test)

Hemoglobin

Hemoglobin

Destruction of fetal red blood cell (phagocytosis of sensitized cells) → Anemia

Breakdown of hemoglobin → Bilirubinemia < Skin → Jaundice / Brain → Kernicterus

• **Fig. 2.49** Etiology of erythroblastosis fetalis (hemolytic disease of the newborn). (Redrawn with permission of Ross Products Division, Abbott Laboratories, from Congenital heart abnormalities [Clinical Education Aid No. 7], 1992.)

Lead Poisoning

Description

Lead poisoning is an environmentally caused blood toxicity resulting from ingestion or inspiration of lead dust or particles.

ICD-10-CM Code   M1A.10X1 *(Lead-induced chronic gout, unspecified site, with tophus [tophi])*
(M1A.10-M1A.19X1 = 24 codes of specificity)
T56.0X1A *(Toxic effect of lead and its compounds, accidental [unintentional], initial encounter)*
T56.0X2A *(Toxic effect of lead and its compounds, intentional self-harm, initial encounter)*
T56.0X3A *(Toxic effect of lead and its compounds, assault, initial encounter)*
T56.0X4A *(Toxic effect of lead and its compounds, undetermined, initial encounter)*
Refer to the physician's diagnosis and then to the current edition of the ICD-10-CM coding manual to ensure the greatest specificity of pathology.

Symptoms and Signs

Children exposed to toxic levels of lead, a poisonous metallic element, exhibit signs of lead poisoning. Some warning signs are loss of appetite, vomiting, irritability, and ataxic gait. Chronic symptoms include anemia, weakness, colic, and peripheral neuritis. Evidence of intellectual developmental disorder resulting from brain damage is possible. A child with acute lead intoxication presents as a medical emergency. The child has symptoms of encephalopathy with vomiting, headache, stupor, convulsions, and coma resulting from cerebral edema (Fig. 2.51).

Patient Screening

Children exhibiting fatigue, headaches, irritability, stomachaches, cramps, muscle and joint pain, and changes in behavior require prompt assessment.

Etiology

Any level of lead in blood is abnormal. Exposure results from breathing or swallowing substances containing lead. The condition has been reported to develop in children who eat flakes of peeling lead paint, drink water from lead pipes, or ingest lead salts in certain foods. Some imported toys have been found to contain lead or are painted with

Rh FACTOR INCOMPATIBILITY OF MATERNAL–FETAL BLOOD

(ERYTHROBLASTOSIS FETALIS, OR HEMOLYTIC DISEASE OF THE NEWBORN)

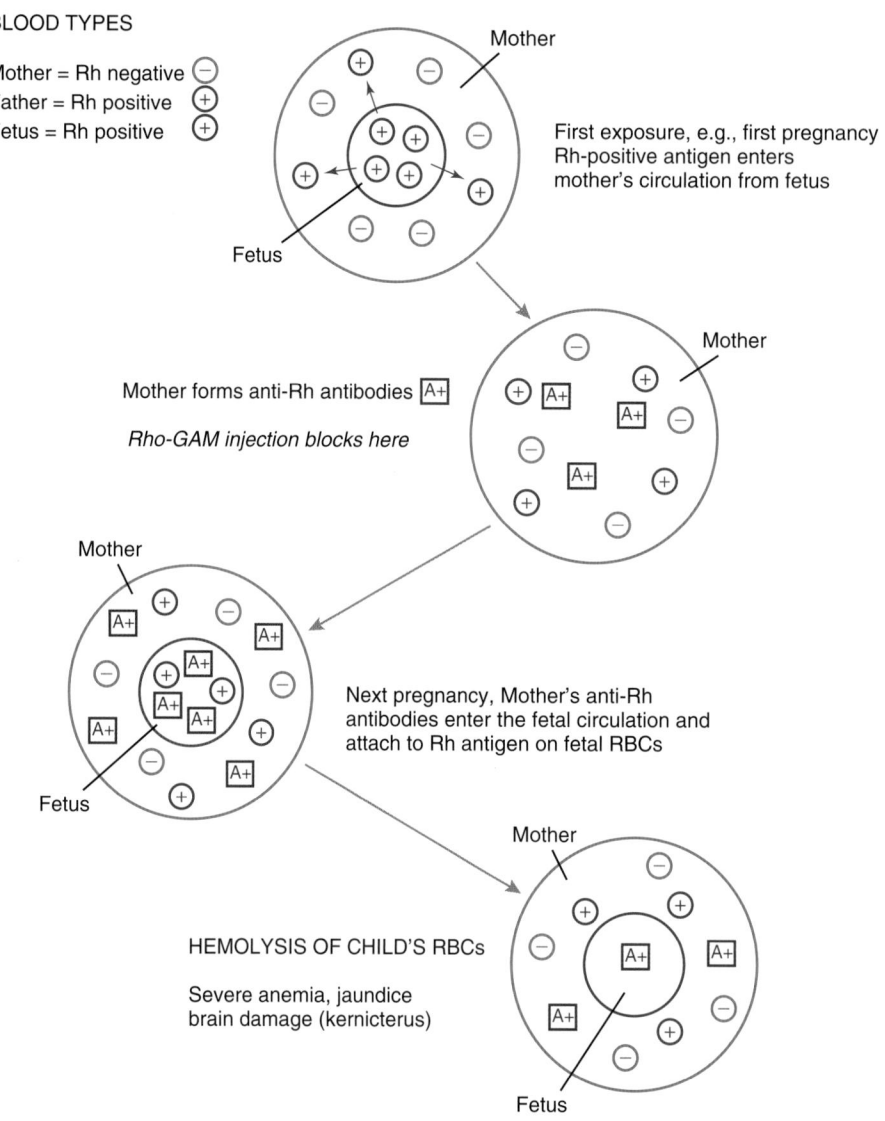

BLOOD TYPES

Mother = Rh negative ⊖
Father = Rh positive ⊕
Fetus = Rh positive ⊕

First exposure, e.g., first pregnancy
Rh-positive antigen enters
mother's circulation from fetus

Mother forms anti-Rh antibodies A+

Rho-GAM injection blocks here

Next pregnancy, Mother's anti-Rh
antibodies enter the fetal circulation and
attach to Rh antigen on fetal RBCs

HEMOLYSIS OF CHILD'S RBCs

Severe anemia, jaundice
brain damage (kernicterus)

• **Fig. 2.50** Rh incompatibility of maternal and fetal blood. *RBCs,* Red blood cells. (From Gould BE: *Pathophysiology for the health professions,* ed 4, St Louis, 2011, Saunders.)

lead-based paint. Lead dust may remain in soil contaminated by exhaust from previous use of leaded gasoline. Lead taken into the body is stored in many tissues; it is released into blood and excreted in urine.

Diagnosis

The history of lead exposure and the presence of symptoms previously listed suggest the diagnosis. Blood tests reveal anemia and a blood lead level greater than 5 μg/dL. Lead excretion through urine is increased. Characteristic changes in the ends of growing bones are noted on radiographs.

Treatment

The source of poisoning first must be eliminated. Subsequent treatment is based on lead level and symptoms.

For patients with levels greater than 25 μg/dL, an attempt may be made to remove the lead from the body by giving substances, known as *chelating agents,* that tie up the lead in a chemically inactive form in the bloodstream while it is transported to the kidneys for elimination. Antiemetics help control nausea and vomiting, and sedation is given for convulsions. After acute therapy, penicillamine (a chelating agent for lead) is given orally for 3 to 6 months.

Prognosis

The prognosis varies, depending on the extent of damage and the promptness in discovering the toxicity. Aggressive intervention and removal of the child from the contaminated environment help prevent additional damage.

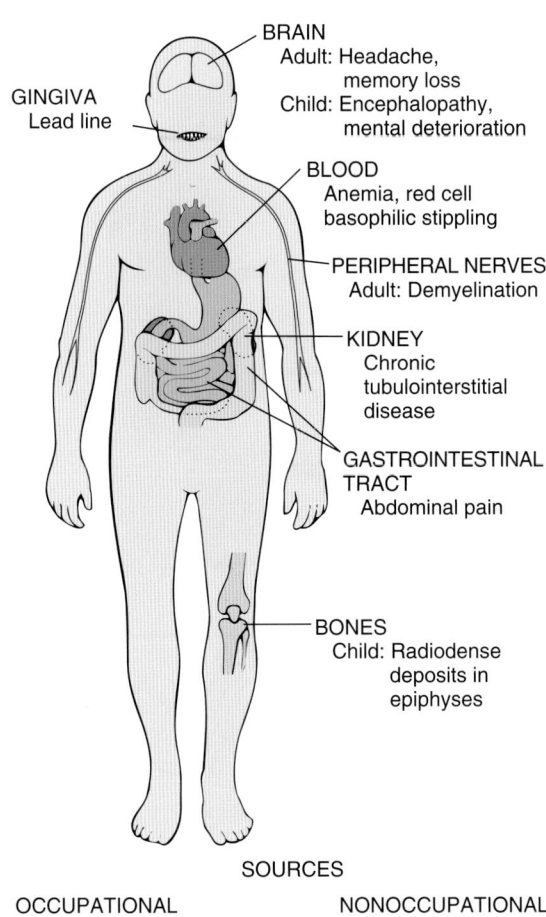

GINGIVA
Lead line

BRAIN
Adult: Headache,
memory loss
Child: Encephalopathy,
mental deterioration

BLOOD
Anemia, red cell
basophilic stippling

PERIPHERAL NERVES
Adult: Demyelination

KIDNEY
Chronic
tubulointerstitial
disease

GASTROINTESTINAL
TRACT
Abdominal pain

BONES
Child: Radiodense
deposits in
epiphyses

SOURCES

OCCUPATIONAL
Spray painting
Foundry work
Mining and extracting lead
Battery burning

NONOCCUPATIONAL
Water supply
Paint dust and flakes
House dust
Urban soil
Newsprint
Automotive exhaust

• **Fig. 2.51** Clinical and pathologic features of lead poisoning. (From Kumar V, Cotran R, Robbins S: *Robbins basic pathology,* ed 8, Philadelphia, 2008, Saunders.)

Prevention

An awareness of the environmental sources of lead, such as lead paint, lead plumbing, and other sources of lead dust is prudent. An act, Title X, or the Lead-Based Paint Hazard Act of 1992, has helped prevent exposure to lead in homes built before 1978 by requiring disclosure of lead-based paint hazards in the home. Dust on vinyl mini-blinds may contain lead deposits. Caution must be used with imported toys that may contain lead or be painted with lead-based paint.

Patient Teaching

Teaching the parents about the hazards of lead poisoning and how to recognize toxic sources is essential.

Miscellaneous Diseases, Syndromes, and Disorders

Reye Syndrome

Description

Reye syndrome is a combination of brain disease and fatty invasion of the inner organs, especially the liver.

ICD-10-CM Code   G93.7 *(Reye's syndrome)*
Refer to the physician's diagnosis and then to the current edition of the ICD-10-CM coding manual to ensure the greatest specificity of pathology.

Symptoms and Signs

This rare syndrome is an acute, often fatal illness that may affect children through age 15 years. The pathogenesis includes a disruption in the urea cycle that causes swelling of the brain, resulting in increased intracranial pressure. The symptoms of Reye syndrome progress through five stages: (1) lethargy, listlessness, irritability, combativeness, vomiting, and hepatic dysfunction; (2) hyperventilation, hyperactive reflexes, hepatic dysfunction, disorientation, convulsions, and delirium; (3) organ changes and coma; (4) deeper coma and loss of cerebral functions; and (5) seizures, loss of deep tendon reflexes, and respiratory arrest.

Patient Screening

Children who begin vomiting 3 to 6 days after a viral illness, such as chickenpox, are possible candidates for Reye syndrome and require immediate assessment and intervention.

Etiology

The cause of Reye syndrome is unknown. However, it typically follows infection with influenza A or B viruses or chickenpox. It has been linked to the use of aspirin during these infections.

Diagnosis

The medical history and the patient's clinical features suggest the disease. Laboratory blood studies show elevated serum ammonia levels. Liver function tests show elevated enzyme levels. Other tests include liver biopsy and CSF analysis.

Treatment

The early recognition and treatment of Reye syndrome has reduced the mortality rate from 90% to 20%. Successful management with early diagnosis involves hospitalization to stabilize the patient, to control cerebral edema, to monitor blood chemistries, to manage seizures, and to provide mechanical ventilation, if needed. Complete recovery is possible.

Prognosis

The prognosis is good with prompt intervention and aggressive treatment.

Prevention

For prevention, the use of nonsalicylate analgesics and antipyretics, such as acetaminophen, is recommended, instead of aspirin.

Patient Teaching

Caution all parents or caregivers that children should not be given aspirin during possible viral infections.

Fetal Alcohol Syndrome

Description

The term *fetal alcohol syndrome* (FAS) describes birth defects and other associated problems in infants born to women who consume alcohol during their pregnancy.

ICD-10-CM Code	P04.3 *(Newborn [suspected to be] affected by maternal use of alcohol)*
	Q86.0 *(Fetal alcohol syndrome [dysmorphic])*

Symptoms and Signs

Intrauterine exposure to sufficient levels of alcohol has been associated with fetal delayed growth, in which the infants are short and below average in weight. Facial characteristics of FAS include smaller eye openings, with eyes spaced widely apart, and a thin upper lip. The infant may experience growth deficiencies and CNS problems. Heart defects, including ASD and VSD, may be present. FAS also is associated with intellectual developmental disorder. The infant may exhibit signs of alcohol withdrawal shortly after birth.

These children may experience learning difficulties, including decreased attention span and memory, visual and auditory problems, and communication difficulties. Poor development of social skills may be present.

Patient Screening

Maternal history and newborn examination usually reveal the condition. Parents seeking medical attention for the child at any stage of development should be scheduled for the earliest possible appointment.

Etiology

FAS is caused when alcohol enters the fetal blood as a result of chronic, excessive use of alcohol by the mother during pregnancy.

Diagnosis

Typical clinical features present in the newborn and a maternal history of chronic alcoholism determine the diagnosis (Fig. 2.52).

Treatment

The treatment depends on the defects present in the newborn. Much of the treatment is supportive because neurologic damage cannot be reversed. Proper nutrition is vital. Because the baby may have a poor sucking reflex, special adaptation may be necessary to ensure proper intake. The psychosocial needs of the infant and the mother must be addressed.

Prognosis

As previously mentioned, neurologic damage cannot be reversed; therefore, the prognosis varies, depending on the amount of neurologic damage sustained.

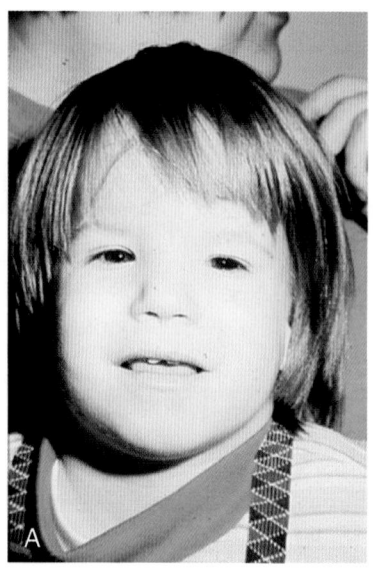

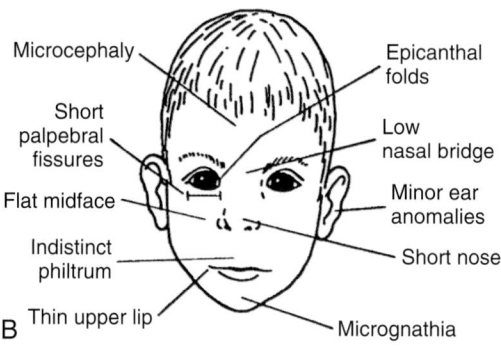

• **Fig. 2.52** (A) Fetal alcohol syndrome (FAS). (B) Affected children typically have features, which, when accompanied by intellectual developmental disorder, are diagnostic of FAS. The features on the left are those most often seen in patients with FAS, whereas those on the right are features that are seen with increased frequency in this population compared with the general population. (From Jones KL, Smith DW, Ulleland CN, et al.: Pattern of malformation in offspring of chronic alcoholic mothers, *Lancet* 1:1267, 1973.)

Prevention

Preventive measures include prenatal care and education. Because experts do not agree on a safe maximum amount of alcohol intake during pregnancy, women generally are advised not to drink during pregnancy.

Patient Teaching

Females should be advised not to drink during pregnancy. In addition, good prenatal care should be emphasized.

Diaper Rash

Description

Diaper rash, considered a contact dermatitis, is evident in the diaper area as an irritation or rash.

ICD-10-CM Code	L22 *(Diaper dermatitis)*

Symptoms and Signs

Diaper rash can vary from mild to severe and can be self-limiting or a chronic source of discomfort to the infant and dismay to the parent or the caregiver. Diaper rash takes multiple forms: from a mild excoriation, or maculopapular rash, to blisters and ulceration.

Patient Screening

Infants and toddlers with diaper rash that does not clear require prompt assessment.

Etiology

Infants with sensitive skin seem to have a hereditary predisposition to diaper rash, or irritant dermatitis. Diaper rash may be triggered by friction or prolonged exposure to moisture, feces, or the ammonia produced by bacterial action on urine. Poorly washed or rinsed diapers and the use of occlusive plastic pants over the diapers may be contributing factors. Poor hygiene or overzealous cleaning could irritate the diaper area.

Diagnosis

One may need to differentiate diaper rash from seborrheic dermatitis, eczema, and secondary skin infection.

Treatment

In addition to frequent diaper changes and proper cleaning and drying of the diaper area, a bland protective agent, such as zinc oxide or hydrated petrolatum, may promote healing. If possible, allowing the infant to remain without a diaper for some time will promote healing. Topical antimicrobial agents are used for secondary skin infection. Cloth diapers should be rinsed of irritating residue.

Prognosis

The prognosis is good.

Prevention

Frequent changing of diapers accompanied by thorough cleansing of the diaper area helps prevent the rash. Leaving the area exposed to air for short periods often will allow the area to dry and helps prevent the rash from returning.

Patient Teaching

Stress the importance of changing the infant's or toddler's diaper on a regular schedule and not leaving the child in a soiled diaper for extended periods. If necessary, demonstrate the method of cleansing the diaper area.

Neuroblastoma

Description

Neuroblastoma, a cancer of the sympathetic nervous system, is the third most common childhood malignancy. It arises from primitive sympathetic ganglion cells.

ICD-10-CM Code	C74.90 (*Malignant neoplasm of unspecified part of unspecified adrenal gland*)
	(C74.0-C74.92 = 9 codes of specificity)

Refer to the physician's diagnosis and then to the current edition of the ICD-10-CM coding manual to ensure the greatest specificity of pathology.

Symptoms and Signs

Neuroblastoma can arise from any site in the sympathetic nervous system, with the adrenal gland and the abdomen being the most common areas. Symptoms include abdominal mass, abdominal pain or fullness, anemia, bone pain, fever, hypertension, and weight loss. Periorbital ecchymosis ("raccoon eyes") is not uncommon (Fig. 2.53).

Patient Screening

When the parents report that their child has an abdominal mass or unexplained fever and weight loss, the child should be evaluated promptly.

Etiology

Most cases of neuroblastoma are diagnosed in the first few years of life. The etiology is unknown, but because of the early age at onset, maternal factors or exposures during pregnancy could play a role.

Diagnosis

Laboratory studies include measurement of urine and serum catecholamine levels, as well as electrolytes and kidney and liver functions. Biopsy of the mass gives a definitive diagnosis. For staging evaluation, bone marrow aspirate and biopsy, radionuclide bone scan, abdominal CT, and chest radiography are all performed. Chest and head CT may be indicated, depending on the patient's symptoms.

Treatment

For patients with low-risk tumors, surgical removal is the only treatment required. For higher-stage tumors, chemotherapy with or without radiation therapy is employed. For children with high-risk disease, high-dose chemotherapy followed by autologous hematopoietic stem cell rescue may be beneficial. Even after therapy is completed, the patient needs to be followed up closely to monitor for

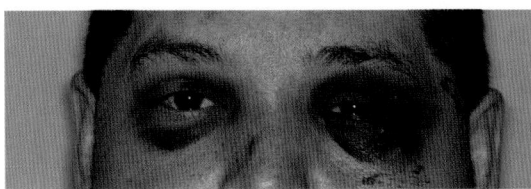

• **Fig. 2.53** Raccoon eyes (periorbital ecchymosis). (From Fonseca RJ, Walker RV, Barber HD, et al: *Oral and maxillofacial trauma*, ed 4, St Louis, 2013, Saunders.)

development of any late effects of treatment, including second malignancies.

Prognosis

The best prognostic indicators include younger age at diagnosis, localized disease, and certain cytogenetic abnormalities. It should be noted that there is a stage 4S that includes children younger than 1 year of age with disseminated disease. This actually confers a better prognosis because these tumors may regress spontaneously without any therapy.

Prevention

There is no known prevention.

Patient Teaching

Work with parents to contact support groups.

Review Challenge

Answer the following questions:

1. List the possible causes of congenital anomalies.
2. What is the purpose of amniocentesis? Describe the procedure.
3. Describe the condition of prematurity, and list its causes. List the associated disorders, identifying their causes, and discuss the treatment options.
4. List some genetic syndromes.
5. What often is a cause of sudden death in a teenage athlete?
6. What is the cause of Down syndrome?
7. Describe neural tube defects, and list the conditions resulting from them.
8. How is hydrocephalus treated?
9. Trace fetal circulation.
10. Explain the difference between cyanotic and acyanotic defects.
11. Name and describe the most common congenital cyanotic cardiac defect.
12. Describe patent ductus arteriosus (PDA) and its treatment.
13. Explain the differences between muscular dystrophy (MD) and cerebral palsy (CP).
14. List the major clinical manifestations of cystic fibrosis (CF).
15. Explain cryptorchidism, how it is treated, and what may happen if left untreated.
16. Explain the symptoms of Wilms tumor.
17. What is congenital pyloric stenosis, and how is it treated?
18. Explain the differences between Klinefelter syndrome and Turner syndrome.
19. Describe the symptoms of chickenpox.
20. Why is it important for parents to follow the recommended schedule of childhood immunizations?
21. Discuss the importance of childhood immunizations, and list the schedule for the first year of life.
22. Describe the symptoms of mumps, and discuss the progression of the disease.
23. What vaccine is important for parents and grandparents to be up to date with?
24. Compare rubeola and rubella.
25. Describe the clinical condition of congenital rubella syndrome.
26. What are symptoms of sudden infant death syndrome (SIDS)?
27. Compare croup and epiglottitis.
28. Why is throat culture important for a child with tonsillitis?
29. What does adenoid hyperplasia cause?
30. Discuss the incidence, etiology, treatment, and risks of asthma.
31. Discuss the types of worm infestations that may occur and how they are treated.
32. Childhood obesity is a major health concern. List some recommended guidelines to assist parents to provide proper nutrition for their children.
33. List the signs of childhood anemia.
34. List the symptoms and signs of anemia; describe the pathology of leukemia.
35. Explain the etiology of erythroblastosis fetalis.
36. Name some warning signs of lead poisoning.
37. Describe the infant born with fetal alcohol syndrome (FAS).
38. List the possible causes of diaper rash.

Real-Life Challenge: Asthma

A 6-year-old male has coughing with audible expiratory wheezes and dyspnea. The child is pale, the skin is moist and cool, and the child has difficulty speaking more than a few words before stopping to catch his breath. His parents state that the difficult breathing had a rapid onset approximately 1 hour earlier when he was playing with the neighbor's dog. The child has a history of previous asthma attacks, primarily after visiting his aunt's home where there are cats.

Assessment of the child shows temperature (T), 98.6°F; pulse (P), 120 beats per minute; and respiratory rate (RR), 40 breaths per minute and labored. Bilateral rales are heard on auscultation, louder on expiration but also present on inspiration. Cromolyn sodium had been prescribed to be taken prophylactically before visits to the aunt's home. The child also has an albuterol sulfate inhaler to be used PRN (as needed). The use of the inhaler has brought no relief.

Questions

1. Which diagnostic procedures would be ordered to reveal the degree of airway obstruction?
2. Which immediate intervention may be ordered to relieve the symptoms and provide comfort to the child?
3. What future testing may be ordered?
4. What is the cause of the dyspnea?
5. List the allergens commonly responsible for asthma attacks.
6. Explain why asthma attacks are considered medical emergencies and what steps should be taken on arrival of a patient experiencing an asthma attack.

Real-Life Challenge: Patent Ductus Arteriosus

A 1-week-old premature infant weighing 1 lb 10 oz begins exhibiting reduced oxygen saturation levels, bradycardia, and cyanosis. The infant's respirations are being maintained with mechanical ventilation. Increased oxygen concentration is required to maintain oxygen saturation levels at 90%. The chest radiograph reveals infant respiratory distress syndrome (IRDS) as resolving. The echocardiogram indicates patent ductus arteriosus (PDA).

Questions

1. Explain the two treatment options, drug therapy and a surgical procedure, used to close the PDA.
2. Explain the complication that could occur as a result of high concentration levels of oxygen.
3. What is the prognosis for the cardiac status of this child once closure has been achieved?
4. Which other congenital cardiac defect may be present?
5. Trace fetal circulation, and explain the role of the ductus arteriosus before birth.

Internet Assignments

1. Go to the Asthma and Allergy Foundation of America website to ascertain and report on recent treatment options for asthma.
2. Go to the Cystic Fibrosis Foundation website to research new treatment options and support systems for patients and their families.

Prepare to discuss the Critical Thinking case study exercises for this chapter that are posted on Evolve.

3

Immunologic Diseases and Conditions

CHAPTER OUTLINE

Orderly Function of the Immune System, 101

Immunodeficiency Diseases, 105

Autoimmune Diseases, 115

    Hematopoietic Disorders, 115

    Renal Disorders, 119

Connective Tissue Diseases, 120

Neurologic Disorders, 128

Vasculitis, 131

LEARNING OBJECTIVES

After studying Chapter 3, you should be able to:

1. Name the functional components of the immune system.
2. List examples of inappropriate responses of the immune system.
3. Characterize the three major functions of the immune system.
4. List the five immunoglobulins and explain complement fixation.
5. Trace the formation of T cells and B cells from stem cells.
6. Explain how T cells and B cells specifically protect the body against disease.
7. Explain the difference between active immunity and passive immunity.
8. Explain the ways that human immunodeficiency virus (HIV) is transmitted.
9. List the guidelines for universal precautions and infection control.
10. Describe the primary absent or inadequate response of the immune system in the following diseases:
    - Common variable immunodeficiency (CVID)
    - Selective immunoglobulin A (IgA) deficiency
    - Severe combined immunodeficiency (SCID) disease
11. Explain the destructive mechanisms in autoimmune diseases.
12. Describe the symptoms and signs of pernicious anemia. Name the primary treatment.
13. Recall the systemic features of systemic lupus erythematosus (SLE). Recall the diagnostic criteria.
14. Detail the pathology of rheumatoid arthritis (RA).
15. Specify the primary objectives of the treatment for RA.
16. List the distinguishing diagnostic features of ankylosing spondylitis.
17. Compare the pathology of multiple sclerosis with that of myasthenia gravis.
18. Describe the pathology of vasculitis in general terms.

KEY TERMS

anticholinesterase (an-tee-koh-lyn-**ES**-ter-ase)
autoimmune (aw-tow-im-**YOON**)
candidiasis (kan-dih-**DIE**-ah-sis)
collagen (**KOLL**-ah-jen)
hematopoietic (hem-ah-toh-poy-**ET**-ik)
hypogammaglobulinemia (hye-poh-gam-a-glob-you-lyn-**EE**-me-ah)
immunocompetent (im-you-no-**KOM**-peh-tent)
immunodeficiency (im-you-no-deh-**FISH**-en-see)
immunoelectrophoresis (im-you-no-ee-lek-troh-foh-**REE**-sis)

immunogen (**IM**-you-no-jen)
immunoglobulin (im-you-no-**GLAHB**-you-lyn)
immunosuppressive (im-you-no-sup-**PRESS**-iv)
keratoconjunctivitis (ker-ah-toh-kon-junk-tih-**VIE**-tis)
lymph (**limf**)
lymphadenopathy (lim-fad-eh-**NOP**-ah-thee)
lymphocyte (**LIM**-foh-sight)
macrophage (**MACK**-roh-fayj)
phagocytes (**FAG**-oh-sights)
phagocytosis (fag-oh-sigh-**TOH**-sis)

Orderly Function of the Immune System

The immune system, a major defense mechanism, is responsible for a complex response of the body to the invasion by foreign substances. The concept of the immune system arose from an observation that a person who recovers from a specific infection does not get sick from that infection again. The person is thereafter "immune" to that particular infectious agent. Immunity is very specific in that a person who has developed immunity to a certain virus, such as the rubella virus, is still susceptible to infection by other viruses, such as the measles virus.

The immune response assists the body in maintaining its functional integrity, and it battles infection by bacteria, viruses, fungi, and parasites. The immune system involves lymphoid tissues classified as primary (thymus and bone marrow) or secondary (tonsils, adenoids, spleen, Peyer patches, appendix, and so on) (Fig. 3.1).

When the immune system reacts appropriately to an antigen and homeostasis is maintained, a person is immunocompetent. If the immune system's response is inappropriate, either too weak or too strong, it results in the disruption of homeostasis. This malfunction in the system is referred to as *immunoincompetence*. Disruption of homeostasis is the cause of many diseases. Inappropriate responses or malfunctioning of the immune system are classified as follows:

- hyperactive responses (e.g., allergies), in which the immune response is excessive and triggered by specific allergens
- immunodeficiency disorders (e.g., acquired immunodeficiency syndrome [AIDS]), in which the immune response is inadequate
- autoimmune disorders (e.g., systemic lupus erythematosus [SLE]), in which the immune response is overactive and misdirected against one's own tissues
- attacks on beneficial foreign tissue (e.g., reaction to blood transfusions or transplanted organ rejection) (see Enrichment box about Transplant Rejection and Fig. 3.2)

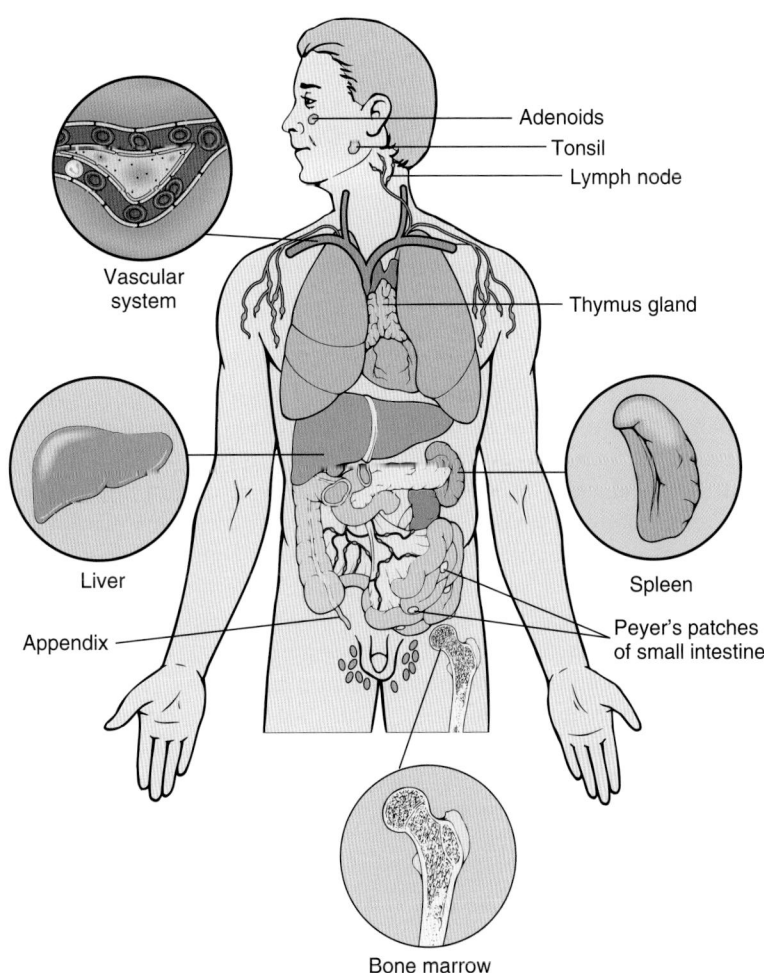

• **Fig. 3.1** Immune system.

Transplant Rejection

Kidney, liver, heart, lung, pancreas, intestines, and corneal tissue all can be replaced with transplants. Skin transplants are used for the treatment of burns. Bone marrow transplantation (BMT) is used to treat many conditions, such as bone marrow failure, leukemia, and aplastic anemia.

To help prevent transplant rejection, donor and recipient are carefully matched for blood type and immunologic characteristics. The recipient is given antirejection (**immunosuppressive**) drugs and steroids to suppress the production of antibodies to the foreign tissue proteins. All homografts (a graft of tissue between two genetically dissimilar individuals of the same species) invariably evoke some level of transplant rejection, which is mediated by antibodies and a delayed cellular immune reaction.

Clinically distinct forms of transplant rejection are recognized:

- Hyperacute reaction occurs during the operation. The transplanted organ must be removed immediately to prevent inevitable complications.
- Acute rejection occurs most often within the first few weeks of transplantation or later when antirejection drugs become ineffectual.
- Chronic rejection evolves slowly over a period of months or years. Vascular injury and inflammation of the tissues and cells of the organ contribute to the ultimate deterioration of the transplanted organ.

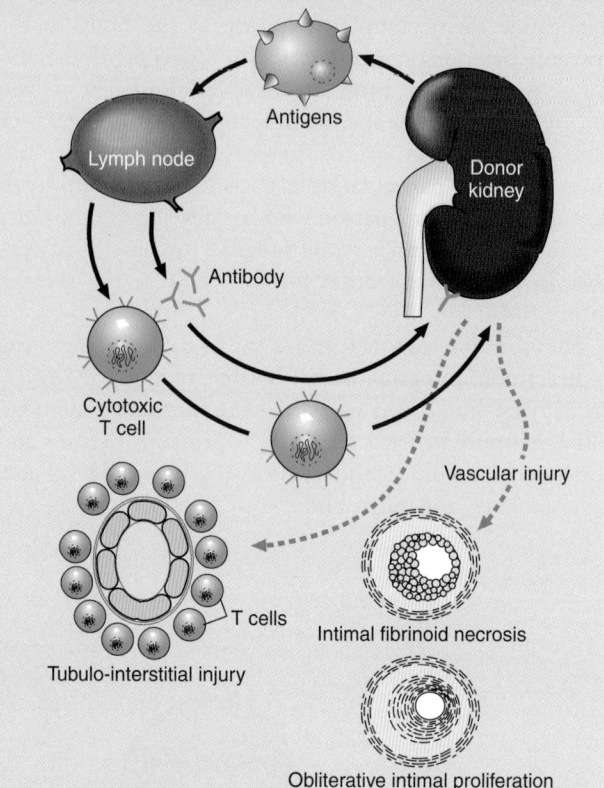

• **Fig. 3.2** Transplant rejection. (Modified from Damjanov I : *Pathology for the health-related professions,* ed 5, St Louis, 2017, Elsevier, Inc.)

The immune response normally is activated whenever foreign substances, or antigens, enter the body by evading its first line of defense—the skin and mucous membranes. The body recognizes the antigen or **immunogen**, usually a protein, as foreign, or nonself, and produces antibodies in response to that specific antigen. Antibody molecules have combining sites on its surface and can combine with threatening cells, such as microorganisms or cancer cells. This forms an antigen–antibody complex that renders the antigen harmless. It is crucial that the immune system be able to differentiate between self and foreign molecules. When this is not the case, autoimmune disease is the result. In autoimmune disease, the body mistakenly recognizes molecules of its own tissues as foreign and then attacks them.

The mechanisms of nonspecific defense involve preformed and fully activated components that launch a nonspecific attack on a foreign organism as soon as it is detected. The main cells involved in nonspecific defense include the following:

- natural killer (NK) cells that kill virus-infected cells and tumor cells by secreting certain toxins
- **macrophages** that phagocytose bacteria, viruses, and other foreign substances

- polymorphonuclear neutrophils (PMNs, or simply *neutrophils*) that also phagocytose bacteria

The development of the components required for immunity begins early in fetal life when the fetal liver produces stem cells, which, in turn, produce all cells of the **hematopoietic** system. Bone marrow assumes this role after birth (Fig. 3.3). Some of the stem cells migrate to the thymus gland, where they become T cells (T lymphocytes), which multiply and develop the capacity to combine with specific foreign antigens derived from viruses, fungi, tumors, or transplanted tissue (Fig. 3.4). Those T cells, coded to recognize self-antigens, are destroyed. The remaining T cells are coded to seek out foreign invaders. The body produces several types of T cells; each has a different function:

- Cytotoxic T cells (killer T cells) directly destroy virus-infected cells, tumor cells, and allograft cells by releasing certain toxins or by inducing apoptosis. These cells also may be referred to as *CD8 cells* because they carry the CD8 glycoprotein on their surface.
- Helper T cells stimulate the B cells to differentiate into plasma cells and to produce more antibodies. They also activate cytotoxic T cells and macrophages. Helper T cells carry the CD4 glycoprotein on their surface.

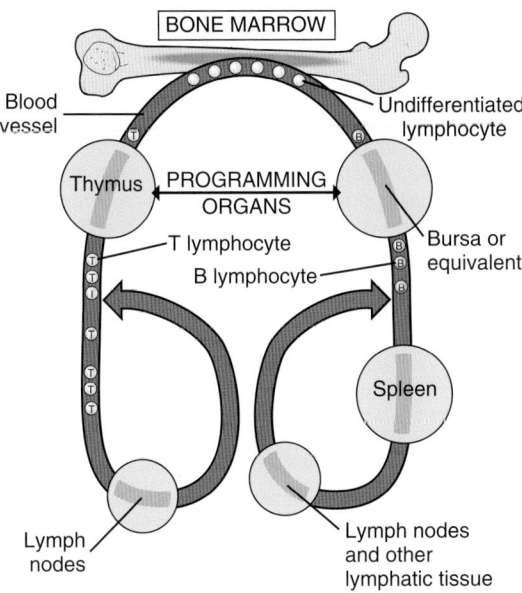

• **Fig. 3.3** Bone marrow formation of lymphocytes.

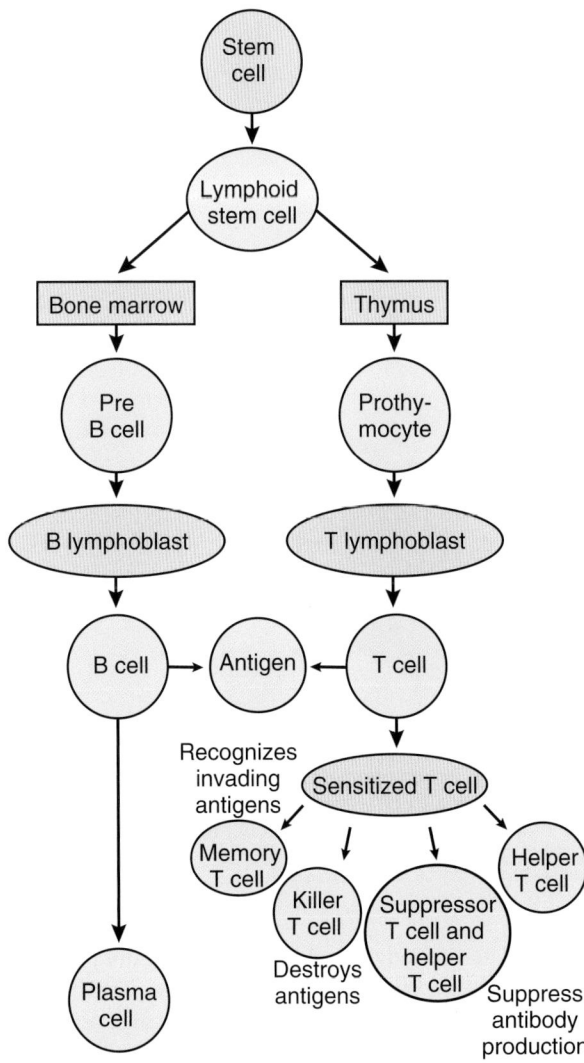

• **Fig. 3.4** T-cell and B-cell formation.

- Suppressor T cells inhibit both B- and T-cell activities and moderate the immune response.
- Memory T cells remain dormant until they are reactivated by the original antigen, allowing a rapid and more potent response years after the original exposure.

T cells are the major component of the type of acquired immunity known as *cell-mediated immunity*. The mononuclear phagocytic system, formerly termed the *reticuloendothelial system,* initiates this immune response. Macrophages, which develop from monocytes, are found in the tissue of the liver, lungs, and **lymph** nodes. These large cells intercept and engulf the foreign invader antigens and then process and present them to the T cells. Cell-mediated immunity defends the body against viral and fungal attacks, mediates graft rejection and tumor cell destruction, and helps or suppresses an antibody-mediated response to infection.

The remaining stem cells develop into B cells (B lymphocytes) to produce the antibody-mediated (humoral) immunity, which protects the body against bacterial and viral infections and reinfections (see Fig. 3.4). Once activated by exposure to an antigen, B cells are stimulated to proliferate and form a clone of cells that respond to that specific antigen. Some B cells become antibody-secreting plasma cells, whereas others become memory B cells, ready for a quick response if the target antigen presents itself again. The plasma cells are responsible for producing antibodies that attach to invading foreign antigens, thus marking the antigens for destruction by other cells of the immune system.

B cells are coated with **immunoglobulins**, giving them the ability to recognize foreign protein and stimulate an antigen–antibody reaction. The five classes of immunoglobulins or antibodies are immunoglobulin M (IgM), IgG, IgA, IgD, and IgE (Table 3.1). These immunoglobulins are usually all present during an antigenic response, although in varying amounts, depending on the stimulant and the health of the patient. Actions of the antigen–antibody complex include the following:

- inactivation of the pathogen or its toxin through direct binding
- stimulation of phagocytosis through complement fixation, the process by which an antibody targets an infected cell for destruction by binding to the cell surface (Phagocytic cells recognize the antibody marker and engulf the infected cell.)

Activation of the complement system (complement fixation) involves several proteins found in plasma or body fluids. The antigen–antibody reaction initiates a series or cascade of reactions that activate the complement system, fixing the complement and consequently permitting the destruction of pathogens by the process of **phagocytosis** or lysis of the pathogen's cell membrane (Fig. 3.5). This activation occurs during an immune reaction mediated by IgG or IgM.

The human body is protected by two types of acquired specific immunity: active immunity and passive immunity. *Active immunity* results when a person has had previous

TABLE 3.1 Classes of Antibodies

Class	Percent of Total	Location	Function
IgG	75–85	Blood plasma	Major antibody in primary and secondary immune responses; inactivates antigen; neutralizes toxins; crosses placenta to provide immunity for newborn; responsible for Rh reactions
IgA	5–15	Saliva, mucus, tears, breast milk	Protects mucous membranes on body surfaces; provides immunity for newborn
IgM	5–10	Attached to B cells; released into plasma during immune response	Causes antigens to clump together; responsible for transfusion reactions in the ABO blood typing system
IgD	0.2	Attached to B cells	Receptor sites for antigens on B cells; binding with antigen results in B-cell activation
IgE	0.5	Produced by plasma cells in mucous membranes and tonsils	Binds to mast cells and basophils, causing release of histamine; responsible for allergic reactions

Ig, Immunoglobulin.
(From Applegate EJ: *The anatomy and physiology learning system,* ed 4, St Louis, 2011, Saunders.)

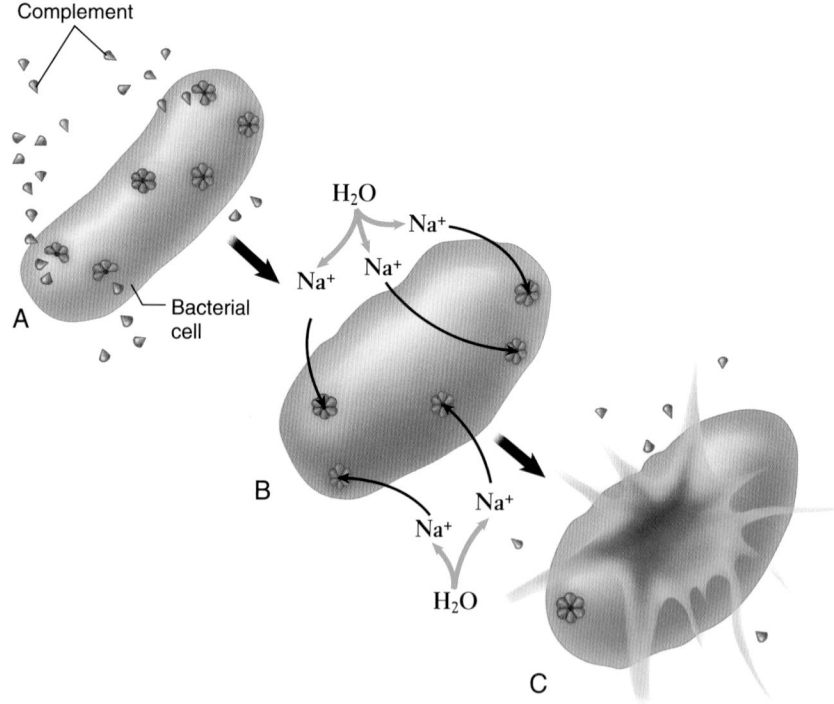

• **Fig. 3.5** Complement Cascade. (A) Complement molecules activated by antibodies form doughnut-shaped complexes in a bacterium's plasma membrane. (B) Holes in the complement complex allow sodium (Na^+) and then water (H_2O) to diffuse into the bacterium. (C) After enough water has entered, the swollen bacterium bursts. This is just one of many functions of the complement proteins. (From Patton KT, Thibodeau GA: *The human body in health and disease,* ed 6, St Louis, 2014, Mosby.)

exposure to a disease or pathogen or when a person receives immunizations against a disease to stimulate the production of a specific antibody. Active immunity affords the person acquired permanent protection. *Passive immunity* bypasses the body's immune response to afford the benefit of immediate antibody availability. A person gains passive immunity by being given immune substances created outside that person's body for temporary immunity, such as antibodies received through the placenta, when breast milk is fed to a child, or when immune globulin, an antibody-containing

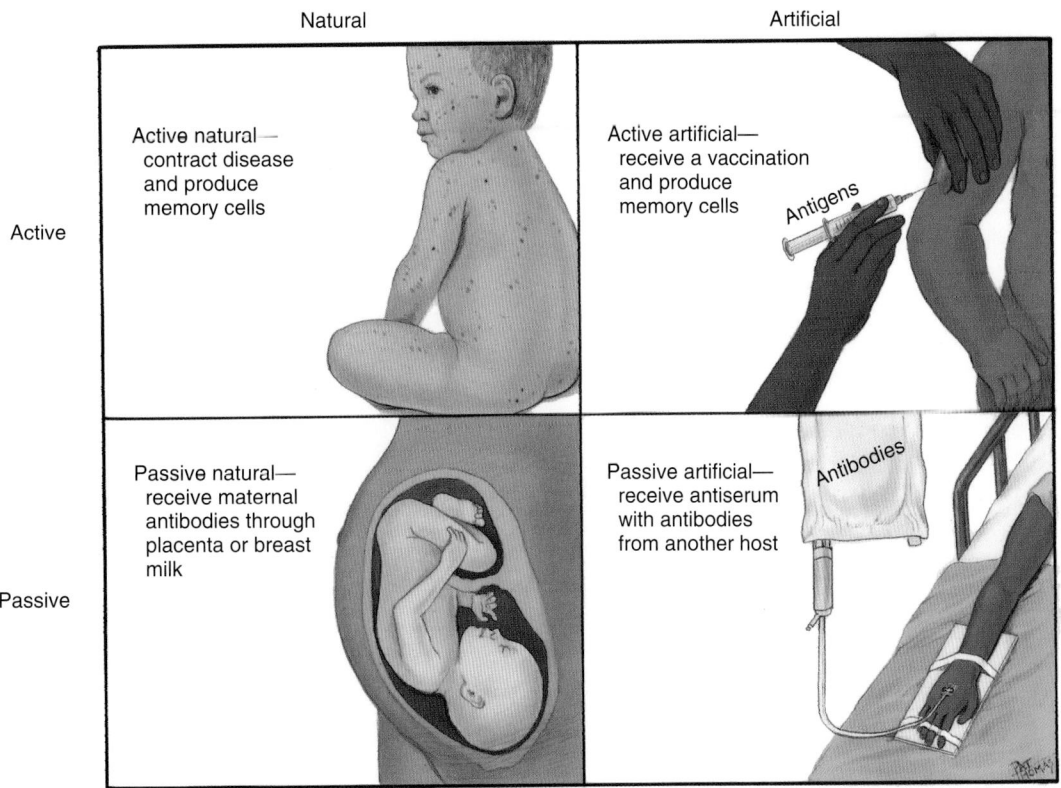

Natural | Artificial

Active

Active natural — contract disease and produce memory cells

Active artificial— receive a vaccination and produce memory cells

Antigens

Passive

Passive natural— receive maternal antibodies through placenta or breast milk

Passive artificial— receive antiserum with antibodies from another host

Antibodies

• **Fig. 3.6** Acquired immunity. (From Applegate EJ: *The anatomy and physiology learning system,* ed 4, St Louis, 2011, Saunders.)

preparation made from the plasma of healthy donors, is given to help a person combat disease (Fig. 3.6).

Immunodeficiency Diseases

An absent or inadequate response of the immune system results in immunodeficiency conditions and increased susceptibility to other diseases and opportunistic infections. **Immunodeficiency** can occur in any of the following major components of the immune system: B cells, T cells, complement, or **phagocytes**. Although the deficiency may be in either the humoral (antibody-related) or the cell-mediated responses, the consequences are similar: The individual does not have the capability to dispose of foreign and harmful substances. In general, an increased susceptibility to bacterial infections results from a B-cell deficiency, whereas recurrent viral, fungal, and protozoan infections are usually caused by decreased T-cell function. Some of the conditions are genetic and present at birth, whereas other defects are not manifested until later in life or are acquired. Acquired immunoincompetence may result from a bacterial or viral insult to the body, malnutrition, or exposure to radiation or certain drugs. The severity of the immunodeficiency disease depends on the type of cell or cells that are affected. It can range from annoying chronic infections to severe life-threatening or fatal conditions.

Acquired Immunodeficiency Syndrome

Description

AIDS is a progressive impairment of the immune system caused by human immunodeficiency virus (HIV). This gradual destruction of the immune system affects many organ systems and is ultimately life-threatening for the person infected.

ICD-10-CM Code   B20 *(Human immunodeficiency virus [HIV] disease)*

Symptoms and Signs

Initially, it is not possible to tell whether people are infected by HIV by simply observing them. They may remain healthy for years during the latent period and may therefore unknowingly transmit the virus to other people. Within 1 to 4 weeks after exposure, the patient may experience a flulike illness with sore throat, fever, and body aches that often lasts about 2 weeks. **Lymphadenopathy**, weight loss, fatigue, diarrhea, and night sweats are common as the clinical course progresses. The body's number of T cells becomes lower and allows for frequent infections, especially opportunistic infections, pneumonia, fever, and malignancies (see the Enrichment box about Malignancies and Common Opportunistic Infections and Conditions in Patients with AIDS, and Figs. 3.7–3.9). Often, in the later stages, encephalopathy and malignancy lead to dementia and death (Fig. 3.10).

◆◆ **ENRICHMENT**

Malignancies and Common Opportunistic Infections and Conditions in Patients with AIDS

- Kaposi sarcoma is an aggressive malignancy of the blood vessels that appears as purple or blue patches on the skin, in the mouth, or anywhere else on the body.
- Lymphomas are cancerous lesions of lymphoid tissues.
- *Pneumocystis carinii* pneumonia (PCP) is a lung infection that can progress to be life-threatening. It is the most common lung disease in persons with AIDS.
- Tuberculosis is a bacterial infection of the lungs or other organs.
- Herpes simplex infection consists of painful blisterlike lesions of the mouth, genitalia, or anus caused by the herpes virus.
- Herpes zoster (shingles) is characterized by clusters of red, blisterlike skin lesions that are distributed along the distribution of an inflamed nerve.
- *Candida albicans* causes a fungal infection of the mucous membranes of the mouth, genitalia, or skin.
- Toxoplasmosis is an infection caused by a protozoan intracellular parasite. A rash and lymphadenopathy can be present, and the central nervous system (CNS), heart, or lungs can become involved.
- Neurologic complications include inflammation of nerves, neuropathy, neoplasms, and AIDS dementia complex.

- Diarrhea is a symptom of a host of bacterial and viral infections of the gastrointestinal (GI) tract, liver, or gallbladder.
- Epstein-Barr virus causes hairy leukoplakia that is characterized by white plaque visible on the tongue.

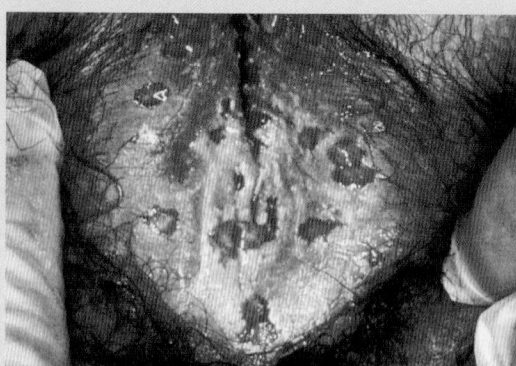

• **Fig. 3.8** Primary perineal herpes with methylene blue stain. (Courtesy the Centers for Disease Control and Prevention, 1992. From Mudge-Grout C: *Immunologic disorders—Mosby's clinical nursing series,* St Louis, 1992, Mosby.)

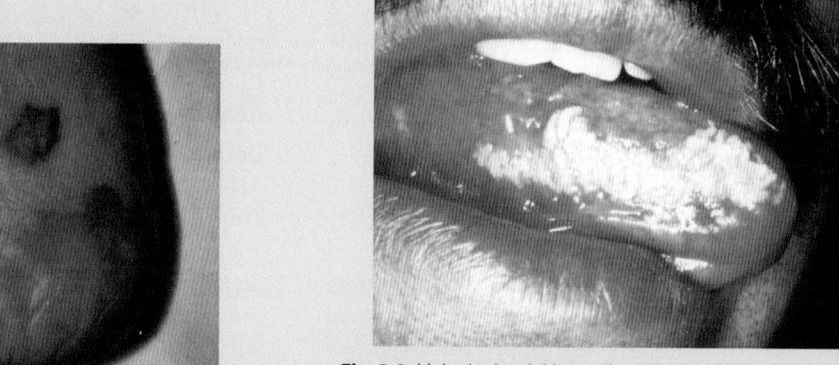

• **Fig. 3.9** Hairy leukoplakia on the tongue of a patient with acquired immunodeficiency syndrome (AIDS). (Courtesy J.S. Greenspan, DDS, University of California-San Francisco. Courtesy the Centers for Disease Control and Prevention, 1992. From Mudge-Grout C: *Immunologic disorders—Mosby's clinical nursing series,* St Louis, 1992, Mosby.)

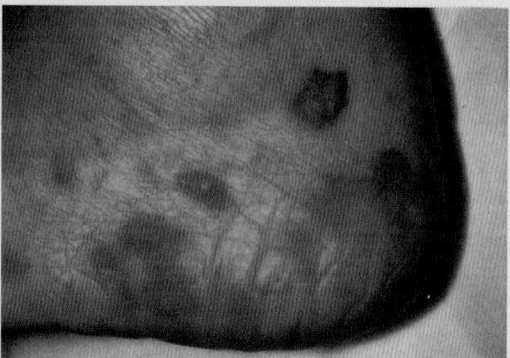

• **Fig. 3.7** Kaposi sarcoma of distal heel and lateral foot. (Courtesy the Centers for Disease Control and Prevention, 1992. From Mudge-Grout C: *Immunologic disorders—Mosby's clinical nursing series,* St Louis, 1992, Mosby.)

Patient Screening

An individual who complains of weight loss, fatigue, swollen glands, night sweats, and/or a persistent flulike syndrome needs an appointment with a physician for a medical evaluation as soon as possible. When an individual reports known HIV exposure through unprotected sexual contact or puncture with a contaminated needle, immediate medical care should be arranged.

Etiology

AIDS is caused by HIV, type 1 or 2 (HIV-1 is found worldwide, and HIV-2 is mainly found in West Africa) retroviruses

that contain RNA; they cannot survive apart from human cells. HIV attacks helper T lymphocytes (CD4 cells), the body's safeguard against tumors, viruses, and parasites. The destruction of T cells and the proliferation of HIV leave the body defenseless against infection and malignancy by reducing cell-mediated immunity. The virus also directly damages the nervous system. AIDS first was recognized in the United States in 1981. Since then, it has become a top killer of young men and a worldwide threat to humankind. It is estimated that more than 35 million people are currently infected by HIV, and more than 36 million have died as a result of the

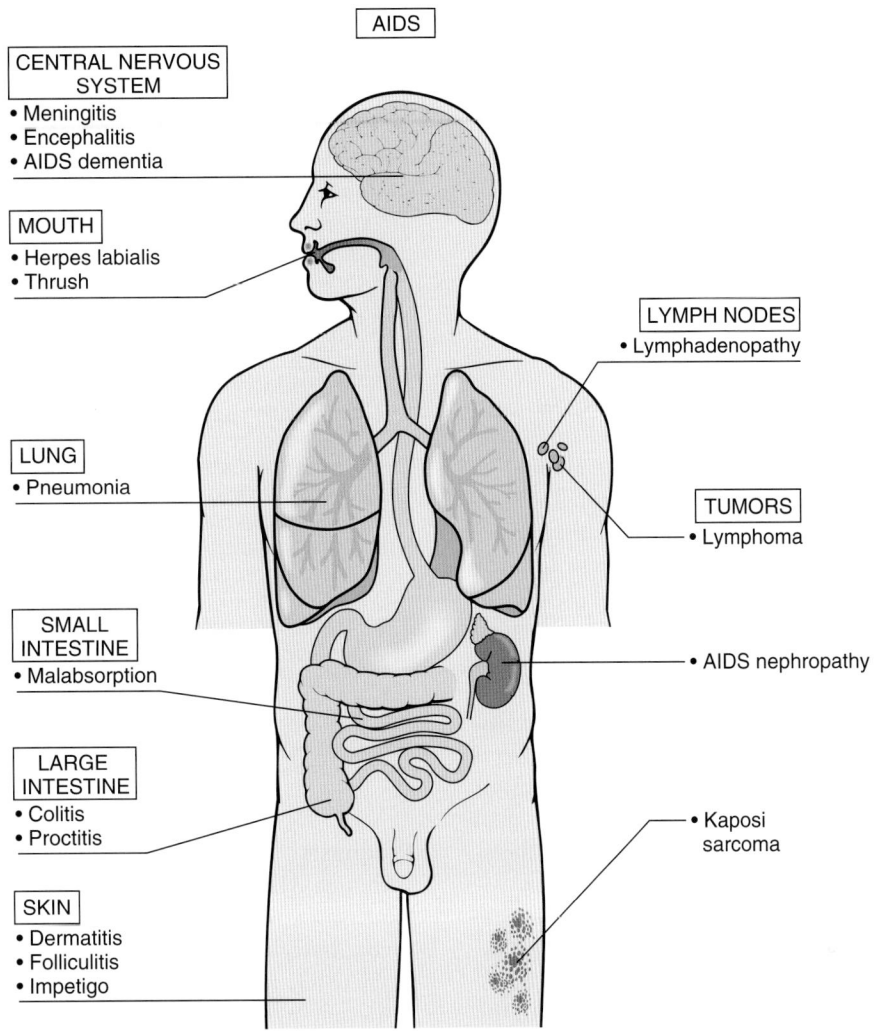

AIDS

CENTRAL NERVOUS SYSTEM
• Meningitis
• Encephalitis
• AIDS dementia

MOUTH
• Herpes labialis
• Thrush

LUNG
• Pneumonia

SMALL INTESTINE
• Malabsorption

LARGE INTESTINE
• Colitis
• Proctitis

SKIN
• Dermatitis
• Folliculitis
• Impetigo

LYMPH NODES
• Lymphadenopathy

TUMORS
• Lymphoma

• AIDS nephropathy

• Kaposi sarcoma

• **Fig. 3.10** Pathologic changes associated with acquired immunodeficiency syndrome (AIDS). (From Damjanov I: *Pathology for the health-related professions,* ed 4, St Louis, 2011, Saunders.)

illness. Without treatment, the time from infection by HIV to death is approximately 10 years. To date, neither a cure nor an effective vaccine has been found for this disease, although the use of highly active antiretroviral therapy (HAART) has significantly prolonged the life span of those infected. According to the Centers for Disease Control and Prevention (CDC) statistics, "An estimated 1.1 million people in the United States had HIV at the end of 2016, the most recent year for which this information is available. In 2016, there were 15,807 deaths among people with diagnosed HIV in the United States. These deaths may be due to any cause."

HIV is spread most readily by direct contact with the blood or semen of an infected person. It is not transmitted by casual contact, such as touching, shaking hands, and hugging. Sexual contact is the primary means of transmission. According to the CDC, most sexually transmitted cases of HIV infection in the United States occur through men having sex with men (MSM); worldwide heterosexual transmission is the primary mode of transmission of HIV. AIDS also can be transmitted through blood and blood products. Infants of infected mothers can contract

the disease in utero through the placenta, during the birth process, and from breast milk. Sharing of needles by intravenous drug users also leads to infection. The risk of transmission of HIV to and from health care workers and patients is minimized by strict adherence to the universal precautions for infection control.

Diagnosis

A common laboratory screening test used to detect the presence of HIV antibodies in blood is enzyme-linked immunosorbent assay (ELISA). If the findings are positive, the test is repeated, and the result is then confirmed by using the Western blot test. A positive result on the p24 antigen test indicates circulating HIV antigen. ELISA results are often negative during the first month of infection, although results of the p24 antigen test or the polymerase chain reaction (PCR) assay may be positive. Rapid HIV antibody testing has become the preferred method of testing because the results are often available within 5 minutes. Although a negative test is regarded as a true negative, a positive result requires confirmatory testing with Western blot. A viral titer and CD4 T-cell count are usually obtained after a positive test result to determine the patient's disease burden and risk for opportunistic infections. Transmission of HIV is possible during all stages of infection, even before it can be detected by laboratory tests, which is called the *window period.*

Home testing kits for HIV have evolved in recent years. The U.S. Food and Drug Administration (FDA) approved an over-the-counter saliva test a few years ago, and individuals can perform these self-tests by using saliva samples and obtain results in less than an hour.

Treatment

Currently, no cure exists for AIDS. After a patient has been diagnosed with it, he or she will undergo periodic measurement of the number of CD4 T cells and the amount of HIV RNA (viral load) present in the bloodstream. These are both markers of disease progression from the initial infection with HIV to the development of AIDS. These numbers can also be used to determine when to begin HAART, although currently, in the United States, it is recommended that HAART be started in all patients with HIV infection irrespective of the CD4 count or the viral load.

HAART consists of a three-drug combination: nucleoside reverse transcriptase inhibitors (NRTIs), and either a non–nucleoside reverse transcriptase inhibitor (NNRTI) or a protease inhibitor (PI). There are currently more than 20 antiretroviral drugs approved for use in HAART; therefore many different drug combinations are possible. Although these drugs have been effective in prolonging life and maintaining the quality of life for patients, they are associated with a number of toxicities and serious side effects, so patients on HAART must be followed up closely. In the later stages of the disease, patients require prophylactic antibiotics. Addressing the psychological needs of the patient with AIDS is essential.

Health care practitioners who are involved in various forms of patient care with exposure to body fluids and blood should follow the principles of infection control and universal precautions (see the Alert box about Infection Control and Universal Precautions). All body fluids and blood from any patient should be handled with extreme care, as if the patient were known to be infected by HIV.

There are many people who are considered to be at high risk for contracting HIV infection. Preexposure prophylaxis, or PrEP, has been effective in reducing the risk of HIV infection by 92% when used consistently every day. The patient should also have appointments with his or her health care provider every 3 months. There are two medications in the pill; tenofovir and emtricitabine, which are labeled under the brand name Truvada.

The results of an 8-year, London-based research study involving almost 1000 gay male couples was released in May 2019. During the 8 years, no partner became infected with HIV even though the couples were not using barrier protection. "A European study of nearly 1000 gay male couples who had sex without condoms—where one partner had HIV and was taking antiretroviral drugs to suppress it—has

found the treatment can prevent sexual transmission of the virus."

> **❗ ALERT!**
>
> **Infection Control and Universal Precautions**
>
> Guidelines: Treat blood and all body fluids as if infected, and remember to use the following precautions:
> 1. Practice frequent and thorough hand washing.
> 2. Report any accidental needlesticks.
> 3. Wear personal protective equipment, including mask or face shield, gown, gloves, and goggles. Change equipment between patients.
> 4. Use caution with laboratory specimens.
> 5. Dispose of contaminated sharps in designated biohazard containers. *Caution:* Do not recap or break needles.
> 6. Use proper linen disposal containers.
> 7. Use clean mouthpieces and resuscitation bags.
> 8. Obtain hepatitis B vaccination to protect against occupational exposure to blood.
> 9. Use proper decontamination techniques.
> 10. Absorb blood spills with paper towels, and then clean the area with soap and water, followed by disinfection of the area with a 1:10 solution of household bleach.

Note: Pathogens can be bloodborne or airborne. Standard precautions, which correlate with universal precautions, are recommended and posted for hospitals and patient care institutions.

Prognosis

Although AIDS is ultimately a fatal disease, the number of Americans dying of AIDS each year has dropped. Treatment strategies that result in better prognosis include use of HAART, use of prophylactic antibiotics, and care by a physician experienced in HIV care.

Prevention

Because HIV is transmitted directly from humans to humans, prevention measures relate to avoiding risk factors for sexually transmitted diseases and practicing infection control through the use of universal precautions. The use of HAART significantly decreases the risk of HIV transmission to an HIV-seronegative sexual partner. Use of condoms and not sharing needles are highly recommended. The drugs used in HAART can be administered as postexposure prophylaxis after a needlestick injury. Patients who test positive for HIV infection should be encouraged to inform their sexual partners because they may be at high risk for contracting the disease.

Patient Teaching

Describe the diagnostic tests, and inform the patient about when to expect test results. Assure the patient of medical confidentiality. It is not prudent to relay test results over the telephone. Make sure that the HIV-positive individual knows how the disease is transmitted. Stress the important aspects of the medication regimen and the dangers of noncompliance. Explain the side effects of the therapeutic drugs, and encourage the patient to contact the health care worker with questions or concerns. Other teaching points include how to minimize infections, the need for lifelong therapy, and the responsibility to inform health care providers about the HIV diagnosis. The psychological, social, and financial ramifications of having HIV require referrals for community support. Eventually referrals will be required to meet a variety of home care needs.

Common Variable Immunodeficiency (Acquired Hypogammaglobulinemia)

Description

Common variable immunodeficiency (CVID) is an acquired B-cell deficiency that results in decreased antibody production and/or function.

ICD-10-CM Code	D83.8 (Other common variable immunodeficiencies)
	D83.9 (Common variable immunodeficiency, unspecified)
	(D83.0-D83.9 = 5 codes of specificity)

Symptoms and Signs

The person with CVID has a history of chronic or recurrent infections, such as pneumonia, bronchitis, sinusitis, and otitis media. Gastrointestinal (GI) disease is often seen with such symptoms as diarrhea, abdominal pain, and weight loss. Lymphadenopathy, splenomegaly, and hepatomegaly often are observed. Chronic lung disease and granulomatous disease are common. CVID is associated with an increased frequency of autoimmune disorders, such as autoimmune hemolytic anemia or immune thrombocytopenia. As the disease progresses, susceptibility to opportunistic and viral infections and malignancies escalates.

Patient Screening

When a child or young teenager is susceptible to frequent infection, it is recommended that an appointment to discuss options be made with the health care provider or that office policy regarding referral to a pediatrician be followed. When the individual, particularly a younger adult, experiences frequent bacterial infections, an appointment for an in-depth medical investigation is indicated.

Etiology

CVID has two peaks of incidence: one between ages 18 and 25 years and a smaller peak between ages 1 and 5 years. Although the exact cause of **hypogammaglobulinemia** is not known, it is thought to be a result of genetic defects leading to immune system dysregulation and a failure of B-cell differentiation. The number of circulating B cells is often normal, but the ability of the B cells to produce all types of immunoglobulins is reduced. Some patients have impaired T-cell signaling as well. Cell-mediated immunity usually remains intact.

Diagnosis

A history of repeated and chronic infections should lead to further investigation of immunoglobulin levels and T-cell quantities. Antibody response to vaccines, when tested, is poor. Hypogammaglobulinemia and IgA and/or IgM deficiency in this clinical setting are indicative of the disease; however, other causes of these findings must be ruled out.

Treatment

Treatment is aimed at preventing infections and implementing early treatment with appropriate antibiotic administration when infections occur. Regular immunoglobulin replacement decreases the number of infections, antibiotic usage, and hospitalizations. Patients should be monitored closely because they are at an increased risk for the development of autoimmune disease and lymphoma. Live virus vaccines are often not given to people known to have CVID. Otherwise, appropriate vaccination is recommended, although vaccine response may be poor.

Prognosis

Although the use of immunoglobulin has improved the prognosis, patients often succumb to chronic lung disease or malignancies. Lower levels of immunoglobulin and a lower percentage of B cells are associated with a poorer prognosis.

Prevention

No methods of prevention are known.

Patient Teaching

Teaching points include steps to take to prevent infection and to ensure good nutrition, adequate rest, and regular follow-up care.

Selective Immunoglobulin A Deficiency

Description

Patients with selective IgA deficiency fail to produce the normal levels of IgA. Selective deficiencies of IgM or IgG have been reported but are rare.

ICD-10-CM Code	D80.2 (Selective deficiency of immunoglobulin A [IgA])
	(D80.0-D80.9 = 10 codes of specificity)

Symptoms and Signs

The majority of patients with IgA deficiency are asymptomatic, perhaps because of a compensatory increase in IgM production in these patients. Those who do experience symptoms have recurrent sinopulmonary infections, GI infections, and/or autoimmune disease. Food allergies are also common. Anaphylactic reactions to blood transfusions may occur. Children with selective IgA deficiency typically exhibit recurrent otitis media, sinusitis, and pneumonia.

Patient Screening

Frequent recurrent infections in a child or adult necessitate an appointment for a medical investigation to determine a possible underlying cause. The patient may also report food allergies and a history of an anaphylactic reaction to blood transfusions. Patients with a family history of IgA deficiency or CVID should be screened.

Etiology

Failure of B cells to produce adequate levels of IgA is the most common immunologic defect in the general population. The most common risk factor for the disease is a family history of either IgA deficiency or CVID.

Diagnosis

In patients who are older than 6 months of age and have recurrent sinopulmonary infections, IgA deficiency should be considered. Levels of immunoglobulins should be measured and should show below-normal levels of circulating IgA but normal IgG and IgM levels. Complete blood count (CBC), complement assay, and vaccine response testing are used to rule out other immunodeficiencies. Because some children with IgA deficiency may spontaneously begin to produce IgA, the diagnosis is not definite until after age 4 years. Appropriate investigations to diagnose autoimmune disease should be done according to the symptoms present.

Treatment

No cure for this condition is known. Treatment is geared toward the prevention and management of infection. Prophylactic antibiotics may be given. If these do not reduce the number of infections, intravenous immune globulin (IVIG) with low concentrations of IgA (to reduce risk of anaphylaxis) may be tried. Patients should be monitored for development of autoimmune disease and progression to CVID. *Patients must be monitored closely when given blood products because of the increased risk of an anaphylactic reaction. Screening for anti-IgA antibodies can help identify those who may have an adverse reaction.*

Prognosis

In most cases, no significant medical problems are expected and the prognosis is good. In some children, slow, spontaneous resolution of the condition may occur.

Prevention

No method of prevention is known.

Patient Teaching

Teaching points include steps to take to prevent infection and to ensure good nutrition, adequate rest, and regular follow-up care. Explain the purpose of prophylactic antibiotic therapy, as prescribed. Encourage patients with severe IgA deficiency to obtain a medical alert bracelet because of the risk for allergic reaction to blood products.

X-Linked Agammaglobulinemia

Description

X-linked agammaglobulinemia (Bruton agammaglobulinemia) is a condition characterized by near absence of serum immunoglobulins and increased susceptibility to infection.

ICD-10-CM Code	D80.0 *(Hereditary hypogammaglobulinemia)*

Symptoms and Signs

The infant with X-linked agammaglobulinemia has absent or near-absent tonsils and adenoids. Lymphadenopathy and splenomegaly are also noticeably missing. They are susceptible to recurrent severe gram-positive infections, including bacterial otitis media, bronchitis, pneumonia, osteomyelitis, and meningitis. Infection with enteroviruses is also common. These are usually first noted between 3 and 18 months of age, when the natural transplacental immunity from the mother has been depleted.

Patient Screening

Recurrent severe bacterial infections in an infant signal the need for in-depth medical investigation to determine the possible underlying cause(s). Follow office policy for referral to a pediatrician, when appropriate.

Etiology

This congenital X-linked disorder affects only males. It is caused by a defect in the Bruton tyrosine kinase *(BTK)* gene, which is normally expressed in B cells during all stages of development. All five immunoglobulin classes are usually absent, along with the absence of circulating B cells and the presence of normal numbers of circulating T cells. This leads to increased infection with encapsulated bacteria and certain viruses. Most affected individuals present with symptoms by 5 years of age, and almost all have symptoms by age 5 years. Around 40% of patients have an affected family member.

Diagnosis

The clinical findings, along with a thorough history including family history of relatives who died of severe infections, suggest X-linked agammaglobulinemia. **Immunoelectrophoresis** indicates decreased levels of serum IgM, IgA, and IgG; however, relying on this method of diagnosis is not valid before the infant is 6 to 8 months of age. Serum antibody titers in response to immunizations are low. Other findings suggestive of this disease are normal T-cell numbers along with low or absent B-cell numbers. It may be useful to assess for the *BTK* gene mutation if there is no significant family history to aid diagnosis. B-cell defects can be detected on newborn screening, but such testing is not routine in most states in the United States at this time.

Treatment

Treatment is directed at improving the child's immune defenses and controlling infections. Intravenous infusions or subcutaneous administrations of immune globulin every 2 to 4 weeks and appropriate antibiotics are administered. *These patients must never be immunized with live virus vaccines, nor should corticosteroids or immunosuppressive drugs be administered.* Killed vaccines should be administered, however, because they may provide T cell–mediated protection for the patient.

Prognosis

Although this condition cannot be cured, regular infusions of immune globulin may provide the patient with a near-normal lifestyle. Affected individuals do tend to miss more days of school or work and are hospitalized more frequently compared with males in the general population, however.

Prevention

No methods of prevention are known, although parents of affected children are encouraged to seek genetic counseling regarding future pregnancies.

Patient Teaching

Discuss the importance of preventing infections. Explain the procedure for immune globulin administrations. Caution the parents about the contraindication for live virus vaccines and immunosuppressive drugs.

Severe Combined Immunodeficiency

Description

Severe combined immunodeficiency (SCID) is a group of disorders that result from a disturbance in the development and function of T cells with or without B cells. Because T-cell signaling is needed for B cells to produce antibody, this leads to an absence of both cell-mediated (T-cell) immunity and antibody-mediated (B-cell) immunity. NK cells may or may not be present. This disease is referred to by some as *Bubble Boy disease*.

ICD-10-CM Code	D81.0 *(Severe combined immunodeficiency [SCID] with reticular dysgenesis)*
	D81.1 *(Severe combined immunodeficiency [SCID] with low T- and B-cell numbers)*
	D81.2 *(Severe combined immunodeficiency [SCID] with low or normal B-cell numbers)*
	D81.89 *(Other combined immunodeficiencies)*
	D81.9 *(Combined immunodeficiency, unspecified)*
	(D81.0-D81.9 = 13 codes of specificity)

Symptoms and Signs

SCID manifests as severe, recurrent infections with bacteria, viruses, fungi, and protozoa; chronic diarrhea; and failure to thrive. This occurs by age 3 to 6 months, when the natural maternal placental immunity begins to be depleted. Common infections are PCP and persistent mucocutaneous candidiasis. Discernible lymphoid tissue (enlarged tonsils, palpable lymph nodes, and so on) may be absent. Abnormal laboratory findings often include hypogammaglobulinemia and very low or absent T cells.

Patient Screening

Abnormal newborn screening results must be followed up. The history of pneumonia in the first weeks of life, followed by frequent, severe infections in the young infant, are indicative of underlying conditions that need a complete medical evaluation. These infections are potentially life-threatening in the infant, and immediate medical care is required. Follow office policy for referral to a pediatrician.

Etiology

Two types of SCID are known: X-linked and autosomal recessive. Both are caused by different genetic mutations that lead to defects in stem cell differentiation into B cells and T cells. These defects result in a disruption in lymphocyte development.

Diagnosis

Testing for SCID is now part of the routine newborn screen in the United States. If the clinical picture indicates suspicion of SCID, many laboratory tests are performed. These include measurement of immunoglobulin levels, antibody titers, and numbers of T cells and B cells. Lymphopenia, with less than 20% of lymphocytes being T cells, is a common finding. T-cell response is also tested. Usually there is absence of the thymic shadow on a chest radiograph.

Treatment

Bone marrow transplantation (BMT) is the only curative treatment for most types of SCID; although gene therapy is being investigated, supportive therapy includes IVIG and prophylaxis for *Pneumocystis jirovecii* and respiratory syncytial virus (RSV). Children with SCID are placed in completely sterile environments to prevent exposure to infectious agents. Live vaccines should not be administered to the patient and his or her caregivers.

Recent experimental approaches to gene therapy have been used for infants with the condition. St Jude Children's Research Hospital has had success with their treatment protocol. The treatment includes stem cells to be implanted in bone marrow by using busulfan to make space for the stem cells to grow. The clinical trial infants are now toddlers and have developed a normal immune system. According to the *New England Journal of Medicine* (April 2019), eight infants were enrolled in the initial treatment study, and they were tracked for 16 months. They showed no unexpected side effects. The previous infections they had all cleared. All of these infants continued to grow at the normal rate and began to produce functional immune cells (T cells, B cells, and NK cells), and they responded to vaccinations.

Although they will continue to be monitored for long-term side effects, the initial treatment is deemed a success.

Prognosis
The clinical trial has had positive effects on the children treated with this protocol. Unless the underlying gene defect is corrected, children with SCID will die of overwhelming infection before age 1 year.

Prevention
No methods of prevention are known, although routine newborn screening aids in a timely diagnosis.

Patient Teaching
Explain the medical interventions used to protect against infection and restore immune response. Refer the parents to available community support organizations that can help with the psychological, physical, and financial burdens precipitated by the infant's prognosis of severe illness and early death. During hospitalizations, encourage the parents to visit and interact with the infant as much as possible. Refer the parents to a genetic counselor.

DiGeorge Anomaly (Thymic Hypoplasia or Aplasia)
Description
DiGeorge anomaly is a congenital condition of immunodeficiency that results from defective development of the pharyngeal pouch system and presents with cardiac anomalies, hypoplastic thymus, and hypocalcemia. In some coding manuals, this disease may be listed as *DiGeorge syndrome.*

ICD-10-CM Code	D82.1 *(DiGeorge's syndrome)*
	(D82.0-D82.9 = 7 codes of
	specificity)

Symptoms and Signs
Children with DiGeorge anomaly often have a set of structural abnormalities. These include abnormally wide-set, downward slanting eyes; low-set ears with notched pinnae; a small mouth (Fig. 3.11); abnormalities of the palate; and cardiovascular defects, such as tetralogy of Fallot. The thymus and parathyroid glands are absent or underdeveloped. The infant exhibits signs of *tetany* resulting from hypocalcemia caused by hypoparathyroidism. Some degree of cognitive impairment often is present. Some patients are susceptible to infections, such as sinopulmonary infections and thrush.

Patient Screening
Infants or children with DiGeorge syndrome anomaly need prompt medical treatment when signs of infection occur.

Etiology
DiGeorge anomaly is the result of abnormal development of the third and fourth pharyngeal pouches during the twelfth week of gestation. This causes the thymus gland to

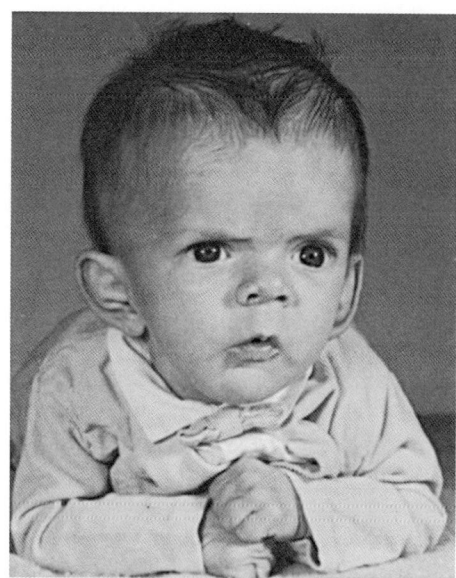

• **Fig. 3.11** Infant with thymic hypoplasia (DiGeorge anomaly). (From Stiehm RS: *Immunologic disorders in infants and children,* ed 5, Philadelphia, 2004, Saunders.)

be underdeveloped or absent, cardiac defects, and parathyroid hypoplasia. This leads to defects in T-cell number function and, in some cases, decreased B-cell function as well. Although some of these children will not be clinically immunodeficient, others will have increased sinopulmonary infections, and up to 1% will have life-threatening SCID as a result of the absent thymus. Most patients with DiGeorge anomaly have a microdeletion on a part of chromosome 22 (22q11.2).

Diagnosis
A definitive diagnosis requires a reduced number of T cells and two of the following three features: cardiovascular defects, hypocalcemia of greater than 3 weeks' duration, and a microdeletion involving chromosome 22 (detected by fluorescence in situ hybridization). Absence, hypoplasia, or abnormal placement of the thymus gland can be detected radiographically.

Treatment
Hypocalcemia should be treated to stabilize the myocardium and to reduce the risk of seizures. Vitamin D and parathyroid hormone replacement therapy are also necessary. Repair of cardiac anomalies may be attempted. Thymic transplantation or BMT may reconstitute immune function in patients with the most severe form of DiGeorge anomaly. Appropriate developmental interventions should be instituted. Safety of administering live vaccines should be determined on a case-by-case basis.

Prognosis
Complete DiGeorge anomaly is usually fatal within the first year of life because of cardiac dysfunction, hypocalcemia,

and/or infection. For some patients with partial DiGeorge anomaly, prognosis depends on the severity of the cardiac and parathyroid defects. Immune function, however, may improve with age and should be monitored regularly.

Prevention
No methods of prevention are known.

Patient Teaching
Congenital structural anomalies, the complications thereof, and the child's susceptibility to infections determine what information is most helpful to parents and caregivers. Procedures, such as those given to treat hypocalcemia, are explained. Referral for genetic counseling may be beneficial.

Chronic Mucocutaneous Candidiasis

Description
Chronic mucocutaneous candidiasis (CMC) refers to a group of disorders characterized by persistent and recurrent candidal (fungal) infections of the skin, nails, and mucous membranes. These disorders are unified by the inclusion of deficient cell-mediated immunity to *Candida* organisms.

ICD-10-CM Code	B37.9 (Candidiasis, unspecified)
	(B37.0-B37.9 = 16 codes of specificity)

Refer to the physician's diagnosis and then to the current edition of the ICD-10-CM coding manuals to ensure the greatest specificity of pathology.

Symptoms and Signs
Symptoms usually develop during the first 2 or 3 years of life or, if late-onset CMC, in young adulthood. Large circular lesions appear on the skin, mucous membranes, nails, or vagina. Sores in the mouth make eating difficult (Fig. 3.12). Recurrent thrush or diaper rash is often the first symptom of the disease in infants. Patients in late stages of the disease experience recurring respiratory tract infections. Associated endocrine disorders or autoimmune conditions can be found depending on the type of CMC. Later onset CMC can be associated with myasthenia gravis, thymoma, or bone marrow abnormalities. Interestingly, systemic *Candida* infections are not seen in these patients.

Syndromes of CMC are:
- chronic oral candidiasis (disease affecting the mucosa of the lips, tongue, and buccal cavity)
- CMC with endocrinopathy (hypoadrenalism, hypothyroidism, hypoparathyroidism, and ovarian failure in females)
- chronic localized candidiasis (cutaneous lesions with hyperkeratosis)
- chronic diffuse candidiasis (widespread infection of the skin, nails, and mucous membranes) (Fig. 3.13)
- candidiasis with thymoma (candidiasis accompanied by hypogammaglobulinemia, neutropenia, aplastic anemia, or myasthenia gravis)

Patient Screening
Frequent, persistent fungal infections of the mouth, skin, or nails in the young child necessitate a prompt appointment with the physician for medical evaluation and to begin treatment.

Etiology
In the immunocompetent individual, *Candida albicans* is a nonpathogenic normal flora. Patients with CMC have a T-cell deficit specific to *Candida* that makes them susceptible to infection. Other T-cell and B-cell functions are usually normal. Mutations in the autoimmune regulator gene *(AIRE)* or the *STAT1* gene have been implicated in CMC pathogenesis. These mutations also lead to susceptibility to various autoimmune diseases.

Diagnosis
Evaluation for CMC is prompted by a history of recurrent *Candida* infections. Potassium hydroxide preparations of scrapings from a lesion show yeast pseudohyphae (a string of atypical fungal cells) when examined under the microscope. Fungal culture grows *Candida*. Blood studies indicate normal T-cell circulation and normal antibody response to all organisms except *Candida*. Patients have normal immunoglobulin

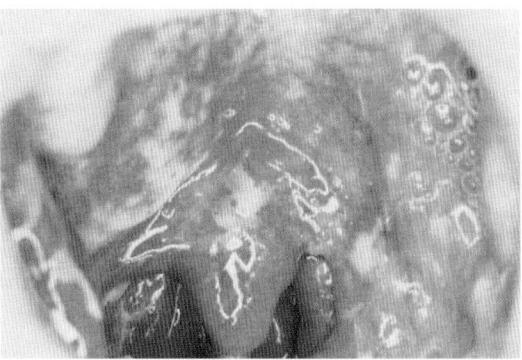

• **Fig. 3.12** Candidiasis. (From Sigler B: *Ear, nose, and throat disorders—Mosby's clinical nursing series,* St Louis, 1994, Mosby.)

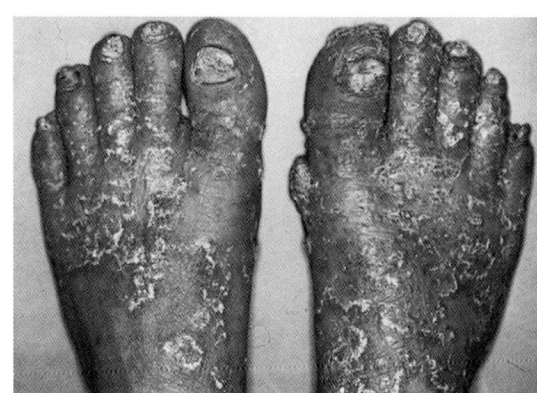

• **Fig. 3.13** Chronic mucocutaneous candidiasis (CMC) of the feet. (From Stiehm RS: *Immunologic disorders in infants and children,* ed 5, Philadelphia, 2004, Saunders.)

levels, normal lymphocyte numbers, and normal response to non-*Candida* antigens. Genetic testing for *AIRE* mutations can be done. Other immunodeficiency diseases need to be ruled out, and all endocrine functions should be evaluated. Any other abnormalities are evaluated according to the organs involved.

Treatment

Treatment is directed at eliminating the infections along with correcting the immunologic defects. Systemic therapy with antifungal agents is the mainstay of treatment. Chronic use of antifungals may prevent recurrences. Transfer factor, a protein of T lymphocytes isolated from donors sensitized to *Candida,* has been shown to increase the immune response to *Candida* in patients with CMC. Topical treatment with antifungal agents appears to improve skin and nail lesions. Associated endocrine or autoimmune disease should be treated appropriately.

Prognosis

Death caused by CMC is unusual because infections are usually localized. Treatment with antifungals has good results, but most patients relapse after cessation of these agents. The associated endocrinopathy or autoimmune disease is usually the major factor affecting prognosis.

Prevention

No method of prevention is known.

Patient Teaching

Give written instructions to the patient or the parents on the medication regimen. Teach comfort measures for mouth lesions, such as a soft diet and the use of a mild mouthwash and a soft toothbrush. Instruct the patient or parents not to delay medical attention for any infections or signs of relapse. Address questions regarding any endocrine involvement, as appropriate to the diagnosis.

Wiskott-Aldrich Syndrome

Description

Wiskott-Aldrich syndrome is a congenital disorder that is characterized by inadequate B- and T-cell function, thrombocytopenia, and eczema.

ICD-10-CM Code	D82.0 *(Wiskott-Aldrich syndrome)*

Symptoms and Signs

The child with Wiskott-Aldrich syndrome experiences eczema, thrombocytopenia with severe bleeding, and an increased susceptibility to bacterial and viral infections. Bleeding manifestations include petechiae, purpura, hematemesis, epistaxis, hematuria, and the more serious GI and intracranial bleeding. In about 50% of patients with Wiskott-Aldrich syndrome, eczema develops in the first year of life. These children are predisposed to the

development of autoimmune disorders (hemolytic anemia, vasculitis, etc.), and lymphoma.

Patient Screening

Severe bleeding manifestations call for immediate assessment and medical care. If the child is being treated for Wiskott-Aldrich syndrome and signs of infection are reported, prompt medical attention is indicated.

Etiology

This rare immunodeficiency disorder is inherited as an X-linked trait affecting only males. It arises from mutations in the gene encoding the Wiskott-Aldrich syndrome protein (WASP), which is expressed in hematopoietic cells. The thymus gland is normal at birth but decreases in size as the child grows up, resulting in decreased B- and T-cell functions. Additionally, metabolic defects in platelet synthesis that cause platelets to be short lived and phagocytes to be incompetent are both present. The average age at diagnosis is 21 months.

Diagnosis

Diagnosis is suspected in a boy with thrombocytopenia and small platelet size, especially when accompanied by eczema and frequent infections. The diagnosis is supported by finding a mutation in *WAS* gene. The numbers of T cells and B cells may be low. Vaccine response may be defective. Regulatory T-cell function is impaired.

Treatment

BMT is the only curative therapy. A high success rate can be expected when the donor is a human leukocyte antigen (HLA)–matched sibling. If BMT is not feasible, then splenectomy may result in an increase in platelet number and size. Additional treatment consists of IVIG and appropriate prophylactic antibiotic therapy. Topical or systemic steroids are used to treat eczema. Trials of gene therapy for Wiskott-Aldrich syndrome are currently underway.

Prognosis

Long-term survival is good for patients who receive a BMT before age 5 years. Patients who undergo splenectomy without BMT have a median survival of 25 years, whereas those who receive neither therapy often die before age 5 years. Bleeding, infections, and malignancy are the main causes of death.

Prevention

No methods of prevention are known.

Patient Teaching

Encourage the parent or caregiver to express concerns about episodes of bleeding. Discuss the signs of bleeding that require emergency care, such as signs of shock. Explain the importance of timely and aggressive treatment for infections. If bone marrow transplantation is scheduled, discuss the procedure and reinforce the physician's explanation of expected results. If the child is experiencing symptoms of eczema, demonstrate the topical application of medication as prescribed.

Autoimmune Diseases

Autoimmune diseases occur when the body's normal immune system mistakenly is misdirected against its own tissues. Autoimmunity is characterized by the presence of abnormal autoantibodies that bind to various portions of the body's own tissues. Tolerance to self-antigens is believed to commence during fetal life. As the body ages and experiences various disease processes or environmental exposures, persons with a variety of genetic risks can have changes in their immune system, because of which the system misidentifies body tissues and develops autoantibodies that result in self-destruction. Present theories consider this state of autoimmunity to be acquired, not congenital; however, certain gene markers identify patients at increased risk for many autoimmune diseases. Currently the specific gene products involved are mostly undetermined.

Autoimmune diseases can occur in many body systems when lymphocytes and antibodies are sensitized to develop against the self, that is, against the constituents of the body's own tissues. The production of the autoantibodies may occur by means of several mechanisms, including disease, injury, metabolic change, and a mutation of immunologically competent cells. Additionally, viral infection, trauma, and certain drugs or chemicals may alter specific body proteins, thereby thwarting recognition resulting in their rejection as if they were foreign proteins. Systems or body tissue particularly affected by autoimmunity and some of the resulting disease entities are listed in Table 3.2.

Hematopoietic Disorders

Autoimmune Hemolytic Anemia

Description

Autoimmune hemolytic anemia is an autoimmune condition in which red blood cells (RBCs) are destroyed by antibodies.

ICD-10-CM Code	D59.0 *(Drug-induced autoimmune hemolytic anemia)*
	D59.1 *(Other autoimmune hemolytic anemias)*
	(D59.0-D59.9 = 9 codes of specificity)

Symptoms and Signs

Autoimmune hemolytic anemia causes the patient to experience fatigue, weakness, chills, fever, dyspnea, and itching. The skin is pale and jaundiced and bruises easily. Additionally the patient may be hypotensive.

TABLE 3.2 Autoimmune Diseases

Body System or Tissue	Disease
Hematopoietic system	Autoimmune hemolytic anemia Pernicious anemia Idiopathic thrombocytopenic purpura (ITP) Idiopathic neutropenia
Kidney	Goodpasture syndrome Immune complex glomerulonephritis
Rheumatoid and collagen	Systemic lupus erythematosus (SLE) Progressive scleroderma (systemic sclerosis) Sjögren syndrome Rheumatoid arthritis (RA) Juvenile rheumatoid arthritis (JRA)
Endocrine system[a]	Graves disease Hashimoto disease (chronic thyroiditis) Type 1 diabetes
Neurologic system	Multiple sclerosis (MS) Myasthenia gravis
Vascular system	Small vessel vasculitis Systemic necrotizing vasculitis

[a]See Chapter 4.

Patient Screening

Schedule a same-day appointment for the patient experiencing the symptoms listed above. Patients with mild or fewer symptoms may be scheduled with less urgency.

Etiology

Because of a misguided immune response, B cell–produced antibodies do not identify RBCs as self, resulting in agglutination of RBCs and an attack on and destruction of the red corpuscles. The two types of hemolytic anemia are warm antibody (agglutinin) anemia and cold antibody (agglutinin) anemia. Warm antibody anemia is associated with an excess of IgG antibodies that react with protein antigens on the RBC surface at body temperature. Although most cases are idiopathic, some may be stimulated by certain drugs (e.g., penicillins), autoimmune diseases (e.g., SLE), or malignancies (especially chronic lymphocytic leukemia). Cold antibody anemia results from fixation of complement proteins on IgM that occurs at colder temperatures (best around 30°F). This type is regularly seen in conjunction with infectious mononucleosis or *Mycoplasma* pneumonia.

Diagnosis

A direct Coombs test indicates antibody-coated RBCs that agglutinate when antiglobulin is added to the medium. Some RBCs appear spherical (spherocytes) as visualized under a microscope; serum bilirubin levels are elevated; and RBC count, platelet count, hemoglobin (Hgb) concentration, and hematocrit usually are all decreased. The reticulocyte (immature RBC) count is usually elevated. Examination of a peripheral blood smear for agglutination of RBCs and flow cytometry may be performed. In mild or sporadic disease, these previously mentioned findings might be less evident.

Treatment

Treatment should first address any underlying disease or drug use that could be causing the hemolytic anemia. Warm and cold antibody anemias are treated differently. In warm antibody anemia, corticosteroids and cytotoxic drugs are administered to reduce antibody production. Splenectomy or IVIG administration may be done to reduce antibody effectiveness. RBC transfusions may be attempted. The most useful therapy in the treatment of cold antibody anemia is avoidance of the cold by dressing warmly even in the summer, wearing gloves and warm hats, and spending the colder months in warmer climates. Plasmapheresis may be helpful in reducing hemolysis.

Prognosis

Anemia resulting from infection or drug use usually abates after the infection resolves or the drug is discontinued. Anemia resulting from other causes is often chronic and poorly responsive to therapy. Warm antibody anemia is generally self-limited in children, disappearing within 1 to 3 months.

Prevention

No methods of prevention are known.

Patient Teaching

Explain the diagnostic tests, and tell the patient when to expect results. If the cause has been determined, explain how the RBCs are being destroyed and how the treatment regimen is expected to help. Discuss expected results from IVIG administration or, if indicated, the removal of the spleen. Instructions on monitoring blood tests can be helpful.

Pernicious Anemia

Description

Pernicious anemia is caused by chronic atrophic gastritis resulting in decreased gastric production of hydrochloric acid and a shortage of intrinsic factor. Additionally the antibodies that are produced are directed against intrinsic factor and parietal cells. These two factors lead to impaired vitamin B_{12} absorption and B_{12} deficiency.

ICD-10-CM Code	D51.0 *(Vitamin B_{12} deficiency anemia due to intrinsic factor deficiency)*
	(D51.0-D51.9 = 6 codes of specificity)

Symptoms and Signs

Patients with pernicious anemia can develop a sore tongue, weakness, and tingling and numbness in the extremities. The lips, tongue, and gums appear pale, whereas the sclera and skin appear slightly jaundiced (Fig. 3.14). Because of the decreased hydrochloric acid production and atrophy of the gastric mucosa, the patient experiences disturbances in digestion, such as anorexia, nausea, vomiting, diarrhea, constipation, flatulence, and weight loss. In this condition, the individual is more vulnerable to infections. Vitamin B_{12} deficiency causes demyelination of the peripheral nerves and eventually the spinal cord. This leads to neuritis, peripheral weakness, numbness, and paresthesia. Ataxia (muscular incoordination), light-headedness, altered vision, tinnitus, and optic muscle atrophy are additional symptoms that may occur as the anemia progresses. CNS changes may cause headaches, irritability, and depression. Reduced Hgb levels cause decreased oxygen-carrying capacity, leading to fatigue, weakness, and lightheadedness. The patient may experience palpitations, dyspnea, tachycardia, premature ventricular contractions, and even congestive heart failure.

Patient Screening

Initially the patient may have insidious and vague symptoms; unless the symptoms are severe, the patient is scheduled for a medical evaluation as soon as it is convenient. Patients complaining of weakness or cardiovascular symptoms (e.g., a rapid heart rate) require prompt medical care. A same-day appointment is scheduled for the patient being treated for pernicious anemia if physical or psychological complications develop.

Etiology

Greater than 90% of patients with pernicious anemia have anti-parietal cell antibodies, which can be cytotoxic to the *parietal* cells. In the majority of patients, anti-intrinsic factor antibodies are also present. Intrinsic factor must be present in the gastric mucosa for vitamin B_{12} absorption to occur. Vitamin B_{12} is necessary for RBC formation, and a deficiency causes RBCs to be deformed and reduced in number. Pernicious anemia is often associated with other autoimmune diseases, such as Graves disease or Hashimoto thyroiditis. It is particularly common in people of Northern European descent ages 40 to 70 years, but it can be seen in any ethnic group.

Diagnosis

Diagnosis is confirmed by the clinical findings and laboratory tests. The Schilling test and/or blood evaluation for the presence of anti-parietal cell or anti-intrinsic factor antibodies is performed. Blood tests reveal a decrease in Hgb level, decreased RBC count, and increased mean cell volume (MCV). The RBCs and the platelets are large and malformed. Bone marrow studies indicate abnormal RBC production and other changes typical of vitamin B_{12} deficiency. Reduced amounts or absence of gastric acid is found on gastric analysis. Hypersegmented neutrophils

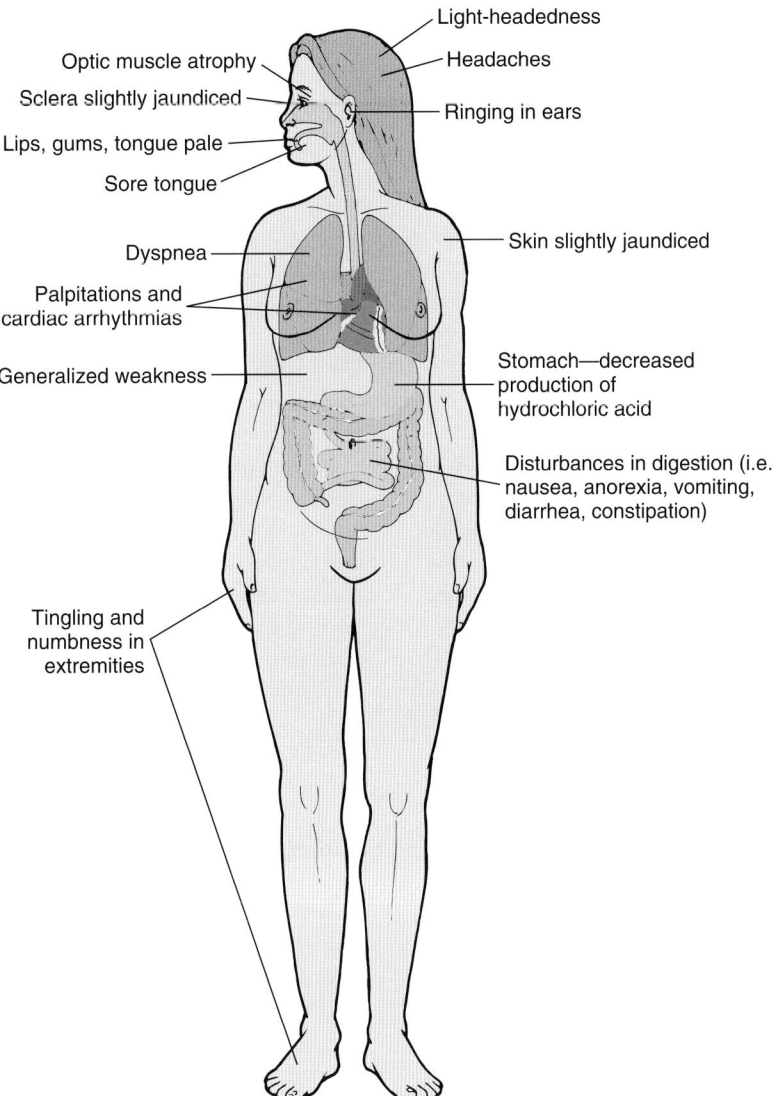

Optic muscle atrophy

Sclera slightly jaundiced

Lips, gums, tongue pale

Sore tongue

Light-headedness

Headaches

Ringing in ears

Skin slightly jaundiced

Dyspnea

Palpitations and
cardiac arrhythmias

Generalized weakness

Stomach—decreased
production of
hydrochloric acid

Disturbances in digestion (i.e.,
nausea, anorexia, vomiting,
diarrhea, constipation)

Tingling and
numbness in
extremities

• **Fig. 3.14** Symptoms and signs of pernicious anemia.

(megaloblasts) on a peripheral blood smear are characteristic. Vitamin B_{12} also is necessary for proper myelin formation; a myelin deficiency can cause damage to the nerves (neuropathy).

Treatment

Initially weekly and then monthly intramuscular injections of vitamin B_{12} are the primary treatment for pernicious anemia, and they are often continued for life. B_{12} is also available in a sublingual form and a nasal spray. Blood replacement may be indicated in severe cases. Supportive measures include adequate rest, gentle nonirritating mouth care, a well-balanced diet high in vitamin B_{12}, and the use of tranquilizers for behavioral problems.

Prognosis

No cure for pernicious anemia is known, but early detection and treatment with vitamin B_{12} maintains a normal hemogram and neurologic function in most patients.

Prevention

No method of prevention for the primary condition is known. Patients who have had extensive gastric surgery also may benefit from vitamin B_{12} replacement because they often cannot produce the intrinsic factor necessary for B_{12} absorption.

Patient Teaching

During the diagnostic phase, give careful instructions about the 24-hour urine collections needed for an accurate Schilling test. If bone marrow studies are ordered, explain the procedure. Once diagnosed, inform the patient that improvement is likely within weeks of treatment and good compliance with the treatment regimen. To promote compliance, explain the importance of lifelong vitamin B_{12} replacement therapy; demonstrate the injection technique to the patient or caregiver, if required. Review signs of any complications that should be reported to the physician.

Idiopathic Thrombocytopenic Purpura

Description
Idiopathic thrombocytopenic purpura (ITP) is an acquired disorder that results from an isolated deficiency of platelets (i.e., other blood counts are normal). It is believed that platelet destruction and/or inhibition of platelet production is the result of autoantibodies against platelets.

ICD-10-CM Code	D69.3 *(Immune thrombocytopenic purpura)* (D69.0-D69.9 = 11 codes of specificity)

Symptoms and Signs
Symptoms are related to an inability of the blood to clot and include spontaneous hemorrhages in skin, mucous membranes, or internal organs. Petechiae, small spiderlike hemorrhages under the surface of the skin (Fig. 3.15), and ecchymoses, larger hemorrhagic areas, are apparent. The patient may experience epistaxis (nosebleeds), GI bleeding, menorrhagia, hematuria, and easy bruising. The clinical symptoms vary with patient age, with older patients exhibiting more severe bleeding symptoms.

Patient Screening
Multiple bruising of unknown cause in a child or an adult requires prompt medical attention. (Note: An event of spontaneous bruising in a child can cause a parent to become extremely alarmed and also precipitates in medical personnel a natural concern about the child's welfare. Care must be taken by medical personnel to avoid judgmental attitudes toward parents unless a sound reason to suspect child abuse has been established.)

Etiology
Thrombocytopenic purpura often is considered idiopathic (of unknown cause), although antibodies that reduce the life of platelets have been found in most cases. Some cases may occur after a viral infection, especially rubella or mumps. Additionally the spleen may be destroying the damaged platelets.

Diagnosis
The diagnosis of ITP is often one of exclusion; therefore other causes of thrombocytopenia must be ruled out first. CBC and peripheral blood smear analysis are performed. The clinical symptoms, along with prolonged bleeding time and reduced platelet count, suggest the diagnosis. The size and shape of the platelets may be abnormal. Circulating platelet time is reduced to hours instead of the normal days. Testing for other diseases, such as HIV infection and SLE, is often performed to rule out other causes of the thrombocytopenia.

Treatment
Corticosteroid administration increases capillary integrity for a short time. IVIG may be administered to increase the platelet count. Anemia needs to be corrected with blood transfusion, and vitamin K administration improves the clotting mechanism. Therapeutic plasma exchange occasionally is attempted. Splenectomy is generally a last resort; however, this treatment is effective. Platelet numbers typically increase rapidly after the procedure. Children are often just given supportive therapy and short-term steroid treatment because ITP in children is usually self-limiting.

Prognosis
Children often experience spontaneous remission of the disease, many times occurring within 2 to 8 weeks of diagnosis. The adult forms are rarely self-limiting. With appropriate treatment, which may be long term, only about 1% of patients die of their disease.

Prevention
No methods of prevention are known.

Patient Teaching
Explain the purpose and procedure of prescribed infusion therapy. The parents of a young child will benefit from reassurance that complete remission is likely. Adults with chronic ITP who fail to respond to initial treatment with corticosteroids may require preoperative instructions for splenectomy.

Immune Neutropenia

Description
The term *immune neutropenia* is used to describe neutropenia, which is a decrease in the number of circulating

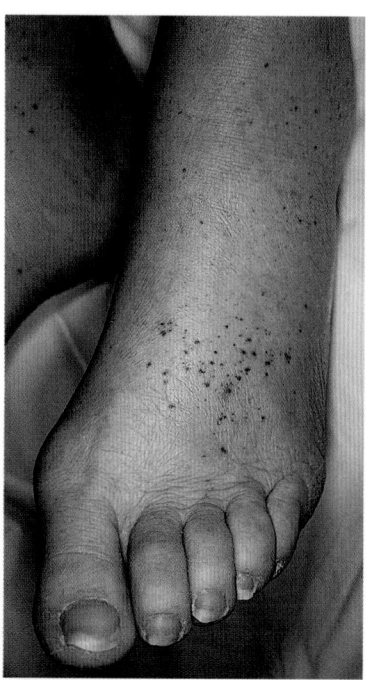

• **Fig. 3.15** Idiopathic thrombocytopenic purpura (ITP). (From *Mosby's dictionary of medicine, nursing and health professionals*, ed 8, St Louis, 2010, Mosby.)

neutrophils usually caused by the production of antineutrophil antibodies.

ICD-10-CM Code   D70.9 *(Neutropenia, unspecified)*
(D70.0-D70.9 = 7 codes of specificity)

Symptoms and Signs
The patient with immune neutropenia experiences malaise, fatigue, weakness, fever, and stomatitis. Recurrent infections are common, especially upper respiratory infections and otitis media in infants.

Patient Screening
Schedule an infant with a respiratory infection for a prompt medical evaluation. Follow office policy regarding referral to a pediatrician. The adult patient complaining of the above symptoms needs a medical evaluation at the first available opportunity.

Etiology
Immune-mediated neutropenia is often associated with an accelerated turnover of neutrophils (increased neutrophil production), but there is an even greater increase in destruction mediated by the antineutrophil antibodies. There is almost complete absence of neutrophils in blood. The neutropenia may be associated with infection, drug exposure, ITP, autoimmune hemolytic anemia, or connective tissue diseases, including SLE and rheumatoid arthritis (RA). A type of immune neutropenia, isoimmune neutropenia, is a rare disorder caused by the transplacental transfer of maternal IgG that reacts with fetal neutrophils. This type of neutropenia usually resolves in 12 to 15 weeks.

Diagnosis
Neutropenia is confirmed by the significantly reduced numbers of neutrophils displayed in a white blood cell (WBC) count. Detection of antineutrophil antibodies is possible in many patients using assays, such as immunofluorescence, agglutination tests, and antiglobulin analysis.

Treatment
Infants with idiopathic neutropenia usually require no specific treatment because their disease typically resolves spontaneously. Children, adults, and infants with severe disease may be treated with corticosteroids, immune globulin, or granulocyte–colony-stimulating factor (G-CSF; a hematopoietic growth factor). Appropriate antibiotics are administered to treat bacterial infections. Transfusions of WBC concentrates may be indicated. Care must be taken to prevent exposure to any type of infection.

Prognosis
In infants, the disease usually resolves spontaneously. Neutropenia in children and adults often follows a benign course, especially with appropriate treatment.

Prevention
No methods of prevention are known.

Patient Teaching
The parents of infants with immune neutropenia can benefit from understanding the relationship between frequent infections and the condition. When treatment is required, explain the effect of immune therapy, transfusion, or the need for antibiotics as prescribed.

Renal Disorders
Goodpasture Syndrome
Description
Goodpasture syndrome (also known as *anti–glomerular basement membrane [GBM] antibody disease*) is an autoimmune kidney disease characterized by the presence of antibodies directed against an antigen in the GBM.

ICD-10-CM Code   M31.0 *(Hypersensitivity angiitis)*
(M31.0-M31.9 = 11 codes of specificity)

Symptoms and Signs
The patient with Goodpasture syndrome experiences acute glomerulonephritis, relatively acute renal failure with proteinuria, anemia, hemoptysis, and hematuria. Systemic complaints may include weight loss, fatigue, and fever.

Patient Screening
Symptoms of acute renal failure, such as scanty urine, blood in urine, and systemic complaints, signal critical illness that requires immediate medical care.

Etiology
The cause of this rare disease is obscure. Antibodies cause complement-mediated tissue damage in the glomerular and alveolar basement membranes, resulting in glomerulonephritis and pulmonary hemorrhage. Progression of the disease may lead to end-stage renal failure.

Diagnosis
The diagnosis is suspected in any patient with acute glomerulonephritis, especially if accompanied by pulmonary hemorrhage and acute renal failure. Detection of anti-GBM antibodies in the serum or the kidney is necessary for definitive diagnosis. This can be done by performing ELISA, immunofluorescence, or renal biopsy. Urinalysis indicates the presence of protein and blood in urine.

Treatment
The treatment of choice is plasmapheresis (to remove anti-GBM antibody) combined with immunosuppressive agents (corticosteroids and cyclophosphamide). The treatment is usually administered for 6 to 12 months. Hemodialysis and

kidney transplantation are the last resorts for severely compromised patients.

Prognosis

Goodpasture syndrome is often self-limiting, and those who survive for a year after the initial diagnosis and maintain intact renal function usually do well. Patient survival during that time correlates with the degree of renal impairment at presentation and the amount of pulmonary involvement. Relapses can occur.

Prevention

No methods of prevention are known. Regular dosing of medication according to prescribed intervals can help minimized chances of reflaring.

Patient Teaching

Explain the purpose and procedure for the diagnostic studies. After the diagnosis has been made, discuss the effects of renal impairment on body systems, as appropriate to the patient's symptoms. Explain the purpose of plasmapheresis and the expected results from the medical regimen. Refer the patient to a dietitian for instruction on how best to maintain optimal nutritional status. Teach the patient how to monitor weight, intake and output of fluids, and warning signs of complications. Encourage questions regarding treatment options as presented by the physician.

Connective Tissue Diseases

The main component of connective tissue, an essential part of all structures in the body, is a fibrous, insoluble protein called collagen. Collagen constitutes 30% of the total body protein.

Connective tissue diseases are autoimmune disorders. In autoimmune disorders, the immune system malfunctions and works against itself. In these connective tissue diseases, the immune system attacks and destroys the collagen, resulting in damage to some of the body's connective tissues. The precise reason for this malfunction of the immune system is unknown, but genetic factors do play some role. The immune system incorrectly identifies the body's own tissues as foreign and attacks them.

No cures for connective tissue diseases are known; treatment is directed at quieting the overactive immune system and reducing inflammation. In some patients, serious damage to the heart, lungs, or kidneys occurs.

Two well-known examples of the many connective tissue diseases are SLE and RA.

Systemic Lupus Erythematosus

Description

SLE, also known as *lupus,* is a chronic, inflammatory autoimmune disease characterized by unusual autoantibodies in the blood that target tissues of the body.

ICD-10-CM Code	M32.10 *(Systemic lupus erythematosus, organ or system involvement unspecified)*
	(M32.0-M32.9 = 10 codes of specificity)

Symptoms and Signs

SLE can inflame and damage connective tissue anywhere in the body. SLE most commonly produces inflammation of skin, joints, nervous system, kidneys, lungs, and other organs. The degree to which any of these tissues are involved varies from patient to patient. A characteristic butterfly rash, or erythema, may be present on the face, spreading from one cheek across the nose to the other cheek (Fig. 3.16A). Similar rashes may appear on other exposed areas of the body. Exposure to the sun can aggravate the rash, a feature known as *photosensitivity.* SLE may begin acutely with fever, fatigue, joint pain, and malaise or may develop slowly over a period of years, with intermittent fever, malaise, joint deformities, and weight loss. Raynaud phenomenon and hair loss are common in SLE. This disease occurs most often in women in their 30s or 40s.

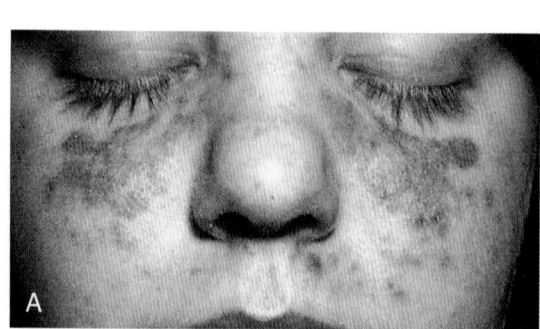
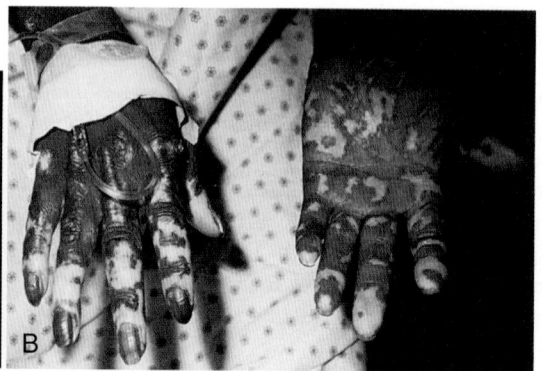

• **Fig. 3.16** (A) Typical butterfly rash of systemic lupus erythematosus (SLE). (B) SLE in black skin. (A, From Goldstein BJ, Goldstein AO: *Practical dermatology,* ed 2, St Louis, 1997, Mosby. Courtesy the Department of Dermatology, University of North Carolina at Chapel Hill. B, From Hill MJ: *Skin disorders—Mosby's clinical nursing series,* St Louis, 1994, Mosby.)

Patient Screening

The manifestation of an unexplained cluster of symptoms, as described earlier, requires a complete medical evaluation. After the initial diagnostic evaluation, follow office policy for referral to a rheumatologist.

Etiology

The cause of SLE is unknown; however, it is thought to be an autoimmune disorder. Genetic, environmental, and hormonal factors may predispose a person to this disease. Events that can precipitate SLE include stress, immunization reactions, pregnancy, and overexposure to ultraviolet light.

Diagnosis

Patients with symptoms of SLE are evaluated for other rheumatic diseases (including RA, dermatomyositis, scleroderma, and Sjögren disease), other autoimmune diseases (including autoimmune hemolytic anemia, autoimmune thyroiditis, and pernicious anemia), and nonautoimmune diseases (e.g., cancer and infections).

The formal diagnosis of SLE can be made if four or more of the following symptoms or positive laboratory tests are present either at the same time or sequentially: a butterfly rash on the face (see Fig. 3.16A), a discoid skin lesion, photosensitivity. Visual appearance of SLE may be impacted by natural skin color. (see Fig 3.16B).

Other symptoms or positive laboratory tests include nasopharyngeal ulceration, polyarthritis without deformity seizures or psychosis, chronic pleuritis or pericarditis, a false-positive serologic test result for syphilis or deoxyribonucleic acid (DNA) or Sm (Smith, an uncharacterized nuclear antigen) antibodies in blood or cardiolipin antibody, greater than 0.5 g of protein in urine in a 24-hour period, the presence of cellular casts in urine, hemolytic anemia, thrombocytopenia, the presence of abnormal antibodies in the bloodstream, and the characteristic leukocytes (WBCs) called *LE cells,* which are not found in the circulation but are created in the laboratory as part of the testing. Diagnostic tests include CBC with differential leukocyte count, platelet count, erythrocyte sedimentation rate (ESR), antinuclear antibody determination, anti-DNA antibody, anti-Sm antibody, and anti-chromatin antibody. The anti-DNA test is the most specific test for SLE, but it is reliably positive more often with active disease.

Treatment

In mild cases, antiinflammatory drugs, including aspirin, nonsteroidal antiinflammatory drugs (NSAIDs), or prednisone, are effective to relieve constitutional symptoms, such as fever and joint pain. Antimalarial agents are commonly added to control skin involvement and arthralgia. For more substantial symptoms, corticosteroids are indicated. Immunosuppressive medications are useful when organ-threatening disease is present. Immunosuppressive agents are also helpful when the patient fails to respond to conventional therapy or when intolerable side effects develop.

The prognosis for SLE varies, depending on the location and degree of organ involvement. It improves with early detection and treatment but remains poor for persons with renal, cardiovascular, or neurologic complications. Morbidity and mortality increases with serious bacterial infection.

Prognosis

The outlook for patients with systemic lupus continues to improve with the development of more accurate monitoring tests and treatments. The prognosis depends on internal organ involvement. Patients with lupus are at a somewhat increased risk for developing cancer as well as heart disease. The cancer risk is most dramatic for blood cancers, such as leukemia and lymphoma, but is also increased for breast cancer.

Prevention

It is essential that patients are diligent in adhering to their medication regimens. Flare-ups of disease can be prevented by not missing doses of prescribed medications and avoiding unnecessary exposure to sunlight.

Patient Teaching

Teaching the patient and the family about the elements of the disease and laboratory testing can beneficially impact the health of patients with lupus. When appropriate, reinforce the physician's advice to avoid stress, decrease exposure to sunlight, cease smoking, and perform moderate exercise.

Scleroderma (Systemic Sclerosis)

Description

Scleroderma is a chronic, progressive disease characterized mostly by sclerosis (hardening) of the skin; scarring of certain internal organs can occur as well. Scleroderma is classified as either diffuse or limited, depending on the extent and location of skin involvement. The diffuse form involves symmetric thickening of the skin of the extremities, face, and trunk, whereas the limited form tends to be confined to the skin of the fingers and face.

ICD-10-CM Code	M34.0 *(Progressive systemic sclerosis)*
	M34.1 *(CR[E]ST syndrome)*
	M34.9 *(Systemic sclerosis, unspecified)*
	(M34.0-M34.9 = 8 codes of specificity)

Symptoms and Signs

Scleroderma is characterized by sclerosis (hardening) and shrinking of the skin and certain internal organs, including the GI tract, heart, lungs, and kidneys. Involved skin becomes taut, firm, and edematous and is firmly attached to the subcutaneous tissue (Fig. 3.17). The skin feels tough and leathery, it may itch, and pigmented patches may occur. Raynaud phenomenon (see Raynaud disease in Chapter 10) is often the first symptom of scleroderma. This is followed by swelling, stiffness, and pain in the joints.

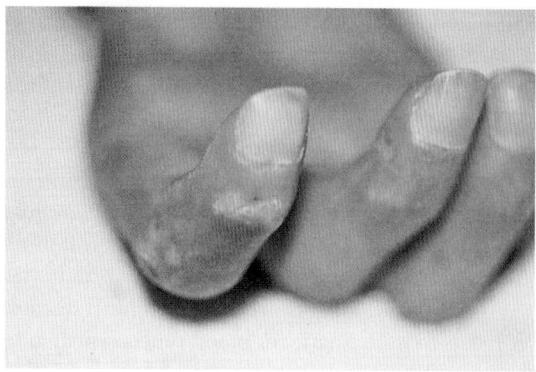

• **Fig. 3.17** CREST (calcinosis, Raynaud phenomenon, esophageal dysmotility, sclerodactyly, and telangiectasia) syndrome of scleroderma. (From Hill MJ: *Skin disorders—Mosby's clinical nursing series,* St Louis, 1994, Mosby.)

Patient Screening

Arrange an appointment for a consultation and medical evaluation to determine options for a person describing unexplained skin changes. Scleroderma can take many forms, affects different parts of the body, and is hard to diagnose.

Etiology

The cause of scleroderma is unknown, but it appears to be an autoimmune disease. It features abnormal activation of scar-forming cells (fibroblasts), vascular endothelial abnormalities, and immune dysregulation. It occurs four times more often in women, especially those 30 to 50 years of age, compared with men.

Diagnosis

A complete history and physical examination are all that are necessary for a diagnosis to be made. Laboratory testing, including Scl-70 and centromere antibodies, can be supportive of the diagnosis. A skin biopsy is only rarely necessary. Blood tests and urinalysis are performed to rule out complications or accompanying conditions. Patients with scleroderma are also evaluated for signs of SLE, polymyositis, Sjögren disease, and hypothyroidism. Lung function testing is helpful to detect pulmonary disease, and echocardiography can be helpful to screen for pulmonary hypertension. Further testing may include high-resolution computed tomography (high-res CT) of the chest and right heart catheterization.

Treatment

No specific treatment for scleroderma is known. A large number of drugs have been tried, including corticosteroids, vasodilators, and immunosuppressive agents, but their effects are merely palliative. Treatment is directed to the area(s) of the body affected. Rheumatology referral is recommended. Physical therapy helps patients maintain muscle strength but does not change the course of joint disease.

Prognosis

The prognosis for patients with scleroderma depends on which organs are affected and the severity of organ involvement. Patients with pulmonary hypertension, interstitial lung disease, and those with uncontrolled blood pressure have a higher risk of mortality.

Prevention

How to prevent scleroderma is not known. Preventing its complications, such as those from Raynaud phenomenon and esophageal reflux, may require medications and lifestyle changes.

Patient Teaching

Teaching the patient and the family about the elements of the disease and laboratory testing can be beneficial to the health of patients with scleroderma. Offer referrals to support groups for individuals coping with chronic disease.

Sjögren Syndrome

Description

Sjögren (pronounced sho'-gren) syndrome is an autoimmune disease that manifests inflammation in the moisture-secreting glands of the body (Fig. 3.18). The result of this glandular problem is dryness in the affected areas.

ICD-10-CM Code	M35.00 *(Sicca syndrome, unspecified)*
	M35.01 *(Sicca syndrome with keratoconjunctivitis)*
	(M35.0-M35.9 = 15 codes of specificity)

Symptoms and Signs

Sjögren syndrome symptoms include xerostomia and keratoconjunctivitis sicca. This dryness of the nasal, oral, and laryngeal pharynx causes difficulty talking, chewing, and

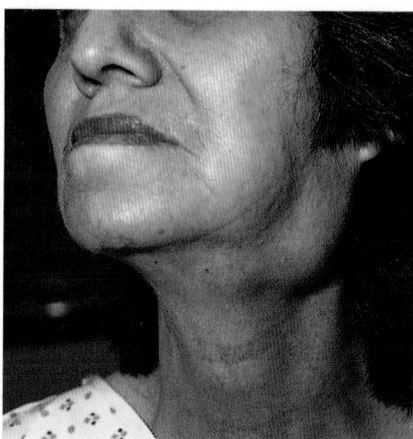

• **Fig. 3.18** Enlargement of the salivary gland in Sjögren syndrome. (From *Mosby's dictionary of medicine, nursing and health professionals,* ed 8, St Louis, 2010, Mosby.)

swallowing. The patient may experience sores on or in the mouth and nose, and dental decay may occur. Sjögren syndrome can follow or precede the onset of RA.

Patient Screening

The onset of symptoms may be insidious or present with much discomfort caused by dryness in the eyes or the oral cavity. When discomfort is present, offer the patient the first available appointment for medical evaluation.

Etiology

The exact cause of Sjögren syndrome is not known. Genetic (inherited) factors seem to play a role in predisposing a person to Sjögren syndrome. It is found more commonly in families that have members with other autoimmune illnesses. Most patients with Sjögren syndrome are females.

Diagnosis

Patients with symptoms of Sjögren syndrome are screened for medication side effects, autoimmune thyroid disease, RA, SLE, sarcoidosis, and scleroderma associated with Sjögren syndrome. Dry eyes can be defined as abnormal results on the Schirmer test for dryness (Fig. 3.19). Enlarged salivary glands may prompt further investigation, including a lower lip biopsy, which may indicate a characteristic infiltration of lymphocytes. Blood studies often demonstrate anemia, decreased WBC count, and elevated ESR. Additional blood testing shows autoantibodies, called *Sjögren syndrome antibodies* (SSA and SSB antibodies), and high rheumatoid factor titers.

Treatment

Treatment is directed toward relieving symptoms, especially for the dryness in the oral cavity and the eyes. Increasing fluid intake, chewing sugarless gum, and using oral sprays help relieve oral dryness. Artificial tears are used in the eyes, and wearing sunglasses is recommended. Sometimes ophthalmologists block the tear ducts with silicone or by cautery to maintain adequate eye moisture. Occasionally prednisone and/or antimalarial medications, such as hydroxychloroquine, are used to lessen the immune inflammation.

Prognosis

Prognosis depends on what complications develop, such as infections in the respiratory tract. A rare complication of Sjögren syndrome is cancer of the lymph glands (lymphoma), for which patients are monitored.

Prevention

Prevention focuses on avoiding irritation of tissues caused by dryness, monitoring for the development of cancer, and the early management of infections.

Patient Teaching

Patients with Sjögren syndrome can benefit by learning about the immune system and precisely how their bodies are affected by the condition. Awareness of the early warning signs of infection can prevent many serious complications. Moisturizing products for the mouth, eyes, and vagina are available over the counter.

Rheumatoid Arthritis

Description

RA is a chronic, inflammatory, systemic disease that affects the joints (Fig. 3.20). It is one of the most severe forms of arthritis, commonly causing deformity and disability. RA affects 1.5 million Americans; women are affected three times more often compared with men. RA may begin at any age, but it most commonly strikes individuals in their 30s and 40s.

ICD-10-CM Code	M06.9 *(Rheumatoid arthritis, unspecified)* (M06.00-M06.9 = 97 codes of specificity)

Symptoms and Signs

RA causes inflammation and edema of the synovial membranes surrounding a joint. Eventually this inflammation spreads to other parts of the affected joint and, if left untreated, has the capacity to destroy cartilage, deform joints,

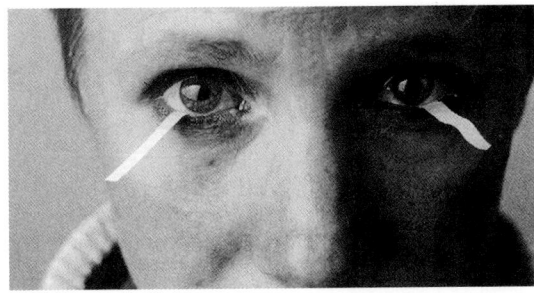

• **Fig. 3.19** Schirmer tear test. (From Mudge-Grout C: *Immunologic disorders—Mosby's clinical nursing series*, St Louis, 1992, Mosby.)

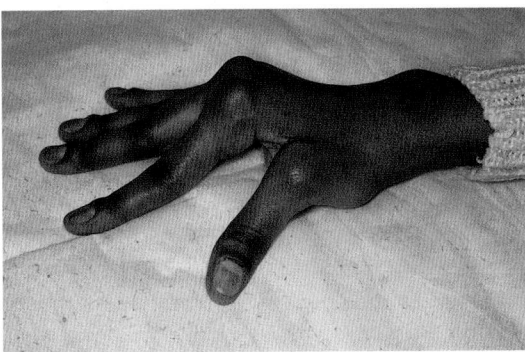

• **Fig. 3.20** Joints affected by rheumatoid arthritis (RA). (From Swartz MH: *Textbook of physical diagnosis, history, and examination*, ed 6, Philadelphia, 2010, Saunders.)

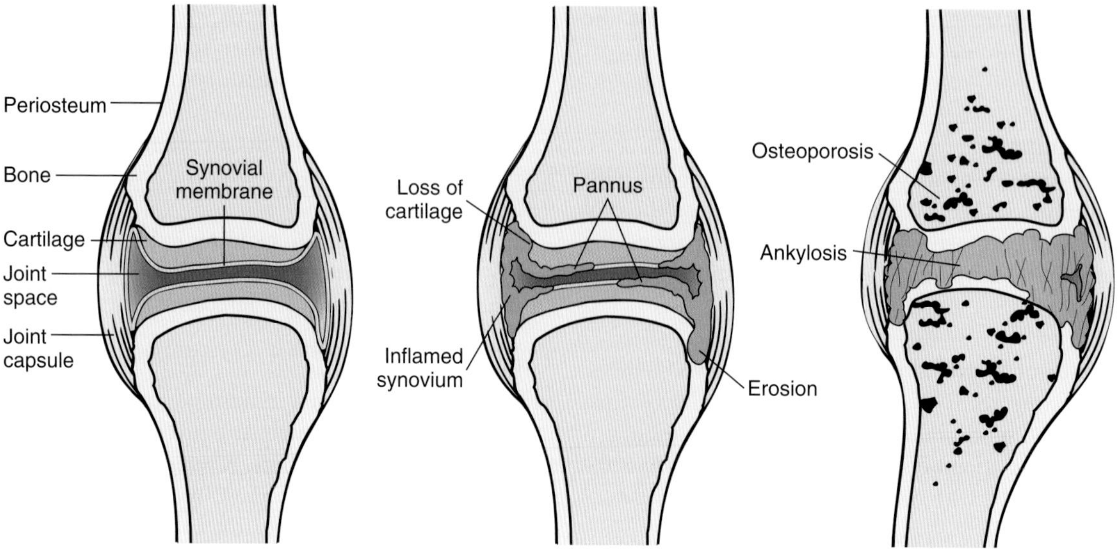

• **Fig. 3.21** Schematic presentation of the pathologic changes in rheumatoid arthritis (RA). The inflammation (synovitis) leads to pannus formation, to obliteration of the articular space, and finally to ankylosis. The periarticular bone shows diffuse atrophy in the form of osteoporosis. (From Damjanov I: *Pathology for the health-related professions,* ed 4, St Louis, 2011, Saunders.)

and destroy adjacent bone (Fig. 3.21). Most commonly, many joints (polyarthritis) on both sides of the body are affected by RA. Occasionally only one or two joints may be affected. When the neck is involved, the spinal cord can be at risk for damage, potentially leading to paralysis or death. RA is called a *systemic disease* because it can affect the entire body. It can cause generalized inflammation around or in the lungs, in the cardiac muscle, in blood vessels, and within the skin layers.

RA may begin without any obvious symptoms in the joints. The person may have unexplained weight loss, fatigue, a persistent low-grade fever, and general malaise. This may accompany or precede joint stiffness, which is noticed especially on wakening and during periods of inactivity. Edema, pain, tenderness, erythema, and warmth in one or more joints occurring in a symmetric pattern gradually emerge as the principal symptoms. Joints typically affected are those of the fingers, wrists, knees, ankles, and toes. RA occurs less often in the spine or the hips, which are more susceptible to osteoarthritis (see the Osteoarthritis section in Chapter 7).

In some patients, the joint symptoms appear suddenly without any precursor symptoms. In other cases, joint symptoms are accompanied by bursitis or anemia. Some persons may have only one mild attack, whereas others may have several episodes that may leave them increasingly disabled.

Patient Screening

RA may have an insidious onset with vague systemic symptoms and joint pain, but occasionally the onset is abrupt. Initially the patient should be seen for diagnostic evaluation. Follow office policy regarding referral to a rheumatologist as soon as possible (see the Enrichment box about Rheumatologist: The Arthritis Doctor).

❖ ENRICHMENT

Rheumatologist: The Arthritis Doctor

A rheumatologist is a medical doctor who specializes in the nonsurgical treatment of rheumatic illnesses, especially arthritis. Rheumatologists have a special interest in unexplained conditions, such as a rash, fever, arthritis, anemia, weakness, weight loss, fatigue, joint or muscle pain, autoimmune disease, and anorexia. They often serve as consultants, acting as detectives for other doctors in evaluating chronic medical problems.

Rheumatologists have particular skills in the evaluation and treatment of the greater than 100 forms of arthritis and rheumatic diseases, including the following:

- rheumatoid arthritis (RA)
- Sjögren syndrome
- osteoarthritis
- psoriatic arthritis
- systemic lupus erythematosus (SLE)
- ankylosing spondylitis (AS)
- gout
- pseudogout
- mixed connective tissue diseases
- fibromyalgia
- osteomyelitis
- osteoporosis
- back pain
- vasculitis
- scleroderma
- Lyme disease
- sarcoidosis
- serum sickness
- reactive arthritis
- Raynaud disease
- growing pains

Pediatric rheumatologists are physicians who specialize in providing comprehensive care to children (as well as their families) with rheumatic diseases, especially arthritis.

(Courtesy William C. Shiel, MD, Mission Viejo, CA.)

Etiology

The exact cause of RA is unknown, although it is thought to be an autoimmune disorder. Heredity may predispose some persons to the disease; in other patients, a viral infection may trigger the disease process.

Diagnosis

Patients with symptoms of RA are first evaluated for SLE, Sjögren syndrome, scleroderma, polymyositis, hormone disorders, cancer, and other possible causes of polyarthritis. Diagnosis is based on a review of the symptoms, patient and family histories, physical examination, radiographic studies, and blood tests that show elevated levels of rheumatoid factor in most patients. Other useful laboratory tests include CBC, synovial fluid analysis, serum protein electrophoresis, ESR, citrulline antibody, and antinuclear antibody titer. Occasionally the diagnosis of RA is achieved only after observation of disease progression for several weeks or months.

Treatment

The primary objectives of treatment are the reduction of inflammation and pain, the preservation of joint function, and the prevention of joint deformity. These require a combination of medication, rest, special exercises, and joint protection. Antiinflammatory medications, including high doses of aspirin, are among the first choices to ease pain and stiffness, to reduce edema, and to control inflammation. NSAIDs are prescribed as an alternative to aspirin. Corticosteroids, by mouth or by local injection, often are given to control acute flare-ups. Even more potent disease-modifying antirheumatic drugs (DMARDs), such as hydroxychloroquine, sulfasalazine (Azulfidine), immunosuppressive agents, and newer biologic response modifiers, may slow the disease process or even stop its progression. These treatments, which can prevent damage, work most effectively when started earlier in the disease. There was a new DMARD drug approved in 2018 for treatment of RA. The drug is baricitinib.

Special splints and other devices to make dressing, bathing, cooking, eating, and performing other daily activities easier often are recommended to prevent, or at least reduce, deformities. Surgery is not often required, but it may be used to correct a deformity, relieve severe pain, and improve range of motion in persons with severe disease. For patients who no longer have adequately functioning joints, replacement with artificial joints may be recommended.

Prognosis

The outlook for patients with RA depends on the adequacy of treatment, which must involve close interaction between the patient and a physician skilled in the management of the disease. Early medical intervention is essential for optimal outcome. Without aggressive treatment directed against the overactive immune system, joint destruction, deformity, and disability are common. In fact, in nearly 25% of patients who present to the rheumatologist, erosive joint damage has already developed. It is optimal to have a rheumatologist involved initially as a member of the health care team.

Prevention

To prevent joint damage, loss of function, and disability, aggressive early medical intervention is mandatory. Earlier treatment is more effective than later treatment. This generally means the early use of DMARDs with or without biologic medications.

Patient Teaching

Patients with RA can benefit by learning about the immune system, joint anatomy, and the pathophysiology of the rheumatoid joint. An understanding of their medications and how their potential side effects are monitored can help ensure compliance and minimize complications. Referral to a physical therapist is helpful for individualized therapeutic exercises. Other supportive measures include splinting of inflamed joints and plenty of sleep each night. Give the patient information about the Arthritis Foundation and its support programs.

Juvenile Idiopathic (Rheumatoid) Arthritis

Description

Juvenile idiopathic arthritis, also referred to as *juvenile rheumatoid arthritis* (JRA), is the most common childhood arthritis and a form of RA that affects children (age < 16 years) and begins most commonly between ages 2 and 5 years.

ICD-10-CM Code	M08.00 *(Unspecified juvenile rheumatoid arthritis of unspecified site)* (M08.0-M08.99 = 121 codes of specificity)

Symptoms and Signs

The three subtypes of JRA are pauciarticular, polyarticular, and systemic (also known as Still disease). Pauciarticular affects no more than four joints and affects girls more than boys at a ratio of 6:1. This form of JRA has the best prognosis, and about 40% of cases fall in this category with onset before a child is 6 years of age. Polyarticular JRV affects more than five joints and affects girls more at a ratio of 2:1. This type also represents 40% of cases and has a better prognosis than systemic onset, but it has the potential to cause delayed growth. Systemic onset can begin at any age and affects boys and girls equally. It represents 20% of all cases. Chronic polyarthritis and involvement of multiple organ systems are key characteristics of this type.

JRA usually involves the large joints; the attacks last for several weeks and tend to lessen in severity with time, usually disappearing completely by puberty (Fig. 3.22).

The child with systemic onset of JRA may have the following symptoms:

- temperature fluctuating from normal or below in the morning rising to around 103°F in the evening

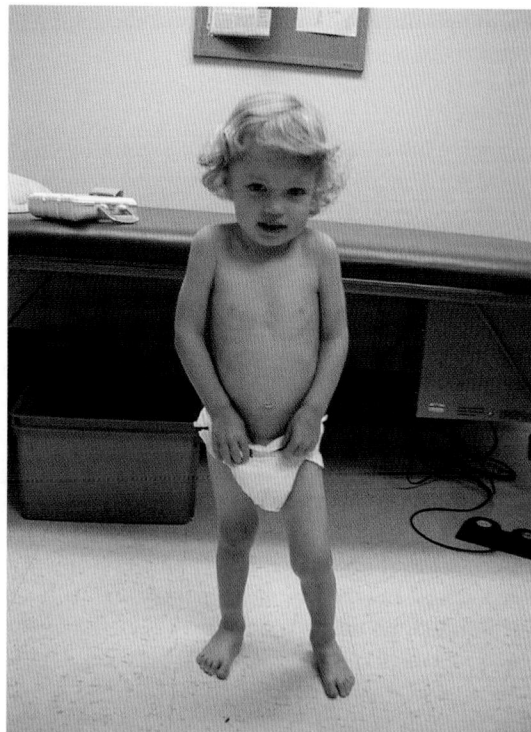

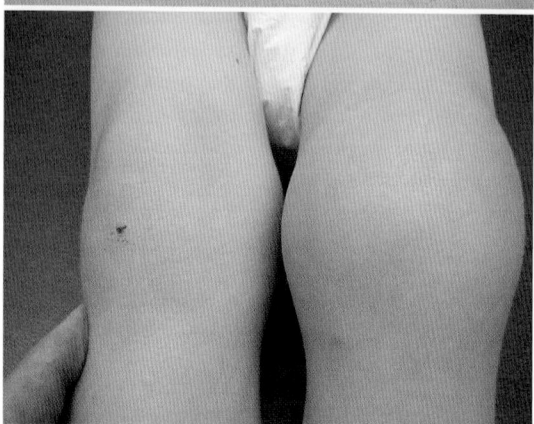

• **Fig. 3.22** Juvenile rheumatoid arthritis (JRA). (From Zitelli BJ, Davis HW: *Atlas of pediatric physical diagnosis,* ed 5, Philadelphia, 2007, Mosby/Elsevier.)

- poor appetite, with resulting weight loss
- a blotchy, salmon-colored rash over the limbs and trunk of the body
- anemia
- swollen, stiff, and painful joints, most commonly involving the neck, elbows, knees, and ankles

Other possible symptoms include red, painful eyes; swollen cervical or axillary lymph glands; irritability; and acute pericarditis. Skeletal development may be impaired if the epiphyseal, or growth, plates of the long bones are damaged because of the inflammation around the joints.

Sites of JRA development vary considerably from child to child, and girls are affected four times more often compared with boys. The inflammation usually develops gradually but can be abrupt. In a few cases, the inflammation in the joints leads to partial or crippling deformity as a result of the recurring attacks. Unlike adult RA, complete remission of JRA occurs in approximately 75% of affected children.

Patient Screening

A young child with fever, rash, and/or swelling and stiffness in the joints should be seen for medical evaluation as soon as possible.

Etiology

The specific cause of JRA is unknown, but it generally is believed that the pathologic changes in the joints are related to an autoimmune disorder. Heredity may play a role in some children, particularly those with spondylitis.

Diagnosis

The diagnosis is based on history and physical examination and the results of blood tests for the rheumatoid factor. Examination may show a lack of growth or delayed physical growth that would be appropriate for the age of the child. Other forms of arthritis that can affect children include spondylitis, the arthritis of inflammatory bowel disease, psoriatic arthritis, and sarcoidosis.

Treatment

Treatment of children with JRA is often similar to that of an adult with RA (see the Rheumatoid Arthritis section). Medication dosages are based on the child's weight. Parents should encourage the child's independence. Participation in school and social activities that do not increase joint pain or cause undue fatigue are also important for the child. A well-balanced diet with plenty of protein is essential. Physical therapy exercises are crucial for minimizing the pain and reducing the crippling effects of arthritis. Braces or splints may be needed to correct growth disturbances and joint contracture. Activity is encouraged.

Prognosis

With proper therapy, children with all forms of arthritis usually improve over time. Indeed, the vast majority of children with arthritis grow up to lead normal lives without significant physical limitations.

Prevention

To prevent joint damage, loss of function, and disability, aggressive early medical intervention is mandatory. This generally means the early use of DMARDs under the guidance of a qualified physician. A physical therapist can play a central role in helping the child maintain optimal function.

Patient Teaching

Patients and families must have as good an understanding of the disease and its management as is possible. Stress the importance of follow-up care and regular eye examinations. The child should be encouraged to be as independent as possible. Give the family information about the Arthritis Foundation and its support programs.

Ankylosing Spondylitis

Description

(AS is a systemic, progressive, inflammatory disease affecting primarily the spinal column.

ICD-10-CM Code   M45.9 *(Ankylosing spondylitis of unspecified sites in spine)* (M45.0-M45.9 = 10 codes of specificity)

Symptoms and Signs

AS commonly affects young men. It is several times more common in men than in women. Typically, it first affects the sacroiliac area of the spine and adjacent soft tissue structures. The patient may have recurring morning low back pain and stiffness that improves with activity. Constitutional symptoms, such as fatigue, weight loss, fever, and/or diarrhea, also may be present at the onset, along with eye pain and photophobia caused by uveitis. Pain and tenderness may be noted over the site of inflammation. The history may include heel pain, inflammatory bowel disease, or family incidence of arthritic conditions. Less often, patients have cervical or thoracic axial pain and stiffness with paraspinal muscular spasm. Peripheral large joints can be involved, particularly in women. Women often have a more mild form of the disease.

As the disease progresses, perhaps over many years, the physical examination can reveal limited range of motion in affected joints resulting from fusion (ankylosis). The inflammation and ossification can progress up the spine, greatly inhibiting the activities of daily life. Eventually, the spinal vertebrae become fused, inflexible, and rigid; the patient's posture exhibits the typical forward flexion of the spine (Fig. 3.23).

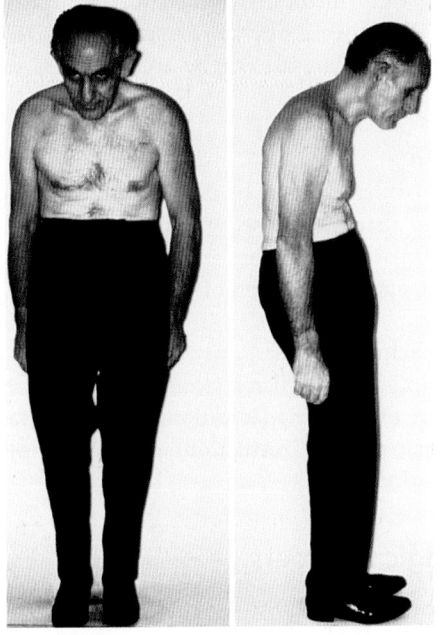

• **Fig. 3.23** Ankylosing spondylitis (AS). (From Seidel HM, Ball JW, Dains JE, et al: *Mosby's guide to physical examination,* ed 7, St Louis, 2011, Mosby/Elsevier.)

Patient Screening

Schedule the patient having back pain and morning stiffness for a medical evaluation. AS is an underdiagnosed cause of low back pain in teens and young adults. Follow office policy for regarding referral to a rheumatologist.

Etiology

The exact cause of AS is not known. Studies support a genetic basis and an association with several genes, including human leukocyte antigen (HLA)-B27. These immunogenic factors may predispose a person to the development of an immune response directed at joint tissue after exposure to particular infectious agents, which have yet to be clearly defined. According to the Spondylitis Association of America: "Identified risk factors that predispose a person to AS include testing positive for the HLA-B27 marker, a family history of AS, and frequent gastrointestinal infections."

Diagnosis

AS shares a number of diagnostic features with other arthritic diseases; thus early clinical diagnosis is often missed, especially in women. The clinical evaluation includes back pain and stiffness, joint pain with limitation of motion, and positive family history. Laboratory results reveal a negative rheumatoid factor and confirm the inflammatory nature of the disease with a mildly elevated ESR or cross-reactive protein (CRP). The HLA-B27 antigen marker is present in the blood of 95% of Caucasian individuals with AS; however, not all patients who are HLA-B27 positive will develop the disorder. According to the Spondylitis Association of America "Scientists suspect that other genes—along with a triggering environmental factor, such as a bacterial infection, for example—are needed to activate AS in susceptible people. HLA-B27 likely accounts for about 30% of the overall risk, but there are numerous other genes working in concert with HLA-B27. Researchers have identified more than 60 genes that are associated with AS and related diseases. Among the newer key genes identified are *ERAP 1, IL-12, IL-17,* and *IL-23.*"

Radiographic evaluation of all areas of symptoms is useful initially and later for monitoring. Characteristic radiographic findings are noted years after the onset and include bilateral sacroiliitis, "squaring" of the vertebrae, fusion of joints, and generalized osteoporosis. These changes produce the classic appearance of a "bamboo spine."

Treatment

No cure for AS is known. The goal of treatment is to relieve pain and swelling with antiinflammatory medication and analgesics. Patients benefit from physical therapy and moderate exercise to maintain good posture and maximize mobility. Surgical procedures are rarely indicated.

Prognosis

The course of AS is variable with periods of remission and episodes of exacerbation. A poorer prognosis is associated with early onset of the disease and male gender. Occasionally the disease takes a severe and rapid course, resulting in systemic complications and severe deformity.

Prevention

No preventive measures for AS are known, but its complications can be prevented or at least lessened with adequate exercise and medications. Because AS is occasionally associated with lung scarring and decreased chest expansion, patients with AS must not smoke.

Patient Teaching

Discuss the importance of maintaining prescribed medication and keeping follow-up appointments. Counsel the patient on individual comfort measures and positional modification in the work environment, as indicated. Stress the importance of moderate, low-impact exercise, such as swimming, to maintain range of motion and good posture. Maintaining healthy weight will prevent the patient from placing additional stress on the joints, and a regular exercise regimen will prevent fusion of the spine. Discuss the progressive nature of the disease, and encourage the patient to contact the local Arthritis Foundation chapter for group support.

Polymyositis

Description

Polymyositis is a disease of muscle that features inflammation of the muscle fibers. The muscles affected are mostly those closest to the trunk or torso. This results in weakness that can be severe. It is a chronic illness with periods of increased symptoms, called *flare-ups* or *relapses,* and decreased symptoms, known as *remissions.*

ICD-10-CM Code	M33.20 *(Polymyositis, organ involvement unspecified)* (M33.00-M33.99 = 16 codes of specificity)

Symptoms and Signs

Muscle weakness is the most common symptom of polymyositis, usually involving the muscles closest to the trunk of the body. The onset can be gradual or rapid. This results in varying degrees of loss of muscle power and atrophy. The loss of strength can be noted as difficulty getting up from chairs, climbing stairs, or lifting above the shoulders. Trouble with swallowing and weakness in lifting the head from the pillow can occur. Occasionally the muscles ache and are tender to the touch. This disease may be accompanied by skin inflammation, in which case it is referred to as *dermatomyositis.* In such cases, a rash may appear and spread over the face, shoulders, arms, and bony prominences (e.g., knuckles, elbows, and knees). Nearly two-thirds of patients with this disease are women. The person with polymyositis may feel generally fatigued and unwell.

Patient Screening

The patient will have diffuse muscle weakness. Schedule the first available appointment for medical evaluation.

Etiology

The cause of polymyositis is unknown; however, it is thought to be an autoimmune disorder. Polymyositis occurs when WBCs, the immune cells of inflammation, spontaneously invade and injure muscles.

Diagnosis

The history and physical examination should include a thorough search for muscle conditions, such as muscular dystrophy, drug toxicity (e.g., toxicity caused by statin cholesterol drugs), thyroid disorder, sarcoidosis, and infections (e.g., HIV infection and parasites). Moreover, because polymyositis can sometimes accompany cancers, an intense screening for underlying cancer is crucial. A medical history and physical examination document weakness. Blood analysis is used to detect elevated levels of muscle enzymes (creatinine phosphokinase [CPK], aldolase, serum glutamate oxaloacetate transaminase [SGOT], serum glutamate pyruvate transaminase [SGPT], and lactate dehydrogenase [LDH]). Electromyography (EMG) demonstrates a typical abnormal pattern of electrical activity in the inflamed muscle, and muscle biopsy confirms the diagnosis.

Treatment

Treatment of polymyositis is directed toward stopping the inflammation and inhibiting the overactive immune system. High doses of steroids usually are prescribed to suppress the inflammation. Immunosuppressive agents, such as cyclophosphamide and methotrexate, as well as IVIG, are also used. Gradually exercise therapy is added to rebuild strength and to prevent muscle atrophy.

Prognosis

Patients ultimately can recover well from the effects, especially with early medical treatment of the disease and its flare-ups. The disease often becomes inactive. Rehabilitation of atrophied muscle can be accomplished with long-term physical therapy.

Prevention

It is essential that patients be diligent in taking their medications and that they closely monitor their muscle symptoms. Optimal outcomes are achieved with intervention at the earliest sign of activation of muscle inflammation.

Patient Teaching

Patients should be instructed clearly about the purpose and importance of regular medications. Physical therapy and occupational therapy instructions play major roles in the recovery process.

Neurologic Disorders

Multiple Sclerosis

Description

Multiple sclerosis (MS) is an inflammatory disease of the CNS. It attacks the myelin sheath, a fatty substance covering most of the nerves in the brain and spinal cord, and ultimately causes scarring (sclerosis) that debilitates the nerves (Fig. 3.24).

ICD-10-CM Code   G35 *(Multiple sclerosis)*

Symptoms and Signs

The sclerosis of nervous tissue prevents the transmission of stimuli to the brain and spinal cord and causes the following sensory and motor abnormalities (Fig. 3.25):

- weakness or numbness in one or more limbs
- optic neuritis
- loss of vision in one eye
- diplopia
- unsteady gait
- vertigo
- difficulty with urination, leading to increased urinary tract infections
- facial numbness or pain
- speech problems
- dysphagia
- hearing loss
- impotence in men
- fatigue
- emotional disturbances, including depression, irritability, and short-temperedness

Patient Screening

Initially a patient with undiagnosed or possible MS may report variable and sporadic symptoms, such as those listed earlier. Schedule an appointment for a clinical evaluation.

Etiology

The cause of MS is unknown. It is thought that the immune system is involved; an inherited trait that increases one's susceptibility to the disease may be a factor as well. A common theory holds that an unknown virus triggers the immune system to turn against the body and attack the myelin, which eventually results in MS. No virus has been conclusively implicated, however. The incidence of MS varies geographically, with the risk increasing as one moves from southern to northern latitude. The risk is also greater in white populations. MS is rare in children; in about two-thirds of cases, it develops in people between ages 20 and 40 years; and it occurs rarely in people older than 60 years of age. MS occurs more often in women than in men.

The most common characteristic of MS is relapse, the onset of clinical dysfunction, followed by a remission during which the symptoms resolve for a period. MS can be defined as one of several types:

- *relapsing-remitting:* Relapses followed by recovery with no progression of neurologic dysfunction between relapses
- *primary-progressive:* Disease progression with no remissions
- *secondary-progressive:* Disease begins as relapsing-remitting but later becomes progressive with few remissions
- *progressive-relapsing:* Progressive disease from the onset, with relapses and disease progression during the period between relapses

Diagnosis

MS can be challenging to diagnose because the symptoms are so variable and sporadic. A physical examination done in the early stages may elicit completely normal findings. Often the diagnosis is determined by eliminating other possible causes of the symptoms. Usually the patient has had two or more distinct episodes of CNS dysfunction with resolution of symptoms between episodes. The diagnosis is made clinically and supported by other test findings. Magnetic resonance imaging (MRI) is the modality of choice for supporting the diagnosis. A characteristic cerebral or spinal plaque is often found. Examination of cerebrospinal fluid (CSF) often results in normal findings, although it may reveal an elevated immunoglobulin levels and oligoclonal bands on an MS panel.

Treatment

Acute attacks are treated with corticosteroids. Those with diagnosed relapsing-remitting disease may be started on medications approved for treatment of this form of MS, including (interferon beta-1a [Avonex, Rebif], interferon beta-1b [Betaseron], glatiramer [Copaxone], and mitoxantrone [Novantrone]). Immunosuppressive therapies may be useful in the treatment of progressive disease (radiation, steroids, immune globulin, and cytotoxic drugs). Newer treatments are biologic medications, such as natalizumab (Tysabri), which can decrease reflare rates and progressive brain injury. Two new drugs, siponimod and cladribine, were approved in 2019 for treating both secondary-progressive MS and relapsing-remitting MS. They are orally administered medications, unlike some of the other more effective injectable treatments, such as Avonex and Betaseron.

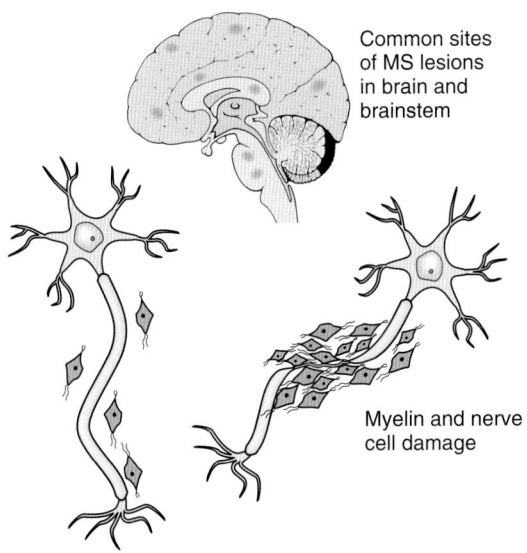

Common sites of MS lesions in brain and brainstem

Myelin and nerve cell damage

• **Fig. 3.24** Myelin degeneration in multiple sclerosis (MS).

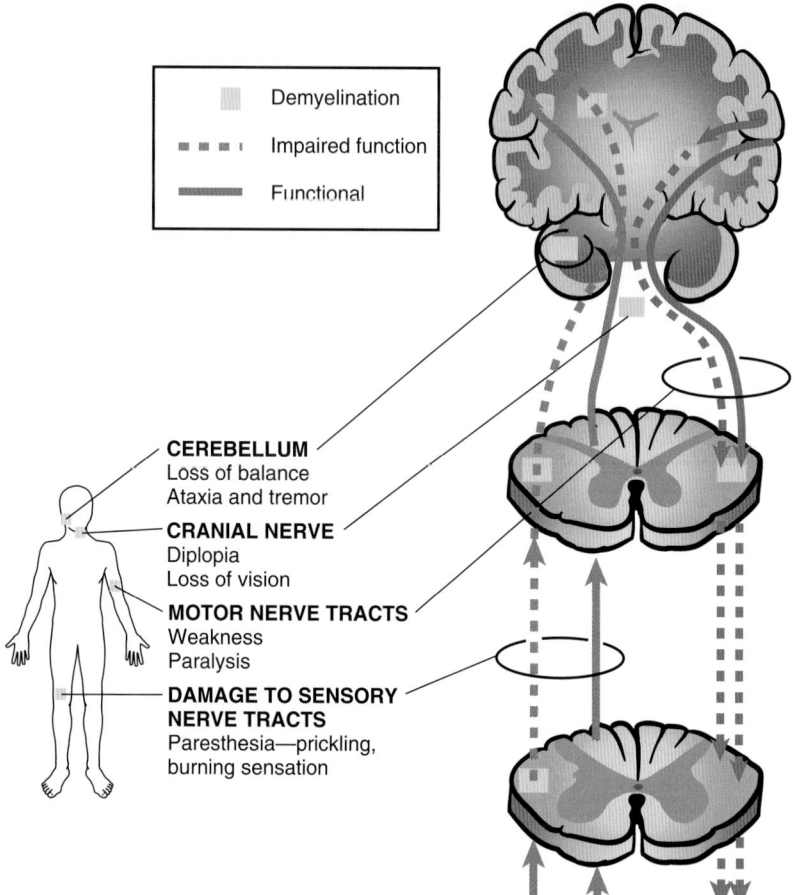

Demyelination

Impaired function

Functional

CEREBELLUM
Loss of balance
Ataxia and tremor
CRANIAL NERVE
Diplopia
Loss of vision
MOTOR NERVE TRACTS
Weakness
Paralysis
DAMAGE TO SENSORY NERVE TRACTS
Paresthesia—prickling, burning sensation

• **Fig. 3.25** Multiple sclerosis (MS)—distribution of lesions. (From Gould BE: *Pathophysiology for the health professions,* ed 4, St Louis, 2011, Saunders.)

Otherwise the disease is treated symptomatically. This may include taking muscle relaxants; taking vitamin supplements to prevent a vitamin B deficiency, which might contribute to nerve damage; undergoing physical therapy to help preserve as much muscle function as possible; wearing braces; and using a cane, walker, or wheelchair. Adequate rest and a well-balanced diet are also important.

Prognosis

No cure for MS is known, and the duration of the disease is variable. Some patients die within a few months after onset of the disease; the average duration is 30 years or longer. Several prognostic indicators are known. A more favorable prognosis is seen in females, with young age at onset, relapsing (rather than progressive) disease, and impairment of sensory pathways as an initial symptom.

Prevention

No method of prevention is known.

Patient Teaching

Describe diagnostic procedures as prescribed, because many will be ordered before the definitive diagnosis is made. Discuss the many possible treatments that address varied symptoms (e.g., speech therapy, assistive devices, bladder training,

physical therapy). Explanations of the possibility of remission and exacerbations are helpful. Discuss the medications that are prescribed and how they will be monitored for side effects. Make referrals to community support groups, such as the National Multiple Sclerosis Society.

Myasthenia Gravis

Description

Myasthenia gravis is a chronic, progressive neuromuscular disease that is caused by autoantibodies to the acetylcholine receptor at nerve synapses.

ICD-10-CM Code	G70.00 *(Myasthenia gravis without (acute) exacerbation)* (G70.00-G70.01 = 2 codes of specificity)

Symptoms and Signs

Myasthenia gravis is characterized by extreme muscular weakness (without atrophy) and progressive fatigue. The onset, although usually gradual, may be sudden, with symptoms of muscular weakness generally appearing first and most noticeably in the face. Drooping eyelids, diplopia, and difficulty with talking, chewing, and swallowing may be the first signs that something is wrong. The degree of weakness varies considerably from hour to hour, day to day, and year to year. Muscle weakness typically occurs late in the day or after strenuous exercise. Short periods of rest characteristically restore muscle function. Muscle weakness is progressive in myasthenia gravis, and eventually paralysis occurs. A myasthenic crisis (sudden inability to swallow and respiratory distress) may be so severe that mechanical ventilation becomes necessary. Prolonged exposure to sunlight, cold, infections, and emotional stress exacerbates the symptoms.

Patient Screening
Abrupt onset of the symptoms listed earlier can be disconcerting to the patient and might be confused with symptoms of stroke. Therefore the patient should receive prompt medical attention.

Etiology
The disease mainly affects women between ages 20 and 40 and men older than 60 years of age. Myasthenia gravis is thought to be caused by an autoimmune mechanism in which a faulty transmission of nerve impulses to and from the CNS occurs, especially at the neuromuscular junction. Autoantibodies against the acetylcholine receptor are found in 80% to 90% of patients. A majority of patients have either thymus hyperplasia or thymoma, and this may play a role in the development of the disease.

Diagnosis
When myasthenia gravis is suspected, a physical examination is done to test for the fatigability of different muscle groups. The Tensilon test, intravenous administration of a short-acting acetylcholinesterase inhibitor, is performed to see whether the administration improves muscle strength. Tests are done to check for the presence of antibodies against the acetylcholine receptor. EMG also may be performed.

Treatment
The treatment of myasthenia gravis is symptomatic and supportive. Treatment choice is largely based on the patient's age and pregnancy status. Restricted activity, complete bed rest for severe cases, and a soft or liquid diet may be necessary. Anticholinesterase drugs are effective initial treatment for the fatigue and muscle weakness, but they become less effective as the condition worsens. Pyridostigmine bromide (Mestinon) is the drug of choice for treatment. If a thymus gland tumor (thymoma) is present, thymectomy is needed. Corticosteroids are effective in patients who have not improved with thymectomy. A useful adjunct to alternate-day therapy with corticosteroids is immunosuppression. Myasthenic crisis is treated with intubation and withdrawal of anticholinesterase medications, followed by reintroduction of the drugs and plasmapheresis.

Prognosis
Unexplained, spontaneous remissions can occur; however, the disease is usually a lifelong condition, characterized by remissions and exacerbations. The prognosis for patients who experience myasthenic crisis has improved over the years, but such an event can still leave many patients who had been independent before the crisis functionally dependent afterward.

Prevention
No methods of prevention are known.

Patient Teaching
Give the patient information about the diagnostic tests prescribed. Explain the medical management of symptoms and what side effects to report. Encourage the patient to take initiative in deciding on his or her own supportive care. List the warning signs of impending myasthenic or cholinergic crisis.

Vasculitis

Vasculitis is inflammation in the walls of blood vessels. The affected vessel becomes necrotic when it is obstructed by a thrombus, and an infarct of adjacent tissue results. Biopsies of an involved vessel can demonstrate the presence of inflammation in the blood vessel wall. Any blood vessel can be involved, and the many forms of vasculitis are each characterized by the particular vessels affected. Vasculitis can be classified into two main types: small vessel vasculitis and systemic necrotizing vasculitis. Each of these types has many subtypes.

Small Vessel Vasculitis
Description
Small vessel vasculitis is the category of vasculitis that primarily affects the capillaries, arterioles, and venules.

ICD-10-CM Code	I77.9 *(Disorder of arteries and arterioles, unspecified)*
	(I77.0-I77.9 = 14 codes of specificity)

Symptoms and Signs
Inflammation of the small vessels causes petechiae (nonblanching), purpura, erythema, ulcerations, and edema; these are found most often on the skin of the lower extremities. Pain and a burning sensation can accompany these lesions. Additionally, depending on the type of small vessel syndrome that the patient experiences, symptoms can include ocular lesions, genital or oral ulcerations, abdominal pain, arthralgia, and weakness.

Patient Screening
The patient with rash, joint pain, fatigue, and weakness needs prompt medical evaluation. Follow office policy regarding referral to a rheumatologist.

Etiology
Although the exact cause is unknown, vasculitis often accompanies other immune disorders. Exposure to certain

chemicals, foreign proteins, medications, foods, and infections has been suggested as possible etiologic factors.

Diagnosis

Diagnosis is confirmed by the histology and often immunofluorescence studies of biopsied tissue. The presence of the immunoglobulins and complement in the blood vessels, as well as the pattern of vascular involvement and the cell types present, can help define the subtype of small vessel vasculitis. Bleeding disorders, anticoagulant medication, and even aspirin can cause skin findings that mimic small vessel vasculitis.

Treatment

Treatment consists of identifying and preventing exposure to the causative agent or managing the underlying disease. Corticosteroid therapy may afford relief; analgesics are prescribed, and rest is encouraged.

Prognosis

The outlook for patients with small vessel vasculitis is generally very good. The condition tends to readily respond to treatment.

Prevention

For those patients who have developed small vessel vasculitis as a result of reaction to certain medications, avoidance of those medications in the future is the key to prevention.

Patient Teaching

The importance of regular medical follow-up and adherence to the medication regimen cannot be overemphasized.

Systemic Necrotizing Vasculitis

Description

Systemic necrotizing vasculitis tends to primarily affect medium and large arteries.

| ICD-10-CM Code | I77.3 (Arterial fibromuscular dysplasia) |
| | I77.8 (Other specified disorders of arteries and arterioles) |

Symptoms and Signs

Systemic necrotizing vasculitis occurs in a number of cutaneous and systemic conditions. Symptoms vary, depending on the body system involved; they can include headaches, fever, weakness, fatigue, malaise, anorexia, and weight loss. Patients also may experience muscle and joint pain, angina, dyspnea, hypertension, and visual disturbances. Impaired tissue perfusion causes ischemic pain in the system or tissues involved. Ulceration of the skin can result. Paralysis of an affected nerve can lead to weakness or numbness.

Patient Screening

Rapid evaluation by a qualified physician experienced in the evaluation and management of vasculitis is crucial.

Etiology

It is not clear how the inflammation and necrosis of blood vessels develop. Each subtype of systemic necrotizing vasculitis has specific clinical features with several probable mechanisms involved. Autoimmune responses play a role and are mediated by cellular and humoral (antibody-related) immunity. Illicit drug use, including cocaine and amphetamines, and hepatitis B and C have been associated with the development of some forms of systemic vasculitis.

Diagnosis

A complete history and a thorough physical examination are important. Comprehensive blood studies, including CBC, ESR, RA factor determination, and serum tests for immunoglobulins, are done. The CBC indicates anemia and usually elevated WBC and platelet counts. The ESR is elevated during the acute stage. The CRP test shows an earlier and more intense increase compared with ESR. When the pulmonary system is involved, chest radiographs show pulmonary infiltrates. Hematuria and proteinuria are present with renal involvement. Aneurysms and myocardial ischemia are indicators of cardiac involvement. Biopsy specimens of involved vessels ultimately confirm the diagnosis by demonstrating the invasion of leukocytes in the blood vessel wall. An alternative to biopsy, in some cases, can be angiography, a radiographic examination of blood vessels.

Treatment

Treatment focuses on decreasing the inflammation of the arteries and improving the function of the affected organs. Treatment addresses the underlying causative factors and systemic involvement. Corticosteroids and analgesics afford relief of the effects of inflammation. Immune-suppressing medications, such as azathioprine and cyclophosphamide, and plasmapheresis are also used to lessen the immune activation. Hypertension is treated with antihypertensive drugs, for example, angiotensin-converting enzyme (ACE) inhibitors. Ocular problems should be closely monitored.

Prognosis

The outlook for patients with systemic necrotizing vasculitis is guarded until the condition is controlled with medications to suppress inflammation and immune activity. This category of vasculitis can permanently damage organs.

Prevention

No method of prevention for systemic necrotizing vasculitis is known, other than avoiding known causes, including cocaine, amphetamines, and hepatitis B and C.

Patient Teaching

The importance of regular medical follow-up, monitoring for signs of activation of disease, and adherence to the medication regimen cannot be overemphasized. Patients with skin damage should be taught good skin care, and those who smoke should be encouraged to stop.

Review Challenge

Answer the following questions:

1. Name the functional components of the immune system.
2. Describe the three major functions of the immune system.
3. List examples of inappropriate responses of the immune system.
4. Explain the difference between active immunity and passive immunity, and give examples for each.
5. Trace the formation of T cells and B cells from stem cells.
6. Explain how T cells and B cells specifically protect the body against disease.
7. List the five immunoglobulins.
8. Explain complement fixation and its importance in the immune system.
9. Describe the invasion of T-helper cells by human immunodeficiency virus (HIV).
10. Explain the ways that HIV infection is transmitted.
11. Discuss the treatment of HIV infection.
12. List the guidelines for universal precautions and infection control.
13. Describe the primary absent or inadequate response of the immune system in the following diseases:
    - common variable immunodeficiency (CVID)
    - selective immunoglobulin A (IgA) deficiency
    - severe combined immunodeficiency (SCID) disease
14. Explain the destructive mechanisms in autoimmune diseases.
15. Describe the symptoms and signs of pernicious anemia. Name the primary treatment.
16. Describe the systemic features of systemic lupus erythematosus (SLE). Recall the diagnostic criteria.
17. Detail the pathology of rheumatoid arthritis (RA).
18. Specify the primary objectives of the treatment for RA.
19. Compare the pathology of multiple sclerosis (MS) to that of myasthenia gravis.
20. Explain the cause of the typical forward flexion of the spine in the patient with advanced ankylosing spondylitis (AS).
21. Discuss the treatment and prognosis for patients with polymyositis.

Real-Life Challenge: Pernicious Anemia

A 46-year-old female patient reports fatigue, loss of appetite with occasional nausea and vomiting, a sore tongue, and weight loss. She also mentions weakness, numbness, and loss of feeling in her hands, lower arms, feet, and lower legs. She has recently experienced lightheadedness, visual disturbances, ringing in the ears, shortness of breath, rapid pulse, and palpitations. In addition, she mentions experiencing headaches, irritability, and depression. Examination shows pale-appearing lips, tongue, and gums. Her skin and sclera appear jaundiced.

Hematology tests reveal reduced hemoglobin, red blood cells (RBCs), white blood cells (WBCs), and platelets and increased mean cell volume (MCV). The RBCs and platelets appear large and malformed. Studies of bone marrow are indicative of abnormal RBC production. Gastric acid is either reduced or absent.

Questions

1. What is meant by pernicious anemia?
2. What is the importance of the intrinsic factor?
3. Why would the patient experience gastrointestinal (GI) type of symptoms?
4. What is the cause of the neurologic symptoms?
5. Why would the patient experience lightheadedness, fatigue, and weakness?
6. How long must the patient continue treatment after the symptoms abate?
7. Why is the patient unable to take the vitamin B_{12} orally?
8. At the present time, what is the cure for pernicious anemia?

Real-Life Challenge: Rheumatoid Arthritis

A 33-year-old woman reports recent onset of pain in the joints of her fingers and hands. She has also experienced weight loss, fatigue, and a persistent low-grade fever. On examination, the joints of the hands and fingers display tenderness, redness, warmth, and swelling. Blood tests indicate an elevated level of the rheumatoid factor. Further observation over a period of a few months shows a continuation of the symptoms with involvement of additional joints. The patient is diagnosed with rheumatoid arthritis (RA).

Questions

1. Compare the incidence of RA in males and females.
2. Compare the symptoms and signs of RA and osteoarthritis (see the Osteoarthritis section in Chapter 7).
3. Describe the projected course of RA that is left untreated.
4. What is the cause of RA?

5. Which diagnostic tests usually are ordered when RA is suspected?
6. Because the primary treatment is to reduce inflammation and pain, preserve joint function, and prevent deformities, what is the usual prescribed treatment?
7. Explain the side effects the patient may experience with nonsteroidal antiinflammatory drug (NSAID) therapy.
8. Explain why early referral to a rheumatologist is recommended.

Real Life Challenge: Ankylosing Spondylitis

A 28-year-old patient complains of lower back pain for several months. She sees her health care provider and is prescribed antiinflammatory medications and physical therapy for muscle strain. The pain continues, and there is no relief after completion of physical therapy. The patient is then referred to an orthopedist. The physician orders a bone scan and also a series of laboratory tests, including the HLA-B27 marker test. The test results are positive for this genetic marker. Which health care provider will need to see the patient with this result? Which disease or disorder may be the source of the patient's pain?

Internet Assignments

1. Explore the Lupus Foundation of America website for breaking news. Learn how to use the website to locate the chapter of the Lupus Foundation nearest to you.
2. Explore the National AIDS Hotline, and report on a top story in the What's New section.
3. Go to the National Multiple Sclerosis Society to identify promising areas of disease research, and list some current clinical trials.

Critical Thinking

1. Why does patient teaching need to be very specific for a patient diagnosed with an immunodeficiency disease?
2. What is the understanding of the "window period" stage of infection with human immunodeficiency virus (HIV)?
3. Explain how autoantibodies cause diseases.
4. What is the relationship between pernicious anemia and shortage of intrinsic factor and the impairment of vitamin B_{12} adsorption?
5. How does the immune system malfunction in connective tissue diseases?
6. Why is scleroderma difficult to diagnose?
7. Which gene is known to be associated with autoimmune disorders, such as ankylosing spondylitis?
8. A patient who has undergone heart transplantation shows immediate signs of organ rejection despite an accurate tissue match prior to the transplantation. What are some of the reasons for this type of rejection?

Prepare to discuss Critical Thinking case study exercises for this chapter that are posted on the Evolve website.

4

Diseases and Conditions of the Endocrine System

CHAPTER OUTLINE

Orderly Function of the Endocrine System, 136
    Bioidentical Hormone Replacement,137
    Pituitary Gland Diseases, 137
    Thyroid Gland Diseases, 143

Parathyroid Gland Diseases, 149
Adrenal Gland Diseases, 152
Endocrine Dysfunction of Pancreas, 154
Precocious Puberty, 159

LEARNING OBJECTIVES

After studying Chapter 4, you should be able to:

1. Describe the importance of hormones and explain some of the critical body functions that they control.
2. List the major glands of the endocrine system.
3. Explain the importance of normal pituitary function.
4. Compare gigantism with acromegaly.
5. Describe the condition of dwarfism and its etiology.
6. Explain the cause of diabetes insipidus.
7. Explain the treatment of a simple goiter.
8. Compare the signs and symptoms of thyroid hypofunction with those of thyroid hyperfunction.
9. List the signs and symptoms of Graves disease.
10. Distinguish between cretinism and myxedema.
11. Describe the signs and symptoms of thyroid malignancy and discuss the most important prognostic factor.
12. Compare and contrast hyperparathyroidism and hypothyroidism.
13. Describe Cushing syndrome and Addison disease.
14. Explain the pathogenesis of diabetes mellitus.
15. Identify the two major types of diabetes mellitus.
16. Distinguish between diabetic coma and insulin shock.
17. Explain the medical management of all three types of diabetes mellitus.
18. Discuss why early recognition of metabolic syndrome offers the patient an advantage to focus on intervention.
19. Explain why hypoglycemia can be a serious medical condition.
20. Define precocious puberty.

KEY TERMS

acidosis (**ass**-ih-**DOE**-sis)
corticotropin (**kor**-tih-ko-**TRO**-pln)
epiphyseal (**eh**-pih-**FEEZ**-e-al)
gonadotropin (**go**-nad-oh-**TRO**-pin)
hyperglycemia (**hye**-per-gli-**SEE**-me-ah)
hyperkalemia (**hye**-per-ka-**LEE**-me-ah)
hypocalcemia (**hye**-poh-kal-**SEE**-me-ah)
hypothalamus (**hye**-poh-**THAL**-ah-mus)
panhypopituitarism (pan-**high**-poh-pih-**TOO**-ih-tair-ism)
polydipsia (pahl-ee-**DIP**-see-ah)

polyphagia (**pahl**-ee-**FAY**-jee-ah)
polyuria (**pahl**-ee-**U**-ree-ah)
pruritus (pruh-**RI**-tus)
radioimmunoassay (ray-dee-oh-**IM**-u-no-**ass**-a)
somatotropin (**soh**-mat-oh-**TROH**-pin)
thyrotoxicosis (**thye**-roh-tox-ih-**KOH**-sis)
thyrotropin (thye-ro-**TRO**-pin)
thyroxine (thye-**ROKS**-in)
triiodothyronine (**try**-eye-oh-doh-**THYE**-row-neen)
vasopressin (**vaz**-oh-**PRES**-in)

Orderly Function of the Endocrine System

Body activities, homeostasis, and the response to stress are communicated and controlled by two distinct but interacting systems: the nervous system and the endocrine system. The systems interact as one system starts, ends, or extends the activity of the other. The nervous system (discussed in Chapter 13) creates an immediate but short-lived response, operating on the principles of electricity through impulse conduction. The endocrine system has a slightly slower onset and a longer duration of action and uses highly specific and powerful hormones to control its response chemically. Hormones are chemical messengers classified as either amino acids (proteins) or steroids.

The endocrine system is composed of many glands scattered throughout the body; these glands secrete unique and potent chemicals called *hormones* directly into the bloodstream (Fig. 4.1). Most hormones direct their action to target glands or tissues at distant receptor sites, thereby regulating critical body functions, such as urinary output, cellular metabolic rate, and growth and development. Hormonal secretions typically are regulated by negative feedback; information about the hormone level or its effect is fed back to the gland, which then responds accordingly (Fig. 4.2).

Certain endocrine glands are stimulated to secrete hormones in response to other hormones. Hormones that stimulate secretion of other hormones are called *tropic hormones.*

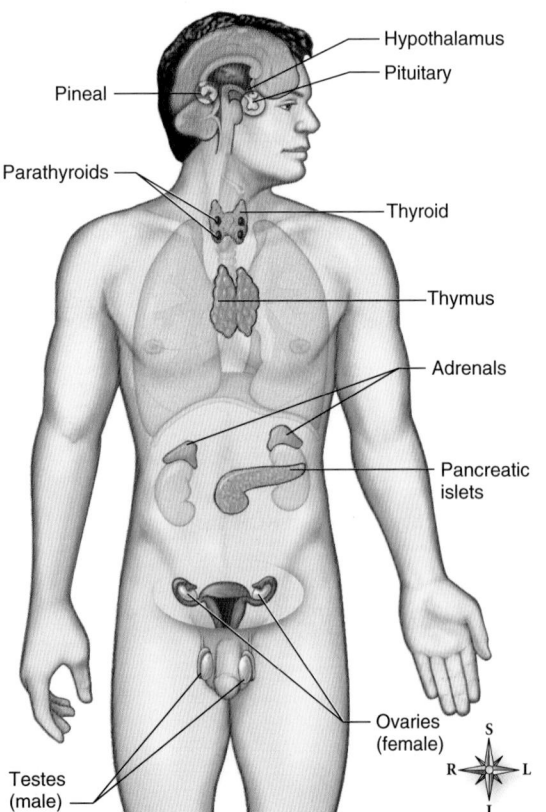

• **Fig. 4.1** Major glands of the normal endocrine system. (From Patton KT, Thibodeau GA: *The human body in health & disease*, ed 6, St Louis, 2014, Elsevier.)

For example, in women, the **gonadotropins** stimulate the synthesis of ovarian hormones. In diagnostic analysis, when excessive hormones are produced by an ectopic source (e.g., a malignant tumor), the tropic hormones are low. Other secreting cells that perform endocrine functions may be scattered in the tissue, such as in the digestive tract, where local hormones regulate the motility and secretions of other hormones. The influence of hormones is of vital importance because they regulate body function to promote health.

Endocrine diseases result from an abnormal increase or decrease in the secretion of hormones. Symptoms of disease vary with the degree of increase or decrease in hormonal secretion and the age of the patient. This divergence from normal hormone quantities may be the result of hyperplasia, hypertrophy, or atrophy of an endocrine gland. Changes in gland size that affect the gland's production and secretion of a hormone often result from an insult to the gland, such as infection, radiation, trauma, surgical intervention, and inflammation. Dysfunction of an endocrine gland is associated with many physical and mental symptoms. Some common symptoms are:

- growth abnormalities
- emotional disturbances or psychiatric problems
- skin, hair, and nail changes
- edema
- hypertension or hypotension
- arrhythmia
- changes in urine output
- muscle weakness and atrophy
- menstrual irregularity or amenorrhea
- impotence or changes in libido
- sterility
- changes in energy level

To appreciate the effect of endocrine gland function on health and disease, review the main glands and their primary hormones (Table 4.1). The pituitary gland, which is intricately connected to the **hypothalamus**, plays a central role in regulating most of the endocrine glands; it has a cascading effect on the glands that it stimulates. The pituitary gland is divided into anterior and posterior lobes; the anterior lobe accounts for about 80% of the gland. The hypothalamus, a part of the brain that also has endocrine functions, controls many activities of the pituitary gland via neural and chemical stimuli. Pituitary dysfunction can affect some or all of the glands that are targets of pituitary hormones, thereby indirectly affecting body structure and function (Fig. 4.3).

Diagnosing endocrine disorders requires correctly matching the patient's symptoms with a specific hormone dysfunction and obtaining laboratory confirmation of overproduction or underproduction of a particular hormone or hormones.

Hormone levels can be detected by using blood serum or plasma, which is collected by the phlebotomy method. Whole blood can also be used when performing blood spot testing, which requires capillary blood. Urine and saliva testing are also methods for evaluating hormone levels.

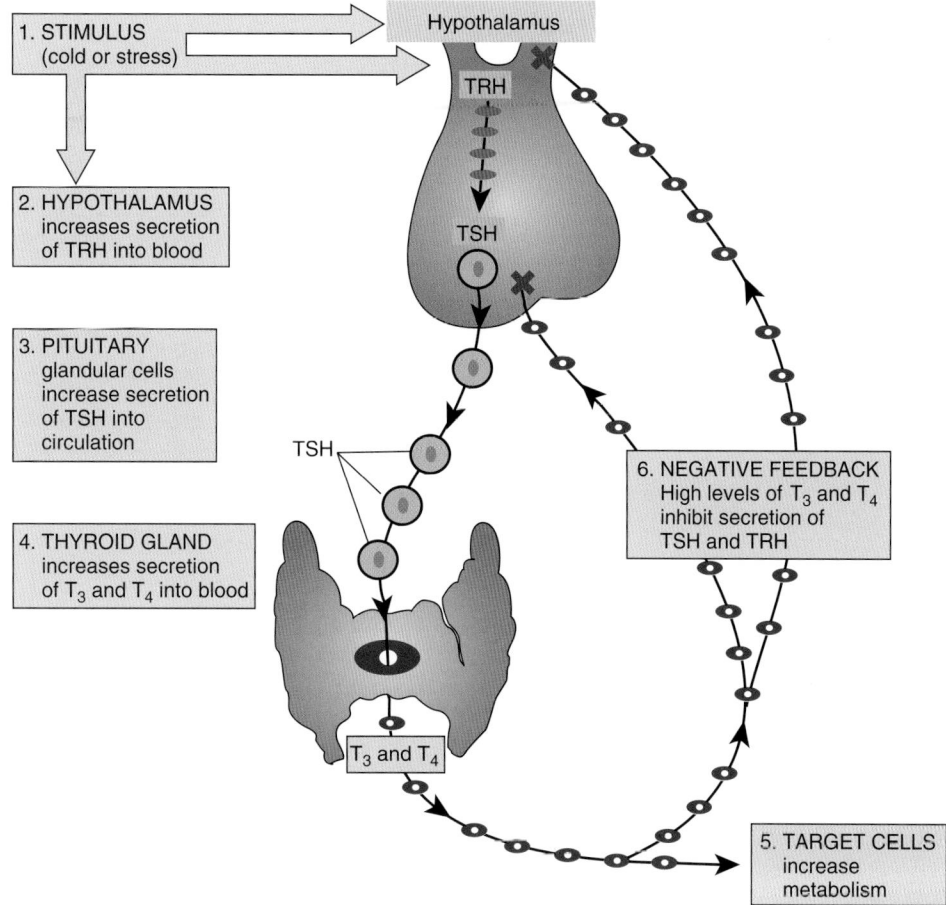

1. STIMULUS
(cold or stress)

Hypothalamus

TRH

2. HYPOTHALAMUS
increases secretion
of TRH into blood

TSH

3. PITUITARY
glandular cells
increase secretion
of TSH into
circulation

TSH

6. NEGATIVE FEEDBACK
High levels of T_3 and T_4
inhibit secretion of
TSH and TRH

4. THYROID GLAND
increases secretion
of T_3 and T_4 into blood

T_3 and T_4

5. TARGET CELLS
increase
metabolism

• **Fig. 4.2** Hypothalamus-pituitary-thyroid gland feedback mechanism with thyroid hormone. *TRH,* Thyrotropin-releasing hormone; *TSH,* thyroid-stimulating hormone; *T_4,* thyroxine; *T_3,* triiodothyronine. (From Gould B: *Pathophysiology for the health professions,* ed 3, Philadelphia, 2006, Saunders.)

Newer research indicates that blood and plasma levels only reflect a small amount of hormones actually being used by the body because these tests measure the levels of circulating hormones rather than the hormones that are available for use by organs. Historically, hormone levels have been measured by serum blood tests by using **radioimmunoassay** (RIA) or immunometric assay (IMA) methodology and occasionally by using a 24-hour urine test. Blood spot testing requires only a drop of blood. Hormone testing can also be accomplished with saliva testing, and patients themselves may even order hormone tests online to check levels with kits that require saliva for testing.

Computed tomography (CT), ultrasonography, and magnetic resonance imaging (MRI) can help determine the type and location of a lesion. Biopsy is performed to determine whether a lesion is malignant.

After an endocrine problem is identified, treatment is initiated to replace the hormone deficit or reduce a lesion by surgical removal or radiation therapy. Newer medical therapies also inhibit the synthesis of hormones. However, therapeutic drugs may have substantial side effects.

Bioidentical Hormone Replacement

Currently hormones called *bioidentical hormones* are available. These hormones are used because they are identical to the hormones in the human body. The companies that make these hormones claim that they are better and that their use has certain advantages over traditional hormone replacement therapy. There may be advantages in some cases and for some patients to use bioidentical hormones, but research has not indicated, at this point, that they are safer or more effective.

Pituitary Gland Diseases

Excess Pituitary Hormones Secretion

Inflammation or tumor of the pituitary gland can lead to a chronic and progressive disease resulting from the excessive production and secretion of pituitary hormones, for example, human growth hormone (hGH). The excessive hGH produces one of two distinct conditions, gigantism or acromegaly, depending on the time of life at which the dysfunction begins.

TABLE 4.1 **Major Endocrine Gland Secretions and Functions**

Endocrine Gland	Hormone	Target Action
Anterior pituitary	Growth hormone (GH)	Promotes bone and tissue growth
	Thyrotropin (thyroid-stimulating hormone [TSH])	Stimulates thyroid gland and production of thyroxine (T_4)
	Corticotropin (adrenocorticotropic hormone [ACTH])	Stimulates adrenal cortex to produce glucocorticoids
	Gonadotropins	
	Follicle-stimulating hormone (FSH)	Initiates growth of eggs in ovaries; stimulates spermatogenesis in testes
	Luteinizing hormone (LH)	Causes ovulation; stimulates ovaries to produce estrogen and progesterone; stimulates testosterone production
	Prolactin (PRL)	Stimulates breast development and formation of milk during pregnancy and after delivery
	Melanocyte-stimulating hormone (MSH)	Regulates skin pigmentation
Posterior pituitary	Vasopressin (antidiuretic hormone [ADH])	Stimulates water resorption by renal tubules; has antidiuretic effect
	Oxytocin	Stimulates uterine contractions; stimulates ejection of milk in mammary glands; causes ejection of secretions in male prostate gland
Thyroid	Thyroid hormone (TH): Thyroxine (T_4) and triiodothyronine (T_3)	Regulates rate of cellular metabolism (catabolic phase)
	Calcitonin	Promotes retention of calcium and phosphorus in bone; opposes effect of parathyroid hormone (PTH)
Parathyroid	PTH	Regulates metabolism of calcium; elevates serum calcium levels by drawing calcium from bones
Adrenal cortex	Mineralocorticoids (MC), primarily aldosterone	Promote retention of sodium by kidneys; regulate electrolyte and fluid homeostasis
	Glucocorticoids (GC): Cortisol, corticosterone, cortisone	Regulate metabolism of carbohydrates, proteins, and fats in cells
	Gonadocorticoids: Androgens, estrogens, progestins	Govern secondary sex characteristics and masculinization
Adrenal medulla	Catecholamines: Epinephrine and norepinephrine	Produce quick-acting "fight or flight" response during stress; increase blood pressure, heart rate, and blood glucose level; dilate bronchioles
Pancreas	Insulin	Regulates metabolism of glucose in body cells; maintains proper blood glucose level
	Glucagon	Increases concentration of glucose in blood by causing conversion of glycogen to glucose
Ovaries	Estrogens	Cause development of female secondary sex characteristics
	Progesterone	Prepares and maintains endometrium for implantation and pregnancy
Testes	Testosterone	Stimulates and promotes growth of male secondary sex characteristics and is essential for erections
Thymus	Thymosin	Promotes development of immune cells (gland atrophies during adulthood)
Pineal gland	Melatonin	Regulates daily patterns of sleep and wakefulness. Inhibits hormones that affect ovaries; other functions unknown

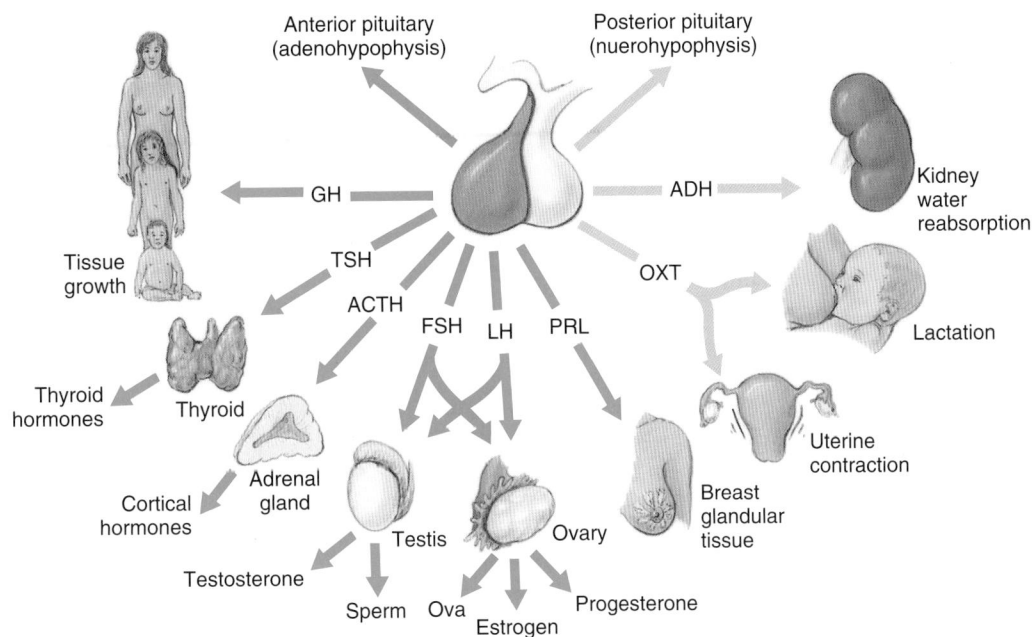

• **Fig. 4.3** The effect of pituitary hormones on target tissues. *ACTH,* Adrenocorticotropic hormone; *ADH,* antidiuretic hormone; *FSH,* follicle-stimulating hormone; *GH,* growth hormone; *LH,* luteinizing hormone; *OXT,* oxytocin; *PRL,* prolactin; *TSH,* thyroid-stimulating hormone. (From Applegate EJ: *The anatomy and physiology learning system,* ed 4, St Louis, 2011, Saunders.)

Gigantism

Description

Gigantism describes an abnormal pattern of growth and stature.

ICD-10-CM Code	E22.0 *(Acromegaly and pituitary gigantism)*

Symptoms and Signs

When the hypersecretion of growth hormone (GH, somatotropin) occurs before puberty, the result is gigantism, a proportional overgrowth of all body tissue (Fig. 4.4). The affected child experiences abnormal and accelerated growth, especially of the long bones, because epiphyseal closure has not begun. Typically an accelerated linear growth prompts an initial investigation in children. Sexual development and mental development are often delayed.

Patient Screening

Symptoms usually appear over time; signs of the condition may be discovered during a routine examination. Follow office policy for referral to an endocrinologist.

Etiology

An anterior pituitary adenoma is often the cause of oversecretion of GH that results in gigantism. Although a genetic link has not been identified, gigantism sometimes affects multiple members of a family. Hypogonadism may lead to tall stature, but not gigantism, by delaying puberty and closure of the epiphyses.

Diagnosis

The clinical picture of abnormal growth in a prepubescent child leads the physician to order diagnostic investigations. Levels of

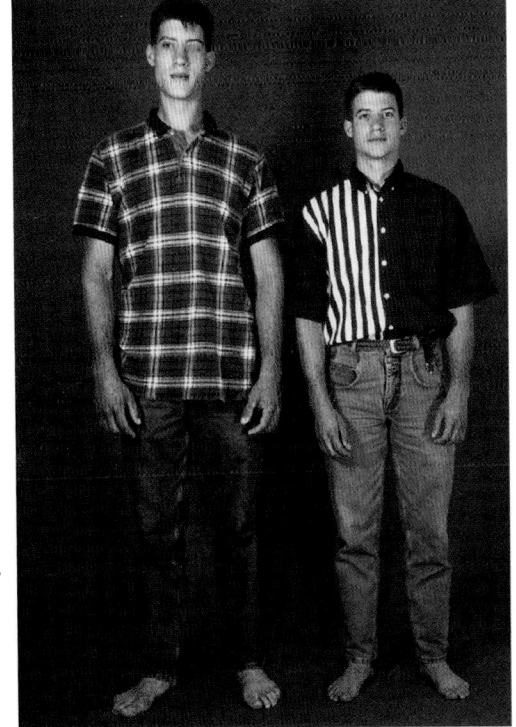

• **Fig. 4.4** Growth hormone (GH) abnormalities. The 22-year-old man on the left with gigantism is much taller than his identical twin on the right (Courtesy Robert F. Gagel, MD, and Ian McCutcheon, MD, University of Texas MD Anderson Cancer Center, Houston, TX. In Black JM, Hawks JH: *Medical-surgical nursing: clinical management for positive outcomes,* ed 8, St. Louis, 2009, Saunders.)

GH are elevated on the laboratory test result. Age-reference norms for insulin-like growth factor 1 (IGF-1) are the best indicators of endogenous secretion of GH. The best imaging study is pituitary MRI; CT can also detect the presence of a pituitary lesion. Bone radiographs show thickening of the cranium, enlargement of the jaws, and elongation of the long bones.

Treatment

The object of treatment is to reduce the amount of GH that is secreted. This is performed ideally through surgery (transsphenoidal approach), with or without the addition of medication or radiation to the pituitary gland to reduce its size (Fig. 4.5). Appropriate gonadal hormones may be needed in children or adolescents exhibiting hypogonadism. Yearly follow-up examinations are recommended.

Prognosis

Correction of the disorder prevents further physical changes.

Prevention

No prevention is known.

Patient Teaching

Explain the diagnostic tests and surgical interventions, as appropriate. Give the child and parents visual aids depicting the pituitary gland and its functions. Emphasize the importance of getting follow-up care and adhering to the dosage schedule for medications.

Acromegaly

Description

Acromegaly is a chronic metabolic condition in adults caused by hypersecretion of GH by the pituitary gland.

ICD-10-CM Code	E22.0 *(Acromegaly and pituitary gigantism)*

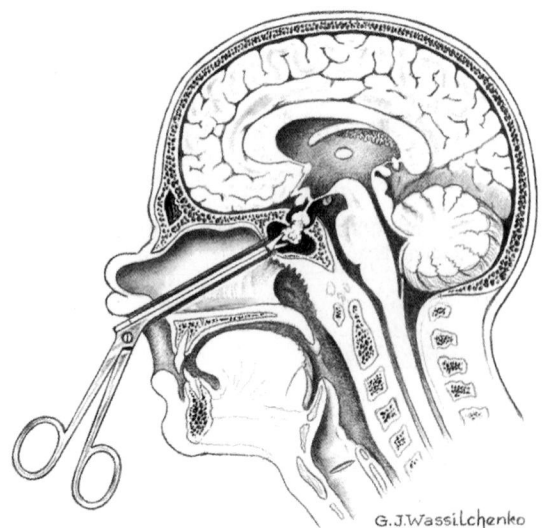

• **Fig. 4.5** Transsphenoidal approach to removing a pituitary tumor. (From Rudy E: *Advanced neurological and neurosurgical nursing*, St Louis, 1984, Mosby.)

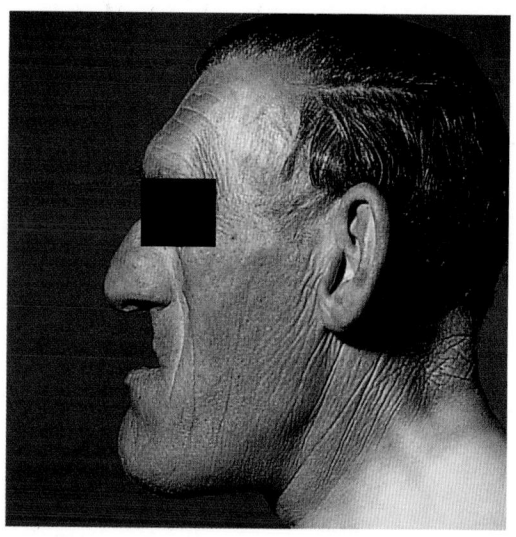

• **Fig. 4.6** Acromegaly. (From Forbes CD, Jackson WF: *Color atlas and text of clinical medicine,* ed 3, London, 2003, Mosby, Elsevier Science Ltd.)

Symptoms and Signs

When hypersecretion of GH occurs after puberty, acromegaly (overgrowth of the bones of the face, hands, and feet) occurs, with an excessive overgrowth of soft tissue because epiphyseal closure has already occurred (Fig. 4.6). It is often seen in those 30 to 40 years of age after they experience years of excess GH. The patient notices that he or she must wear larger gloves, shoes, or both. Excessive jaw growth causes larger spaces between teeth. The individual may experience joint pain resulting from osteoarthritis and a host of other clinical problems in the body systems.

Patient Screening

Symptoms usually appear over time; signs of the condition may be discovered during a routine examination. Follow office policy for referral to an endocrinologist.

Etiology

As with gigantism, a pituitary tumor or adenoma often is the cause of acromegaly. It affects women and men with equal frequency.

Diagnosis

The clinical picture of abnormal thickening of the bones of the face, hands, and feet leads the physician to order diagnostic tests. Levels of GH and IGF-1 are elevated. In conjunction, another reliable test is the glucose tolerance test because increased glucose levels cause failure of suppression of GH levels. As with gigantism, MRI of the pituitary and CT can detect the presence of a pituitary lesion.

Treatment

The object of treatment is to reverse or prevent tumor mass effects and reduce the amount of GH secreted. Correcting the disorder prevents further disfigurement and reduces the mortality that results from excess GH. This is performed ideally through surgery (transsphenoidal approach), with or without the addition of medication or radiation to the pituitary gland to reduce its size (see Fig. 4.5). The success of medical therapies depends on the response of the tumor cells to the intervention.

Prognosis

Acromegaly causes an increase in mortality, mostly as a result of cardiovascular and cerebrovascular diseases. Reduction in the levels of GH is associated with improvement in symptoms and signs.

Prevention

No prevention is known.

Patient Teaching

Offer visual aids, including videos when available, that explain the anatomy and function of the pituitary gland and its hormones. Reinforce the physician's explanation of the cause and treatment of acromegaly. Explain the purpose of the required diagnostic tests. Describe the surgical procedures, if appropriate. Explain the medication dosage schedule and the possible adverse effects to report. Encourage the patient to express concerns and questions about changes in body image.

Hypopituitarism

Description

Hypopituitarism is a condition caused by a deficiency or absence of any of the pituitary hormones, produced by the anterior pituitary lobe.

ICD-10-CM Code	E23.0 (Hypopituitarism)
	(E23.0-E23.7 = 6 codes of specificity)

Symptoms and Signs

Because the anterior pituitary secretes several major hormones, the syndrome can be complex and marked by metabolic dysfunction, sexual immaturity, or delayed growth. Physical findings vary, depending on the specific hormone deficiency. A deficiency of pituitary hormones that stimulate other endocrine glands can result in the atrophy of those glands. When thyrotropin (thyroid-stimulating hormone [TSH]) secretion is reduced, the functioning of the thyroid gland is affected, and the patient experiences symptoms of hypothyroidism. When the secretion of corticotropin (adrenocorticotropic hormone [ACTH]) dwindles, salt balance and nutrient metabolism are affected. Gonadotropin deficiency impairs sexual functions, including sexual development, menstruation, and libido.

Hypopituitarism causes delayed growth in children. Headache and blindness are signs of tumor infringement on the optic nerve.

Patient Screening

Symptoms of the complex syndromes associated with this disorder usually have an insidious onset. Schedule a complete medical evaluation, and follow office policy for referral to an endocrinologist.

Etiology

The cause of hypopituitarism may be a pituitary tumor or a tumor of the hypothalamus. Some causes are congenital deficiencies, and some are acquired. In some instances, hypopituitarism results from damage to the pituitary gland caused by radiation or surgical removal or from ischemia of the gland caused by infarct, tumor, or basilar skull fracture. If the ischemia is severe and not reversed, permanent destruction of glandular tissue begins. Destruction of the entire anterior lobe results in panhypopituitarism, a decline in multiple anterior pituitary hormone secretion. The condition is most common in women, and sometimes the cause is unknown.

Diagnosis

When the patient has the clinical symptoms of hyposecretion of any of the anterior pituitary hormones, a complete medical evaluation is necessary to detect partial or selective hormone deficiencies and to pinpoint the diagnosis. A history of head trauma, previous radiation, or a surgical procedure to the gland or nearby tissue contributes to the diagnosis. Plasma levels of all or some of the pituitary hormones are low. Radiographic films of the skull, cranial CT, and MRI are used to identify the tumors. The clinical investigation must rule out diseases of the target glands themselves.

Treatment

The age of the patient, the severity and type of deficiency, and the underlying cause of hypopituitarism determine the course of treatment. When neoplasia is the cause, removal of the tumor alleviates the symptoms. Replacement therapy with hormonal supplements, including thyroxine (T$_4$), cortisone, sex hormones, or somatropin (hGH), is usually effective. Hormone levels must be continually monitored during hormone replacement therapy.

Prognosis

The prognosis varies because of the many possible causes of hypopituitarism and the complex functions of the pituitary gland itself.

Prevention

No prevention is known.

Patient Teaching

Give the patient visual aids depicting the pituitary gland, and describe the features of the major pituitary hormones. Explain the diagnostic procedures and any planned surgical intervention. Emphasize the importance of following any instructions given by the endocrinologist regarding hormone replacement therapy, and list the warning signs of overreplacement. Emphasize the importance of follow-up visits to monitor the results of therapy and adjust the dosage.

Dwarfism

Description

The deficiency of pituitary GH in children results in short stature. Dwarfism is generally defined as an abnormal underdevelopment of the body in children, with adult height reaching only 4 feet 10 inches or less.

ICD-10-CM Code   E34.3 *(Short stature due to endocrine disorder)*

Symptoms and Signs

Hyposecretion of the pituitary gland hormones, especially GH, results in delayed growth. As a result, the child is extremely short, with a body that is small in proportion (see Fig. 4.4). The prepubescent child does not develop secondary sex characteristics. The condition may be linked to other defects and a varying degree of intellectual developmental disorder.

Patient Screening

Children deficient in GH require regular follow-up appointments during therapy. Follow office policy for referral to an endocrinologist.

Etiology

Dwarfism can be congenital, the result of a cranial tumor, or hemorrhage after the birth process. Occasionally there is no identifiable cause. A deficiency of the growth hormone–releasing hormone (GH-RH) produced by the hypothalamus is termed *secondary hypopituitarism* and results from head trauma, tumor, or infection.

Diagnosis

Physical examination shows that the child fails to grow at a normal rate and is short in stature. The child's general health appears to be good. However, secondary tooth eruption is delayed, and fat deposits may be noted in the lower trunk area. Persistently low serum GH levels are found. CT may confirm the presence of a cranial tumor.

Treatment

Somatotropin (hGH) is administered until the child reaches a height of 5 feet. These children also may need replacement thyroid and adrenal hormones when multiple hormone deficiencies are found to exist. As they approach puberty, sex hormones are administered, if necessary.

Prognosis

Clinical manifestations of GH deficiencies depend on the time of onset and the degree of hormone deficiency. GH replacement is effective in children with well-documented GH deficiency. Treatment is essential to help reach final adult height. Safety for long-term GH administration indicates negligible adverse effects.

Prevention

Known causes are not preventable; but common precautions may be taken to prevent head trauma and infection.

Patient Teaching

Give the patient and family visual aids, using e-learning media when available, to familiarize them with the pituitary gland and the hormones that affect growth and maturation.

Explain the regimen of GH treatment, which may include frequent injections, and emphasize the importance of patient compliance to achieve the desired therapeutic goal.

Diabetes Insipidus

Description

Diabetes insipidus is a disturbance of water metabolism, resulting in extreme thirst and excessive secretion of dilute urine.

ICD-10-CM Code   E23.2 *(Diabetes insipidus)*

Symptoms and Signs

Diabetes insipidus is a deficiency in the release of **vasopressin** (antidiuretic hormone [ADH]) by the posterior pituitary gland, resulting in the excretion of copious amounts of dilute urine (**polyuria**). The patient experiences excessive thirst (**polydipsia**), fatigue, and symptoms of dehydration, including dry mucous membranes, hypotension, dizziness, and poor skin turgor. The onset of symptoms may be abrupt.

Patient Screening

An abrupt onset of excessive thirst and excessive urination, together with the symptoms of dehydration, merits prompt medical attention.

Etiology

In diabetes insipidus, the posterior pituitary gland releases reduced amounts of vasopressin. The condition may be hereditary, or it may be the result of an insult to the hypothalamus or to the pituitary gland resulting from head trauma, cerebral edema, or an intracranial lesion. Nephrogenic diabetes insipidus results from renal tubular resistance to the action of vasopressin. More common in men than in women, this disease may occur in childhood or early adulthood. In many cases, the cause is unknown. When the amount of vasopressin is insufficient, the distal tubules of the nephron do not reabsorb water from the filtrate back into the bloodstream; consequently, the volume of urine is excessive.

Diagnosis

The presence of polyuria and polydipsia leads the clinician to investigate the composition of urine through laboratory tests. Urinalysis that reveals almost colorless urine that has a low specific gravity (<1.005) suggests diabetes insipidus as a diagnosis. To confirm the diagnosis of diabetes insipidus, the patient is given the water-restriction test, during which the kidneys exhibit inability to concentrate urine despite the patient being deprived of fluid intake for several hours. When the urine concentration (osmolality) is stable on consecutive measurements or blood osmolality is above normal, vasopressin (ADH) is administered. Urine volume is compared with specific gravity. Reduced output and increased specific gravity of urine after the administration of vasopressin indicate diabetes insipidus.

Treatment

Treatment consists of vasopressin injections, nasal spray, or oral desmopressin acetate (trade name DDAVP). In nephrogenic diabetes insipidus, thiazide diuretics act by inducing mild volume depletion. In the kidneys, hypovolemia induces an increase in proximal sodium and water resorption, diminishing water delivery to the vasopressin-sensitive collecting tubules, thus reducing urine output. Any underlying cause should be identified and treated. When the excessive diuresis is the result of trauma to the pituitary gland, the symptoms begin to subside as the insult resolves.

Prognosis
Patients who are bedridden or unable to drink enough water to compensate for urinary loss of water can become dangerously dehydrated.

Individuals with uncomplicated diabetes insipidus respond to treatment and return to a normal life.

Prevention
The causes and contributing factors cannot be prevented.

Patient Teaching
Give the patient guidelines for monitoring fluid intake and output to ensure adequate water replacement. Instruct the patient to notify the physician of any increase in symptoms, including weight loss or gain. Demonstrate the procedure of checking the specific gravity of urine. Discuss the side effects or toxic effects of the prescribed medications.

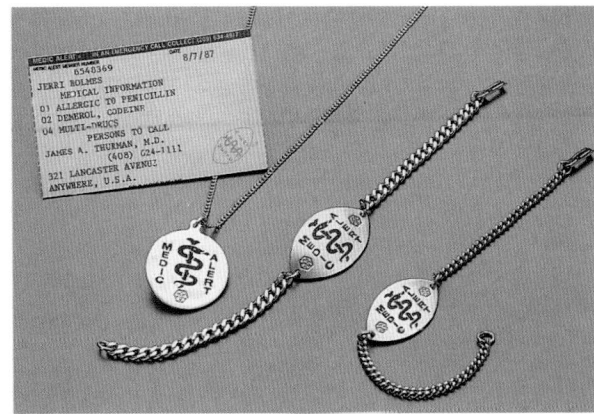

• **Fig. 4.7** Medical alert bracelet.

Encourage the patient to wear a medical alert bracelet (Fig. 4.7).

Thyroid Gland Diseases

Thyroid diseases present as functional disturbances that produce excessive or reduced secretions of thyroid hormones—thyroxine (T_4) and triiodothyronine (T_3)—and mass lesions of the thyroid. Table 4.2 lists types of thyroid diseases and their signs and symptoms. Fortunately, diseases of the thyroid gland may be resolved through medical and surgical interventions.

TABLE 4.2 Comparison of Hypothyroid and Hyperthyroid Disorders

	Hypofunction of Thyroid	Hyperfunction of Thyroid
Names or types	Congenital, untreated can become cretinism or thyroid dwarfism	Hyperthyroidism
	Myxedema coma	Thyrotoxicosis
	Hashimoto thyroiditis	Graves disease: autoimmune with or without exophthalmos
	Iodine deficiency: simple goiter	Toxic nodular hyperplasia
	Idiopathic hypothyroidism	Toxic adenoma, thyroid tumors
Symptoms and signs	Decreased activity, sleepiness, lethargy	Restlessness, irritability, easy fatigability, nervousness
	Reduced mental alertness, easy fatigability	Tremors
	Dry skin and hair, decreased sweating	Moist skin, increased sweating
	Cold intolerance	Heat intolerance
	Bradycardia	Tachycardia and palpitations
	Constipation	Diarrhea
	Weight gain	Weight loss, increased appetite
	Edema, bloated face, puffy eyelids	Polydipsia
	Poor circulation, extremity edema	Loss or thinning of hair
	TSH levels increased	TSH levels decreased
	T_3, T_4 levels decreased	T_3, T_4 levels increased
	I^{131} uptake decreased	I^{131} uptake increased

I131, Radioactive iodine; *T_3*, triiodothyronine; *T_4*, thyroxine; *TSH*, thyroid-stimulating hormone.

The thyroid gland is the endocrine organ that most often produces pathology. Under the control of TSH from the pituitary gland, the thyroid gland produces two types of hormones: T_4 and T_3. Iodine in the diet is necessary for the synthesis of thyroid hormone. Released into systemic circulation, thyroid hormones affect the metabolism of all body tissues, the function of the pituitary gland's essential GH, and many body systems. The size and superficial location of the thyroid gland in the neck make it uniquely available for inspection and palpation. A goiter is often the first sign of thyroid disease.

Simple Goiter

Description

The term *goiter* refers to any enlargement of the thyroid gland usually evidenced by a swelling in the neck.

ICD-10-CM Code	E04.0 *(Nontoxic diffuse goiter)*
	OR
	E01.2 *(Iodine-deficiency related (endemic) goiter, unspecified)*
	(E01.0-E01.8 = 4 codes of specificity)
	E04.9 *(Nontoxic goiter, unspecified)*

Disorders of the thyroid gland are coded according to the underlying pathology. Refer to the physician's diagnosis and then to the current edition of the ICD-10-CM coding manual to ensure the greatest specificity of pathology.

Symptoms and Signs

Simple goiter, or hyperplasia of the thyroid gland, may be asymptomatic in the early stages. The patient, who is usually a female, may be unaware of the condition until the anterior aspect of the neck enlarges with conspicuous swelling of the thyroid gland, called a *goiter* (Fig. 4.8). As the hyperplasia increases, it presses on the esophagus, producing difficulty swallowing, and occasionally it can enlarge further, pressing onto the trachea and producing dyspnea. Weight loss despite a hearty appetite, heat intolerance, tachycardia, anxiety, and increased sweating may be reported by the patient when there is excessive production of thyroid hormones.

Patient Screening

The patient who complains of enlargement in the area of the thyroid gland, with or without accompanying discomfort in the area, should be scheduled for a thorough patient history and physical examination.

Etiology

Simple, or nontoxic, goiter results from deficiency of iodine in the diet. Iodine is necessary for the synthesis of both T_3 and T_4. Together known as *thyroid hormone,* these are produced by the thyroid gland. The inadequate

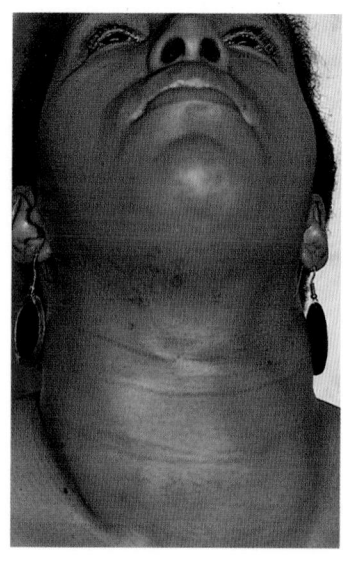

• **Fig. 4.8** Goiter (From Swartz MH: *Textbook of physical diagnosis,* ed 4, Philadelphia, 2002, Saunders.)

blood level of thyroid hormone causes the anterior pituitary gland to increase its secretion of thyrotropin (TSH). Thyrotropin keeps attempting to stimulate the thyroid gland to produce thyroid hormone. This continued stimulation, in turn, causes the thyroid gland to increase in size.

In the past, there were high rates of simple goiter among people living in geographic regions where the soil had low levels of iodine and where seafood was not readily available. The regular addition of iodine in salt and the advent of rapid refrigerated transport of seafood and fresh vegetables from areas where soil and water iodine levels are high have reduced the endemic aspects of this condition. Simple goiter can be exacerbated as a result of ingestion of large amounts of goitrogenic foods, such as cassava and cabbage, or drugs, such as lithium.

Diagnosis

Diagnosis is made by examination of the neck, noting the enlargement of the thyroid gland (goiter). Blood studies indicate elevated thyrotropin levels and occasionally reduced levels of T_3 and T_4. Measurement of radioactive iodine uptake by the thyroid gland is often helpful in determining the cause of the abnormality. Thyroid ultrasonography can confirm the presence of thyroid nodules.

Treatment

Treatment in the early stages is simple: the administration of one drop per week of saturated solution of potassium iodide. Prevention calls for the addition of iodine to the diet; there are no longer any iodine-deficient areas in the United States because of the introduction of iodized salts. There has been an increase in the use of sea salt for seasoning foods. Sea salt has some iodine but not as much as table salt, which has added iodine. Sporadic goiter requires avoidance of goitrogenic drugs or food. Thyroid hormones, such as T_4, sometimes help.

Prognosis
The prognosis is good when treatment to reduce the goiter is successful. When a large goiter is unresponsive to treatment, a subtotal thyroidectomy may be required.

Prevention
Adequate dietary intake of iodized salt (150–300 μg of iodine) prevents this deficiency. Some individuals should be advised to avoid goitrogenic drugs or foods. Examples of goitrogenic foods include broccoli, cauliflower, turnips, Brussels sprouts, cabbage, and radishes.

Patient Teaching
Instruct the patient to take the prescribed thyroid hormone medication at the same time each day to maintain a constant level of the medication in blood. Make sure the patient and the family know the symptoms of the adverse effects of a thyroid preparation that should be reported to the physician: palpitations, increased pulse rate, anxiety, insomnia, sweating, and tremors.

Hashimoto Thyroiditis
Description
Hashimoto thyroiditis (chronic lymphocytic thyroiditis) is a chronic disease of the immune system that attacks the thyroid gland.

ICD-10-CM Code	E06.3 (Autoimmune thyroiditis) (E06.0-E06.9 = 7 codes of specificity)

Symptoms and Signs
The condition occurs in women eight times as often as in men, is most common between ages 45 and 65 years, and is the leading cause of goiter and hypothyroidism. The outstanding clinical feature is the gradual and painless lumpy enlargement of the thyroid gland, which causes a feeling of pressure in the neck and may result in difficulty with swallowing. Symptoms of hypothyroidism, such as sensitivity to cold, weight gain, fatigue, depression, and mental apathy, appear as the disease progresses.

Patient Screening
Schedule a physical examination for a patient with a "lump in the throat" or a swelling in the neck. Follow office policy for referral to an endocrinologist.

Etiology
Heredity plays a prominent role in Hashimoto thyroiditis. Antibodies appear to destroy thyroid tissue instead of stimulating it. The gland enlarges as a result of an inflammatory process, with infiltration by lymphocytes and plasma cells. As a result, gland tissue is replaced by fibrous tissue, and a significant number of patients with Hashimoto thyroiditis become hypothyroid.

Diagnosis
Serum TSH levels are elevated in patients with hypothyroidism. Autoantibodies against thyroid tissue, such as thyroid peroxidase antibodies (TPOs), are found in blood. In Hashimoto thyroiditis, characteristic changes can be seen in the thyroid gland through needle biopsy and examination of the gland tissue, but these procedures are not necessary.

Similarly, a radioactive iodine uptake scan will show a low uptake, but it usually is not needed to make the diagnosis.

Treatment
The treatment is lifelong replacement of thyroid hormones in patients with hypothyroidism. This also prevents further growth of the goiter.

Prognosis
Mild hypothyroidism is common and usually responds well to thyroid replacement therapy.

Prevention
No prevention is known.

Patient Teaching
Explain each diagnostic test and procedure. Generate print-on-demand electronic materials, when possible, as teaching tools. Review the purpose and dosage schedule of the prescribed medication and the adverse effects to report. Emphasize the importance of follow-up visits to monitor the thyroid replacement therapy. Encourage the patient to expect improvement in symptoms with treatment.

Hyperthyroidism
Graves Disease
Description
Graves disease, a condition of primary hyperthyroidism, occurs when the entire thyroid gland hypertrophies, resulting in a diffuse goiter and an overproduction of thyroid hormones.

ICD-10-CM Code	E05.00 (Thyrotoxicosis with diffuse goiter without thyrotoxic crisis or storm) OR E05.0 (Thyrotoxicosis with diffuse goiter) (E05.0-E05.91 = 14 codes of specificity)

Refer to the physician's diagnosis and then to the current edition of the ICD-10-CM coding manual to ensure the greatest specificity of pathology.

Symptoms and Signs
Overproduction of thyroid hormone causes increased metabolism and multisystem changes. The patient has rapid heartbeats and palpitations, nervousness, excitability, and

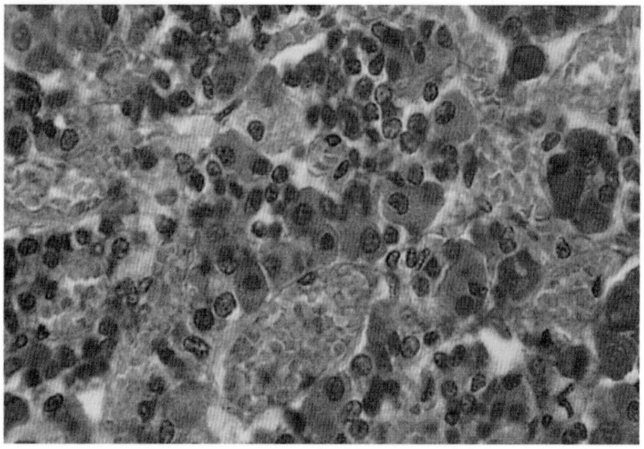

• **Fig. 4.9** Graves disease. (From Goldman L, Schafer AI: *Goldman's Cecil medicine,* ed 24, vol. 2, Philadelphia, 2012, Saunders.)

insomnia. Despite excessive appetite and food consumption, the patient loses weight. Profuse perspiration and warm, moist skin cause the person to be intolerant of hot weather. Other symptoms include muscular weakness and nail changes (onycholysis). General hyperactive behavior, tremor, and loss of hair are noted. Sometimes the eyes develop exophthalmos, an outward protrusion, which gives the patient a staring expression (Fig. 4.9), and sometimes skin changes called *dermopathy* are noted. A sudden exacerbation of symptoms may signal thyrotoxicosis, or thyroid storm, resulting from exaggerated thyroid hormone levels, can be life-threatening.

Patient Screening

A patient with mild or vague symptoms should be scheduled for a medical history and a physical examination. An acute manifestation of severe symptoms (e.g., notable tachycardia, manic behavior, vomiting, confusion, or coma) can indicate a life-threatening condition. Prompt consultation with the physician is necessary.

Etiology

Graves disease is believed to be an autoimmune response. Antibodies to thyroid antigens stimulate the hyperactivity of the thyroid gland. There is a familial predisposition that strongly suggests genetic causation.

Diagnosis

Taking the clinical picture and a thorough history are the first steps in the diagnosis. Serum T_3 and T_4 levels are elevated, and TSH levels are low. A thyroid scan is diagnostic and shows an increased uptake of radioiodine. Blood tests may reveal elevated levels of certain antithyroid immunoglobulins, such as thyroid-stimulating immunoglobulin (TSI).

Treatment

The goal of treatment is to reduce the formation and secretion of thyroid hormone. Treatment begins with the administration of antithyroid drugs, such as propylthiouracil and methimazole (Tapazole) to block the synthesis of thyroid hormones. β-Blockers, such as propranolol hydrochloride

(Inderal) and atenolol (Tenormin), are given to treat the tachycardia. Alternative treatments include radioactive iodine therapy or surgery (thyroidectomy), which is used to reduce the activity of the thyroid gland, although surgery is almost never done for this condition in the United States. Patients require ongoing medical supervision to monitor thyroid hormone levels. Some patients need help coping with the anxiety and physical discomfort associated with Graves disease.

Prognosis

Therapeutic intervention almost always restores the balance of thyroid hormone in the body and relieves symptoms. Some patients are more difficult to treat, especially older patients with concomitant underlying heart disease, and complications may arise. However, some patients experience spontaneous remission. Relapses do occur; thus lifelong follow-up is recommended.

Prevention

Graves disease being hereditary in nature, the precise triggering factors are not understood, so prevention remains unidentified.

Patient Teaching

Give the patient visual aids that explain the location and function of the thyroid gland. Offer appropriate computer-based health education, when possible. Explain the effects of hyperthyroidism on the body and on emotional stability. Discuss the diagnostic procedures and their purposes. Explain the dosage schedule of medications and the adverse effects to report. Give preoperative and postoperative instructions, as appropriate. Emphasize the importance of follow-up appointments to monitor treatment. Special instructions are required for skin care and eye care.

Hypothyroidism

Hypothyroidism, a very common condition, refers to any state in which thyroid hormone production is below normal. There are several possible causes that must be considered, including familial tendency. At first, the symptoms may be subclinical or subtle and take time, even years, to be noticed. Fatigue; cold intolerance; constipation; and dry, flaky skin may be experienced initially (see Table 4.2). A simple blood test measures the level of TSH secreted by the pituitary gland and the levels of the thyroid hormones (T_3 and T_4). An increase of TSH and below-normal levels of T_3 and T_4 or free T_4 are indicative of the condition. With proper diagnosis of hypothyroidism, the patient can be treated with hormone replacement and expect excellent results. In most cases, lifelong treatment with a form of T_4 (levothyroxine) is indicated, along with careful monitoring for therapeutic blood levels. Failure to treat the condition can lead to an increase in symptoms and/or severity of the disease.

Although more common in women, hypothyroidism can strike either gender and at any age. Much of the world's population lives at high risk in iodine-deficient areas, resulting in congenital hypothyroidism, a cause of mental deficiency.

Cretinism

Description

Cretinism is a congenital hypothyroidism developing in infancy or early childhood.

> ICD-10-CM Code   E00.9 *(Congenital iodine-deficiency syndrome, unspecified)*
> (E00.0-E00.9 = 4 codes of specificity)

Symptoms and Signs

Cretinism is a congenital hypothyroid condition in which the thyroid gland is absent or thyroid hormone is not synthesized by the thyroid gland; this causes intellectual developmental disorder and delayed growth in the infant or young child. The child develops as a dwarf, is stocky in stature, and has a protruding abdomen. Other physical characteristics include a short forehead, a broad nose, and small wide-set eyes with puffy eyelids; a wide-open mouth with a thick, protruding tongue; an expressionless face; and dry skin. The sex organs fail to develop. A lack of muscle tone contributes to inability to stand or walk.

Patient Screening

Follow office policy for referral of newborns or children with endocrine conditions or with suspected developmental disorders.

Etiology

An error in fetal development may cause the thyroid gland to fail to develop or to function. The patient may have congenital absence of one of the enzymes necessary for T_3 and T_4 synthesis. Maternal thyroid deficiency or antithyroid drugs taken during pregnancy may be an etiologic factor. Cretinism occurs in areas where the diet is deficient in iodine.

Diagnosis

Blood test results showing the absence or abnormally low amount of T_4 in the presence of an elevated TSH level indicate cretinism. A thyroid scan confirms the absence of thyroid tissue. If cretinism is not detected during the neonatal period, the infant will be slow to smile and intellectual developmental disorder will occur.

Treatment

Early treatment with thyroid hormone promotes normal physical growth but may not prevent intellectual developmental disorder. This replacement therapy must continue throughout the life of the patient.

Prognosis

The prognosis is good when cretinism is discovered early in life and T_4 replacement is begun. Even skeletal abnormalities are reversible with treatment. The condition may be associated with other endocrine abnormalities.

Prevention

The use of iodized salt greatly reduces the incidence of cretinism in a population. Public education about the importance of good prenatal care that manages any maternal endocrine disease is important.

Patient Teaching

Explain the importance of regular monitoring of the therapeutic response to hormone replacement. The response to the hormone replacement takes time; give the parent reasonable expectations for the child taking the medication. Giving the parents and/or caregivers educational materials and referrals to support their individual needs provides a blended learning experience.

Myxedema and Myxedema Coma

Description

Myxedema (hypothyroidism) is a disease characterized by clinical manifestations associated with a low metabolic rate caused by thyroid hormone deficiency.

Myxedema coma is the result of severe untreated hypothyroidism exacerbated by an acute event, such as myocardial infarction, infection, or the use of sedatives.

> ICD-10-CM Code   E03.9 *(Hypothyroidism, unspecified)*
> (E03.0-E03.9 = 8 codes of specificity)

Symptoms and Signs

Severe hypothyroidism with significant reduced levels of T_4 and T_3, especially in the older adult, leads to a slowing of function in multiple organs. Excessive fatigue, muscular weakness, loss of hair, weight gain, constipation, and intolerance to cold are common symptoms. The skin is dry and scaly, and there is puffiness of the hands and face, in addition to an enlarged tongue (Fig. 4.10). Sometimes the term *myxedema* is also used synonymously with severe hypothyroidism. Rarely does it progress to myxedema coma when severe

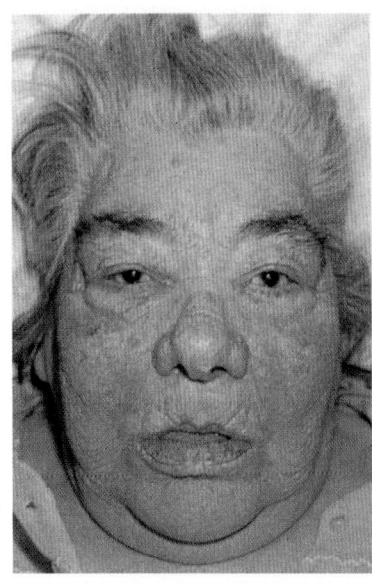

• **Fig. 4.10** Myxedema facies. (From Patton KT, Thibodeau G: *Human body in health & disease,* ed 7, St. Louis, 2018, Mosby.)

hypothyroidism is accompanied by signs of hypothermia and altered mental status: slurred speech and drowsiness, followed by profound lethargy or even unconsciousness. Myxedema coma is a medical emergency because it has a high mortality rate. This is best treated at the intensive care unit.

Patient Screening

Complaints vary, depending on age at onset. When a parent reports slowing of physical and mental activities in a child or an adult reports the same, an appointment for a complete physical examination is needed. Keep in mind that the symptoms may mimic depression.

Etiology

The thyroid gland's ability to synthesize T_4 is impaired. This can be the result of reduced amounts of thyrotropin, radiation destruction of the thyroid gland, surgical removal of the gland without T_4 replacement therapy, tumor, or failure of the thyroid gland to function. The disorder also may be secondary to failure of the pituitary to produce thyrotropin. A common cause for hypothyroidism in women is Hashimoto thyroiditis.

Diagnosis

The clinical features of myxedema in the adult or the delayed physical and mental development in the child may lead the physician to order diagnostic tests. Blood studies indicate abnormally low levels of thyroid hormones (total T_4, total T_3, and free T_4) and, in most cases, significantly elevated TSH levels. Rarely is the TSH level low as a result of a pituitary condition.

Treatment

The goal of medical management is to achieve normal thyroid function with the lowest possible dose. The patient should be told that replacement therapy is required for the rest of his or her life.

Myxedema coma is treated as an emergency. Levothyroxine sodium (T_4), a therapeutic agent, is administered orally or intravenously. Additionally, it is important to treat any coexisting medical condition, including adrenal insufficiency, with corticosteroids.

Prognosis

The response to hormone replacement therapy is usually good, and the symptoms improve. If myxedema coma develops, the mortality is high.

Prevention

Endocrinologists and other health care providers recommend screening (testing for TSH levels) in identified high-risk groups and at age 35 years and every 5 years thereafter as part of a periodic health examination.

Patient Teaching

Patients on medications should be taught the importance of taking the medication at the same time each day on an empty stomach and recognizing the signs of overmedication. Inform the patient that a clinical response to the medication may take several weeks to appear and that blood tests will be required to monitor for therapeutic blood levels of the medication. Demonstrate and encourage periodic self-examination of the thyroid gland. Use customized electronically generated educational materials, when available, to reinforce the treatment plan.

Thyroid Cancer

Description

Thyroid cancer is a neoplasm of the thyroid gland. The term includes primary thyroid tumors, thyroid lymphoma, and metastases from breast, colon, kidney, or skin cancers to the thyroid gland.

ICD-10-CM Code	C73 *(Malignant neoplasm of thyroid gland)*

Refer to the physician's diagnosis and then to the current edition of the ICD-10-CM coding manuals to ensure the greatest specificity of pathology.

Symptoms and Signs

Thyroid malignancies often do not cause symptoms until the disease is advanced. Signs of cancer include palpation of a hard, painless lump or nodule on the thyroid gland, vocal cord paralysis, obstructive symptoms, and cervical lymphadenopathy. Some patients exhibit dysphagia or hoarseness resulting from compression of the upper aerodigestive tract. A rapidly enlarging neck mass may be a sign of anaplastic thyroid cancer.

Patient Screening

When patients complain of persistent hoarseness, difficulty swallowing, or a painless lump in the neck, schedule an appointment with the physician as soon as possible.

Etiology

Thyroid cancer accounts for a small percentage of all thyroid nodules. Other causes include multinodular goiter, Hashimoto thyroiditis, cysts, and follicular adenomas. The four main types of thyroid cancer are papillary (small nipplelike projections), follicular (saclike ball of cells), medullary (affecting the interior portion of the gland), and anaplastic (loss of differentiation of cells). Papillary and follicular carcinomas are the most common and occur mainly between ages 30 and 60 years. Anaplastic tumors are rare and occur mainly in patients older than 60 years of age. Women are nearly three times more likely to have thyroid cancer compared with men. Relatives of patients with thyroid cancer have a 10-fold higher incidence of thyroid cancer, which indicates a genetic basis for tumor susceptibility. Previous head and neck radiation exposure, especially in early childhood, is the only other established risk factor. A diet deficient in iodine may contribute to follicular cancer. Although 80% of cases of medullary carcinoma are sporadic, some are caused by inherited genetic mutations, resulting in multiple endocrine neoplasia (MEN) type 2, a rare, heritable disorder characterized by various types of endocrine tumors. Inherited medullary cancer usually presents in the third decade of life.

Diagnosis

Thyroid nodules are usually discovered by the patient, found incidentally on physical examination, or detected by a radiologic procedure done for another reason. TSH is measured in all patients with thyroid nodules. Fine-needle aspiration (FNA) and histologic examination of the nodule tissue are needed to confirm the diagnosis and type of cancer. Medullary thyroid carcinomas often secrete calcitonin and occasionally secrete carcinoembryonic antigen (CEA), both of which can serve as tumor markers. Patients with this type of thyroid cancer should undergo testing for mutations in the *RET* gene to evaluate for MEN type 2. Tests used for staging include CT or ultrasonography of the neck and chest radiography. All anaplastic tumors are considered stage IV tumors and require a positron emission tomography (PET) to better determine the extent of tumor spread (see Chapter 1 for discussion of staging of cancer).

Treatment

The primary therapy mode for papillary, follicular, and medullary thyroid cancers is surgery. Most patients undergo total thyroidectomy with removal of any involved lymph nodes, followed by the administration of radioiodine to destroy any remaining thyroid tissue and tumor and to image any recurrent disease. Aggressive initial therapy yields lower rates of local and regional recurrence and lower overall mortality. Thyroid surgery is associated with the risk of vocal cord paralysis resulting from damage to the recurrent laryngeal nerve and the risk of hypoparathyroidism. After surgery, patients are started on T_4 therapy to prevent TSH stimulation of tumor growth and to prevent hypothyroidism. However, excessive T_4 therapy carries risks of accelerated bone loss, atrial fibrillation, and cardiac dysfunction, so the amount of T_4 administered is carefully regulated. Because thyroid cancers are largely resistant to conventional chemotherapy, new agents are being investigated to treat this disease. Tyrosine kinase inhibitors can be used to delay progression in patients with metastatic disease.

Anaplastic tumors are the most aggressive form of thyroid cancers. They are resistant to most therapy. Nonsurgical treatment (e.g., radiotherapy and/or chemotherapy) may prolong survival. Total thyroidectomy is indicated to reduce symptoms caused by the tumor mass if the disease is confined to the local area.

Most recurrences of any type of thyroid neoplasm appear within 5 years of initial treatment, although they can occur decades afterward. All patients should undergo a physical examination and measurement of serum thyroglobulin, TSH, and T_4 levels periodically after treatment. Patients with medullary thyroid cancer with preoperatively elevated levels of calcitonin and/or CEA should have the levels of these tumor markers measured periodically as well.

Prognosis

Most patients with differentiated thyroid carcinomas have a very good prognosis. The most important prognostic factors are age at diagnosis, size of the primary tumor, and the presence of tissue invasion or metastases. The overall 5-year survival rate based on individuals diagnosed between 2008 and 2014 for localized papillary, follicular, and medullary thyroid cancers is greater than 99%. For localized anaplastic tumors, the 5-year survival rate is 30%.

If the cancer has spread to other organs or tissues close to the thyroid gland, it is referred to as *regional thyroid cancer.* Five-year survival rate for regional follicular cancer is 96%, and the 5-year survival rate for regional papillary thyroid cancer is 99%. Five-year survival rate for individuals with regional medullary cancer is 91%, and those with regional anaplastic cancer have a poor 5-year survival rate of 13%.

If thyroid cancer metastasizes and spreads to other distant organs, the percentage for 5-year survival drops. Anaplastic and medullary cancers spread more frequently compared with follicular or papillary tumors. The 5-year survival rate for metastatic papillary thyroid cancer is 78%, and that for metastatic follicular thyroid cancer is 56%. Individuals with metastatic medullary thyroid have a projected life expectancy rate of 37% after 5 years, and individuals diagnosed with anaplastic thyroid cancer have a life expectancy rate of 3% after 5 years.

Prevention

Patients who have been exposed to radiation should receive follow-up screening for thyroid cancer, depending on their estimated risk level. Those at low risk should undergo thyroid palpation every year or every other year. Those at high risk should undergo annual palpation and thyroid ultrasonography on a regular basis. Those at high risk usually have been exposed to high-dose radiation of the thyroid at a young age.

Patient Teaching

Give the patient preoperative instructions, and encourage the patient to ask questions about the risks the surgeon identifies. Tell the patient what to expect after surgery, including symptoms of low calcium or a temporary loss of voice. Explain postoperative instructions, including hormone therapy, chemotherapy, and/or radiotherapy, as prescribed by the physician. Refer the patient to the attending physician for questions about the prognosis after treatment. Emphasize the need for follow-up appointments, and review the schedule for these appointments.

Parathyroid Gland Diseases

The parathyroid glands are found on the back of the thyroid gland (Fig. 4.11). They secrete parathyroid hormone (PTH), the main hormone the body uses to maintain calcium homeostasis. Blood calcium levels are regulated by a feedback loop to maintain a normal calcium level. Disorders of parathyroid secretion result in serious disturbances throughout the body.

Hyperparathyroidism

Description

Hyperparathyroidism is a condition caused by overactivity of one or more of the four parathyroid glands and results in the overproduction of PTH.

ICD-10-CM Code	E21.3 *(Hyperparathyroidism, unspecified)*
	(E21.0-E21.5 = 6 codes of specificity)

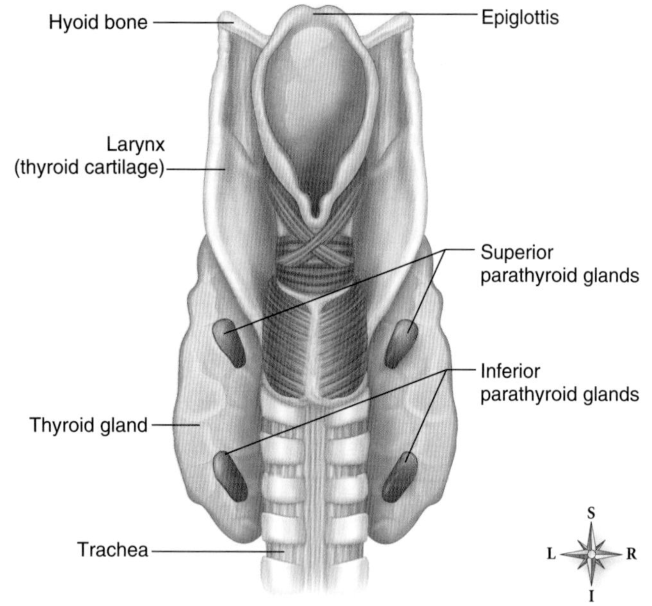

Hyoid bone

Epiglottis

Larynx
(thyroid cartilage)

Superior
parathyroid glands

Inferior
parathyroid glands

Thyroid gland

Trachea

S

L — R

I

• **Fig. 4.11** Parathyroid glands. (From Patton KT, Thibodeau GA: *Anthony's textbook of anatomy & physiology,* ed 20, St Louis, 2013, Mosby.)

Symptoms and Signs

Hyperparathyroidism increases the breakdown of bone from the skeletal system (demineralization), which results in excessive calcium in blood (hypercalcemia). Hypercalcemia produces the symptoms of hyperparathyroidism. Hypercalcemia reduces the irritability of nerve and muscle tissues, and this causes the patient to experience muscle weakness and atrophy, gastrointestinal pain, and nausea. High serum calcium levels can produce conduction defects in the heart. An increased deposit of calcium in soft tissue causes low back pain and renal calculi. Bone tenderness, arthritis type of pain, and easy fracturing of the bones are the result of demineralization of the bone (Fig. 4.12).

Patient Screening

Some patients may have vague symptoms, such as fatigue, weakness, or mental disturbance. Schedule a complete physical examination. The patient experiencing symptoms of hypercalcemia is very ill and requires prompt medical intervention.

Etiology

The cause of primary hyperparathyroidism is increased activity of the parathyroid gland, usually as a result of an excessive growth of one of the parathyroid glands (adenoma) or an

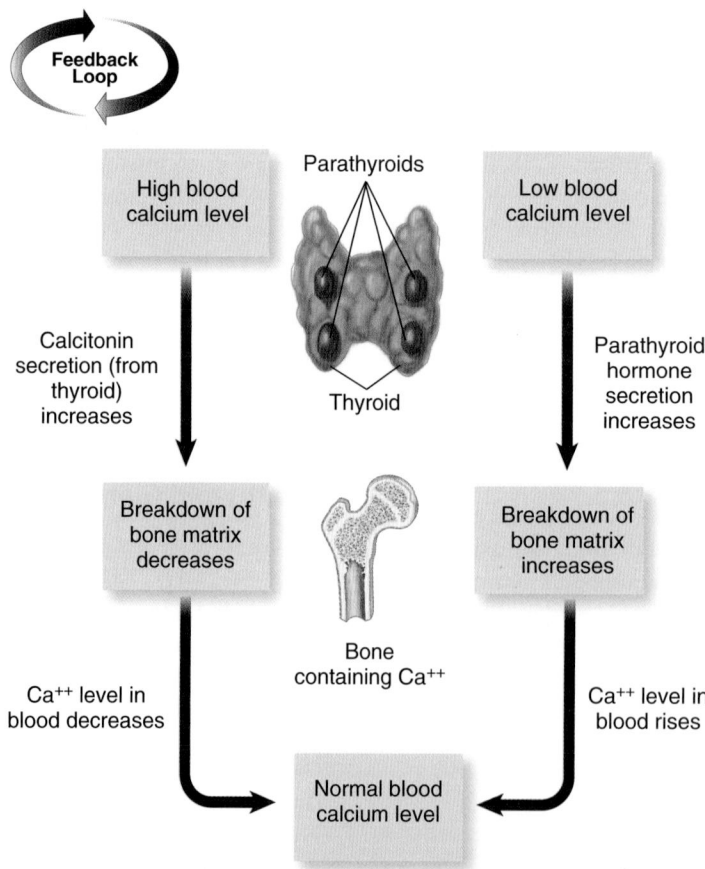

Feedback
Loop

Parathyroids

High blood
calcium level

Low blood
calcium level

Calcitonin
secretion (from
thyroid)
increases

Parathyroid
hormone
secretion
increases

Thyroid

Breakdown of
bone matrix
decreases

Breakdown of
bone matrix
increases

Bone
containing Ca++

Ca++ level in
blood decreases

Ca++ level in
blood rises

Normal blood
calcium level

• **Fig. 4.12** Regulation of blood calcium levels. Calcitonin and parathyroid hormones (PTHs) have antagonistic (opposite) effects on calcium concentration in blood. (From Patton KT, Thibodeau GA: *Anthony's textbook of anatomy & physiology,* ed 20, St Louis, 2013, Mosby.)

idiopathic hyperplasia of the gland. The incidence rises sharply after age 40 years and is twice as common in women. Secondary hyperparathyroidism may be caused by an increased secretion of PTH induced by a low level of serum calcium or serum vitamin D as a result of renal disease or other disorders.

Diagnosis

Serum intact PTH (iPTH) level is elevated with an increased calcium level and reduced phosphorus levels in serum. The alkaline phosphatase levels tend to be increased, and urine calcium is high. Low bone mineral density, especially at sites richer in cortical bone (i.e., femoral neck and forearm), is noted through the appearance of bone on radiographic films.

The demineralization of bones leads to osteoporosis and can be detected by dual-energy x-ray absorptiometry (DEXA, a bone density test).

Treatment

The treatment plan for hyperparathyroidism varies with the cause and is highly individualized. If the hypersecretion of PTH is caused by an adenoma, the tumor can now be removed by minimally invasive parathyroid surgery. If hyperplasia is the cause of the hypersecretion, usually three and a half of the four glands are removed. When the condition is secondary, the underlying cause must be treated and blood serum calcium levels reduced. Drugs that increase the excretion of calcium by the kidneys or inhibit the reabsorption of calcium from bone may be used.

Prognosis

After successful surgery, calcium replacement prevents **hypocalcemia** and allows skeletal remineralization in patients with bone disease.

Prevention

No prevention is known.

Patient Teaching

Use an educational video or a DVD as a visual aid to explain the location and function of the parathyroid glands. Explain hyperparathyroid disease and the treatment plan. Fractures can occur easily, and the patient is advised to take care to avoid trauma. Give preoperative and postoperative instructions, as indicated. Explain the dosage schedule for prescription medication and the adverse side effects to report. Caution against using over-the-counter medications containing excessive calcium. Refer the patient to a dietitian, as required.

Hypoparathyroidism

Description

Hypoparathyroidism is the condition in which the secretion of PTH by the parathyroid glands is greatly reduced.

ICD-10-CM Code	E20.9 *(Hypoparathyroidism, unspecified)*
	(E20.0-E20.9 = 4 codes of specificity)

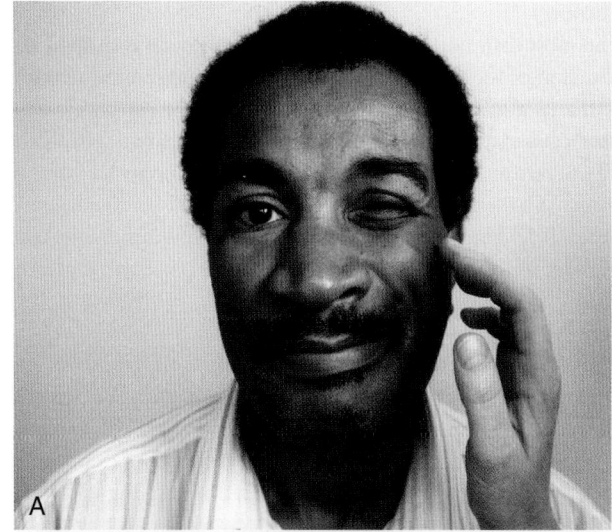
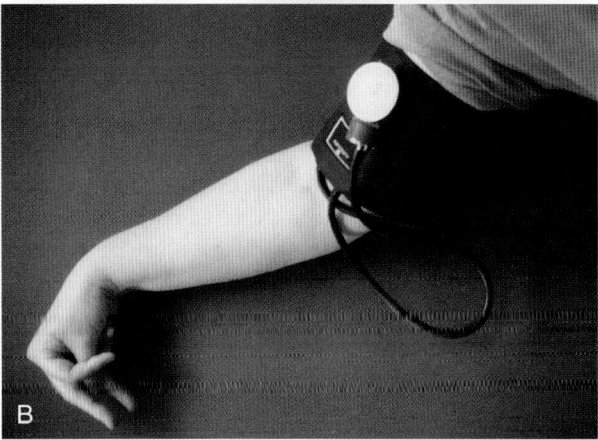

• **Fig. 4.13** Signs of Hypocalcemia. (A) Chvostek sign (facial twitch). (B) Trousseau sign (carpopedal spasm). (From Ignatavicius DD, Workman ML: *Medical-surgical nursing: patient-centered collaborative care,* ed 8, St Louis, 2016, Saunders.)

Symptoms and Signs

PTH increases the blood calcium level by stimulating bone demineralization and increasing absorption of calcium in the digestive tract and the kidneys. When the level of this hormone is insufficient, circulating levels of calcium are reduced, resulting in hypocalcemia, with the occasional possibility of excessive deposits of calcium into tissue. A consequence of the hypocalcemia is a hyperexcitable nervous system, resulting in an overstimulation of the skeletal muscles (Fig. 4.13). Initial symptoms include numbness and tingling of fingertips, toes, ears, or nose, followed by muscular spasms or twitching of the hands and feet. Tetany, or severe, sustained muscular contractions, may develop. The patient may experience emotional changes, confusion, and irritability. Sustained hypocalcemia leads to laryngospasm, arrhythmias, respiratory paralysis, and death.

Patient Screening

Acute, symptomatic hypocalcemia requires emergency treatment.

Etiology

The most common cause of hypoparathyroidism is surgical destruction of the parathyroid glands. Accidental surgical removal of the parathyroid gland during thyroidectomy can induce hypocalcemia. Acquired hypoparathyroidism can result from injury to one or more of the parathyroid glands, ischemia from an infarct, accidental radiation, neoplasia, or various disease processes. The condition may result from an autoimmune genetic disorder or from a congenital absence of the parathyroid glands.

Diagnosis

The clinical picture of neuromuscular hyperexcitability along with a history of possible insult to the parathyroid glands leads the physician to further investigation. The presence of the Trousseau phenomenon is a sure indication of hypocalcemia. Blood studies indicate reduced serum calcium levels and increased serum phosphate levels. Electrocardiography shows increased QT and ST intervals. PTH levels are reduced.

Treatment

Calcium replacement therapy with vitamin D reduces hypocalcemia. This replacement therapy usually is given for life unless the condition is reversible. In the case of a life-threatening deficiency (tetany), calcium gluconate is administered intravenously. The patient is encouraged to follow a high-calcium diet.

Prognosis

Reversible forms of the condition respond to appropriate treatment. Some cases are transient.

Prevention

No prevention is known.

Patient Teaching

Answer questions about the location and function of the parathyroid gland. Explain hypocalcemia and the way it affects the nervous system. Refer the patient to a dietitian, as indicated. Emphasize the importance of follow-up care to monitor renal function and serum calcium levels.

Adrenal Gland Diseases

Cushing Syndrome

Description

Cushing syndrome is a condition of chronic hypersecretion of the adrenal cortex, which results in excessive circulating cortisol levels.

ICD-10-CM Code	E24.0 *(Pituitary-dependent Cushing's disease)*
	E24.2 *(Drug-induced Cushing's syndrome)*
	E24.3 *(Ectopic ACTH syndrome)*
	E24.8 *(Other Cushing's syndrome)*
	E24.9 *(Cushing's syndrome, unspecified)*

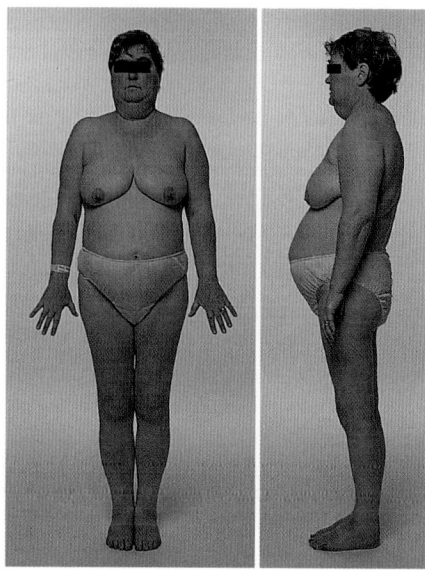

• **Fig. 4.14** Clinical manifestations in a patient with Cushing syndrome. (From Forbes CH, Jackson WF: *Color atlas and text of clinical medicine,* ed 3, St Louis, 2003, Elsevier Science Limited/Mosby.)

Symptoms and Signs

The patient with Cushing syndrome experiences fatigue, muscular weakness, weight gain, and changes in body appearance. Fat deposits form in the scapular area (buffalo humps) and in the trunk, causing a protruding abdomen (Fig. 4.14). Salt and water retention result not only in hypertension and edema but also in the characteristic moon face noted in the patient with Cushing syndrome. The patient may show clinical evidence of hyperlipidemia, hyperglycemia, osteoporosis, and atherosclerosis. Changes in mood and cognition and decreased short-term memory are common. The skin becomes thin, has a tendency to bruise easily, and develops red or purple striae (stretch marks). The individual is predisposed to infection as a result of suppression of the immune response. Other symptoms include excessive hair growth, amenorrhea, and impotence.

Patient Screening

Early manifestations include weight gain, hypertension, and emotional instability. These symptoms warrant a medical evaluation. Follow office policy for referral to an endocrinologist.

Etiology

Excessive levels of circulating cortisol can be caused by hyperplasia of the adrenal gland, excessive secretion of corticotropin (ACTH) from the pituitary gland, a tumor of the adrenal cortex, or production of corticotropin in another organ (e.g., cancer cells in the lungs). Iatrogenic factors, such as prolonged administration or large doses of glucocorticoids used to treat other diseases, can induce Cushing syndrome.

Diagnosis

The typical picture of the moon face, buffalo hump, and gross obesity of the trunk, particularly the abdomen, leads the physician to further investigation. Continuous elevation of serum cortisol levels is found in Cushing syndrome. Free cortisol levels are elevated in a 24-hour urine collection. CT or MRI may detect adrenal tumors.

Treatment

Treatment of Cushing syndrome depends on the cause of the over secretion of cortisol. When a tumor is the cause, surgical removal or radiation of the tumor in the pituitary gland or adrenal gland is indicated. Drug therapy to suppress ACTH secretion can be used separately or as an adjunct to radiation.

Prognosis

The prognosis depends on the underlying cause. Without treatment, or when the condition is caused by ectopic carcinoma, the prognosis is poor.

Prevention

Generally there is no prevention; however, the patient on large doses of glucocorticoids is monitored closely.

Patient Teaching

Appropriate computer-based health education about Cushing syndrome can be helpful, when available, for patient teaching. If surgery is indicated, give the patient information about the procedures and what to expect after surgery. Give careful instructions about medication if hormone replacement is planned; the medication must be taken exactly as directed and never discontinued abruptly. Refer the patient to a dietitian, as indicated. Teach the patient about recognizing symptoms of adrenal hypofunction: apathy, fatigue, weakness, and syncope.

Addison Disease

Description

Addison disease is partial or complete failure of adrenocortical function.

ICD-10-CM Code	E27.1 *(Primary adrenocortical insufficiency)*
	E27.2 *(Addisonian crisis)*
	E27.40 *(Unspecified adrenocortical insufficiency)*
	(E27.0-E27.9 = 8 codes of specificity)

Symptoms and Signs

Addison disease, adrenal insufficiency or hypoadrenalism, gradually manifests as symptoms of fatigue, weakness, anorexia, agitation, confusion, weight loss, and gastrointestinal disturbances. A typical bronze skin color is exhibited. The patient can experience cardiovascular difficulties, including irregular pulse, reduced cardiac output, and orthostatic (postural) hypotension. Depression, anxiety, and emotional distress are often experienced. Reduced levels of aldosterone cause inability to retain salt and water. When dehydration, hyperkalemia (high blood potassium level), and electrolyte imbalance occur, the condition is life-threatening.

Patient Screening

The onset is usually gradual over weeks or months. However, in acute cases when complications, such as fever, profound weakness, or confused behavior, prompt the call for medical attention, life-threatening conditions may follow, requiring emergency care.

Etiology

The onset of Addison disease is usually gradual, with progressive destruction of the adrenal gland and reduction in its important hormones. The destruction can result from an autoimmune process, tuberculosis, hemorrhage, fungal infections, neoplasms, or surgical resection of the gland. There are familial tendencies. The disease also can be secondary to hypopituitarism, in which there is reduced output of corticotropin.

Diagnosis

Blood and urine cortisol levels are low, as are serum sodium and fasting glucose levels. Serum potassium, blood urea nitrogen, lymphocyte, and eosinophil levels and hematocrit are elevated. Sometimes adrenal calcification is identified on radiographs.

Treatment

Treatment includes replacement of the natural hormones with glucocorticoid and mineralocorticoid drugs and correction of salt and potassium levels. Hormone replacement therapy with close medical supervision must continue for life. The patient must be educated about the symptoms of overdosing and underdosing and the role of stress and infection in Addison disease. Insufficiency or a sudden decrease in adrenocortical hormone levels, such as from sudden withdrawal of glucocorticoid therapy, can result in a life-threatening emergency, called an *addisonian crisis*.

Prognosis

Early diagnosis and strict adherence to the treatment regimen can result in a good prognosis, and the patient's resistance to infection and general well-being can be maintained (Fig. 4.15).

Prevention

There is no known prevention. After diagnosis, the individual with adrenal hypofunction requires lifelong steroid replacement.

Patient Teaching

The goal of patient teaching is good compliance to prevent adrenal crisis and to promote general well-being. Refer the patient to a dietitian to ensure adequate nutrient and fluid intake. Give the patient instructions on recognizing the signs of electrolyte imbalance or adrenal crisis. Give careful instructions on taking medications, and warn the patient not to discontinue medications abruptly. Emphasize the importance of getting follow-up care from the health care provider. Explain the value of wearing a medical alert bracelet.

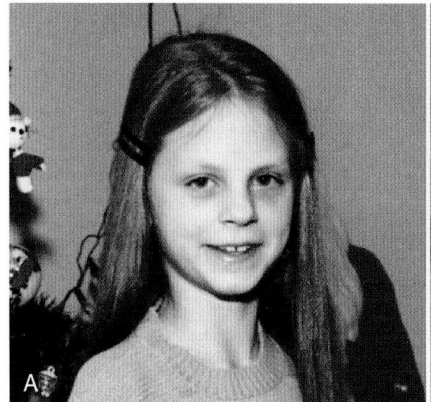
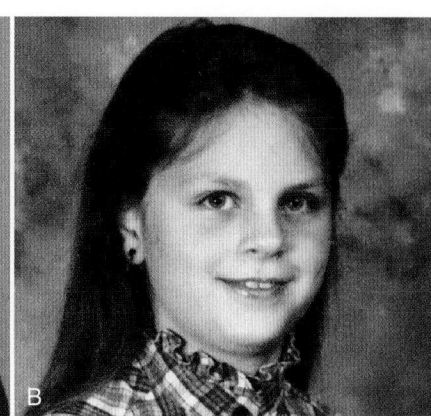

• **Fig. 4.15** (A) Young girl with adrenocortico-tropic hormone (ACTH) deficiency shows wasting and pallor rather than excessive bronzing. (B) The same girl after therapy. (From Zitelli BJ, Davis HW: *Atlas of pediatric physical diagnosis,* ed 6, Philadelphia, 2012, Mosby.)

Endocrine Dysfunction of Pancreas

Diabetes Mellitus

Description

Diabetes mellitus is a chronic disorder of carbohydrate, fat, and protein metabolism caused by inadequate production of insulin by the pancreas or faulty use of insulin by the cells.

ICD-10-CM Code	E11.9 *(Type 2 diabetes mellitus without complications)*
	(E08.0-E13.9 = 205 codes of specificity)

Diabetes mellitus is coded in the fourth digit according to clinical manifestations and with a fifth-digit modifier for non–insulin-dependent or insulin-dependent state. Refer to the physician's diagnosis and then to the current edition of the ICD-10-CM coding manual to ensure the greatest specificity of pathology.

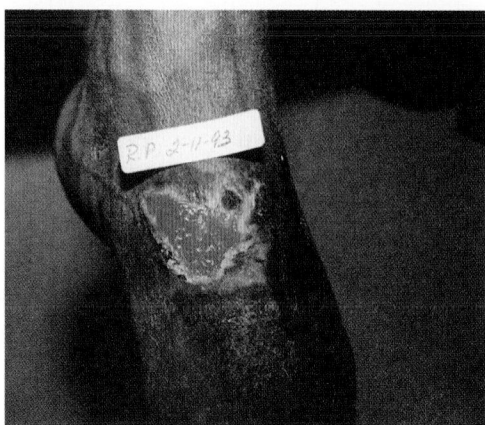

• **Fig. 4.16** Diabetic ulcer, dorsal aspect of the foot. (From Hill MJ: *Skin disorders—Mosby's clinical nursing series,* St Louis, 1994, Mosby.)

Symptoms and Signs

The functional pancreas secretes insulin and maintains glucose levels within a precise range. Insulin normally reduces blood glucose levels by transporting glucose into the cells for use as energy and storage as glycogen. A reduction in insulin results in **hyperglycemia** and deprives cells of fuel. Cells begin to metabolize fats and proteins; this process allows wastes called *ketone bodies* to accumulate in the blood (ketosis). Ketonuria develops as excess ketone bodies are excreted in urine. This leads to **acidosis**. Hyperglycemia is at the root of the principal symptoms: polyuria, **polyphagia**, polydipsia, weight loss, and fatigue. The patient may have **pruritus**, especially in the genital area, and a fruity odor to the breath may be noted when ketosis occurs in type 1 diabetes. Diagnostic tests of blood and urine point to the common signs of diabetes mellitus.

There are two primary forms of diabetes mellitus:

1. Type 1 (formerly known as *juvenile onset diabetes* or *insulin-dependent diabetes mellitus [IDDM]*) has an early, abrupt onset, usually before age 30 years, with little or no insulin being secreted by the patient, and can be difficult to control.
2. Type 2 (formerly known as *adult onset diabetes* or *non–insulin-dependent diabetes mellitus [NIDDM]*), the most common form, has a gradual onset in adults older than 30 years of age, and more often in people older than 55 years of age. In this form, some pancreatic function remains, permitting control of symptoms by dietary management; in addition, an oral hypoglycemic medication is often prescribed.

Untreated or poorly managed diabetes has many systemic complications: retinopathy, which leads to blindness; neuropathy; renal failure; atherosclerosis leading to myocardial infarction; and cerebrovascular accidents. Hyperglycemia delays healing and impairs resistance to infection. Patients with diabetes require careful attention to foot care to prevent the damage that can result from circulatory disorders and infections (Fig. 4.16). Improved glycemic control and adequate blood pressure and lipids control prevent diabetic complications.

Patient Screening

Individuals known to be at high risk require screening for the signs of diabetes as part of regular medical checkups. Known patients with diabetes having warning signs of diabetic coma or insulin reaction need instructions for immediate medical intervention (Table 4.3). Anyone complaining of weight loss, excessive thirst, excessive hunger, and frequent urination needs a prompt appointment for diagnostic evaluation.

Etiology

The disease is often familial but may be acquired. Metabolic abnormalities can induce the diabetic disease process, causing insulin resistance, abnormal insulin secretion by the

TABLE 4.3   Warning Signs and Interventions for Diabetic Coma and Insulin Reaction

Diabetic Coma	Insulin Reaction
Causes	
Undiagnosed diabetes	Excessive insulin
Skipped insulin dose	Delayed meal
Excessive food	Insufficient food
Infection or stress	Excessive exercise
Symptoms and Signs	
Slow onset	Rapid onset
Thirst	Hunger
Increased urination	Trembling and paleness
Nausea and vomiting	Feeling of faintness
Abdominal pain	Cold sweat
Drowsiness	Headache
Lethargy	Anxiety
Flushed appearance	Rapid heartbeat
Dry skin	Irritability
Fruity breath odor	Impaired vision
Dehydration	Hypoglycemia
Heavy respirations	Confusion
Dilated, fixed pupils	Seizures
Hyperglycemia	Loss of consciousness
Ketoacidosis	
Loss of consciousness	
Coma	
Intervention	
Give insulin, fluids, and salt.	If awake, give simple sugar, candy, orange juice, or soda.
If severe, give intravenous fluids, insulin, and sodium bicarbonate.	If unconscious, give intravenous dextrose or glucagon.

pancreas, or inappropriate glucose production by the liver. Both forms of diabetes are linked genetically. In type 1 diabetes, an infection early in life may trigger an autoimmune process that produces antibodies that destroy the β-cells of the pancreas. Type 2 tends to occur in older, overweight adults. Destruction of the pancreas by tumor, trauma to the pituitary gland, or other endocrine disorders can induce diabetes mellitus. Some drugs also may suppress insulin production. Some genetic disorders render the body's insulin receptors insensitive to insulin.

Diagnosis

The diagnosis of diabetes mellitus is straightforward, beginning with a patient history. The patient is assessed carefully for the cardinal symptoms. At least two positive tests of fasting blood plasma glucose and the presence of glucose and acetone in the urine confirm the diagnosis. Other tests include blood insulin level determination and an ophthalmic examination for diabetic retinopathy. Glycated hemoglobin testing is also used to determine the range of the patient's glucose level over the preceding 2 to 3 months before the test is collected.

Treatment

The goal of treatment is to normalize blood glucose levels and thus prevent complications. Management of diabetes is multifactorial, including a well-balanced diet closely integrated with insulin administration or oral medication, exercise, blood and urine testing, and hygienic measures. Patient compliance and education are vital to the control of symptoms and complications.

Patients with type 1 diabetes require insulin replacement therapy that correlates closely with calculated carbohydrate intake on a regular schedule. Methods of insulin delivery include injection, insulin pump therapy (see the Enrichment box about Insulin Pump Therapy), and insulin pens. Insulin preparations can be short-acting, intermediate-acting, long-acting, or premixed insulins. Researchers are investigating other insulin delivery methods. Patients with type 2 diabetes usually do not necessarily require insulin injections to control blood glucose levels. Their therapeutic regimen includes restricted caloric intake and exercise or oral hypoglycemic medications.

◆ ENRICHMENT

Insulin Pump Therapy

More recent technology offers an alternative to multiple insulin injection regimens for patients with type 1 diabetes as well as some patients with type 2 diabetes on insulin. The insulin pump is a small computerized device that delivers small doses of insulin at regular intervals 24 hours a day. The pump is programmed to deliver fast-acting insulin at a rate calculated for that individual. Some devices function to monitor the blood sugar level as well. It is necessary to test the blood sugar level throughout the day and then enter the data into the pump. Then adjustments to accommodate food intake and balance the delivery of insulin to maintain proper blood sugar can be realized.

An insulin pump unit is about the size of a beeper or smaller. These devices are clipped to a belt or directly applied to the skin. Insulin is delivered from small cartridges within the pump either directly through the skin via a microscopic cannula or through a plastic cannula inserted and secured into tissue just under the skin. The pump is monitored by the patient or, in the case of a child or a very sick patient, by a trained caregiver. This trained observer can monitor the functioning of the unit and can help distinguish between symptoms of hyperglycemia or hypoglycemia. An insulin pump requires a prescription from a physician.

There are lifestyle benefits and more freedom for many patients with diabetes who can manage their own care in this way with fewer side effects. Management of diabetes in children and teenagers who respond well to training in the use of an insulin pump can achieve tighter blood sugar control and reduce the risk for long-term complications in patients with diabetes.

Various forms of oral drug therapy currently are used to treat type 2 diabetes. The sulfonylureas and the meglitinide drugs (oral hypoglycemic drugs), such as glipizide (Glucotrol), glyburide (DiaBeta or Micronase), repaglinide (Prandin), and nateglinide (Starlix), stimulate the pancreas to produce insulin. These medications are usually taken once or twice a day, and blood glucose levels must be monitored on a strict schedule. Because sulfonylureas stimulate the pancreas to increase insulin production, the increased insulin levels tend to lower blood glucose levels, often resulting in symptoms and complications of hypoglycemia.

Metformin (Glucophage) works in several ways. It primarily prevents the liver from producing hepatic glucose but also helps enhance the benefits of the available insulin. Under normal circumstances, metformin hydrochloride does not elevate blood insulin levels and therefore does not produce hypoglycemia. See the Alert box for special information and warnings about Antidiabetic Agents.

ⓘ *ALERT!*

Antidiabetic Agents: Information and Warnings

Metformin (Glucophage), an antidiabetic agent used for type 2 diabetes, should not be taken by patients with a history of kidney disease, congestive heart failure, liver disease, or alcoholism. Patients should be instructed to stop taking metformin before undergoing any imaging procedures with injectable contrast agents. Patients needing a procedure to place stents will have to wait 3 days until it is safe for an iodine dye to be in blood.

A rare but serious side effect of metformin is lactic acidosis. It is a rare side effect and is seen in patients with renal failure, liver failure, and congestive heart failure.

The symptoms and signs of lactic acidosis are weakness, fatigue, unusual muscle pain, dyspnea, unusual stomach discomfort, dizziness or lightheadedness, and bradycardia or cardiac arrhythmias. With any of these symptoms, the patient should stop metformin immediately and contact the physician.

Rosiglitazone maleate (Avandia) was transiently removed from the U.S. market because of heart disease risks but was recently reinstituted. Pioglitazone (Actos) is in the same class as Avandia, but when compared in a separate safety study, it did not show any increased risk of cardiovascular disease. Patients should talk to their health care professionals if they have concerns.

Acarbose (Precose), an α-glucosidase inhibitor, works in the gastrointestinal tract to delay the digestion of carbohydrates and lengthens the time needed to convert carbohydrates to glucose, mainly affecting blood sugar levels after eating. An annoying side effect is the formation of intestinal gas and resulting flatus.

Rosiglitazone (Avandia) and Pioglitazone (Actos) belong to the thiazolidinedione class of drugs. They work as insulin sensitizers by binding to the peroxisome proliferator–activated receptors (PPARs) of cells, making them more responsive to insulin.

Pramlintide (Symlin) is an injectable drug, which resembles human amylin produced by the pancreas. It has four mechanisms of action. Symlin inhibits glucagon production (therefore reduces hepatic glucose production), delays gastric emptying, increases pancreatic insulin production, and reduces appetite.

The mechanism of action of incretin hormones is similar to that of pramlintide (Symlin). It increases the production of insulin right after eating, inhibits postprandial hepatic glucose production, delays gastric emptying, and induces satiety. Exenatide (Byetta, Bydureon) and liraglutide (Victoza) are the injectable medicines in the class of drugs called *incretin mimetics.*

Incretin hormones regulate glucose levels through the mechanism of action mentioned above. They are broken down within minutes in the bloodstream by enzymes called *DPP IV.* A new class of oral drugs called *DPP IV inhibitors* inhibit this enzyme and therefore regulate blood glucose. Sitagliptin (Januvia), saxagliptin (Onglyza), linagliptin (Tradjenta), and alogliptin (Nesina) are the approved medications in this class of drugs.

Bromocriptine (Cycloset) works by increasing dopamine receptor activity in the morning, and this lowers blood sugar without increasing insulin levels. The drug is taken once each morning when dopamine levels are low.

Sodium-glucose linked transporter 2 (SGLT2) inhibitors prevent the function of sodium-dependent glucose transport proteins in the kidney to reabsorb filtered glucose. This leads to reduction of blood glucose levels and concomitant loss of calories and therefore weight. Canagliflozin (Invokana) and dapagliflozin (Farxiga) are the first approved drugs within this class.

Early implementation and use of combination medications seems to be the most effective way to treat patients with diabetes. The goal is to normalize glucose control by optimizing hemoglobin A1c (HbgA1c) while avoiding hypoglycemia.

Prognosis

People with diabetes mellitus are now living longer than in the past. When people with diabetes mellitus practice appropriate self-care, the symptoms are eased, blood glucose levels are controlled, and there are fewer complications and fewer hospitalizations. Without treatment and when blood sugar levels remain high over a long period, the eyes, blood vessels, kidneys, and nerves sustain serious damage.

Prevention

The precise causal mechanism of diabetes mellitus remains unknown; however, screening for diabetes mellitus is recommended for those with risk factors, such as genetic susceptibility, obesity, a history of gestational diabetes, and age 45 years or greater. Prediabetes has been identified as a risk factor for progression to type 2 diabetes. Education about lifestyle changes known to delay the onset of diabetes is an appropriate prevention strategy when the blood glucose level is higher than normal (see the Alert box about Prediabetes).

Prediabetes

Prediabetes is defined as a blood glucose level moderately elevated but not high enough to meet the diagnostic values indicating diabetes. When this condition is identified, it is considered a risk factor for the later development of type 2 diabetes. Prediabetes is considered a significant health problem itself. Many health risks are associated with prediabetes, such as hypertension, abnormal cholesterol, obesity, and increased risk for cardiovascular disease. It is important to help those showing signs of prediabetes understand their risk of progressing to type 2. There are known steps that can be taken to reduce or prevent this progression.

Lifestyle intervention with weight management, nutritional interventions, and exercise can be challenging but effective first steps in the prevention of diabetes. These lifestyle changes must be maintained by the patient taking responsibility for his or her self-care decisions; however, positive social support from an individual or a group increases the success of compliance and health. Recently, the Centers for Disease Control and Prevention (CDC) authorized the establishment of a National Diabetes Prevention Program.

Patient Teaching

Diabetes control is monitored daily mainly by measuring blood glucose levels through the use of a device for that purpose, a glucose meter. (The manufacturer of the glucose meter may have a website that demonstrates the use and care of a glucose meter.) These monitoring techniques are taught to patients so that they can use them at home. With experience, the patient can interpret the results and make simple modifications in insulin dosage and caloric intake to maintain precise blood glucose control.

The Continual Glucose Monitoring System may be a supplement for traditional glucose monitoring. The system consists of a sensor inserted via needle, and a transmitter device. Each sensor is single-use and is designed to remain in place for 7 consecutive days. Sensors are sold in packs of five, along with a transmitter that is reusable and rechargeable. There is a monthly charge for monitoring via a smartphone/smartwatch app.

The product is designed for insertion into the abdomen or the back of the forearms.

- The sensor is placed into an insertion device they refer to as a *serter*.
- The base of the serter is placed flat against the skin. Two buttons on the serter are pressed simultaneously to insert the sensor (via a needle) under the skin.
- The insertion needle is then removed, leaving only the sensor and the transmitter in place.
- The sensor is then taped in place.
- The sensor transmits via Bluetooth to a smartphone/smartwatch app.
  - The app can be configured to receive alerts from the sensor based on glucose reading parameters the patient sets up.
  - The app can be configured to prepare report data to track long-term continual glucose reading results.

Patients may have to commit to twice-daily traditional glucose monitoring, in addition to using this system.

All patients with diabetes are encouraged to reach and maintain the appropriate body weight. In addition, patients must be taught that the balance between insulin and glucose requirements is upset easily by trauma and infection. Regular medical supervision is encouraged, especially for insulin-dependent patients. Patients and caregivers are taught the proper techniques of insulin administration; special training in the use of an insulin pump is offered, when appropriate. The patient and his or her family members must be educated to recognize the symptoms of diabetic coma (high blood glucose with the release of ketone levels) and insulin shock (excessive insulin) and to take immediate action to correct these serious complications (see Table 4.3).

The patient must understand the importance of preventing infection and injury. Give the patient written material that explains the importance of skin care, foot care, and dental care. Instruct the patient to carry some form of fast-acting sugar, such as glucose tablets, to combat the onset of hypoglycemia. Advise the patient to obtain a medical alert bracelet (see Fig. 4.7). Refer the patient to counseling and support to help him or her adapt to the challenges of a long-term disease.

✕ NOTE

A more accurate assessment of overall blood glucose control may be obtained with the glycosylated hemoglobin test (designated HgbA1c). The test is performed every 3 months, and there are no dietary or medication restrictions.

Gestational Diabetes

Description

Gestational diabetes mellitus (GDM) is a condition of damaged ability to process carbohydrate that has its onset during pregnancy.

ICD-10-CM Code	O99.810 *(Abnormal glucose complicating pregnancy)* (O99.810-O99.815 = 3 codes of specificity)

Symptoms and Signs

GDM is detected between 24 and 28 weeks of pregnancy. The pregnant patient may be asymptomatic, or she may exhibit the usual signs of diabetes mellitus: polyuria, polydipsia, and polyphagia. Routine blood or urine screening, performed during each prenatal visit, indicates the presence of excessive glucose.

Patient Screening

The pregnant female exhibiting the onset of the above symptoms is scheduled for a same-day appointment. With a prior diagnosis of GDM, prompt medical attention is necessary for any increase in symptoms or onset of new complaints. Strict adherence to scheduled follow-up appointments is important for careful monitoring.

Etiology

Increased destruction of insulin by the placenta plays a role in causing GDM. There is reduced effectiveness of maternal insulin during pregnancy. The fetus takes its glucose from the mother, stressing the balance of glucose production and glucose use. Elevated levels of estrogen and progesterone block the action of insulin. Risk factors include a family history of diabetes, obesity, and age greater than 25 years.

Diagnosis

The first indication of GDM is the presence of glucose in urine demonstrated on a routine prenatal urine glucose test. Fasting blood glucose determination indicates elevated levels of glucose. Other serum tests are the glucose tolerance test, 2-hour postprandial (oral glucose tolerance) test, and glycated hemoglobin test. Elevations above normal levels yield a positive diagnosis.

Treatment

Treatment is started as soon as possible to preserve a healthy pregnancy. The medical management of GDM is similar to the treatment of any type of diabetes, with close surveillance of mother and fetus because of the increased risk of complications, control of the diet, and limits on the intake of simple sugars. Consistent moderate exercise, such as walking, is encouraged. Oral hypoglycemic agents may be prescribed, or insulin may be indicated. The patient is instructed to monitor blood glucose levels frequently with fingersticks and blood glucose testing. If delivery of the infant and placenta does not terminate the condition, the therapeutic diabetic regimen must continue.

Prognosis

The risk of cesarean delivery and neonatal complications, including large body size and hypoglycemia, is increased. The condition usually disappears right after delivery. Of the women who have had GDM, 30% to 40% develop type 2 diabetes within 5 to 10 years of GDM.

Prevention

GDM is a common enough complication of pregnancy to warrant regular monitoring of glucose levels in urine and blood during the pregnancy.

Patient Teaching

Emphasize the importance of regular prenatal checkups to monitor weight, proper nutrition, and blood glucose levels. This is even more important for women who have a family history of diabetes. Teach self-monitoring of blood glucose and insulin administration, as required. Dietary management depends on the severity of the disease and the amount of insulin therapy required. Make sure the patient has instructional material on the specific prescribed diet, or refer her to a dietitian. Offer reassurance that the condition can be managed with close monitoring and good compliance with the treatment plan.

◆ ENRICHMENT

Metabolic Syndrome

Metabolic syndrome (also known as *syndrome X*) is a collection of signs and/or conditions that together may increase an individual's risk for type 2 diabetes and cardiovascular disease. Early recognition of this syndrome can help determine suitable interventions to correct the individual mechanisms of metabolic syndrome.

Metabolic syndrome has five main components:
1. Central obesity, defined as a collection of excess fat around the abdomen (a waist circumference of greater than 35 inches for women and greater than 40 inches for men)
2. Increased blood pressure, that is, greater than 130/85 mm Hg in men or women
3. Abnormal triglyceride levels above 150 mg/dL
4. Abnormal high-density lipoprotein (HDL) cholesterol levels below 40 mg/dL
5. Fasting glucose levels above 100 mg/dL

These components, especially obesity, have metabolic consequences. Although the exact cause is not known, poor nutrition and inadequate physical exercise contribute to the risk factors of metabolic syndrome. Recognition of metabolic syndrome offers a patient the opportunity to focus on interventions that may prevent the premature onset of cardiovascular disease and/or type 2 diabetes.

Hypoglycemia

Description

Hypoglycemia is an abnormally low glucose level in the blood.

ICD-10-CM Code	E16.2 *(Hypoglycemia, unspecified)*
	(E16.0-E16.2 = 3 codes of specificity)

Symptoms and Signs

Hypoglycemia, a deficiency of glucose (sugar) in blood, can be a serious condition. It occurs when excessive insulin enters the bloodstream or when the glucose release rate falls below tissue demands. This condition may occur despite adequate food intake. Symptoms include sweating, nervousness, weakness, hunger, dizziness, trembling, headache, and palpitations. Because glucose is the primary fuel of the brain, the consequences of hypoglycemia can be severe. Extremely low blood glucose levels can cause central nervous system manifestations, including confusion, visual disturbances, behavior that may be mistaken for drunkenness, stupor, coma, and seizures. Hypoglycemic syndromes are classified as drug-induced (the most common) or non–drug-induced.

Patient Screening

An individual with severe symptoms of acute reactive hypoglycemia requires emergency medical attention. For the individual experiencing milder episodes of hypoglycemia, an appointment should be scheduled as early as possible for diagnostic evaluation of the cause. Follow office policy for referral of an infant or child to a pediatrician.

Etiology

The major cause of drug-induced hypoglycemia is insulin overdose in a subject with diabetes. Failure to eat a meal or excessive exercise also can trigger hypoglycemia in the insulin-dependent patient with diabetes. A person with a significantly elevated blood alcohol level can experience alcoholic hypoglycemia. Sulfonylureas can induce hypoglycemia. Non–drug-induced hypoglycemia can result from fasting, delayed or excessive secretion of insulin by the pancreas, adenoma or carcinoma of the pancreas, gastrointestinal disorders, or various hereditary or endocrine disorders.

Diagnosis

Diagnosis requires evidence that the symptoms correlate with a low blood glucose level and can be remedied by raising the blood glucose level. The glucometer can be used as a quick screening test to detect abnormally low blood glucose levels in patients with symptoms of hypoglycemia. The blood glucose level is further evaluated through the glucose tolerance test. Typically fasting plasma glucose level can be as low as less than 45 mg/dL after a period of fasting. The diagnosis of hypoglycemia is commonly defined as blood glucose level less than 50 mg/dL. Typically, hypoglycemia is only significant when it is associated with symptoms. Thus when symptoms of hypoglycemia occur together with a documented low glucose level and the symptoms promptly resolve with the administration of glucose, a diagnosis of hypoglycemia can be made. Hypoglycemia is uncomplicated when the initial assessment suggests a probable cause, such as a history of insulin use, excessive ingestion of alcohol, and the use of sulfonylureas in treatment.

Treatment

In acute hypoglycemia, the priority is to restore the normal blood glucose level through intravenous infusion of glucose. The hormone glucagon also may be given to counteract the effects of insulin. As the patient's condition is stabilized, a complex carbohydrate and protein snack is given to keep the blood glucose level within normal limits. When hypoglycemia is associated with a tumor, surgery may be required. The diet is modified to correct hereditary fructose intolerance or gastrointestinal conditions that provoke the symptoms.

Prognosis

The underlying cause of hypoglycemia dictates the long-term management of the disorder. In most cases, the signs and symptoms of hypoglycemia resolve with ingestion of food or glucose to increase the glucose level in blood. Severe, prolonged hypoglycemia can cause irreversible brain damage.

Prevention

The most common cause of episodic hypoglycemia is prevented by proper adjustment of diet, insulin, and exercise in the individual with diabetes. Insulin-dependent patients benefit from conscientious application of self-management skills.

Patient Teaching

Teach the patient to watch for signs of hypoglycemia. Instruct the insulin-dependent patient with diabetes to be always prepared to counter an attack of hypoglycemia by carrying glucose tablets to take at the first sign of hypoglycemia. Address the effects of alcohol intoxication and adverse reactions to medications on hypoglycemia, as appropriate. Refer the patient to a dietitian as indicated.

Precocious Puberty

Precocious Puberty in Boys

Description

Precocious puberty in boys is defined as the onset of puberty before age 9 years.

ICD-10-CM Code	E30.1 *(Precocious puberty)*
	E30.8 *(Other disorders of puberty)*
	(E30.0-E30.9 = 4 codes of specificity)

Symptoms and Signs

Precocious, or earlier-than-expected, sexual maturity in the male manifests as early development of secondary sex characteristics, gonadal development, and spermatogenesis. The patient's history may include altered growth pattern or emotional disturbances. Pubic hair and facial hair begin to grow, the gonads and the penis increase in size, and sebaceous gland activity increases. Male puberty normally begins between ages 13 and 15 years; onset before 9 years of age is considered precocious.

Patient Screening

Schedule a physical examination with the health care provider. Then follow office policy regarding referral to an endocrinologist.

Etiology

Idiopathic precocity may be transmitted genetically. The hypothalamus normally initiates puberty by stimulating the pituitary gland. Because the pituitary gland secretes vital gonadotropic hormones that stimulate the testes to produce sex hormones, many problems involving sexual development can be traced to pituitary dysfunction. Intracranial pituitary or hypothalamic neoplasia can cause excessive or premature secretion of gonadotropin. Testicular tumors and other endocrine disorders can induce precocious development. The history may reveal inadvertent ingestion of sex steroids through therapeutic medications or deliberate ingestion of sex steroids.

Diagnosis

Obvious physical and emotional signs of precocity are noted. Diagnostic tests include MRI, blood tests for elevated hormone levels, brain scan, skull and bone radiographic studies, chromosomal karyotype studies, and testing of blood for male hormone levels.

Treatment

The therapy depends on the cause of precocious puberty. When condition is idiopathic, no specific treatment may be needed. One treatment is to take hormones to suppress sexual maturation until the appropriate time for the onset of puberty. Gonadotropin-releasing hormone (GnRH) agonists, medications that inhibit androgen action (spironolactone), inhibit androgen synthesis (ketoconazole), or block the conversion of androgens, have been used. When the cause is testicular tumor or brain tumor, the treatment is more invasive, and the prognosis is guarded. Other endocrine disorders may require lifelong hormone therapy.

Prognosis

Early diagnosis and treatment of true precocious puberty offers a positive outcome. More complicated cases have a guarded prognosis.

Prevention

In almost all cases, no prevention is known.

Patient Teaching

Emphasize the importance of following the exact medication regimen and keeping follow-up appointments. Refer the patient to genetic counseling and psychological support, as indicated by the treatment plan.

Precocious Puberty In Girls

Description

Precocious puberty in girls is defined as the onset of puberty before age 8 years.

| ICD-10-CM Code | E30.1 *(Precocious puberty)* |
| | E30.8 *(Other disorders of puberty)* |

Symptoms and Signs

Precocious, or earlier-than-expected, sexual maturity in the female is marked by increased growth rate, breast enlargement, and the appearance of pubic hair and underarm hair before age 8 years; the onset of menstruation (menarche) may occur before age 10 years. Ovarian function makes pregnancy a possibility. Emotional problems may occur.

Patient Screening

Schedule a physical examination with the health care provider. Then follow office policy regarding referral to an endocrinologist.

Etiology

In most cases, precocious puberty in girls is idiopathic, without associated abnormalities. Uncommon causes include intracranial tumors, encephalopathy, meningitis, and endocrine disorders. The ingestion of oral contraceptives and other estrogen-containing drugs is a rare cause. Hormone-secreting ovarian or adrenal neoplasms are infrequent causes.

Diagnosis

Blood serum levels of follicle-stimulating hormone (FSH), luteinizing hormone (LH), and sex steroids are in the normal adult range. Urinalysis of hormone levels and excretion of 17-ketosteroids show elevated levels. Other diagnostic studies to determine the cause include ultrasonography, CT, and MRI.

Treatment

As in male precocity, the treatment of precocious female puberty depends on the cause. Tumors, if treatable, may require surgery or radiation. Hormone therapy may be used to suppress the secretion of gonadotropins and to prevent menstruation in true precocious puberty. The girl and her family may benefit from mental health counseling to develop coping skills for handling emotional problems. Parents must understand that physical maturity may occur with psychological immaturity and that precocious puberty does not necessarily trigger sexual behavior.

Prognosis

The outcome depends on the early diagnosis and treatment of true precocious puberty; certain causes prompt a more guarded prognosis.

Prevention

In almost all cases, no prevention is known.

Patient Teaching

Emphasize the importance of following the exact medication regimen and keeping follow-up appointments. Provide a referral for psychological support as indicated by the treatment plan.

Review Challenge

Answer the following questions:
1. Name the major glands of the endocrine system.
2. What are some ways in which the endocrine system affects health and disease?
3. Describe two conditions that are the result of increased production and secretion of pituitary human growth hormone (hGH).
4. What pathologic changes may result from hypopituitarism? Why is the age of the individual significant?
5. What causes diabetes insipidus?
6. What causes the thyroid gland to enlarge in the patient with a simple goiter?
7. Which hypothyroid condition (or chronic thyroiditis) is thought to be caused by autoimmune factors?
8. Describe the signs and symptoms of Graves disease.
9. What disease may be induced by prolonged administration or large doses of corticosteroids?
10. What are the possible causes of Addison disease?
11. Compare the cause and treatment of type 1 and type 2 diabetes mellitus.
12. Distinguish between diabetic coma and insulin shock.
13. How are hypoglycemic syndromes classified?
14. Name the important prognostic factors for thyroid malignancy.

15. What are the possible causes of precocious puberty in boys and girls?

16. Which benefits do bioidentical hormones provide versus traditional hormone replacement therapy?

Real-Life Challenge: Hypothyroidism

A 40-year-old female reports tiredness, loss of hair, and weight gain. She has not had a menstrual period for 3 months. Her skin appears dry and scaly. On questioning, the patient reports episodes of constipation and being unable to tolerate cold. Her speech is somewhat slow and slurred. A blood test for thyroid functioning shows low thyrotropin levels. Thyroid scan shows no uptake of iodine. The diagnosis for this patient is hypothyroidism.

Questions

1. Severe untreated hypothyroidism with onset at maturity can lead to *myxedema coma.* What is the term describing hypothyroidism with onset in infancy or early childhood?
2. What causes the insidious onset of the various complaints and conditions of the patient with hypothyroidism?
3. What can be the cause of the reduced production of thyroxine (T_4) by the thyroid gland?
4. Hormone replacement is the usual drug therapy of choice. Research levothyroxine sodium (Synthroid), and explain its side effects.
5. For patient teaching, how long will the patient be instructed to take the medication?

Real-Life Challenge: Diabetes Mellitus

A 50-year-old man became lethargic and drowsy with flushed dry skin after eating a large meal. His family became concerned when he was difficult to rouse and had a fruity odor to his breath. He was transported to an emergency facility, where he gave a history of extreme thirst, hunger, and frequent urination. He recently had an upper respiratory infection that was slow to clear. Adult-onset diabetes mellitus is suspected.

Questions

1. Which blood test would be ordered?
2. Identify normal results of blood glucose and glycated hemoglobin levels.
3. What are some of the possible causes of adult-onset type 2 diabetes mellitus?
4. In addition to the symptoms previously described, what else might be observed?
5. What determines the course of the treatment prescribed?
6. Why is glucose level monitoring important?
7. What patient teaching should be considered?
8. Why is diet important?
9. Explain how insulin works.
10. What is the therapeutic action of the sulfonylureas?
11. How does metformin (Glucophage) reduce blood glucose levels?

Internet Assignments

1. Choose a related topic (an endocrine disorder) from the National Institute of Diabetes, and research the latest health information on that topic. Review the easy-to-read and/or Spanish-language options.
2. Visit the American Thyroid Association website, and report on a recent public health statement related to the treatment of thyroid disease.

Critical Thinking

1. What factors are considered essential in the diet plan for the insulin-dependent patient with diabetes?
2. Discuss the circumstances that can cause diabetic coma in a patient with diabetes. What circumstances can cause insulin shock?
3. What are the clinical manifestations in the patient with Cushing syndrome caused by excessive levels of circulating cortisol? Which gland(s) may be responsible for the disease? Why must the patient on large doses of glucocorticoids for another disease be monitored for Cushing syndrome?
4. Why is it wise for patients with endocrine diseases (e.g., diabetes, thyroid gland disease, or hypoglycemia) to wear a medical alert bracelet?
5. What known medical history information indicates a high risk for thyroid cancer?

Prepare to discuss Critical Thinking case study exercises for this chapter that are posted on Evolve.

5

Diseases and Disorders of the Eye and Ear

CHAPTER OUTLINE

Disorders of the Eye, 163

Functioning Organs of Vision, 163

Refractive Errors, 166

Nystagmus, 167

Strabismus, 168

Disorders of the Eyelid, 169

Disorders of the Globe of the Eye, 175

Cancer of the Eye, 184

Disorders of the Ear, 185

Functioning Organs of Hearing, 185

Disorders of Conduction, 186

Meniere Disease, 193

Benign Paroxysmal Positional Vertigo, 193

Labyrinthitis, 194

Ruptured Tympanic Membrane (Ruptured Eardrum), 195

Cholesteatoma, 196

Mastoiditis, 197

Sensorineural Hearing Loss, 198

Cancer of the Ear, 199

LEARNING OBJECTIVES

After studying Chapter 5, you should be able to:

1. Recall and define the four main refractive errors of vision.
2. Compare the pathology and etiology of nystagmus with those of strabismus.
3. Name the possible causes of conjunctivitis.
4. List the possible causes of "dry eye syndrome."
5. List the causes of cataracts.
6. Explain the importance of early treatment of glaucoma.
7. Characterize the visual disturbance caused by macular degeneration.
8. Explain the susceptibility of patients with diabetes to diabetic retinopathy.
9. Explain why early diagnosis and treatment are important in retinal detachment.
10. Using a diagram or an anatomic model, describe the process of hearing.
11. Compare conductive hearing loss with sensorineural hearing loss.
12. List the symptoms of otitis externa.
13. Describe the treatment of otitis media.
14. Explain the signs and symptoms of Meniere disease.
15. Describe the symptoms of benign paroxysmal positional vertigo.
16. Discuss the importance of preventing sensorineural hearing loss.

KEY TERMS

amblyopia (**am**-blee-**OH**-pee-ah)
blepharitis (**blef**-ar-**RIE**-tis)
cryotherapy (kry-o-**THER**-ah-pee)
diplopia (dih-**PLO**-pee-ah)
iridotomy (ir-ih-**DOT**-oh-me)
labyrinth (**LAB**-ih-rinth)
macula (**MACK**-you-la)
meibomian (my-**BO**-mee-an)
myringotomy (mir-in-**GOT**-oh-me)

otoscopy (oh-**TOSS**-ko-pee)
retinopathy (**ret**-ih-**NOP**-ah-thee)
seborrhea (seb-oh-**RHEE**-ah)
sensorineural (**sen**-so-ree-**NEU**-rol)
tinnitus (tih-**NIE**-tus)
tonometry (tohn-**AHM**-eh-tree)
tympanoplasty (**tim**-pan-oh-**PLAS**-tee)
vertigo (**VER**-tih-go)

Disorders of the Eye

Functioning Organs of Vision

Focusing a clear image on the retina is vital for good vision. The functional process of vision takes place in the presence of light in the following manner: (1) An image is formed on the retina; (2) the rods and cones are stimulated; and (3) nerve impulses are conducted to the brain. The area of the brain that involves the sense of sight is much larger than the areas involved in the other senses. Before discussing the pathophysiology of ocular disease, a review of the complex structure of the eye is in order (Fig. 5.1).

The eyeball, similar in shape to a sphere, is composed of a wall of primary structures in three concentric layers—the sclera, the choroid, and the retina—and is connected to the brain by way of the optic nerve.

The sclera, the outermost layer, consists of tough fibrous connective tissue that is visible as the white of the eye. Attached to the sclera are the six extrinsic muscles that move the eye (Table 5.1). The cornea, the colorless transparent structure on the front of the eye, is continuous with the sclera on the anterior aspect of the globe. This transparent structure uses its curvature to help focus the light rays as they enter the eye.

Next to the sclera is the middle layer of tissue called the *choroid*. This layer is continuous with the ciliary body and the iris. These vascular structures supply the tissues of the eye with oxygen and nutrients. Anteriorly, the choroid joins the ciliary body, which contains ciliary muscles used to

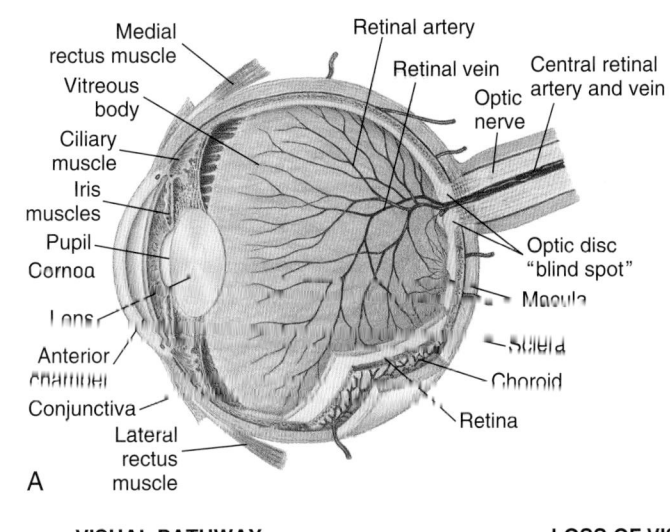

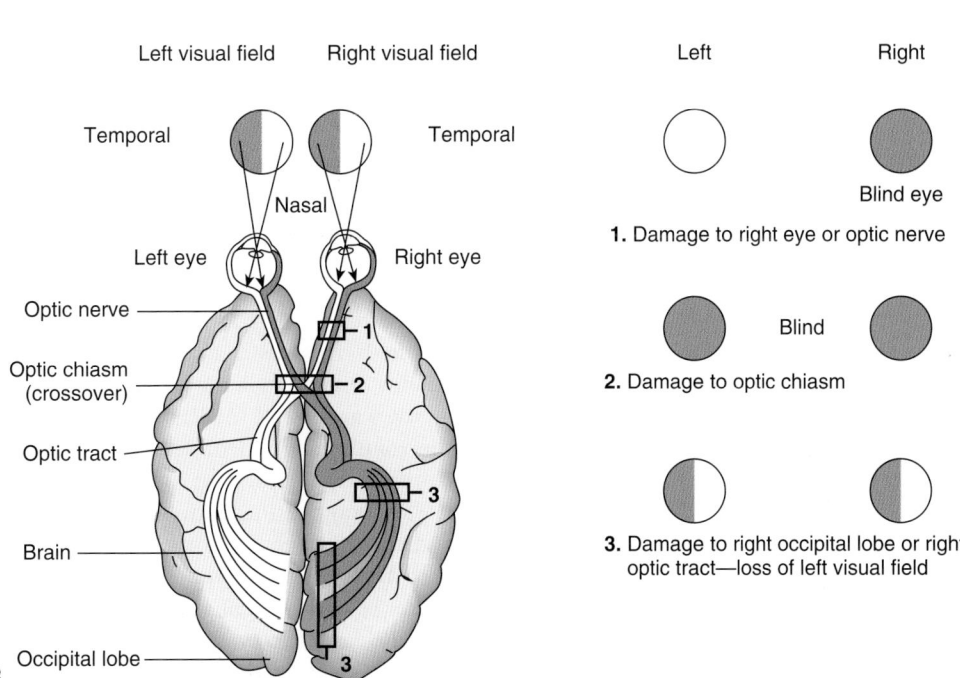

• **Fig. 5.1** (A) Anatomy of the human eye. (B) The visual pathway. (A, From Seidel HM, et al: *Mosby's guide to physical examination,* ed 8, St Louis, 2014, Mosby. B, From Gould B: *Pathophysiology for the health professions,* ed 3, St Louis, 2006, Mosby.)

TABLE 5.1 Muscles of the Eye

Muscle	Function	Cranial Innervation
Extrinsic Muscles of the Eye		
Inferior rectus	Rotates eyeball downward and medially; adducts	Oculomotor nerve (CN III)
Lateral rectus	Rotates eye laterally; abducts eyeball	Abducens nerve (CN VI)
Medial rectus	Rotates eye medially; adducts eyeball	Oculomotor nerve (CN III)
Superior rectus	Causes eye to look up	Oculomotor nerve (CN III)
Inferior oblique	Rotates eyeball upward and outward; abducts	Oculomotor nerve (CN III)
Superior oblique	Rotates eyeball downward and outward; abducts	Trochlear nerve (CN IV)
Intrinsic Smooth Muscles of the Eye		
Ciliary muscle	Regulation of lens shape for close vision	Oculomotor (CN III)
Iris (radial muscles)	Sympathetic stimulation; dilation of pupil	Oculomotor (CN III)
Iris (circular muscles)	Parasympathetic stimulation; contraction of pupil	Oculomotor (CN III)

CN, Cranial nerve.

focus the lens of the eye. The ciliary processes in the ciliary body secrete aqueous humor, the fluid found in the anterior portion of the eye. The ciliary body is connected by suspensory ligaments to the biconvex, transparent lens of the eye. Contraction of the ciliary muscles causes the suspensory ligaments to relax. The lens then bulges, allowing the focusing that is necessary for close vision.

Also attached to the ciliary body is the iris, or colored portion of the eye, which helps regulate the amount of light entering the eye. In a brightly lit environment, the iris contracts, causing the opening in the center of the iris, the pupil, to become smaller. In limited light conditions, the iris relaxes and the pupil enlarges, permitting more light to enter the eye.

The innermost layer, covering the posterior three-quarters of the eye, is called the *retina.* The retina is a light-sensitive layer made up of photo-receptive cells called *rods* and *cones.* The rods function best in dim light, thereby enabling night vision, whereas the cones function in bright light and also detect color and fine detail. Within the rods and cones, the image initiates a chemical reaction and sends messages through the nerve fiber layer of the retina to the optic nerve. The optic nerve penetrates the fibrous layers at the optic disc and continues on to the brain. The optic disc contains no receptor cells and often is called the *blind spot* of the eye. The optic nerve transmits the image to the portion of the brain that is used for vision. The brain interprets the impulses from each eye and produces a single three-dimensional image. The macula lutea, a yellow spot, lies lateral to the optic disc. In the center of the macula lutea is the fovea centralis, the area that produces the sharpest image.

Covering the anterior externally visible portion of the sclera is a thin, transparent membrane called the *conjunctiva.* It begins at the edge of the cornea, extends over the exposed sclera, and folds anteriorly to line the inside portion of the

lids. This creates both a superior cul-de-sac and an inferior cul-de-sac, where the conjunctiva reflects images from the sclerae to the lids. The space between the iris, the colored portion of the eye, and the anterior clear cornea is called the *anterior chamber.* The fluid occupying the anterior chamber is a watery substance called the *aqueous humor,* which is produced by the ciliary body. The fluid exits the anterior chamber through the trabecular network, a drainage system located at the junction of the base of the iris and the cornea. Appropriate pressure within the eye is maintained by the aqueous humor, which ultimately enters the general circulation of the body. The large cavity behind the lens is the vitreous body; it contains a jellylike fluid called the *vitreous humor,* which helps maintain the globular shape of the eyeball.

The internal lens of the eye is elastic and therefore can focus images whether viewed close by or at a distance. The focusing is accomplished by contraction and relaxation of the muscles of the ciliary body. This action makes it possible for the lens to assume either a more rounded spherical shape or a flatter elongated shape, depending on the focus length required. The lens is attached to the ciliary body by small strands of tissue called *zonules.* These are attached at points all the way around the lens. When the ciliary body relaxes, the zonules are pulled, causing flattening of the lens, the configuration needed for focusing on a distant image.

Light rays are the key to sight. The light rays enter the eye and pass through the cornea, aqueous humor, lens, and finally the vitreous humor. These rays can travel in a straight line or be bent at an angle. The process of bending light rays is known as *refraction.* The cornea and the lens are capable of bending or refracting the light rays so that they can be focused on the retina. The image that forms on the retina is reversed both in the up/down and right/left directions. The image is turned right side up and forward in the brain as the brain interprets the visual concept. Another step in the process of vision involves accommodation. Adjustments must be made in the eye to facilitate the image in relation to the viewer's distance from the object. The process of accommodation involves changing the shape of the lens, making it either flatter or thicker. The ciliary muscle and the suspensory ligaments contract and relax in opposition to accomplish this task.

The intrinsic muscles of each eye respond to light levels and change the size of the pupil to regulate the amount of light that enters the eye and reaches the retina. Each eye has six extrinsic muscles that control the movements of the eye; these muscles pull on the eyeballs, making the two move together to converge on one visual field (see Table 5.1). Normally, the eyes work together in unison, so an assessment of the functioning of these muscles often is included in a neurologic assessment. Table 5.2 summarizes the functions of the major parts of the eye.

Some eye disorders are signs of systemic diseases, such as hypertension, diabetes mellitus, or certain autoimmune arthritic diseases. Common symptoms of eye diseases and conditions that should be called to the attention of the physician include the following:
- redness of the eye;
- pain, itching, or burning in or around the eye;
- swollen red eyelids;
- drainage from the eyes;
- lesions/sores in or around the eyes;
- visual disturbances;
- unequal pupils, sudden loss of vision, persistent pain, or other symptoms associated with eye injury;
- repetitive, involuntary movements of the eye.

Diagnostic tests for eye diseases and conditions include the following:
- eye charts, such as the Snellen chart, to measure visual acuity;
- visual field tests to check central and peripheral vision;
- tonometry to measure intraocular pressure (IOP);
- eye cultures to identify viral or bacterial infectious agents;
- dilation to directly view the posterior structures of the eye, including the retina and the optic nerve;
- electronystagmography (ENG) to measure the direction and degree of nystagmus;
- electroretinography to measure electric activity of the retina in response to flashing of light;
- fluorescein angiography to assess the vasculature of the eye;
- optical coherence tomography (OCT) scans to capture three-dimensional images and to measure the dimensions of structures in the posterior chamber, such as epiretinal membranes and optic discs;
- ocular and orbit ultrasonography, another excellent method to detect and evaluate many diseases and conditions of orbital and posterior orbital structures.

Many systemic medications taken for a variety of diseases can have ocular side effects. Thus it is important for patients taking certain systemic medications to be monitored periodically for ocular toxicity. These include hydroxychloroquine (Plaquenil) used in the treatment of lupus and rheumatoid arthritis, ethambutol used in the treatment of tuberculosis, and steroids used in the treatment of various conditions.

TABLE 5.2 Functions of the Major Parts of the Eye

Structure	Function
Sclera	External protection
Cornea	Light refraction
Choroid	Blood supply
Iris	Light absorption and regulation of pupillary width
Ciliary body	Secretion of vitreous fluid; in addition, its smooth muscles change the shape of the lens
Lens	Light refraction
Retinal layer	Light receptor that transforms optic signals into nerve impulses
Rods	Means of distinguishing light from dark and perceiving shape and movement
Cones	Color vision
Central fovea	Area of sharpest vision
Macula lutea	Blind spot
External ocular muscles	Movement of the globe
Optic nerve (cranial nerve II)	Transmission of visual information to the brain
Lacrimal glands	Secretion of tears
Eyelid	Eye protection

Refractive Errors

Refractive errors are the most common cause of diminished visual acuity. Refractive errors that result in the eye being unable to focus light effectively on the retina are identified as hyperopia, myopia, astigmatism, and presbyopia.

Hyperopia (Farsightedness)

Description

Hyperopia (farsightedness) occurs when light that enters the eye is focused behind the retina rather than on the retina, requiring refocusing by the internal lens or the use of an external corrective lens to reposition the viewed object on the retina to sharpen the image. With this condition, near vision is particularly impaired. Hyperopia occurs when the eyeball is abnormally short, as measured from front to back (Fig. 5.2).

ICD-10-CM Code	H52.03 *(Hypermetropia, bilateral)* (H52.00-H52.03 = 4 codes of specificity)

Myopia (Nearsightedness)

Description

Myopia (nearsightedness) is the result of light rays entering the eye being focused in front of the retina, causing blurred vision. Near objects can be seen clearly, but distant objects are blurry, and the image being viewed cannot be sharpened by the internal lens of the eye. Myopia occurs when the eyeball is abnormally long, as measured from front to back (Fig. 5.3).

ICD-10-CM Code	H52.13 *(Myopia, bilateral)* (H52.10-H52.13 = 4 codes of specificity)

Astigmatism

Description

Astigmatism is an irregular focusing of the light rays entering the eye. It usually is caused by the cornea not being spherical. The front of the cornea may be more egg-shaped than spherical, thereby causing light rays to be unevenly or diffusely focused across the retina. This causes some images to appear clearly defined, whereas others appear blurred.

ICD-10-CM Code	H52.209 *(Unspecified astigmatism, unspecified eye)* (H52.20-H52.229 = 12 codes of specificity)

Refer to the physician's diagnosis and then to the current edition of the ICD-10-CM coding manual to ensure the greatest specificity of pathology.

Presbyopia

Description

Presbyopia is the inability of the internal lens of the eye to focus on near objects due to the loss of elasticity of the lens. This condition is related to aging and usually starts in people in their mid-40s.

ICD-10-CM Code	H52.4 *(Presbyopia)*

Symptoms and Signs

The primary symptoms of a refractive error are blurred vision and eye fatigue, which can lead to squinting, frequent rubbing of the eyes, and headaches.

Patient Screening

Schedule a comprehensive refractive examination for a patient complaining of changes in visual acuity or clearness or sharpness of visual perception.

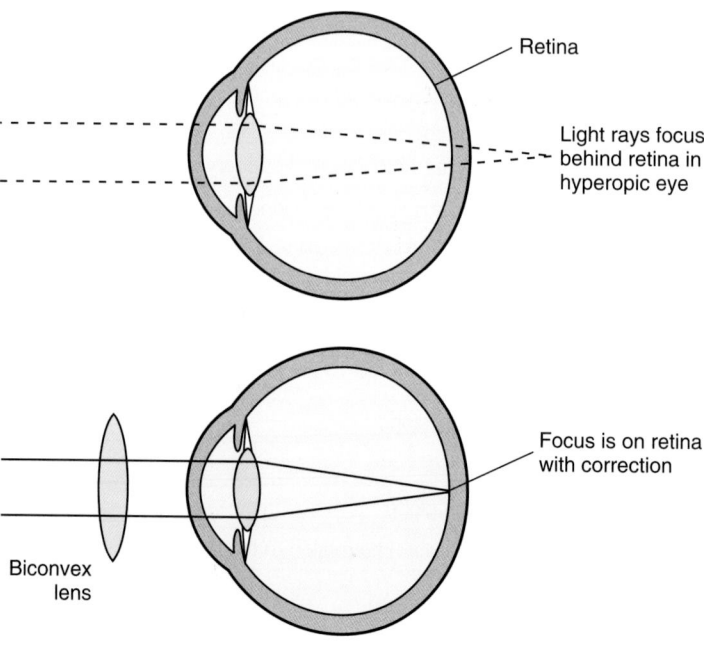

• **Fig. 5.2** Hyperopia and correction.

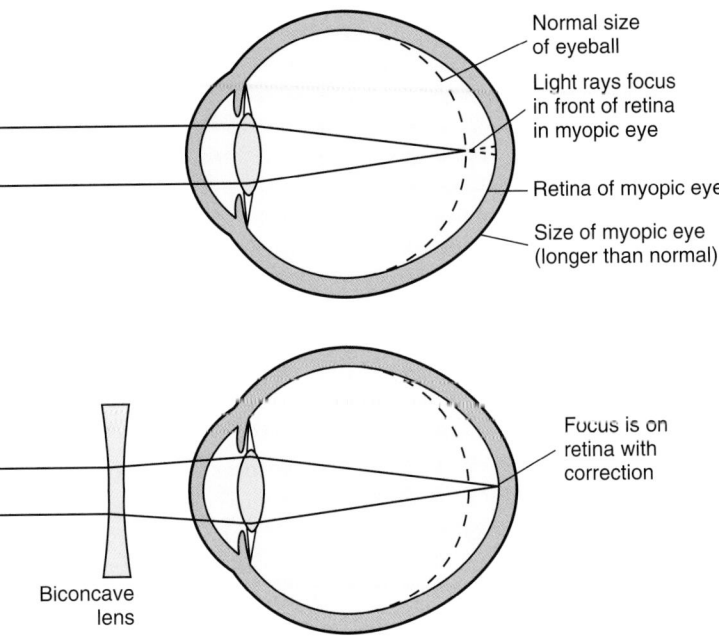

• **Fig. 5.3** Myopia and correction.

Etiology
Some refractive errors seem to be familial, which suggests a genetic link. Others may be linked to prolonged close work.

Diagnosis
Eye health history and tests for visual acuity and refraction are used to diagnose refractive errors. For children, usually the pupils are dilated with eye drops, and the eyes are then evaluated for refractive error with a retinoscope. The optimal lens adjustment needed to correct the deficit is determined by having the patient look through a series of corrective lenses of different powers.

Treatment
Correcting refractive errors involves fitting the patient with artificial lenses in the form of eyeglasses or contact lenses or performing corrective surgery. Radial keratotomy, a surgical procedure used to reshape the eye, has been replaced by laser surgery, which results in more precise visual correction and has fewer complications. The following refractive surgical procedures can be done to correct myopia, hyperopia, and astigmatism: laser-assisted in-situ keratomileusis (LASIK), astigmatic keratotomy (AK), photorefractive keratotomy (PRK), laser thermal keratoplasty (LTK), conductive keratoplasty (CK), and intraocular contact lenses (lens permanently placed in the eye).

Prognosis
Excellent results can be expected with correctly prescribed eyeglasses or contact lenses. Elective refractive surgical procedures can benefit those individuals who are medically eligible. The risks for complications are generally low.

Prevention
Refractive errors, in general, cannot be prevented.

Patient Teaching
When a patient is to have refractive surgery, describe the procedure and advise the patient as to when to expect visual recovery, how to use preoperative and postoperative medications, and when return to a regular work schedule is likely. Explain the importance of follow-up visits to monitor progress.

Nystagmus

Description
Nystagmus is involuntary, repetitive, rhythmic movements of one or both eyes.

ICD-10-CM Code	H55.00 *(Unspecified nystagmus)*
	(H55.00-H55.09 = 6 codes of
	specificity)

Refer to the physician's diagnosis and then to the current edition of the ICD-10-CM coding manual to ensure the greatest specificity of pathology.

Symptoms and Signs
Any repetitive or involuntary movement of one or both eyes is a sign of nystagmus. The eye movements can be horizontal, vertical, circular, or a combination of these. Blurred or decreased vision also can be associated with nystagmus.

Patient Screening
Schedule a comprehensive ophthalmic examination for a patient complaining of changes in visual acuity or of any

involuntary or "jerky" movements of the eye. *Acquired nystagmus always necessitates a complete neurologic evaluation.*

Etiology

Spontaneous nystagmus can be congenital or acquired. Congenital nystagmus is manifested before age 6 months to 1 year and is the most common type. Acquired nystagmus results when a disease process produces lesions in the brain or inner ear. Alcohol use and abuse of certain drugs also may cause this condition. Brain tumors and cerebrovascular lesions can cause nystagmus, or it may instead be the result of abnormal development of the nervous system.

Diagnosis

Nystagmus usually can be diagnosed clinically by external examination of the eyes and observation of any involuntary movements. Other, more specific, complex tests are available as well, when needed for definitive diagnosis.

Treatment

Acquired nystagmus is managed by treating the underlying cause of the condition. Congenital nystagmus often can be lessened by using the Kestenbaum procedure, in which the eyes are surgically rotated toward the null point of the eye.

Prognosis

The outcome of acquired nystagmus depends on the treatment of the underlying cause. Surgical intervention for congenital nystagmus attempts to minimize nystagmus when the eyes are looking straight ahead.

Prevention

No specific method of prevention is known.

Patient Teaching

In acquired nystagmus, the patient benefits from understanding the underlying cause and treatment of the nystagmus. Parents of the child with congenital nystagmus are given support and clear explanations about the condition and the surgical treatment, if indicated.

Strabismus

Description

Strabismus, a visual defect of misalignment, is failure of the eyes to look in the same direction at the same time, which primarily occurs because of weakness in the nerves stimulating the muscles that control the position of the eyes (Fig. 5.4).

ICD-10-CM Code	H51.9 *(Unspecified disorder of binocular movement)* (H51.0-H51.9 = 9 codes of specificity)

Refer to the physician's diagnosis and then to the current edition of the ICD-10-CM coding manual to ensure the greatest specificity of pathology.

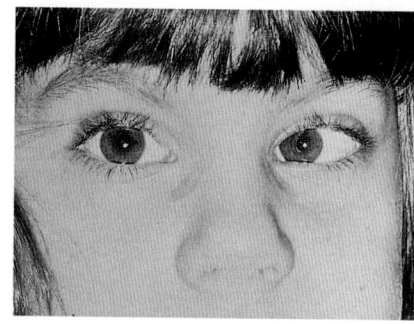

• **Fig. 5.4** Strabismus. (From Zitelli BJ, Davis HW: *Atlas of pediatric physical diagnosis,* ed 6, Philadelphia, 2012, Mosby.)

Symptoms and Signs

In esotropia (convergent strabismus, or cross-eye), both eyes turn inward; in exotropia (divergent strabismus, or wall-eye), both eyes turn outward. With either form, the main symptom is diplopia if strabismus is acquired in adulthood. Diplopia is usually not present when the strabismus is congenital.

Patient Screening

Schedule a comprehensive ophthalmic examination for a patient complaining of changes in visual acuity, clearness or sharpness of visual perception, or double vision. Parents may report the noted appearance of "crossed eyes" in an infant or young child.

Etiology

Esotropia usually develops in infancy or early childhood and may be associated with amblyopia. Amblyopia is reversible until the visual pathways fully develop at about age 7 to 8 years. In almost all cases, esotropia that develops in adults is caused by a condition or disease elsewhere in the body. The brain, the cranial nerves (CNs), or the muscles themselves are affected. These diseases and conditions include diabetes mellitus, temporal arteritis, muscular dystrophy, high blood pressure, trauma, aneurysm, or an intracranial lesion.

Diagnosis

To discover the underlying cause, the physician performs a complete ophthalmic examination and orders various appropriate radiographic studies and blood tests.

Treatment

Strabismus should be treated as soon as possible. Early intervention is the key. Corrective glasses, treatment to minimize or prevent amblyopia, or surgery to restore the eye muscle balance may be used in the course of the treatment. In some cases, preventing amblyopia involves covering the fixing eye to force the child to use the deviating eye.

Prognosis

In most cases, children respond well to early treatment. The prognosis of adults with acquired strabismus depends on the underlying cause.

Prevention

No specific method of prevention is known. Normal development of visual pathways begins in early childhood with appropriate retinal stimulation. Amblyopia may be prevented or at least minimized by early diagnosis and intervention.

Patient Teaching

Give parents of children with strabismus an explanation of the condition and the cause, if known. Parents are taught how to apply an eye patch. Reinforce the importance of early treatment to help prevent visual loss. The adult with acquired strabismus can benefit from an explanation of the relationship of the eye condition to the identified underlying cause.

Disorders of the Eyelid

Hordeolum (Stye)

Description

Hordeola (styes) are acute, painful abscesses of an eyelash follicle or in a sebaceous gland of the eyelids (Fig. 5.5).

ICD-10-CM Code	H00.019 *(Hordeolum externum unspecified eye, unspecified eyelid)*
	(H00.011-H00.029 = 14 codes of specificity)
	H00.029 *(Hordeolum internum unspecified eye, unspecified eyelid)*
	H00.039 *(Abscess of eyelid unspecified eye, unspecified eyelid)*
	(H00.031-H00.039 = 7 codes of specificity)

Symptoms and Signs

Styes occur most often at the outside edge of the lid. Pain, swelling, redness, and formation of pus at the site are the main symptoms of a stye. Patients may report a feeling of having "something in the eye."

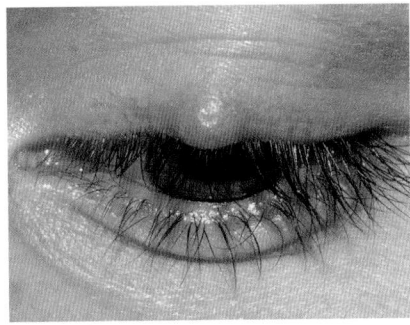

• **Fig. 5.5** Acute hordeolum of upper eyelid. (From Palay DA, Krachmer JH: *Ophthalmology for the primary care physician,* St Louis, 1997, Mosby.)

Patient Screening

Patients complaining of a lesion of the eyelid, with or without purulent drainage, require an appointment with their health care provider for an examination of the affected area. Follow office policy for referral to an ophthalmologist.

Etiology

Often styes are the result of a staphylococcal infection and can be associated with and secondary to blepharitis (see the Blepharitis section).

Diagnosis

Visual examination alone is usually sufficient for making the diagnosis.

Treatment

To hasten drainage, warm compresses over a period of days may be applied to the eye as soon as the inflammation is evident. Topical antibiotics are also effective at shortening the duration of symptoms. If surrounding soft tissue becomes infected (cellulitis), oral antibiotics may be needed. If persistent, these lesions need to be surgically drained.

Prognosis

Hordeola are usually self-limiting infections; thus the prognosis is good, but recurrence can be common.

Prevention

Lid hygiene and warm compresses can prevent recurrence.

Patient Teaching

Instruct the patient regarding the correct technique of applying an eye compress as prescribed. Inform the patient about the correct application and usage of topical or systemic antibiotic therapies.

Chalazion

Description

A chalazion is a small, firm, nonmobile, painless, subcutaneous nodule on the margin or body of the eyelid; it occurs with occlusion of the meibomian glands.

ICD-10-CM Code	H00.19 *(Chalazion unspecified eye, unspecified eyelid)*
	(H00.11-H00.19 = 7 codes of specificity)

Symptoms and Signs

A chalazion can vary in size, from being barely visible to being the size of a pea. Chalazia can become infected, producing redness, swelling, and pain (Fig. 5.6).

Patient Screening

A brief visual examination by an ophthalmologist is sufficient for the diagnosis of a chalazion.

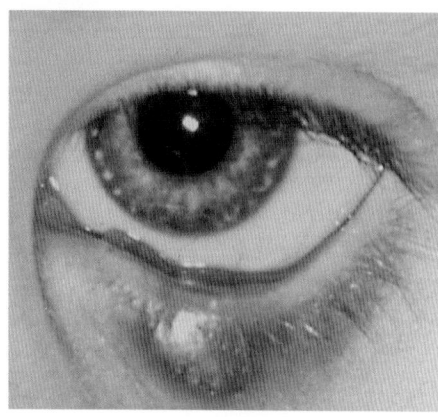

• **Fig. 5.6** Chalazion. (From Zitelli BJ, Davis HW: *Atlas of pediatric physical diagnosis,* ed 6, Philadelphia, 2012, Mosby.)

Etiology

Chalazia are caused by a blockage of fluid originating from one of the meibomian glands, which lubricate the eyelid margin.

Diagnosis

Visual examination and patient history are all that is necessary to make the diagnosis.

Treatment

Small chalazia usually disappear spontaneously over a month or two with regular application of warm compresses. Resolution may be facilitated by topical antibiotic treatment. Antibiotic therapy may vary from gentamicin or tobramycin to azithromycin or quinolone drops.

Isolated recurrent chalazia may respond to corticosteroid injection. Larger chalazia may not spontaneously disappear and may need to be removed surgically. This is a minor procedure that often can be done in the ophthalmologist's office in an outpatient setting.

Prognosis

Complete resolution is expected, but chalazia can be recurrent.

Prevention

Lid hygiene and warm compresses can help prevent recurrence.

Patient Teaching

The patient may be told a chalazion is not infectious. If surgical removal is recommended, reassure the patient that the procedure is minor.

Keratitis

Description

Keratitis is any inflammation or infection of the cornea.

| ICD-10-CM Code | H16.9 *(Unspecified* |
| | *keratitis)* |

Keratitis has many forms and therefore many ICD-10-CM codes. Refer to the physician's diagnosis and then to the current edition of the ICD-10-CM coding manual to ensure the greatest specificity of pathology.

Symptoms and Signs

Symptoms are decreased visual acuity, irritation, tearing, photophobia, and mild redness of the conjunctiva. Pain or numbness of the cornea may soon follow and is a significant sign.

Patient Screening

The patient experiencing the symptoms listed earlier is scheduled for a prompt ophthalmic examination. Follow office policy for referral to an ophthalmologist.

Etiology

Keratitis often is caused by an infection resulting from herpes simplex virus. This is especially likely when the keratitis is preceded by an upper respiratory infection (URI) with facial cold sores (see the Herpes Simplex [Cold Sores] section in Chapter 8). Certain bacteria (i.e., *Pseudomonas aeruginosa* or *Neisseria gonorrhoeae*) and fungi also can be responsible for keratitis. Contact lens wear substantially increases the risk of bacterial keratitis, especially for those who sleep with lenses in place. Other forms of keratitis can be caused by corneal trauma or by exposure of the cornea to dry air or intense light, as occurs during welding. Cultures may be taken to identify the causative organism.

Diagnosis

Examination of the cornea with use of a slit lamp confirms the diagnosis. Medical history may indicate a recent URI, and visual acuity may be decreased.

Treatment

To avoid internal spread of the infection, urgent treatment is necessary. The administration of a broad-spectrum antibiotic or an antiviral agent can effectively eradicate the infection, depending on which type of organism is the causative agent. Ophthalmic moisturizing ointments and eye drops may be prescribed for symptomatic relief. An eye patch may be needed to relieve discomfort caused by photophobia. However, this is contraindicated in cases of fungal infection or contact lens wear.

Prognosis

Prompt treatment of the condition decreases the risk of ulceration that can erode the cornea and cause formation of scar tissue that may interfere with vision.

Prevention

Following the recommended instructions for contact lens wear and care, such as proper handling and cleaning of the lenses, can reduce the risk of infection. Avoiding hand-to-eye contact can lessen transfer of infection to the eye from contaminated medication, makeup, or contact lenses.

Patient Teaching

Explain how infections can be transferred to the eyes by the fingers. Encourage contact lens wearers to adhere to strict hand hygiene. Teach the patient the proper technique for instillation of ophthalmic ointment and eye drops as prescribed; emphasize the importance of proper hand washing. Inform the patient of the increased risk of keratitis with wearing contact lenses while sleeping.

Blepharitis

Description
Blepharitis is inflammation of the margins of the eyelids involving hair follicles and glands.

ICD-10-CM Code H01.009 (Unspecified blepharitis unspecified eye, unspecified eyelid)
(H01.001-H01.029 = 21 codes of specificity)
H01.019 (Ulcerative blepharitis unspecified eye, unspecified eyelid)
H01.029 (Squamous blepharitis unspecified eye, unspecified eyelid)

Refer to the physician's diagnosis and then to the current edition of the ICD-10-CM coding manual to ensure the greatest specificity of pathology.

Symptoms and Signs
Blepharitis causes persistent redness and crusting on and around the eyelids (Fig. 5.7). Symptoms may include itching, burning, or foreign body sensation. The conditions are usually bilateral and symmetric. In severe cases, eyelashes can fall out, and the patient may experience persistent irritation of the eyes.

Patient Screening
The patient experiencing irritation of the eyelids with crusts, itching, and burning needs a prompt clinical evaluation.

Etiology
The ulcerative form of blepharitis is usually the result of a staphylococcal infection. Nonulcerative blepharitis can be caused by allergies or exposure to smoke, dust, or chemicals.

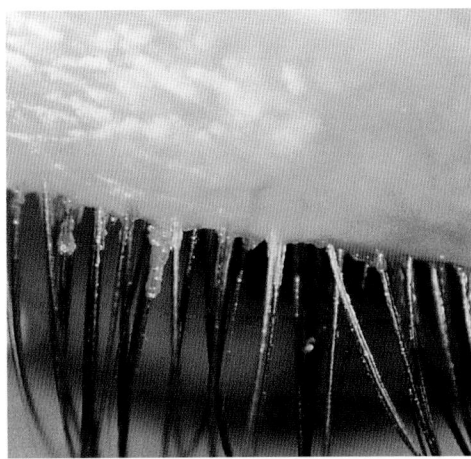

• **Fig. 5.7** Blepharitis. (From Zitelli BJ, Davis HW: *Atlas of pediatric physical diagnosis,* ed 6, Philadelphia, 2012, Mosby.)

This condition also can be secondary to seborrhea of the eyelid's sebaceous glands, and often the patient has a history of repeated hordeola (see the Hordeolum [Stye] section) and chalazia (see the Chalazion section).

Diagnosis
Visual examination of the eyelids and the presence of collarettes (tiny scales) can determine the presence of staphylococci.

Treatment
Use of warm wet compresses and cleansing of the lids with a mild solution of baby shampoo and water generally resolves the inflammation within 14 days. If the condition has not resolved in that time, a physician should be consulted. Antibiotic ophthalmic ointments (bacitracin or erythromycin) may be needed in more severe cases.

Prognosis
The condition can sometimes be resistant to treatment and may become chronic if not properly treated. Untreated chronic cases may lead to corneal and conjunctival inflammation.

Prevention
It is prudent to protect the eyes from infection by adhering to proper hygiene.

Patient Teaching
Describe eyelid hygiene, which includes rigorous cleaning of the eyelids and lashes with a clean warm washcloth daily. Teach the patient the proper technique for instilling ophthalmic ointment and eye drops as prescribed; emphasize the importance of hand washing before the procedure. Some patients benefit from the use of medicated shampoos for seborrheic dermatitis.

Entropion

Description
In the case of entropion, the eyelid margins (more often the margin of just the lower lid) turn inward, causing the lashes to rub the conjunctiva (Fig. 5.8).

ICD-10-CM Code H02.009 (Unspecified entropion of unspecified eye, unspecified eyelid)
(H02.001-H02.059 = 42 codes of specificity)

Refer to the physician's diagnosis and then to the current edition of the ICD-10-CM coding manual to ensure the greatest specificity of pathology.

Symptoms and Signs
The patient has the sensation of a foreign body in the eye, tearing, itching, and redness. Chronic irritation of the conjunctiva may cause conjunctivitis (see the Conjunctivitis section). Entropion can also damage the cornea, causing epithelial defects and vision problems, if not corrected.

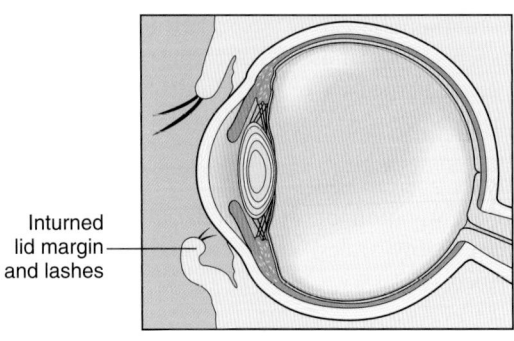

Inturned lid margin and lashes

• **Fig. 5.8** Entropion.

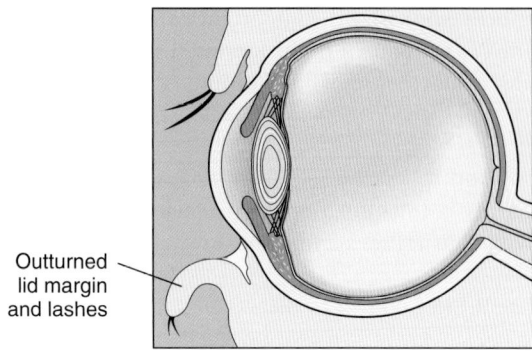

Outturned lid margin and lashes

• **Fig. 5.9** Ectropion.

Patient Screening

Schedule an appointment for the patient reporting the discomforting symptoms mentioned earlier.

Etiology

Entropion most often affects older people. With aging, the soft tissue on the lower eyelids loses elasticity, causing the eyelids to turn inward, thereby allowing the lashes to irritate the conjunctiva and the cornea.

Diagnosis

Visual examination reveals an inversion of the eyelid. The lashes are visible on the conjunctiva, as is the redness that results from the irritation.

Treatment

For persistent irritation, the patient should be seen by a physician. A minor surgical procedure on the eyelid usually corrects the problem.

Prognosis

Surgical treatment usually corrects the problem.

Prevention

No specific method of prevention is known.

Patient Teaching

To avoid infection, advise the patient not to rub the eyes. If surgery is required to correct the condition, explain the minor procedure.

Ectropion

Description

Ectropion is a condition in which the lower eyelid everts from the eyeball and the exposed surface of the eyeball and the lining of the eyelid become dry and irritated (Fig. 5.9).

| ICD-10-CM Code | H02.109 *(Unspecified ectropion of unspecified eye, unspecified eyelid)* |

Refer to the physician's diagnosis and then to the current edition of the ICD-10-CM coding manual to ensure the greatest specificity of pathology.

Symptoms and Signs

Eversion of the eyelid exposes the conjunctival membrane lining the eyelid. Tears are diverted away from the tear duct and run down the cheeks instead. The patient reports dryness in the eye and tearing.

Patient Screening

Schedule a medical evaluation for a patient experiencing the symptoms listed earlier.

Etiology

This condition usually occurs in older adults as a result of decreased elasticity of the lower eyelid. A scar on the eyelid or cheek that contracts and pulls the eyelid downward can cause a cicatricial ectropion.

Diagnosis

The problem can be detected easily by visual examination, and a history of symptoms confirms the diagnosis.

Treatment

Ectropion rarely disappears without treatment; therefore a physician should be consulted. A minor surgical procedure is all that is needed to correct the condition.

Prognosis

If it is not treated, ectropion can cause the development of corneal ulcers and permanent damage to the cornea.

Prevention

No method of prevention is known.

Patient Teaching

Assure the patient, who often is elderly, that a minor surgical procedure can correct the problem. Teach the patient the proper technique for instilling ophthalmic ointment and eye drops as prescribed; emphasize the importance of hand washing before performing the procedure.

Blepharoptosis

Description

Blepharoptosis, also called *ptosis,* is a permanent drooping of the upper eyelid, such that it partially or completely covers the eye (Fig. 5.10).

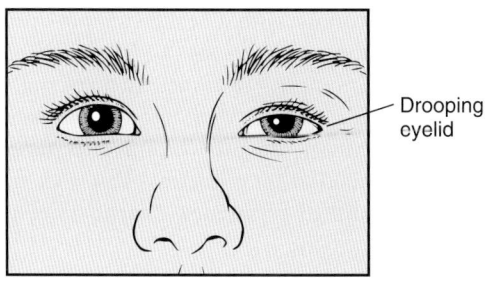

• **Fig. 5.10** Blepharoptosis.

ICD-10-CM Code   H02.409 (*Unspecified ptosis*
                                  of unspecified eyelid)
Refer to the physician's diagnosis and then to the current
edition of the ICD-10-CM coding manuals to ensure the
greatest specificity of pathology.

Symptoms and Signs

Blepharoptosis usually affects one eye, but both can be involved. The condition can vary in severity throughout the day. Blepharoptosis can occur at any age, is often familial, and, if severe, obstructs the vision of the affected eye.

Patient Screening

When vision is affected, or a previously normal upper eyelid has begun to droop, a physician should be consulted. Schedule the first available appointment.

Etiology

This condition is caused either by weakness of CN III or weakness of the muscle that raises the eyelid. Blepharoptosis also can occur when the muscle of the eyelid or the nerve that controls the muscle is damaged. Several diseases, such as muscular dystrophy and myasthenia gravis, can cause ptosis.

Diagnosis

In addition to an ophthalmic examination, blood tests and imaging may be ordered to rule out underlying disease.

Treatment

An operation can be performed to elevate the eyelid position, or in the case of myasthenia gravis, systemic medication may be prescribed.

Prognosis

Successful treatment of any underlying disease should help correct the blepharoptosis.

Prevention

No specific method of prevention is known.

Patient Teaching

Explain the relationship between the ptosis and the underlying disease, if known. If surgery is scheduled, describe the procedure to the patient, and provide written postoperative instructions, if appropriate.

Conjunctivitis

Description

Inflammation of the conjunctiva, the mucous membrane that covers the anterior portion of the eyeball and also lines the eyelids, is called *conjunctivitis*.

ICD-10-CM Code   H10.9 (*Unspecified conjunctivitis*)
                                (H10.01-H10.9 = 68 codes of
                                  specificity)
Refer to the physician's diagnosis and then to the
current edition of the ICD-10-CM coding manual to
ensure the greatest specificity of pathology.

Symptoms and Signs

Conjunctivitis can be either unilateral or bilateral and is common. Symptoms include redness, swelling, foreign body sensation, and itching of the conjunctiva. The eyes may tear excessively and be extra sensitive to light. In the case of infectious conjunctivitis, a discharge ranging from watery to hyperpurulent can be present. This condition ("pink eye") is highly contagious (Fig. 5.11).

Vernal conjunctivitis can be caused by extreme allergies or sensitivity or by irritation by contact lenses. This type of conjunctivitis appears as bumps or cobblestones when the eyelid is turned up.

Patient Screening

Schedule a prompt ophthalmic examination for the patient presenting with swollen, red, itchy eyes.

Etiology

Conjunctivitis can be caused by infection, most commonly viral or bacterial, and also by irritation resulting from allergies or chemicals. Infections often are transmitted when contaminated fingers, washcloths, or towels touch the eyes. Conjunctivitis can also be produced through sexual contact with someone who has a sexually transmitted disease.

Diagnosis

Ophthalmic examination reveals inflammation of the conjunctiva. To identify bacterial or viral organisms, samples of

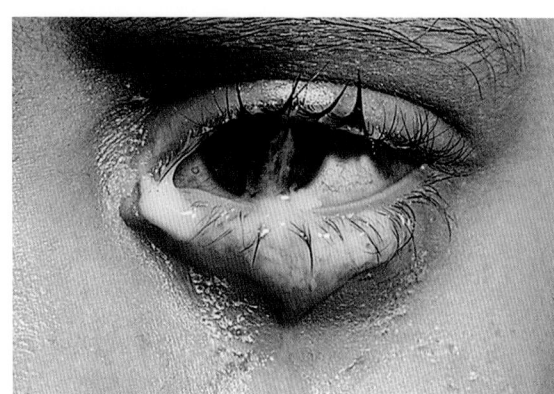

• **Fig. 5.11** Purulent conjunctivitis. (From Stein HA, Stein RM, Freeman MI: *The ophthalmic assistant: a text for allied and associated ophthalmic personnel,* ed 10, St Louis, 2018, Elsevier.)

the discharge can be taken for culture and sensitivity tests, although this is rarely necessary.

Treatment

The treatment varies, depending on the causative agents. The eyes should be kept free from discharge. This can be accomplished with cool compresses applied to the eyes. For bacterial infections, topical or systemic antibiotics are prescribed.

Prognosis

Except in severe instances, conjunctivitis is usually not a serious condition, although recurrences are common. Usually, 1 to 2 weeks of treatment clears up this type of infection. Viral infections usually are self-limiting.

Prevention

If the determined cause is irritants or allergens, avoiding the offending agents can result in resolution of the symptoms. Infectious conjunctivitis can be controlled by having the patient avoid contaminated washcloths and refrain from touching the eyes with contaminated fingers.

Patient Teaching

Give the patient written instructions on how to apply cool compresses and on the dosage schedule to be followed for medications. Teach the patient the proper technique for instilling ophthalmic ointment and eye drops as prescribed; emphasize the importance of hand washing before performing the procedure. When an oral antibiotic is ordered, advise the patient to be sure to take the entire course of medication.

Keratoconjunctivitis Sicca (Dry Eye Syndrome)

Description

Keratoconjunctivitis sicca (dry eye syndrome) is a condition in which tears do not furnish the eyes with ample lubrication. Dry eye syndrome is uncomfortable and may cause irritation of the eye.

ICD-10-CM Code	H04.12 (Dry eye syndrome)
	H04.123 (Dry eye syndrome of bilateral lacrimal glands)
	H04.129 (Dry eye syndrome of unspecified lacrimal gland)

Symptoms and Signs

Symptoms include a feeling of having a foreign object in the eyes; scratchy, burning, or stinging sensation in the eyes; sensitivity to light; blurred vision; and/or redness of the eyes. Additionally, the individual may experience difficulty with nighttime driving or with the wearing of contact lenses.

Patient Screening

Individuals reporting scratchiness accompanied by visual difficulty require prompt assessment. Schedule an appointment that same day, or consult with a health care provider to add the patient to the schedule as a "work in" so that they can be seen promptly. In some cases, referral to their ophthalmologist or a facility where prompt assessment can occur may be necessary after the health care provider has made a recommendation for a referral. This, too, may vary according to established versus new-patient office protocol and guidelines.

Etiology

Lack of adequate tear production often is the cause. Aging, many medical conditions, medications, damage to the tear glands as the result of radiation or inflammation, or temporary damage related to laser eye surgery. Increased tear evaporation may be caused by blinking less often than usual, dry air, wind, smoke, or structural eyelid problems.

Risk factors include being a female, being older than 50 years of age, wearing contact lenses, and consuming a diet low in vitamin A.

Diagnosis

The diagnosis is made from patient history and symptoms along with an examination of the eyes.

Treatment

Treatments include the application of over-the-counter eye drops. Medications, including cyclosporin ophthalmic emulsion (Restasis) and lifitegrast ophthalmic solution (Xiidra), may be prescribed. Recommendations for relief include some changes in lifestyle, such as avoiding environments with smoke, wind, and dry air. Contact lens wearers should follow instructions regarding length of time for wearing.

Prognosis

Instillation of eye drops will possibly be lifelong. Smokers may need to smoke less or avoid secondhand smoke. If lifestyle changes are made, symptoms may be reduced.

Prevention

The patient should follow instructions for wearing of contact lenses and avoid environments of dry air, wind, and smoke.

Patient Teaching

Instruct patients in the correct way to apply eye drops to prevent the possibility of eye injury or contamination of the solution. Patients should be instructed to not touch the tip of the applicator to the surface of the eye. Emphasize the importance of hand washing before performing the procedure.

Recommend situations where air is not blowing directly into the eyes. Have the patient establish a routine of using artificial tears on a regular basis; attempt to have more humid environment by adding moisture to the air; and take breaks when performing long tasks with eyes (reading, computer use).

Disorders of the Globe of the Eye

Corneal Abrasion or Ulcer

Description

A corneal abrasion is the painful loss of surface epithelium, or outer layer of the cornea. Corneal ulceration is infection of the cornea.

ICD-10-CM Code	S05.00XA *(Injury of conjunctiva and corneal abrasion without foreign body, unspecified eye, initial encounter)*
	H18.829 *(Corneal disorder due to contact lens, unspecified eye)*
	(H18.821-H18.829 = 4 codes of specificity)

Symptoms and Signs

The transparent outer covering of the eye is called the *cornea.* Because of its location, it is susceptible to injury and infection. Symptoms of abrasion and ulcer include pain, redness, and tearing. The patient may describe a sensation of having something foreign in the eye constantly and may report vision impairment as well. The patient may have a history of having had a foreign body in the eye or of recent ocular trauma.

Patient Screening

The patient with corneal abrasion may experience significant persistent pain in the eye. Prompt medical care is indicated. The physician should be consulted for instructions immediately after documenting a thorough history of any chemicals the eye has been exposed to. Follow office policy for referral to an ophthalmologist.

Etiology

Abrasions may be caused by foreign bodies being trapped between the cornea and the eyelid; by direct trauma to the cornea, such as being poked by a fingernail; or by the wearing of contact lenses that are scratched or poorly cleaned. Poorly fitting contact lenses also can cause corneal abrasions. If abrasions are not treated promptly, an ulcer can develop. A corneal ulcer is always a serious problem, and the patient should be referred to an ophthalmologist immediately in such cases. Individuals working on the underside of a vehicle should always wear eye protection. Frequent injuries may be from rust falling off the underside of the vehicle. Upon examination, a rust ring may be identified, requiring attention as well as removal of the rust particle.

Diagnosis

The diagnosis is confirmed by the presence of characteristic symptoms as well as by a visual examination of the patient. Corneal abrasions and ulcerations stain with fluorescein, which makes them readily detectable. In addition, corneal ulcers also demonstrate an opaque area on the cornea that represents the infiltrate of immune cells.

Treatment

If a foreign body is present, it must be removed promptly to prevent further ulceration and infection. An ophthalmic antibiotic ointment or drops are often prescribed to prevent a secondary infection in cases of corneal abrasion. Application of an eye dressing may be needed to promote healing if an abrasion is present. The dressing reduces movement of the cornea against the eyelid. Corneal ulcers need to be treated with intensive broad-spectrum antibiotic therapy immediately.

Prognosis

Most corneal abrasions heal spontaneously. Early treatment of corneal ulcers results in healing and regeneration of tissue. Complications can include secondary infection and scarring of tissue that may necessitate corneal transplantation.

Prevention

Abrasions can be prevented by wearing protective eyewear while working in hazardous situations or when engaging in sports that might put a person at risk for ocular injuries. Avoiding overnight wear of contact lenses can help prevent the development of corneal ulcers.

Patient Teaching

Teach the patient the proper care of an eye dressing and the technique for instilling ophthalmic ointment and eye drops, as prescribed; emphasize the importance of hand washing before performing the procedure. Stress the importance of keeping follow-up appointments to monitor the treatment of corneal ulcers. Contact lens should be avoided during healing and may be used once the abrasion has resolved and the provider has given approval for contact lens use.

Episcleritis/Scleritis

Description

Inflammation of the episclera (the external surface of the sclera) is called *episcleritis*; inflammation of the deeper sclera, the white outermost covering of the eyeball, is called *scleritis*. Episcleritis occurs far more commonly than scleritis.

ICD-10-CM Code	H15.009 *(Unspecified scleritis, unspecified eye)*
	(H15.001-H15.099 = 28 codes of specificity)
	H15.109 *(Unspecified episcleritis, unspecified eye)*
	(H15.101-H15.129 = 12 codes of specificity)

Refer to the physician's diagnosis and then to the current edition of the ICD-10-CM coding manual to ensure the greatest specificity of pathology.

Spontaneous Subconjunctival Hemorrhage

A spontaneous subconjunctival hemorrhage is the result of a small blood vessel rupturing underneath the surface of the conjunctiva. All or a portion of the white part of the eye (sclera) appears bright red (Fig. 5.12). This event is usually painless and observed when looking in the mirror. It can be the result of an episode of violent sneezing or severe coughing, vomiting, straining. It also may be the result of trauma to the eye. Often the cause cannot be determined. The condition usually resolves spontaneously within 10 days to 2 weeks.

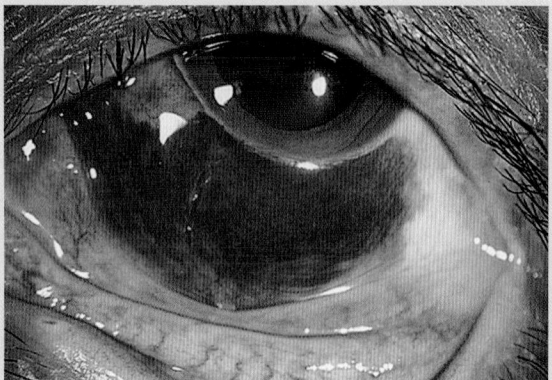

• **Fig. 5.12** Subconjunctival hemorrhage (From Stein HA, Stein RM, Freeman MI: *The ophthalmic assistant: a text for allied and associated ophthalmic personnel,* ed 10, St Louis, 2018, Elsevier.)

Symptoms and Signs

Episcleritis usually affects only one eye and presents as redness and irritation in an isolated portion of the eye. Scleritis can affect either one or both eyes; symptoms include intense redness in one or more areas of the sclera and are more commonly associated with pain and blurred vision. Inflammation can occur in the posterior portion of the eye, which may cause some loss of vision. If scleritis is left untreated, perforation of the globe and loss of the eye are possible outcomes.

Patient Screening

Eye pain and redness indicate the need for an ophthalmic examination as soon as possible.

Etiology

Episcleritis is usually not associated with any other concomitant systemic disease. Scleritis, however, is often associated with autoimmune disorders, such as rheumatoid arthritis (see the Rheumatoid Arthritis section in Chapter 3), and certain digestive disorders, including Crohn disease (see the Crohn Disease [Regional Enteritis] section in Chapter 8) or ulcerative colitis.

Diagnosis

The patient should see an ophthalmologist as soon as possible if symptoms develop. A thorough ophthalmic examination is needed, and blood tests may be necessary to determine any underlying causes. Diagnostic evaluation may include ultrasonography, magnetic resonance imaging (MRI), or both to identify infectious or autoimmune connective tissue disease.

Treatment

Episcleritis and mild cases of scleritis usually respond well to instillation of topical steroid eye drops. Artificial tears and lubricating ophthalmic ointments may be used for palliative relief. For severe cases, immunosuppressive drugs may be prescribed. Perforation of the sclera, which is rare, necessitates surgical repair called *scleroplasty.*

Prognosis

The prognosis is good for mild cases.

Prevention

No method of prevention is known.

Patient Teaching

Teach the patient the proper technique for instilling ophthalmic ointment and eye drops as prescribed; emphasize the importance of hand washing before performing the procedure. If surgery is required, use visual aids (if possible) to describe the anatomy of the eye to the patient, and explain the surgical repair procedure. Describe the postoperative regimen and stress the importance of follow-up care.

Cataract

Description

Cataract is opacification of the natural lens of the eye.

ICD-10-CM Code	H26.9 *(Unspecified cataract)*
	(H25.011-H26.9 = 92 codes of specificity)

Additional digits are required. Refer to the physician's diagnosis and then to the current edition of the ICD-10-CM coding manual to ensure the greatest specificity of pathology.

Symptoms and Signs

Cataracts usually develop slowly and gradually reduce visual acuity. The primary symptom is the deterioration of vision in the affected eye. The patient may report poor night vision, yellowing or fading of colors, loss of brightness of color, and the need for bright light for reading. In advanced cases, the cataract may become readily visible, giving the pupil a white, opaque appearance and blocking light, thereby impairing vision (Fig. 5.13).

Patient Screening

Cataracts often are noted during a routine ophthalmic examination. Patients reporting changes in visual acuity and/or glare should be given the first available appointment for an ophthalmic examination. Follow office policy for referral to an ophthalmologist. Although many patients are of the

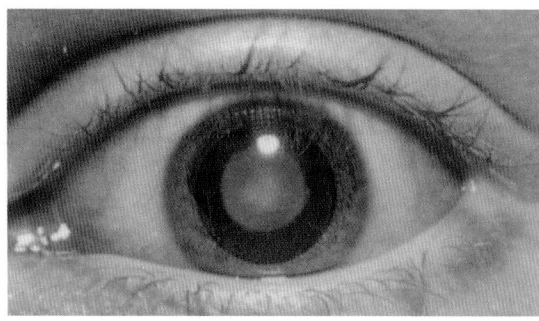

• **Fig. 5.13** Cataract. (From Black JM, Hawks JH, Keene AM: *Medical-surgical nursing: clinical management for positive outcomes*, ed 8, Philadelphia, 2009, Saunders. Courtesy Ophthalmic Photography, University of Michigan WK Kellogg Eye Center, Ann Arbor, MI.)

aging population, cataracts can develop in some younger patients also.

Etiology
The most common cause of cataracts is opacification of the lens caused by the aging process, and in the United States, the condition is present in about 50% of persons age greater than 75 years. According to the National Eye Institute, "the risk of cataract increases with each decade of life starting around age 40. By age 75, half of white Americans have cataract. By age 80, 70% of whites have cataract compared with 53% of blacks and 61% of Hispanic Americans." The numbers vary from one ethnic group to another.

Cataracts may be congenital or result from ocular trauma, drug toxicity (prolonged high-dose corticosteroid administration), or systemic diseases, such as diabetes mellitus, or as a complication of other ocular diseases. Long-term, unprotected exposure to sunlight is considered causative as well. Prevalence of cataracts often is familial; however, they also are a common condition in the general population.

Diagnosis
Examination by an ophthalmologist should be considered if vision becomes distorted or seems to be deteriorating. Ophthalmoscopy, with dilation of the eye and a slit-lamp examination, confirms the presence of a cataract.

Treatment
Treatment depends on the amount of visual impairment and the age, health, and occupation of the patient. Surgery is advised when the cataracts begin to interfere with the lifestyle of the patient. The most common method of removing a cataract is phacoemulsification. In extracapsular surgery, the nucleus, or center, of the cataract is removed in one piece. This necessitates a larger incision and more sutures. With phacoemulsification, an ultrasonic probe vibrates to break up the cataract, which subsequently is aspirated through the small incision. With this method, often no sutures are required for wound closure.

In both extracapsular cataract extraction and phacoemulsification, the posterior capsule of the lens is left in place.

This membrane helps support an artificial lens, which is placed into the eye after removal of the cataract. Often the posterior membrane becomes cloudy after surgery, and this again reduces visual acuity. If this does occur, a laser can be used to make an opening in the center of the cloudy membrane, thus immediately restoring good vision. This outpatient procedure is called *YAG capsulotomy* and entails local anesthesia.

Prognosis
After cataract surgery, the patient will need a change in eyeglass prescription. Cataract surgery currently is quite successful; however, as with all surgery, significant complications are possible, especially when other ocular diseases exist.

Prevention
Cataracts are primarily associated with the aging process, and no method of prevention is known. It is prudent for patients and physicians to consider the risk of cataracts associated with drug toxicity from certain medications.

Patient Teaching
Explain the preoperative tests and medications that are prescribed. Emphasize the importance of hand washing before performing the procedure. Give the patient written instructions regarding the technique for instilling eye drops and all other medications, how to apply the eye shield carefully, and any limitation of activities during recovery. Stress the importance of regular follow up visits.

Glaucoma
Description
Glaucoma is damage to the optic nerve in the presence of elevated IOP.

ICD-10-CM Code	H40.9 *(Unspecified glaucoma)* (H40.0-H42 = 67 codes of specificity)

Additional digits are required. Refer to the physician's diagnosis and then to the current edition of the ICD-10-CM coding manual to ensure the greatest specificity of pathology.

Glaucoma is one of the major causes of blindness. It is more common in patients older than 60 years of age; however, it can occur at any age. The ciliary body in the eye continually produces fluid called *aqueous humor*. This fluid circulates freely between the posterior and anterior chambers of the eye and passes through the trabecular meshwork and drains into the general circulation. Several different pathologic causes and abnormalities in fluid drainage lead to glaucoma. Risk factors include age greater than 60 years, nearsightedness, blood relatives with glaucoma, and African American descent.

The many types of glaucoma include chronic open-angle, acute angle-closure, secondary, and congenital (Fig. 5.14). Secondary glaucoma results from a specific disease in the eye

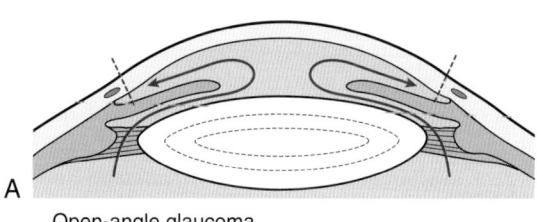

A
Open-angle glaucoma

B
Closed-angle glaucoma

• **Fig. 5.14** Glaucoma (A) In open-angle glaucoma, the obstruction occurs in the trabecular meshwork. (B) In closed-angle glaucoma, the trabecular meshwork is covered by the root of the iris or adhesions between the iris and the cornea. (From Damjanov I: *Pathology for the health-related professions,* ed 4, St Louis, 2011, Saunders.)

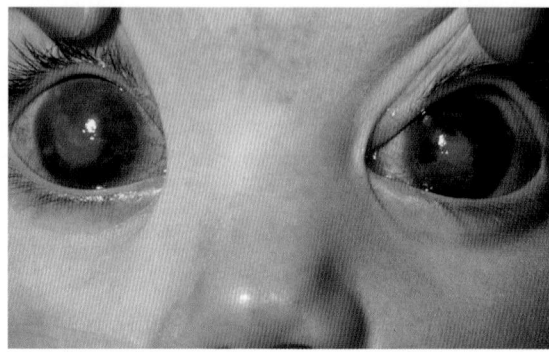

• **Fig. 5.15** Congenital glaucoma. Note enlargement of the eyes. (From Krachmer JH, Palay D. *Cornea atlas,* ed 3, Philadelphia, 2014, Elsevier.)

and can occur after trauma or neovascularization in the anterior chamber and may occur after diabetes. Infantile glaucoma or congenital glaucoma causes the eye to distend and resemble the eye of an ox (Fig. 5.15).

Patient Screening

Encourage patients, especially those with the risk factors listed earlier, to have regular ophthalmic examinations and appropriate testing. Patients reporting the onset of headaches, changes in visual acuity, photophobia, nausea and vomiting, and/or eye pain need to see their ophthalmologist immediately; their condition should be treated as an emergency.

Chronic Open-Angle Glaucoma

ICD-10-CM Code   H40.10 (*Unspecified open-angle glaucoma*)
Refer to the physician's diagnosis and then to the current edition of the ICD-10-CM coding manual to ensure the greatest specificity of pathology.

Symptoms and Signs. Chronic open-angle glaucoma, a silent disease, is the most common form of glaucoma and is the most treatable cause of blindness. Patients can have open-angle glaucoma for a significant period before symptoms appear. By the time symptoms do appear, considerable damage usually has occurred. The best way to detect glaucoma is by having periodic routine ophthalmic examinations, which include IOP readings and optic nerve evaluations. If the IOP is somewhat elevated or the optic nerve shows signs of enlarging, glaucoma needs to be considered as a possibility. If chronic open-angle glaucoma goes untreated, the patient experiences characteristic loss of vision. The central vision may remain clear for a considerable period. However, if the condition progresses, the central vision is also lost, causing complete blindness.

Etiology. In chronic open-angle glaucoma, a block at the level of the trabecular meshwork impairs aqueous humor reabsorption. Chronic open-angle glaucoma can occur secondary to trauma, even years later. Overuse of topical steroids also can cause the condition. Risk factors include family history, the aging process, diabetes mellitus, ocular trauma, and obesity. Among blacks, glaucoma is the leading cause of blindness.

Diagnosis. The diagnosis of open-angle glaucoma is determined by patient history, ophthalmic examination with tonometry, examination of the optic nerves, and visual field analysis.

Treatment. Early treatment of glaucoma is essential; if not treated promptly, the disease can lead to blindness, because any vision lost as a result of the disease generally cannot be regained. This condition usually is treated with medication to decrease the production of aqueous humor (carbonic anhydrase inhibitors, beta-blockers, and alpha-adrenergic agents) or increased uveoscleral outflow (prostaglandin analogues). Different types of laser treatment, including argon laser trabeculoplasty (ALT) and selective laser trabeculoplasty (SLT), also can be beneficial in opening the drainage system; occasionally, trabeculectomy or drainage implantation is necessary to bypass the drainage system. Fortunately, most of the time, chronic open-angle glaucoma can be controlled with eye drops.

> ✴ **NOTE**
>
> Beta-blockers used in glaucoma treatment can cause a rise in blood levels as the beta-blockers are absorbed through the tear duct. Eye drops in this class have been shown to affect heart rate and blood pressure and worsen symptoms of asthma. Beta-blockers are contraindicated in patients who suffer from heart failure.

Acute Angle-Closure Glaucoma

ICD-10-CM Code   H40.20 (*Unspecified primary angle-closure glaucoma*)
Refer to the physician's diagnosis and then to the current edition of the ICD-10-CM coding manual to ensure the greatest specificity of pathology.

Symptoms and Signs. Acute angle-closure glaucoma usually is associated with blurred vision, severe eye pain, headaches, and redness of the eye. The patient becomes photophobic and sees "halos" around light. With the full attack of acute glaucoma, the symptoms persist and become worse. Often severe pain develops and is associated with nausea and vomiting. The cornea of the eye becomes hazy because of the elevated pressure. The elevation of pressure in acute angle-closure glaucoma is usually significantly higher than that associated with chronic open-angle (simple) glaucoma. If acute angle-closure glaucoma is left untreated, the patient can lose his or her vision.

Etiology. In acute angle-closure glaucoma, the mouth or opening of the drainage system is narrow and can close completely, causing a substantial increase in the IOP during a short time.

Diagnosis. The diagnosis is made on the basis of the patient's history and a notable increase in the IOP. With a special lens called a *goniolens,* the ophthalmologist can directly view the opening of the drainage system to determine whether it is open or closed. The eye is usually red, and the cornea can be hazy.

Treatment. Treatment of acute angle-closure glaucoma is done primarily by laser iridotomy, which creates a small opening in the iris, allowing the filtering angle to open. Often the IOP is lowered with medication before the laser treatment. However, the definitive treatment of angle-closure glaucoma is virtually always a laser iridotomy.

Prognosis. The prognosis depends on the type of glaucoma, how early the condition is recognized and treatment is begun, and patient compliance with therapeutic regimens. Untreated glaucoma is a major cause of blindness.

Prevention. Regular ophthalmic examinations with testing appropriate to age and risk factors are recommended.

Patient Teaching. Explain the type of glaucoma and the treatment regimen. Teach the patient the proper technique for instilling ophthalmic ointment and eye drops as prescribed; emphasize the importance of hand washing before performing the procedure. Review the symptoms and signs that should be reported to the physician: severe eye pain, headache, blurred vision, halos, nausea, and vomiting. Stress the importance of good compliance with the medication regimen and follow-up care. Provide referrals for support services.

Macular Degeneration

Description
Macular degeneration is progressive deterioration or breakdown of the macula of the retina.

ICD-10-CM Code	H35.30 *(Unspecified macular degeneration [age-related])* (H35.30-H35.389 = 24 codes of specificity)

Refer to the physician's diagnosis and then to the current edition of the ICD-10-CM coding manual to ensure the greatest specificity of pathology.

Symptoms and Signs
The area of the retina near the optic nerve in the center of the field of vision that defines fine details is known as the *macula lutea.* An early symptom of macular degeneration may be a mild distortion of central vision. As the condition progresses, the patient may describe seeing wavy lines when looking at lines that are straight and/or seeing semiopaque spots in the visual field. The condition is usually painless, develops slowly, and does not affect the peripheral vision. In most cases, both eyes are affected, either at the same time or one right after the other. As the condition worsens, reading and activities that require sharp vision become impossible. Eventually, the central vision may disappear altogether. Age-related macular degeneration (AMD) is the most common cause of blindness among white persons in the United States.

Patient Screening
Macular degeneration is often considered to be age related; therefore the mature adult is encouraged to have regular ophthalmic examinations. Patients reporting changes in visual acuity or loss of sharpness in central vision are scheduled for a prompt ophthalmic examination. Follow office policy for referral to an ophthalmologist.

Etiology
Age, genetic factors, and prolonged exposure to bright light are all causative factors. Macular degeneration usually is caused by degenerative changes in the pigment epithelium of the retina. Atrophic changes in the macula constitute dry macular degeneration; this is the more common type. The presence of abnormal fragile and hemorrhage-prone blood vessels can develop behind the macula and convert the disease to its wet form. Hemorrhage may occur when these abnormal vessels break and damage the retina. The result is loss of central vision.

Diagnosis
The diagnosis of macular degeneration is made after a thorough examination with dilation by an ophthalmologist. In nonexudative or dry macular degeneration, pigmentary changes are seen in the macular area, and drusen deposits are evident (Fig. 5.16A). In cases suspicious for wet macular degeneration, fluorescein angiography detects the presence and leakage of abnormal blood vessels.

Treatment
No definitive medical cure is known; however, a recent study has shown that vitamin supplements, especially vitamins C and E, beta-carotene, and zinc, can help slow the deterioration of moderate dry macular degeneration. The wet form of this disease may be treated with traditional laser photocoagulation, photodynamic laser therapy, or the injection of antiangiogenic factors. Intraocular injection with an anti–vascular endothelial growth factor (anti-VEGF) has become standard for the treatment of wet AMD. Clinical trials and new technology are providing new information that is being used to direct changes in the way the disease is

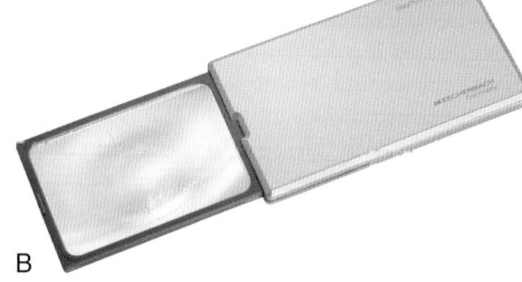

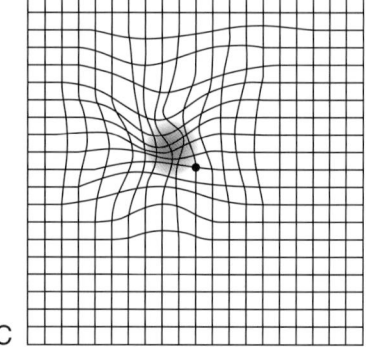

• **Fig. 5.16** (A) The black arrows point to the drusen bodies in the image. Drusen bodies. (B) Handheld magnifier. (C) Amsler grid showing visual changes. (A, From Seidel HM, et al: *Mosby's guide to physical examination,* ed 7, St Louis, 2011, Mosby. Courtesy Dr. Robert P. Murphy. B, Courtesy Eschenbach Optik, http://www.eschenbach.com. C, From Harding M, et al: *Lewis's medical-surgical nursing,* ed 11, St. Louis, 2020, Elsevier.)

being managed. Visual aids, such as handheld magnifiers (see Fig. 5.16B) and closed-circuit television, also may be beneficial. The patient is given an Amsler grid for home monitoring of visual changes that need to be reported (see Fig. 5.16C).

Prognosis

No cure is known, and the success of treatment has been limited; however, new treatment methods will hopefully provide a more positive prognosis in the future.

Prevention

Signs of early macular degeneration (tiny drusen) can be seen by the ophthalmologist during an eye examination before the patient is symptomatic. Taking a vitamin therapy called *AREDS* and protecting the eyes from ultraviolet rays and bright light are considered prudent measures. It has been suggested that smoking is a risk factor.

Patient Teaching

Patients benefit from an explanation of why their vision and depth perception have changed and how they can use visual aids to improve vision. Explain and demonstrate the use of the Amsler grid for home monitoring. Instruct the patient to contact the physician immediately if a sudden worsening of vision is experienced or any changes are noted on home Amsler grid monitoring. Stress the importance of follow-up appointments as suggested by the physician. The patient's family should also be included in patient teaching, and simulation glasses may be helpful in education of the patient's family members on exactly what their family member sees. Driving will become difficult, and the patient will need a strong support group to adapt to his or her limitations.

Diabetic Retinopathy

Description

Diabetic retinopathy is pathologic alterations of the retinal blood vessels and the pathologic proliferation of retinal vessels.

ICD-10-CM Code	E13.319 *(Other specified diabetes mellitus with unspecified diabetic retinopathy without macular edema)*
	E11.311 *(Type 2 diabetes mellitus with unspecified diabetic retinopathy with macular edema)*
	E11.36 *(Type 2 diabetes mellitus with diabetic cataract)*
	E11.39 *(Type 2 diabetes mellitus with other diabetic ophthalmic complication)*
	(E11.31-E11.39 = 12 codes of specificity)

Refer to the physician's diagnosis and then to the current edition of the ICD-10-CM coding manual to ensure the greatest specificity of pathology.

Symptoms and Signs

Diabetic retinopathy is characterized by microaneurysm, hemorrhages, dilation of retinal veins, macular edema, and the formation of abnormal new vessels (neovascularization). This condition usually occurs in both eyes, affecting the sharpness and clarity of vision. Diabetic retinopathy is a major cause of acquired blindness in the United States.

Patient Screening

The patient with diabetes is encouraged to have frequent ophthalmic examinations, at least annually. Any sudden change in visual acuity is to be reported to the primary care physician and the ophthalmologist immediately. Available new technology has been successful in helping health care providers identify potential problems during regular examinations at the office. The RetinaVue is a handheld device that makes images of the retina. Many providers are now screening patients in the medical office and referring them to the ophthalmologist when this test identifies irregular images. This has been particularly helpful in populations of patients with diabetes who are not seeing their eye doctors for regular examinations as needed. Referrals are made from the health care provider's office, and patients follow up with the specialists.

Etiology

Diabetic retinopathy usually occurs about 8 to 10 years after the onset of diabetes mellitus. It occurs most often in those with diabetes who do not control their blood glucose levels, but all persons with diabetes are susceptible. Diabetes causes poor circulation in the retinal blood vessels and may cause leakage of exudate into the retina. Sometimes fragile new blood vessels (neovascularization) can grow and lead to leakage of blood into the vitreous humor. This may greatly reduce vision. In some cases, the blood is reabsorbed by the choroid; however, persistent vitreous hemorrhage necessitates surgical intervention (Fig. 5.17). There are four stages of this type of eye disorder, each one being progressively

worse than the other. Mild nonproliferative, moderate nonproliferative, severe nonproliferative, and proliferative. Proliferative diabetic retinopathy can result in retinal detachment and permanent blindness.

Diagnosis
Complete ophthalmoscopic examination detects the retinal effects of diabetes. As with other ocular disorders, a thorough ophthalmic examination should be done regularly, especially when diabetes is a factor.

Treatment
Treatment will depend on the severity of the retinopathy. In mild cases, the patient may be monitored closely before treatment begins. Treatment with laser photocoagulation is usually effective in controlling retinopathy. Panretinal photocoagulation may also be used. Shrinking and scarring of the abnormal vessels occurs with this scatter laser treatment. The condition has a tendency to recur, but with treatment and tight control of blood sugar, vision often may be maintained. In cases of vitreous hemorrhage or proliferative disease, a vitrectomy may be necessary. Intravitreal steroid injection is also beneficial.

Prognosis
Diabetic retinopathy can be controlled with treatment; however, the prognosis is guarded.

Prevention
Maintaining tight blood glucose control can prevent the onset of diabetic retinopathy and can improve any existing retinopathy.

Patient Teaching
Stress the importance of good diabetic care, especially good blood glucose control, to help prevent the complication of diabetic retinopathy and possible loss of vision.

Retinal Detachment

Description
Retinal detachment is elevation (separation) of the retina from the choroid (Fig. 5.18).

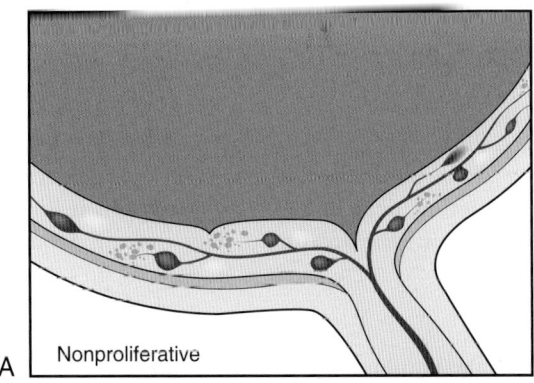
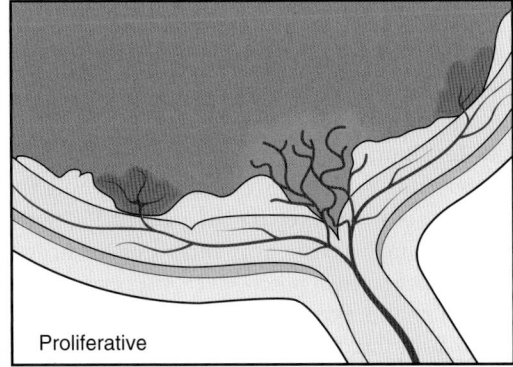

• **Fig. 5.17** Diabetic Retinopathy. (A) Nonproliferative retinopathy shows edema, microaneurysm, and exudates. (B) Proliferative retinopathy shows new blood vessel formation. (From Damjanov I: *Pathology for the health-related professions*, ed 4, St Louis, 2011, Saunders.)

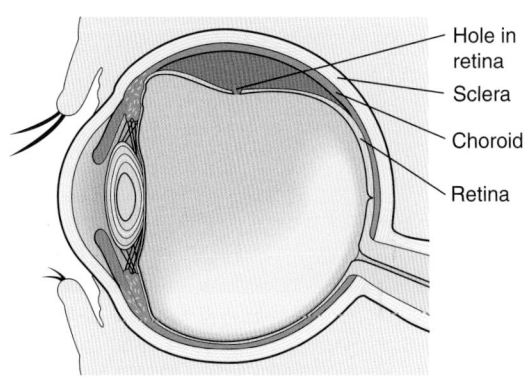

• **Fig. 5.18** Retinal detachment.

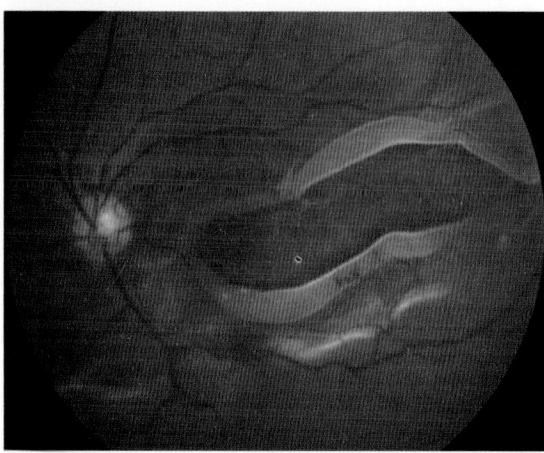

• **Fig. 5.19** Large retinal tear with associated retinal detachment. (From Kanski J, Bowling B: *Clinical ophthalmology—a systematic approach*, ed 7, Edinburgh, 2011, Saunders.)

ICD-10-CM Code	H33.20 *(Serous retinal detachment, unspecified eye)* (H33.20-H33.23 = 4 codes of specificity)

Refer to the physician's diagnosis and then to the current edition of the ICD-10-CM coding manual to ensure the greatest specificity of pathology.

Symptoms and Signs

Retinal detachment may be partial or complete and usually is associated with a retinal tear or a hole in the retina (Fig. 5.19). Early symptoms of detachment consist of the patient seeing many new floaters and light flashes. This persists and worsens and is followed by seeing a dark shadow that extends from the periphery inward. This may begin in either the lower or upper field of vision or in one of the side fields of vision. If the detachment extends to the central retina, the central vision also is blocked. The detachment often happens suddenly and without pain (Fig. 5.20).

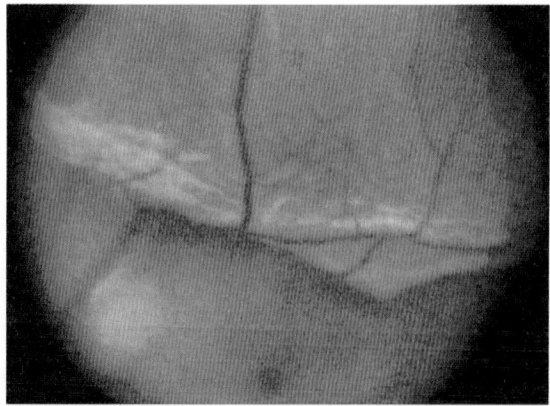

• **Fig. 5.20** Retinal detachment. Folding of the retina, which is in focus anteriorly. (From Stein HA, Stein RM, Freeman MI: *The ophthalmic assistant: a text for allied and associated ophthalmic personnel*, ed 10, St Louis, 2018, Elsevier.)

Patient Screening

The patient reporting light flashes, painless changes in vision, and visualization of new floating spots is brought to the physician's attention for an immediate dilated examination.

Etiology

Certain retinal detachments are commonly associated with severe diabetic retinopathy. People who are extremely near-sighted are more susceptible to retinal detachments compared with the general population. Ocular trauma or retinal atrophy also can predispose a person to retinal detachment. A retinal detachment usually begins with a tear in the retina. Fluid then leaks under the retina and separates it from the choroid. After the retina is separated from the choroid, that portion of the retina no longer functions visually. As the retina continues to detach, more and more vision is lost.

Diagnosis

An ophthalmoscopic examination readily reveals the retinal detachment.

Treatment

Early treatment is advised; intervention is imperative. Treatment of a retinal detachment consists of either photocoagulation or surgery. This should be done without delay to prevent additional portions of the retina from detaching. If the detachment has extended to the macula, the central retina, permanent reduction in central acuity often occurs. Photocoagulation or cryotherapy can be used to treat retinal tears if no significant detachment occurs. Photocoagulation is a relatively simple procedure, which can be used to seal retinal tears before the development of retinal detachment. Early diagnosis is important in such cases. The treatment may include a period of bed rest.

Prognosis

Irreversible blindness can result from untreated retinal detachment.

Prevention

No specific method of prevention is known.

Patient Teaching

Use visual aids to explain the condition and the treatment to the patient. Prepare the patient for postsurgical procedures and treatments, including instruction on wearing a protective patch over the eye, taking pain medications, and executing measures to prevent raising IOP. Explain the importance of bed rest, if ordered. Teach the patient the proper technique for instilling ophthalmic ointment and eye drops as prescribed. Emphasize the importance of hand washing before performing the procedure.

Uveitis

Description

Uveitis denotes inflammation of the uveal tract, including the iris, ciliary body, and choroid.

> ICD-10-CM Code   H20.9 *(Unspecified iridocyclitis)*
> *Refer to the physician's diagnosis and then to the current edition of the ICD-10-CM coding manual to ensure the greatest specificity of pathology.*

Symptoms and Signs

Uveitis may be either unilateral or bilateral. Pain, photophobia, blurred vision, and redness can occur. The photophobia is often pronounced.

Patient Screening

Having a complete ophthalmic examination performed as soon as possible is necessary for a patient experiencing the symptoms mentioned earlier. Follow office policy for referral to an ophthalmologist.

Etiology

Uveitis can be associated with autoimmune disorders; juvenile rheumatoid arthritis (see Chapter 3) and ankylosing spondylitis (see Chapter 3) are especially likely to be associated with uveitis. Infections, such as syphilis, tuberculosis, toxoplasmosis, and histoplasmosis or inflammatory bowel disease, also may be causative. Often an exact cause for uveitis cannot be determined.

Diagnosis

A complete examination with the slit lamp is necessary for the diagnosis to be made. To detect some forms of disease, skin tests for tuberculosis, toxoplasmosis, and histoplasmosis may be needed. Certain blood tests also may aid in confirming the diagnosis.

Treatment

Treatment is specific for the particular type of uveitis and consists largely of topical or, in severe cases, systemic steroid use. Any underlying cause should be treated. Cycloplegic agents that cause paralysis of the ciliary muscle are often beneficial in reducing the pain associated with ciliary inflammation.

Prognosis

The prognosis is variable, depending on the clinical type and the underlying cause.

Prevention

No method of prevention is known.

Patient Teaching

Use visual aids to demonstrate what structure(s) of the eyes are involved in the inflammation. Explain the medical treatment.

Teach the patient the proper technique for instilling ophthalmic ointment and eye drops as prescribed; emphasize the importance of hand washing before performing the procedure.

Exophthalmos

Description

Exophthalmos is abnormal protrusion of the eyeballs.

> ICD-10-CM Code   H05.20 *(Unspecified exophthalmos)*
> (H05.20, H05.241-H05.269 = 13 codes of specificity)
> Q15.8 *(Other specified congenital malformations of eye)*
> (Q15.0-Q15.9 = 3 codes of specificity)
> *Refer to the physician's diagnosis and then to the current edition of the ICD-10-CM coding manual to ensure the greatest specificity of pathology.*

Symptoms and Signs

Exophthalmos exposes an abnormally large amount of the anterior eye. Patients report dryness and a gritty feeling in the affected eye or eyes. They also may note double vision and eye movement restriction. In severe cases, vision becomes seriously blurred.

Patient Screening

Schedule a prompt appointment for a complete medical evaluation and ophthalmic examination. Follow office policy for referral to an ophthalmologist.

Etiology

Exophthalmos is caused by multiple factors, including enlarged extraocular muscles, retrobulbar mass, or edema of the soft tissue that lines the bony orbit of the eye. This condition may be associated with hyperthyroid, hypothyroid, or euthyroid (normal thyroid) status (see the Hyperthyroidism section in Chapter 4). Sudden unilateral onset is usually a sign of retrobulbar hemorrhage or inflammation.

Diagnosis

A complete ophthalmic examination, along with blood tests, radiographic studies, computed tomography (CT), and echography, are done to determine the underlying cause.

Treatment

The diagnosis determines the therapy. If the condition is caused by hyperthyroidism, the underlying disorder needs to be corrected. Severe cases may require surgical decompression of the orbit, and systemic steroids are beneficial in controlling edema.

Prognosis

The prognosis depends on the successful treatment of the underlying cause.

Prevention

No method of prevention is known.

Patient Teaching

Explain how exophthalmos relates to the underlying cause as diagnosed. Explain the purpose and dosage schedule of prescribed medication. Give emotional support, because the patient is likely to be distressed by the cosmetic effect of "bulging eyeballs."

Cancer of the Eye

Description

Cancer of the eye may involve the globe (ocular tumors), the orbit (the bone surrounding the orbital cavity and the soft tissues and muscles that lie between the globe and the bone), the optic nerve, or the eyelids. Neoplasms may be benign, malignant, or metastatic from another location (secondary tumors).

ICD-10-CM Code	C69 *(Malignant neoplasm of eye and adnexa)* (C69.00-C69.92 = 27 codes of specificity)

Neoplasms of the eye must be specified for location and type. Therefore it is not possible to list all applicable ICD-10-CM codes for neoplasms of the eye. Refer to the physician's diagnosis and then to the current edition of the ICD-10-CM coding manual to ensure the greatest specificity of pathology.

Symptoms and Signs

Tumors of the eyelid generally present as visible lesions (see Chapter 6 for a discussion of basal cell carcinoma [BCC], squamous cell carcinoma [SCC], and malignant melanoma lesions). Seborrheic keratosis presents as a skin tag (skin projection) on the eyelid. Ocular melanoma may present as a growing pigmented spot on the iris. Secondary eye tumors are usually associated with pain, which distinguishes them from most primary eye cancers.

Patient Screening

Patients reporting visible lesions around or "in" the eye, or those experiencing any unusual appearance or movement of the eye(s), with or without pain, need a timely appointment for a medical evaluation and an ophthalmic examination. In addition, infants and young children should be evaluated for leukokoria (white pupil) and strabismus at well-child examinations and referred urgently to an ophthalmologist, if noted.

Etiology

Ocular tumors include retinoblastoma, the most common primary malignancy of the eye in children, representing 3% of all childhood cancers (Fig. 5.21), and ocular (or

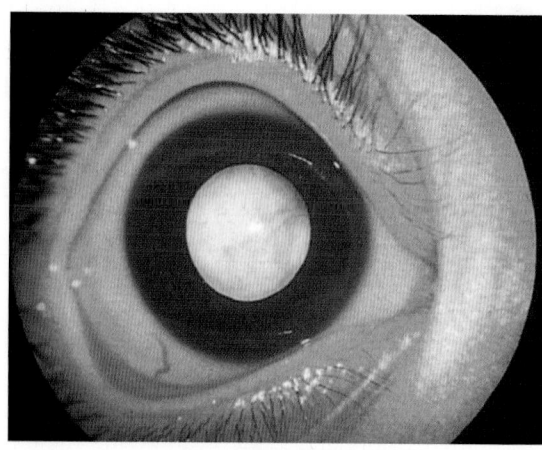

• **Fig. 5.21** Retinoblastoma. (From Michelson JB, Friedlaender MH: *The eye in clinical medicine,* London, 1996, Times Mirror International.)

uveal tract) melanoma and intraocular lymphoma, the most common ocular tumors in adults. Retinoblastoma is a neoplasm of the retina affecting around 1 in 16,000 children. In approximately 40% of cases, it is due to a heritable mutation on chromosome 13. Most cases of ocular melanoma are found in Caucasians. Orbital tumors are more rare and include rhabdomyosarcoma (malignant) and capillary hemangioma (benign) in children and cavernous hemangioma (benign) in adults.

Eyelid tumors include skin cancers (usually caused by sun exposure of the eyelid) and benign squamous papillomas (caused by human papillomavirus [HPV] infection). BCC is the most common malignant eyelid tumor (85% to 90% of eyelid lesions). Eyelid melanoma, on the other hand, accounts for only 1% of eyelid tumors, but greater than 65% of all deaths are caused by neoplasms of the eyelid. Optic pathway glioma is a low-grade tumor of the optic nerve that usually occurs in children under age 20 years. Approximately 2800 new cases of primary eye cancer occur each year, and 320 deaths result from this type of cancer. The most common tumor of the eye is cancer that has metastasized to the eye. The most common sites of origin are the lung in men and the breast in women, but many other types of cancer also are known to metastasize to the eye.

Diagnosis

The lesions of ocular melanoma may be first identified on routine eye examination, but ultrasound helps make the diagnosis. Eyelid tumors are diagnosed after biopsy of the lesion. Other types of eye tumors may be seen on funduscopic examination and MRI. With or without a biopsy (depending on the tumor type and location), these are used for diagnosis and evaluation of the extent of disease. Additionally, CT and chest radiograph may be done for staging. Patients with retinoblastoma should have molecular genetic testing done in case they have a heritable form of the disease.

Treatment

Treatment may involve excision of the tumor, eyeball removal, radiation therapy, chemotherapy, or laser therapy. Treatment of secondary eye cancer rarely improves patient survival, but chemotherapy or radiation therapy may be given for palliation of symptoms.

Prognosis

Overall 5-year survival rate for patients with primary eye neoplasms is generally good but largely depends on tumor type, size, and stage at diagnosis. There may be vision loss, depending on the treatment used. Although greater than 90% of children survive retinoblastoma with appropriate treatment, they are at risk for developing secondary malignancies, especially osteosarcoma, later in life.

Prevention

No methods of prevention are known for orbital and ocular eye tumors. Siblings and children of patients with retinoblastoma should have frequent evaluations by an ophthalmologist, because the disease can be hereditary. The skin neoplasms of the eyelid may be prevented by wearing sunglasses and wide-brimmed hats to reduce sun exposure of that area.

Patient Teaching

Information given to the patient is determined by the type of neoplasm, the treatment, and the prognosis. Patients, or the parents of children, benefit from clear explanations of all ongoing diagnostic and therapeutic procedures. In all cases, emotional support is imperative. Referral for genetic counseling is helpful for families of patients with the heritable form of retinoblastoma.

Disorders of the Ear

Functioning Organs of Hearing

The ear is the organ of balance and the organ of hearing. The ear is composed of three sections: the outer ear, the middle ear, and the inner ear (Fig. 5.22).

The outer section is made up of the external ear, also called the *pinna* or *auricle,* and the external auditory canal. The latter's function is to collect sound waves, or vibrations, from the air or environment and channel them to the tympanic membrane (eardrum), which then begins to vibrate.

The middle section contains the tympanic membrane and three ossicles (tiny bones) called the *malleus* (hammer), the *incus* (anvil), and the *stapes* (stirrup). Also in the middle ear is a canal, called the *eustachian tube,* which leads to a cavity (the pharynx) at the back of the nose. At the innermost region of the middle ear is the oval window, the opening to the inner ear. The middle ear receives the sound waves from the vibrating eardrum and relays them along the three bones to the oval window (see Fig. 5.22).

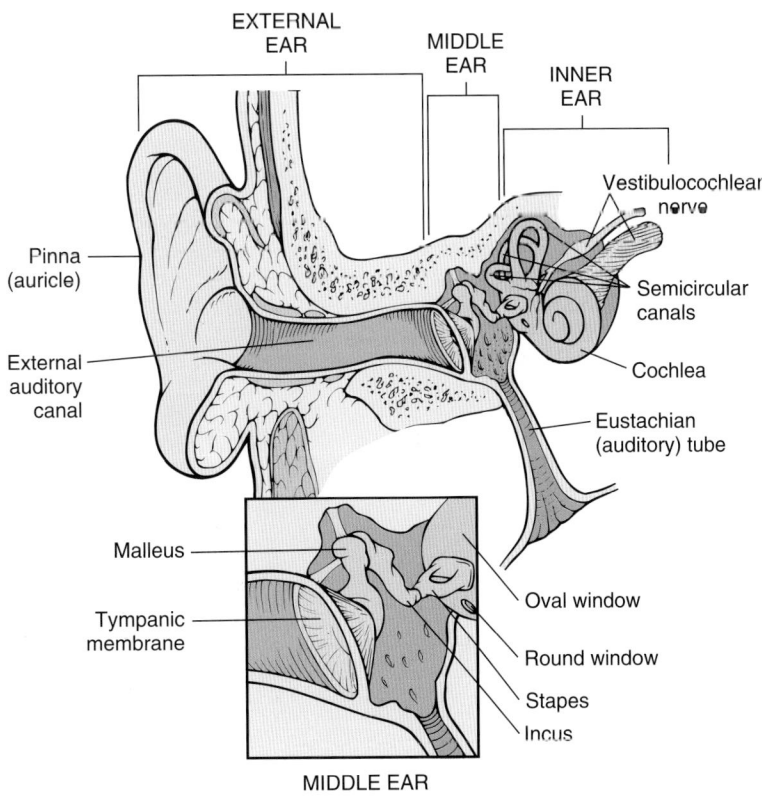

• **Fig. 5.22** Normal ear.

The inner ear contains two membrane-lined chambers, each filled with fluid, called the *cochlea* and the labyrinth. The cochlea contains tiny hairs that change the sound waves in the fluid into nerve impulses, which then are transmitted to the brain via the auditory nerve. The labyrinth is responsible for maintaining balance. It consists of three connected tubes bent into half circles, called the *semicircular canals.* Their function is to detect movement of the head and relay this information to the brain.

Common symptoms of ear diseases and conditions that should receive attention from health care professionals include the following:

- hearing loss
- ear pain or pressure
- tinnitus (ringing or buzzing noise)
- vertigo (dizziness)
- nausea and vomiting

Hearing loss or deafness is denoted as two basic types: conductive loss and sensorineural loss. Conductive deafness is caused by an impairment of the eardrum or bones in the middle ear, which conduct sound waves to the cochlea in the inner ear. Sensorineural deafness, or nerve deafness, results from impairment of the cochlea or the auditory nerve (see the Enrichment box about Cochlear Implants).

Central deafness results when the central nervous system (CNS) cannot interpret impulses because of a cerebrovascular accident (CVA) or brain tumor (see the Alert box about Ototoxicity for chemical causes of temporary or permanent hearing loss).

Disorders of Conduction

Impacted Cerumen

Description

Impacted cerumen is atypical accumulation of cerumen in the canal of the outer ear. The "earwax" that has accumulated hardens and has a tendency to prevent sound waves from reaching the tympanic membrane (eardrum), resulting in decreased hearing (Fig. 5.24).

ICD-10-CM Code	H61.23 *(Impacted cerumen, bilateral)*
	(H61.20-H61.23 = 4 codes of specificity)

Symptoms and Signs

The normal soft, yellowish brown, waxlike secretion produced by the glands of the external ear canal is called *cerumen,* or earwax. If this secretion accumulates excessively, gradual loss of hearing may occur, and the patient may have

---

❖ ENRICHMENT

Cochlear Implants

Individuals who experience severe sensorineural hearing loss that is not helped by hearing aids may have partial hearing restored by means of cochlear implants. Cochlear implants are electronic devices that use minute electrical currents to stimulate the auditory nerve and help the currents travel to the auditory cortex to be perceived as sound.

Cochlear implant systems are complex and include an electrode array, a receiver, a speech processor, a transmitting coil, and a microphone. The electrode array is placed surgically in the cochlea, and the receiver is implanted and fixed to the skull behind the mastoid bone. The surgical incision is allowed to heal for 4 to 6 weeks, after which the external components (the microphone, transmitting coil, and speech processor) are fitted to the patient. Fitting includes calibration of the transmitting coil and programming of the speech processor. Auditory and speech training are provided to the implant recipient.

Cochlear implants do not restore normal hearing; however, they can improve a deaf person's functioning in a hearing world. Candidates for the implants are selected carefully and should have a severe to profound bilateral sensorineural hearing loss and be older than 2 years of age. Many still employ lip reading and American Sign Language (ASL) as adjunct therapies to communicate.

An alternative implant device uses the principle of bone conduction to conduct sound waves to the inner ear. The bone conduction system is for individuals who experience conductive hearing loss, mixed, or single-sided hearing loss. Sound waves are transmitted to the inner ear by bone conduction bypassing outer or middle ear problems. A bone conduction system has

an internal bone conduction implant (BCI) that is placed entirely subcutaneously. It contains a magnet to hold the externally placed audio processor above the BCI. The audio processor consists of a battery, microphones, and a digital processor. Fig. 5.23 shows cochlear implants.

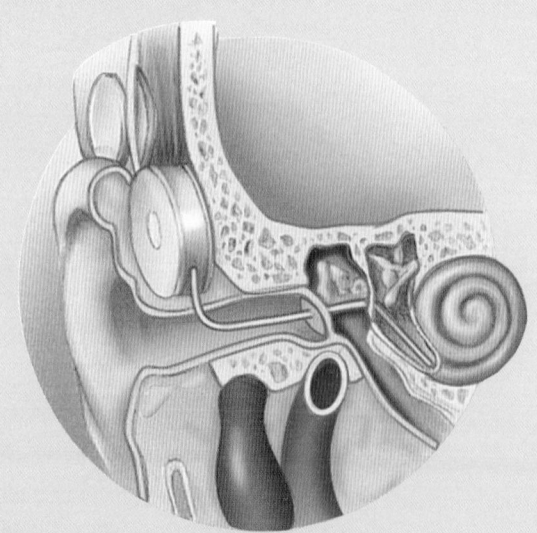

• **Fig. 5.23** Cochlear implant. (From Patton KT, Thibodeau GA: *The human body in health & disease,* ed 6, St Louis, 2014, Elsevier.)

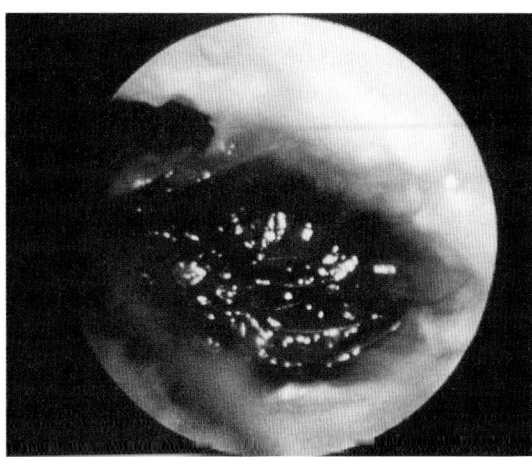

• **Fig. 5.24** Impacted cerumen. (From Sigler B: *Ear, nose, and throat disorders—Mosby's clinical nursing series,* St Louis, 1994, Mosby.)

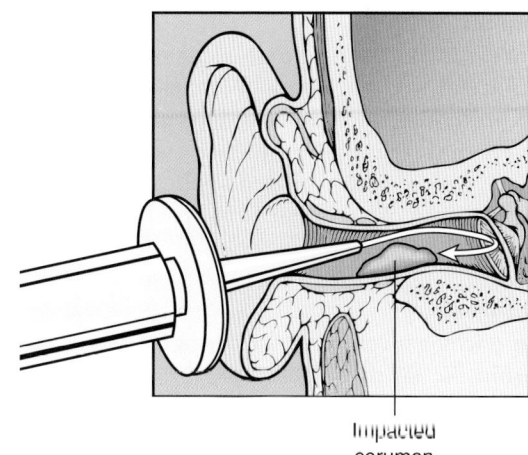

Impacted cerumen

• **Fig. 5.25** Irrigation of the ear for impacted cerumen. Irrigation of the ear also is used to remove foreign bodies.

ⓘ ALERT!

Ototoxicity

Ototoxicity occurs when a drug or chemical causes damage to CN VIII (acoustic nerve) or to the inner ear, resulting in temporary or permanent hearing loss or disturbances in balance. Symptoms and signs of ototoxicity usually have an insidious onset and include tinnitus, a feeling of fullness or pressure in the ears, hearing loss, vertigo, and occasionally nausea.

Drugs that can cause ototoxicity include salicylates (aspirin and aspirin-containing products); nonsteroidal antiinflammatory drugs (NSAIDs); certain antibiotics (aminoglycosides, erythromycin, and vancomycin); loop diuretics (furosemide [Lasix], bumetanide [Bumex], and ethacrynic acid [Edecrin]); chemotherapeutic agents (cisplatin, vincristine, and vinblastine); quinines (quinidine and quinine); and heavy metals, including mercury and lead.

The physician should be notified of any of the aforementioned symptoms when the individual is taking or going to receive any of the previously mentioned medications.

Discontinuing aspirin, aspirin-containing products, and NSAIDs often reverses the ototoxic effects of these drugs.

Any of the other drugs should not be discontinued unless so ordered by the physician. Quinine ototoxicity, like aspirin-induced ototoxicity, usually can be reversed when the medication is stopped. Large dosages of antibiotics that may be ototoxic usually are administered in life-threatening situations.

Chemotherapeutic agents are monitored for any ototoxic side effects. In normal dosages, the loop diuretics usually have very few ototoxic side effects; it is when they are given in massive doses for treatment of acute kidney failure or acute hypertension that ototoxicity may occur.

Environmental chemicals include, but are not limited to, butyl nitrite, carbon disulfide, hexane, styrene, toluene, trichloroethylene, and xylene.

Once damage has occurred, it cannot be reversed. Hearing loss may be helped somewhat by hearing aids or cochlear implants. When the patient experiences loss of balance, physical therapy may be needed to help the patient regain the ability to balance.

a feeling that the ear is plugged and may experience tinnitus or sometimes an earache (otalgia). Impacted cerumen is a common cause of conductive hearing loss.

Patient Screening

Individuals complaining of ear pain should be seen as soon as possible. Many times, the only complaint is one of reduced hearing level. Schedule an appointment as soon as possible. Referral to an audiologist may be indicated. Awareness of the incidence of impacted cerumen may come about during a routine examination or during the course of an office visit for some other reason.

Etiology

Abnormal accumulation of cerumen can be caused by dryness and scaling of the skin or by excessive hair in the ear canal. Some people have abnormally narrow ear canals, which may predispose them to this condition.

Diagnosis

The physician or specialist does an otologic examination, and the patient history of symptoms confirms the diagnosis.

Treatment

If impacted cerumen is found, it must be removed. If the cerumen adheres to the wall of the ear canal, it may have to be softened first with oily drops or hydrogen peroxide and then irrigated with water to accomplish removal (Fig. 5.25). Any hearing loss caused by the impaction is alleviated after removal of cerumen.

Prognosis

The prognosis for removal is positive. Hearing usually improves once the ear canal is clear of the impacted earwax. Recurrence is likely, so periodic examinations may be necessary.

Prevention
Prevention includes routine cleansing of the ear canal by the primary care physician or an ear care specialist. Other prevention includes avoiding placing any object in the ear canal that may push the earwax down into the ear canal. Use of cotton-tipped applicators in the ear is often the cause of cerumen being packed into the ear canal.

Patient Teaching
Patient teaching involves reinforcement of not putting anything into the ear that would have the ability to push or pack the earwax down into the outer ear canal. Providing written information concerning proper ear care to the patient and family is helpful.

Infective Otitis Externa
Description
Inflammation of the external ear canal is called *otitis externa*. This condition is usually accompanied by an infectious process.

ICD-10-CM Code	H60.399 *(Other infective otitis externa, unspecified ear)*

(H60.391-H60.399 = 4 codes of specificity)
H60.00 *(Abscess of external ear, unspecified ear)*
(H60.00-H60.03 = 4 codes of specificity)
H60.10 *(Cellulitis of external ear, unspecified ear)*
(H60.10-H60.13 = 4 codes of specificity)
H60.319 *(Diffuse otitis externa, unspecified ear)*
(H60.311-H60.319 = 4 codes of specificity)
H60.329 *(Hemorrhagic otitis externa, unspecified ear)*
(H60.321-H60.329 = 4 codes of specificity)
H60.399 *(Other infective otitis externa, unspecified ear)*
(H60.391-H60.399 = 4 codes of specificity)

Designation by the physician of any special circumstances determines the applicable code. Refer to the physician's diagnosis and then to the current edition of the ICD-10-CM coding manual to ensure the greatest specificity of pathology.

Symptoms and Signs
Severe pain; a red, swollen ear canal; hearing loss; fever; and pruritus are common symptoms of otitis externa. Drainage from the ear may be either watery or purulent.

Patient Screening
Individuals reporting pain in the ear accompanied by drainage require prompt attention.

Etiology
Accumulation of cerumen in the ear canal, when mixed with water, acts as a culture medium for bacteria or fungi. Otitis externa also may be caused by dermatologic conditions, such as seborrhea and psoriasis. Trauma to the ear canal, caused by attempts to clean or scratch inside the ear with a foreign object or frequent use of earphones and earplugs or hearing aids can predispose a person to the development of otitis externa.

Diagnosis
An otologic examination and a history of symptoms confirm the diagnosis (Fig. 5.26). If a bacterial infection is suspected, a culture of the material found in the canal may be needed to determine how to properly treat the infection.

Treatment
The ear canal must be kept clean and free from water. Antibiotic or steroid eardrops and systemic antibiotics may be prescribed, depending on the severity. Otitis externa tends to recur and can become chronic.

Prognosis
The prognosis is positive with treatment. Chronic otitis externa may develop with repeated irritation by earphones, earplugs, or hearing aids.

Prevention
Preventive measures include keeping the ear clean and dry. It is important to also keep earphones, earplugs, and hearing aids clean. Additionally, the use of another person's earphones or earplugs is discouraged. If this is a usual practice, any shared object placed in the ears should be disinfected before use.

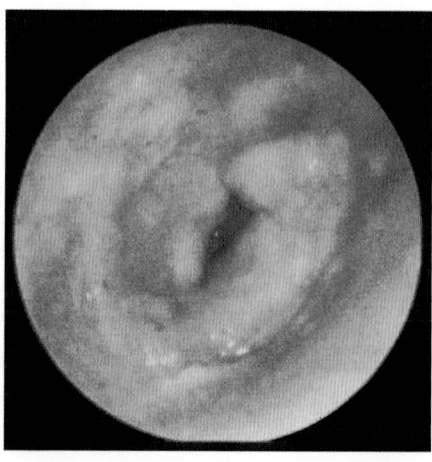
• **Fig. 5.26** External otitis.

Patient Teaching

Provide the patient or family with pictures of the anatomy of the ear. Demonstrate how moisture trapped in the ear by earphones, earplugs, or hearing aids can contribute to infective otitis externa. Explain why sharing of objects that are placed in the ear may cause infective otitis externa.

Swimmer's Ear

Description

Inflammation and resulting infection of the outer ear canal after water has been entrapped during swimming is termed *swimmer's ear*.

ICD-10-CM Code	H60.339 *(Swimmer's ear, unspecified ear)* (H60.331-H60.339 = 4 codes of specificity)

Symptoms and Signs

Similar to infectious otitis externa, severe pain; a red, swollen ear canal; hearing loss; fever; and pruritus are common symptoms of swimmer's ear. Any drainage from the ear may be either watery or purulent. Typically, the onset of the condition occurs after the patient has been swimming.

Patient Screening

Individuals reporting pain in the ear accompanied by drainage require prompt attention.

Etiology

Accumulation of cerumen in the ear canal when mixed with water, as during swimming, acts as a culture medium for bacteria or fungi.

Diagnosis

An otologic examination and a history of symptoms confirm the diagnosis. If a bacterial infection is suspected, a culture of the material found in the canal may be needed to determine how to properly treat the infection.

Treatment

It is important for the ear canal to be kept clean and to be dried after swimming. Antibiotic or steroid eardrops and systemic antibiotics may be prescribed, depending on the severity of the condition. Swimmer's ear tends to recur and can become chronic for those with repeated exposure to water, as in swimming.

Prognosis

Prognosis is positive with treatment. Swimmer's ear has a tendency to recur with subsequent exposure to water during swimming or other water-related activities.

Prevention

Preventive measures include keeping the ear clean and dry. Ear plugs may be used during water activities and swimming.

Thorough drying of the ear canal after exposure to water is important.

Patient Teaching

Provide the patient or family with pictures of the anatomy of the ear. Demonstrate how moisture in the ear can contribute to swimmer's ear. Encourage compliance with any drug therapy prescribed and also to report any symptoms of swimmer's ear as early as possible for treatment.

Otitis Media

Description

Otitis media is inflammation of the normally air-filled middle ear with the accumulation of fluid behind the tympanic membrane (eardrum), occurring either unilaterally or bilaterally.

ICD-10-CM Code	H65.90 *(Unspecified nonsuppurative otitis media, unspecified ear)* (H65.90-H65.93 = 4 codes of specificity) H66.009 *(Acute suppurative otitis media without spontaneous rupture of eardrum, unspecified ear)* (H66.001-H66.009 = 8 codes of specificity)

Refer to the physician's diagnosis and then to the current edition of the ICD-10-CM coding manual to ensure the greatest specificity of pathology.

Symptoms and Signs

Otitis media is the most common reason for visits to physicians by children and also can be experienced by adults.

Otitis media is classified as either serous or suppurative, according to the composition of the accumulating fluid. In serous (nonsuppurative) otitis media, the fluid is relatively clear and sterile. With suppurative otitis, the fluid is purulent. Symptoms vary according to the type. With serous otitis media, the only symptoms may be a feeling of fullness or pressure and some degree of impaired hearing. Suppurative otitis media, also referred to as *acute otitis media,* however, is painful and usually has sudden onset. General symptoms, such as infection, fever, chills, nausea, and vomiting, usually accompany this type. Children often rub or pull at the affected ear and lean the head sideways toward the affected side. Dizziness can be a symptom in either type. Muffled hearing may be present, or a significant loss of hearing may occur.

Patient Screening

The febrile individual or child experiencing ear pain and possible diminished hearing requires prompt assessment and pain relief. If it is not possible to see the patient the same day as the initial phone contact, refer the patient to another medical care facility where prompt assessment can be provided.

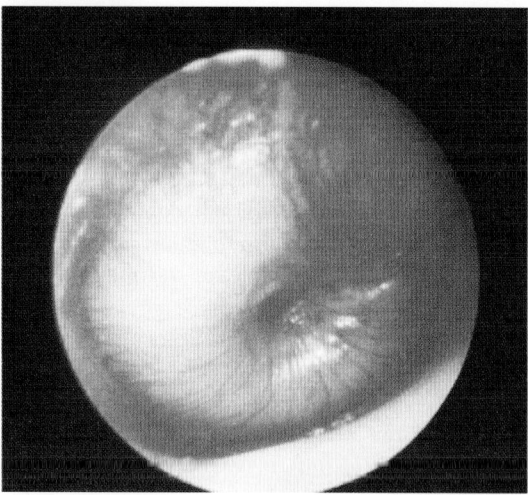

• **Fig. 5.27** Acute otitis media. (From Sigler B: *Ear, nose, and throat disorders—Mosby's clinical nursing series,* St Louis, 1994, Mosby.)

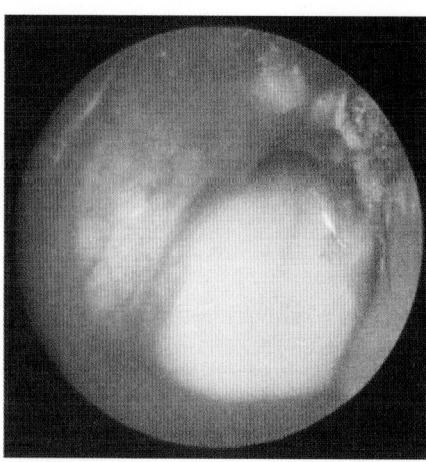

• **Fig. 5.29** Suppurative otitis media. (From Sigler B. *Ear, nose, and throat disorders—Mosby's clinical nursing series,* St Louis, 1994, Mosby.)

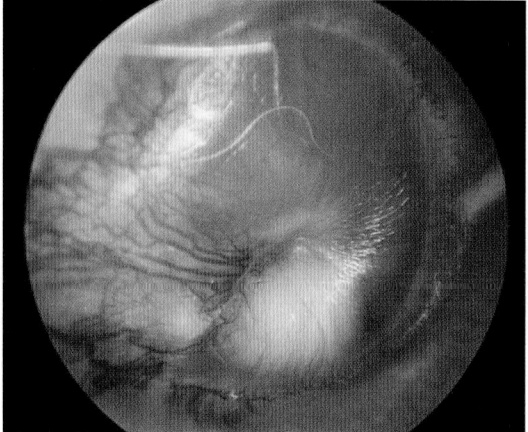

• **Fig. 5.28** Chronic otitis media. (From Damjanov I, Linder J: *Pathology: a color atlas,* St Louis, 1999, Mosby.)

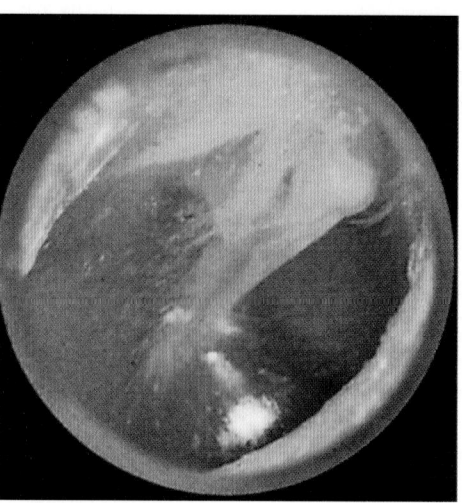

• **Fig. 5.30** Normal tympanic membrane. (From Seidel HM, et al: *Mosby's guide to physical examination,* ed 7, St Louis, 2011, Mosby. Courtesy Richard A. Buckingham, Otolaryngology, Abraham Lincoln School of Medicine, University of Illinois, Chicago, IL.)

Etiology

Serous otitis media may be either acute or chronic. With acute serous otitis media (Fig. 5.27), the cause is usually a virus from a URI that has spread through the eustachian tube into the middle ear. It can occur spontaneously or may result from an allergic reaction. Chronic otitis media (Fig. 5.28) can develop from an acute attack, hypertrophy of the adenoids, or chronic sinus infections. Suppurative otitis media (Fig. 5.29) is caused by bacteria, which also can enter the middle ear through the eustachian tube from the nose or throat or from a ruptured tympanic membrane. This condition often follows a bout of influenza or mumps. Variations in the normal structure of the eustachian tube can predispose a person to this disease. Often an allergic response is responsible for swelling of the eustachian tube and the resulting otitis media.

Diagnosis

Otoscopy reveals the presence of a fluid-filled middle ear. The normally pearl-gray eardrum (Fig. 5.30) is inflamed and may be bulging. Fluid bubbles may be visible through the membrane. If a culture of the fluid taken from the ear shows bacteria and the white blood cell (WBC) count is elevated, suppurative otitis media is present. Audiometry may reveal mild to severe hearing loss. Measurement of the pressure in the middle ear with a tympanogram provides the physician with an estimation of how well the eustachian tube is functioning.

Treatment

Analgesics and decongestants may be ordered to provide pain relief and to promote drainage in both types of otitis media. Oral or topical antibiotics are ordered for cases of suppurative otitis media. In severe cases or in patients who fail to respond to medical treatment, surgical evacuation of the fluid (**myringotomy**) is necessary to prevent permanent hearing loss and the possible development of mastoiditis (see the Mastoiditis section) or a cholesteatoma (see the Cholesteatoma section). To keep the middle ear filled with air and to prevent fluid from accumulating, myringotomy tubes (Fig. 5.31) may need to be inserted after the myringotomy (Fig. 5.32). Diagnosis and treatment of any allergic response involved is necessary. Removal of hypertrophic adenoids is a therapeutic measure.

Prognosis

Prognosis is positive with drug therapy. Otitis media often recurs; thus any indication of returning symptoms requires prompt attention. Surgical intervention with placement of myringotomy tubes usually helps promote a positive outcome. Identification of allergic-mediated responses and removal of enlarged adenoids is also helpful for a positive outcome.

Prevention

Prompt treatment of URI helps prevent the occurrence of otitis media. When the otitis is a result of an upper respiratory allergic reaction, diagnosis and control of allergic response is helpful, as is the surgical removal of hypertrophied adenoids.

Patient Teaching

If surgery is scheduled, provide patients and family with information regarding the care of the ear with myringotomy tubes in place. Stress the importance of drug therapy compliance and completion of the prescribed antibiotic regimen.

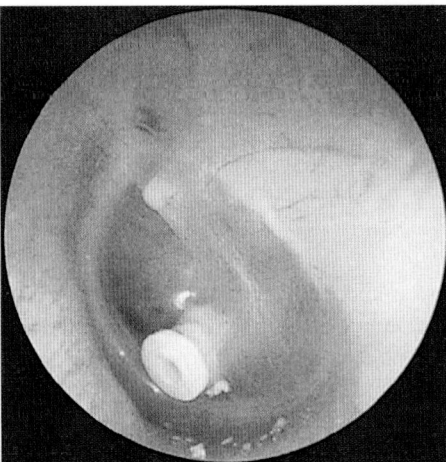

• **Fig. 5.31** Myringotomy tube. (From Fireman P, Slavin RG: *Atlas of allergies,* ed 3, London, 2003, Gower Medical Publishing.)

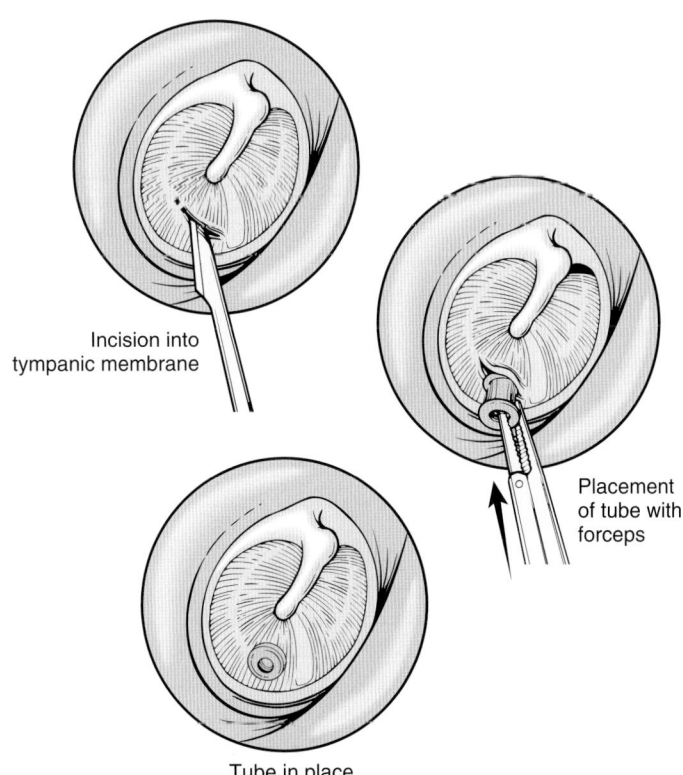

Incision into tympanic membrane

Placement of tube with forceps

Tube in place

• **Fig. 5.32** Myringotomy and insertion of a tympanoplasty tube as a treatment for otitis media.

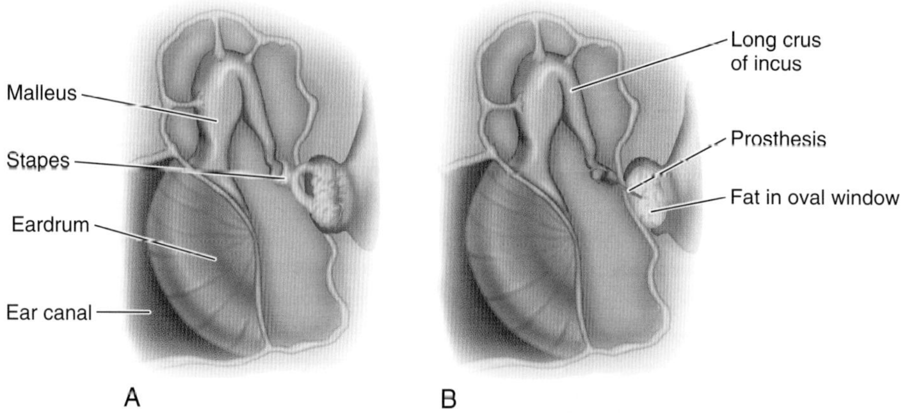

• **Fig. 5.33** Illustration of Otosclerosis Showing Bones Fusing. (A) Pre-intervention of otosclerosis. (B) Post-intervention treatment for otosclerosis with prosthesis insertion. (From Black JM, Hawks JH: *Medical-surgical nursing: clinical management for positive outcomes,* ed 8, St Louis, 2009, Saunders.)

Otosclerosis

Description

Otosclerosis, an abnormal bone growth in the middle ear, primarily affects the stapes, the third bone or ossicle of the middle ear, as the individual ages. Movement of the ossicles is impaired, which causes diminished conduction of sound waves and resulting hearing loss (Fig. 5.33).

| ICD-10-CM Code | H80.93 *(Unspecified otosclerosis, bilateral)* (H80.00-H80.93 = 20 codes of specificity) |

Designation by the physician of any special circumstances determines the applicable code. Refer to the physician's diagnosis and then to the current edition of the ICD-10-CM coding manual to ensure the greatest specificity of pathology.

Symptoms and Signs

With this condition, an abnormal growth of spongy bone forms around the oval window, causing ankylosis of the stapes, the third ossicle (small bone) in the middle ear.

Ankylosis produces conductive deafness because the ossicles cannot conduct the sound vibrations as they enter the ear. Symptoms of otosclerosis are tinnitus and a gradual hearing loss of low or soft sounds, which may be unilateral at first but usually affects both ears at some point. Patients usually report not being able to hear as well with the affected ear when talking on the telephone. Relatives may notice that patients turn their heads to hear well. Otosclerosis is a young person's disease, with onset usually beginning after puberty and before age 35 years.

Patient Screening

Individuals requesting an appointment for evaluation of decreased hearing are scheduled for the next available appointment that is convenient for them. It is important to realize that patients experiencing hearing loss may be anxious.

Etiology

Otosclerosis is idiopathic, but there is evidence of familial tendency, suggesting genetic factors. The condition seems to be more prevalent in women and can be aggravated by pregnancy.

Diagnosis

A diagnosis of otosclerosis is made by the physician using an audiogram, the patient history, and otoscopy. The audiogram shows a moderate to severe hearing loss, especially for loss in the low range.

Treatment

The only treatment that cures otosclerosis is a surgical procedure called *stapedectomy*. A stapedectomy involves the removal of the diseased stapes and replacement with a prosthesis. The composition of the prosthesis may be metal or a ceramic or plastic material. Use of ceramic or plastic is likely because these materials facilitate visualization with MRI for the purpose of diagnosing and because of the inability to perform an accurate test of the patient's hearing if the prosthesis is made of metal. If the condition is bilateral, only one ear is operated on at a time so that the success of the procedure can be evaluated. Generally, hearing improves soon after the surgery. A recent procedure, stapedotomy, is performed with laser, which creates a hole in the stapes permitting placement of a prosthetic device. If surgery is not an option for the patient, a hearing aid can be tried.

Prognosis

Surgical intervention usually has a positive outcome.

Prevention

Because this is an idiopathic condition, no method of prevention is known.

Patient Teaching

Provide patients and families with information concerning postsurgical care for surgical intervention. Assist patients and families in locating and contacting community support groups for those with diminished hearing.

Meniere Disease

Description

Meniere disease is a chronic disease of the inner ear that affects the labyrinth.

ICD-10-CM Code	H81.09 (Ménière disease, unspecified ear)
	(H81.01-H81.09 = 4 codes of specificity)

There are specific codes for various states and sites of Ménière disease. Once the physician has established the pathologic evolvement of Meniere's disease, refer to the physician's diagnosis and then to the current edition of the ICD-10-CM coding manual to ensure the greatest specificity of pathology.

Symptoms and Signs

Meniere disease is marked by a recurring syndrome of vertigo, tinnitus, progressive hearing loss, and a sensation of fullness or pressure in the affected ear. Symptoms have a sudden onset. Nausea, vomiting, tinnitus, sweating, and loss of balance can follow an acute attack of vertigo. Some individuals may be subjected to nystagmus, whereas others may experience an unusual sensitivity to noises (hyperacusis). These attacks can last from a few hours to several days and may become increasingly serious with each recurrence. Meniere disease usually affects just one ear, but both ears may become involved eventually. The disease usually manifests in individuals 40 to 50 years of age.

Patient Screening

Individuals reporting symptoms of vertigo, tinnitus, progressive hearing loss, and the sensation of fullness and pressure in the ear require prompt assessment and intervention. If an appointment time is not immediately available, refer the patient to an emergency facility for evaluation. Suggest that the patient not drive.

Etiology

The cause of this disease is unknown; however, the disease process seems to involve destruction of the tiny hair cells inside the cochlea. It recently has been postulated that an increase in endolymph may cause the membranous labyrinth to dilate, creating the symptoms. Predisposing factors for Meniere disease are middle ear infections, head trauma, dysfunction in the autonomic nervous system, noise pollution, and premenstrual edema.

Diagnosis

The presence of four core symptoms (recurring vertigo, tinnitus, progressive hearing loss, and a sensation of fullness [aural fullness] in the ear) suggests the diagnosis of Meniere disease. Additional testing with audiometry; balance studies; radiographic studies, including MRI; and ENG may be necessary. Electrocochleograph (EcoG) studies, a recent addition to the available diagnostic techniques, are used to measure inner ear fluid pressure.

Treatment

For acute attacks of Meniere disease, the physician usually prescribes medication to control the nausea, vomiting, and dizziness. Long-term treatment could include following a salt-free diet; restricting fluid intake; and using diuretics, meclizine, and mild sedatives. Limiting the amount of caffeine and alcohol in the diet and stopping smoking may be recommended. Patients are encouraged to avoid stressful situations if possible. If the disease does not respond to dietary restrictions and medications, surgical intervention may be needed. Surgical destruction of the affected labyrinth, using ultrasound, relieves the symptoms but also causes permanent hearing loss unless the cochlea is preserved.

Prognosis

No cure for Meniere disease is known. The goal of treatment is to improve or control symptoms. This condition has a tendency to recur.

Prevention

At the present time, no etiology has been established, and therefore no preventive measures have been identified. Prompt treatment of otitis media is a prudent action and hopefully can ameliorate the condition.

Patient Teaching

Provide patients and family with information regarding the condition and its possible outcomes. Assist patients and families with locating and contacting appropriate community resource agencies for those with decreased hearing. Encourage patients to make changes in their lifestyles, such as avoiding caffeine and alcohol, stopping smoking, and avoiding possible stressful situations. Caution the patients not to drive or operate machinery while symptoms persist.

Benign Paroxysmal Positional Vertigo

Description

Benign paroxysmal positional vertigo (BPPV) is usually a vestibular system disorder. Patients complain of a spinning sensation, which becomes worse with movement of the head. They also may complain of a feeling that their surroundings are moving.

ICD-10-CM Code	H53.139 (Sudden visual loss, unspecified eye)
	(H53.131-H53.139 = 4 codes of specificity)

Symptoms and Signs

Patients with BPPV experience a spinning sensation with movement of the head. The dizziness experienced is that the room is spinning while the body is still; this is a false sensation. With closed eyes, the individual feels that the body is moving, and with the eyes open, the surroundings appear to be spinning. Nausea, vomiting, involuntary eye movement, and difficulty standing or walking may be present. The patient may report a feeling of dizziness, light-headedness, unsteadiness, and feeling faint. Although most of the episodes of vertigo are transient, lasting from 3 to 10 seconds (or slightly longer), the patient may experience an episode that feels much longer. Most report onset with change of position, turning over in bed, moving the head side to side, bending over, getting out of bed or a chair, and when looking up.

Patient Screening

An individual experiencing vertigo is usually in distress and will request prompt medical attention. Schedule the first available appointment. Advise the patient not to drive and to find assistance with transportation.

Etiology

The spinning sensation usually is the result of balance or equilibrium disorders. Normal functioning of the vestibular system occurs with movement of the head, causing transmission of impulses to the labyrinth in the inner ear. The labyrinth contains the three semicircular canals that are surrounded by fluid. This transmission of impulses causes a subsequent transmission to the vestibular nerve, which then transmits the impulse to the brainstem and the cerebellum. The brainstem and the cerebellum are responsible for the coordination of balance, movement, consciousness, and blood pressure. When the system is not functioning properly, problems with equilibrium, dizziness, light-headedness, and balance disorders occur. Head trauma may be a causative factor. Occasionally otitis media may be a precursor. Free-floating carbonate crystals that find their way into the semicircular canals may be the cause of the vertigo. Additional causes may be a viral infection, vascular in origin, or as an isolated symptom of unknown cause.

Diagnosis

Diagnosis is made from the history and examination. In addition to the false sensation of the room spinning or the patient spinning, nystagmus (involuntary eye movements) may be present. An audiogram or other means of hearing testing are used to determine the patient's level of hearing. Many times, the hearing is decreased. Lack of coordination may be detected, along with weakness and unsteadiness in the legs. Additional testing to rule out CNS involvement may include head CT, MRI of the head, or magnetic resonance angiogram (MRA) of the brain's blood vessels. Another test is caloric stimulation, where, using a syringe, cool water followed by warm water is gently flushed against the eardrum to test eye reflexes. In a normal test, no abnormal eye movements are observed. During the test, BPPV can be detected if the eyes show involuntary movement from side to side. Blood tests may be ordered to rule out other disease conditions.

Treatment

Antihistamines (meclizine [Antivert, Dramamine]), anticholinergics (scopolamine [Scopace]), and benzodiazepines (prochlorperazine [Compazine]) may be prescribed to reduce the symptoms of positional vertigo. Exercises, such as the individual repeatedly turning the head from side to side, may also be helpful.

Prognosis

When the condition is benign, medication often will control the symptoms, as will the prescribed exercises. Often the vertigo resolves with time.

Prevention

There is no prevention for this condition.

Patient Teaching

Encourage the patient to take the medications as prescribed. Also instruct on how to perform the prescribed exercises. Caution the patient not to drive or operate machinery while symptoms persist.

Labyrinthitis

Description

Labyrinthitis is inflammation or infection of the labyrinth of the inner ear.

ICD-10-CM Code	H83.09 (*Labyrinthitis, unspecified ear*)
	(H83.01-H83.2X9 = 12 codes of specificity)

Additional digits are required. Once the physician has designated the pathology and type of labyrinthitis, refer to the physician's diagnosis and then to the current edition of the ICD-10-CM coding manual to ensure the greatest specificity of pathology.

Symptoms and Signs

The labyrinth is a group of three fluid-filled chambers (the semicircular canals) in the inner ear that control balance (Fig. 5.34). Inflammation or infection of these chambers is called *labyrinthitis.* The onset of infection is often acute and is associated with fever, with temperatures of 100°F to

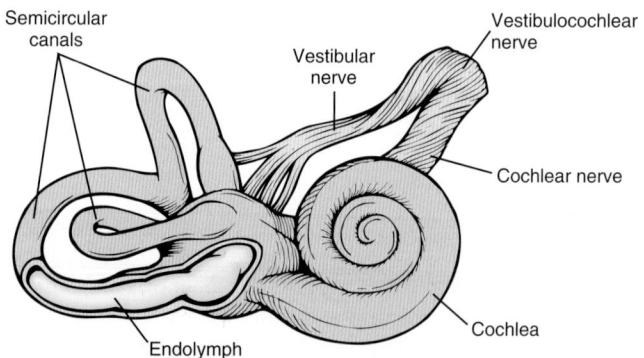

• **Fig. 5.34** Labyrinth or inner ear. Labyrinthitis is caused by a disturbance in the fluid in the semicircular canals.

101°F. The main symptom of this disease is extreme vertigo. Balance is affected, and nausea and vomiting may occur in some cases. The individual with labyrinthitis may experience tinnitus, loss of hearing in one ear, and difficulty focusing the eyes.

Patient Screening

Individuals reporting sudden onset of fever, vertigo, balance problems, and nausea and vomiting require prompt assessment. Refer the patient to an emergency facility for assessment to rule out a severe neurologic infection.

Etiology

Labyrinthitis is usually the result of a virus but can be caused by a bacterial infection that has spread from the middle ear. It also may be a result of meningitis.

Diagnosis

The diagnosis of labyrinthitis is based on the results of several tests, including audiometry and blood, neurologic, caloric, and possibly imaging studies.

Treatment

Bed rest for several days may be necessary. Prescriptions for a tranquilizer, an antiemetic agent, and an antibiotic may be necessary if a bacterial infection is present. Antihistamines and/or corticosteroids also may be prescribed. When properly treated, labyrinthitis is not a dangerous condition; however, it can be debilitating, and the labyrinth is a delicate and easily damaged organ.

Prognosis

In most cases, labyrinthitis completely clears up within 1 to 3 weeks; however, a result of bacterial labyrinthitis may be permanent hearing deficiency or loss and/or balance problems.

Prevention

Prevention involves prompt medical treatment for otitis media or any other ear infection.

Patient Teaching

Stress the importance of seeking medical attention for ear infections. Provide written information about the condition. Encourage the patient to rest and be still when symptoms occur, to avoid sudden change of position, to avoid bright lights, and to try not to read while symptomatic.

Ruptured Tympanic Membrane (Ruptured Eardrum)

Description

Any type of tear or injury to the eardrum causes a breach in the integrity of the membrane. This may be the result of pressure, force, or insult from the exterior aspect, or it may be caused by increased pressure within the middle ear.

ICD-10-CM Code   H72.90 *(Unspecified perforation of tympanic membrane, unspecified ear)*
(H72.00-H72.93,
H73.811-H73.93 = 48
codes of specificity)
Refer to the physician's diagnosis and then to the current edition of the ICD-10-CM coding manual to ensure the greatest specificity of pathology.

Symptoms and Signs

Symptoms of a ruptured tympanic membrane (eardrum) are usually slight pain and partial loss of hearing and may include a slight discharge or bleeding from the ear. Buzzing in the ear and/or facial weakness or dizziness may be experienced. When an infectious process is involved, the drainage usually is purulent in nature. These symptoms may last only a few hours. The major risk is that an infection may develop in the middle ear.

Patient Screening

Individuals calling with complaints of diminished hearing, pain in the ear, ear infections, history of abrupt force or pressure being incurred, and drainage from the ear require prompt assessment.

Etiology

The four most common causes of a ruptured eardrum are insertion of a sharp object into the ear canal, an abrupt explosion (including lightning strikes), a severe middle ear infection, and a blow to the ear. A ruptured eardrum also can occur as a result of a fractured skull. The eardrum occasionally ruptures spontaneously.

Diagnosis

A visual examination of the ear with an otoscope confirms the diagnosis of a ruptured eardrum (Fig. 5.35). Purulent drainage is usually present during an episode of suppurative otitis media complicated by rupture of the tympanic membrane (Fig. 5.36). Audiometry also may be used.

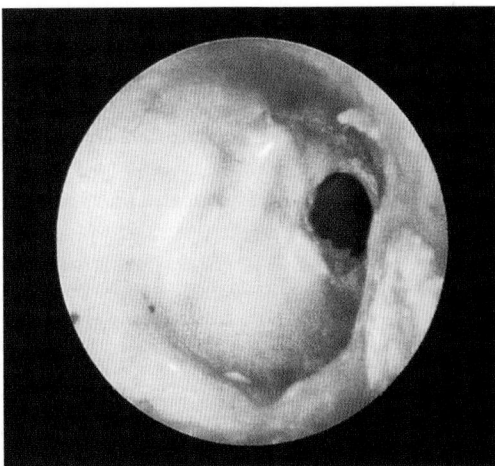

• **Fig. 5.35** Ruptured tympanic membrane. (From Sigler B: *Ear, nose, and throat disorders—Mosby's clinical nursing series,* St Louis, 1994, Mosby.)

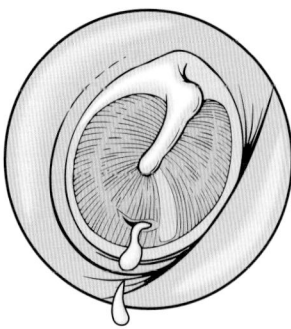

• **Fig. 5.36** Ruptured tympanic membrane with purulent discharge.

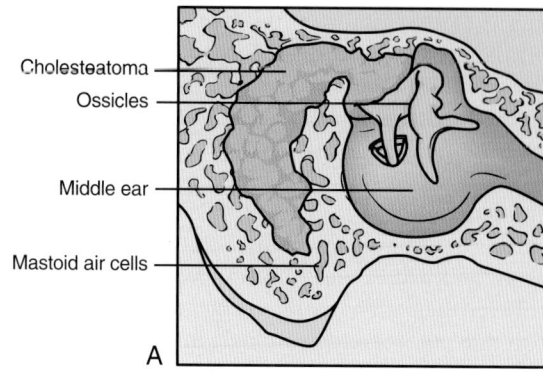

Mastoid air cells and cholesteatoma

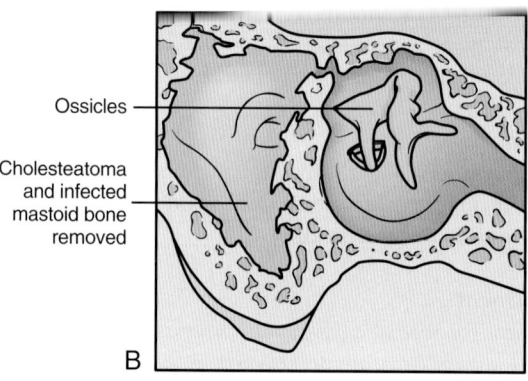

Mastoid bone with air cells and cholesteatoma removed

• **Fig. 5.37** Illustration of Cholesteatoma. (A) Pre-intervention for cholesteatoma. (B) Post-intervention for cholesteatoma. (From Phillips N: *Berry & Kohn's operating room technique,* ed 12, St Louis, 2013, Mosby.)

Cholesteatomas are located at various sites in the ear and therefore have specific codes for various sites. Refer to the physician's diagnosis and then to the current edition of the ICD-10-CM coding manual to ensure the greatest specificity of pathology.

Treatment

An antibiotic may be prescribed to prevent infection, and a patch may be applied to the eardrum to aid healing and to improve hearing. This procedure is similar to a tympanoplasty (tympanoplasty involves actual grafting of tissue for eardrum repair). Analgesics may be prescribed for pain.

Prognosis

Prognosis is good after treatment of the underlying cause. The eardrum heals naturally in about 1 to 2 weeks. After the eardrum has healed, hearing loss is minimal.

Prevention

Prompt intervention in otitis media may help prevent buildup of pressure in the middle ear. It is not possible to prevent many environmental causes of otitis media.

Patient Teaching

Provide an explanation and demonstration of the mechanism of ruptured tympanic membrane. Encourage patients and families to seek early treatment for otitis media.

Cholesteatoma

Description

A cholesteatoma is a pocket of skin cells located in the middle ear, normally shed by the eardrum and that collect into a cystlike mass or ball and become infected. As the infected material accumulates, the bone lining the middle ear cavity erodes, and the ossicles become damaged (Fig. 5.37).

ICD-10-CM Code	H71.20 *(Cholesteatoma of mastoid, unspecified ear)*
	H71.21 *(Cholesteatoma of mastoid, right ear)*
	H71.22 *(Cholesteatoma of mastoid, left ear)*
	H71.23 *(Cholesteatoma of mastoid, bilateral)*
	H71 *(Cholesteatoma of middle ear)*
	(H71.00-H71.93 = 20 codes of specificity)

Symptoms and Signs

The most common symptom of cholesteatoma is mild to moderate hearing loss. A purulent substance may drain from the affected ear, and earache, headache, vertigo, and some weakness of the facial muscles also may be present.

Patient Screening

Individuals with cholesteatomas usually have a history of otitis infections and are scheduled for routine reassessments. Often the condition is recognized during a routine follow-up examination. As with other ear conditions, drainage from the ear and diminished hearing require prompt assessment. The patient should be scheduled for the next available appointment on the day the patient calls.

Etiology

This condition often begins to develop in infancy, or it may be the result of chronic ear infection. The eustachian tube from the middle ear to the pharynx either fails to open properly or becomes blocked with material from recurring middle ear infections (see the Otitis Media section). As a result, this normally air-filled chamber develops a weak vacuum, causing the eardrum to become retracted. This forms the pocket in the eardrum that allows the cholesteatoma to develop.

Diagnosis
Patient history, otoscopy, and audiometry enable the physician to make the diagnosis. Radiographic studies, including CT, also may be useful, and a culture of the purulent drainage may be necessary to determine the most effective antibiotic for treatment.

Treatment
If the cholesteatoma is discovered early, before eroding begins, it can be removed fairly simply by a thorough cleaning of the middle ear cavity. Inflation of the eustachian tube may produce some improvement, and treatment with steroids and antibiotics helps prevent recurrence. If the cholesteatoma is discovered in an advanced stage, its removal becomes much more complicated. Damage to the middle ear structures may be extensive, necessitating surgical reconstruction of these structures. Complications may include deafness in one ear, persistent ear drainage, and vertigo. Badly damaged hearing may be improved with the use of a hearing aid. Additional complications may include erosion into the facial nerve with resulting facial paralysis and/or labyrinthitis. Untreated, a cholesteatoma erodes the roof of the middle ear cavity, making the development of an epidural abscess or meningitis possible.

Prognosis
Surgical intervention usually leads to a positive outcome.

Prevention
Early development of the condition begins in infancy. Prompt attention to otitis infections and problems of eustachian tube drainage helps delay the onset of this condition. Total prevention is not considered possible.

Patient Teaching
Encourage parents of children with chronic otitis media to schedule routine examinations that include audiology testing. Explain the origin and progression of the condition so that families have an understanding of how early intervention can help relieve this condition.

Mastoiditis

Description
Mastoiditis, whether acute or chronic, is inflammation of the mastoid bone, or mastoid process.

ICD-10-CM Code　　H70.90 (Unspecified mastoiditis, unspecified ear)
(H70.001-H70.13, H70.811-H70.93 = 28 codes of specificity)

H70.009 (Acute mastoiditis without complications, unspecified ear)
H70.10 (Chronic mastoiditis, unspecified ear)
Refer to the physician's diagnosis and then to the current edition of the ICD-10-CM coding manual to ensure the greatest specificity of pathology.

Symptoms and Signs
The mastoid is a round process of the temporal bone that can be felt immediately behind each ear and is porous or honeycombed in appearance. Pain and occasionally edema are present over and around the mastoid. Fever and chills, as well as headache and hearing loss, may be present. Some may experience drainage from the affected ear. A profuse discharge from the external canal is likely because of the middle ear involvement.

Patient Screening
Individuals reporting discharge from the ears accompanied by fever, chills, and pain in the mastoid region require prompt assessment. Schedule an appointment that same day, or if none is available, refer the patient to a facility where prompt assessment is possible.

Etiology
Acute mastoiditis is the result of neglected acute otitis media. Common causative organisms are *Streptococcus pneumoniae*, *Haemophilus influenzae*, and *Moraxella catarrhalis*. Less common causes are group A streptococci and *Staphylococcus aureus*. Chronic mastoiditis, necessitating radical or modified radical mastoidectomy, is associated with cholesteatoma.

Diagnosis
The diagnosis is made from patient history; otoscopy; audiometry; radiographic studies, including radiographs and CT of the mastoid; and the results of blood and culture studies.

Treatment
The treatment is based on the results of the sensitivity studies. Antibiotic or sulfonamide therapy is prescribed. Mastoiditis not responding to this treatment necessitates a surgical procedure, called *simple mastoidectomy*, to prevent further complications and to preserve hearing. Radical mastoidectomy may be needed for chronic mastoiditis.

Prognosis
Prognosis is variable and depends on the degree of infection, extent of tissue involvement, and response to antibiotic and drug therapy. Surgical intervention usually corrects chronic involvement. Recurrence may occur when the infection is nonresponsive to antibiotic treatment. Complications may include partial or complete hearing loss of the affected ear. Additionally, there may be destruction of the mastoid bone, facial paralysis, and even meningitis. In severe nonresponsive cases, an epidural abscess may result, along with spread of the infection to the brain.

Prevention

Because acute mastoiditis is the result of neglected acute otitis media, prompt medical intervention for otitis media is essential in preventing complications.

Patient Teaching

Stress the importance of prompt medical treatment of otitis media and completion of the prescribed antibiotic regimen.

Sensorineural Hearing Loss

Description

In sensorineural hearing loss (deafness), also often referred to as *occupational hearing loss,* sound waves reach the inner ear but are not perceived because the nerve impulses are not transmitted to the brain.

ICD-10-CM Code	H90.5 *(Unspecified sensorineural hearing loss)* (H90.3-H90.8 = 8 codes of specificity)

Refer to the physician's diagnosis and then to the current edition of the ICD-10-CM coding manual to ensure the greatest specificity of pathology.

Symptoms and Signs

Symptoms include tinnitus and partial to severe hearing loss.

Patient Screening

Sensorineural hearing loss usually has an insidious onset. Many times, the hearing loss is detected during a routine medical examination or preemployment screening. An abrupt onset of hearing loss is possible after exposure to a sudden loud explosive type of noise or nearby lightning strike. Consider the anxiety level of these individuals when making an appointment for prompt assessment.

Etiology

The cause of sensorineural hearing loss is nerve failure or damage to the cochlea or the auditory nerve (CN VIII, or vestibulocochlear cranial nerve). This can be the result of the aging process (Table 5.3); however, loud music, machinery noise, or sometimes the side effects of medications—including aminoglycosides (tobramycin), loop diuretics, aspirin, or antimetabolites (methotrexate)—can cause such damage at any age (Fig. 5.38). Other causes include mumps, measles, syphilis, meningitis, suppurative labyrinthitis, or viral infections. In addition, physical trauma from fracture of the temporal bone may be a causative factor.

Diagnosis

The patient history and audiometry findings are usually all that is needed to make the diagnosis. Physicians are concerned that sensorineural hearing loss, tinnitus, and vertigo may be symptoms of a space-occupying mass, such as a tumor or an aneurysm; therefore these symptoms are investigated further to rule out such masses.

Treatment

Regardless of the amount of damage to the cochlea, steps must be taken to prevent further damage. Reducing noise levels by implementing measures, such as turning down the volume on loud music and wearing ear protectors at rock concerts or in work areas with high noise levels, can prevent further or future damage to the ears.

Prognosis

Sensorineural hearing loss that is caused by damage to the cochlea is irreversible. Prevention is essential.

Prevention

No method of preventing hearing loss that results from the aging process is known. Prevention of exposure to constant and extensive loud noise is essential in the prevention of sensorineural hearing loss. Use of ear protection at rock

TABLE 5.3	Changes In Hearing Caused By Aging[a]
Changes in Structure	**Changes in Function**
Cochlear hair cell degeneration	Inability to hear high-frequency sounds (presbycusis, sensorineural loss); interferes with understanding speech; hearing may be lost in both ears at different times
Loss of auditory neurons in spiral ganglia of organ of Corti	Inability to hear high-frequency sounds (presbycusis, sensorineural loss); interferes with understanding speech; hearing may be lost in both ears at different times
Degeneration of basilar (cochlear) conductive membrane of cochlea	Inability to hear at all frequencies but more pronounced at higher frequencies (cochlear conductive loss)
Decreased vascularity of cochlea	Equal loss of hearing at all frequencies (strial loss); inability to disseminate localization of sound
Loss of cortical auditory neurons	Equal loss of hearing at all frequencies (strial loss); inability to disseminate localization of sound

[a]Hearing loss affects about one-third of older people.

(From McCance KL, Huether SE: *Pathophysiology: the biological basis for disease in adults and children,* ed 6, St Louis, 2010, Mosby.)

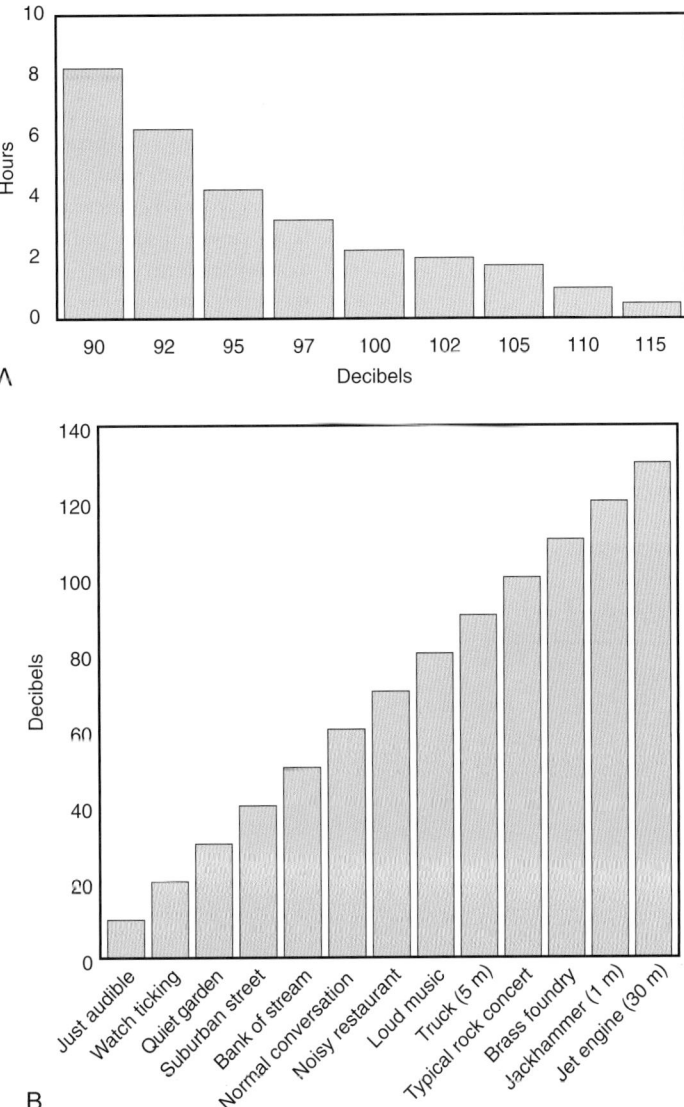

• **Fig. 5.38** (A) Maximum occupational noise exposure (in hours per day) allowed by U.S. Occupational Safety and Health Administration (OSHA) regulations. (B) Examples of decibel levels in everyday situations.

concerts and in work areas with high noise levels is helpful. It is prudent to limit the use of medications that affect the auditory nerve, when possible.

Recommended noise exposure limit is 85 decibels for an 8-hour time average, and any level above this is considered a risk factor for sensorineural hearing loss.

Patient Teaching

Provide patients with information about noise pollution and preventive measures that can be taken, including wearing ear protection when exposure to loud noise is possible. Stress the importance of avoiding high volume on the radio or other audio equipment. Discuss sources of everyday noise pollution.

Cancer of the Ear

Description

Tumors of the ear can occur in any part of the ear and may be benign or malignant. They include skin cancers of the external ear, ceruminal gland neoplasms, acoustic and facial neuromas, and glomus tumors. Many cancers from other locations in the body may metastasize to the ear, resulting in secondary ear cancer.

ICD-10-CM Code	D49.2 (Neoplasm of unspecified behavior of bone, soft tissue, and skin)
	C41.0 (Malignant neoplasm of bones of skull and face)
	C79.89 (Secondary malignant neoplasm of other specified sites)

Neoplasms of the ear must be specified for location and type. Therefore it is not possible to list all applicable codes for neoplasms of the ear. Refer to the physician's diagnosis and then to the current edition of the ICD-10-CM coding manual to ensure the greatest specificity of pathology.

Symptoms and Signs

Symptoms of these neoplasms commonly include progressive hearing loss, chronic otic discharge, a visible mass or lesion on ear examination, loss of equilibrium, and tinnitus. Some cancers, such as SCC of the middle ear, are quite painful. Glomus tumors cause a pulsatile tinnitus, that is, hearing a pulsing sound in the ear that has the tumor, as a result of the tumor pressing on the bones of hearing.

Patient Screening

Symptoms may have an insidious onset with recognition of diminished hearing being thought of as troublesome rather than an acute symptom. Drainage from the ear, loss of equilibrium, and tinnitus require prompt assessment. Schedule patients with these symptoms for the next available appointment on the day of call. It is also important to consider the anxiety experienced by these patients and their families with the onset of these symptoms.

Etiology

Benign tumors of the ear include acoustic neuromas, facial neuromas, and glomus tumors. Acoustic neuroma arises from CN VIII, whereas facial neuroma is a tumor of the facial nerve. These tumors put pressure on the nerve fibers as they expand, causing hearing loss or facial paralysis, respectively, among other symptoms. Glomus tumors are the most common tumors of the middle ear and arise from the glomus bodies (tiny structures that serve as baroreceptors) (Fig. 5.39).

The most common malignant tumors of the external ear are the skin cancers: BCC and SCC (see Chapter 6 for further discussion of these skin cancers). Another type of

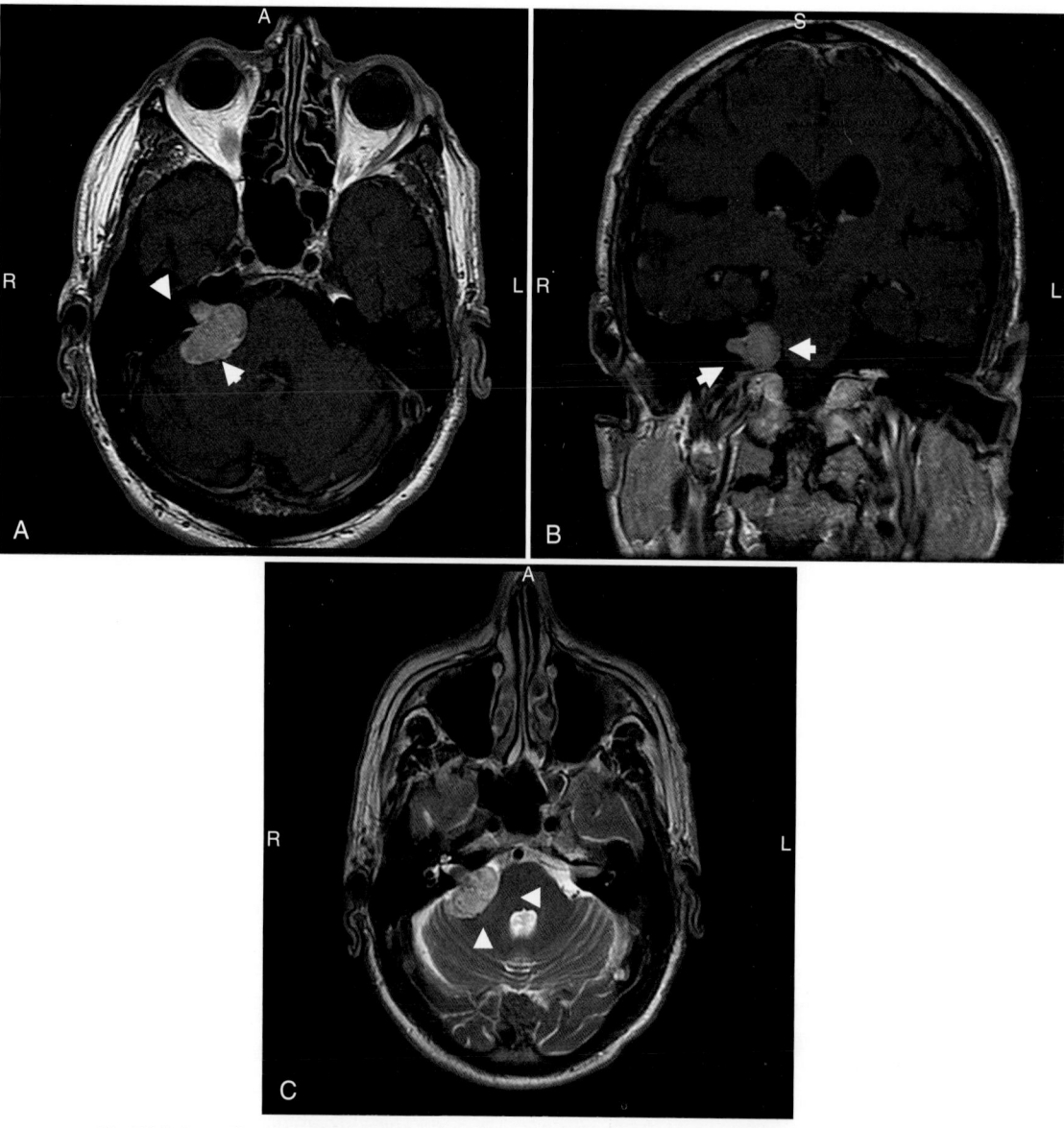

• **Fig. 5.39** Acoustic neuroma magnetic resonance T1-weighted axial. (A) and coronal (B) and T2-weighted axial (C) images show considerable contrast enhancement of the right-sided lesion (arrows and arrowheads). Note the normal neural structures on the left. (From Eisenberg RL, Johnson NM: *Comprehensive radiographic pathology*, ed 7, St Louis, 2021, Elsevier.)

tumor found in the external auditory canal is the ceruminal gland neoplasm, a tumor arising from the glands producing cerumen, which can be either malignant or benign. Malignant tumors of the middle ear are very uncommon. SCC may arise in this location because of chronic inflammation of the middle ear, or mastoid.

Diagnosis

Tumors of the ear are often first identified because of the symptoms they cause. Examination of the ear may reveal a BCC or SCC lesion, a mass in the external ear canal, or evidence of one of the other neoplasms. Biopsy is often performed to confirm the nature of the lesion, and CT and MRI are used to evaluate the extent of disease (see Fig. 5.39).

Treatment

Treatment for all of these tumors is surgical excision. Radiation therapy is used if the tumor is known to be aggressive. A nerve graft may be performed after surgical excision of a neuroma.

Prognosis

Prognosis for many of these tumors is good after the patient receives appropriate treatment. However, SCC of the middle ear has a very poor prognosis because it is often at an advanced stage at the time of diagnosis.

Prevention

No methods for prevention of most ear neoplasms are known. The skin cancers of the external ear may be prevented by reducing sun exposure of that area.

Patient Teaching

Encourage patients to be compliant with prescribed therapy. Provide information for postoperative care of any surgical excision site.

Review Challenge

Answer the following questions:

1. How does the process of normal vision take place?
2. List the three structures of the wall of the eye.
3. What is the function of the iris?
4. Discuss the function of the ciliary body.
5. What are the four main errors of refraction?
6. What is the difference between nystagmus and strabismus?
7. Name a common etiologic factor in hordeolum and blepharitis.
8. What are the pressing symptoms and signs of conjunctivitis? Is the condition contagious?
9. How is dry eye syndrome treated?
10. Name some possible causes of corneal abrasions.
11. How do cataracts interfere with vision?
12. Differentiate between the two primary types of glaucoma.
13. How is diabetic retinopathy detected and treated?
14. Explain the pathology involved in retinal detachment. How is this condition treated?
15. What are the possible causes of exophthalmos?
16. What is the primary symptom of refractive errors?
17. Name the etiologic factors of macular degeneration.
18. What is the best way to help control diabetic retinopathy?
19. Describe some ways cancer can affect the eye and adjacent structures.
20. Describe the three separate parts of the ear.
21. How does impacted cerumen cause deafness?
22. Precisely define *otitis media*. How is it classified? How is it diagnosed?
23. What is myringotomy?
24. What symptoms may an individual with Meniere disease experience?
25. Name the major symptom of labyrinthitis.
26. List common causes of a ruptured eardrum.
27. What causes occupational deafness?
28. List major symptoms of otitis media.
29. Define *otosclerosis*.
30. Which cranial nerve is damaged causing ototoxicity?
31. Which device can be used in the medical office to screen patients for diabetic retinopathy?

Real-Life Challenge: Acute Angle-Closure Glaucoma

A 61-year-old man has sudden onset of blurred vision, head and eye pain, and nausea and vomiting. Upon questioning, he admits to seeing "halos" around lights and being especially sensitive to light. The physician examination confirms blurred vision and photosensitivity. Intraocular pressure (IOP) measures greater than 20 mm Hg on the tonometer.

The patient is diagnosed with acute angle-closure glaucoma and referred to an ophthalmologist for immediate treatment.

Questions

1. Compare the symptoms of chronic open-angle glaucoma and acute angle-closure glaucoma.
2. Compare the reason for a buildup of IOP in chronic open-angle glaucoma and acute angle-closure glaucoma.
3. What history would suggest this patient is at risk for glaucoma?
4. Which type of treatment would you expect the ophthalmologist to institute?

5. If this were chronic open-angle glaucoma, which types of medications would you expect to be prescribed?

6. How would these medications help treat the disorder?
7. What is the danger of untreated glaucoma?

Real-Life Challenge: Otitis Media

An 18-month-old male child has been brought to the physician's office by his parents who say that he has been fussy and crying for the past 10 hours. The mother says she is having difficulty getting him to eat, and she has noticed that he sits with his head held to the right side. He has a history of a cold in the past few days with a runny nose and watering eyes.

Examination reveals a temperature of 103°F, pulse of 116 beats per minute, and respirations of 32 breaths per minute. The otoscopic examination is used to evaluate the condition of the tympanic membranes. The physician examines the left ear first, a method employed to see what the asymptomatic

ear looked like. It reveals a normal translucent pearl-gray tympanic membrane. Examination of the right or symptomatic ear discloses a red, bulging eardrum. The mucous membrane of the nasal passages appears inflamed, as does the back of the throat.

An antibiotic (amoxicillin trihydrate [Amoxil] 125 mg four times daily [q.i.d.] × 10 days) is prescribed. The parents are instructed to give acetaminophen or ibuprofen (Motrin) for a temperature greater than 101°F and to call if the fever and pain persists beyond 24 hours. The child is scheduled for a follow-up visit in 1 week.

Questions

1. Why is it important to note that the child sits with his head held to the side?
2. What effect does the elevated temperature have on the other vital signs?
3. Why did the physician examine the left eardrum first?
4. What patient teaching would you offer the parents about the medication suggested for the elevated temperature?
5. What patient teaching would you offer the parents about the antibiotics?
6. Why are treatment and follow-up important?
7. Which surgical procedure may be indicated?
8. What long-term effects may the child experience if the otitis does not respond to treatment?

Real-Life Challenge: Sensorineural Hearing Loss

A 54-year-old retired male police officer presents with complaints that his hearing has diminished over the past few years. He is accompanied by his wife, who says he does not hear what she says any more. She states that this has been getting progressively worse, but she has noted that he is turning up the sound on the television so loud that she cannot stand it. She also says that he cannot hear the phone ring. Additionally, she reports that he does not hear what she is saying and confuses that information.

On examination, audiometry indicates a loss of hearing. The patient has difficulty hearing the examiner's commands or

questions. He also complains of ringing in his ears (tinnitus). The patient has had a few experiences of dizziness or vertigo.

The physician attempts to discover a possible source of the condition and also to rule out other conditions, including tumors or aneurysms. The patient confirms previous exposure to extensive gun firing on a range without adequate ear protection. He also has worked in a machine shop where presses punch out metal objects on dies. Treatment includes reducing the source of damage, including reduction of noise levels. The reduction can be obtained by turning down the television volume and wearing ear plugs.

Questions

1. What is the significance of the wife's complaints?
2. Why would an audiometric examination have been necessary?
3. What might have been some of the sources of the hearing loss?
4. What is the significance of shooting without adequate ear protection?
5. What will be the outcome if noise levels are reduced?
6. Why is it important for the physician to rule out a tumor or aneurysm?

Internet Assignments

1. Research facts about aging and vision by exploring the website of the American Foundation for the Blind (AFB). Choose a subject that considers older individuals and vision loss.
2. Visit the National Institute on Deafness and Other Communication Disorders website, choose the *News*

and Events option, and research a current subject, such as new state guidelines for screening infant hearing.
3. Research a current topic, such as the danger of using illegal contact lenses, by visiting the American Academy of Ophthalmology website.

Critical Thinking

1. Your latest *Glamor* magazine has an article written by a clinician suggesting that women replace their mascara product with a fresh unit at least once a month. It is also recommended never to share the mascara unit with someone else. What is the concern behind these suggestions?
2. Why must close attention be paid to any changes in vision reported by a patient with age-related macular degeneration (AMD) before you schedule an appointment or contact the physician?
3. During an examination for employment, a small lesion is noted on the eyelid. The patient dismisses it as unimportant because it is not painful. What would be your necessary response, and why?
4. Discuss effects of otitis media on school attendance of children.

5. Encourage a discussion about the psychological effect of otitis media.
6. Encourage a discussion as to how benign paroxysmal positional vertigo (BPPV) affects an individual's life.
7. Encourage a discussion about the causes of tympanic membrane rupture. Also promote discussion of teaching children not to place anything in their ears (use the example "nothing smaller than your elbow").
8. Encourage discussion of complications resulting from mastoiditis.
9. Encourage students to write a teaching plan for prevention of sensorineural hearing loss.
10. Prepare to discuss Critical Thinking case study exercises for this chapter that are posted on Evolve.

6

Diseases and Conditions of the Integumentary System

CHAPTER OUTLINE

Orderly Functioning of the Integumentary System, 205

Dermatitis, 205

Urticaria, 211

Psoriasis, 212

Rosacea, 213

Acne Vulgaris, 214

Herpes Zoster (Shingles), 215

Impetigo, 217

Furuncles and Carbuncles, 218

Cellulitis, 219

Dermatophytoses, 220

Decubitus Ulcers, 222

Scabies and Pediculosis, 223

Benign and Premalignant Tumors, 225

Skin Carcinomas, 227

Abnormal Skin Pigmentation, 231

Alopecia (Baldness), 234

Corns and Calluses, 236

Verrucae (Warts), 236

Folliculitis, 237

Deformed or Discolored Nails, 238

Paronychia, 238

Necrotizing Fasciitis, 239

LEARNING OBJECTIVES

After studying Chapter 6, you should be able to:

1. Explain the functions of the skin.
2. Recognize common skin lesions.
3. Describe how seborrheic dermatitis affects the skin.
4. Discuss the possible causes of contact dermatitis, atopic dermatitis, and psoriasis.
5. Describe the treatment of acne vulgaris.
6. Explain the pathologic course of herpes zoster.
7. Name the etiology of impetigo.
8. Explain why the treatment of cellulitis is important.
9. Cite examples of the classifications of fungal infections of the skin.
10. List preventive measures for decubitus ulcers.
11. Name the two most common parasitic insects to infest humans. Describe how infestation can occur.
12. Name two common premalignant tumors.
13. Differentiate the three types of skin cancer.
14. Describe the guidelines for avoiding excessive sun exposure.
15. List some conditions that are caused by the abnormal development or distribution of melanocytes.
16. Name some possible causes of alopecia.
17. State the cause of warts.
18. List some of the likely causes of deformed or discolored nails.

KEY TERMS

bulla (**BUL**-la)
cellulitis (sell-you-**LIE**-tis)
comedo (**KOM**-ee-doe)
dermatome (**DER**-mah-tome)
electrodesiccation (ee-leck-tro-**des**-ih-**KAY**-shun)
erythema (**eh**-rih-**THEE**-ma)
exudate (**EKS**-you-date)
exudative (**EKS**-you-**day**-tive)
fissure (**FIS**-ur)

keratolytic (ker-ah-toe-**LIT**-ik)
keratosis (ker-ah-**TOE**-sis)
nevus (**NEE**-vus)
papule (**PAP**-youl)
plaques (**plaks**)
sebaceous (seh-**BAY**-shus)
vesicle (**VES**-ih-kl)
vesicular (veh-**SIK**-you-lar)
wheal (**WHEEL**)

Orderly Functioning of the Integumentary System

The system comprising the skin and its accessory organs (hair, nails, and glands) is called the *integumentary system.* The skin, one of the largest organs, protects the body from trauma, infections, and toxic chemicals. When exposed to sunlight, the skin synthesizes vitamin D. Within the skin are millions of tiny nerve endings called *receptors.* These receptors sense touch, pressure, pain, and temperature. In addition to the skin's roles in protection, sensation, and synthesis of vitamin D, it assists in the regulation of body temperature and in excretion.

The skin has three main structural layers (Fig. 6.1). The epidermis (outer layer) is a thin, cellular, multilayered membrane that is responsible for the production of keratin and melanin. The dermis, or corium (middle layer), is a dense, fibrous layer of connective tissue that gives skin its strength and elasticity. Within the dermis are blood and lymph vessels, nerve fibers, hair follicles, and sweat and sebaceous glands. The third layer is the subcutaneous layer, a thick, fat-containing section that insulates the body against heat loss.

Skin diseases frequently are manifested by cutaneous lesions, or alterations of the skin surface (Table 6.1). The diagnosis of a cutaneous disease often is based on the appearance of a specific type of lesion or group of lesions (Fig. 6.2).

Common presenting symptoms that need attention from health care professionals include:
- cutaneous lesions or eruptions
- pruritus (itching)
- pain
- edema (swelling)
- erythema (redness)
- inflammation

Many skin conditions are known to be aggravated by stress. Cosmetically, the skin is important to appearance. Much time and money are spent pursuing "beauty" and disguising the aging of the skin. Patients with skin conditions may feel anxious about their appearance. The treatment of many skin diseases is tedious, requiring strict compliance. Patient education and psychological support reduce the patient's anxiety and encourage good adherence to the treatment plan.

Dermatitis

Inflammation of the skin, or dermatitis, occurs in many types or forms. They all manifest as pruritus, erythema, and the appearance of various cutaneous lesions. The more common forms are seborrheic dermatitis, contact dermatitis, and atopic dermatitis (eczema). All forms of dermatitis can be acute, subacute, or chronic.

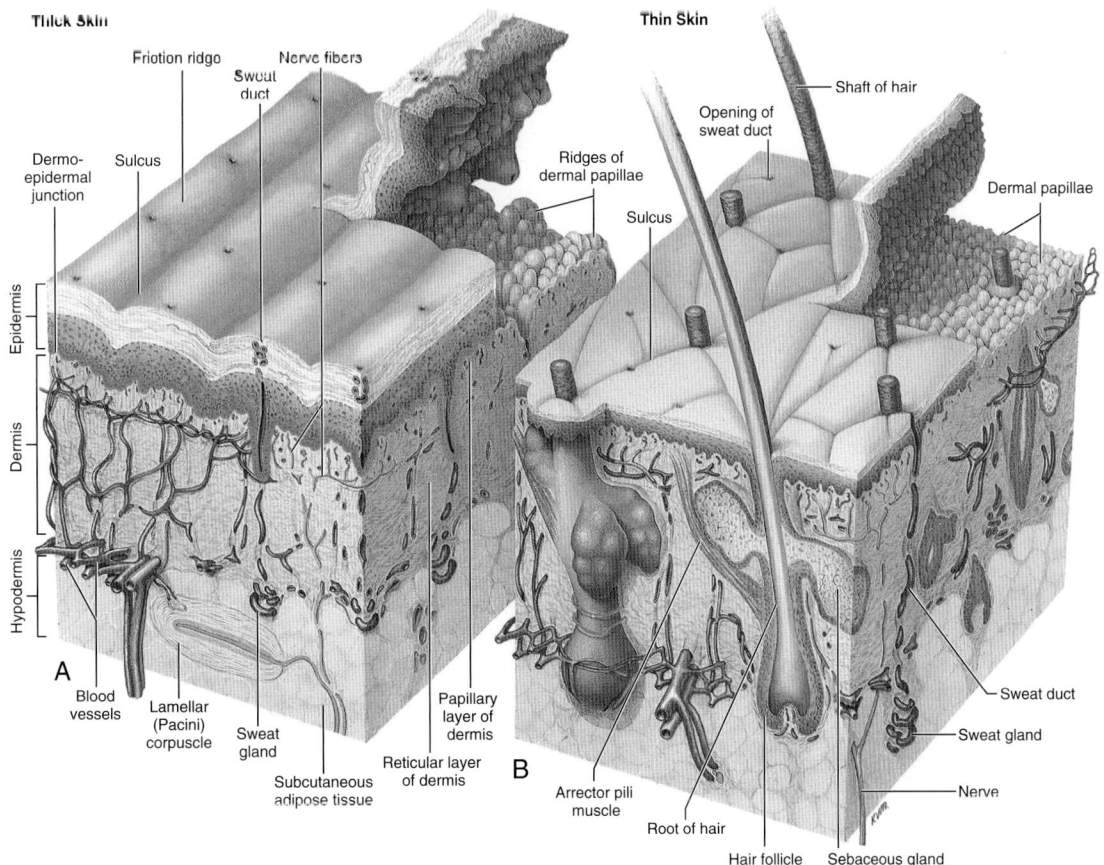

• **Fig. 6.1** Normal skin. (From Patton KT, Thibodeau GA: *Anatomy and physiology,* ed 9, St Louis, 2016, Mosby.)

TABLE 6.1 Description of Some Skin Lesions

Skin Lesion	Description
Macule	Small, flat circumscribed lesion of a color different from that of normal skin
Papule	Small, firm, elevated lesion
Nodule	Palpable elevated lesion; varies in size
Pustule	Elevated erythematous lesion, usually containing purulent exudate
Vesicle	Elevated, thin-walled lesion containing clear fluid (blister)
Plaque	Large, slightly elevated lesion with flat surface, often topped by scale
Crust	Dry, rough surface or dried exudate or blood
Lichenification	Thick, dry, rough surface (leather like)
Keloid	Raised, irregular, and increasing mass of collagen resulting from excessive scar tissue formation
Fissure	Small, deep, linear crack or tear in skin
Ulcer	Cavity with loss of tissue from the epidermis and dermis, often weeping or bleeding
Erosion	Shallow, moist cavity in epidermis
Comedo	Mass of sebum, keratin, and debris blocking the opening of a hair follicle

(From Gould B: *Pathophysiology for the health professions,* ed 3, Philadelphia, 2006, Saunders.)

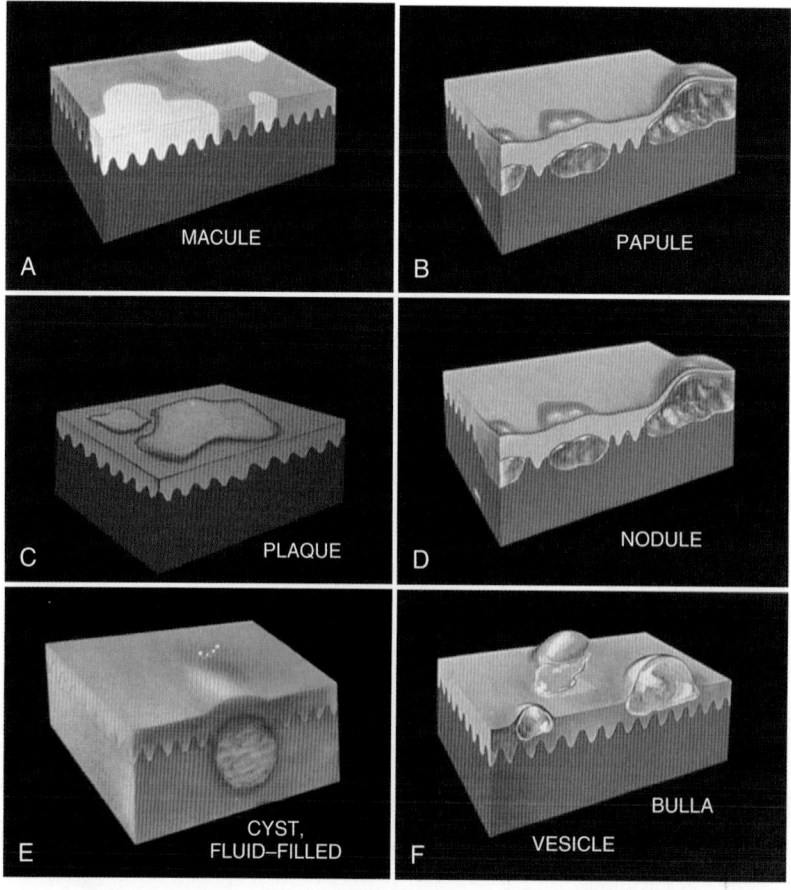

• **Fig. 6.2** Skin lesions. (A) Macule. A flat, colored lesion that may be white (hypopigmented), brown (hyperpigmented), or red (erythematous and purpuric). (B) Papule. A small elevated lesion less than 0.5 cm in diameter. (C) Plaque. A plateaulike elevated lesion greater than 0.5 cm in diameter. (D) Nodule. A marblelike lesion greater than 0.5 cm in depth and diameter. (E) Cyst. A nodule filled with either liquid or semisolid material. (F) Vesicle and bulla. Blisters containing clear fluid. Vesicles are less than 0.5 cm in diameter, and bullae are greater than 0.5 cm in diameter.

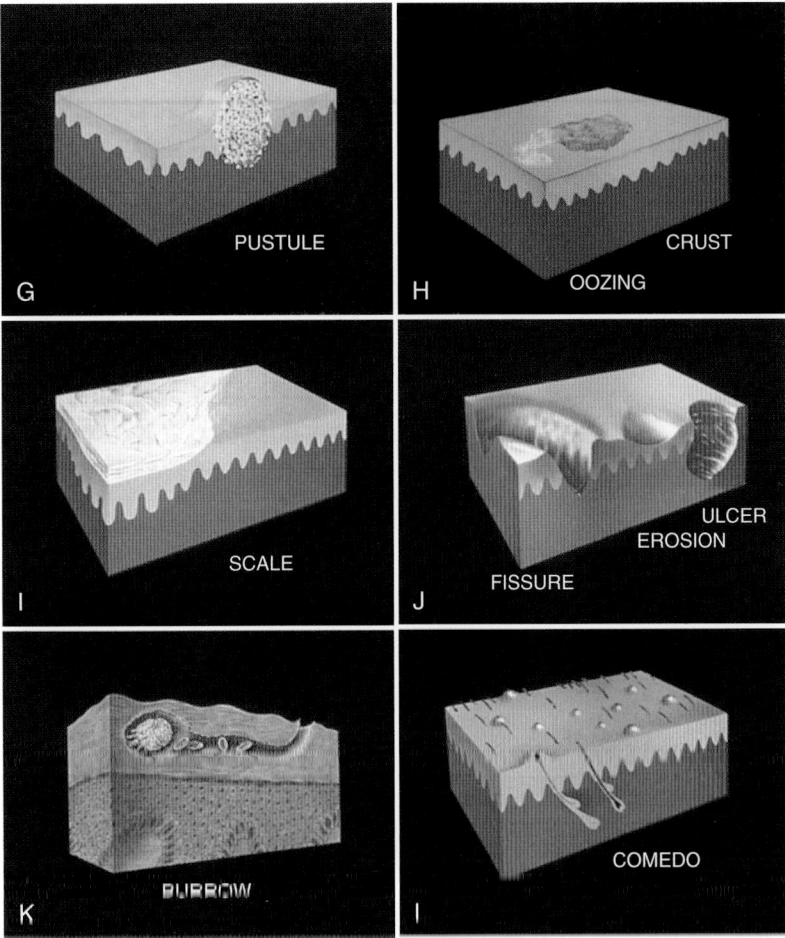

• Fig. 6.2, cont'd (G) Pustule. A vesicle containing purulent or cloudy fluid. (H) Crust. Liquid debris dried on the skin's surface, resulting from ruptured vesicles, pustules, or bullae. (I) Scale. A thickened outer layer of skin that is dry and whitish colored. (J) Fissure, erosion, and ulcer. A fissure is a thin tear. An erosion is a wide but shallow fissure. An ulcer involves the epidermis and dermis. (K) Burrow. A tunnel or streak caused by a burrowing organism. (L) Comedo. A lesion of acne. (From Marks JG, et al: *Lookingbill & Marks' principles of dermatology*, ed 4, Philadelphia, 2006, Saunders.)

Seborrheic Dermatitis

Description

Seborrheic dermatitis, one of the most common skin disorders, is an inflammatory condition of the sebaceous, or oil, glands.

ICD-10-CM Code	L21.9 *(Seborrheic dermatitis, unspecified)*
	(L21.0-L21.9 = 4 codes of specificity)
	L21.0 *(Seborrhea capitis)*
	L20.83 *(Infantile [acute] [chronic] eczema)*
	(L20.81-L20.9 = 6 codes of specificity)
	L21.8 *(Other seborrheic dermatitis)*

Symptoms and Signs

Seborrheic dermatitis is marked by a gradual increase in the amount of, and a change in the quality of, sebum, which is produced by the sebaceous glands. The inflammation occurs in areas with the greatest number of sebaceous glands. These include the scalp, eyebrows, eyelids, sides of the nose, the area behind the ears, and the middle of the chest. Affected skin is reddened and covered by yellowish, greasy-appearing scales. Itching may occur but is usually mild.

Seborrheic dermatitis can occur at any age but is most common during infancy, when it is called *cradle cap*. Cradle cap (Fig. 6.3) usually clears without treatment by age 8 to 12 months. Seborrheic dermatitis occurs at a higher rate in adults with disorders of the central nervous system, such as Parkinson disease. Patients who are recovering from stressful medical conditions, such as a myocardial infarction (heart attack); patients who have been confined to hospitals or nursing homes for long stays; and those who have immune system disorders, such as acquired immunodeficiency syndrome (AIDS), appear to be more prone to this disorder. More intense forms of seborrheic dermatitis can be seen in patients with psoriasis (see the Psoriasis section). Mild forms are mainly cosmetic problems that can be easily treated or may disappear spontaneously.

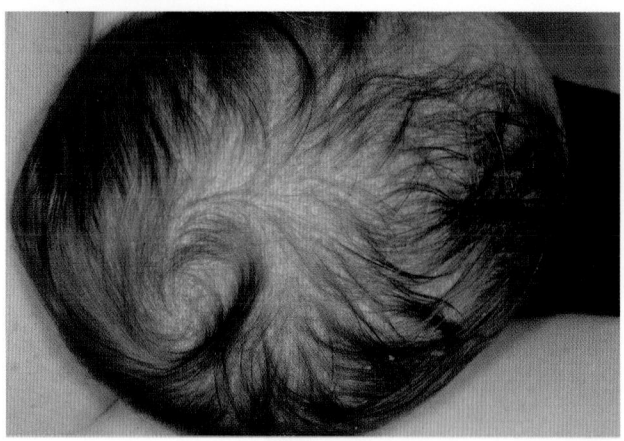

• **Fig. 6.3** "Cradle cap," the most frequent form of seborrheic dermatitis in infants. The condition often begins in the first 2 to 3 weeks of life and usually disappears by age 12 months. (From Paller SA: *Hurwitz clinical pediatric dermatology: A textbook of skin disorders of childhood and adolescence*, ed 4 Philadelphia, 2012, Saunders.)

Patient Screening

This condition has a gradual onset. The irritation becomes troublesome, and the patient or a parent calls to request an appointment. Schedule the patient to be seen at the earliest convenient time or the next available appointment.

Etiology

This condition is idiopathic; however, heredity may predispose an individual to the condition, and emotional stress may be a precipitating factor. Evidence suggests that this skin disorder may be perpetuated or intensified by the yeastlike organism *Pityrosporum,* which is normally found on the skin in small numbers. Whether diet or food allergies play a role in the development of seborrheic dermatitis in infants is still unknown.

Diagnosis

In most patients, blood, urine, and allergy tests are not necessary. In the rare case of chronic seborrheic dermatitis that does not respond to treatment, skin biopsy or more extensive testing may be performed to rule out the possibility of another disease.

Treatment

One of the more effective methods of treatment is the use of a low-strength cortisone or hydrocortisone cream applied topically to the affected area. *Caution:* Prolonged use of these medications should be avoided because of the possible side effects of steroids. When the scalp is involved, causing dandruff, frequent use of nonprescription shampoos containing tar, zinc pyrithione, selenium sulfide, sulfur, and salicylic acid also is recommended. Patients not responding to these treatments should consult a dermatologist, who can prescribe stronger medications.

Treatment of cradle cap involves gentle massage of the scalp to loosen scales and improve circulation. When scales are present, shampooing daily with a mild soap is recommended. After the scales disappear, shampooing may be done twice a week. Care should be taken to rinse off all soap. The child's hair should be brushed with a soft brush after shampooing and several times during the day. When the scales do not loosen easily, mineral oil can be applied to the scalp and a warm cloth used to cover the child's scalp for approximately 1 hour. The temperature of the cloth must be monitored so that it does not cool down too much and reduce the child's body temperature. The scalp should be shampooed and dried. If this treatment is not successful in removing the scales, the physician may prescribe a lotion or cream to be applied to the child's scalp.

Prognosis

Most episodes resolve with treatment. Those who do not respond positively should be referred to a dermatologist for additional drug therapy. Whether treated or not, this condition tends to recur.

Prevention

No prevention is known.

Patient Teaching

Teach the patient to properly apply the prescribed medication. For infants with cradle cap, instruct the parents to shampoo the scalp daily and perhaps gently massage the area with a toothbrush.

Contact Dermatitis

Description

Contact dermatitis is an acute inflammation response of the skin triggered by an exogenous chemical or substance.

ICD-10-CM Code	L25.9 *(Unspecified contact dermatitis, unspecified cause)* (L25.0-L25.9 = 8 codes of specificity)

Contact dermatitis has more than one form and therefore more than one ICD-10-CM code. The general code is L25.9 for the ICD-10-CM. Refer to the physician's diagnosis and then to the current edition of the ICD-10-CM coding manual to ensure the greatest specificity of pathology and any appropriate modifiers. A list of some of the specific codes follows:

Contact Dermatitis:

ICD-10-CM Code	L24.0 *(Irritant contact dermatitis due to detergents)*
	L24.1 *(Irritant contact dermatitis due to oils and greases)*
	L24.2 *(Irritant contact dermatitis due to solvents)*
	L25.1 *(Unspecified contact dermatitis due to drugs in contact with skin)*
	L25.3 *(Unspecified contact dermatitis due to other chemical products)*
	L25.4 *(Unspecified contact dermatitis due to food in contact with skin)*

L25.5 *(Unspecified contact dermatitis due to plants, except food)*
L56.0 *(Drug phototoxic response)*
L56.1 *(Drug photoallergic response)*
L56.2 *(Photocontact dermatitis [berloque dermatitis])*
L25.8 *(Unspecified contact dermatitis due to other agents)*
L25.9 *(Unspecified contact dermatitis, unspecified cause)*

Symptoms and Signs

Contact dermatitis is caused either by the action of irritants on the skin's surface or by contact with a substance that causes an allergic response. Symptoms include erythema, edema, and small vesicles that ooze, itch, burn, or sting (Fig. 6.4).

Patient Screening

The patient reporting symptoms of contact dermatitis feels the characteristic itching, burning, and stinging. These patients should be scheduled at the earliest possible time on the same day they call. If this is not possible, the prudent step for patient comfort is to refer the patient to another facility.

Etiology

Many substances can induce contact dermatitis, including plants, such as poison ivy, oak, or sumac. Poison ivy may be spread as an airborne irritant by burning plants. Other irritants are dyes used in soaps and facial and toilet tissues, other dyes, latex, furs, preservatives, drugs, detergents, cleaning compounds, cosmetics, chemicals, acids, and certain metals (e.g., nickel) used to make jewelry. Solar radiation and other forms of radiation, including exposure through a tanning bed, may cause the dermatitis. If an irritant remains in constant contact with the skin, the dermatitis spreads.

Contact dermatitis develops in three ways:

1. It can develop through irritation, either chemical or mechanical, such as by latex gloves and wool fibers. If the irritant is strong, a single exposure may cause a severe inflammatory reaction.

2. Contact dermatitis may develop through sensitization. This means that the first contact with a substance causes no immediate inflammation. However, after the skin becomes sensitized, future contact or exposure results in inflammation.

3. Another interesting but uncommon mechanism for the development of this form of dermatitis is photoallergy. Some chemicals found in perfumes, soaps, suntan lotions containing para-aminobenzoic acid (PABA), or medications (e.g., tetracycline) can sensitize the skin to sunlight. The next time the individual uses the products and is exposed to sunlight, a rash develops.

Diagnosis

Diagnosis of a contact dermatitis is based on the appearance of the affected area; medical history, including prior outbreaks and their locations; and identification of the specific irritant or allergen with a patch test.

Treatment

If a patient has come in contact with a known irritant, thoroughly cleaning the skin surface should be the first step. This should be followed by the topical application of a corticosteroid cream. An oral steroid, such as methylprednisolone (Medrol) or prednisone, may be prescribed for 6 to 12 days, with a decreasing dosage. Some physicians believe that 6 days is typically not a long enough treatment for many contact dermatitis conditions. Poison plant dermatitis nearly always needs at least 12 days of medication. Sometimes dermatitis rebounds after short-course steroids.

Prognosis

The prognosis varies, depending on the amount of skin area involved and the likelihood of the causative agent being removed. The response to drug therapy is usually positive when combined with removal of the offending substance.

Prevention

Identification of the offending or causative substance is primary in preventing recurrences. After the substance is identified, contact must be avoided. Should accidental contact occur, immediate intervention by removing the source and seeking drug therapy may reduce the intensity of the condition.

Patient Teaching

Encourage patients to avoid substances or situations that trigger contact dermatitis. Give information about proper methods of cleansing the skin, affected clothing, and bed linens after contact with offending substances. Instruct patients to refrain from scratching affected skin to prevent additional damage or infection from developing in the skin tissue.

Atopic Dermatitis (Eczema)

Description

Atopic dermatitis (eczema) is a chronic inflammation of the skin that tends to occur in patients with a family history of allergic conditions.

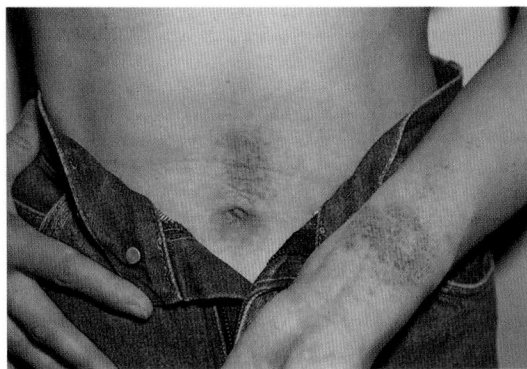

• **Fig. 6.4** Contact dermatitis. (From Marks JG, et al: *Lookingbill & Marks' principles of dermatology*, ed 4, Philadelphia, 2006, Saunders.)

ICD-10-CM Code
L20.0 *(Besnier's prurigo)*
L20.81 *(Atopic neurodermatitis)*
L20.82 *(Flexural eczema)*
L20.84 *(Intrinsic [allergic]*
eczema)
L20.89 *(Other atopic dermatitis)*

Symptoms and Signs

A rash, with vesicular and exudative eruptions in children and dry, leathery vesicles in adults, develops (Figs. 6.5 and 6.6). The rash occurs in a characteristic pattern on the face, neck, elbows, knees, and upper trunk of the body and is accompanied by pruritus.

Patient Screening

When the individual calls for an appointment, consider the discomfort that he or she is experiencing, and schedule the patient to be seen at the earliest possible time. If a prompt appointment is not possible, referral to another facility is indicated.

Etiology

Eczema is an idiopathic disease. The tendency of this condition to develop is inherited, and an allergic connection is

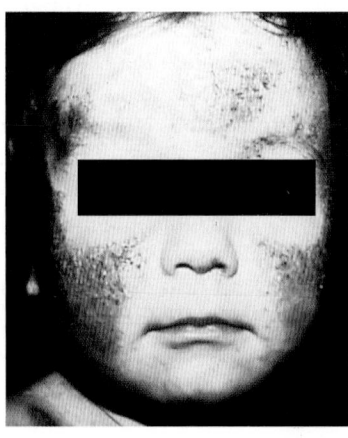

• **Fig. 6.5** Infantile atopic dermatitis. (From Zitelli BJ, Davis HW: *Atlas of pediatric physical diagnosis,* ed 6, Philadelphia, 2012, Mosby.)

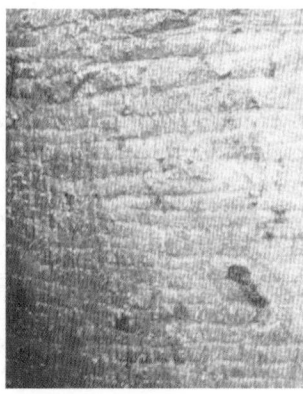

• **Fig. 6.6** Atopic dermatitis. (From Marks JG, et al: *Lookingbill & Marks' principles of dermatology,* ed 4, Philadelphia, 2006, Saunders.)

assumed. Eczema in some infants is believed to be traceable to sensitivity to milk, orange juice, or some other foods.

A flare-up of eczema can be triggered by stress, anxiety, or conflict. Stress actually can make the condition worse. Climate, especially sudden or extreme changes in temperature, can affect or aggravate the condition. Eczema may improve in summer and flare up in winter. Wool clothing or blankets in contact with the skin may also cause a flare-up of the condition. Skin barrier disruption associated with transepidermal water loss from frequent bathing and/or hand washing without moisturizing is also an important trigger factor. Eczema in babies usually subsides by age 2 years. The rash may resolve during adolescence or persist into adulthood. Eczema generally tends to improve over time.

Diagnosis

A medical history, including a family history, along with examination of the skin, confirms the diagnosis. Occasional skin testing for specific allergies is indicated to identify underlying causes.

Treatment

The main objective in treating atopic dermatitis is reducing the frequency and severity of eruptions and relieving the pruritus. Simple atopic dermatitis may be treated with skin moisturizers, sunlight therapy, vitamin D, or calcipotriene. Unfortunately, no medications can eliminate eczema. Topical ointments and creams containing a cortisone derivative are the primary treatment for eczema. In addition, three unique new nonsteroidal antiinflammatory drugs (NSAIDs), tacrolimus (Protopic) and pimecrolimus (Elidel), and Eucrisa, a phosphodiesterase type 4 (PDE4) inhibitor, are prescribed specifically to treat eczema. A newer class of injectables to block interleukin 4 (IL-4) and IL-13 (brand name Dupixent) is considered a biologic agent. Local and systemic medications, such as antihistamines, tranquilizers, and other sedatives, may be prescribed to prevent or control the pruritus. Secondary bacterial or viral infections can result from scratching of the rash or lesions. A secondary bacterial infection is the most common complication. The physician usually prescribes an antibiotic to control the infection. A more serious complication of eczema can be caused by infection by certain viruses, especially herpes simplex virus.

Prognosis

Reduction in the frequency and severity of eruptions and relief from pruritus are the positive outcomes. There is no cure, and eczema cannot be eliminated with medications. Medications are prescribed to control the itch–scratch cycle that aggravates the condition. Many occurrences resolve spontaneously but recur later.

Prevention

As an idiopathic disease with a tendency to be inherited and possibly with an allergic connection, eczema has no known prevention. An attempt should be made to prevent the secondary bacterial or viral infections that result from scratching of the rash or lesions.

Patient Teaching

Teach the patient about the importance of not scratching the involved area. In young adults and older people, explain how scratching aggravates the condition. Daily bathing, followed by application of unscented emollients, should be encouraged. Use of soap should be avoided, except in body folds, and hot baths should be avoided as well.

Urticaria

Description

Urticaria, or hives, is associated with severe itching followed by the appearance of redness and an area of swelling (wheal) in a localized area of skin (Figs. 6.7A and B).

ICD-10-CM Code	L50.9 (Urticaria, unspecified)

Urticaria has more than one form and therefore more than one ICD-10-CM code. The general code for urticaria is L50.9 for the ICD-10-CM. Refer to the physician's diagnosis and then to the current edition of the ICD-10-CM coding manual to ensure the greatest specificity of pathology and any appropriate modifiers. Some of the specific codes follow:

ICD-10-CM Code	L50.0 (Allergic urticaria)
	L50.1 (Idiopathic urticaria)
	L50.2 (Urticaria due to cold and heat)
	L50.3 (Dermatographic urticaria)
	L50.4 (Vibratory urticaria)
	L50.5 (Cholinergic urticaria)
	L50.6 (Contact urticaria)
	L50.8 (Other urticaria)
	L50.9 (Urticaria, unspecified)

Symptoms and Signs

Hives of various sizes can erupt as a few lesions anywhere on the skin and often are scattered over the body or mucous membrane. In gastrointestinal involvement, the patient complains of abdominal colic. When hives develop in the pharyngeal mucosa, the airway can become obstructed, causing asphyxiation. When the swelling involves deeper tissues, the condition is called *angioedema* and is more serious. Urticaria is common, often acute, and self-limiting, lasting a few hours. In other cases, hives continue over months or years, becoming a chronic condition. Patient complaint of itching is a significant symptom.

Patient Screening

Hives can develop into a life-threatening condition if they involve the respiratory system. Anyone experiencing respiratory difficulties should be brought into the emergency medical system for immediate assessment and intervention. Cutaneous symptoms make the individual very uncomfortable, and the patient should be seen immediately or referred to another facility for prompt assessment.

Etiology

Urticaria affects the dermis and results from an acute hypersensitivity and the release of histamine. This causes local inflammation and vasodilation of capillaries with substantial edema. Allergic reactions to food (e.g., shellfish, strawberries, or peanuts); drugs (e.g., penicillin), or insect stings (frequently by bees) are some common causes. Infection can cause an attack of hives, as can some inhalants, sunlight, and temperature extremes. Sometimes the cause is not identified.

Diagnosis

Visual inspection of the urticaria is diagnostic. A prior episode in conjunction with a particular exposure to a known allergen is significant in the patient's history. If the medical history offers no clues to the cause, sensitivity testing and blood tests for antibodies may help identify the causative agent.

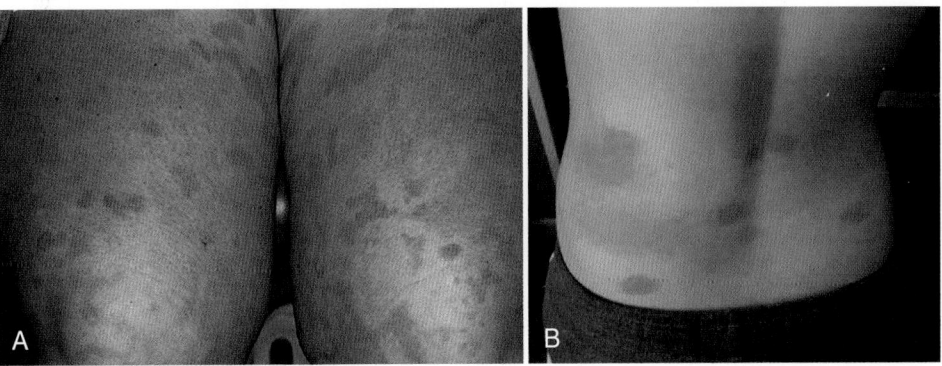

• **Fig. 6.7** (A) Urticaria. (B) Hives as experienced by a 19 year-old female, (A, From Murphy GF, Herzberg AJ: *Atlas of dermatopathology*, Philadelphia, 1996, Saunders. B, Courtesy Margaret Frazier, 2019.)

Treatment

If known, the antigenic factor is removed and then avoided, if possible. Antihistamines bring quick relief of symptoms. An injection of epinephrine is used in more severe cases.

In persistent cases, a course of prednisone or methylprednisolone is therapeutic. A variety of corticosteroid creams or ointments may be used also.

Prognosis

Immediate drug therapy usually resolves the allergic response, and the hives disappear. Another exposure to the same allergen will probably elicit the same response, so the triggering allergen must be avoided.

Prevention

Prevention depends on identifying the offending allergen and avoiding it.

Patient Teaching

Teach patients the importance of avoiding the causative allergen and seeking proper and prompt medical intervention during recurrence of the condition.

Psoriasis

Description

Psoriasis is a chronic skin condition marked by thick, flaky, red patches of various sizes, covered with characteristic white, silvery scales (Fig. 6.8).

ICD-10-CM Code	L40.0 *(Psoriasis vulgaris)*
	L40.1 *(Generalized pustular psoriasis)*
	L40.2 *(Acrodermatitis continua)*
	L40.3 *(Pustulosis palmaris et plantaris)*
	L40.4 *(Guttate psoriasis)*
	L40.8 *(Other psoriasis)*

Psoriasis has more than one form and therefore more than one code. Refer to the physician's diagnosis and then to the current edition of the ICD-10-CM coding manual to ensure the greatest specificity of pathology.

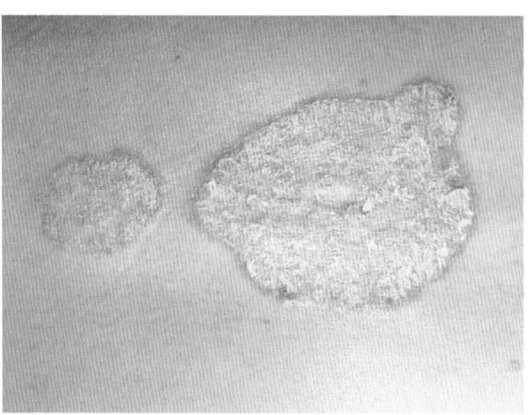

• **Fig. 6.8** Psoriasis. (From Marks JG, et al: *Lookingbill & Marks' principles of dermatology,* ed 4, Philadelphia, 2006, Saunders.)

Symptoms and Signs

Psoriasis is an inflammatory chronic and recurrent skin condition with silvery scales. These scales develop into dry plaques (see Fig. 6.2C), sometimes progressing to pustules (see Fig. 6.2G). They usually do not cause discomfort but might cause a slight itch or soreness. Affected skin typically appears dry, cracked, and encrusted. The most common areas where psoriasis develops are the scalp; the outer sides of arms and legs, especially elbows and knees; and the trunk of the body. In addition, the palms of hands and the soles of feet may be affected. In some patients, psoriasis spreads to the nail beds, causing the nails to thicken and crumble. Psoriasis plaques can also develop in areas of physical trauma (Koebner phenomenon). Psoriasis can occur at any age but is more common between ages 10 and 30 years. It is noninfectious and does not affect general health.

Patient Screening

Symptoms of psoriasis are troublesome. For the patient calling for an appointment for these symptoms, the next convenient appointment should be scheduled.

Etiology

The cause of psoriasis is unknown, but it seems to be genetically determined. Psoriasis may be an autoimmune disorder and is more common among white individuals. Psoriasis is now identified as an autoimmune disorder. Precipitating factors for the development of psoriasis include hormonal changes, such as those occurring with pregnancy, climate changes, emotional stress, and a period of generally poor health. Some drugs, including lithium, beta-blockers, and NSAIDs, are suspected of exacerbating psoriasis.

Diagnosis

The white, silvery scales of psoriasis are recognizable, making the condition easy to diagnose. Careful history taking, observation of the skin, or skin biopsy may help when the scales are not evident, as with patients who bathe and scrub frequently. Scratching of the lesions reveals the telltale scales.

Treatment

The goal of treatment is to reduce inflammation and to slow the rapid growth of skin cells that cause the condition. Keeping the involved skin moist and lubricated is beneficial. Treatment options include exposure to ultraviolet (UV) light to help delay cell reproduction;, use of a psoralens medication (methoxsalen) in combination with UV light; application of topical steroid creams/ointments; application of coal tar preparations; application of cream containing retinoids (vitamin A derivative); administration of low-dosage antihistamines; and oatmeal baths. Additional treatments may involve application of creams containing synthetic vitamin D analogues (calcipotriene 0.005%). Severe cases of psoriasis may require chemotherapy with methotrexate (Trexall, Rheumatrex) or acitretin (Soriatane), cyclosporine (Neoral), or the use of etretinate (Tegison), which is related to vitamin A. *Caution:* Pregnant women and nursing mothers should never take methotrexate, acitretin, or etretinate. Cyclosporine is in the U.S. Food and Drug Administration (FDA) pregnancy category C. Antibiotics also may be prescribed. A new group of medications known as *monoclonal antibodies* and *fusion proteins (biologics)* have recently been approved in the treatment of psoriasis. However, long-term safety with this class of medications has yet to be determined.

Recently a new drug, ustekinumab (Stelara), has been marketed as being more effective than etanercept (Enbrel) for the treatment of psoriasis. However, both drugs are considered quite dangerous and may not be considered for treatment unless the psoriasis is quite severe.

Prognosis

No cure for psoriasis is known, but it is controllable. Remissions and exacerbations occur often, and the condition may require lifelong treatment. Advise patients to consider counseling for stress reduction, because stress may cause recurrence of the disorder.

Prevention

The condition has an autoimmune etiology; thus no prevention is known. Keeping the skin moist and lubricated; avoiding cold, dry climates; preventing stress and anxiety; limiting alcohol intake; and not scratching and picking at the skin help prevent recurrence of the condition.

Patient Teaching

Explain the concept of exposure to UV light and methods of timing the exposure. Demonstrate application of steroid creams, coal tar preparations, and other skin creams.

Rosacea

Description

Rosacea, a chronic inflammatory disorder of the facial skin, causes redness primarily of the areas that manifest blushing or flushing.

ICD-10-CM Code	L71.0 (Perioral dermatitis)
	L71.1 (Rhinophyma)
	L71.8 (Other rosacea)
	L71.9 (Rosacea, unspecified)

Symptoms and Signs

The onset of rosacea is insidious and often is mistaken for a change in complexion, sunburn, or even acne. The redness becomes more noticeable and does not go away. The skin then may begin exhibiting dryness and pimples that may become inflamed or filled with pus. In addition, small blood vessels of the cheeks and face enlarge and show through the skin as red lines even after the redness diminishes (Figs. 6.9 and 6.10). Small knobby bumps occasionally appear on the nose, causing it to look swollen, mostly in the male with rosacea.

There are four major types of rosacea. The signs and symptoms vary from one form to the other. Ocular rosacea,

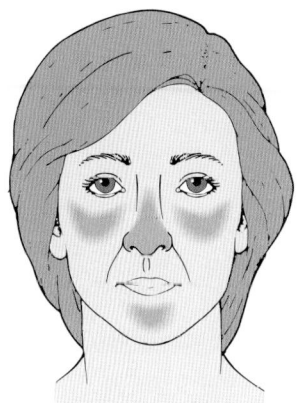

• **Fig. 6.9** Rosacea.

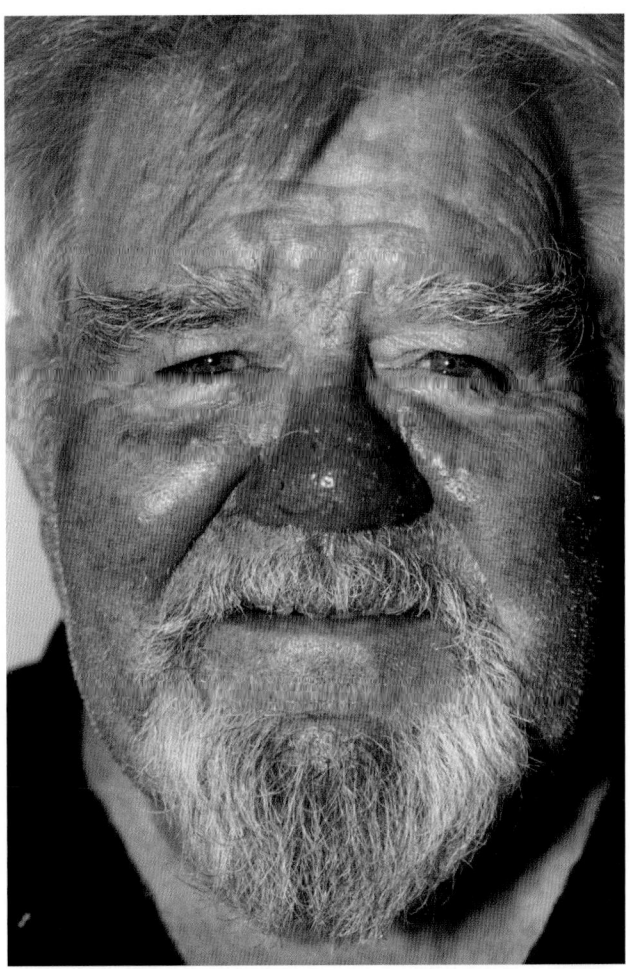

• **Fig. 6.10** Rosacea papules and pustules superimposed on background of erythema. (From Marks JG, et al: *Lookingbill & Marks' principles of dermatology,* ed 4, Philadelphia, 2006, Saunders.)

an inflammatory eye condition, is a less common form of rosacea. The blood vessels in the sclera become inflamed, and the eyelids appear to be reddened and swollen, often with small bumps that are inflamed and eyelashes that fall out. The individual may experience a burning or gritty feeling in the eyes. The eyes have a bloodshot appearance (Fig. 6.11).

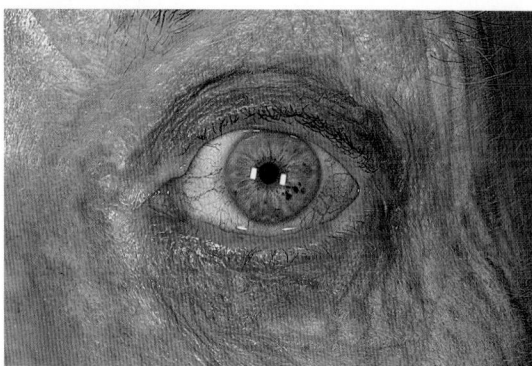

• **Fig. 6.11** Patient with ocular rosacea. (From Habif TP, et al: *Skin disease diagnosis and treatment,* ed 3, St Louis, 2011, Saunders.)

Etiology

The etiology of rosacea, a chronic and often cyclic condition, is unknown. A possible correlation with the frequency of the individual's blushing or facial flushing has been suggested. Those with lighter complexions appear to have a greater incidence of the disorder, which possibly may be inherited. Rosacea is not considered infectious or contagious and is not spread through skin contact. The etiology of ocular rosacea also is unknown.

Diagnosis

Rosacea is diagnosed on the basis of a history of facial blushing and flushing. Although rosacea often has many of the same symptoms as acne, the individual experiencing episodes of rosacea does not have the blackheads or whiteheads (**comedones**) typical of acne. A dermatologist should be consulted for a definitive diagnosis.

Ocular rosacea is diagnosed on the basis of a history of chronically bloodshot eyes, and examination of the eyes usually reveals inflammation and debris on the margins of the eyelids.

Treatment

Rosacea has no cure, but symptoms can be controlled through medical treatment with azelaic acid 15% (Finacea); metronidazole cream 1%; sodium sulfacetamide; topical antibiotics (erythromycin and clindamycin); and lifestyle changes. The patient is urged to identify situations that cause him or her to blush or experience facial flushing and attempt to avoid these triggers. These events may be different for various rosacea sufferers, so the patient would be wise to avoid sunlight, hard exercise, extreme heat or cold, stress, spicy foods, hot drinks, and alcohol. Sun exposure, hot weather, cold weather, and wind all have been identified as triggers, as have abrupt changes of season and weather extremes. The physician may prescribe medications to control the redness. Antibiotics (minocycline, doxycycline, or tetracycline) are prescribed in some cases. For stubborn cases, the redness can also be treated with laser surgery. Mild cleansers should be used, and moisturizers that do not contain alcohol or drying agents should be applied routinely. Use of a sunscreen helps. Consistent treatment is necessary to prevent flare-ups. A topical gel, Mirvaso, works

by constricting the blood vessels, thereby decreasing the appearance of redness.

The treatment of ocular rosacea is similar to the treatment of facial rosacea and includes daily cleansing of eyelids with a form of diluted non-tearing shampoo. If the individual is not allergic, antibiotics (minocycline, doxycycline, or tetracycline) are prescribed sometimes.

Prognosis

As previously mentioned, rosacea has no cure, but the patient may be able to control the symptoms with medical treatment and lifestyle modifications. Similar to facial rosacea, ocular rosacea has no cure.

Prevention

The etiology is unknown, so prevention is not possible. Identifying situations with the potential to cause blushing or facial flushing and avoiding these triggers are helpful. Avoiding sunlight, hard exercise, extreme heat or cold, stress, spicy foods, hot drinks, and alcohol also helps. The patient is urged to avoid triggers, such as exposure to the sun, hot weather, cold weather, wind, abrupt changes of seasons, and weather extremes.

Patient Teaching

Work with patients to identify the causative factors, and discuss ways to avoid these factors. Assist them in locating and contacting support groups for patients with this disorder.

Acne Vulgaris

Description

Acne vulgaris is an inflammatory disease of the sebaceous glands and hair follicles. **Papules**, **pustules**, and comedones are usually present (Fig. 6.12).

ICD-10-CM Code	L70.1 *(Acne conglobata)*
	L70.8 *(Other acne)*
	L70.9 *(Acne, unspecified)*

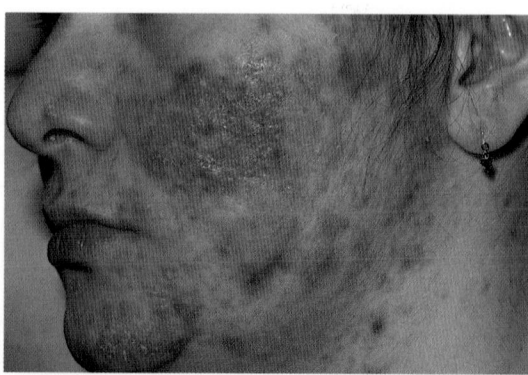

• **Fig. 6.12** Acne. Inflammatory acne is characterized by erythematous papules and pustules with the possibility of eventual scarring. (From Cotran R, et al: *Robbins pathological basis of disease,* ed 6, Philadelphia, 1999, Saunders.)

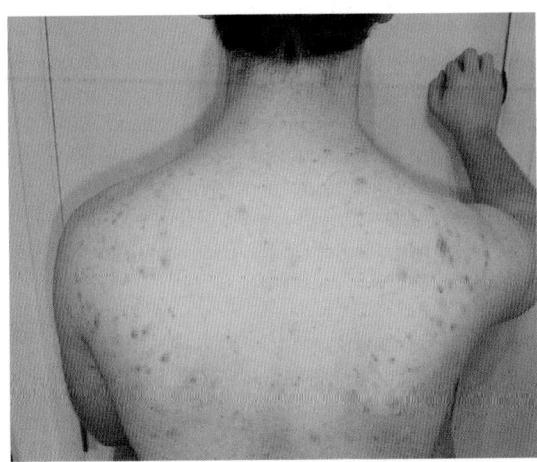

• **Fig. 6.13** Photo of teenage acne. (Courtesy David Frazier, 2003.)

Symptoms and Signs

Acne vulgaris is marked by the appearance of papules, pustules, and comedones (see Fig. 6.2B, G, and L). Deeper, boil-like lesions, called *nodules,* sometimes can occur. Scars may develop if the chronic irritation and inflammation continue for a long period. Acne is found most often on the face but can also occur on the neck, shoulders, chest, and back (Fig. 6.13). Acne can appear at any age but is more common in adolescents. In girls, it is usually at its worst between ages 14 and 17 years. In boys, it reaches its peak in the late teens.

Patient Screening

Many calls requesting appointments for treatment of acne type of conditions will be for teenagers. Acne is not a medical emergency, but an individual experiencing its symptoms may be feeling emotional stress. Therefore the physician should schedule the next available appointment for these patients.

Etiology

The cause of acne vulgaris is unknown. Research on the cause, however, links it to hormonal changes of adolescence that affect the activity of the sebaceous glands. Hereditary tendencies also are known to be predisposing factors. Precipitating factors may include food allergies, endocrine disorders, psychological factors, fatigue, and the use of steroid drugs.

Sebum, an oily substance produced by the sebaceous glands, reaches the skin surface through the hair follicle. Overproduction of the oil seems to stimulate the follicle walls, causing a faster shedding of skin cells. This causes the cells and sebum to stick together and to form a plug, which promotes the growth of bacteria in the follicles. This is the process by which pimples and nodules form.

Diagnosis

Examination of the characteristic lesions and patient history confirm the diagnosis.

Treatment

Therapy may include the use of topical or systemic antibiotics or both. Topically applied **keratolytic** agents may prove appropriate for many cases of acne. Topical application of medications chemically related to vitamin A (e.g., tretinoin [Retin-A] and adapalene) reduces the skin's natural oils and promotes drying and peeling of the acne lesions. Benzoyl peroxide gels are also effective. Antibiotics are prescribed to kill bacteria residing on the skin or in the lesions. Long-term antibiotic use for acne treatment, however, may have side effects. Often combination therapy, including benzoyl peroxide, topical antibiotics, and retinoids, is the most effective.

For severe acne, isotretinoin (Accutane) may be indicated. Isotretinoin helps reduce the amount of sebum the body produces. Low-dose estrogen is prescribed to balance hormone levels. Optimal results usually are obtained by incorporating medications. Caution must be taken in the use of isotretinoin because it may produce serious psychological side effects, including depression, psychosis, and even suicide. Pregnant or nursing mothers should never take isotretinoin. Isotretinoin is a vitamin A derivative that is administered under an FDA program called IPLEDGE. Providers (physicians, nurse practitioners), patients, and pharmacists must participate in the IPLEDGE program for use of this agent. A newer treatment of intralesional dilute steroid injection can be done. This usually results in significant decreased size and erythema in a matter of hours but can cause a depression.

Prognosis

The prognosis varies, depending on the extent of the acne and the individual's compliance with the medication regimen, including all topical and ingested medications prescribed.

Prevention

The etiology is unknown, so no prevention is known.

Patient Teaching

Give patients information about acne and its care. Teach patients the methods of applying dermal medications. Encourage patients to report any side effects resulting from oral medications. Emphasize the importance of not squeezing any pimples or pustules. In addition, emphasize the importance of good hand washing after touching involved skin areas.

Herpes Zoster (Shingles)

Description

Herpes zoster, or shingles, is an acute inflammatory dermatomal eruption of extremely painful vesicles.

ICD-10-CM Code	B02.9 *(Zoster without complications)*
	(B02.0-B02.9 = 16 codes of specificity)

Herpes zoster has more than one form and location and therefore more than one code. Refer to the physician's diagnosis and then to the current edition of the ICD-10-CM coding manual to ensure the greatest specificity of pathology.

Symptoms and Signs

Shingles occurs in a bandlike unilateral pattern along the course of the peripheral nerves or dermatomes that are affected, and it does not cross the midline of the body (Fig. 6.14). Pain, often in the form of burning or tingling, begins about 2 or 3 days before the appearance of the lesions and sometimes is accompanied by a fever. The eruptions begin as a rash that rapidly develops into vesicles. The skin that overlies the affected dermatome or dermatomes becomes reddened and blistered. These vesicles often are grouped on a reddened area of the skin. After several days, the vesicles appear pustular, develop a crust, and then develop a scab.

The incubation period is 7 to 21 days. The duration of the disease, from onset to recovery, is usually 10 days to 5 weeks. If all the vesicles appear within 24 hours, the total duration is usually shorter. Although the commonly affected site is the skin overlying thoracic dermatomes (see Fig. 6.14), any area of the body may be affected. Shingles occasionally occurs on the face, neck, and scalp. When nerves supplying the eye are involved, the disease may cause serious damage to the eye structure.

Patient Screening

Patients experiencing the onset of herpes zoster often experience excruciating pain in the affected area. Prompt assessment and intervention are required. An appointment should be scheduled as soon as possible for the day of the call. When no appointment is available, refer to a facility where the patient can be seen promptly. Drug therapy beginning immediately helps reduce the severity of symptoms.

Etiology

The cause is varicella-zoster virus (VZV), which is the same virus that causes chickenpox. For unknown reasons, after lying dormant in the dorsal root ganglia, it becomes reactivated in later years. Stress appears to be a precipitating factor.

Diagnosis

Shingles (Fig. 6.15) is diagnosed by its characteristic pattern and painful vesicles. One can confirm the diagnosis by culturing the virus from vesicle scrapings. A blood sample containing VZV antibodies also aids in the diagnosis.

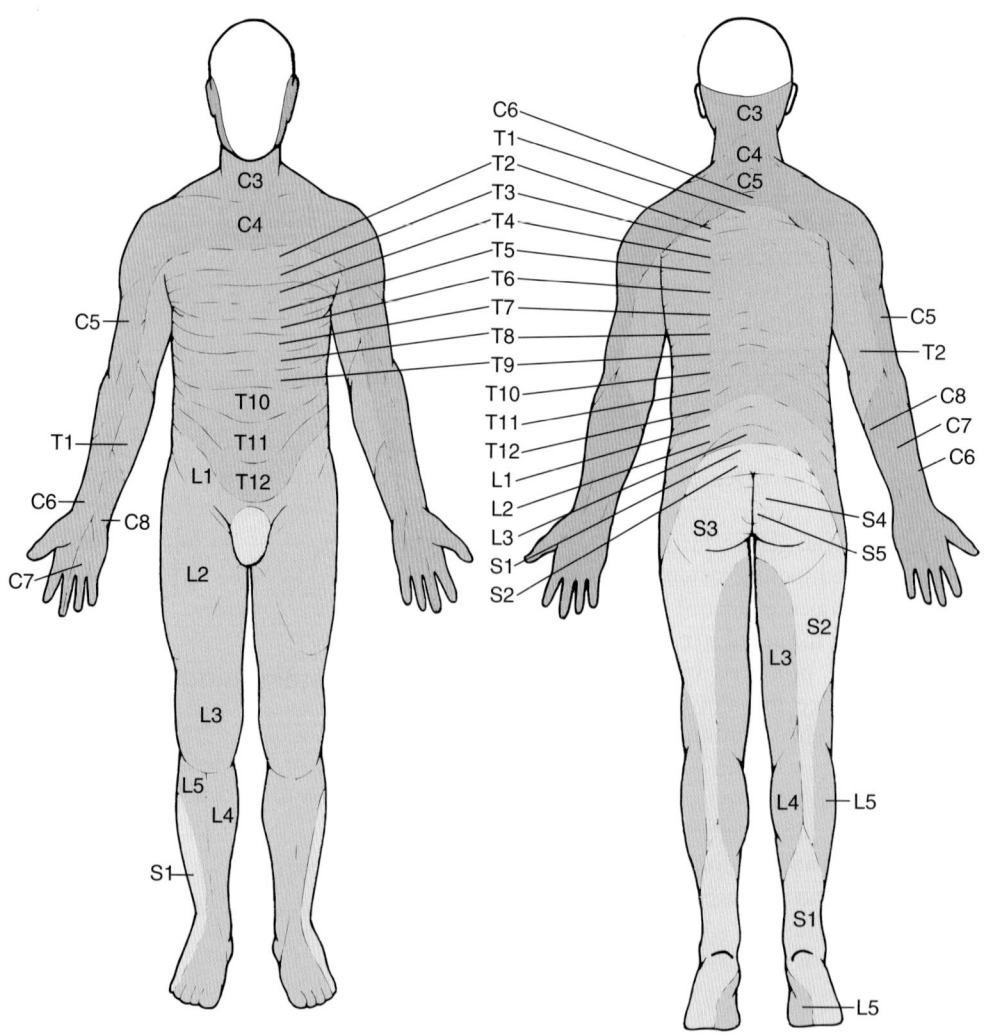

• **Fig. 6.14** Dermatomes.

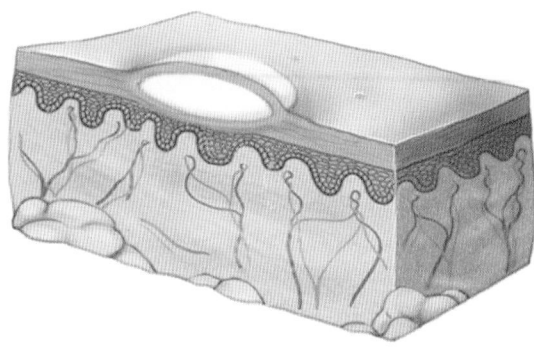

• **Fig. 6.15** Illustration of blisters of shingles. (From Brooks ML, Brooks DL. *Exploring medical language: a student-directed approach*, ed 8, St Louis, 2012, Mosby.)

Although shingles can affect any age group, those older than 55 years of age are more frequently affected.

Treatment

Treatment of shingles is directed toward making the patient comfortable. Analgesics, mild tranquilizers or sedatives, antipruritics, steroids (e.g., methylprednisolone, prednisone, and betamethasone [Celestone Soluspan]), and a drying agent to be applied directly to the vesicles may be prescribed. Acyclovir (Zovirax) used orally, parenterally, or topically also is prescribed and is quite effective. Other antiviral agents that may be prescribed include Famciclovir (Famvir), valacyclovir (Valtrex), or foscarnet sodium (Foscavir). Antibiotic therapy may be necessary to prevent secondary infections. If the eye is affected, early treatment with idoxuridine is necessary. An ophthalmologist should supervise the latter therapy. Topical treatment with capsaicin cream may provide relief in some cases. Caution is advised because capsaicin may burn when applied. There is also anecdotal evidence that certain essential oils applied to the vesicles can provide pain relief.

When the pain is intolerable, injections of lidocaine and nerve block agents may be attempted. If these steps do not provide relief, permanent nerve blocks via alcohol or nerve resection may be used as a last resort. Shingles occasionally recurs at later dates.

Prognosis

Most cases resolve within a month. A common complication for some patients is postherpetic neuralgia (PHN). This chronic pain may persist from a month to years after the skin lesions have healed. Patients with chronic PHN may be treated with gabapentin (Neurontin) and are often referred to pain clinics for treatment.

Prevention

A vaccine for herpes zoster, Zostavax, is now available. A newer vaccine, Shingrix, was introduced in 2017 and is now the preferred vaccine. This is a relatively new vaccine, and its success is still under study. Other than vaccination with Zostavax and Shingrix, no prevention is currently known. Research is being conducted to determine the effectiveness of the chickenpox vaccine in preventing subsequent incidence of shingles. Shingles is not contagious, but exposure to fluid in the blisters by an individual who has never had chickenpox may cause chickenpox in that individual. Immunocompromised patients and pregnant women should avoid contact with individuals diagnosed with shingles.

Patient Teaching

Give patients information about the disorder. Encourage patients to take their medications, including pain medications, as prescribed.

Impetigo

Description

Impetigo is a common, contagious, superficial skin infection. It manifests with early vesicular or pustular lesions that rupture and form thick yellow crusts (Fig. 6.16).

ICD-10-CM Code	L01.00 *(Impetigo, unspecified)*
	(L01.00-L01.09 = 5 codes of specificity)
	L01.03 *(Bullous impetigo)*

Impetigo has more than one form or location and therefore more than one code. Refer to the physician's diagnosis and then to the current edition of the ICD-10-CM coding manual to ensure the greatest specificity of pathology.

Symptoms and Signs

Impetigo lesions, a honey-colored crust, usually develop on the legs and are found less often on the face, trunk, and arms. Small vesicles are surrounded by a circle of reddened skin and usually are accompanied by pruritus. Adjacent lesions may develop as a result of autoinoculation resulting from scratching, but systemic symptoms are uncommon. Ulcerations with erythema and scarring also may result from scratching or abrading of the skin.

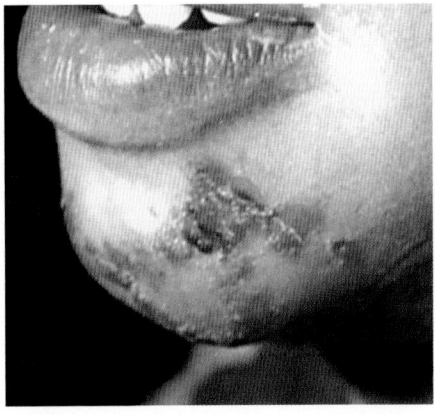

• **Fig. 6.16** Impetigo. (From Marks JG, et al: *Lookingbill & Marks' principles of dermatology*, ed 5, Philadelphia, 2014, Saunders.)

Patient Screening

Discovering the impetigo infection can be distressing to the individual or to the parent of an affected child. Urgent attention also is needed because impetigo can spread among children or other contacts. Because of the contagious nature of impetigo, the child's school may require immediate attention to the situation. Schedule the next available appointment for the patient, and if none is available that day or the next, refer the patient to an open facility (emergency department or clinic) for prompt assessment and treatment.

Etiology

Impetigo is caused by either *Streptococcus* or *Staphylococcus aureus*. The infection is thought to originate from insect bites, scabies infestation, poor hygiene, anemia, malnutrition, and impairment in skin integrity related to eczema. It is also highly contagious and so may be spread among children in schools or in the childcare environment. Cases of impetigo are common in temperate climates and occur more often in warm weather.

Diagnosis

The diagnosis is based on the appearance of the characteristic lesions. To differentiate impetigo from other skin diseases, the Tzanck test and Gram staining may be useful.

Treatment

Systemic use of antibiotics and proper cleaning of lesions two or three times a day are effective treatments for impetigo. Mupirocin ointment (Bactroban) or cream, along with penicillin, cephalexin, erythromycin, or dicloxacillin, is used in the treatment. Avoiding infected individuals is essential.

Prognosis

With treatment, the prognosis is good. Most children recover without difficulty.

Prevention

Good hygiene is essential in preventing impetigo. Frequent and thorough hand washing is the first line of defense, as in many contagious conditions. Instruct children not to share towels, bedding, clothing, or other personal items.

Patient Teaching

Give parents or caregivers information about impetigo and the ways it spreads. Encourage them to teach children about the importance of good hygiene.

Furuncles and Carbuncles

Description

A furuncle, or boil, is a pus-containing abscess that involves the entire hair follicle and adjacent subcutaneous tissue. A carbuncle is either an unusually large furuncle or multiple furuncles that develop in adjoining follicles, connected by many drainage canals.

ICD-10-CM Code	L02.92 (Furuncle, unspecified)
	L02.93 (Carbuncle, unspecified)
	(L02.01-L02.93 = 56 codes of specificity)

Furuncles and carbuncles are coded by the site or location. The code above is for unspecified site. Refer to the physician's diagnosis and then to the current edition of the and ICD-10-CM coding manual to ensure the greatest specificity of pathology.

ICD-10-CM Code	L02.02 (Furuncle of face)
	L02.03 (Carbuncle of face)
	L02.12 (Furuncle of neck)
	L02.13 (Carbuncle of neck)
	L02.221 (Furuncle of abdominal wall)
	L02.222 (Furuncle of back [any part, except buttock])
	L02.223 (Furuncle of chest wall)
	L02.224 (Furuncle of groin)
	L02.225 (Furuncle of perineum)
	L02.226 (Furuncle of umbilicus)
	L02.229 (Furuncle of trunk, unspecified)
	L02.231 (Carbuncle of abdominal wall)
	L02.232 (Carbuncle of back [any part, except buttock])
	L02.233 (Carbuncle of chest wall)
	L02.234 (Carbuncle of groin)
	L02.235 (Carbuncle of perineum)
	L02.236 (Carbuncle of umbilicus)
	L02.239 (Carbuncle of trunk, unspecified)
	L02.429 (Furuncle of limb, unspecified)
	L02.439 (Carbuncle of limb, unspecified)
	L02.529 (Furuncle of unspecified hand)
	L02.539 (Carbuncle of unspecified hand)
	L02.33 (Carbuncle of buttock)
	L02.429 (Furuncle of limb, unspecified)
	L02.439 (Carbuncle of limb, unspecified)
	L02.629 (Furuncle of unspecified foot)
	L02.639 (Carbuncle of unspecified foot)
	L02.821 (Furuncle of head [any part, except face])
	L02.828 (Furuncle of other sites)
	L02.831 (Carbuncle of head [any part, except face])
	L02.838 (Carbuncle of other sites)

Symptoms and Signs

Furuncles begin as the inflamed hair follicle becomes infected and the infection extends beyond the follicle. The affected area is red, swollen, and painful (Fig. 6.17). Eventually, over several days, the pus-filled abscess either bursts through the skin or, less often, discharges internally. In either case, the pain is relieved and the boil heals. Erythema and edema may persist at the site for several more days or weeks.

Boils are extremely common. They can affect almost everyone at some time. Carbuncles are much rarer. Both boils and carbuncles tend to recur.

Patient Screening

The individual reporting the symptoms of a furuncle or carbuncle will convey the degree of urgency to be seen. Give the patient some possible appointment times and schedule to his or her convenience. When the patient reports pain and swelling, offer the next available appointment.

Etiology

The most common cause of furuncles and carbuncles is bacterial infection with *Staphylococcus*, usually *S. aureus*. Both are localized infections and usually heal uneventfully. Predisposing factors include diabetes mellitus, nephritis, immunodeficiency, intravenous (IV) drug abuse, and other underlying diseases (e.g., digestive or gastrointestinal conditions). However, many have no underlying medical disease. In some cases, furuncles and carbuncles result from poor resistance to infection or from poor hygiene.

Diagnosis

The diagnosis is made by observing the characteristic lesion. An abscess may be cultured to isolate the causative organism. If recurring boils are a problem, the physician may order blood and urine analyses to rule out any underlying disease.

Treatment

Applying hot compresses every few hours helps relieve the discomfort and hasten the draining. Surgical incision and drainage (I&D) may be necessary. Antibiotic (cephalexin [Keflex] or dicloxacillin) treatment also may be needed for several weeks. There has been an increase in methicillin-resistant *S. aureus* (MRSA) as a causative agent in recurring carbuncles. If MRSA is suspected, culture and alternative antibiotic therapy is recommended; either a sulfa-based antibiotic or doxycycline can be effective against most MRSA infections.

Prognosis

Most furuncles and carbuncles resolve with I&D and antibiotic therapy.

Prevention

Prevention requires thorough cleansing of the skin and application of good hand washing techniques. Patients should be urged not to squeeze the lesions.

Patient Teaching

Give patients information on skin infections and how they spread. Demonstrate good hand washing techniques.

Cellulitis

Description

Cellulitis is an acute, diffuse, bacterial infection of the skin and subcutaneous tissue.

ICD-10-CM Code	L03.90 *(Cellulitis, unspecified)*
	L03.91 *(Acute lymphangitis, unspecified)*
	(L03.011-L03.91 = 86 codes of specificity)

Cellulitis appears in many forms and locations and thus has more than one code. Refer to the physician's diagnosis and then to the current edition of the ICD-10-CM coding manual to ensure the greatest specificity of pathology.

Symptoms and Signs

Cellulitis occurs most often in the lower extremities, but any part of the body can be affected. Clinically erythema and pitting edema develop, and the skin becomes tender and hot to the touch (Fig. 6.18). The infection develops and spreads gradually over a couple of days. Red lines or streaks may appear proximal to the infection and run along lymph vessels to nearby lymph glands. If the lymph glands become edematous, systemic symptoms of fever and malaise may be present.

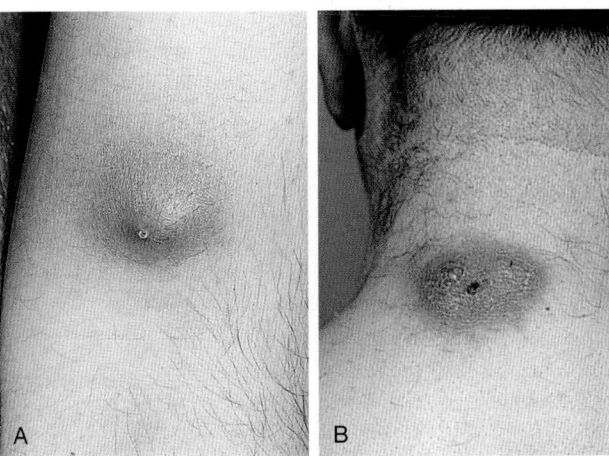

• **Fig. 6.17** (A) Furuncle. (B) Carbuncle. (A, From LaFleur B: *Exploring medical language: a student-directed approach,* ed 9, St Louis, 2014, Mosby; B, From Lawrence CM, Cox NH: *Physical signs in dermatology: color atlas and text,* London, 1993, Mosby Europe.)

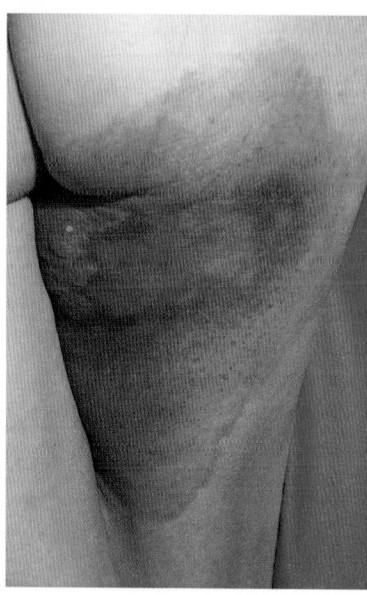

• **Fig. 6.18** Cellulitis. (From Marks JG, et al: *Lookingbill and Marks' principles of dermatology,* ed 4, Philadelphia, 2006, Saunders.)

Patient Screening

An individual reporting symptoms of edematous skin, reddened, and hot along with streaks of red radiating from the site, requires prompt assessment. If the individual cannot be seen in the office within a few hours, refer him or her to a medical facility where prompt and immediate evaluation and treatment may be obtained.

Etiology

The cause of cellulitis is either *Streptococcus* or *Staphylococcus,* which enters the skin's surface via a small cut or lesion. The bacteria produce enzymes that break down the skin cells. As a result of the release of enzymes, the infection spreads locally. These enzymes prevent body responses that normally would reduce local spread of infection by closing off the site.

Diagnosis

An examination of the affected body part, a check for pitting edema and other symptoms, and a blood culture aid the physician in making the diagnosis.

Treatment

The affected limb should be immobilized and elevated. Cool magnesium sulfate (Epsom salt) solution compresses may be used for discomfort. Warm compresses should be applied to increase circulation to the affected part. Systemic antibiotics, with penicillin being the drug of choice, are prescribed for the infection. Aspirin, NSAIDs, or acetaminophen alone or in combination with codeine is given for pain. Acetaminophen combinations with narcotics is also an option. Hospitalization is indicated when cellulitis is severe.

Prognosis

The prognosis is good with prompt intervention and drug therapy. Hospitalization with IV drug therapy often is required to achieve a positive outcome.

Prevention

Good hand washing is essential for prevention. Attention to small nicks and cuts helps prevent this infection.

Patient Teaching

Give patients information about skin infections and the importance of seeking medical attention promptly for an infected cut or scrape.

Dermatophytoses

Description

Dermatophytosis (tinea) is a chronic superficial fungal infection of the skin.

ICD-10-CM Code	B35.9 *(Dermatophytosis, unspecified)*
	(B35.0-B35.9 = 9 codes of specificity)

There are many codes for dermatophytosis, depending on site. Refer to the physician's diagnosis and then to the current edition of the ICD-10-CM coding manual to ensure the greatest specificity of pathology.

Symptoms and Signs

Dermatophyte infections are classified by the body region they inhabit. All dermatophytosis lesions are characterized by an active border and are marked by scaling with central clearing. Dermatophytosis occurring on the scalp is called *tinea capitis;* the body, *tinea corporis;* the nails, *tinea unguium;* the feet, *tinea pedis* (athlete's foot); and the groin region, *tinea cruris.*

Patient Screening

Dermatophytosis is troublesome, worrisome, and annoying. The individual calling for an appointment for these symptoms should be seen at the next convenient appointment.

Tinea Capitis

ICD-10-CM Code	B35.0 *(Tinea barbae and tinea capitis)*

Tinea capitis is characterized by round, gray, scaly lesions on the scalp (Fig. 6.19). It is contagious and often epidemic among children. The infected child may have a slight pruritus of the scalp or may be asymptomatic. It is rarely seen in adults.

Tinea Corporis (Ringworm)

ICD-10-CM Code	B35.9 *(Dermatophytosis, unspecified)*

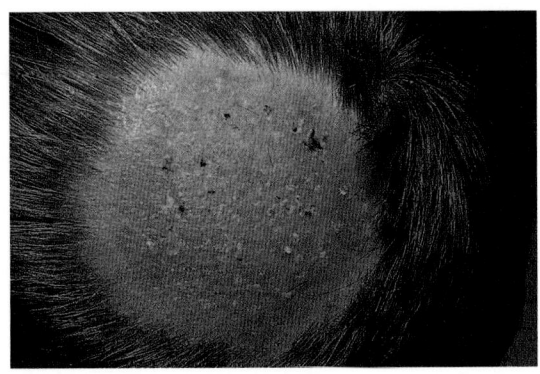

• **Fig. 6.19** Tinea capitis. (From Callen J, et al: *Color atlas of dermatology,* ed 1, Philadelphia, 1993, Saunders.)

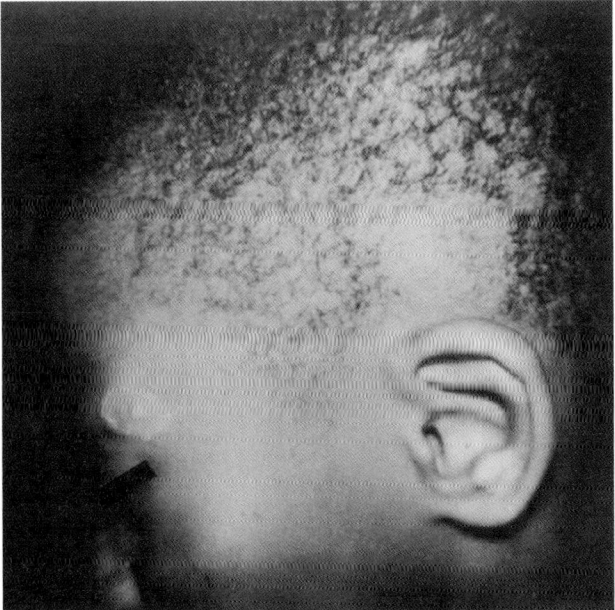

• **Fig. 6.20** Tinea corporis (ringworm). (From Mahon CR, et al: *Textbook of diagnostic microbiology,* ed 5, Philadelphia, 2015, Saunders.)

Tinea corporis is characterized by lesions that are round, ringed, and scaled with vesicles (Fig. 6.20). This infection can occur in anyone who has skin contact with infected domestic animals, especially cats. It is more common in rural settings and in hot and humid climates. It can also be the result of autoinoculation from infections in other parts of the body, such as tinea pedis or tinea capitis, or of contact with contaminated soil.

Tinea Unguium

ICD-10-CM Code	B35.1 *(Tinea unguium)*

Tinea unguium frequently begins at the tip of toenails, affecting one or more nails at a time. It also can affect fingernails, but this is less common. The affected nail or nails appear hypertrophic or thickened, brittle, and lusterless.

Tinea Pedis (Athlete's Foot)

ICD-10-CM Code	B35.3 *(Tinea pedis)*

Tinea pedis is characterized by intense burning, stinging pruritus between the toes and on the soles of feet (Fig. 6.21). The skin can become inflamed, dry, and peeling; and fissures (see Fig. 6.2J) may develop. This condition is rare in children.

Tinea Cruris (Jock Itch)

ICD-10-CM Code	B35.6 *(Tinea cruris)*

Tinea cruris is characterized by raised, red, pruritic vesicular patches, with well-defined borders, located in the groin area (Fig. 6.22). It can be associated with athlete's foot and occurs more often in adult men. Flare-ups are frequent in summer months and are aggravated by physical activity, perspiration, and tight-fitting clothes.

Etiology

Dermatophytosis is caused by several species of fungi that can invade the skin or nails, especially if the integrity of the skin is compromised. The infection is transmitted by direct contact with the fungus or its spores.

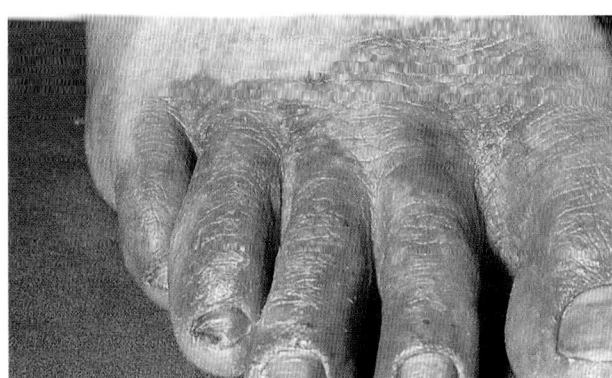

• **Fig. 6.21** Tinea pedis (athlete's foot). (From Gawkrodger D: *Dermatology,* ed 5, New York, 2012, Churchill Livingstone.)

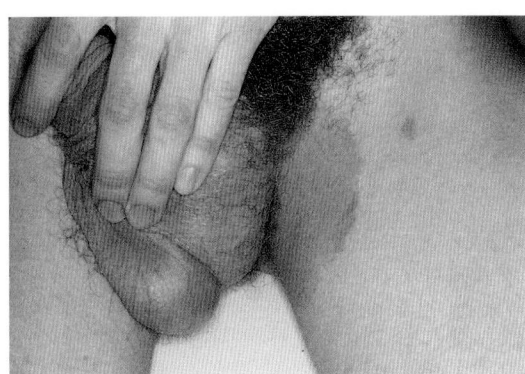

• **Fig. 6.22** Tinea cruris (jock itch). (From Callen J, et al: *Color atlas of dermatology,* ed 1, Philadelphia, 1993, Saunders.)

Diagnosis

The diagnosis is based on the appearance and location of the lesions. To isolate the causative fungus, culture of the lesions is necessary.

Treatment

Antifungal medications are prescribed either for topical application (ointment) or for oral use, depending on the severity of the infection. Selenium sulfide 2.5% (Selsun shampoo) is usually prescribed for treatment of tinea capitis, whereas terbinafine hydrochloride (Lamisil), butenafine (Lotrimin Ultra), and fluconazole (Diflucan) are normally prescribed for treatment of tinea pedis, tinea corporis, and tinea cruris, respectively. The affected skin must be kept as clean and dry as possible, clothing should be loose-fitting and clean, and exercise should be limited to prevent excessive perspiration. Because all forms of dermatophytosis tend to be persistent and chronic, meticulous management is needed to correct this condition.

Prognosis

The prognosis is good with treatment that includes drug therapy and good skin care; however, because the condition tends to be chronic, recurrence is likely.

Prevention

Wearing loose-fitting cotton clothing helps prevent the condition. The patient must dry the skin after bathing or swimming, with special attention to drying the skin between the toes and in the folds of the skin. Use of a blow dryer on low setting can aid in drying the area thoroughly.

Patient Teaching

Give the patient information about the disorder. Encourage the patient to dry the skin after exposure to moisture, especially in the areas between the toes and in the folds of the skin. Explain the importance of wearing cotton clothing that absorbs moisture from the body. Advise patients with diabetes and those with compromised peripheral circulation to seek medical attention for athlete's foot.

Decubitus Ulcers

Description

A decubitus ulcer, commonly called a *pressure ulcer* or *bed sore,* is a localized area of dead skin that can affect the epidermis, dermis, and subcutaneous layers (Fig. 6.23).

ICD-10-CM Code	L89.90 (Pressure ulcer of unspecified site, unspecified stage) (L89.000-L89.95 = 151 codes of specificity)

Skin ulcers can occur in many locations. Refer to the physician's diagnosis and then to the current edition of the ICD-10-CM coding manual to ensure the greatest specificity of pathology.

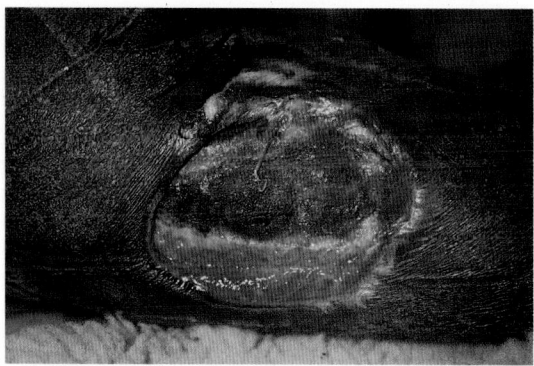

• **Fig. 6.23** Decubitus ulcer. (From Callen J, et al: *Color atlas of dermatology,* ed 1, Philadelphia, 1993, Saunders.)

Symptoms and Signs

An early sign of a decubitus ulcer is shiny, reddened skin appearing over a bony prominence in individuals with prolonged immobilization. Other signs that eventually occur include blisters, erosions, necrosis, and ulceration. If the decubitus ulcer becomes infected, a foul-smelling, purulent discharge is present. Pain may or may not accompany a decubitus ulcer.

Patient Screening

Most patients experiencing decubitus ulcers are confined to a bed or are generally immobile. These patients may not be capable of going to the office for a visit and therefore are seen in the hospital, nursing care facility, or home. Make arrangements for those who are immobile to be visited by a physician in their environments. Schedule an appointment for the mobile patient to be seen at the earliest available time.

Etiology

Decubitus ulcers are caused by impairment or lack of blood supply to the affected area of skin. This is the result of constant pressure against the surface of the skin, as seen in people who are debilitated, paralyzed, or unconscious.

Diagnosis

Visual examination of the ulcer is sufficient for a diagnosis. If infection is suspected, culture and sensitivity testing may be needed to isolate the causative organism.

Treatment

If not treated vigorously, the ulcer progresses from a simple erosion of the skin to complete involvement of all layers of skin. Eventually the ulcer extends to the underlying muscle and bone tissue, and osteomyelitis and/or gangrene may result.

Topical agents that have proved effective in the treatment of decubitus ulcers include absorbable gelatin sponges, granulated sugar, karaya gum patches, antiseptic irrigations, débriding agents, and antibiotics (when infection is present).

Prognosis

The prognosis is fair. Resolution and healing of the lesion depends on the patient's general health and potential for mobility and removal of pressure on the lesion site.

Prevention

Preventive measures include frequent inspection of the skin for signs of breakdown; alleviation of pressure points over bony prominences; good skin care; early ambulation, when possible; position changes every 2 hours; passive range-of-motion exercises; and the use of special pads and mattresses.

Patient Teaching

Most teaching is directed to the caregivers. Encourage preventive measures and prompt reporting of any signs of impending skin breakdown.

Scabies and Pediculosis

Description

Itch mites (scabies) and lice (pediculosis) are the two most common parasitic insects to infest humans. Human scabies infestations are caused by the human itch mite, *Sarcoptes* *scabiei* (Fig. 6.24A). The three species of human lice are the head louse, *Pediculus humanus capitis* (Fig. 6.25A); the body louse, *P. humanus corporis;* and the pubic, or crab, louse, *Phthirus pubis* (Fig. 6.26A). Lice resemble insects, but they are wingless parasites with sucking mouths to feed on human blood. They prefer to lay their eggs on body hair but also lay them in folds of clothing.

ICD-10-CM Code	B85.2 *(Pediculosis, unspecified)*
	(B85.0-B85.4 = 5 codes of specificity)
	B86.0 *(Scabies)*
	B85.0 *(Pediculosis due to Pediculus humanus capitis)*
	B85.1 *(Pediculosis due to Pediculus humanus corporis)*
	B85.3 *(Phthiriasis)*

Scabies and lice codes should be confirmed for accuracy with a coding manual. Refer to the physician's diagnosis and then to the current edition of the ICD-10-CM coding manual to ensure the greatest specificity of pathology.

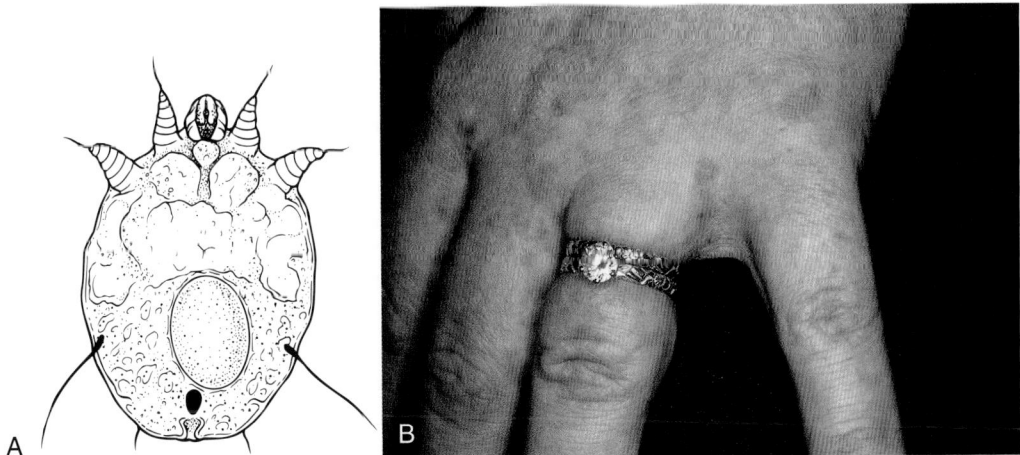

• **Fig. 6.24** (A) Itch (scabies) mite. (B) Scabies rash. (A, From Callen J, et al: *Color atlas of dermatology,* ed 1, Philadelphia, 1993, Saunders. B, From James WD, et al: *Andrews' diseases of the skin,* ed 11, Philadelphia, 2011, Saunders.)

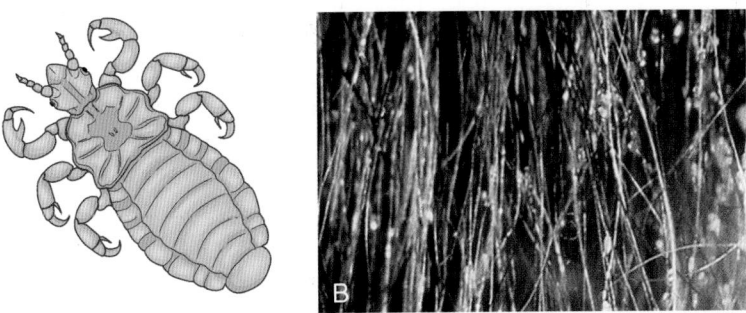

• **Fig. 6.25** (A) Pediculus humanus capitis (head louse). (B) Lice in hair. (From Lissauer T, et al: *Illustrated textbook of paediatrics,* ed 4, London, 2012, Mosby.)

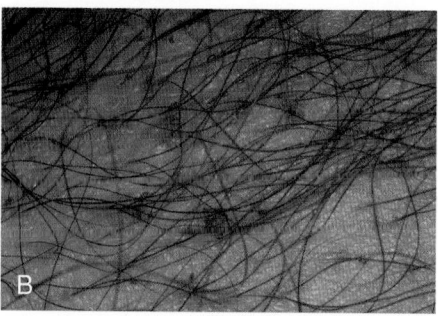

• **Fig. 6.26** (A) Phthirus pubis (pubic, or crab, louse). (B) Pubic lice rash. (From Long SS, et al: *Principles and practice of pediatric infectious diseases,* ed 4, Philadelphia, 2012, Saunders.)

Symptoms and Signs

Both scabies and pediculosis are *highly* contagious. They produce intense pruritus and a sensation of something crawling on the skin. With scabies, the most common symptom is a rash (see Fig. 6.24B) accompanied by intense itching that worsens at night. Scabies can occur anywhere on the body but usually is found on the hands, breasts, armpits, waistline, and the genital area. Lice also can produce a rash or wheals, but the most common sign or symptom is the presence of nits (eggs) on hair shafts, skin, or clothing (see Figs. 6.25B and 6.26B).

Patient Screening

Patients reporting symptoms of scabies or lice should be seen as soon as possible. The infestation in children may have been detected at a child care facility or school. These children must be assessed, and treatment must be prescribed and started as soon as possible. Although not a life-threatening condition, scabies or lice can be spread to others through close contact, and the offending mites and lice should be brought under control quickly.

Etiology

Itch mites and lice can infest anyone at any age. Both are spread easily from person to person via close physical contact. Transmission occurs most often among children playing together, family members, and sexual partners. In addition to physical contact, transmission may occur indirectly via infected clothing, bed sheets, towels, and hair combs or brushes. Although the scabies mite can infest other mammals, it is not transmitted from pets to humans. Pubic lice, however, have been known to infest dogs and then migrate to humans. Both scabies and pediculosis are common in overcrowded areas that have inadequate facilities and where personal hygiene is poor.

Diagnosis

Visual examination can identify lice and nits on the hair, body, and clothing. Other skin disorders, such as atopic dermatitis (see the Atopic Dermatitis (Eczema) section), contact dermatitis (see the Contact Dermatitis section), and psoriasis (see the Psoriasis section), must be ruled out when scabies is suspected. A similar rash occurring about the same time in several family members should suggest scabies.

Treatment

The goals of treatment of scabies and pediculosis are to remove the mites, lice, and nits; to eliminate the pruritus; to provide emotional support to the patient, family, and contacts; and to treat the environment to prevent reinfestation.

To kill head lice, a special shampoo (lindane shampoo and permethrin creme rinse) must be used and then repeated in 7 to 10 days to ensure that all nits are dead. The patient must follow this with meticulous combing with a special fine-toothed comb to remove the nits. Body lice are removed with soap and water or the same shampoo used for head lice. Pubic lice may be treated with shampoo, creams, or lotions. Directions must be followed when using these special shampoos, because they may have residual toxic effects. Nonprescription treatments for head lice include permethrin, pyrethrins, or piperonyl butoxide. Prescription treatments include permethrin, malathion, or lindane, as well as ivermectin and spinosad for resistant cases.

Scabies treatment includes the use of special shampoos, creams (permethrin cream [Elimite]), sulfur preparations, and topical steroids. Because of the intense pruritus and the scratching associated with scabies and lice infestations, secondary infections may occur, necessitating treatment with oral antibiotics.

With both scabies and pediculosis, family members and others who have had direct contact with the infected person must be treated as well. All clothing and bedding belonging to the infected person must be washed in hot water or drycleaned. Any furniture that the person has been using also should be cleaned either with a surface cleaner or by vacuuming.

Prognosis

The prognosis is good with treatment and appropriate disinfection or decontamination of clothing, bedding, and furniture. Those who have had contact with the patient must be made aware of the infestation and be treated in a similar manner to prevent reinfestation.

Prevention

Prevention is difficult with the close social contact among people. Recommend that family members, including children, not share hats and hair-grooming equipment. Infestation by pubic lice is considered a sexually transmitted disease (STD), and suggested precautions are discussed in Chapter 12.

Patient Teaching

Give patients written information about recognizing scabies and lice. Pictures of the offending organisms help in their recognition. Explain the importance of laundering clothing and bedding appropriately. Emphasize the importance of notifying all persons in contact with the patient about the infestation so that they can seek treatment. Teach the correct methods of using shampoos or scabicides.

Benign and Premalignant Tumors

Description

Noncancerous growths or tumors of the skin fall into two categories: benign and premalignant. Benign tumors are usually a cosmetic problem only. Premalignant tumors must be identified and treated as early as possible to prevent them from developing into malignancies. Common benign and premalignant tumors include seborrheic keratoses, dermatofibromas, keratoacanthomas, keloids and hypertrophic scars, epidermal (sebaceous) cysts, acrochordons (skin tags), actinic keratoses, and nevi.

Symptoms and Signs

Symptoms and signs vary according to the conditions experienced. Moles are the most common premalignant tumors. Following is a discussion of the conditions.

Patient Screening

Although benign tumors are usually only a cosmetic problem, they still present a source of anxiety to the patient. Premalignant tumors require early identification and treatment to prevent their development into malignancies. Recognize the patient's anxiety level, and schedule an appointment at the earliest convenient time.

Seborrheic Keratosis

ICD-10-CM Code   L82.0 (Inflamed seborrheic
                          keratosis)
                    (L82.0-L82.1 = 2 codes of
                          specificity)
                    L82.1 (Other seborrheic keratosis)

Seborrheic keratoses are benign growths originating in the epidermis, clinically appearing as tan-brown, greasy papules or plaques (see Fig. 6.2B and C) and having the appearance of being pasted onto the skin (Fig. 6.27). They are, for the most part, asymptomatic but may cause pruritus, especially in older people. These usually painless lesions may be black, brown, yellow, or other colors and may be located on the

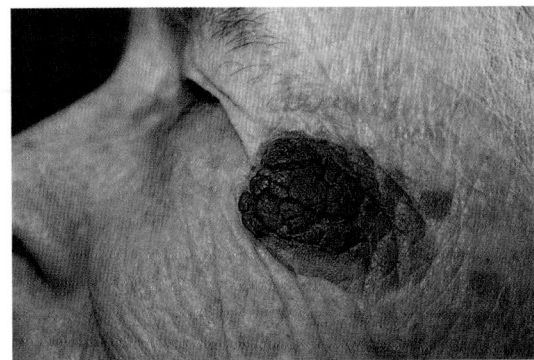

Fig. 6.27 Seborrheic keratosis. (From Callen J, et al: *Color atlas of dermatology,* ed 1, Philadelphia, 1993, Saunders.)

face, chest, back, shoulders, or other areas. Additionally, the lesions may have a rough, wartlike texture and may have a slightly elevated flat type of surface. The cause of seborrheic keratoses is unknown, and although they have no potential for developing into malignancy, they should be differentiated from other potentially malignant tumors. The appearance of a sudden increase in the number or size of these growths on uninflamed skin could indicate the presence of an internal malignancy, most commonly of the stomach.

Dermatofibroma

ICD-10-CM Code   D23.9 (Other benign neoplasm
                          of skin, unspecified)
                    (D23.0-D23.9 = 18 codes of
                          specificity)
Dermatofibromas can have more than one site
    and therefore more than one code. Refer to the
    physician's diagnosis and then to the current edition
    of the ICD-10-CM coding manual to ensure the
    greatest specificity of pathology.

Dermatofibromas are benign and asymptomatic and can be found on any part of the body, particularly on the front of the lower leg. They are most often seen in young adults and are more common in women. These lesions are thought to be caused by fibrous reactions to viral infections. These growths also can be caused by a reaction to insect bites and trauma. Dermatofibromas are scaly, hard growths that are slightly raised and pinkish brown (Fig. 6.28).

Keratoacanthoma

ICD-10-CM Code   D48.5 (Neoplasm of
                          uncertain behavior of skin)

Keratoacanthoma is a benign epithelial growth that may be caused by a virus and generally is seen in people in their 60s. The growth is a smooth, red, dome-shaped papule with a central crust that usually appears singly but may occur in multiple numbers (Fig. 6.29). Keratoacanthoma can disappear spontaneously, but scarring is common. It must be differentiated from squamous cell carcinoma (SCC).

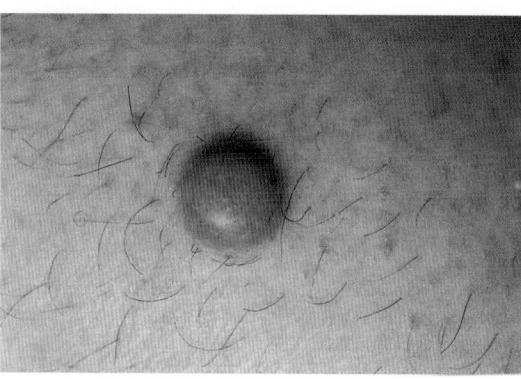

• **Fig. 6.28** Dermatofibroma. (From Callen J, et al: *Color atlas of dermatology,* ed 1, Philadelphia, 1993, Saunders.)

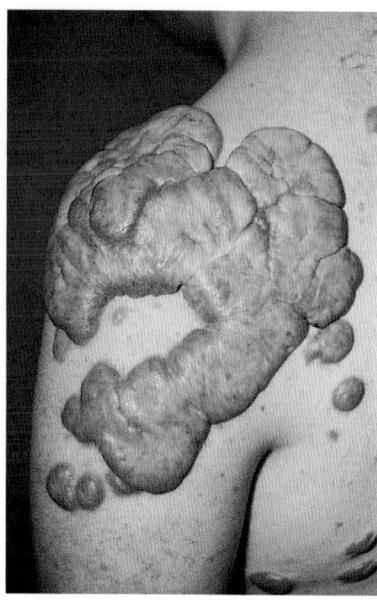

• **Fig. 6.30** Keloid. (From Callen J, et al: *Color atlas of dermatology,* ed 1, Philadelphia, 1993, Saunders.)

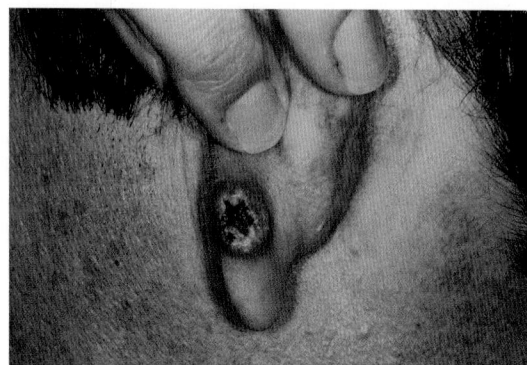

• **Fig. 6.29** Keratoacanthoma. (From Callen J, et al: *Color atlas of dermatology,* ed 1, Philadelphia, 1993, Saunders.)

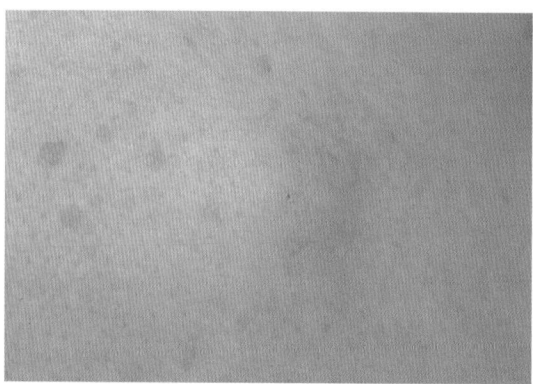

• **Fig. 6.31** Epidermal (sebaceous) cyst. (From Marks JG, et al: *Lookingbill and Marks' principles of dermatology,* ed 4, Philadelphia, 2006, Saunders.)

Keloids and Hypertrophic Scars

ICD-10-CM Code	L91.0 *(Hypertrophic scar)*
	(L91.0-L91.9 = 3 codes of specificity)

Keloids and hypertrophic scars occur secondary to trauma or surgery. A keloid first appears normal, but after several months, it becomes noticeably larger and thicker (Fig. 6.30). Keloids are harmless, but they can cause pruritus and sometimes deformities. They are more common in dark-skinned people. Keloids extend beyond the wound site and do not regress spontaneously. Hypertrophic scars, however, do not extend but stay confined to the site, and they generally regress over time. Keloids can be addressed surgically.

Epidermal (Sebaceous) Cyst

ICD-10-CM Code	L72.12 *(Trichodermal cyst)*

Sebaceous cysts develop when a sebaceous gland slowly fills with a thick fluid. This process can take many years but is usually painless and harmless. Some cysts, usually small ones, have a blackhead in the pore connecting the cyst to the skin's surface. Larger cysts most often are closed on the surface. The cysts are palpable and moveable and range in size from millimeters to several centimeters (Fig. 6.31). Sebaceous cysts commonly are found on the scalp, on the face, at the base of the ears, and on the chest. They also can develop in any area of the body that contains sebaceous glands. If bacteria enter the pore, the cyst becomes infected and enlarges, and inflammation and tenderness occur. The cyst eventually may burst, releasing a foul-smelling pus. Inflammation recedes, but the cyst remains and can become reinfected at another time.

Acrochordon (Skin Tag)

ICD-10-CM Code	L90.9 *(Atrophic disorder of skin, unspecified)*
	(L90.0-L90.9 = 9 codes of specificity)
	L91.9 *(Hypertrophic disorder of the skin, unspecified)*

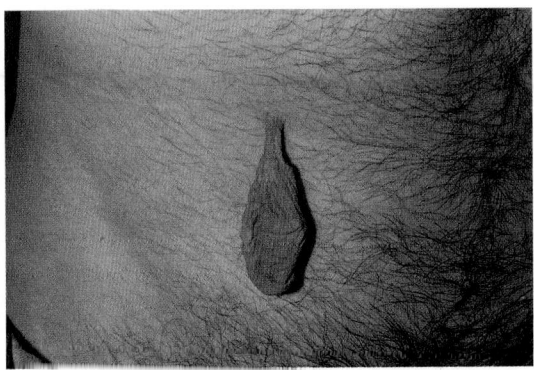

• **Fig. 6.32** Acrochordon (skin tag). (From Callen J, et al. *Color atlas of dermatology*, ed 1, Philadelphia, 1993, Saunders.)

Acrochordons are common benign skin growths or tags. Painless and usually caused by friction, they are found mainly in the axilla, on the neck, and on inguinal areas of the body. They can be brown or skin colored, flat or slightly elevated, and are attached to the body by a short stalk (Fig. 6.32).

Actinic Keratosis

ICD-10-CM Code L57.0 *(Actinic keratosis)*

Actinic keratoses are common premalignant lesions and are seen on sun exposed areas of the body. They are caused by long-term exposure to the UV portion of sunlight, and their numbers increase with age. Light-skinned people have a higher risk. Actinic keratosis initially appears as an area of rough, vascular skin, which later forms a yellowish brown, adherent crust (Fig. 6.33).

Etiology

The causes vary, depending on the type of lesion.

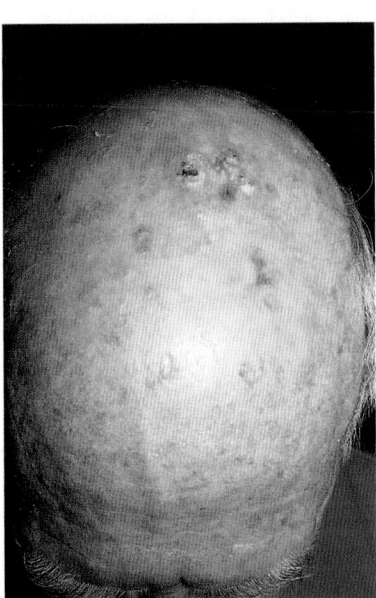

• **Fig. 6.33** Actinic keratoses. (From Callen J, et al: *Color atlas of dermatology*, ed 2, Philadelphia, 2000, Saunders.)

Diagnosis

The diagnosis of these lesions is made through visual examination; biopsy may be necessary to confirm the findings.

Treatment

Treatment of these lesions varies, depending on the specific type of lesion. Seborrheic keratoses are treated with cryosurgery and curettage. Dermatofibromas can be surgically excised if symptomatic. Keratoacanthoma is treated with surgical excision, adrenocorticosteroids applied topically, and, for multiple lesions, oral isotretinoin and etretinate. Keloids and hypertrophic scars are treated with corticosteroids injected into the lesion once every 4 weeks or with surgery and scar compression. Epidermal, or sebaceous, cysts are excised surgically and treated with antibiotics, if infected. Acrochordons (skin tags) also are treated with excisional surgery. Actinic keratosis is treated with topical agents, tretinoin (Retin-A) alone or in combination with fluorouracil, and with curettage and desiccation.

Prognosis

The prognosis varies, depending on the condition, the duration of the condition, the amount of skin involved, and the physical condition of the patient. Biopsy reports will indicate the possible outcome.

Prevention

Most of these lesions cannot be prevented. Avoiding direct exposure of the skin to sunlight helps prevent keratoacanthoma and actinic keratosis. The use of sunscreen is encouraged.

Patient Teaching

Give patients information about various benign and premalignant tumors. Encourage consistent use of sunscreen and regular evaluation of suspicious skin lesions by a physician. Explain that many patients are referred to a dermatologist for follow-up care.

Skin Carcinomas

Collectively, the skin cancers, basal cell carcinoma (BCC), SCC, and malignant melanoma, represent the most common type of malignancy. In fact, BCC is the most prevalent form of cancer worldwide. Because BCC and SCC usually do not metastasize, they often are not included on most cancer registries. Left untreated, however, these nonmelanoma skin cancers can be extremely locally destructive and can invade nerves, lymphatics, blood vessels, cartilage, and bone.

Nonmelanoma Skin Cancers

Description

BCC and SCC affect more than 3 million Americans each year. BCC arises in the basal (deepest) layer of the epidermis, and SCC arises in the epithelial (outer) layer.

ICD-10-CM Code

(Refer to the Neoplasm Table in the current edition of the ICD-10-CM coding manual)

Skin cancers are coded by body site and type. Refer to the physician's diagnosis and then to the current edition of the ICD-10-CM coding manual to ensure the greatest specificity of pathology. A morphology code is also required and is listed in the current edition of the coding manual.

Symptoms and Signs

BCC and SCC lesions can appear anywhere on the body. The most common sites are the sun-exposed areas: face, scalp, ears, back, chest, arms, and back of the hands. About 70% of BCC lesions occur on the face (25%–30% on the nose) (Fig. 6.34). The BCC skin lesion can appear several ways:

- A shiny bump or nodule that is pearly white, pink, red, or translucent. Blood vessels may appear on the surface;
- A sore that bleeds, heals, and recurs. It may be associated with ulceration and crusting;
- A reddish, irritated area, usually on the back, shoulders, extremities, or chest that may or may not be painful or cause pruritus;
- A smooth growth with an indented center and elevated, rolled edge, or border; and
- A scarlike area, often with poorly defined edges, that is white, yellow, or waxy in appearance.

SCC lesions often present as a crusted or scaly area with a red, inflamed base; as a growing tumor; as a nonhealing ulcer; or as a raised, firm papule (Fig. 6.35). Hyperkeratosis is an important feature that distinguishes SCC from BCC. The ulcerated lesions may be painful.

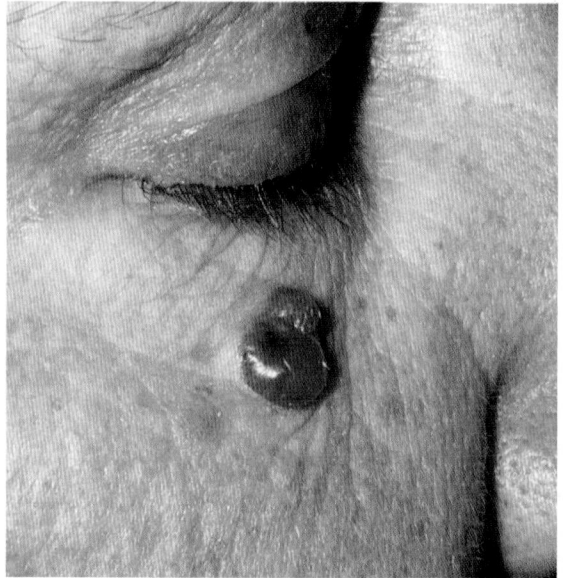

• **Fig. 6.34** Basal cell carcinoma (BCC). (From James WD, et al: *Andrews' diseases of the skin,* ed 11, Philadelphia, 2011, Saunders.)

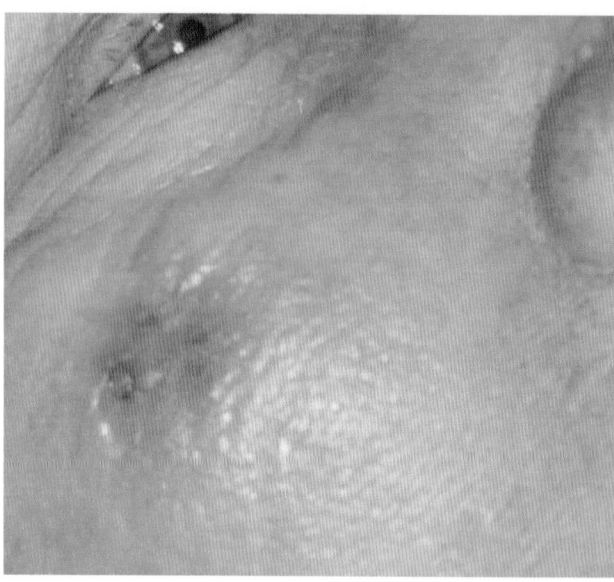

• **Fig. 6.35** Squamous cell carcinoma (SCC) of the nose. (From Pfenninger JL, Fowler GC: *Pfenninger and Fowler's procedures for primary care,* ed 3, Philadelphia, 2011, Saunders.)

Patient Screening

Patients reporting any of the following should be scheduled to be seen at the next available appointment: skin lesions, such as a sore that bleeds, heals, and recurs; a reddish, irritated area, usually on the back, shoulders, extremities, or chest, that may or may not be painful or cause pruritus; or a smooth growth with an indented center and elevated, rolled edge or border or a scarlike area, often with poorly defined edges, that is white, yellow, or waxy in appearance. Although most of these conditions at an early stage are not life-threatening, the patient's anxiety probably is quite high. Giving the patient the earliest possible appointment for assessment and treatment of the condition is a prudent approach to total patient care.

Etiology

These forms of skin cancer can develop in anyone, especially those with a history of sun exposure. It is thought that recent sun exposure is the major risk factor for SCC, whereas childhood and adolescent sun exposure is the major risk for BCC. People at highest risk for both carcinomas have fair skin and light-colored hair and eyes. Chronic exposure to the UV radiation in sunlight has two main effects that can lead to tumor formation: (1) It causes mutations in deoxyribonucleic acid (DNA); and (2) it suppresses the skin's immune system, weakening its ability to fight any tumors that do form. Additional risk factors include therapeutic radiation treatment, immunosuppression, and chronic exposure to arsenic. Rare genetic syndromes, such as basal cell nevus syndrome, also increase the risk of nonmelanoma skin cancer. SCC often arises from actinic keratosis or chronically inflamed skin resulting from scar tissue or burns. Smoking increases the risk of development of these carcinomas. Although nonmelanoma skin cancers are not likely to metastasize, some forms of SCC are more aggressive and will spread to distant locations in the body. Both types will cause local destruction if left untreated.

Diagnosis

Unusual skin lesions are often identified by the patient or by the physician on examination of the skin. A biopsy (usually a punch biopsy) of the lesion is required for definitive diagnosis. Patients with SCC should have a lymph node examination to assess for nodal metastases. Those with high-risk SCC may also require computed tomography (CT), magnetic resonance imaging (MRI), or positron emission tomography (PET) examinations to evaluate for disease spread. SCC is staged according to the TNM (tumor–node–metastasis) staging system.

Treatment

Treatment consists of conventional or Mohs (surgery with intraoperative histologic evaluation) surgical excision (90% of cases), cryosurgery (tissue destruction by freezing), electrodesiccation (tissue destruction by heat), and curettage (ED&C), or radiation therapy. Topical therapy may include 5-fluorouracil or imiquimod. Systemic chemotherapy is reserved for those with distant metastases or locally advanced disease.

Patients should be monitored closely for 5 years after treatment to check for recurrence, metastasis, or a new skin cancer.

Prognosis

The overall 5-year survival rate for nonmelanoma skin cancer is 95%. SCC carries a worse prognosis if it occurs on the lip, ear, or scalp or is larger than 2 cm in diameter. About 50% of patients develop another skin cancer within 5 years. Although BCC carries an excellent prognosis because it rarely metastasizes, around 40% of patients with one BCC develop another lesion within 5 years. Having nonmelanoma skin cancer increases the risk of getting another BCC or SCC and of developing malignant melanoma.

Prevention

Minimizing sun exposure, especially during childhood, is the key to prevention, because people generally receive most of their lifetime UV exposure before adulthood. Any suspicious skin lesions should be evaluated by a physician.

Patient Teaching

Give patients written information about skin cancer. Help them find additional resources for more information. After excision of any lesion, give the patient information about care of the site. Encourage consistent use of sunscreen on exposed skin, and recommend that the patient limit the duration of exposure. Emphasize the importance of regular follow-up examinations.

Malignant Melanoma

Description

Malignant melanoma is the most serious of the three types of skin cancer, but it is not as common. It arises in epidermal melanocytes, cells that make the brown pigment melanin.

ICD-10-CM Code   C43.9 *(Malignant melanoma of skin, unspecified)*

Symptoms and Signs

Most melanomas occur as solitary lesions. They can be found anywhere on the skin but are most common on the backs in men and the legs in women. The most common symptom is change, either a newly pigmented area of the skin or a change in a mole that may have been present since birth or childhood (Fig. 6.36). Changes that may indicate the presence of malignant melanoma are:
- change in size, especially sudden or continuous enlargement
- change in color, especially multiple shades of tan, brown, and black; mixing of red, white, and blue; or spreading of color from the border into adjacent skin
- change in shape, especially the development of an irregular, notched border of an area with a previously regular border
- change in the elevation of a previously flat pigmented area
- change in the surface: scaliness, erosion, oozing, crusting, or bleeding

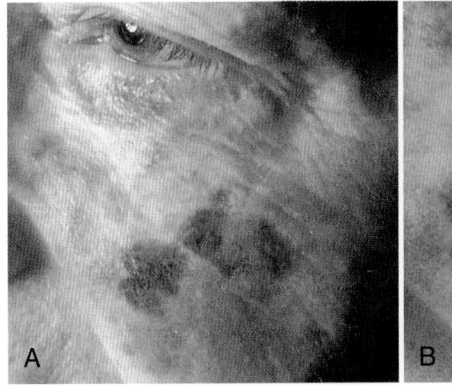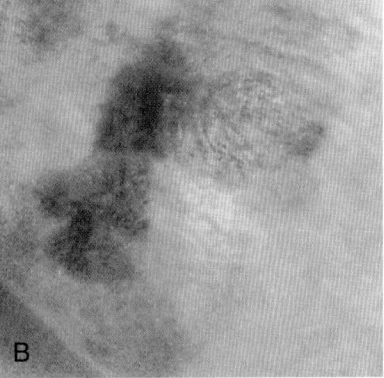

• **Fig. 6.36** (A) A fully developed malignant melanoma of the left cheek in an older man. (B) Close-up of the lesion. (From Rigel DS, et al: *Cancer of the skin,* ed 2, London, 2012, Saunders.)

- change in the surrounding skin: redness, swelling, or the development of colored areas adjacent to, but not part of, the pigmented area
- change in sensation: tenderness, pain, or pruritus
- change in consistency: softening or hardening

These changes are incorporated into a list known as the ABCDEs of melanoma (see the Enrichment box).

◆ ENRICHMENT

ABCDEs of Malignant Melanoma

- A = Asymmetry (lack of equality in the diameter)
- B = Border (notched, scalloped, or indistinct)
- C = Color (uneven, variegated ranging from tan, brown, or black to red and white)
- D = Diameter (usually greater than 6 mm)
- E = Evolving (any change in size, shape, color, elevation, or another trait; or any new symptom, such as bleeding, itching, or crusting)

Patient Screening

Patients who report the previous warning signs or symptoms should be seen at the next available appointment. Consider that the patient's anxiety level is probably quite high. Giving the patient the earliest possible appointment for assessment and treatment of the condition is a prudent approach to total patient care.

Etiology

Risk factors for melanoma include a sun-sensitive skin type (fair skin, light-colored hair and eyes, and skin that burns easily), history of severe sunburn (especially during childhood), geographic location closer to the equator, and use of tanning beds. Intermittent, intense exposures to UV light increase the risk more compared with continuous exposure. Apart from sun/UV radiation exposure, other factors that make certain people more prone to malignant melanoma are:

- a family history of malignant melanoma
- a previous case of malignant melanoma or nonmelanoma skin cancer
- having many atypical (irregular shape or color) moles
- xeroderma pigmentosum, a genetic disorder associated with defects in DNA repair, leading to multiple skin cancers at a young age

Diagnosis

If a patient observes any of the ABCDE warning signs or notices an unusual growth, he or she should see a physician immediately. Greater than 50% of melanomas are first identified by the patient. Biopsy, usually excisional biopsy, is needed for histologic diagnosis and for staging. Staging is performed on the basis of the results of a full physical examination, chest radiography, liver function tests, and serum lactate dehydrogenase (LDH) measurement. If distant metastases are expected, CT, MRI, and PET may be ordered. For patients with advanced melanoma, biopsy specimens may be tested for certain genetic mutations, such as mutation of the *BRAF* gene, which may help guide therapy choices.

Treatment

The treatment of choice is complete excision of the cancerous lesion with wide margins. Sentinel lymph node biopsy is often performed, with complete lymph node dissection if the sentinel node tests positive. Immunotherapy and targeted chemotherapy are becoming the mainstays of treatment for advanced melanoma. The goal of immunotherapy is to boost the body's own immune system to destroy cancer cells. Immunotherapeutic agents currently being used include ipilimumab, interferon-α, and interleukin-2. Recently drugs that specifically target the BRAF protein have been approved for the treatment of melanoma in individuals whose tumor harbors *BRAF* mutation. Many other targeted drugs are currently in clinical trials. Conventional chemotherapy and radiation therapy are still used in many cases.

Prognosis

The overall 5-year survival rate for all stages of melanoma is around 90%, although the presence of distant metastasis reduces this rate to only 15% to 20%. Poorer prognosis is associated with the presence of an ulcerated lesion, axial location of the melanoma, higher number of positive lymph nodes, age greater than 60 years, and male gender. The level of the S-100 protein, a tumor marker, can be used to determine the prognosis, with high levels after melanoma resection indicating a worse prognosis. In addition, the prognosis can be accurately correlated with tumor thickness (called *Breslow thickness*). The correlation ranges from a thickness of less than 0.5 mm carrying a 10-year survival rate of 96% to a thickness of greater than 4 mm carrying a 10-year survival rate of 54%.

Prevention

Increased awareness of skin cancer and education about the dangers of excessive sun exposure greatly can improve the prevention and early detection of skin carcinomas and save lives. Adults should perform regular skin self-examinations. People at very high risk (those with familial melanoma syndromes, multiple atypical or common moles, or excessive sun exposure) should see their physicians for periodic whole-body examinations to look for early melanoma lesions. Patients who have had melanoma require close, regular follow-up to screen for recurrence.

Patient Teaching

As with BCC and SCC, give the patient written information about skin cancer. Help the patient find additional sources of information. After excision of any lesion, give the patient information about care of the site. Encourage consistent use of sunscreen on exposed skin, and recommend limiting the time of exposure. Emphasize the importance of regular follow-up examinations. Encourage patients to ask questions about the effects of chemotherapy and radiation therapy.

See the Enrichment box for guidelines for protecting the skin against excessive sun exposure, and see Chapter 15 for a discussion of sunburn, including the latest FDA information about recent changes in sunscreen labeling and recommended use.

ENRICHMENT

Guidelines for Protecting the Skin Against Excessive Sun Exposure

- Avoid sunlight between 10 AM and 3 PM, when ultraviolet (UV) rays are the strongest.
- Plan outdoor activities for early morning or late afternoon.
- Wear protective clothing, especially a hat.
- Use a sunscreen with a sun protection factor (SPF) of at least 15, applied 15 to 30 minutes before exposure and again after getting wet, especially after swimming.

! ALERT!

Tanning Beds

The cancer division of the World Health Organization recently listed tanning beds as definitive cancer causers. Ultraviolet (UV) radiation emitted from both the sun and tanning beds was identified as a causative agent in cancers, particularly skin cancers. The use of tanning beds has been shown in studies to increase the risk of melanoma.

Abnormal Skin Pigmentation

Description

The skin normally contains special cells called *melanocytes* that produce melanin, a black pigment that gives color to the skin. Several conditions cause the melanocytes to develop abnormally or to be distributed abnormally. Melanocytes sometimes are fewer in number or less active than normal. This results in a pale area of skin that does not tan when exposed to sunlight. When melanocytes are more numerous or more active than normal, it results in a darker area of skin that tans easily. These abnormal conditions include albinism, vitiligo, melasma (chloasma), nevi (moles), seborrheic warts, pityriasis, and abnormal suntan.

Patient Screening

Abnormal skin pigmentation presents a cosmetic problem. For the individual calling for an appointment for these symptoms, the next convenient appointment should be scheduled.

Albinism

ICD-10-CM Code	E70.29 *(Other disorders of tyrosine metabolism)*
	(E70.20-E70.29 = 3 codes of specificity)
	E70.30 *(Albinism, unspecified)*
	(E70.30-E70.39 = 14 codes of specificity)
	E70.8 *(Other disorders of aromatic amino-acid metabolism)*

Albinism is a rare inherited condition in which the melanocytes are unable to produce melanin. The patient is pale skinned, with white hair and generally pink or pale blue eyes (Fig. 6.37). A rare disorder occurring in all races, albinism often is accompanied by eye problems. Eye problems may include myopia, hyperopia, astigmatism, nystagmus, strabismus, and photophobia. Patients with albinism must avoid the sun to prevent their eyes and skin from burning. This genetic disorder has no cure, but many of the eye problems can be treated. Counseling may help the child or young adult deal with social problems created by a general lack of understanding about the disorder.

Vitiligo

ICD-10-CM Code	L80 *(Vitiligo)*

Possibly an autoimmune condition, vitiligo produces pale irregular patches of skin, often evenly located on one side of the body (Fig. 6.38). The patches may enlarge, shrink, or stay the same size. Vitiligo can occur on any area of the body and affects all races. Vitiligo often follows a stressful incident. Vitiligo has no cure, but cosmetics may be used to cover the affected skin areas. Patients with vitiligo should be encouraged to use sunscreen.

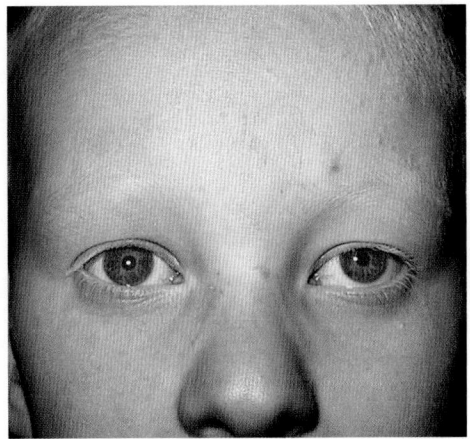

- **Fig. 6.37** Albinism. (From Zitelli BJ, Davis HW: *Atlas of pediatric physical diagnosis,* ed 6, Philadelphia, 2012, Mosby.)

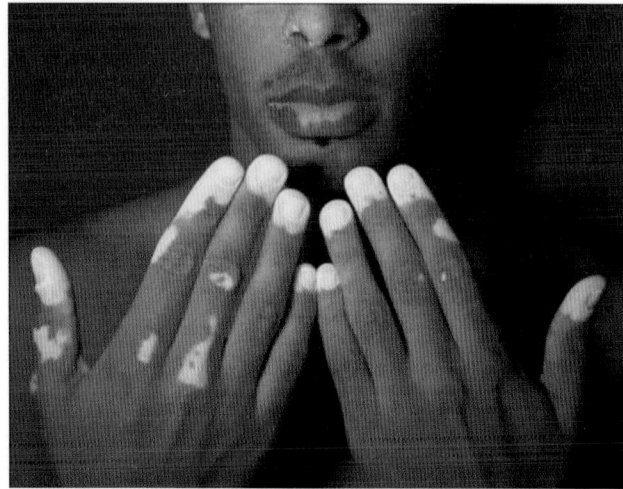

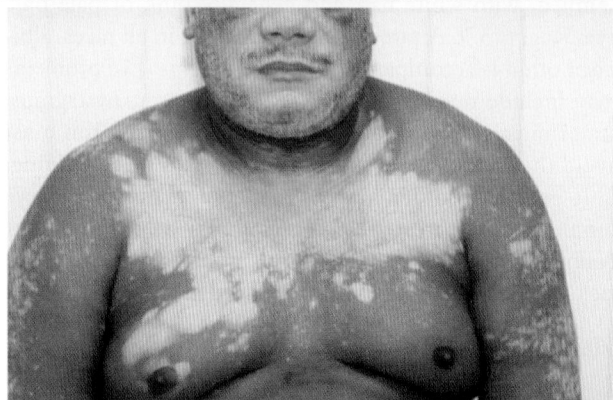

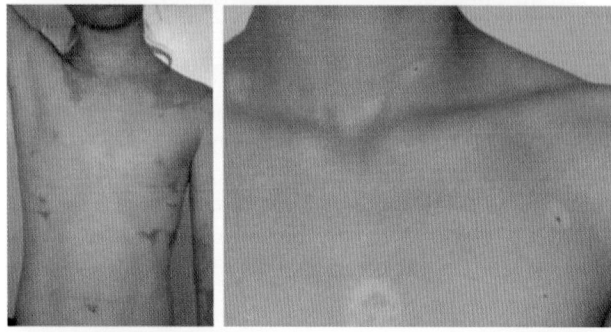

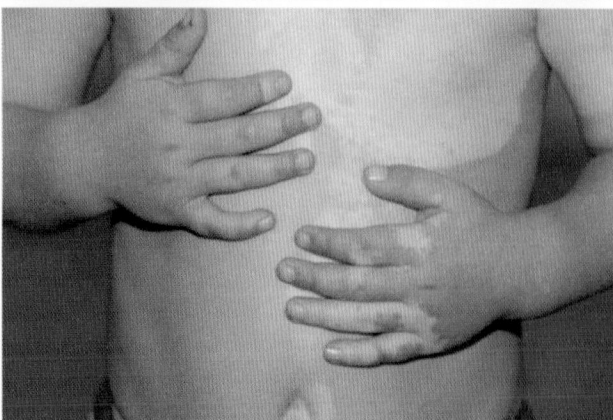

• **Fig. 6.38** Vitiligo. (From Ezzedine K, et al: Vitiligo. *Lancet,* 2015; 386(9988):74–84.)

Melasma (Chloasma)

ICD-10-CM Code   L81.8 *(Other specified disorders of pigmentation)*
(L81.0-L81.9 = 10 codes of specificity)

Melasma occurs in some women during hormonal changes, such as during pregnancy or with oral contraceptive use. Patches of darker skin develop on the face, especially over the cheeks (Fig. 6.39). This condition disappears after childbirth or when the oral contraceptive use is discontinued.

Hemangiomas

ICD-10-CM Code   D18.00 *(Hemangioma unspecified site)*
(D18.00-D18.09 = 5 codes of specificity)
Hemangiomas are coded by sites and types. Refer to the physician's diagnosis and then to the current edition of the ICD-10-CM coding manual to ensure the greatest specificity of pathology.

Hemangiomas are benign lesions of proliferating blood vessels in the dermis that produce a red, blue, or purple color. Examples of hemangiomas are the **nevus** flammeus (port wine stain), which is dark red to purple and usually is located on the face (Fig. 6.40A); the strawberry hemangioma, which is bright red and has a protruding, rough surface (see Fig. 6.38B); and the cherry hemangioma, which is red to purple and is a smooth, dome-shaped, small papule that is 2 to 5 mm in diameter (see Fig. 6.40C).

Nevi (Moles)

ICD-10-CM Code   *(Refer to Neoplasm, Skin, Benign in the current edition of the ICD-10-CM coding manual)*
There are many codes for nevus. Refer to the physician's diagnosis and then to the current edition of the ICD-10-CM coding manual to ensure the greatest specificity of pathology.

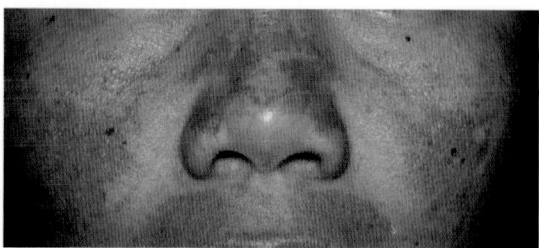

• **Fig. 6.39** Melasma (chloasma). (From Marks JG, et al: *Lookingbill & Marks' principles of dermatology,* ed 4, Philadelphia, 2006, Saunders.)

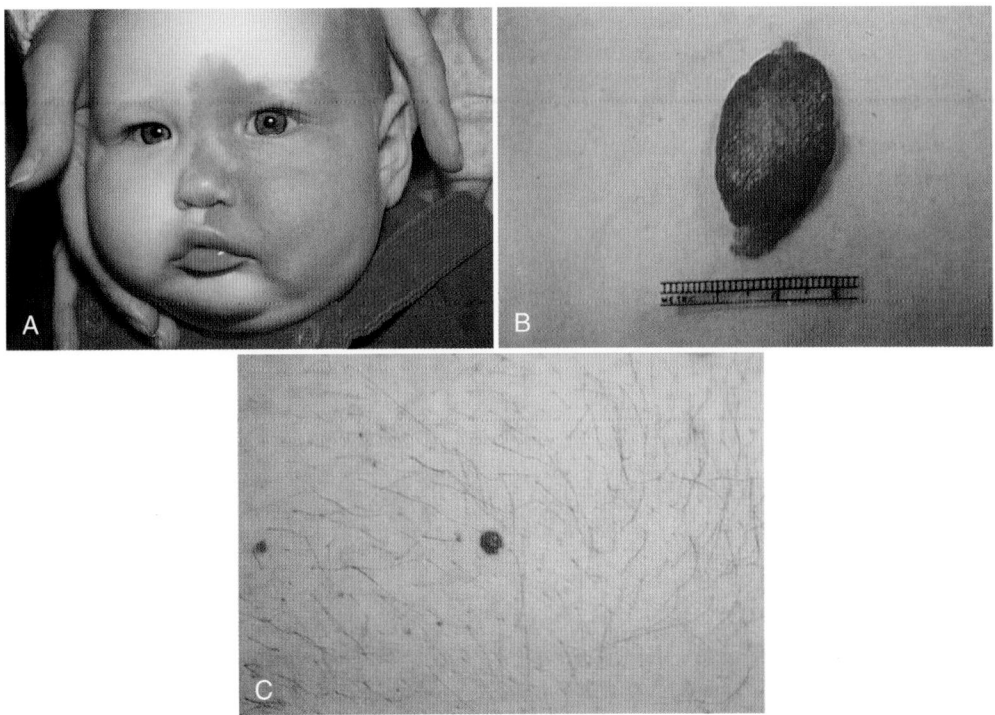

• **Fig. 6.40** (A) Port wine stain. (B) Strawberry hemangioma. (C) Cherry hemangioma. (A, From Zitelli BJ, Davis HW: *Atlas of pediatric physical diagnosis,* ed 6, Philadelphia, 2012, Mosby. B and C, From Marks JG, et al: *Lookingbill and Marks' principles of dermatology,* ed 4, Philadelphia, 2006, Saunders.)

Moles are small dark areas of skin composed of dense collections of melanocytes (Fig. 6.41); some may contain hair. A mole occasionally may become malignant (see the Malignant Melanoma section).

Pityriasis

ICD-10-CM Code   L30.5 *(Pityriasis alba)*
*Pityriasis may be coded according to location or form.
Refer to the physician's diagnosis and then to the
current edition of the ICD-10-CM coding manual to
ensure the greatest specificity of pathology.*

Pityriasis is a fungal infection that causes patches of flaky, light, or dark skin to develop on the trunk of the body. This is an uncommon condition. There are many types of pityriasis, with some leaving permanent changes to the skin color.

Abnormal Suntan

ICD-10-CM Code   L57.8 *(Other skin changes
                        due to chronic exposure
                        to nonionizing radiation)*

Abnormal suntan is an unspecified adverse effect resulting from a proper drug, medicinal, or biologic substance properly administered. Some drugs and certain diseases, such as Addison disease, can produce a suntan even without exposure to sunlight.

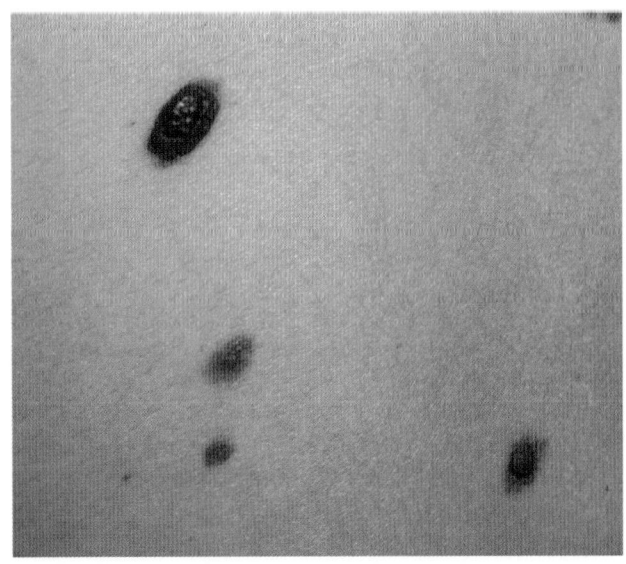

• **Fig. 6.41** Brown and tan nevi showing variation in appearance. (From Marks JG, et al: Lookingbill and *Marks' principles of dermatology,* ed 4, Philadelphia, 2006, Saunders.)

Etiology

The causes of abnormal skin pigmentation vary, depending on the abnormality.

Diagnosis

Most of these conditions are harmless, and visual examination by a physician confirms the diagnosis. Moles may cause concern, especially if size or shape has changed. The physician may recommend biopsy to rule out a malignancy.

Treatment

When any of these conditions produce skin color variations, nonprescription depigmenting creams may be used to lighten the affected skin. Vitiligo may be improved with UV lamp treatments combined with drug therapy. Pityriasis can be cured with application of antifungal ointments. Moles can be removed surgically, and other skin blemishes can be covered by using special cosmetics. Laser surgery may be used to treat hemangiomas.

Prognosis

The prognosis varies, depending on the condition and its extent. When drug therapy and surgical intervention are not appropriate or successful, cosmetics may be used to conceal the pigmentation problem.

Prevention

The etiology varies, so prevention varies as well. Hereditary conditions cannot be prevented. Most of these conditions occur without warning.

Patient Teaching

Help patients locate and use the available resources for their condition. Support groups often are available for certain cases. Encourage patients to recognize their self-worth.

Alopecia (Baldness)

Description

Alopecia is loss or absence of hair, especially on the scalp.

ICD-10-CM Code	L65.9 *(Nonscarring hair loss, unspecified)*

(L65.0-L65.9 = 5 codes of specificity)
Refer to the physician's diagnosis and then to the current edition of the ICD-10-CM coding manual to ensure the greatest specificity of pathology.

ICD-10-CM Code	L63.2 *(Ophiasis)*
	L63.8 *(Other alopecia areata)*
	L65.0 *(Telogen effluvium)*
	L65.8 *(Other specified nonscarring hair loss)*
	L66.0 *(Pseudopelade)*
	L66.2 *(Folliculitis decalvans)*
	L66.8 *(Other cicatricial alopecia)*

(L66.0-L66.9 = 7 codes of specificity)

Symptoms and Signs

Alopecia can be either temporary or permanent. It can appear gradually, as with aging, or suddenly, occurring all at once or in patchy areas, as with alopecia areata (Fig. 6.42).

Patient Screening

Alopecia is a troublesome and worrisome condition. It also may be the sign of an underlying health problem. Schedule an appointment for this patient to be seen when convenient for all involved.

Etiology

In most cases, baldness is a result of the aging process or heredity. It can, however, be a consequence of certain systemic illnesses, such as thyroid diseases, iron deficiency anemia, syphilis, or an autoimmune disease. Certain forms of dermatitis (see the Dermatitis section) also can cause alopecia. Chemotherapy, radiation therapy used to treat

---

◆ ENRICHMENT

Cosmetic Dermatology

Procedures may be performed in a dermatology office. They may include surgical and nonsurgical procedures, skin resurfacing, and application/prescription of anesthesia-type products. Some advanced offices may perform face lifts, blepharoplasty, rhinoplasty, otoplasty, lip implants, and facial liposuction. Collagen replacement and fat transfer procedures help decrease wrinkle depth.

Botulinum toxin (BTX), Botox (Allergan, Inc.), and Dysport (Ipsen, Slough, UK) have been approved by the FDA for the treatment of facial wrinkles (glabellar lines). Contraindications for these applications are Eaton-Lambert syndrome, amyotrophic lateral sclerosis (ALS) or myasthenia gravis, and a history of sensitivity to human albumin.

Injectable fillers (ranging from temporary to permanent) may be used for treating wrinkles and scars and for augmentation of the lips and other tissues. Microdermabrasion, dermabrasion,

and chemical peels are used for varying degrees of skin ablation, ranging from superficial skin conditions to tattoos, photoaging, and scarring. Laser treatments are used to treat photoaging, tattoos, pigmentation, vascular lesions, and acne scarring. There are nonablative procedures to treat fine lines and wrinkles by using radiofrequency resurfacing therapy that utilizes heat energy. Other treatments use a cooling process that kills fat cells to help with weight reduction.

Warning

Patients should be made aware of any dangers of any of these procedures and that there are no guarantees that any of them will provide the expected results. Caution must be used if any general type of anesthesia is being used for an outpatient procedure.

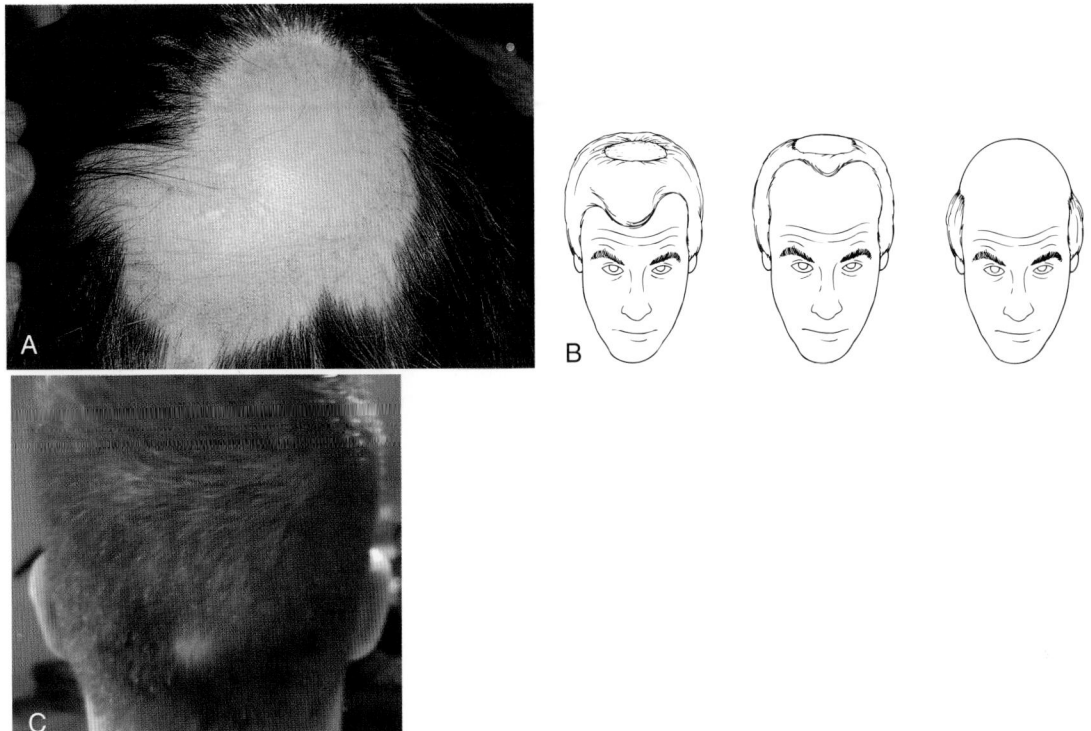

• **Fig. 6.42** (A) Alopecia areata. (B) Androgenetic alopecia (male pattern baldness). (C) Twenty-six-year-old male with patches of baldness that has been treated with steroids. (A and B, from Callen J, et al: *Color atlas of dermatology,* ed 2, Philadelphia, 2000, Saunders. C, Courtesy Margaret Frazier 2019.)

cancer, and some other types of medications may lead to thinning and loss of hair. Hair often grows back after treatment has been completed. More often, however, hair loss is not attributed to any specific disease process.

In men, alopecia tends to be part of the aging process and follows a familial pattern on the mother's side. The typical pattern is for the front hairline to recede and for the hair on the top of the head to thin. In some men, these areas eventually meet, leaving hair on only the sides of the head. This pattern of hair loss is called *androgenetic alopecia* (male pattern baldness) (see Fig. 6.42). Most women experience a gradual, but slight, loss of hair throughout life. Some women experience thinning of hair about 3 months post partum. This is a fairly common occurrence and corrects itself within a few months.

Loss of hair in oval patches without signs of inflammation is often the result of alopecia areata. It is most commonly seen on the scalp but can affect other hair-bearing areas, such as the eyebrows, beard, arms, or legs. Duration of hair loss is weeks to months and often spontaneous regrowth occurs. It is thought to be an autoimmune disease. A more severe but rare form of alopecia causes permanent hair loss over the entire body, including the eyebrows and eyelashes.

Diagnosis
Visual examination may be all that is needed for the diagnosis, but the cause should also be investigated. Blood and thyroid studies are needed to rule out thyroid disease and anemia. Sometimes punch biopsy is performed if scarring is present.

Treatment
Treatment of alopecia varies, depending on the cause. Effective treatment of any underlying disease usually restores hair growth to normal. To treat male pattern baldness, minoxidil (Rogaine) preparations used topically in cream and spray forms have shown promise. Finasteride (Propecia), is a drug therapy, but it should not be taken by women of child-bearing age because it may have teratogenic effects on their male offspring. Other options include wearing a toupee or wig or undergoing hair transplantation. Transplantation is effective for certain types of hair loss, especially male pattern baldness, but transplantation and the use of minoxidil are expensive and can have side effects. Minoxidil must be continued indefinitely, or hair will begin to fall out again. Alopecia areata can be treated with superpotent topical steroids or intralesional injection of triamcinolone.

Prognosis
The prognosis varies, depending on the cause. Alopecia resulting from the aging process or heredity will not resolve. As previously stated, treatment of an underlying medical cause may result in improvement.

Prevention
No prevention is known for alopecia.

Patient Teaching

Those who have baldness resulting from the aging process or heredity should be encouraged to accept the condition. Offer information about alopecia and permanent or temporary hair replacement.

Corns and Calluses

Description

Corns and calluses are extremely common, localized hyperplastic areas of the stratum corneum layer of the epidermis.

ICD-10-CM Code	L84 *(Corns and callosities)*

Symptoms and Signs

Corns have a glassy core, are small (less than one-fifth of an inch), are more painful than calluses, and develop on the toes. Calluses are larger (up to 1 inch) and commonly develop on the ball of the foot and the palm of the hand. Tenderness and pain over the affected area are the common symptoms.

Patient Screening

Patients with corns and calluses usually report painful feet when requesting an appointment. Schedule the next available appointment that is convenient for all involved.

Etiology

Both conditions may result from pressure or friction caused by ill-fitting shoes, orthopedic deformities, or faulty weight bearing. People who play stringed instruments and manual laborers are prone to calluses caused by repeated trauma to the affected area. In addition, people with impaired circulation in their feet resulting from peripheral neuropathy (sometimes caused by diabetes mellitus) are more prone to corns and calluses.

Diagnosis

It is unusual for corns and calluses to become so painful that the patient needs to consult a physician. When the patient does consult a physician, a physical examination of the affected area and brief history are sufficient for diagnosis.

Treatment

Relieving pressure and friction points as soon as possible is the goal of treatment. Many self-help measures, such as pads and sponge rings, chemical agents to soften and loosen corns, and pumice stone to rub off dead skin resulting from calluses, are available on the market. If these treatments are ineffective, a physician can trim the corn or callus surgically or with strong chemicals. *Caution:* Patients with diabetes mellitus should not use self-help measures but should seek the help of a podiatrist to treat corns and calluses.

Prognosis

Most corns and calluses resolve with treatment and removal of the offending pressure source.

Prevention

Properly fitting shoes help prevent corns and calluses. Some calluses caused by repeated trauma cannot be prevented.

Patient Teaching

Give patients information about the etiology of corns and calluses. Recommend the wearing of proper footwear. Encourage patients with diabetes and those with impaired circulation to seek professional foot care on a regular basis.

Verrucae (Warts)

Description

Verrucae are elevated growths of the epidermis that result from hyperplasia (Fig. 6.43).

ICD-10-CM Code	B07.9 *(Viral wart, unspecified)*
	(B07.0-B07.9 = 3 codes of specificity)

Warts have several codes. Refer to the physician's diagnosis and then to the current edition of the ICD-10-CM coding manual to ensure the greatest specificity of pathology.

Symptoms and Signs

Warts are a cutaneous manifestation of human papillomavirus (HPV) infection. The three most often seen types are common warts, plantar warts, and flat warts. Of the several types of warts, the most common is the common wart, which represents approximately 70% of all cutaneous warts. This wart is a small, hard, white or pink lump with a cauliflower-like surface. Inside the wart are small, clotted blood vessels that resemble black splinters.

A verruca can develop anywhere on the body but is most likely to appear on the hands or the soles of the feet. For the most part, the wart is painless, but a wart on the sole of a foot (plantar wart) can feel as if there is a stone in the shoe. Pruritus also can accompany a wart. Verrucae are common among teenagers and children, but no serious health risks are associated with these warts.

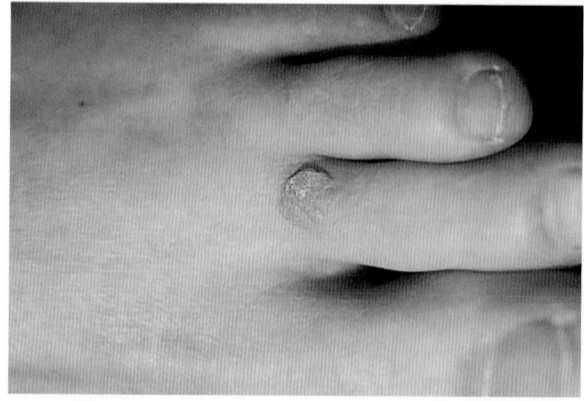

• **Fig. 6.43** Verruca (common wart). (Courtesy Department of Dermatology, School of Medicine, University of Utah, Salt Lake City, Utah.)

Etiology

Warts are caused by viruses and are spread by touch or contact with the skin shed from a wart. Each of the types of viruses known to cause warts tends to infect a different part of the body.

Diagnosis

Diagnosis is made on visual examination. There are two types of warts for which a physician should be consulted. One is penile or vulvar warts, and the other is a wart that develops after age 45 years. What looks like a wart actually could be a serious skin condition, such as skin cancer.

Treatment

Most warts disappear naturally over time. Many self-help remedies are available in the form of paints, creams, or plasters. These medications contain chemicals that destroy the abnormal skin cells, but they also damage the surrounding healthy cells. Care must be taken to minimize soreness. Warts located on the face or genitals should not be treated with these chemicals. A physician can remove persistent warts by surgical excision, cryosurgery, or electrodesiccation. Treatment is often painful and prolonged.

Prognosis

With medical intervention, the prognosis for most warts is good. Some warts tend to recur.

Prevention

Warts are contagious, and a wart may shed cells along with the virus when it is touched. Prevention of genital warts is discussed in Chapter 12.

Patient Teaching

Give patients information about warts and how they are spread. Advise them to wear shower shoes when using a public bathing facility.

Folliculitis

Description

Folliculitis is an inflammatory reaction of the hair follicles that produces erythemic, pustular lesions (Fig. 6.44).

ICD-10-CM Code	L66.3 (Perifolliculitis capitis abscedens)
	L73.8 (Other specified follicular disorders)
	(L73.0-L73.9 = 5 codes of specificity)

Symptoms and Signs

The pustules of folliculitis occur individually and do not combine. They usually are found on the thighs and buttocks but can also occur in the beard area and on the scalp. Some patients may report mild discomfort, mainly because

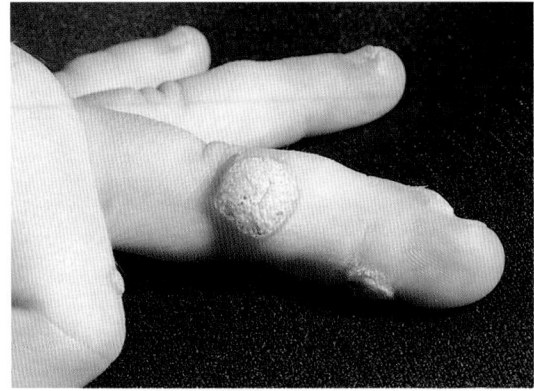

• **Fig. 6.44** Folliculitis. (From Callan J, et al: *Color atlas of dermatology*, ed 1, Philadelphia, 1993, Saunders.)

of pruritus, associated with the pustules, but folliculitis is usually asymptomatic.

This is a relatively common condition that affects primarily young adults. It can be chronic or recurrent.

Patient Screening

As with many other skin disorders, folliculitis is a troublesome and worrisome condition. Schedule the next available appointment for the patient.

Etiology

Folliculitis is a bacterial infection caused by *S. aureus*. The bacteria enter the skin through the opening of the hair follicle and cause a low-grade infection within the epidermal layer. Shaving with a straight razor is a common precipitating factor.

Diagnosis

The diagnosis of folliculitis is based on the presence of hairs within the pustular lesions. It is confirmed when a culture of the purulent material shows the presence of *S. aureus*.

Treatment

For most mild cases of folliculitis, a topical antiseptic cleanser, such as povidone-iodine (Betadine), used daily or every other day for several weeks, helps manage the problem. More extensive involvement requires a systemic antibiotic, such as erythromycin, taken four times a day for 10 days, or cephalexin taken twice daily, in addition to the topical cleansers.

Folliculitis occasionally results in the development of a furuncle that requires incision and drainage (see the Furuncles and Carbuncles section).

Prognosis

With treatment, the prognosis is good.

Prevention

Use of a straight razor should be avoided. Good hygiene always helps combat any infectious condition.

Patient Teaching

Give patients information about the disorder. Encourage them not to squeeze any pustules.

Deformed or Discolored Nails

Description

Nails with any unusual thickening, shape, or color that deviates from normal are classified as deformed or discolored nails.

ICD-10-CM Code	L60.9 (Nail disorder, unspecified)
	(L60.0-L62 = 9 codes of specificity)

Symptoms and Signs

Any unusual thickening, color variation, and change in the shape of either the fingernails or the toenails can be symptoms of an underlying disease or disorder.

Patient Screening

Patients reporting deformities, odd shapes, or discoloration of nails are usually scheduled for an appointment that fits their convenience. The physician must remember that any sudden deviation from normal may be the result of an underlying disease process.

Etiology

Injury to the nail bed caused by continuous pressure from ill-fitting shoes or poor circulation caused by arteriosclerosis can lead to thickening of the whole nail. Many disorders can produce nail deformities. Psoriasis, lichen planus, and chronic paronychia can cause the end of the nail to separate from the underlying skin. Bacteria can enter this space and make the nail turn a blackish green. Iron deficiency anemia can cause spooning of the nails. Congenital heart disorders and lung cancer can cause clubbing, or knobby ends of the fingers or toes, and then cause the nails to grow around these ends.

Nail discoloration is caused by many illnesses. With anemia, the nail bed appears pale. A person with chronic hepatic disease has white nail beds. Small, black, splinterlike areas appear under the nails with infections of the cardiac valves, systemic lupus erythematosus, and dermatomyositis.

Vitamin or mineral deficiencies and injury to a nail may cause one or more white patches to develop in the nail. The nail of the big toe sometimes can curve under at the sides and dig into the skin, causing pain as it grows. This is known as an *ingrown toenail*.

Diagnosis

Examination of the affected nail or nails and a medical history may be all that is needed for a diagnosis. A blood chemistry profile detects any underlying condition or illness.

Treatment

Deformities and discolorations caused by underlying illnesses resolve when the illness is corrected. Nails damaged by injury usually grow back in or grow out again in about 9 months. The patient can practice several self-help measures with an ingrown toenail, such as wearing loose-fitting shoes, keeping the area clean and dry to prevent infection, and cutting the nail straight across the top. If these measures do not help, the patient should see a physician. The physician can remove the ingrowing edge of the nail and the toe's nail fold and apply a chemical to the edge to relieve the discomfort and prevent the edge from growing in again. When the discoloration is caused by a fungus, terbinafine hydrochloride (Lamisil) may be prescribed.

Prognosis

As previously mentioned, deformities and discolorations caused by underlying illnesses usually resolve when the illness is corrected. Nails damaged by injury usually grow back in or grow out again in about 9 months. Treatment for ingrown toenails usually has a positive outcome.

Prevention

Trimming toenails straight across helps prevent ingrown toenails. Malformations of the nails often are the result of injury to the nails or nail beds or the sequela to certain disease processes and cannot be prevented.

Patient Teaching

Give patients information about proper care and trimming of nails. Encourage those with ingrown toenails to select shoes with sufficient space for the toes.

Paronychia

Description

A paronychia is an infection of the skin around a nail.

ICD-10-CM Code	L03.019 (Cellulitis of unspecified finger)
	(L03.011-L03.019 = 3 codes of specificity)

There are several codes listed for paronychia, so refer to the physician's diagnosis and then to the current edition of the ICD-10-CM coding manual to ensure the greatest specificity of pathology. Additional codes are required to identify the causative organism.

Symptoms and Signs

With acute paronychia, the cuticle or nail fold becomes edematous, red, and painful. If the cuticle lifts away from the base of the nail, purulent material may be expressed from beneath. When the nail fold is affected, a blister of pus called a whitlow develops beside the nail (Fig. 6.45). Chronic infections produce similar symptoms, and often several nails are affected. With the cuticle lifted, the nail roots no longer are protected and become damaged. This produces deformed or discolored nails.

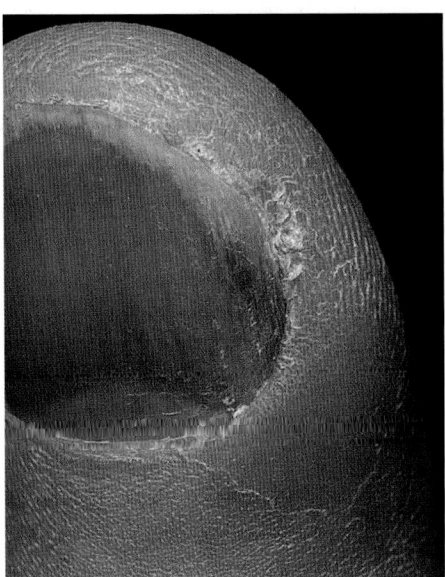

• **Fig. 6.45** Paronychia. (Modified from Jarvis C: *Physical Examination and Health Assessment,* ed 5, St Louis, 2007, Saunders.)

Patient Screening

The patient experiencing paronychia may also feel pain in the hand. If an immediate appointment cannot be scheduled, refer the patient to a medical facility that can provide prompt assessment and treatment.

Etiology

The infection may be caused by bacteria or fungi. Bacteria usually cause acute infections, whereas fungi usually cause chronic infections. The chronic infections develop slowly and are less painful but are also more persistent. Paronychia occurs particularly in people who have their hands in water for long periods.

Diagnosis

A physician can diagnose a paronychia on examination of the affected areas and with a history of the symptoms. A culture of the **exudate** is needed to identify a bacterial or fungal origin.

Treatment

Antibiotics correct a bacterial infection, and if the infection is chronic, an antifungal cream or paint (ciclopirox [Penlac]) is prescribed.

Prognosis

Drug therapy usually helps resolve the infection. Several months of treatment may be required for the swelling to subside and the raised cuticle to return to normal.

Prevention

Encourage use of the proper hand washing technique, along with thorough drying of the hands after washing or being in water for extended periods.

Patient Teaching

Demonstrate the proper hand washing technique. Emphasize the importance of drying hands after exposure to water.

Necrotizing Fasciitis

Description

Necrotizing fasciitis is a bacterial infection. The infection spreads systemically and can cause death.

ICD-10-CM Code	M72.6 Necrotizing Fasciitis

Symptoms and Signs

Early symptoms include swollen and red areas of the skin, severe pain that can radiate from the red area (Fig. 6.46). Swelling is common, and the patient may have a fever. Later symptoms are changes in skin color, blisters, black spots on the skin, ulcers, purulent drainage, fatigue, dizziness, nausea, and diarrhea.

Patient Screening

A break in the skin is usually present and allows bacteria to enter the patient's body. However, in some cases, the pathogen does not enter through a break in the skin.

Etiology

According to the Centers for Disease Control and Prevention (CDC), group A *Streptococcus*, referred to as *flesh-eating bacteria*, is the most common cause of necrotizing fasciitis, but there are other bacteria that can cause the condition.

Diagnosis

Laboratory work to identify the cause of the infection and imaging studies of the affected area are used to diagnose the

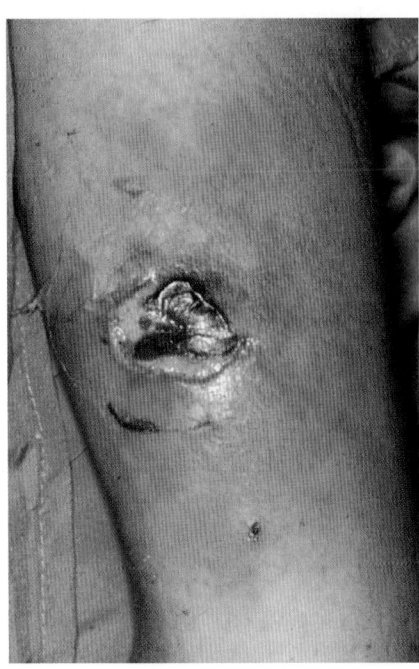

• **Fig. 6.46** Necrotizing fasciitis. (Courtesy J. H. Brien.)

condition, along with biopsy of the affected tissue to determine the cause.

Treatment

Necrotizing fasciitis is treated with IV antibiotics, and surgery may also be performed to remove affected tissue and prevent spread of the infection. Prompt treatment is important in preventing death.

Prognosis

Necrotizing fasciitis can lead to serious complications, including loss of limbs as a result of damage and scarring. This can lead to shock, organ failure, and sepsis. One in three people with die as a result of the infection, even with treatment.

Prevention

Cleaning and caring for wounds and keeping the skin free from bacteria are ways to prevent skin infections of all types. Washing with antibacterial soap to remove pathogens is one measure. Covering open wounds with clean bandages helps prevent the spread of bacteria. For a deep wound or puncture, consultation with a physician is recommended. Avoiding swimming in lakes, pools, and rivers when having open wounds is also recommended.

Patient Teaching

Patient should follow-up with the physician and take all medications as prescribed and report any change in the condition of the skin as the wound heals.

Review Challenge

Answer the following questions:

1. What are the functions of the integumentary system?
2. What is the difference between a macule and a cyst? A plaque and a fissure? A comedo and a pustule?
3. How is cradle cap related to seborrheic dermatitis?
4. What factors might induce the inflammation of contact dermatitis?
5. How is the skin likely to appear in a person diagnosed with atopic dermatitis?
6. What are general symptoms and signs of urticaria?
7. Where on the body are the lesions of psoriasis most likely to appear?
8. Where does rosacea usually appear?
9. What treatment might the physician prescribe for acne vulgaris?
10. What is the clinical course of herpes zoster?
11. Because impetigo is contagious, what actions may a school decide to take?
12. Describe symptoms and signs of cellulitis, and discuss where the condition usually manifests itself.
13. Are there any conditions considered predisposing to furuncles and carbuncles? If so, what are they?
14. How are dermatophytoses classified?
15. What are the early signs of a decubitus ulcer?
16. What is the comprehensive treatment plan for a human scabies infestation or for lice?
17. What are two of the most common premalignant skin tumors?
18. What is the common cause of actinic keratosis?
19. Name the two nonmelanoma skin cancers, and identify the most common sites for nonmelanoma skin cancers.
20. What is the most serious type of skin cancer? What are the characteristics of such a lesion?
21. What are tanning beds reported to cause?
22. Besides the aging process, what are other possible causes of alopecia?
23. What are the ABCDEs of malignant melanoma?
24. What are the special cells that control skin color called?
25. What is the cause of albinism?
26. What is the cause of vitiligo?
27. What is the primary cause of melasma?
28. What is folliculitis?
29. What is the cause of warts?
30. Describe the long-term complications of necrotizing fasciitis.

Real-Life Challenge: Shingles

A 57-year-old woman has severe pain in the left occipital region, on the left side of her neck, and in the left scapular region. The onset was approximately 36 hours ago. She describes the pain as intermittent, sharp, shooting, and severe. She has been taking ibuprofen for the pain, with little relief. She noticed small blisters forming along the painful areas in the last few hours. She is afebrile and appears quite uncomfortable.

On examination, small blisterlike eruptions are noted along the left side of the neck, left anterior shoulder, and clavicular area. Some eruptions also appear at the base of the skull just in the hairline. These eruptions do not cross the midline on either the front or back of the body.

The patient is diagnosed with shingles, along the C-2, C-3, and C-4 peripheral nerves or the dermatome area. On questioning, the patient confirms having had chickenpox in childhood when she was about 8 years of age.

Medications prescribed include famciclovir (Famvir) 500 mg three times daily for 7 days. Acyclovir (Zovirax) cream also was prescribed for topical application to the affected areas and hydrocodone bitartrate with acetaminophen (Vicodin) for pain.

Questions

1. What is the significance of the previous occurrence of chickenpox?
2. What is the causative agent of chickenpox? Of shingles?
3. Why is the fact that the eruptions do not cross the midline important?
4. Identify other medications that may be prescribed for shingles.
5. What might the patient expect as an outcome of this condition?
6. What is meant by postherpetic neuralgia (PHN)?

Real-Life Challenge: Malignant Melanoma

A 35-year-old, fair-skinned woman has noticed the enlargement of a mole on her right lower arm. The mole has been present as long as she can remember. In the past month, it appears to have doubled in size and has become darker.

The patient admits to having been exposed to direct sunlight for the past several years. She lives in southern Texas and spends several hours a day in the sun while doing garden work. She has not consistently applied sunscreen to her lower arms and hands.

Visual examination shows a slightly elevated, 7-mm, irregularly shaped, dark, multicolored lesion on the dorsal aspect of the right lower arm, about 3 inches above the wrist. Closer examination shows the lesion to be asymmetric, with a notched border.

Family history reveals that the patient's mother had three lesions removed from her arms and face that were diagnosed as malignant melanoma. In addition, two maternal aunts have had malignant melanomas. One aunt recently died as a result of metastatic cancer. The patient remembers having incurred several sunburns with blistering as a child.

Surgical excision of the lesion is performed, and biopsy confirms the diagnosis of malignant melanoma. The patient is referred to an oncologist for possible chemotherapy.

Questions

1. What characteristics in the patient suggest that she may have malignant melanoma?
2. What symptoms distinguish malignant melanoma from basal cell or squamous cell carcinoma?
3. What is the prognosis for a patient with malignant melanoma, such as this patient?
4. What patient teaching would you offer to patients about extensive exposure to sunlight?
5. What is the importance of a good family history?
6. Why was the patient referred to an oncologist?
7. Would this patient be a candidate for further surgical procedures? If so, what procedures would be performed, and why?
8. List the warning signs of malignant melanoma.

Real-Life Challenge: Rosacea

A 70-year-old man is seen in the office for what he says is a change in his complexion. He presents with a reddened skin color on his face as well as pimples. A significant redness is noted on his cheeks and across the nose. On close examination, the small blood vessels in this area appear enlarged and show through the skin as red lines. The nose appears swollen, showing some small knobby bumps. This man is a businessman in the community, and his wife states that she has heard rumors that he has problems with excessive drinking and that his business is failing because of that. She also states that when he gets flustered or embarrassed, his face gets redder. The patient says that his younger grandchildren are becoming fearful of him.

Questions

1. What characteristics that are common in rosacea does this patient exhibit?
2. What might be the cause of this condition?
3. The grandchildren's mother is concerned that his condition may be contagious. What can be done to ease her concerns?
4. What treatment is available for this condition?
5. What outcome can the patient expect with treatment?
6. What would you advise the patient to avoid?

Internet Assignments

1. Research actinic keratosis at the American Academy of Dermatology, and write a report on its association with squamous cell carcinoma.
2. Research the incidence of malignant melanoma and its treatment at The Melanoma Research Foundation. Investigate the mortality and morbidity rates of this condition.

3. Research the statistics for Group A streptococcus in association with necrotizing fasciitis.

4. Prepare to discuss Critical Thinking case study exercises for this chapter that are posted on Evolve.

Critical Thinking

1. List the five functions of the skin.
2. Which layer of the skin gives it strength and elasticity?
3. List manifestations of dermatitis.
4. Discuss the feelings of parents of an infant who had just been diagnosed with "cradle cap."
5. Describe sensitization in relationship to dermatitis.
6. Discuss the psychological effects of eczema and of psoriasis on patients.
7. When can hives become a life-threatening condition?
8. Discuss the possible psychological effects of rosacea experienced by the patient.
9. Discuss some of the options individuals, especially the youth, may attempt to cure or prevent acne.
10. How is herpes zoster cured?
11. Discuss how schools handle the issue of children with impetigo.
12. What is the importance of good hand washing in dermatologic conditions?
13. Discuss the prevention of dermatophytosis.
14. How can decubitus ulcers be prevented?
15. Discuss the contagious state of scabies and pediculosis.
16. Why is it important to have seborrheic keratosis evaluated by a professional?
17. What are the two common types of nonmelanoma skin cancers?
18. Explain differences in melanoma and nonmelanoma skin cancers.
19. Discuss the emotional response of the patient who has just been told of the diagnosis of malignant melanoma.
20. Discuss the various skin pigment disorders.
21. Discuss psychological aspects of alopecia.
22. Explain how you would feel if diagnosed with a skin disorder that affected your appearance.

7

Diseases and Conditions of the Musculoskeletal System

CHAPTER OUTLINE

The Musculoskeletal System, 244

Fibromyalgia, 247

Spinal Disorders, 248

Osteoarthritis, 252

Lyme Disease, 254

Bursitis, 255

Osteomyelitis, 256

Gout, 257

Paget Disease (Osteitis Deformans), 259

Marfan Syndrome, 260

Musculoskeletal Tumors, 261

Osteoporosis, 263

Osteomalacia and Rickets, 265

Hallux Valgus (Bunion), 265

Hallux Rigidus, 266

Hammer Toe, 267

Traumatic and Sports Injuries, 268

LEARNING OBJECTIVES

After studying Chapter 7, you should be able to:

1. List the functions of the normal skeletal system.
2. Discuss the specifics of a physical examination when fibromyalgia is suspected.
3. Distinguish among the pathologic features of lordosis, kyphosis, and scoliosis.
4. Describe the signs and symptoms of the most common form of arthritis.
5. Explain the importance of early diagnosis and treatment of Lyme disease.
6. Discuss the prevention of bursitis.
7. Describe the clinical picture of osteomyelitis and explain how it is treated.
8. Explain why joint disability results from gout.
9. Describe the treatment of bone tumors, both benign and malignant.
10. Describe the disability that results from advanced osteoporosis.
11. Explain why osteomalacia is termed *a metabolic bone disease.*
12. Distinguish between hallux valgus and hallux rigidus.
13. Explain the causes of fractures (broken bones) and how fractures are classified.
14. Explain what the term *phantom limb* refers to.
15. Differentiate between a strain and a sprain.
16. Explain the importance of proper treatment of dislocations.
17. Recall the medical term for "frozen shoulder."
18. Describe the cause of shin splints.
19. List some factors that contribute to the development of plantar fasciitis.
20. Explain how torn meniscus is treated.
21. Describe the signs and symptoms of rotator cuff tears.

KEY TERMS

avulsion (ah-**VUL**-shun)
bursae (**BURR**-see)
calcitonin (**kal**-sih-**TOE**-nin)
crepitation (krep-ih-**TAY**-shun)
fascia (**FASH**-ee-ah)
hematopoiesis (**heem**-ah-toe-poy-**EE**-sis)

meniscus (meh-**NIS**-kuss)
metatarsophalangeal (**met**-ah-**tar**-so-fah-**LAN**-jee-al)
ossification (**oss**-ih-fih-**KAY**-shun)
osteogenesis (**oss**-tee-oh-**JEN**-eh-sis)
synovial (sin-**OH**-vee-al)
tenorrhaphy (teh-**NOR**-ah-fee)

The Musculoskeletal System

Muscles, bones, ligaments, tendons, cartilage, and the joints they form provide a supportive and functional framework for the body that allows flexibility of movement and protects the internal organs. The tissues of the musculoskeletal system also give shape to the body, act partially as a storage-and-supply area for minerals, and serve as sites for the formation of blood cells.

When the tissues are unable to perform their usual functions because of trauma, rheumatic, inflammatory, or degenerative conditions, a person's physical support, protection, mobility, and ability to perform normal activities are affected. Trauma is a major cause of musculoskeletal disorders; automobile accidents and injuries (strains, sprains, dislocations, and fractures) are the leading causes of disabilities and death.

All muscles are composed of a basic cellular unit called the *muscle fiber,* which is made of protein. Muscles of the skeleton are collections or masses of tissue that cover bones, providing bulk to the body while also helping to hold body parts together and to move joints (Fig. 7.1). These skeletal muscles make up approximately 40% of the total body mass.

All movement, including the movement of the body itself and of the internal organs, is performed by muscle tissue. The three types of muscle tissues, defined histologically, are striated (skeletal), nonstriated (smooth), and cardiac (Fig. 7.2). Muscles are also classified as either voluntary or involuntary. Skeletal muscle is voluntary and is under the control of the conscious mind; this includes the muscles used to move the extremities, which are stimulated by nerves at the request of the brain. The point of attachment of a muscle to a stationary bone is referred to as the *origin of the muscle,* and the point of attachment to a bone that is moved by the muscle is referred to as its *insertion* (Fig. 7.3). When a muscle contracts, the insertion moves toward the origin. Smooth muscle and heart muscle are involuntary and function without conscious control or awareness. Examples are the muscles of the intestines, which move food through the bowels, and cardiac muscles, which move blood throughout the chambers of the heart.

The skeletal system is composed of 206 bones. These serve to provide an important support system for the many body parts, enabling a person to assume various body postures (Fig. 7.4). In coordination with muscles and joints, bones assist in body movement.

Some bones encase and protect specific organs (e.g., the skull protects the brain, the rib cage protects the heart and lungs, and the vertebrae protect the spinal cord). Blood cells are formed in bone marrow inside the bones in a process called **hematopoiesis.**

Bones are not lifeless structures but, instead, are structures infused with living cells arranged in a hard framework of minerals (calcium and phosphorus). Bone cells are continuously forming new bone; bone formation is counterbalanced by bone reabsorption or breakdown. Normally the balance of these two processes prevents bones from

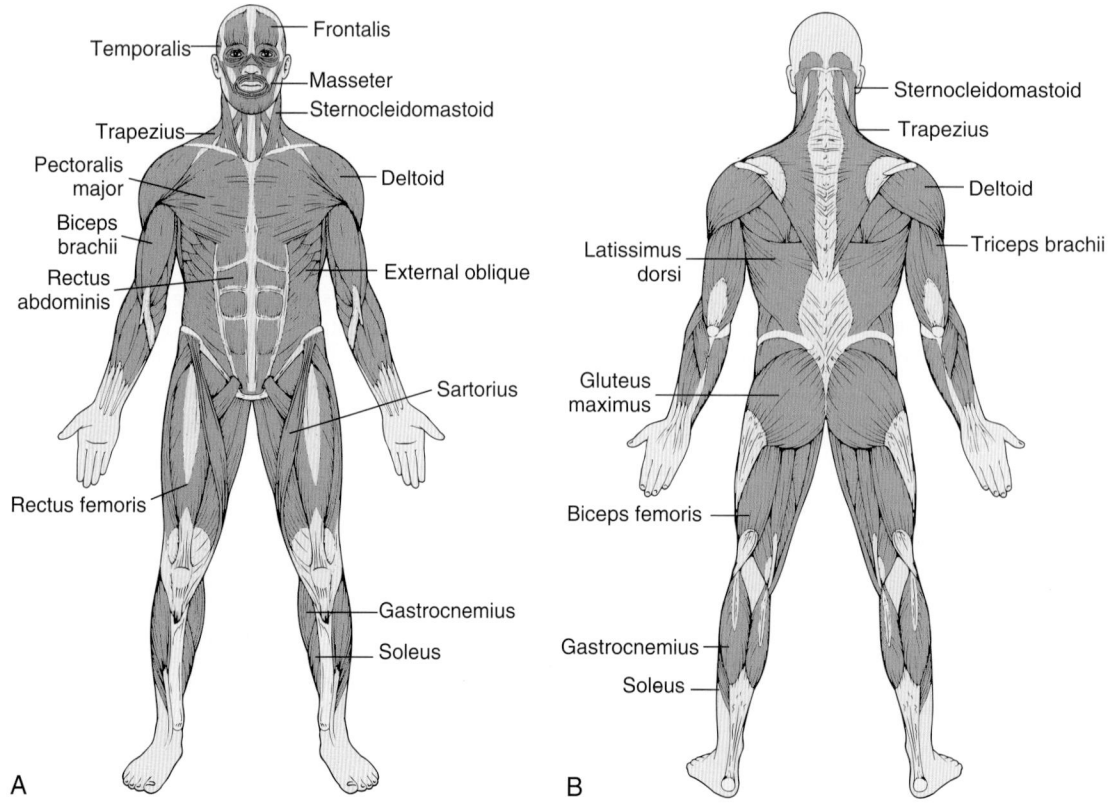

A   B

• **Fig. 7.1** Normal Muscular System. (A) Anterior view. (B) Posterior view.

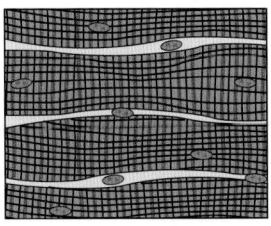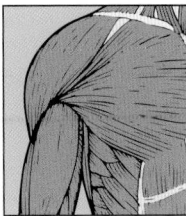

Striated (skeletal) muscle

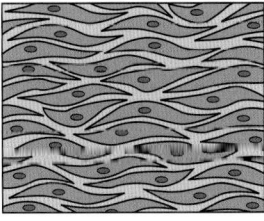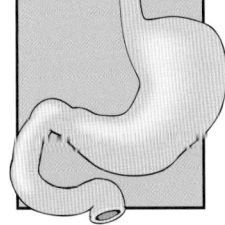

Nonstriated (smooth) muscle

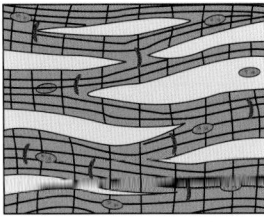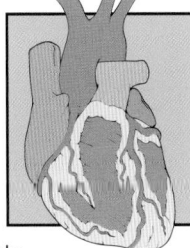

Cardiac muscle

• **Fig. 7.2** Types of muscles.

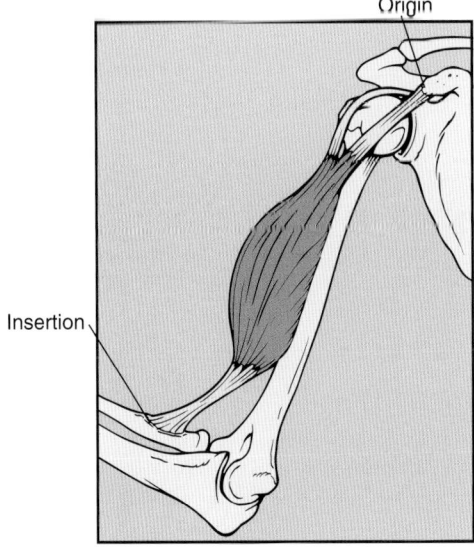

• **Fig. 7.3** Insertion and origin of a muscle.

becoming excessively thick, as in Paget disease of bone, or too thin, as in osteoporosis. This balance also serves to maintain the normal blood level of calcium and phosphorus in the body.

Bones are complete organs; they are composed mainly of connective tissue with a rich supply of blood vessels and nerves. They develop through a process called osteogenesis,

and the complete skeleton is formed by the end of the third month of fetal age. The fetal skeleton is composed of cartilage tissue, which is replaced gradually by bone cells in a process called ossification. Ossification depends on adequate supplies of calcium and phosphorus getting to the bone tissue.

Several different types of bone make up the skeleton. Long bones are strong and have broad ends and large surface areas for muscle attachment. They are found in the humerus (arm), the ulna and radius (forearm), the femur (thigh), and the tibia and fibula (leg). Short bones have small, irregular shapes and include the carpal (wrist) and tarsal (ankle) bones. Flat bones cover soft body parts; they include the scapula (shoulder), ribs, and pelvic bones. Sesamoid bones are small and rounded and are found near joints. The patella (kneecap) is the largest sesamoid bone.

Joints, or articulations, are body structures in which bones are joined or the surfaces of two bones come together for the purpose of creating motion. With the help of ligaments, joints hold bones firmly together yet allow movement between them. Joints are classified by the type of material found between bones: fibrous, cartilaginous, and synovial. Joints also are classified according to the degree of movement (Fig. 7.5) they can make. Immovable (synarthrodial) joints (e.g., suture joints between the bones of the skull) are connected by fibrous tissue; slightly movable (amphiarthrodial) joints (e.g., the intervertebral joints and the pubic symphysis) are connected by cartilage; and freely movable (diarthrodial) joints (e.g., the knee and the elbow) are called *synovial joints* because they are lined with the fluid-producing synovial membrane. Also within synovial joints are bones; cartilage that covers the ends of bones; ligaments that hold bones together; a joint capsule containing synovial fluid, blood, and lymph vessels; and nerves.

Most joints are of the freely movable type. The amount or degree of movement that a joint has is referred to as its *range of motion* (ROM). Only the freely movable joints can execute a wide range of movements; examples are the shoulder, wrist, and hip.

Ligaments are tough, dense, fibrous bands of connective tissue that hold bones together, either around a joint capsule (e.g., the hip joint) or across a joint (e.g., the knee [Fig. 7.6]). They allow movement in some directions while restricting it in other directions, thereby providing some stability. Injury to ligaments can occur in several ways; they can be overstretched and sustain partial or complete tears (sprains) or be torn completely loose from their attachment to a bone, an injury called avulsion. They can also be loosened by the inflammation caused by inflammatory arthritis.

Tendons are tough strands, or cords, of dense connective tissue. They serve to attach muscles to bones and other parts (see Fig. 7.6). Tendons are nonelastic and are capable of withstanding great forces from contracting muscles without sustaining damage. Injury to a tendon is called *strain*.

Fascia is a specialized flat band of tissue located just below the skin that covers and separates underlying tissues,

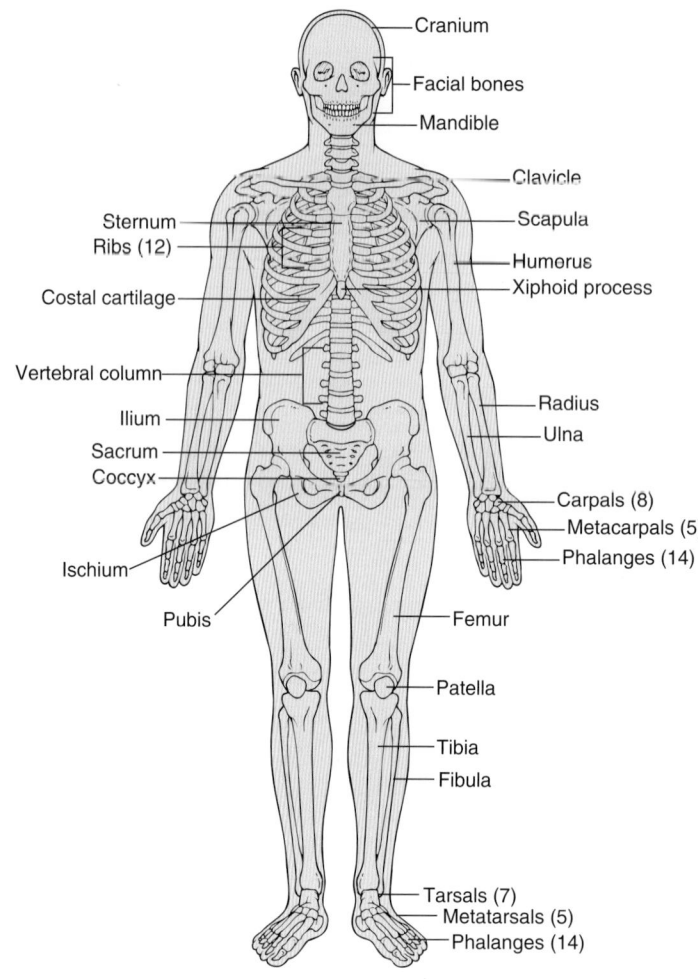

• **Fig. 7.4** Normal skeletal system, anterior view.

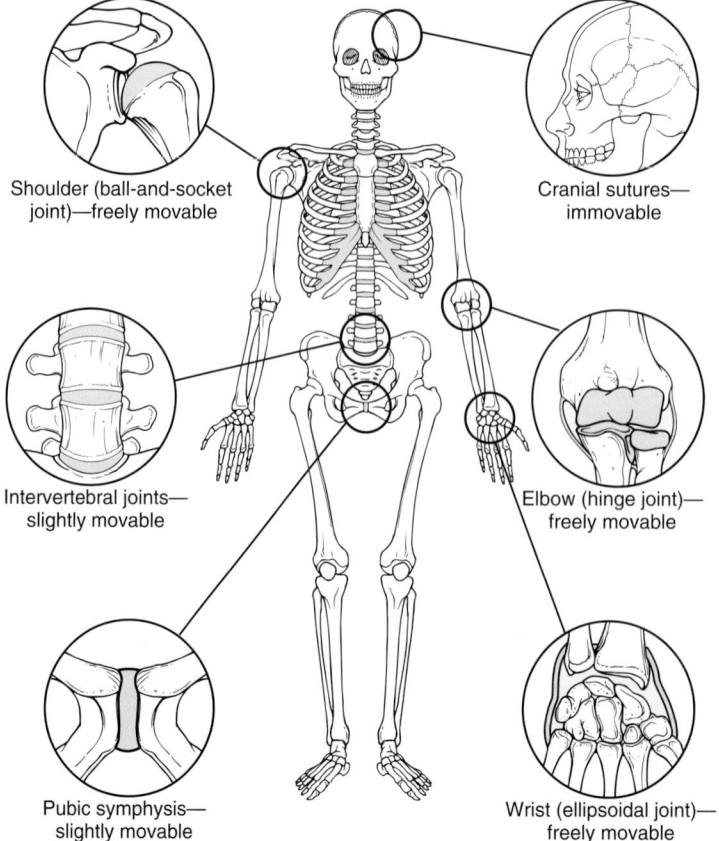

• **Fig. 7.5** Examples of types of joints.

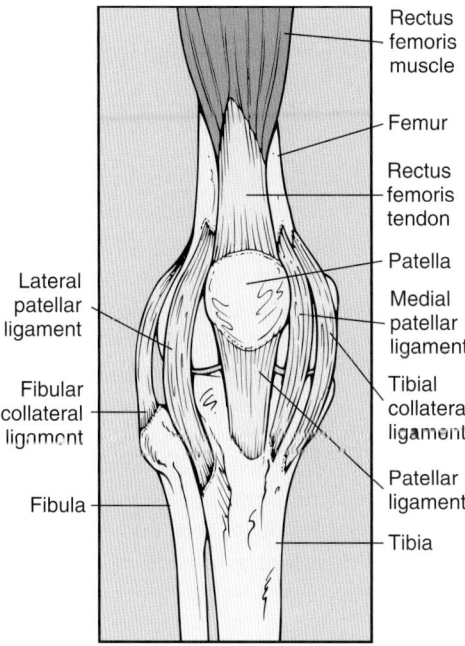

• **Fig. 7.6** Ligaments and tendons of the knee joint.

commonly muscle layers. Inflamed or injured fascia is referred to as *fasciitis.*

Cartilage is a semismooth, dense, supporting connective tissue that is found at the ends of bones. It forms a cap over the ends of bones and provides support and protection when bones are engaged in weight-bearing activities. Cartilage absorbs the energy force of weight pressed or thrust against joints to prevent injury to joints, bones, and the cartilage itself; in effect, it functions as a "shock absorber." To remain healthy, cartilage at the joints must receive nutrients from the joint fluid and maintain normal joint movement and weight-bearing activities.

Also necessary for the functioning of the musculoskeletal system are the bursae, closed sacs or cavities of synovial fluid lined with a synovial membrane. Positioned between tissues, such as tendons, bones, and ligaments, bursae make it possible for these tissues to glide over each other without creating friction. Bursae are located in the shoulder, elbow, and knee joints.

Another substance found throughout the musculoskeletal system is a fibrous protein called *collagen.* Collagen constitutes 30% of the total body protein and is the major supporting element, or glue, in the connective tissues between the cells that holds them together. In adults, collagen makes up one-third to one-half of the total body protein (see the Connective Tissue Diseases section in Chapter 3).

Fibromyalgia

Description
Fibromyalgia is a chronic pain condition associated with stiffness and tenderness that affects muscles, tendons, and joints throughout the body. Fibromyalgia is also characterized by restless sleep, depression, fatigue, anxiety, and bowel dysfunction.

ICD-10-CM Code	M60.9 *(Myositis, unspecified)* (M60.000-M60.19 = 64 codes of specificity; M60.8-M60.9 = 26 codes of specificity) M79.1 *(Myalgia)* M79.7 *(Fibromyalgia)*

Symptoms and Signs
Fibromyalgia, one of the most common diseases affecting muscles, causes chronic pain in the muscles and soft tissues surrounding joints. Fatigue is extremely common in patients with this condition. Often symptoms include diffuse aching or burning in the muscles, stiffness, disturbed sleep patterns, poor concentration, irritability, and depression. Patients may note extreme tenderness of various areas of the body. Other nonspecific symptoms include headaches, jaw pain, and sensitivity to odors, bright lights, and loud noises. Some patients experience symptoms of irritable bowel syndrome or "spastic colon," including nausea, diarrhea, constipation, or abdominal pain with gas and distention. Urinary symptoms, when present, include urinary urgency or frequency brought on by bladder spasms and irritability. Often patients wake up feeling tired, even if they have slept all through the night. Others sleep lightly and wake up during the night.

Patient Screening
For the patient complaining of persistent fatigue and unexplained muscle pain and tenderness, schedule an appointment at the earliest convenience.

Etiology
The cause of fibromyalgia is unknown. Patients experience pain in response to stimuli that are normally not perceived as painful. Fibromyalgia appears to be linked to changes in how the brain and spinal cord process pain signals. Researchers have found elevated levels of a nerve growth factor and a chemical signal, called *substance P,* in the spinal fluid of patients with fibromyalgia. The amount of serotonin, a chemical produced in the brain and that affects nerves, is relatively low in these patients. Furthermore, those with fibromyalgia experience impaired non–rapid eye movement (non-REM) sleep, which likely explains the common feature of waking up feeling fatigued and unrefreshed. The onset of fibromyalgia is sometimes associated with psychological distress, trauma, and infection. The condition may be aggravated by poor posture, inappropriate exercise, weight, and smoking.

Diagnosis
Many medical conditions can cause pain in multiple areas of the body, thus mimicking fibromyalgia. Blood testing and physical examination are important to *exclude* some conditions, such as hypothyroidism, hypoparathyroidism, other muscle diseases, bone diseases, viral infections, and cancer.

There are no specific laboratory or imaging studies that can be used to diagnose fibromyalgia. Testing is done only to exclude other causes of chronic muscle pain. The diagnosis of fibromyalgia is made purely on clinical grounds and is based on thorough history and physical examination and the patient's symptoms.

Historically, fibromyalgia was diagnosed if a patient had widespread tenderness and pain or aching commonly in at least 11 of 18 specific tender points (Fig. 7.7). The problem with these criteria is that the symptoms sometimes come and go. The patient may have 11 symptoms one day and then 4 the next.

According to the Mayo Clinic, newer diagnostic criteria are being used. It includes:

1. widespread pain lasting at least 3 months
2. presence of other symptoms, such as fatigue, waking up tired, and trouble thinking
3. no other underlying condition that might be causing the symptoms

Treatment

Although no cure for fibromyalgia is known, treatment can help alleviate symptoms and restore function. Treatment involves patient education, stress reduction, physical activity, and medications. Attempts are made to reduce pain and improve the quality of sleep. Medications that can improve sleep patterns may be prescribed, such as low doses of the antidepressant amitriptyline (Elavil). Newer treatments include pregabalin (Lyrica), duloxetine (Cymbalta), and milnacipran (Savella). For muscle and joint soreness, nonsteroidal antiinflammatory drugs (NSAIDs) and/or muscle relaxants can be helpful. Stress reduction, relaxation techniques, massage therapy, acupressure, and exercise also have been found to be beneficial. Exercises that are helpful in reducing pain include walking, biking, swimming, or water aerobics.

Prognosis

With good understanding of the concepts of the symptoms and methods of treatment available, patients generally can control their condition and return to normal function. Despite potentially disabling body pain, patients with fibromyalgia do not develop musculoskeletal damage or deformity. Fibromyalgia also does not cause damage to internal body organs.

Prevention

To prevent initiating or worsening symptoms, patients should work toward minimizing stressful situations; perform aerobic exercise regularly; and, under the guidance of their health care professionals, consider taking medications that can lessen symptoms.

Patient Teaching

Optimal management of fibromyalgia involves maximizing the patient's understanding of all known concepts of the illness. The patient and the health care provider then develop the ideal treatment strategy, which is customized for each patient and involves a dynamic balance of patient education, exercise, stress reduction, and medication.

Spinal Disorders

The normal curves of the spine are important because they provide a strong supportive structure to the body. Additionally, the spine provides the necessary balance to stand, walk, and even hold the head up straight. The ribs and internal organs are suspended from the spine in the front; the hips and legs are attached to the lower spine.

The following text includes a discussion of three relatively common abnormal curvatures of the spine: lordosis, kyphosis, and scoliosis.

Lordosis

Description

Lordosis is an exaggerated inward curvature of the spine. Lordosis is sometimes referred to as a *swayback* or *saddleback deformity.*

ICD-10-CM Code	M40.40 *(Postural lordosis, site unspecified)*
	(M40.40-M40.57 = 8 codes of specificity)

Symptoms and Signs

The lumbar spine normally curves inward. This normal anterior curve of the lumbar spine can become exaggerated by a variety of conditions. Excessive inward curvature, or lordosis, occurs as the person compensates for added abdominal girth caused by pregnancy, obesity, or large

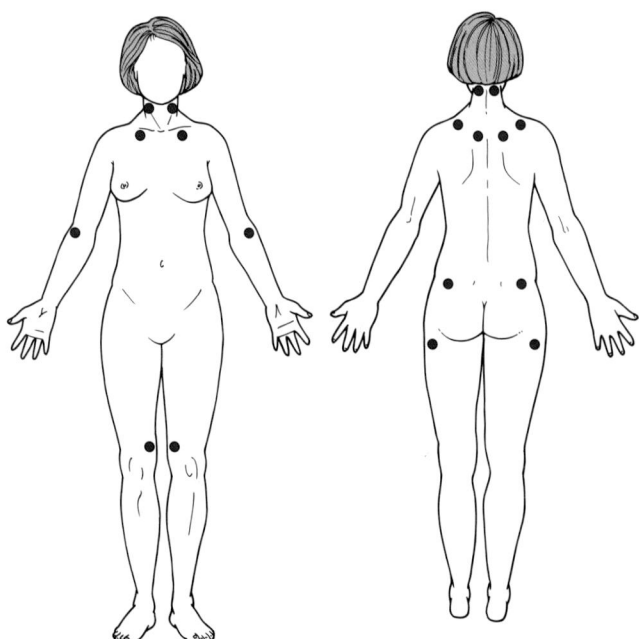

• **Fig. 7.7** Eighteen tender points used to diagnose fibromyalgia.

abdominal tumors. Lordosis also can occur developmentally for unknown reasons. Lordosis may cause no symptoms, or the patient may experience low back pain because of strains on the muscles and ligaments. Compared with the normal spine posture (Fig. 7.8), lordosis results in a protruding abdomen and buttocks and an arched lower back (Fig. 7.9).

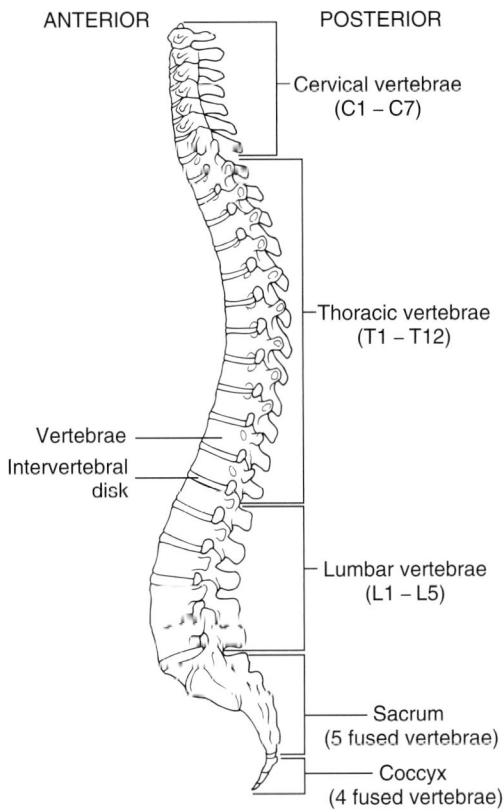

• **Fig. 7.8** Normal spine.

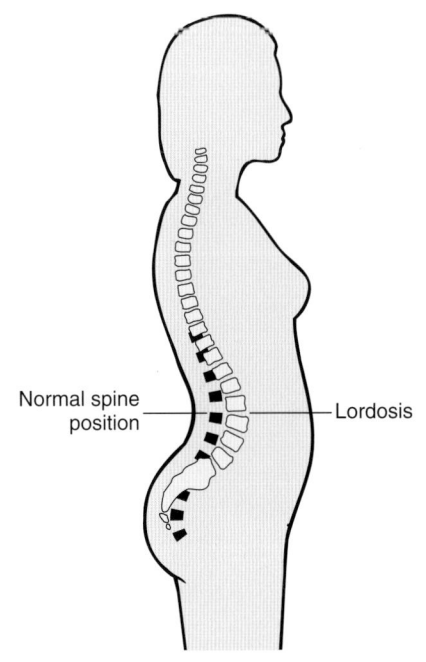

• **Fig. 7.9** Lordosis.

Patient Screening

For the patient complaining of persistent low back pain, but no history of injury or symptoms of infection, schedule the first convenient appointment.

Etiology

Excessive abdominal weight gain and mass cause an individual to compensate by unconsciously tightening the muscles in the lower back to maintain balance when standing. Lordosis often is noted in prepubescent girls. One possible cause is rapid skeletal growth that occurs without the necessary natural stretching of the posterior soft tissues. Osteoporosis, with resulting loss of bone mass, may cause lordosis in the older population.

Diagnosis

Patients who have persistent low back pain should be evaluated for degenerative and congenital diseases of the spine, inflammation of the spine (spondylitis), and conditions involving adjacent internal organs, such as the kidneys, prostate gland, aorta, and pancreas.

Observation of the spine in various postures and examination of the lower spine are the primary steps in diagnosis. When the condition is a result of pregnancy, no additional information usually is required to make the diagnosis. Further investigation can include radiographic studies to determine the extent of lordosis, along with a thorough history and physical examination to discover the underlying cause of the condition.

Treatment

When lordosis is caused by pregnancy, delivery usually resolves the condition. When obesity is the cause, weight loss and exercises to strengthen abdominal muscles are beneficial. Performing pelvic tilt exercises and maintaining good posture help correct the condition. Progressive untreated lordosis can lead to degenerative lumbar disk disease or ruptured lumbar disks. Additional treatment of the condition can include the use of a brace. For severe lordosis, spinal fusion and displacement osteotomy are considered. This latter procedure requires the surgical division of a vertebra, with shifting of the bone segments to change the alignment of, or alter weight-bearing stress on, the spine.

Prognosis

Lordosis may never cause symptoms, but patients who do have symptoms usually respond to conservative management techniques.

Prevention

Optimal prevention measures center on developing ideal posture habits, exercises, and support devices, such as braces and lumbar support when seated.

Patient Teaching

Patients can benefit from a brief review of the normal anatomy of the affected areas, particularly addressing the spine and the paraspinous musculature, as well as specific exercise instructions. Recommendations on proper posturing and adjustments to their specific sitting environments can be extremely valuable.

Kyphosis

Description

Kyphosis is abnormal outward curvature of the spine (convexity backward).

ICD-10-CM Code	M40.00 *(Postural kyphosis, site unspecified)*
	M40.209 *(Unspecified kyphosis, site unspecified)*
	(M40.00-M40.299 — 19 codes of specificity)

Symptoms and Signs

Kyphosis, an excessive posterior curve of the thoracic spine, often has an insidious onset and is asymptomatic until the hump becomes obvious. As the curve progresses, the patient may begin to experience mild pain, fatigue, tenderness along the spine, and decreasing mobility of the spine. The shoulders appear rounded, and the head protrudes forward (Fig. 7.10A).

Patient Screening

For the individual complaining of persistent upper back pain, without history of injury or symptoms of infection, schedule an appointment at his or her convenience.

Etiology

Kyphosis that occurs in very young children has no specific cause and is believed to be developmental. Adolescent kyphosis usually is related to Scheuermann disease, a degenerative deformity of the thoracic vertebrae (see Fig. 7.10B). Additional disease processes that contribute to the occurrence of kyphosis include tumors or tuberculosis of the vertebral bodies and ankylosing spondylitis. Collapse of vertebrae from the weakened bone of osteoporosis is often responsible for the hunchback (dowager's hump) that develops in the older person, particularly in postmenopausal women. Wearing away of the anterior portion of the vertebrae in a wedge type of manner (anterior wedging) or deterioration of the vertebrae, from whatever cause, results in the excessive curvature with kyphosis.

Diagnosis

Visual inspection of the spine discloses the excessive curve in the thoracic region. Radiographs and bone scans document the concave curvature of the thoracic spine, along with the wedging of the anterior aspect of the vertebral bodies (see Fig. 7.10B). Patients with osteoporosis experience loss of bone density.

Treatment

Exercises to strengthen the muscles and ligaments are prescribed. Back braces also are used to stabilize the condition. The underlying cause must be determined and treated. When other measures fail to produce results and when the respiratory and cardiac systems are compromised, spinal

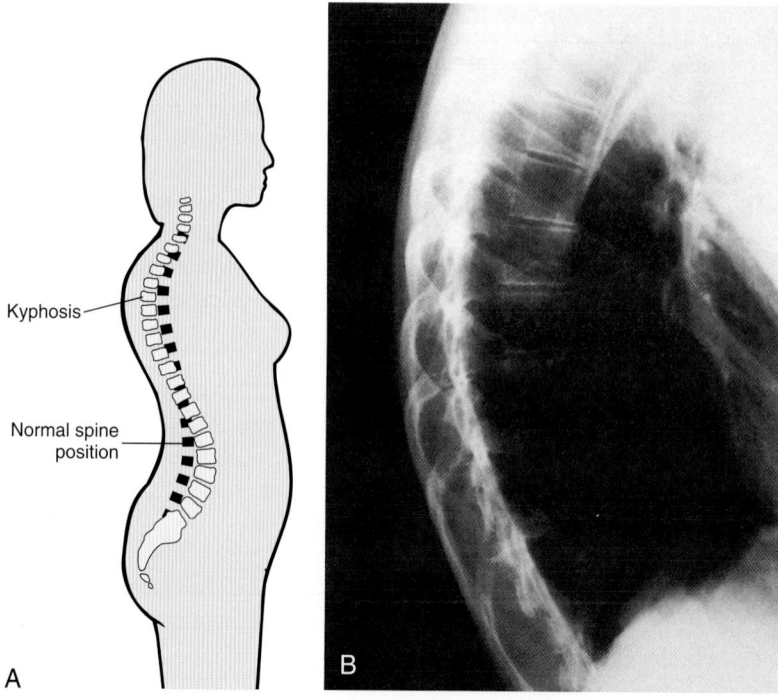

Kyphosis

Normal spine position

A

B

• **Fig. 7.10** (A) Kyphosis. (B) Kyphosis associated with Scheuermann disease. (From Mourad LA: *Orthopedic disorders—Mosby's clinical nursing series,* St Louis, 1991, Mosby.)

fusion, with instrumentation and temporary immobilization, is performed. Kyphosis that is caused by a sudden collapse of a vertebra because of osteoporosis is sometimes treated with a new procedure called *vertebroplasty*, in which bone cement is inserted within the vertebra to maintain the reestablished vertebral height and to reduce pain.

Prognosis
The outlook for patients with kyphosis depends on the cause. Optimal outcome results from accurate diagnosis and early treatment.

Prevention
Optimal prevention measures center on developing ideal posture habits, exercises, and support devices, such as braces and back support when seated. Medications may be needed for osteoporosis, pain, or inflammation of the spine.

Patient Teaching
Patients with kyphosis who are found to have significant osteoporosis should be instructed regarding exercise programs, calcium and vitamin D supplementation, and prescription medications.

Scoliosis

Description
Scoliosis is lateral (sideways) curvature of the spine. Scoliosis typically is congenital, but some diseases also can cause it.

ICD-10-CM Code	M41.20 *(Other idiopathic scoliosis, site unspecified)*
	(M41.00-M41.9 = 55 codes of specificity)
	Q67.5 *(Congenital deformity of spine)*
	Q76.3 *(Congenital scoliosis due to congenital bony malformation)*
	Q76.425 *(Congenital lordosis, thoracolumbar region)*
	Q76.426 *(Congenital lordosis, lumbar region)*
	Q76.427 *(Congenital lordosis, lumbosacral region)*
	Q76.428 *(Congenital lordosis, sacral and sacrococcygeal region)*

Symptoms and Signs
Scoliosis, the lateral curvature of the spine, often has an insidious presentation, possibly going unnoticed for years before detection. In women, for example, the first indication is often unequal bra strap lengths. The patient, usually an adolescent female, reports back pain, fatigue, and sometimes shortness of breath on exertion. Observation of the back reveals lateral curve of the spine, one shoulder higher than

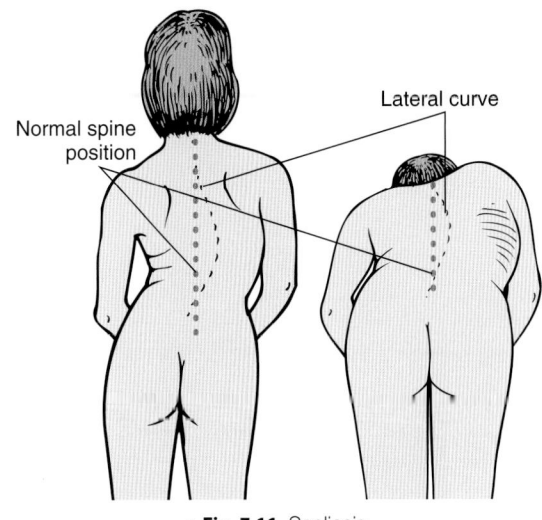

• **Fig. 7.11** Scoliosis.

the other, one scapula more prominent than the other, one hip higher than the other, and when the patient bends over, an enlarged muscle mass on one side of the back (Fig. 7.11).

Patient Screening
Referrals may come from school scoliosis screening programs that have detected possible scoliosis.

Etiology
Idiopathic scoliosis is the most common form; however, the cause is postulated to be genetic in some cases. Other suggested causes of scoliosis are deformities of the vertebrae; uneven leg lengths; and muscle degeneration or paralysis from diseases, such as poliomyelitis, cerebral palsy, and muscular dystrophy.

Diagnosis
Patients with scoliosis are evaluated for muscle disease and weakness, congenital conditions, neurologic disorders, and degeneration of the bones and disks of the spine. Diagnosis is made from visual examination of the back, which reveals uneven shoulder and hip heights, a prominent scapula on one side, an enlarged muscle mass on one side, and a definite torsional curve of the vertebral column. It is important to examine the lengths of the lower limbs, because discrepancy of the leg lengths can lead to spinal curvature. Radiographs not only confirm the diagnosis but also provide the physician with the means to measure the degree of curvature. This is also useful for long-term monitoring (Fig. 7.12).

Treatment
Treatment depends on the extent and cause of the curvature. Mild scoliosis is treated with exercise to strengthen the weak muscles. Bracing of the back with a Milwaukee brace, a Boston brace, a molded plastic clamshell jacket, or a Wilmington brace, along with an exercise program, is the suggested course of treatment for the growing girl or boy.

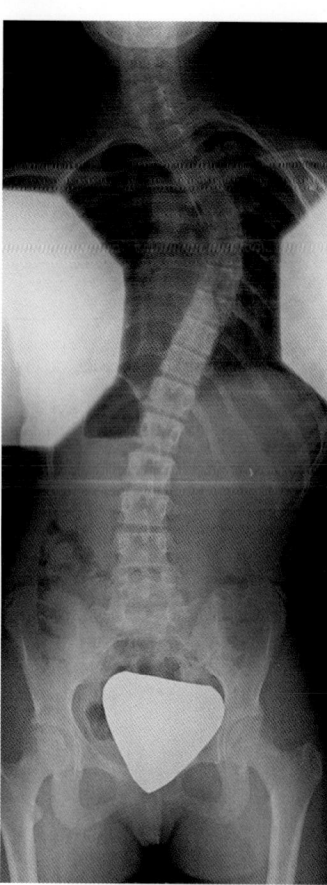

• **Fig. 7.12** A radiograph showing pronounced scoliosis. (Courtesy Texas Scottish Rite Hospital for Children, Dallas, TX.)

This bracing may take from 2 to 5 years to prevent further curvature. Curves that do not respond to the bracing or that are severe (> 40 degrees) need surgical intervention to decrease the curve and to realign and stabilize the spine. These procedures include fusion of the vertebrae and internal fixation with instrumentation by means of rods, wires, or plates and pedicle screws. Some patients are placed in body casts or plastic jackets to maintain the integrity of the fixation until the fusion heals. The respiratory and cardiac systems may be compromised if the curvature is left untreated.

Prognosis

The outlook for patients with scoliosis depends primarily on the severity of the curvature. Optimal outcome results from accurate diagnosis and early treatment.

Prevention

Prevention measures center on developing ideal posture habits, performing beneficial exercises, and wearing support devices, such as the braces described above. Timely surgical intervention is crucial for severely affected children.

Patient Teaching

Posture training, regular use of proper bracing, and instructions for avoiding stresses to the affected spine are essential for ideal management. Children with significant scoliosis should avoid aggressive contact sports, such as football and rugby.

Osteoarthritis

Description

Osteoarthritis is a type of arthritis that results from the breakdown and eventual loss of the cartilage of one or more joints.

ICD-10-CM Code	M15.9 *(Polyosteoarthritis, unspecified)*
	(M15.0-M15.9 = 7 codes of specificity)
	M19.90 *(Unspecified osteoarthritis, unspecified site)*
	(M19.01-M19.93 = 49 codes of specificity)

Osteoarthritis is coded according to the site affected. Refer to the physician's diagnosis and then to the current edition of the ICD-10-CM coding manual for most accurate specificity.

Symptoms and Signs

Osteoarthritis, also known as *degenerative joint disease* or *degenerative arthritis,* is, by far, the most common form of arthritis. It develops as a result of normal wear and tear on the joints and is most common in older adults, being almost universal in those older than 75 years of age. Osteoarthritis occurs mainly in the large weight-bearing joints, especially the knees and hips (Fig. 7.13). There is a tendency for the smallest joints at the ends of the fingers to be affected by spur formation, which leads to the classic bony enlargement referred to as a *Heberden node.* To a lesser degree, involvement of the joints of the fingers at the proximal interphalangeal (PIP) joints (Bouchard nodes, Fig. 7.14), that is, wrists, elbows, and ankles, can occur. Degenerative changes in the spinal vertebrae and the joints of the pelvis can lead to abnormal curvature and local pain. A very common location of osteoarthritis is at the base of the thumbs.

The onset of osteoarthritis is usually insidious, and the symptoms vary with the severity of the disease. Some of the common symptoms are joint soreness, aching, and stiffness, especially in the morning and with changes in the weather; edema; dull pain; and deformity. Stiffness is noted, particularly after the patient has been immobile for a period. Clicking or crackling sounds (crepitation) often are heard with joint movement. Decreased ranges of motion, joint instability, and an increase in pain with use of the joints are also common.

Patient Screening

When a patient develops a persistent joint problem, a thorough history and physical examination are essential. Schedule the first available appointment. Follow office policy for a subsequent referral to a rheumatologist.

Etiology

The exact cause in most osteoarthritis cases is unknown, but it appears to be generally associated with aging. The tendency toward developing osteoarthritis is sometimes

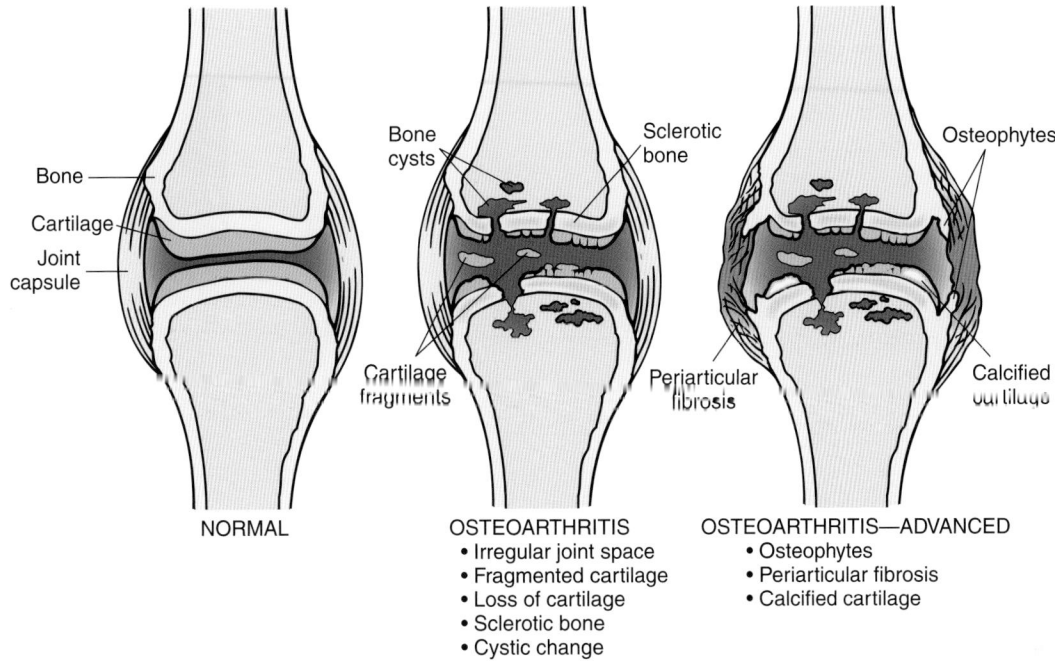

NORMAL

OSTEOARTHRITIS
• Irregular joint space
• Fragmented cartilage
• Loss of cartilage
• Sclerotic bone
• Cystic change

OSTEOARTHRITIS—ADVANCED
• Osteophytes
• Periarticular fibrosis
• Calcified cartilage

• **Fig. 7.13** Schematic presentation of the pathologic changes in osteoarthritis. Fragmentation and loss of cartilage denude the subchondral bone, which undergoes sclerosis and cystic change. Osteophytes form on the lateral sides and protrude into the adjacent soft tissues, causing irritation, inflammation, and fibrosis. (From Damjanov I: *Pathology for the health professions,* ed 4, St Louis, 2012, Saunders.)

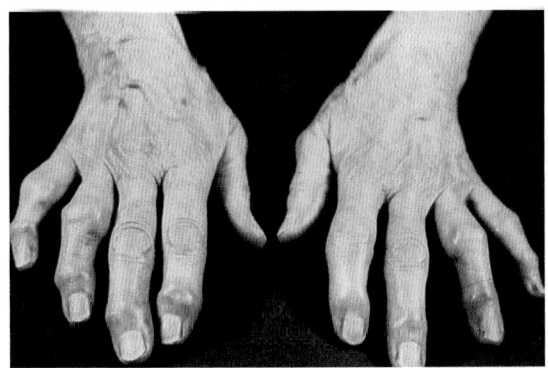

• **Fig. 7.14** Bouchard nodes. (From Monahan FD, et al: *Phipps' medical-surgical nursing,* ed 8, St Louis, 2007, Mosby.)

inherited. In some persons, osteoarthritis may follow injury to the joint or be associated with hormonal disorders or underlying diseases, such as diabetes and obesity.

Diagnosis

Patients must be evaluated to exclude other forms of arthritis, and any underlying diseases or conditions must be detected as well. The diagnostic investigation begins with physical examination and patient history. Radiographs, computed tomography (CT) scans, and magnetic resonance imaging (MRI) scans confirm the presence and document the severity of osteoarthritis. Plain radiography can be very helpful for excluding other causes of pain in a particular joint. Radiography can also measure the severity of the osteoarthritis and assist in deciding when surgical intervention should be considered.

Treatment

Because osteoarthritis cannot be cured, the goal of treatment is to reduce inflammation, to minimize pain, and to maintain functioning joints. Treatment of osteoarthritis involves physical and drug therapy, nutritional management, and supportive care. Surgery also may be needed in severe cases. Physical therapy includes ROM exercises, alternation of moist heat and cold applications, massage therapy, and the use of elastic bandages and splints for limb support. Drug therapy can include the use of analgesics, muscle relaxants, and NSAIDs. Intraarticular steroid injections may be used for specific or individual joints. Intraarticular hyaluronic acid can be used to reduce pain in affected knee joints. Fish oils have been suggested to have some antiinflammatory properties. Food supplementation with glucosamine and chondroitin may reduce pain and stiffness in some patients. For supportive care, it may be necessary to use a cane, walker, braces, or crutches to lessen the strain on some joints. (Always examine cane tips to be certain that they are not dangerously worn out!) Restricting physical activity or resting the affected joints also may be necessary. Surgery for osteoarthritis may involve total joint replacement. Joints commonly replaced are the base of the thumb, the hip, and the knee. Ankle, wrist, elbow, and shoulder joints also can be replaced. Joint fusion may be done to increase the stability of the cervical and lumbar vertebrae.

Prognosis

The outlook for patients with osteoarthritis depends primarily on the severity and location of the involved joints. Optimal outcome results from accurate diagnosis and early management.

Prevention

Avoiding injury and reinjury to joints is important in preventing osteoarthritis. Persons with flaccid (overstretched) ligaments may require support devices to engage in some activities. Early contact with health care professionals can optimize long-term health.

Patient Teaching

Providing specific guidance on food supplementation, medications, and proper exercise can significantly improve the quality of life for these patients.

Lyme Disease

Description

Lyme disease is an infectious disease caused by *Borrelia burgdorferi,* a spirochete bacterium. Ticks that bite the skin spread Lyme disease by injecting the bacterium from their gut into the human body when securing a blood meal. Lyme disease can affect the skin, joints, heart, and nervous system.

ICD-10-CM Code	A69.20 *(Lyme disease, unspecified)* (A69.20-A69.29 = 5 codes of specificity)

Symptoms and Signs

Lyme disease, also known as *Lyme arthritis,* was first detected in 1975 in Lyme, Connecticut, in the United States. Lyme disease is more prevalent in the northeast part of the United States, especially New York, New Jersey, Connecticut, District of Columbia, Maine, Maryland, Massachusetts, Minnesota, New Hampshire, Pennsylvania, Rhode Island, Vermont, Virginia, West Virginia, and Wisconsin, where large areas of forests and fields provide a habitat for ticks. The disease has been found throughout the world.

Lyme disease can occur in any age group, and no one is immune to the infection. Approximately half of all patients with Lyme disease have a characteristic red, itchy rash with a red circle center resembling the bull's eye on a target (target lesion) (Fig. 7.15A) early in the illness. Lyme disease can masquerade as arthritis and cause influenza-like symptoms, such as headache, fever, fatigue, joint pain, and general malaise. If the person does not seek medical attention for the symptoms, late complications of muscle weakness, paralysis, and neurologic conditions (e.g., learning difficulties, excessive fatigue, and muscle coordination problems) can develop as the bacterium spreads unchecked internally. Encephalitis, gastritis, or carditis may develop in some patients.

Patient Screening

Early detection of Lyme disease is imperative because treatment can eliminate the risk of more significant organ-threatening consequences. In areas where the deer tick is prevalent and/or the patient reports a "target lesion," a visual inspection and diagnostic laboratory tests are necessary. Likewise, if a patient reports flulike symptoms 2 to

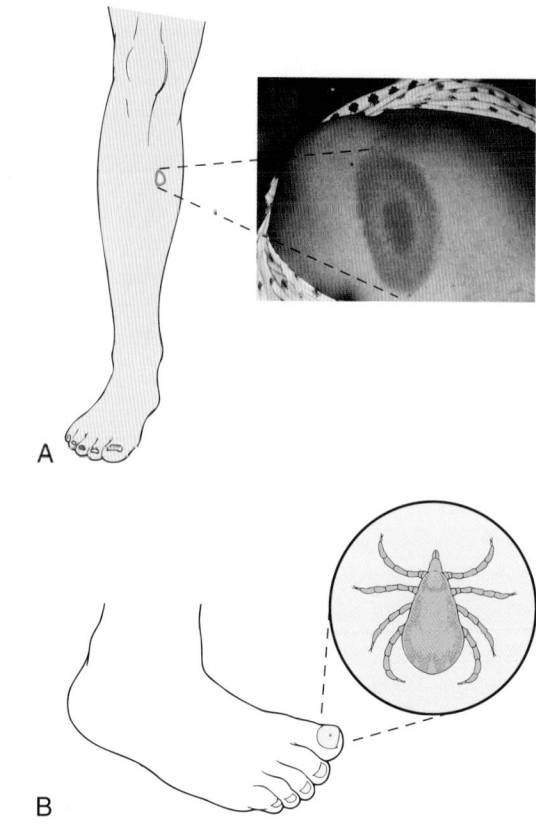

• **Fig. 7.15** (A) Target lesion of Lyme disease. (B) Tick that causes Lyme disease. (From Stone DR, Gorbach SL: *Atlas of infectious diseases,* Philadelphia, 2000, Saunders.)

4 weeks after sustaining a tick bite, an appointment for prompt diagnostic evaluation is indicated.

Etiology

Lyme disease is caused by *Borrelia burgdorferi,* a spirochete bacterium, which is transmitted to humans by a bite from a small tick (see Fig. 7.15B), which is carried by mice or deer vectors. *Borrelia burgdorferi* is prevalent in the United States. In Europe, the prevalent bacterium is *Borrelia afzelii,* which also causes Lyme disease. The disease is usually transmitted to humans while they are camping or hiking in the woods, fields, or other areas that ticks inhabit. After infiltrating the skin, the bacterium can infect internal organs of the body, causing a variety of symptoms, which often leads to delay in making the correct diagnosis.

Diagnosis

The evaluation of patients with the nonspecific symptoms of early Lyme disease, such as headache, fever, fatigue, joint pain, and general malaise can be exhaustive. A complete history, physical examination, and laboratory tests are important for excluding other infectious diseases, forms of arthritis, immune diseases, muscle diseases, and even cancer.

The diagnosis of Lyme disease can be based on physical examination (the discovery of a tick on the skin), the presence of the classic target lesion, and the patient's history. Confirmation is made on the basis of positive test results for the Lyme antibodies or by directly identifying the bacterium in the infected skin via biopsy, if necessary.

Treatment

Treatment of Lyme disease begins with removal of the tick if it is found on the skin or clothing. Early treatment is imperative, because treatment in the early stages of disease leads to a complete cure with simple oral antibiotics. The drug of choice for Lyme disease is doxycycline. Alternatively, the Centers for Disease Control and Prevention (CDC) also recommends amoxicillin or cefuroxime. Lyme disease in the later stages requires intravenous antibiotics, such as ceftriaxone or penicillin, to cure the disease. Antipyretics are given for headache and fever. Bed rest is necessary if neurologic symptoms are present, and physical therapy is prescribed for impaired musculoskeletal mobility. Joint symptoms are often treated with antiinflammatory medications and hydroxychloroquine.

Prognosis

Lyme disease is curable with antibiotics. The outlook for patients with Lyme disease is a function of how early it is detected. Early-stage Lyme disease involves a minor skin rash with muscle ache that easily resolves with antibiotics. Later-stage Lyme disease can cause residual damage to the joints, heart, or nervous system. Optimal outcome results from accurate diagnosis and early treatment.

Prevention

Avoiding tick bites is the best prevention against Lyme disease. In locations known to harbor ticks, one should wear long clothing to protect the skin. All clothing first and then the entire body, including the scalp, should be carefully examined to detect the presence of ticks after being in high-risk areas. Close inspection of children and pets is especially important. Ticks can be removed gently with tweezers and saved in a jar in case identification is needed later. Bathing the skin and scalp and washing clothes after possible exposure to ticks may not only prevent the bite but also subsequent transmission of the disease. Vaccines were once available, but these have been removed from the market. Further studies of vaccines are needed.

Patient Teaching

Community awareness of tick avoidance measures is essential for prevention. Patients who develop Lyme disease should be instructed to closely follow the specific instructions regarding therapeutic medications provided by their qualified health care professionals.

Bursitis

Description

Bursitis is inflammation of a bursa. A bursa is a tiny fluid-filled sac that functions as a gliding surface to reduce friction between tissues of the body. Bursae are found between muscles and tendons and cover bony prominences to facilitate movement. They can become inflamed, infected, or traumatized.

The major bursae are located adjacent to the tendons of the large joints, such as the shoulders, elbows, hips, and knees.

ICD-10-CM Code	M71.50 *(Other bursitis, not elsewhere classified, unspecified site)*
	(M71.10-M71.19 = 24 codes of specificity; M71.50-M71.58 = 20 codes of specificity)
	M70.039 *(Crepitant synovitis [acute] [chronic], unspecified wrist)*
	(M70.031-M70.049 = 6 codes of specificity)
	M70.30 *(Other bursitis of elbow, unspecified elbow)*
	(M70.30-M70.32 = 3 codes of specificity)
	M70.40 *(Prepatellar bursitis, unspecified knee)*
	(M70.40-M70.52 = 6 codes of specificity)

Symptoms and Signs

The classic symptoms of bursitis are tenderness, pain when moving the affected part, flexion and extension limitation, and edema at the site of inflammation. The most frequently affected bursae are those of the shoulder (Fig. 7.16), elbow, knee, hip, and between the tendons and muscles of the tibia. Point tenderness may be present, in which case the patient actually can point to the spot of greatest tenderness. If bursae are continually or chronically irritated and inflamed, calcifications can develop. In addition, adhesions can occur around an affected bursa, which limits the movement of the tendons.

Patient Screening

Pain, swelling, or limitation of motion in any joint, with or without previous injury, requires an appointment for

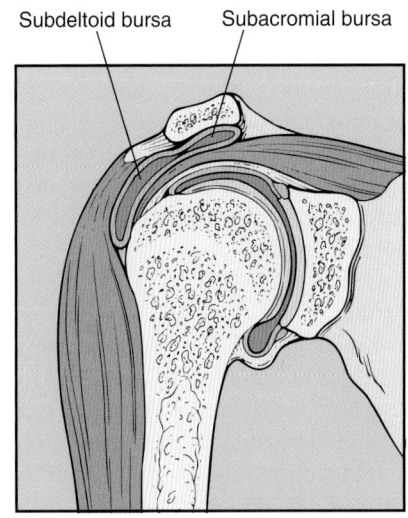

• **Fig. 7.16** Bursae of the shoulder.

diagnostic evaluation. Early treatment and relief from pain are important measures.

Etiology

Bursitis can result from continual or excessive friction between the bursae and the surrounding musculoskeletal tissues. Systemic diseases (e.g., gout and rheumatoid arthritis) and infection can lead to the development of bursitis. In addition, repeated trauma from overuse of a joint can cause bursitis (see the Cumulative Trauma section in Chapter 15).

Diagnosis

Bursitis is generally a straightforward diagnosis that can be made after evaluating information gained from the history and physical examination. However, in patients with bursitis that is not associated with injury, possible underlying gout or arthritis should be considered. In patients with abrasion or puncture wounds of the overlying skin, infection also must be considered. ROM may be impaired, and the pain is acute. MRI indicates an enlarged bursa, and radiographs may show calcified deposits at the affected site when the bursitis is chronic. Aspiration of fluid from an inflamed bursa can assist in diagnosing gouty or infectious bursitis (septic bursitis).

Treatment

The treatment for traumatic bursitis may include avoidance of activities until acute pain subsides, the application of moist heat, immobilization of the affected part, the use of aspirin or acetaminophen for pain, the administration of NSAIDs (e.g., ibuprofen and indomethacin), and local injection of a corticosteroid. If infection is present, drainage of the inflamed bursa and the use of antibiotics specific to the infectious microbe are critical. Active ROM exercises to prevent adhesions and to maintain or regain motion are needed after the acute pain subsides. Surgical excision of the bursa and any accompanying calcified deposits can be required for either chronic noninfectious or infectious bursitis.

Prognosis

Bursitis is curable. With treatment and proper attention to any underlying cause, the outlook is excellent.

Prevention

Actions that initiate or promote tissue inflammation, such as repetition of a throwing motion in the case of shoulder bursitis, prolonged leaning on the elbow in the case of elbow bursitis, or prolonged kneeling in the case of knee bursitis should be avoided.

Patient Teaching

Patients can benefit from being given specific information regarding the cause of the inflamed bursa and from instructions regarding aggravating factors to avoid. It is important to help the patient understand that the bursitis problem is adjacent to, but not involving, the joint. The joint should otherwise be unharmed. For any recurrent inflammation, patients should be instructed to immediately apply ice packs to the area so that inflammation can be minimized. Those with past infectious bursitis should notify their physician's office.

Osteomyelitis

Description

Osteomyelitis (Fig. 7.17) is a serious infection of bone that requires aggressive antibiotic treatment.

ICD-10-CM Code	M86.9 (Osteomyelitis, unspecified)
	(M86.00-M86.9 = 189 codes of specificity)

Refer to the physician's diagnosis and then the current edition of the ICD-10-CM coding manual for greatest specificity of site and stage (acute or chronic) of bone infection.

Symptoms and Signs

Inflammation, swelling, localized heat, redness, pain, and local tenderness over and around the affected bone are

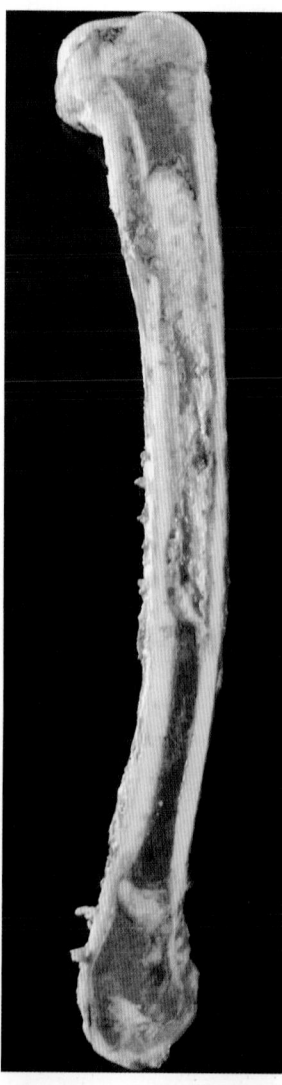

• **Fig. 7.17** Osteomyelitis. (From Cooke RA, Stewart B: *Colour atlas of anatomical pathology,* ed 3, London, 2003, Churchill Livingstone.)

characteristic signs of osteomyelitis. Other symptoms of osteomyelitis include chills, fever, sweating, and malaise. As the infection progresses, a purulent material called *subperiosteal abscess* may develop, causing pressure and eventual fracturing of small pieces of the bone. These fractured, dead pieces of bone may, in turn, become surrounded by the purulent material and form a sequestrum.

The most commonly involved bones in osteomyelitic infections are the upper ends of the humerus and tibia, the lower end of the femur, and occasionally the vertebrae.

Osteomyelitis most often begins as an acute infection; however, it can remain undetected for months or years and evolve into a chronic condition. Both the acute and chronic forms can present the same clinical picture.

Patient Screening
Patients with localized bone inflammation and pain must be evaluated for possible fractures and bone tumors before the diagnosis of osteomyelitis can be ascertained.

Etiology
Staphylococcus aureus is the bacterial organism responsible for 90% of osteomyelitic infections. Streptococcal bacteria account for the next largest number of infections. Rarely, viruses and fungi also have been known to cause osteomyelitis. Osteomyelitis can develop when bloodborne pathogens are deposited in the metaphyseal area of a bone after physical trauma or surgery.

Diabetes mellitus or peripheral vascular disease may predispose individuals to the development of osteomyelitis, as can the presence of prosthetic hardware (e.g., rods, screws, and plates within bone) and total joint replacement. Osteomyelitis in infants and children develops as a secondary infection from streptococcal pharyngitis (strep throat). Persons with sickle cell disease, immunodeficiency, or malignancies are also at increased risk for the development of osteomyelitis.

The possible development of osteomyelitis must be the concern of any person who has an open wound, sore (strep) throat, or a systemic infection that could be transmitted to the bones.

Diagnosis
Aspiration and culture of material taken from the site of the infection are essential to isolating the causative organisms. Blood culture, white blood cell (WBC) count, and erythrocyte sedimentation rate (ESR) are also helpful for determining diagnosis and monitoring treatment. MRI, CT, or bone scanning aid in determining the site and extent of acute or chronic infection.

Treatment
Osteomyelitis usually requires extensive, long-term antibiotic treatment with follow-up care to prevent recurrent infections. Parenteral or locally administered antibiotics (e.g., aqueous penicillin, cephalosporin, and ampicillin), at a dosage specific to the patient's age and the pathogenic organism involved, are needed. Additional measures include increased intake of proteins and vitamins A, B, and C to promote cell regeneration; bed rest, as needed, to conserve energy; control of chronic conditions (e.g., diabetes); immobilization of the affected part to prevent fracture of weakened bones; and analgesics. Surgical drainage to remove purulent material and sequestrum also may be necessary, along with bone grafting. Hyperbaric oxygen treatments may prove beneficial as well.

Prognosis
Osteomyelitis is curable. The long-term outcome depends on the amount of bone and/or joint damage as a result of the infection. Damaged bone can lead to deformity and impaired function, especially if growth plates are affected in children.

Prevention
For most patients, osteomyelitis cannot be prevented because it occurs randomly. However, patients with diabetes mellitus, sickle cell disease, or impaired immune systems should be particularly diligent about reporting to their doctors any signs of infections.

Patient Teaching
Patients must be instructed on the specific details and importance of their antibiotic management. Long-term antibiotic treatments administered intravenously can require special catheters, such as a peripherally inserted central catheter (PICC), which must be cared for according to specific guidelines.

Gout

Description
Gout is a chronic disorder of uric acid metabolism that manifests as an acute, episodic form of arthritis; chronic deposits of uric acid forming hard nodules in tissues; and/or kidney impairment or stones.

ICD-10-CM Code	M10.9 *(Gout, unspecified)*
	(M1a.00-M10.9 = 243 codes of specificity)

Gout is coded according to site and type of pathologic involvement. Refer to the physician's diagnosis and then to the current edition of the ICD-10-CM manual for greatest specificity.

Symptoms and Signs
Gout involves an overproduction or decreased excretion of uric acid and urate salts. This leads to high levels of uric acid in blood and also in the synovial fluid of joints. Deposits of other urate compounds can be found in and around the joints of extremities, often leading to joint deformity and disability (Fig. 7.18).

Typically, gout affects the first metatarsal joint of the great toe (podagra), causing severe to excruciating pain when an attack occurs. The joints of the feet, ankles, knees,

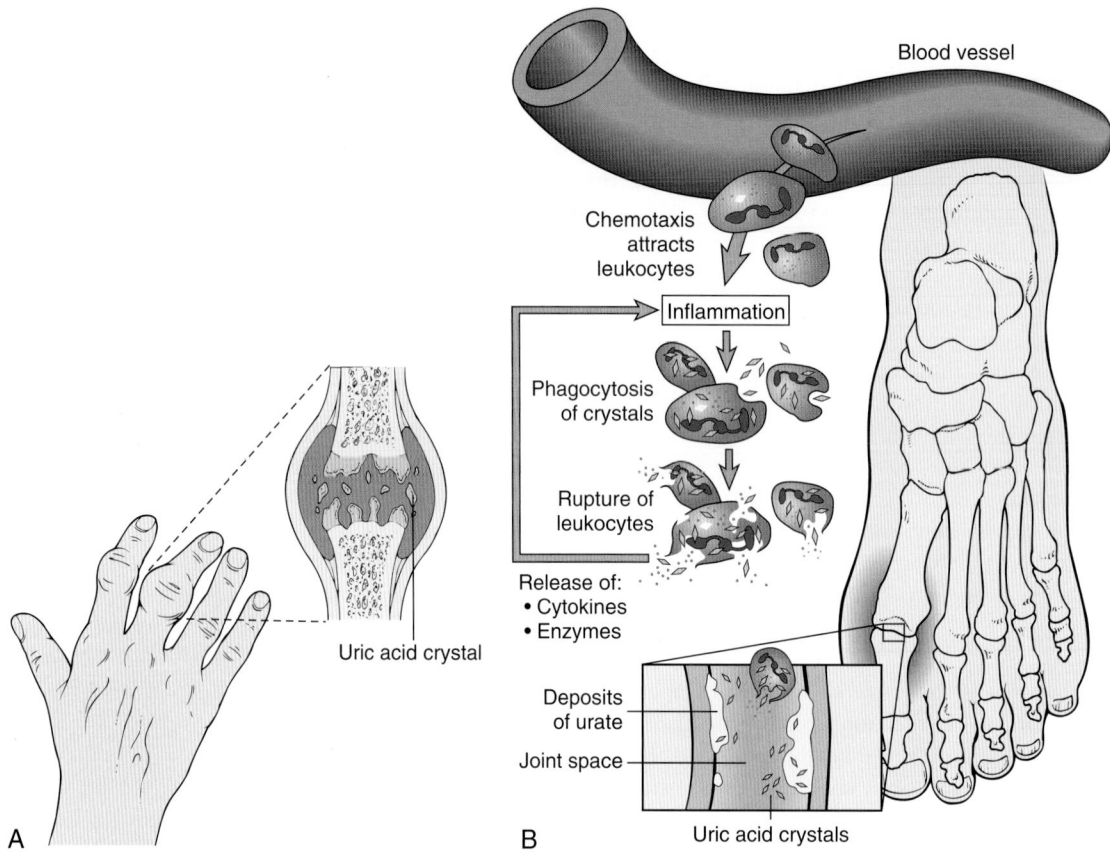

• **Fig. 7.18** (A) Gout. (B) Gouty arthritis. Deposits of uric acid crystals in the connective tissue have a chemotactic effect and cause exudation of leukocytes into the joint. The inflammation most often affects the metatarsophalangeal (MTP) joint. (From Damjanov I: *Pathology for the health professions,* ed 4, St Louis, 2012, Saunders.)

and even hands also can be affected. Pain usually peaks after several hours and then subsides gradually. A slight fever, chills, headache, or nausea may accompany an acute attack. Between attacks, the person is characteristically free from any symptoms. Gout also is characterized by renal dysfunction, hyperuricemia, and renal calculi (kidney stones).

The disease is uncommon in children; gout generally appears in males after puberty. Men are affected more often compared with women. In women, gout generally appears after menopause. Gout also can develop secondary to cell breakdown resulting from drug therapy, especially with chemotherapy for malignant diseases (e.g., leukemia).

Patient Screening

The patient with gout may complain of severe, acute joint pain and possibly mild systemic symptoms. Schedule an urgent appointment (especially if acute gouty arthritis is present) so that treatment can begin and medication that will relieve the pain can be prescribed.

Etiology

The cause of this disorder is most often an inherited abnormality of metabolism. It may result from a deficiency of enzymes needed to completely metabolize purines in foods for excretion from the kidneys. This incomplete metabolism leads to the buildup of uric acid in the tissues of the body.

Uric acid is a breakdown product of purines that are digested in foods. Renal gout is caused by some forms of kidney dysfunction. The body may produce levels of uric acid that are normal, but kidney function is insufficient to remove the product from blood. Excessive weight gain, leukemias and lymphomas, and certain drugs, including diuretics and tuberculosis medications, also can precipitate gout.

Diagnosis

Patients with new-onset joint inflammation are evaluated to exclude many types of arthritis, such as rheumatoid arthritis, spondylitis, reactive arthritis, and joint infection. Microscopic examination of aspirated synovial joint fluid or material from soft tissue uric acid deposits (called *tophi*) demonstrates the presence of urate crystals (see Fig. 7.18B) and proves the diagnosis. A serum uric acid test can indicate hyperuricemia, though up to one-third of patients with acute gout will have a normal uric acid level. Radiographs may be used to assess the amount of damage to the affected joints.

Treatment

General treatment of an acute attack of gout can involve bed rest to lessen pressure on affected joints, immobilization of the affected limb, and the application of cold packs to the inflamed joints, if the patient is able to tolerate the pressure of an ice bag. An NSAID, colchicine (Colcrys), or corticosteroids taken orally or injected into the gouty area are options that can reduce inflammation. Dietary modifications include a low-purine diet and adequate fluid intake. Dairy products have been shown to reduce the frequency of attacks of gouty arthritis. For chronic gout, after the acute attack has subsided, the patient may be given antihyperuricemic medications, such as probenecid (Benemid), allopurinol (Zyloprim), febuxostat (Uloric). Gradual weight reduction can be helpful for those patients who are overweight.

Prognosis

With proper management, potential damage to bones and joints can be avoided. Chronic gouty deposits of uric acid (tophi) can be difficult to treat, so if the tophi do not shrink with medication, they can be surgically resected.

Prevention

Limiting alcohol intake, avoiding dehydration, and eating a proper (low-purine, high-dairy) diet are keys to the prevention of gout attacks.

Patient Teaching

Patients should understand that early measures to treat inflammation, such as ice packs and antiinflammatory medication, may help them avoid prolonged pain and dysfunction. Specific dietary instructions should be given to any patient with gout.

Paget Disease (Osteitis Deformans)

Description

Paget disease is a chronic bone disorder that typically results in enlarged, deformed bones resulting from irregular breakdown and formation of bone tissue. Paget disease can cause bones to weaken and may result in bone pain, arthritis, bone deformities, and fractures. Paget disease is also known as *osteitis deformans*.

ICD-10-CM Code	M88.9 *(Osteitis deformans of unspecified bone)* (M88.0-M88.9 = 27 codes of specificity)

Symptoms and Signs

In patients with Paget disease, affected areas of bone produce new bone tissue faster than the old bone can be broken down. Paget disease occurs characteristically in two stages. The initial stage is called the *vascular stage*. Bone tissue is broken down, but the spaces left are filled with blood vessels and fibrous tissue instead of new strong bone. In the second, or *sclerotic*, stage, the highly vascular fibrous tissue hardens and becomes similar to bone, but it is fragile instead of being strong (Fig. 7.19). This can lead to pathologic fractures.

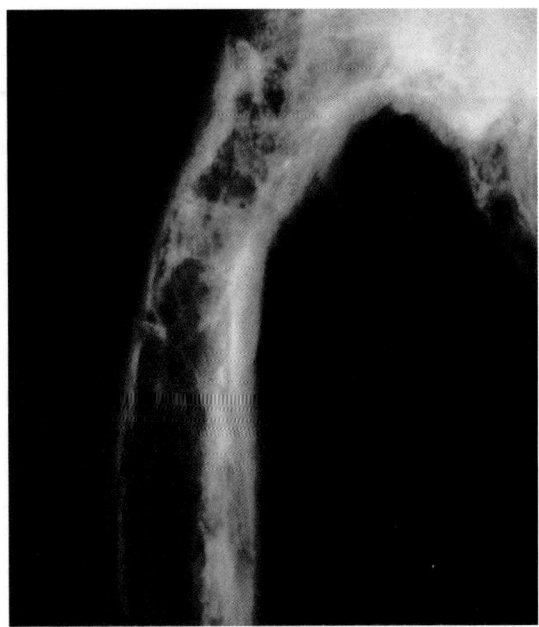

• **Fig. 7.19** Paget disease (osteitis deformans). (From Browner B, Jupiter J, Trafton P: *Skeletal trauma: basic science, management, and reconstruction,* ed 3, Philadelphia, 2003, Saunders.)

This disease can occur in a part of one bone, all of one bone, or many bones throughout the skeletal system. The most common sites of the disease are the pelvis and the tibia. Other sites often affected are the femur, spine, skull, and clavicle. Paget disease usually affects individuals older than 40 years of age and becomes increasingly more common with advancing age.

Paget disease often causes no symptoms. When symptoms do occur, they usually include local bone pain. The pain can become disabling. Aching is almost continuous and is often worse at night. Some patients may have edema or deformity in one of the bones or may notice that they need a larger hat size because the bones of the skull have enlarged. If the ossicles of the ear are involved, hearing loss or deafness may occur. Other complications of Paget disease can include frequent fractures, spinal cord injuries, hypercalcemia, renal calculi, and rarely, bone sarcoma, a serious form of cancer.

Patient Screening

A patient having bone pain must be evaluated for fracture and infection of bone along with blood calcium and alkaline phosphatase levels.

Etiology

The cause of Paget disease is not known.

Diagnosis

Physical examination and history of the patient's symptoms are needed. The physician then orders several tests and blood work. Radiographic imaging, bone scanning, and possibly bone marrow biopsy assist in the diagnosis. Blood analysis will indicate an elevated serum concentration of alkaline phosphatase, and urinalysis reveals elevated hydroxyproline concentration. Both these findings are produced by the high rate of bone production.

Treatment

Patients with Paget disease who have no symptoms require no treatment. With symptoms, treatment options include analgesics, antiinflammatory drugs, cytotoxic agents, or injections of a hormone called calcitonin. Calcitonin is produced naturally by the thyroid gland and works with parathyroid hormone (parathormone) and vitamin D to regulate the level of calcium in blood. Increased amounts of calcitonin can reduce pain for some patients and prevent bone loss. Eating a high-protein, high-calcium diet, with vitamin D supplementation, may be advised as well. Newer treatments include bisphosphonate medications, such as alendronate (Fosamax), risedronate (Actonel), tiludronate, pamidronate (Aredia), and zoledronic acid (Reclast).

Prognosis

In most patients with Paget disease, few, if any, symptoms are noted. If needed, medications can relieve persistent bone pain. Complications including hypercalcemia, fractures, heart failure, gout, and bone cancer (sarcoma) can lead to increased morbidity.

Prevention

Patients with Paget disease should receive 1000 to 1500 mg of calcium, adequate exposure to sunshine, and at least 400 units of vitamin D daily. This is especially important for patients being treated with bisphosphonates. Patients with a history of kidney stones should discuss calcium and vitamin D intake with their physician.

Patient Teaching

Exercise is an important part of maintaining skeletal health, as are avoiding weight gain and maintaining joint mobility. Because undue stress on affected bones should be avoided, patients should discuss any planned exercise program with their physician before beginning.

Marfan Syndrome

Description

Marfan syndrome is a group of inherited conditions featuring abnormal connective tissue with weakness of blood vessels and excessive length and flexibility of the extremities (Fig. 7.20).

ICD-10-CM Code	Q87.40 *(Marfan's syndrome, unspecified)* (Q87.40-Q87.43 = 5 codes of specificity)

Symptoms and Signs

Marfan syndrome is characterized by abnormally long extremities and digits. Additional deformities include subluxation of the lens of the eyes and heart and vascular

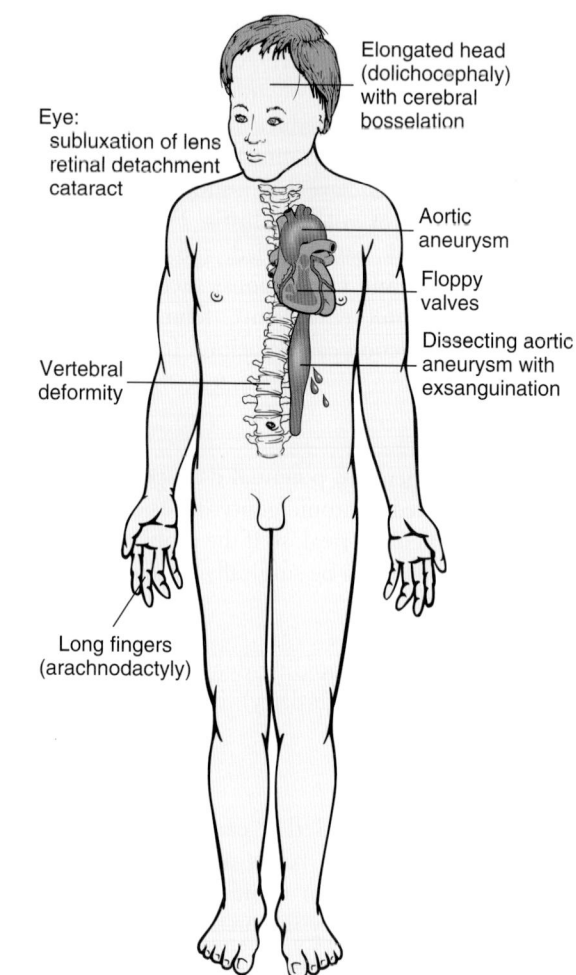

• **Fig. 7.20** Typical features of Marfan syndrome. (From Damjanov I: *Pathology for the health professions,* ed 4, St Louis, 2012, Saunders.)

anomalies. This condition may go undetected until harmful complications are precipitated. The person with Marfan syndrome is tall and slender and has long, narrow digits. An asymmetry of the skull may be noted. Visual difficulties are encountered when lens dissociation occurs. Scoliosis is another manifestation. Joints can be hyperextensible in those with Marfan syndrome. Mitral valve prolapse and thickening of the heart valves and aortic aneurysm may be present but frequently go undetected (see the Valvular Heart Disease section in Chapter 10). Often the first indication of the syndrome occurs during exercise that precipitates rupture of an aortic aneurysm, with catastrophic results.

Patient Screening

A patient diagnosed with Marfan syndrome may develop serious complications of the eyes or cardiovascular system requiring immediate medical attention. Defer to the health care professional for direction.

Etiology

This syndrome is an autosomal dominant genetic disorder. The affected gene is on the long arm of chromosome 15. The defective gene can be inherited as follows: The child of a person who has Marfan syndrome has a 50% chance of inheriting the gene. The defective gene determines the structure of fibrillin, a protein that is an important component of connective tissue. Although everyone with Marfan syndrome has the same defective gene, not everyone experiences the same symptoms. This is referred to as *variable expression* of the gene.

Diagnosis

Patients with Marfan syndrome may sometimes be confused with those who have homocystinuria (an amino acid disorder) because connective tissue abnormalities and abnormal movement of the lens of the eye are present in both conditions. A person with Marfan syndrome is born with the disorder, although it may not be diagnosed until later in life. The diagnosis is made on the basis of family history, physical examination findings of abnormal length of the limbs and lens abnormality in the eye, and results of tests of the heart and blood vessels. Diagnosis of the syndrome in early childhood is possible when the lens dissociation and mitral valve prolapse anomalies are detected. The clinical picture of a rapid growth spurt and scoliosis, coupled with the visual disturbance and mitral valve prolapse, leads to further investigation. Echocardiographic measurements of the aortic diameter aid in detecting potential aortic dissection. Patients at risk for impending aortic dissection may be asymptomatic, or may experience chest pain that is tearing in nature and radiates to the neck, back, and arms.

Treatment

Treatment involves controlling excessive height with hormones before puberty, preventing glaucoma, controlling blood pressure, and preventing aortic dissection. Ophthalmic examinations should be conducted on a routine basis to detect any problem at an early stage. Monitoring blood pressure and maintaining it at a normal level are essential. Close observation of aortic status is necessary, and surgical replacement of diseased portions may be indicated. Aortic and mitral valves may need to be replaced surgically. Echocardiography is used on a regular basis to assess the status of the aorta.

Prognosis

The major risks to life are rupture of blood vessels, particularly the aorta. Patients can be disabled because of severe spine abnormalities and joint dislocations.

Prevention

The key measures to prevent complications include avoiding elevated blood pressure and trauma that could cause bleeding or bone and joint injury. Evaluation and monitoring of the status of the aorta and heart valves by echocardiography is essential.

Patient Teaching

Patients should be educated about the anomalies in their own anatomy and physiology so that they will understand the need to minimize high-risk activities and to report any signs of problems to their health care providers. Genetic counseling may be helpful.

Musculoskeletal Tumors

Description

Musculoskeletal tumors are abnormal growths, whether benign or malignant, within muscles or bones. Benign neoplasms are much more common than malignant tumors.

Bone Tumors

Description

The term *bone tumor* describes any abnormal growth, whether benign or malignant, in bone. The definition includes chondrogenic (from cartilage), osteogenic (from bone), and fibrogenic (from fibrous tissue) tumors.

ICD-10-CM Code	(Refer to the Neoplasm table in the current edition of the ICD-10-CM coding manual.)

Neoplasms of the bone are coded according to anatomic site, classified as benign or malignant, or designated as unspecified. Refer to the physician's diagnosis and then to the current edition of the ICD-10-CM coding manual for greatest specificity.

Symptoms and Signs

With bone tumors, pain is the most common presenting complaint. It is often worse at night or with exercise. A parent may notice a child beginning to limp or curtailing physical activity. Painful soft tissue swelling may be evident as the neoplasm enlarges. Patients with Ewing sarcoma often have systemic symptoms, such as fever, fatigue, and pallor caused by anemia.

Sometimes bone tumors produce no symptoms and are detected incidentally when radiographic imaging is performed for some other reason. Radiographic studies can reveal osteonecrosis or increased ossification and calcification. Different types of malignant tumors have characteristic radiographic findings. Osteosarcoma has a "sunburst" appearance on the radiograph. The Ewing sarcoma lesion has an "onion skin" appearance. Chondrosarcomas have a lobular pattern.

The bone tumor weakens the bone and makes it susceptible to fracture when subjected to the slightest strain. This is called a *pathologic fracture* (see Fig. 7.28I). A pathologic fracture is often one of the first indications of the presence of metastases to bones, and it commonly occurs in the acetabulum or the proximal femur.

Patient Screening

Bone pain, with or without local swelling, requires a timely medical evaluation. Systemic symptoms also may be present and indicate the need for the earliest possible appointment.

Etiology

Malignant tumors may be primary or secondary in origin. Primary tumors are most commonly found in adolescents, often during the adolescent growth spurt. Males are affected more often than females. Metastatic, or secondary, tumors in bones occur more often than do primary tumors and are more common in older age groups. Cancers that commonly metastasize to bones include breast, lung, prostate, thyroid, and kidney cancers. The bones affected most often are the pelvis, vertebrae, ribs, hip, femur, and humerus. Risk factors for primary bone tumors include prior chemotherapy, radiation therapy, or a history of Paget disease or other benign bone lesions.

Osteosarcoma is the most common type of primary bone neoplasm (Fig. 7.21). Osteosarcoma develops most often in the distal femur, followed by the proximal tibia and the humerus. Metastasis to the lung within 2 years of treatment is common. Ewing sarcoma most often involves the pelvis and the lower extremity and can extend into soft tissues. Both often metastasize to the lungs. Metastases to the lungs and other bones occur early in the disease. Chondrosarcoma often arises in the pelvis and proximal femur. It primarily affects individuals between ages 30 and 60 years. Chondrosarcoma grows more slowly compared with other malignant tumors of the bone and is locally invasive.

Diagnosis

The diagnosis is made on the basis of findings from a complete patient history, physical examination, laboratory studies, and diagnostic procedures. Many studies, including radiography, radionuclide bone scanning or positron emission tomography (PET), CT, and MRI greatly aid in determining the diagnosis and in evaluating the extent of disease. For Ewing sarcoma, bone marrow aspiration is performed to check for metastasis to bone marrow. Other markers may be useful in identification of tumor type. Osteosarcomas generally have an elevated serum alkaline phosphatase level, whereas in Ewing sarcoma, the level of lactate dehydrogenase (LDH) can be elevated. Biopsy is necessary for definitive diagnosis and for staging purposes. Bone cancers are often staged by using a system based on the tumor grade, tumor site, and presence of metastases.

Treatment

Bone tumors, whether benign or malignant, are treated with surgical excision. The surrounding muscle, bone, and other tissue are often removed also, and bone grafting may be needed. The goal is to perform limb-sparing surgery, but tumor location and extent may necessitate amputation. Isolated metastases to the lungs may be amenable to surgical resection as well. Surgery alone is enough to treat benign tumors, whereas treatment of malignant neoplasms usually includes administration of chemotherapy and/or radiation therapy. Treatment choice depends on tumor type. For example, Ewing sarcoma is usually chemosensitive, whereas chondrosarcomas are generally chemoresistant.

Prognosis

The prognosis depends largely on tumor type, extent of disease at presentation, and anatomic location. Poor prognostic indicators are a high-grade tumor, large tumor size, and presence of metastasis. A high LDH level at diagnosis often correlates with a poor prognosis in Ewing sarcoma.

Prevention

Prevention is difficult because few risk factors have been identified. Bone pain and masses should be evaluated promptly to reduce the risk of complications, such as fractures, deformity, and need for amputation. No type of routine screening is recommended, even for those with risk factors for bone tumors, such as Paget disease or prior radiation therapy.

Patient Teaching

Patients and families require specific instructions regarding the use and rehabilitation of the involved extremities. Managing the timing and intensity of weight bearing with leg involvement, for example, is crucial for avoiding injury.

Muscle Tumors

Description

Neoplasms of muscle include benign tumors or malignant sarcomas that may arise at any site in the body. The most commonly affected areas are the buttocks, groin, extremities, head and neck region, trunk, and retroperitoneum.

ICD-10-CM Code	(Refer to the Neoplasm table in the current edition of the ICD-10-CM coding manual.)

Neoplasms of the muscle are coded according to anatomic site, classified as benign or malignant, or designated as unspecified. Refer to the physician's diagnosis and then to the current edition of the ICD-10-CM coding manual for greatest specificity.

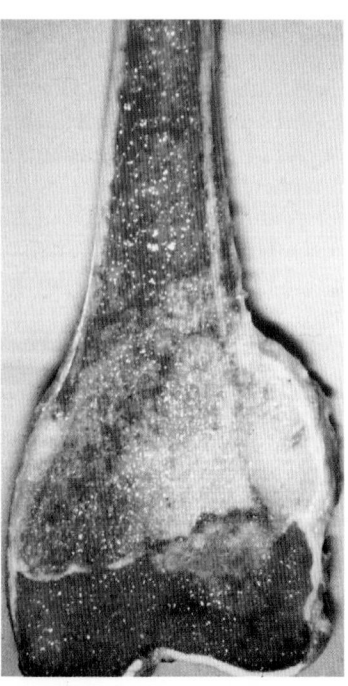

• **Fig. 7.21** Osteosarcoma. (From Kumar V, et al: *Robbins basic pathology*, ed 8, Philadelphia, 2008, Saunders.)

Symptoms and Signs

Skeletal muscle tumors often present as a painless lump of a few weeks' or months' duration, often with erythema of the overlying skin. In some instances, pain and tenderness may be present secondary to pressure effects on a nerve from the mass. Smooth muscle tumors often cause pain in and/or bleeding from the organ affected. For example, a uterine leiomyoma may cause abnormal uterine bleeding. At times, benign tumors are asymptomatic and are discovered incidentally on physical or radiographic examinations.

Patient Screening

A child or adult with a lump or painless swelling in a muscle should be scheduled for a visual inspection and medical evaluation.

Etiology

Muscle neoplasms are often benign and not life-threatening (e.g., leiomyomas [tumors of smooth muscle] and rhabdomyomas [tumors of striated muscle]). Malignant tumors (e.g., leiomyosarcomas and rhabdomyosarcomas) often grow and metastasize rapidly. Malignant muscle tumors grow by local extension and infiltration along tissue planes. In contrast to primary bone tumors, muscle sarcomas occur most often in patients older than 50 years of age. The exception is the small peak of incidence of rhabdomyosarcoma in early childhood. Risk factors include radiation treatment for previous cancer and exposure to carcinogenic chemicals.

Diagnosis

MRI is the most effective imaging technique for muscle tumors. Radiography or CT of the chest is performed to look for metastasis to the lungs. Biopsy (usually core-needle biopsy) can compromise subsequent treatment and should be carefully planned by using the information from imaging studies. Bone marrow aspiration is performed if a malignant tumor is present. The most common staging system used is a variation of the TNM (tumor–node–metastasis) system that also incorporates grade and tumor depth into the stage grouping. See Chapter 1 for information about the staging and grading systems used to assess malignant neoplasms.

Treatment

Surgical resection of the tumor is performed for all tumors, benign or malignant. For benign tumors, complete surgical resection is usually all that is required for treatment. For sarcomas, surgery is often combined with radiation therapy. Chemotherapy is used as an adjunct to surgery in children with rhabdomyosarcoma. Resection of pulmonary metastases may offer survival benefit and possible cure. Because lung metastasis can be clinically silent, follow-up imaging studies are indicated for all patients after initial treatment.

Prognosis

Prognosis worsens significantly with increasing tumor grade. Other poor prognostic indicators include deep anatomic tumor location, large tumor size, and presence of metastases. The 5-year survival rate for malignant tumors varies widely, depending on tumor subtype and grade.

Prevention

No methods of prevention are known.

Patient Teaching

Explain the scheduled diagnostic procedures to the patient, and describe what is normally experienced during the tests. Tell the patient when to expect the results. If surgery is necessary, explain the preoperative and postoperative procedures. Address patient concerns if the tumor is malignant, within the guidelines suggested by the physician. Give a full explanation of the radiation and chemotherapy regimens and what side effects may occur. Offer sensitive support to parents when the patient is a child, and make appropriate referrals for additional support.

Osteoporosis

Description

Osteoporosis is a condition characterized by loss of the normal bone density. Osteoporosis leads literally to porous bone that can be described as being compressible, like a sponge, rather than being dense, like a brick (Fig. 7.22).

ICD-10-CM Code	M81.0 *(Age-related osteoporosis without current pathological fracture)*

Osteoporosis may be coded according to cause or onset. Refer to the current edition of the ICD-10-CM coding manual for greatest specificity.

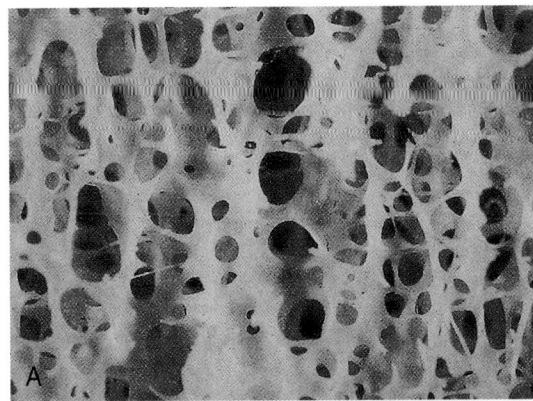
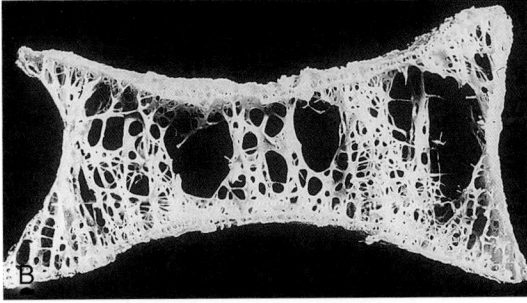

• **Fig. 7.22** (A) Normal metacarpal bone. (B) Osteoporotic metacarpal bone. (From Long BW, Frank ED, Ehrlich RA: *Radiography essentials for limited practice,* ed 4, St Louis, 2013, Elsevier.)

Symptoms and Signs

Osteoporosis is a condition in which there is wasting or deterioration of bone mass and density. It occurs more often in women, especially postmenopausal women, than in men. Women who are small boned, who are of northern European or Asian descent, who smoke, and who have a family history of the disease have the greatest risk for osteoporosis.

Unless it occurs in the vertebrae or the weight-bearing bones, osteoporosis usually does not produce symptoms. Osteoporosis is a silent disease until a bone break causes pain. Spontaneous fractures, especially in the vertebrae of the mid-to-lower thoracic spine, and loss of height are the most common signs (Fig. 7.23).

Patient Screening

Patients with risk factors should undergo bone density testing. Unrecognized osteoporosis may be first discovered when the patient sustains a fracture. Emergency care is required for breathing difficulty, severe pain, protrusion of bone through the skin, or numbness in a limb.

Etiology

Osteoporosis is the most common metabolic bone disease. It is caused by the imbalance between the breakdown of old bone tissue and the production of new bone. Metabolic bone diseases primarily originate from hormonal or dietary factors or disuse, but trauma also may cause the development of this condition. Osteoporosis can be caused by radiation treatments, malabsorption, smoking, alcohol abuse, calcium-wasting nephropathy, immobility, and chronic disease, such as rheumatoid arthritis. Senile and postmenopausal osteoporosis, usually resulting from lack of estrogen, are the most common forms. Osteoporosis also can result from use of medications, such as heparin, phenytoin, and the cortisone

medications prednisone and prednisolone. Males with a low testosterone level are at risk for osteoporosis.

Diagnosis

Patients with spontaneous bone fracture are screened for cancer in the involved bone by using radiographic testing. When osteoporosis is detected, patients are further evaluated for hormone imbalances, kidney disease, diet inadequacy, intestinal malabsorption, and use of certain medications, including cortisone medications, such as prednisone and prednisolone.

The diagnosis of osteoporosis is based on the results of blood serum studies, radiography, urinalysis, CT, and bone scanning. The best test for osteoporosis is dual energy x-ray absorptiometry (DEXA). If more specific diagnostic data are needed, bone biopsy may be ordered.

Treatment

Osteoporosis can cause permanent disability if not arrested, and treatment varies, depending on the cause. Increased dietary intake of calcium, calcium carbonate, calcium carbonate with sodium fluoride, phosphate supplements, and vitamins, especially vitamin D, may be prescribed. Estrogen replacement therapy may be used for postmenopausal osteoporosis. Alternatives to estrogen replacement therapy are bisphosphonate medications, such as alendronate sodium (Fosamax), risedronate (Actonel), ibandronate (Boniva), or zoledronate (Reclast). Calcitonin (Miacalcin) nasal spray and parathyroid hormone (Forteo) are other options in certain situations. Exercise can help minimize osteoporosis by slowing the loss of calcium. Moderate exercise in the form of walking, swimming, or use of a stationary bicycle is best. Physical therapy exercises for persons who are immobilized or paralyzed are necessary. If, however, the bones have become brittle, exercise of any type may be limited. To alleviate pain and muscle spasms, analgesics and muscle relaxants may be prescribed.

Prognosis

The outlook for patients with osteoporosis depends on many factors, including age and mobility, severity of bone loss, underlying causes, and complications related to fractures. The prognosis improves when the underlying causes are identified and treatment is provided.

Prevention

Prevention is absolutely the key to osteoporosis management. Bone density testing should be performed in all women older than 65 years of age, in all postmenopausal women with risk factors for osteoporosis, and postmenopausal women who sustain fractures. Women should consult their clinicians regarding adequate calcium intake and regular exercise programs.

Patient Teaching

Patients must be instructed regarding diets that promote bone health, smoking cessation, calcium and vitamin D intake, and exercise programs. Fall risk education can prevent fractures.

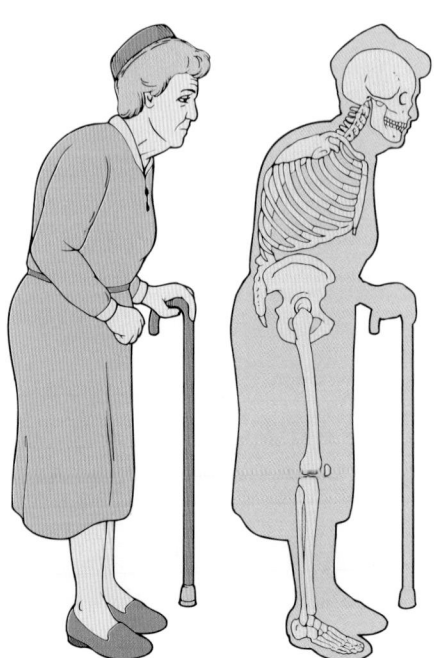

• **Fig. 7.23** Typical posture in osteoporosis.

Osteomalacia and Rickets

Description

Osteomalacia is a bone disease characterized by defective mineralization.

ICD-10-CM Code	M83.9 *(Adult osteomalacia, unspecified)*
	(M83.0-M83.9 = 8 codes of specificity)

Additional codes may be required to identify the nature or cause of osteomalacia. Refer to the physician's diagnosis and then to the current edition of the ICD-10-CM coding manual for greatest specificity.

Symptoms and Signs

Osteomalacia causes bones to become increasingly soft, flexible, and deformed. When the disorder occurs in children, it impacts the growing skeleton and is called *rickets* (Fig. 7.24). In adults, it usually is referred to as *osteomalacia*.

Early symptoms may include general fatigue; progressive stiffness; tender, painful bones; backaches; muscle twitches and cramps; and difficulty standing up. As the disease progresses, the patient may experience fractures, bowing of the legs, chest deformity, and shortening of the spine leading to an overall reduction in height.

Patient Screening

The early symptoms mentioned above require an appointment for a medical assessment.

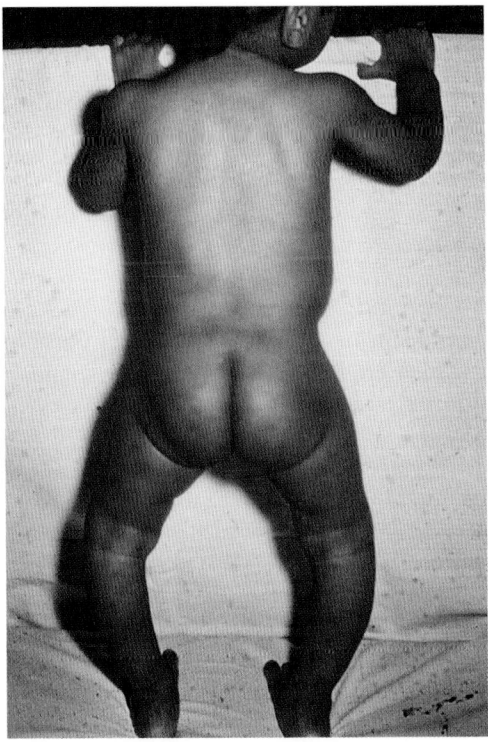

• Fig. 7.24 Rickets. (From Kumar V: *Robbins basic pathology,* ed 9, Philadelphia, 2013, Saunders.)

Etiology

Osteomalacia is a metabolic bone disease resulting from deficiency or ineffective use of vitamin D, which is essential for proper bone formation. Without adequate vitamin D, the body cannot absorb and use the bone-building minerals (calcium and phosphorus).

Other causes of this disorder may include an inadequate exposure to sunlight, which prevents the body from synthesizing its own vitamin D; intestinal malabsorption of vitamin D; and chronic renal diseases.

Diagnosis

Children with skeletal abnormalities suggestive of rickets are evaluated for genetic disorders and disease of the kidneys and bowels. Adults with osteomalacia are screened for metabolism disorders, as well as kidney and bowel disease.

The diagnosis of osteomalacia can involve a series of blood tests (e.g., serum calcium, serum alkaline phosphatase, vitamin D levels, and ESR), radiographic studies, bone scanning, and possibly bone biopsy.

Treatment

Treatment involves vitamin D supplementation and adding dietary vitamin D, calcium, and calcitonin. Exposure to sunlight increases vitamin D metabolism and absorption, especially in older persons. Any underlying disorder causing the deficiency, such as kidney or bowel disease, must be treated.

Prognosis

The outlook for patients with osteomalacia depends, to a great extent, on how early the condition is detected. The severity of the disorder, underlying causes, and complications, such as fractures, are all important factors affecting the long-term outlook.

Prevention

Prevention focuses on early diagnosis and prevention of bone injury.

Patient Teaching

Patients are instructed regarding vitamin D and calcium metabolism, dietary requirements, and the role of ultraviolet radiation in sunlight for producing natural vitamin D within the body.

Hallux Valgus (Bunion)

Description

A bunion is a localized area of enlargement of the inner portion of the first metatarsophalangeal (MTP) joint at the base of the big toe (Fig. 7.25).

ICD-10-CM Code	(M20.10-M20.12 = 3 codes of specificity)

Symptoms and Signs

Bunions cause progressive enlargement of the inner aspect of the first MTP joint. This can be associated with local

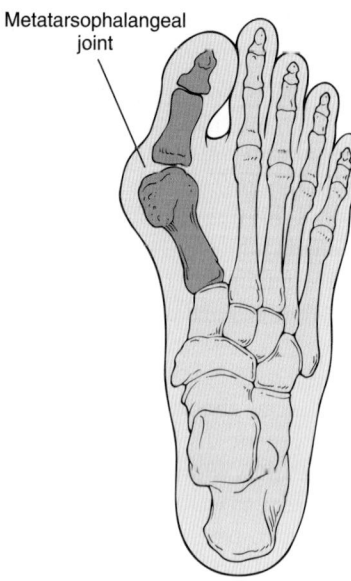

Metatarsophalangeal joint

• **Fig. 7.25** Bunion (hallux valgus).

inflammation and pain. If an adjacent inflamed bursa develops, secondary to pressure and inflammation at the joint, it can become even more painful. At times, the great toe may override or undercut the second toe. This causes crowding of the other toes and the possible development of hammer, claw, or mallet toes. Bunion development is more common in women and adolescent girls.

Patient Screening

Schedule an appointment for a visual examination for a patient complaining of a painful large toe.

Etiology

A bunion is often the result of a foot disorder known as *hallux valgus,* in which the great toe is positioned toward the midline of the body. The condition has been associated with rheumatoid arthritis. A flatfoot also contributes to hallux valgus and the development of a bunion because of the fallen, or dropped, longitudinal arch of the foot. The wearing of improperly fitting or high-heeled shoes aggravates hallux valgus. There is also a familial tendency for developing this condition. Bunions are common in ballet dancers.

Diagnosis

Patients with bunions are evaluated for underlying forms of arthritis, particularly osteoarthritis, rheumatoid arthritis, and gout. Footwear should be closely scrutinized. Physical examination of the foot, along with history of the symptoms, may be sufficient for the diagnosis. Radiographic studies confirm the lateral displacement of the great toe and any degenerative arthritic joint changes.

Treatment

Management of a bunion can include wearing shoes with a roomy "toe box" to avoid crowding the toes together;

wearing shoes with lower heels; using padding between the toes or around the bunion to relieve pressure; applying ice to the bunion to reduce the inflammation and lessen the pain; and resting the affected joints.

Analgesic medications (e.g., aspirin and acetaminophen) are given for pain. Intraarticular (joint) injections of a corticosteroid may be helpful as well.

There are many different surgical procedures for the treatment or correction of hallux valgus. Bunionectomy, osteotomy, and arthroplasty are the more common procedures.

Prognosis

With proper footwear, bunions often can be tolerated without surgical intervention. For those with persistent pain, surgical treatments can be curative.

Prevention

Proper footwear to minimize trauma to the toe and MTP joint is essential for the best outcome.

Patient Teaching

Patients can benefit by learning about the anatomy of the foot and the affected joint. They should be alerted to the risk for secondary infection if the bunion is abraded by footwear; if such is the case, antibiotics are instituted, if needed.

Hallux Rigidus

Description

Hallux rigidus is a stiff big toe that develops as a result of degeneration of the cartilage of the first MTP joint.

ICD-10-CM Code	(M20.20-M20.22 = 3 codes of specificity)

Symptoms and Signs

Hallux rigidus causes pain and loss of motion in the joint. The MTP joint becomes painful, stiff, and swollen. The onset may be insidious, with the limitation of movement being gradual.

Patient Screening

An appointment for visual inspection and possibly radiographic studies are indicated for a patient complaining of pain in the large toe.

Etiology

Degeneration of the MTP joint can occur as a result of injury or underlying arthritis, such as osteoarthritis. Over time, constant wear and tear on the joint or repetitive minor trauma to the joint causes the articular cartilage of the joint to degenerate, resulting in raw bone surface rubbing against raw bone surface. This degenerative arthritic type of process allows for the formation of bone spurs or osteophytes in the joint space that restrict joint motion.

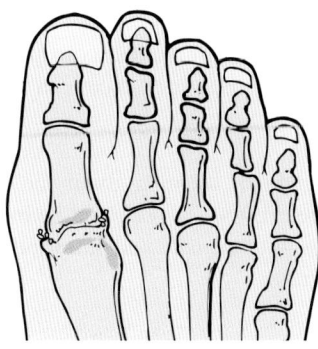

• **Fig. 7.26** Hallux rigidus.

Diagnosis

Diagnosis is made from a history of pain, either continuous or when walking, and restriction of motion of the MTP joint of the great toe. Physical examination usually reveals a straight hallux with an enlarged and tender joint with limited dorsiflexion (Fig. 7.26). Radiographic studies confirm the degenerative process and the joint space being diminished. Advanced conditions may cause chips of the cartilage in the joint space, which may eventually calcify.

Treatment

Conservative treatment includes drug therapy with antiinflammatory medications and wearing of shoes with thick, hard soles and low heels. When surgical intervention is indicated, cheilectomy to remove bone spurs and degenerative changes of the joint is considered. During cheilectomy, a portion of the dorsal aspect of the metatarsal head also is removed. This is followed by rehabilitation with ROM exercises. When the progression of the condition is extensive, arthrodesis, or fusion of the joint, may be the only method of pain relief. Some surgeons may perform arthroplasty to replace the destroyed joint with a plastic prosthesis or an artificial joint. The problem with this procedure is that the lifetime of the joint usually is limited, possibly necessitating future procedures.

Prognosis

With proper footwear and medication to relieve intermittent pain, hallux rigidus often can be tolerated without surgical intervention. For those with persistent pain, surgical treatments can be curative.

Prevention

Proper footwear to minimize trauma to the toe and MTP joint is essential for the best outcome.

Patient Teaching

Patients can benefit by learning about the anatomy of the foot and the affected joint. Repeated impact loading of the affected joint can lead to progressive worsening.

Hammer Toe

Description

Hammer toe is a condition in which the toe bends upward like a claw because of an abnormal flexion of the PIP joint; it can occur in any one of the four lesser toes (Fig. 7.27A).

ICD-10-CM Code	M20.40 (Other hammer toe(s) [acquired], unspecified foot)
	(M20.40-M20.42 = 3 codes of specificity)

Symptoms and Signs

Hammer toe most often occurs in the second toe and with hyperextension of the MTP joint. This deformity can be painful and often causes abrasion and inflammation where the flexed toe rubs against footwear. It can lead to the formation of a corn on the top of the affected toe and callus formation on the sole of the foot and tip of the involved toe.

Patient Screening

Patients with hammer toe are evaluated for underlying forms of arthritis, such as rheumatoid arthritis and psoriatic arthritis.

Etiology

Many factors may contribute to the occurrence of hammer toe. Although a congenital tendency of a long second metatarsal bone may exist, often shoes that are too short and have pointed toes or high heels may be the contributing factor. Nerves supplying the muscles of the toe are subjected to repeated insult, resulting in muscle imbalance in the foot and the development of hammer toe. Underlying arthritis from such diseases as rheumatoid arthritis and psoriatic arthritis can lead to the formation of hammer toes.

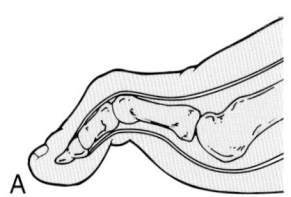

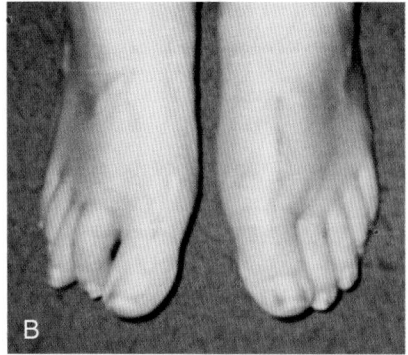

• **Fig. 7.27** (A) Hammer toe. (B) Hammer toe of second lesser toe, right foot.

Diagnosis

History of pain in the affected toe along with visual inspection is usually sufficient for determining diagnosis (see Fig. 7.27 B). Imaging studies confirm the diagnosis and rule out certain forms of arthritis.

Treatment

If the patient comes in early in the onset of symptoms, often switching to shoes that fit properly and allow enough space for the second toe can reverse the process, and the toe will eventually straighten. Splinting of the affected toe and performing therapeutic exercises can be helpful. The more advanced conditions when a contracture exists require surgical arthroplasty and possible fusion of the PIP joint (see Fig. 7.27C).

Prognosis

Proper footwear and monitoring for secondary infection improve the outcome. For those with persistent pain and irritation, surgical treatments can be curative.

Prevention

Proper footwear to minimize trauma to the toe is essential for the best outcome. Box-toed shoes can be very helpful.

Patient Teaching

Patients can benefit by learning about the anatomy of the foot and the affected toe. They should be instructed on the care of the foot and toenails and monitoring for signs of secondary infection.

Traumatic and Sports Injuries

Fractures

Description

Fractures, or broken bones, are caused by stress on the bone resulting from a traumatic insult to the musculoskeletal system, severe muscle spasm, or bone disease. They can occur in any bone in the body and are classified by the nature of the fracture, which is the result of the mechanism of injury (Fig. 7.28A–O).

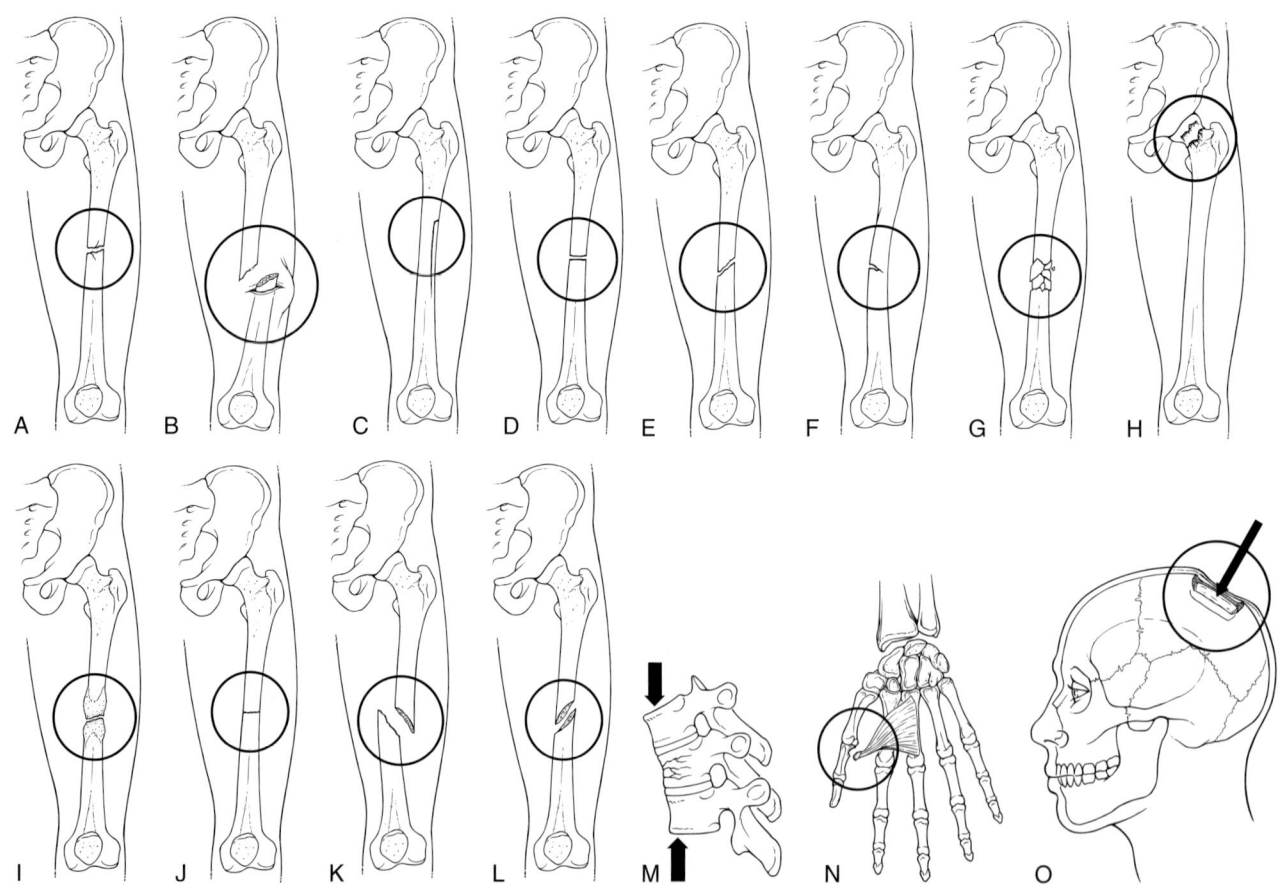

• **Fig. 7.28** Types of Fractures. (A) Closed, or simple. The overlying skin is intact. (B) Open or compound. The skin overlying the bone ends is not intact. (C) Longitudinal. The fracture extends along the length of the bone. (D) Transverse. The fracture is at right angles to the axis of the bone. (E) Oblique. The fracture extends in an oblique direction. (F) Greenstick. The fracture is on one side of the bone; the other side is bent. (G) Comminuted. The bone is splintered or crushed. (H) Impacted. The fractured ends of the bone are driven into each other. (I) Pathologic. The fracture results from weakening of the bone by disease. (J) Nondisplaced. The bone ends remain in alignment. (K) Displaced. The bone ends are out of alignment. (L) Spiral. The fracture results from a twisting mechanism, causing the break to wind around the bone in a spiral. (M) Compression. Excessive pressure causes the bone to collapse. (N) Avulsion. Tearing away of a muscle or a ligament is accompanied by tearing away of a bone fragment. (O) Depression. Bone fragments of the skull are driven inward.

ICD-10-CM Code   S codes that require 7 digits
Fractures are classified and coded according to site, type, multiple fractures of sites, and cause of injury, and subclassified by factors such as the occurrence of complications and late effects. Refer to the physician's diagnosis and then the current edition of the ICD-10-CM coding manual for greatest specificity.

Fractures are described by specific names or by location:

- Colles fracture is fracture of the distal head of the radius, with possible involvement of the ulnar styloid. Colles fractures usually result from a fall in which the person attempts to break the fall with an extended arm and open hand. Pain and swelling are experienced. Treatment includes closed reduction of the fracture and immobilization of the arm, including the elbow, with a cast.
- Fracture of the humerus involves an obvious displacement of the bone of the upper arm along with shortening of the extremity and an abnormal mobility of the upper arm. Closed reduction of the fracture is followed by immobilization in a hanging arm cast and sling and swathe.
- Fracture of the pelvis is usually the result of severe trauma, such as from a motor vehicle accident or a fall, but can occur spontaneously in patients with osteoporosis. Complications of this fracture include lacerated colon, paralytic ileus, bladder and urethral injury, and intrapelvic hemorrhage. Treatment includes bed rest, possible immobilization with a pelvic sling or skeletal traction, and open reduction and repair.
- A fractured hip is usually the result of a fall. This fracture occurs most often because of underlying osteoporosis in women older than 60 years of age. An outward rotation along with a shortening of the affected extremity is noted. Repair is accomplished with surgery that involves the insertion of a prosthesis or pins, or both.
- Fracture of the femoral shaft is more common in young adults and usually is the result of a severe direct impact related to motor vehicle accidents or severe trauma. A notable angulation deformity and shortening of the affected leg is present. The patient is unable to move the knee or hip. The fracture is stabilized by skeletal traction or internal fixation with a rod or plate and screws.
- Fracture of the tibia results from a strong force exerted on the lower leg that causes soft tissue damage in addition to the fracture. Open or closed reduction is employed, followed by immobilization with a cast.
- Vertebral fracture in the neck can be the result of acceleration–deceleration trauma. Immediate immobilization is imperative to prevent spinal cord damage and resulting paralysis. Thoracic and lumbar vertebrae can be fractured often as a result of a fall and landing directly on the buttocks or may be associated with osteoporosis. Immobilization may be followed by surgical repair and possible insertion of surgical hardware (rods, plates) for stabilization.
- In some cases, a less invasive orthopedic procedure called *vertebroplasty* can be used to repair fractured and compressed vertebrae. Bone cement is injected into the area of compression to seal and stabilize the fracture.

- Basilar skull fracture is fracture of the floor of the cranial vault (see Fig. 13.11 in Chapter 13). It is usually the result of massive trauma to the head caused by a motor vehicle accident.
- LeFort fracture, a bilateral horizontal fracture of the maxilla, often results when the face is forced against the steering wheel in a motor vehicle accident.
- In Pott fracture, the lower part of the fibula is fractured. The lower tibial articulation sustains serious injury.
- Clavicular fracture is fracture of the clavicle (collar bone). It is a common sports injury, commonly occurring in bicycling accidents and often in children of all ages.

Symptoms and Signs

Pain accompanies most fractures. Edema, tenderness, discoloration, and inability to move the affected part follow. In some instances, deformity of the affected part is noted. The location of the fracture and the type of the fracture are determining factors in the symptoms and signs.

Patient Screening

Severe pain, deformity, inability to move an extremity, bone protruding through the skin, numbness or tingling in a joint, or difficulty breathing are indications for emergency care.

> **NOTE**
>
> In some diseases, fractures are not associated with injury but are "spontaneous fractures."

Etiology

Any force, external or internal, that disrupts the continuity of the bone causes a fracture. Diseases such as neoplasms, tuberculosis of bone, Paget disease, and osteoporosis cause pathologic fractures, which occur without significant external trauma.

Diagnosis

The major issues in assessing patients' injuries include defining the extent and location of the fracture and any complications resulting from the fracture and also detecting any underlying disease of bone. A complete history and physical examination are followed by radiographic studies of the affected structure. Bone scanning and MRI aid in determining diagnosis. Any underlying pathologic change is investigated and diagnosed; sometimes this requires bone biopsy.

Treatment

Treatment depends on the location, severity, type, and cause of the fracture, as described earlier. Simple fractures of the long bones are reduced and immobilized. Compound fractures are cleaned, débrided, reduced, and immobilized (tetanus status must be checked in the case of a compound fracture). Immobilization is accomplished by splinting (including the use of posterior splints), casting, taping, and external or internal fixation. Internal fixation (open reduction) includes the use of surgically implanted pins, wires, rods, plates, screws, or other devices. Some fractures are placed in traction to hold the ends of the bones in proper alignment until healing takes place.

Prognosis

The outlook depends on the location severity of the fracture, complications, and the presence of an underlying disease. Fractures that damage the epiphyseal plate (growth plate) in the child may have long-term residual effects, such as stunted growth or osteoarthritis.

Prevention

Wearing protective gear when playing contact sports and engaging in conditioning exercises can decrease the risk for fractures.

Patient Teaching

Patient education should be focused on appropriate conditioning programs to prevent future fractures. After a fracture, instructions to the patient regarding cast or brace care, activity limitations, and gradual rehabilitation exercises are essential.

To ensure optimal rehabilitation of the involved body areas, explain the exact condition and the long-term goals to the patient.

 ENRICHMENT

Amputation

Most limb amputations involve the legs and are necessary because of peripheral vascular disease caused by atherosclerosis and consequent gangrene. Trauma, malignancy, and congenital defects are additional reasons for amputation of limbs and digits. Amputations can also be necessitated by crushing injuries, open fractures, frostbite, and thermal or electrical burns. Infection and malignancy also may necessitate amputations. The extent of the amputation can range from removal of a portion of a digit to complete disarticulation at the hip or shoulder.

Rehabilitation is important and is attempted as soon as possible to afford the patient independence. Many customized prostheses are available for both upper and lower extremities.

Complications of fractures include compartment syndrome, in which the circulation to the area is compromised because of edema; nonunion and malunion of bones; infection; necrosis; fat emboli; and pulmonary emboli.

 ENRICHMENT

Phantom Limb and Phantom Limb Pain

Phantom limb sensation is an unpleasant complication that sometimes follows an amputation, especially of a leg, and is difficult to treat. It is the feeling that the limb still is attached. Phantom limb pain of the leg can present as a burning sensation of the foot or as a feeling of having the toes stepped on, even though no limb exists.

Both conditions usually disappear with time and with the realization that the limb is gone. Phantom limb pain may necessitate injection or removal of troublesome nerve endings that are located in the stump.

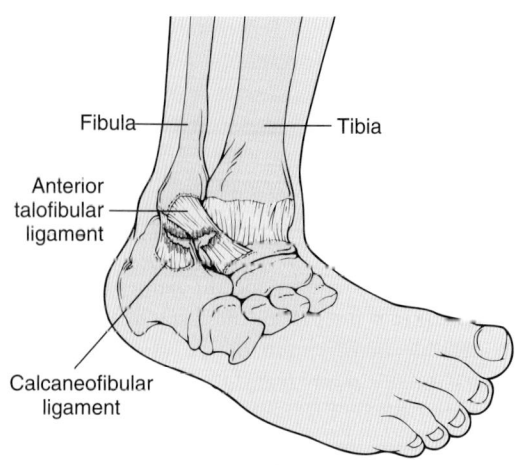
• **Fig. 7.29** Ankle sprain.

Strains and Sprains

Description

A strain is an injury of a tendon, muscle, or other tissue resulting from overuse, overstretching, or excessive forcible stretching of the tissue beyond its functional capacity.

A sprain is an acute tear of a ligament (Fig. 7.29). Sprains are classified as first-, second-, or third-degree, or -grade, sprains.

> ICD-10-CM Code   S codes that require 7 digits
> *Strains and sprains are classified and coded according to such factors as site, occurrence of injury, and involvement of adjacent structures. Refer to the physician's diagnosis and then the current edition of the ICD-10-CM coding manual for greatest specificity.*

Symptoms and Signs

Strains and sprains can be acute injuries or can be the result of chronic overuse (cumulative trauma). Symptoms may include localized pain, weakness, numbness, and possibly edema around the site of the injury. With both strain and sprain injuries, using, moving, or bearing weight on the affected limb or part is difficult or sometimes nearly impossible for the patient. Sprains may include damage to blood vessels and nerves; edema; ecchymosis; and sharp, transient pain. When sprains and strains are caused by chronic overuse, they typically cause stiffness, tenderness, and soreness.

Patient Screening

Ankle injury accompanied by obvious deformity, bone protruding through the skin, or bleeding requires emergency care. Schedule a same-day appointment for an individual with a painful ankle injury that involves inability to bear weight or walk.

Etiology

Strains and sprains can be caused by acute trauma (e.g., sports injury or automobile accidents) or cumulative trauma (e.g., overuse, as in occupational or sports-related injuries).

Diagnosis

A physical examination and medical history of a recent injury resulting from physical activity, an accident, or repetitive overuse may suggest the diagnosis. Patients with obvious significant physical trauma should be evaluated for possible associated fractures. Radiographic studies are ordered to rule out the possibility of a fracture.

Treatment

The treatment of both strains and sprains is similar and depends on the degree, or grade, of the injury. The sprain, being the more serious injury, requires more intense treatment. Treatment of sprains and strains includes elevation and rest of the affected limb and the application of cold pack or ice to control edema. Immobilization of the limb with an elastic bandage, soft cast, or splint may be necessary. Analgesics and possibly antiinflammatory agents are used to control pain and inflammation. Surgery may be indicated if the injury involves a large tear or if it heals improperly.

Prognosis

Healing of a strain or sprain usually takes 2 to 4 weeks, or longer with the more serious degrees of strain or sprain. The outlook is best when the patient participates in a progressive rehabilitation program.

Prevention

Recognizing personal physical limitations, following safety precautions, and taking time to warm up the muscles with slow, easy stretching before engaging in exercise or physical activity all help prevent sprains and strains. Sometimes support bracing is necessary when engaging in strenuous activities after incurring one of these injuries.

Patient Teaching

Encourage compliance with the treatment plan and rehabilitation program. Discuss the importance of the preventive measures mentioned above to avoid reinjury.

Dislocations

Description

A dislocation is the forcible displacement of a bone from its joint, thereby causing loss of joint function (Fig. 7.30).

> ICD-10-CM Code   S codes that require 7 digits
> *Dislocations are coded according to site, type (e.g.,
>   open or closed), occurrence of injury, and nature
>   (e.g., congenital, pathologic, recurrent). Refer to the
>   physician's diagnosis and then the current edition of
>   the ICD-10-CM coding manual for greatest specificity.*

Symptoms and Signs

A joint that is dislocated appears misshapen, is extremely painful, and rapidly becomes edematous, ecchymotic, and immovable. Injury to the ligaments and capsule of the joint is present. Other symptoms are a function of the extent of

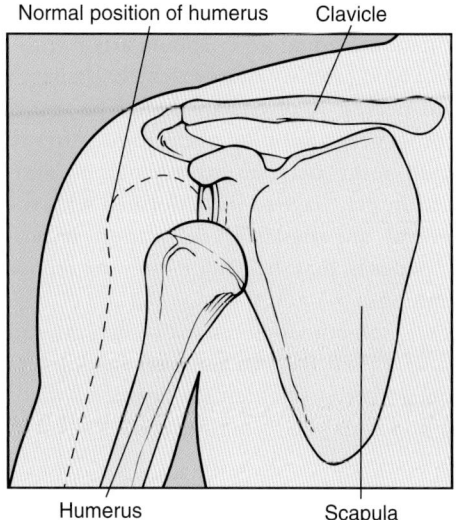

Normal position of humerus   Clavicle

Humerus   Scapula

• **Fig. 7.30** Dislocation of the shoulder.

damage to the surrounding tissues, nerves, and blood vessels.

Dislocation of spinal vertebrae can result in damage to the entire spinal cord and cause numbness, tingling, or paralysis below the injured area. A dislocation of a shoulder or hip can damage the nerve supply and cause paralysis of the limb. Some joints that have been dislocated tend to be susceptible to developing osteoarthritis in later years.

Patient Screening

Traumatic dislocations require *immediate* emergency medical care.

Etiology

The cause of a dislocation is usually a severe injury (e.g., a fall, automobile accident, or sports-related trauma) that exerts force great enough to tear the joint ligaments. Occasionally the injury that causes the dislocation also causes a fracture.

Dislocations not caused by injury may result from congenital weakness of the joint structures or from a complication of arthritis. They can happen repeatedly, without apparent cause, to a joint already weakened by an earlier injury. Jaw and shoulder joints are especially susceptible to recurring dislocations.

A rare congenital cause of recurrent dislocations is the inherited connective tissue disorder Ehlers-Danlos syndrome, which is characterized by joint hypermobility and skin laxity.

Diagnosis

The obvious abnormal appearance of the affected joint, the history of the injury, and physical examination may be all that are necessary to determine the diagnosis. A radiographic study can confirm whether a dislocation has occurred and whether any fractures are present. Patients also must be evaluated for nerve and blood vessel injuries.

Treatment

An untrained individual never should attempt to reduce a dislocation; doing so may cause extensive damage to blood vessels and nerves. A physician should be seen immediately for proper repositioning of the joint. After that time, a dislocated joint may be so edematous and painful that reduction may have to be performed with the patient under general anesthesia. If dislocation is a recurring problem, patients may be taught how to reposition the joint themselves.

Surgery is sometimes necessary to achieve satisfactory reduction. If a joint has become weakened from repeated dislocation, surgery to tighten the ligaments that hold the adjoining bones may be recommended.

Prognosis

The outlook for a dislocated joint depends on the amount of damage to the tissues of the joint and the overall strength of the adjacent muscles. Surgical procedures can stabilize the joint but sometimes limit ROM.

Prevention

Persons who have suffered a dislocation to a joint may require use of stabilization splints when engaging in activities. Repeated dislocation is potentially damaging to the joint.

Patient Teaching

Teaching the proper use of splinting devices and proper timing of resumption of activities is essential for the optimal outcome.

Adhesive Capsulitis (Frozen Shoulder)

Description

Adhesive capsulitis is a condition in which a shoulder is significantly limited in its ROM as a result of inflammation, scarring, thickening, and shrinkage of the capsule that surrounds the normal shoulder joint. Adhesive capsulitis is commonly called *frozen shoulder*.

ICD-10-CM Code	M75.00 *(Adhesive capsulitis of unspecified shoulder)* (M75.00-M75.02 = 3 codes of specificity)

Symptoms and Signs

Adhesive capsulitis presents as a shoulder that has become stiff and painful, making normal movement impossible. The pain can be either localized in the shoulder itself or spread out, encompassing the upper arm or neck. It is often severe enough to disrupt sleep. Symptoms become gradually worse during the first few months after injury and then remain at a constant degree of discomfort for a couple more months, and finally a period of gradual improvement begins. With time, the pain subsides, but the mobility of the shoulder often remains permanently impaired, or frozen.

Patient Screening

Regular follow-up appointments are important for patients undergoing treatment for adhesive capsulitis.

Etiology

Adhesive capsulitis is caused by inflammation of the capsule of the joint with secondary scarring. It usually begins after a slight injury or minor problem, such as bursitis or tendinitis, which prevents normal use of the joint. Disuse of the shoulder leads to more and more stiffness and increased disuse. For unknown reasons, adhesive capsulitis occurs more frequently in patients with diabetes.

Diagnosis

The symptoms alone are usually enough to identify this condition. However, a review of the patient history may indicate a recent injury that precipitated bursitis or tendonitis. Patients with adhesive capsulitis are evaluated for underlying arthritis, injury, and diabetes.

Radiographic tests can be helpful for detecting underlying problems in the shoulder and can demonstrate calcification that would indicate past chronic inflammation.

Treatment

A stiff shoulder must be kept in motion, as much as possible, to prevent permanent immobility. A physical or occupational therapist may be needed to teach and assist the patient with ROM exercises. Analgesics, antiinflammatory agents, and often an injection of a steroid medication into the joint are needed. If adhesive capsulitis is severe and persistent, the physician may suggest shoulder manipulation, under general anesthesia, to increase mobility.

Prognosis

The outlook for a patient with adhesive capsulitis depends on the severity and duration of the condition and the presence of underlying joint disorders. Longstanding adhesive capsulitis tends to be less responsive to treatments.

Prevention

Persons who have had chest surgery, including heart and breast procedures, should, as soon as appropriate, perform upper body exercises to minimize the risk of developing adhesive capsulitis.

Patient Teaching

Patients are instructed on the details and importance of ROM exercises to restore joint function. Avoiding reinjury to the shoulder is key for optimal outcome.

Severed Tendon

Description

Tendons are long, fibrous cords that connect muscles to bones (e.g., the Achilles tendon connects the gastrocnemius muscle to the calcaneus bone at the back of the heel). A severed tendon is torn completely into two sections and thus prevents the muscle from performing its function of moving a body part.

ICD-10-CM Code   T14.90 *(Injury, unspecified)*
Note: This code is for use only when no documentation is available that identifies the specific injury. This code is not for use in the inpatient setting.

Symptoms and Signs

A severed tendon produces immediate, severe pain, inflammation, and immobility of the affected parts (Fig. 7.31).

Patient Screening

Injury followed by pain and immobility of the affected area requires urgent medical care.

Etiology

The cause of a severed tendon is an injury or laceration. It involves the forearm, hand, calf of the leg, or foot. The injury may extend partially or completely through one or more tendons.

Diagnosis

Physical examination of the injured site and the patient's inability to move the affected parts are usually sufficient for determining the diagnosis. A radiographic study can be used to detect an accompanying bone fracture. A person with a severed tendon must be closely evaluated for possible infection and foreign objects or materials in the wound site.

Treatment

Tendons are under tension, so if they become severed, the two ends snap away from each other and are difficult to retrieve. A surgeon may suture the two ends of the tendon together (**tenorrhaphy**) immediately or may wait for the injury to heal, depending on the extent of the injury. A large incision may be necessary to locate the ends of the tendon to expose and retrieve the tendon before the tenorrhaphy can be attempted. To repair the damaged tendon, it may be necessary to insert a piece of tendon from elsewhere in the body.

The outcome of tendon repair is usually satisfactory. However, in some cases, the affected parts may be stiff and have less mobility after the surgery than before the injury. Physical therapy ensures as much mobility as possible.

Prognosis

The prognosis depends on the tendon involved and the results of surgery. Infection complicates the outcome. Permanent muscle atrophy can result from tendon damage.

Prevention

Persons with lacerated tendons should receive tetanus vaccination.

Patient Teaching

Patients are instructed on the details of rehabilitation and progressive exercise, beginning with gentle ROM exercises.

Shin Splints

Description

Shin splints are a painful condition involving inflammation of the periosteum, the extensor muscles in the lower leg, and the surrounding tissues.

ICD-10-CM Code   S83.90XA *(Sprain of unspecified site of unspecified knee, initial encounter)*
(S83.001(A)(D)(S)-S83.92XX(A)(D)(S) = 118 codes of specificity)
S86.919A *(Strain of unspecified muscle(s) and tendon(s) at lower leg level, unspecified leg, initial encounter)*
(S86.101(A)(D)(S)-S86.999(A)(D)(S) = 60 codes of specificity)

Symptoms and Signs

Inflammation, edema, pain, and tenderness along the inner aspect of the tibia are common symptoms of shin splints. The pain worsens with exercise and then disappears with rest. Shin splints occur most commonly during the first weeks of a new exercise program or after a sudden increase in the amount of exercise in an ongoing program.

This disorder is especially common in sports and fitness enthusiasts who jog, run, or engage in high-impact aerobics and is most often bilateral.

Patient Screening

A physical examination is required to evaluate the cause of pain and identify tenderness along the tibia.

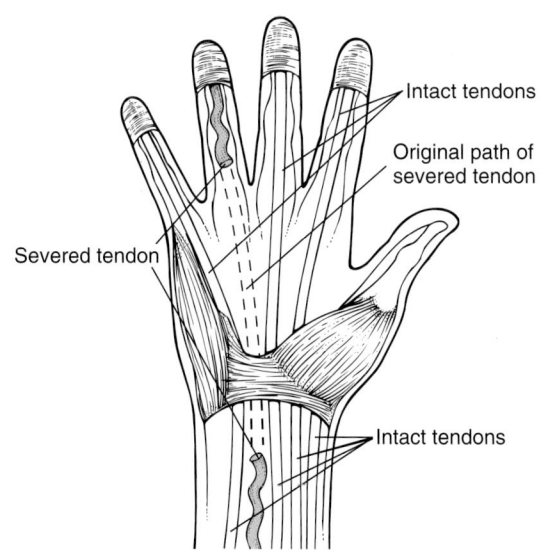

• **Fig. 7.31** Severed tendon of the hand.

Etiology

Overuse and overpronation are the most common factors that predispose an individual to shin splints. Pronation of the foot is an inward rotation of the ankle that causes the inner arch of the foot to sag and the ankle joint to tip upward (Fig. 7.32). All people pronate when they walk to some degree; however, excessive pronation places abnormal stress on the calf muscles. This leads to the development of shin splints and tendon and ligament strain around the ankles and knees.

Improper conditioning and running on hard surfaces also can contribute to the development of shin splints.

Diagnosis

The diagnosis is based on physical examination and a history of pain that worsens with exercise and disappears after rest. A patient with symptoms of shin splints also can have stress fracture of the tibia bone. This can be detected with bone scanning and is considered when pain and tenderness are severe and persistent.

Treatment

The key to successful treatment of shin splints is rest. Applications of ice or heat, or both alternately, are essential in the treatment. Aspirin or prescription NSAIDs may be ordered to relieve the pain and to reduce inflammation. Gradually, physical therapy with specific stretching exercises can be helpful. Specially designed shoes to correct overpronation or the use of an orthotic device in existing shoes may be recommended.

Prognosis

The prognosis is generally very good for complete recovery, although this can sometimes be prolonged for serious athletes. Shin splints are painful but not dangerous, unless they are ignored and consequently result in stress fractures.

Prevention

Proper conditioning and gradual stretching of the legs before exercise, jogging or running on grass or other soft surfaces, performing aerobic exercises on mats, and ensuring that exercise shoes are well padded for arch support can help prevent this condition.

Patient Teaching

Patient education is focused on proper footwear and conditioning and gradual return to exercise while incorporating a stretching and strengthening program.

Plantar Fasciitis (Calcaneal Spur)

Description

Plantar fasciitis, also known as *calcaneal* or *heel spur syndrome,* is an inflammatory response at the bottom of the heel bone (calcaneus). There the flat tissue (fascia) that acts like a bowstring for the arch of the foot attaches to the bottom of the heel.

ICD-10-CM Code	M72.2 *(Plantar fascial fibromatosis)*

Symptoms and Signs

Plantar fasciitis is a common problem among people who are active in sports, especially runners. The problem begins as a dull, intermittent pain on the bottom of the foot and can progress to a sharp, persistent pain. Characteristically the pain is worse on getting out of bed and taking the first few steps in the morning, after sitting for a time, after standing or walking, and when beginning a sporting activity. Plantar fascia injury also can occur at the midsole or near the toes.

The plantar fascia is a thick, fibrous material on the bottom of the foot. It is attached to the calcaneus, fans forward toward the toes, and acts like a bowstring to maintain the arch of the foot.

Patient Screening

Patients complaining of significant foot or heel pain (usually not associated with trauma) require the first available appointment to determine the cause and begin treatment as soon as possible.

Etiology

Plantar fasciitis usually occurs when part of the inflexible fascia is repeatedly placed under tension (e.g., when running). This constant tension causes an inflammatory response, usually at the point where the fascia is attached to the calcaneus. The result is pain and the development of the spur.

Factors contributing to the development of plantar fasciitis include:
- flat (pronated) feet
- high-arched, rigid feet
- toe running or hill running
- running on soft terrain (e.g., sand)
- poor shoe support
- sudden increase in activity level
- sudden weight increase

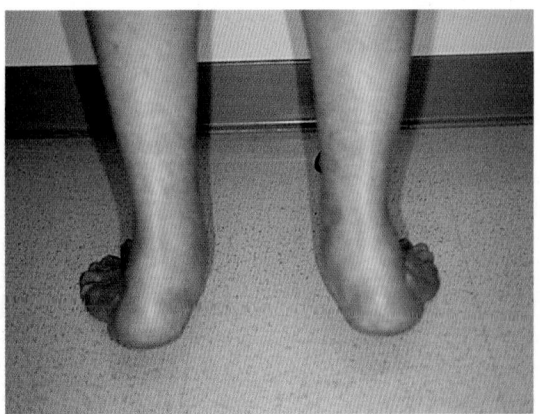

• **Fig. 7.32** Excessive pronation of the foot. (From Seidel HM, et al: *Mosby's guide to physical examination,* ed 7, St Louis, 2003, Mosby.)

- increasing age
- familial tendency
- possible underlying disease

The inflammatory response at the calcaneus can produce spike-like projections of new bone called *calcaneal* (heel) *spurs* (Fig. 7.33A). They do not cause the initial pain, nor do they cause the initial problem; they are a result of the problem.

Diagnosis

Physical examination and the patient history of symptoms usually provide sufficient information for making the diagnosis. The bottom of the foot is typically very tender, typically at the heel. Radiographs sometimes show the spur (see Fig. 7.33B). Patients with plantar fasciitis are evaluated for possible reactive arthritis, inflammatory bowel disease, ankylosing spondylitis, and diffuse idiopathic skeletal hyperostosis.

Treatment

The initial treatment of heel spurs consists of resting, applying ice to the sore area, taking antiinflammatory or analgesic medication, using heel pads (doughnut-shaped pads that equalize and absorb the shock on the heel and ease pressure on the plantar fascia), and wearing a shoe with good arch support. Sometimes local cortisone injection can reduce inflamed tissues. In addition, the physician may tape the foot to maintain the arch and help take some of the tension off the plantar fascia. Shoe inserts called *orthotics* also may be prescribed.

After the inflammation has subsided, physical therapy to strengthen the small muscles of the foot can begin. If done regularly, this helps prevent reinjury. Surgery rarely is required for the correction of heel spurs. It is considered only if all forms of more conservative treatment fail and the pain still is incapacitating after several months of treatment. When performed, surgery involves removing the bone spur and releasing the plantar fascia.

Prognosis

The prognosis is generally very good in response to conservative management. Surgical procedures are usually not required.

Prevention

The key to prevention is the use of proper footwear. Any underlying associated medical condition should be optimally managed.

Patient Teaching

Understanding the anatomy of the foot and what causes the condition can benefit affected individuals as they undertake measures to promote healing.

Ganglion

Description

A ganglion is a benign, saclike swelling, or cyst, that is filled with a colorless, jellylike fluid. A ganglion is formed from the tissue that lines a joint or tendon.

ICD-10-CM Code	M67.40 *(Ganglion, unspecified site)*
	(M67.40-M67.49 = 24 codes of specificity)

Symptoms and Signs

A ganglion most commonly develops on the back of the wrist as a single smooth lump, just under the surface of the skin (Fig. 7.34). It can, however, develop near other joints, such as around the ankle joint, behind the knee, and on the fingers. Ganglia may appear as multiples or in clusters. Most are about the size of a pea, but others may grow as large as an inch or more in diameter. Ganglia may be soft

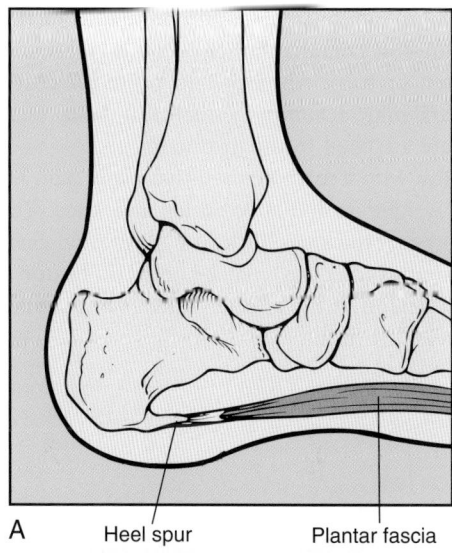
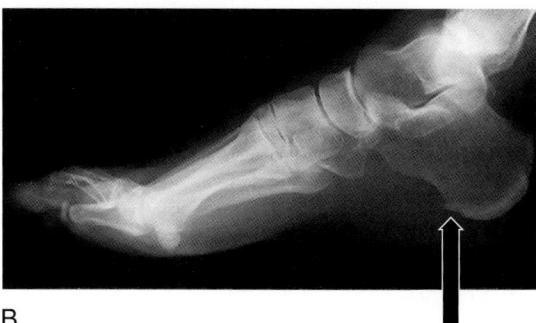

• **Fig. 7.33** (A) Calcaneal (heel) spur. (B) Radiographic appearance.

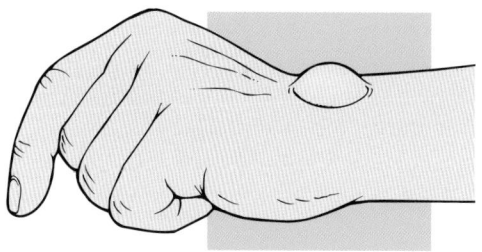

• **Fig. 7.34** Ganglion.

to the touch or firm, and they are usually either painless or only somewhat bothersome. Pain may occur when moving the wrist from a wrist ganglion, especially if the growth is large or inflamed.

Patient Screening
A visual examination by the health care provider is indicated for a cystic swelling on a joint.

Etiology
Although sometimes ganglia are caused by repetitive minor injuries, the underlying cause usually is unknown. A ganglion is sometimes a sign of arthritis of the adjacent joint. Whatever triggers the ganglion's development, it usually arises either in the joint capsule or in a tendon sheath.

Diagnosis
The primary concern in evaluating a patient with a ganglion is whether or not underlying arthritis is present. A ganglion usually can be diagnosed by palpation and by observation of the appearance of the lump and the characteristic site. If in doubt, the physician can perform needle aspiration to withdraw some of the fluid for laboratory analysis.

Treatment
If the ganglion does not cause pain and is not large enough to cause disfigurement or to interfere with wrist function, treatment is unnecessary. However, if the ganglion is causing pain, disfigurement, or impairment of the ROM, several options are available. The physician may try to rupture the ganglion by applying firm pressure. Needle aspiration may be used to remove as much fluid as possible, followed by instillation of a steroid, such as cortisone, or a sclerosing solution that helps prevent recurrences. The physician may recommend a surgical procedure called *ganglionectomy* to remove the ganglion.

Ganglia that originate in the wrist joint may be difficult to remove completely and therefore tend to recur. Even after surgical excision, approximately 10% recur. Over a period of months, ganglia often disappear spontaneously.

Prognosis
Ganglia are usually harmless and do not impair function.

Prevention
The key to prevention is the identification of underlying arthritis.

Patient Teaching
Simple reassurance that the condition can be resolved along with an explanation of the nature of the ganglion is generally helpful to patients.

Torn Meniscus
Description
A **meniscus** is a semilunar cartilage found in the knee joint. There are two menisci within the joint, a medial and a lateral (Fig. 7.35). A tear of the meniscus is a crack or fissure that is usually a result of wear or injury.

ICD-10-CM Code	S83.209A *(Unspecified tear of unspecified meniscus, current injury, unspecified knee, initial encounter)*
	S83.30XA *(Tear of articular cartilage of unspecified knee, current, initial encounter)*

Symptoms and Signs
The medial meniscus is larger and more restricted in movement than the lateral meniscus and therefore is injured more often or torn. Anterior and posterior cruciate ligament tears may accompany meniscal tears because the menisci are attached to the ligaments.

A person with a torn meniscus has acute pain when putting full weight on the affected leg and knee. The person may report that the knee "locks" or "gives way." Snapping or clicking sounds (crepitus) may be heard on flexion or extension. Full flexion of the affected knee may be difficult, and pain increases with full extension.

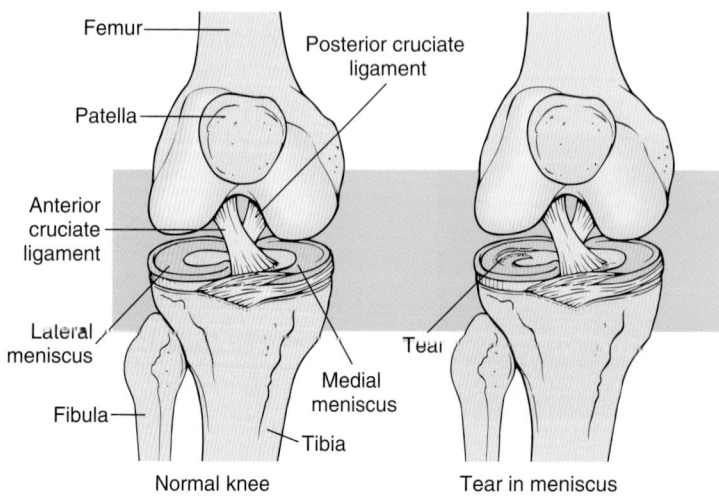

Femur
Posterior cruciate ligament
Patella
Anterior cruciate ligament
Lateral meniscus
Medial meniscus
Fibula
Tibia
Tear

Normal knee   Tear in meniscus

• **Fig. 7.35** Torn meniscus.

Patient Screening

Patients experiencing acute knee pain should be seen by the health care professional as soon as possible.

Etiology

Most torn menisci are related to sports injuries. Participants in football, baseball, and soccer are especially susceptible to this type of injury. Tears in the meniscus usually result from sudden twisting or external rotation of the leg while the knee is flexed.

Diagnosis

Patients with symptoms suggestive of a meniscal tear are evaluated for ligament injury and arthritis of the affected joint. Physical examination of the knee indicates the limitation of movement. Radiographic studies and MRI, which is the preferred procedure, are ordered; MRI may show the exact injury to the meniscus and, if any, to the ligaments.

Treatment

The injured knee should be immobilized immediately and elevated, with ice applied to slow bleeding and edema. No weight bearing should be allowed, and the physician should be seen as soon as possible. Antiinflammatory or analgesic medications are often needed.

The treatment of a torn meniscus might only require physical therapy. Surgical repair can be done arthroscopically with the patient under an anesthetic, unless injury to the cruciate ligaments also has occurred. Ligament tears require more extensive surgery to expose and repair them. Total excision or partial excision of the torn meniscus is called *meniscectomy*. Total meniscectomy usually is not done because it predisposes the knee to degenerative changes and instability.

Prognosis

Meniscal tears respond very well to surgical treatments.

Prevention

The key to prevention is the early care of the underlying arthritis.

Patient Teaching

A customized, extensive, progressive exercise rehabilitation program begins after the immediate postoperative period and continues over the subsequent months.

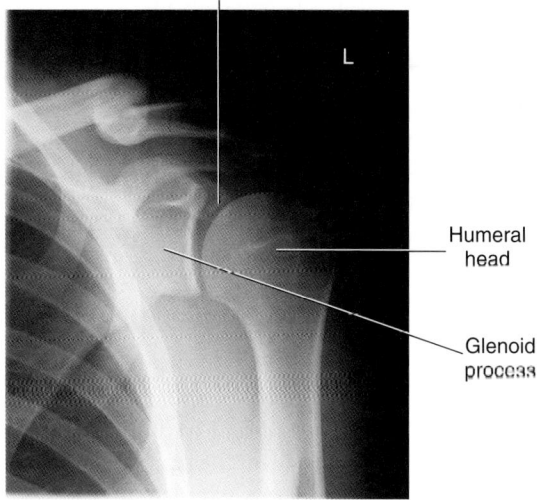

• **Fig. 7.36** Structures of the shoulder. (From Long BW, Frank ED, Ehrlich RA: *Radiography essentials for limited practice,* ed 4, St Louis, 2013, Elsevier.)

Rotator Cuff Tears

Description

The four tendons of the rotator cuff, formed by the muscles of the shoulder, partially surround the head of the humerus and stabilize it in the glenoid cavity or socket (Fig. 7.36). The infraspinatus muscle rotates the humerus externally, and the subscapularis muscle rotates the humerus internally. Other muscles with tendons that form the rotator cuff are the supraspinatus and the teres minor. Tears in any of the rotator cuff tendons limit the function of the shoulder.

ICD-10-CM Code   S43.429A *(Sprain of unspecified rotator cuff capsule, initial encounter)* (S43.421-S43.429 = 3 codes of specificity)

Symptoms and Signs

Tears in the tendons of the rotator cuff muscles can produce an immediate snapping sound and acute pain. The person may be unable to abduct the arm. ROM becomes limited to varying degrees, depending on the severity of the particular tear.

❖ ENRICHMENT

Arthroscopy

Arthroscopy is a surgical procedure used to examine the structures within a joint by using a tubelike viewing instrument called an *arthroscope*. The arthroscope is a small tube that contains optical fibers and lenses. It is passed through tiny incisions in the skin into the joint to be examined. The arthroscope is connected to a video camera that allows the interior of the joint to be seen on a display monitor. The size of the arthroscope used varies with the size of the joint being examined.

Arthroscopy can be used for diagnosis and/or treatment. When procedures are performed in addition to examining the joint with the arthroscope, this is referred to as *arthroscopic surgery*. A number of procedures are done in this fashion. When a procedure can be done arthroscopically instead of using traditional open surgical methods, it usually causes less tissue trauma and therefore results in less pain. This tends to promote a quicker recovery.

Arthroscopy is performed by orthopedic surgeons, typically in an outpatient setting. After the procedure, patients usually can return home and begin a rehabilitation program.

Patient Screening

Patients having acute shoulder pain and limited mobility of the shoulder require medical attention as soon as possible.

Etiology

Tears can result from acute trauma (most common) or from degenerative changes with age. Calcium deposits may develop in the insertion sites because of the degenerative changes and may predispose the tendons to tears or rupture. Also steroid injections into the tendon areas can predispose them to tears or rupture.

Diagnosis

Diagnosis is based on physical examination findings and patient history. The shoulder may have limited and painful ROM. Confirmation is made on the basis of an arthrogram or an MRI scan. Patients are screened for bursitis and arthritis of the shoulder.

Treatment

Acute pain is managed with pain-relieving medications. Acetaminophen is given for moderate pain, and antiinflammatory medications are given for inflammation. With rest and conservative therapy, including gradual physical therapy, minor tears can heal with restoration of function.

Significant acute tendon tears are surgically repaired immediately to preserve strength of the muscles and to restore motion of the shoulder. After surgery, the affected arm is placed in a shoulder immobilizer or abduction splint for a number of weeks. Extensive, active exercises are begun when the cast is removed.

Prognosis

Minor tears can heal in response to conservative measures. Major tears require surgical repair.

Prevention

Conditioning and stretching exercises are the best prevention for rotator cuff tears.

Patient Teaching

Rubber band shoulder exercises and stretching are keys to long-term rehabilitation of the rotator cuff. A customized, extensive, progressive exercise program begins after the immediate postoperative period and continues over the subsequent few months.

Review Challenge

Answer the following questions:
1. What are the functions of the normal skeletal system?
2. What procedures are employed in diagnosing scoliosis?
3. What pathology is characteristic of osteoarthritis?
4. The symptoms of Lyme disease mimic which disease?
5. Are any preventive measures recommended for Lyme disease?
6. What is the clinical picture of a patient with osteomyelitis?
7. What metabolite forms crystals in the joints in gout?
8. Which disease is characterized by irregular breakdown and formation of bone tissue?
9. What would the treatment plan for a patient with osteoporosis include?
10. How is vitamin D deficiency related to osteomalacia?
11. What specific findings from a physical examination are typical of fibromyalgia?
12. What causative factors contribute to hallux valgus (bunion)? Hallux rigidus? Hammer toe?
13. How are fractures classified?
14. How would you describe Colles fracture?
15. What is meant by the term *phantom limb*?
16. What methods are used to immobilize fractures?
17. Why is a sprain considered more serious than a strain?
18. What joints are more susceptible to dislocation?
19. What conditions result in adhesive capsulitis ("frozen shoulder")?
20. What is the relationship of overpronation to shin splints?
21. Under what conditions might plantar fasciitis (spur syndrome) develop?
22. What acute symptoms is a person with torn meniscus likely to describe? A person with rotator cuff tear?

Real-Life Challenge: Osteoporosis

A 72-year-old woman recently experienced bandlike, midthoracic back pain after a minor fall. Imaging studies confirmed fractures of T-7 and T-8 vertebrae. Measurements in this small-boned woman revealed loss of 1 inch in height, with the current measurement being 5 feet 1 inch compared with 5 feet 2 inches at the last physical examination 14 months ago. Serum calcium is elevated. The computed tomography (CT) scan indicates osteoporosis.

According to history, the patient does not include many dairy products in her diet and takes no dietary supplements. In addition, she has never taken any form of estrogen replacement and does not exercise regularly.

Questions

1. In what type of individual would you expect to find the greatest incidence of osteoporosis?
2. What bones other than vertebrae are prone to fractures in osteoporosis?
3. Why would serum calcium be elevated in osteoporosis?
4. What is meant by the description of osteoporosis as a metabolic bone disease?

5. What should be included in a diet to prevent or slow the onset of osteoporosis?
6. Why is daily exercise important in preventing osteoporosis?

7. What type of drug therapy may be prescribed for the patient?

Real-Life Challenge: Lyme Disease

A 27-year-old man has been experiencing flulike symptoms for 4 days. He reports headache, fatigue, joint pain, and "just not feeling well." Vital signs are temperature of 102.28° F, pulse of 96, respirations of 20, and blood pressure of 132/86 mm Hg. Physical examination reveals two areas on the left lower leg that have a fading red rash in a circle type of pattern. The center of each circle is pale, and there is a possible spot at the center of each.

Questioning discloses that the patient was deer hunting 5 days ago, walking through tall grass. He remembers experiencing itching on the lower left leg. Lyme disease is suspected. A blood test to detect antibodies to the spirochete *Borrelia burgdorferi* is ordered. Antibiotics and acetaminophen for the fever, pain, and aches are prescribed. The patient is encouraged to rest and return for a recheck in a few days.

Questions

1. In what region of the United States would you expect this patient to live?
2. What precautions should be taken by people who will be out walking in tall grass?
3. What should individuals who think they have been bitten by a tick do as soon as they discover the bite?

4. If Lyme disease is not diagnosed in its early stages, what complications may develop?
5. What is the causative agent of Lyme disease?
6. Discuss the prevention of Lyme disease.

Real-Life Challenge: Fibromyalgia

A 23-year-old female has been diagnosed with fibromyalgia. She complained of chronic pain in the muscles and soft tissue surrounding joints. Additionally she mentioned feeling fatigued most of the time and a diffuse aching or burning in the muscles along with stiffness. She also experienced headaches, some jaw pain and sensitivity to odors, bright lights, and loud noises. Disturbances in sleep patterns were experienced on a regular basis.

1. Along with the chronic muscle pain and restless sleep, what other symptoms may the patient experience?

2. Although the cause of fibromyalgia is unknown, what might be a possible cause?
3. How is rapid eye movement (REM) sleep affected?
4. What is a key factor in the diagnosis of fibromyalgia?
5. State some beneficial options other than drug therapy that may help this patient.
6. What may help provide a more positive outcome for the patient?

Internet Assignments

1. Visit the American Lyme Disease Foundation website to research the latest statistics on Lyme disease; also gather information on other tickborne diseases.

2. Research the "News and Events" page at the National Osteoporosis Foundation website, and report on the recent findings.

Critical Thinking

1. How would you approach discussing bursitis, possible causes, and the treatment plan as prescribed by the physician with a patient just diagnosed with the condition?
2. Gout is a disease known to be extremely painful. In an acute attack, the treatment can be extensive. What does the treatment typically involve? Explain the importance of empathy and patience during the patient teaching phase.
3. Why should a patient with a chronic arthritic condition be strongly encouraged to comply with the treatment plan and keep all follow-up appointments?

4. Discuss the kinds of muscle tumors and the variety of diagnostic procedures used to determine the type and extent of the treatment required.
5. What are the differences between an ankle strain and an ankle sprain? Describe some prevention measures.
6. What is a necessary assessment on patients with open injuries?

Prepare to discuss Critical Thinking case study exercises for this chapter that are posted on Evolve.

8

Diseases and Conditions of the Digestive System

CHAPTER OUTLINE

Orderly Function of the Digestive System, 281

Disorderly Function of the Digestive System, 281

    Diseases and Conditions of the Oral Cavity and Jaws, 281

Diseases of the Gastrointestinal Tract, 295

Diseases of the Liver, Biliary Tract, and Pancreas, 322

Disorders of Nutrient Intake and Absorption, 332

LEARNING OBJECTIVES

After studying Chapter 8, you should be able to:

1. Explain the process of normal digestion and absorption.
2. Discuss the importance of normal teeth and a normal bite.
3. Describe the presenting symptoms of temporomandibular joint disorder (TMD).
4. Compare the etiology of herpes simplex with the etiology of thrush.
5. Describe the treatment of oral leukoplakia.
6. Describe the treatment of gastroesophageal reflux disease (GERD).
7. Explain the clinical significance of Barrett esophagus.
8. Name a serious complication of esophageal varices.
9. Describe the pathology of peptic ulcers and identify the etiology.
10. Explain the diagnosis of gastric cancer.
11. List the symptoms a patient with appendicitis may experience.
12. Describe hiatal hernia.
13. Distinguish the types of abdominal hernias.
14. Explain the differences between the pathology of Crohn disease and that of ulcerative colitis.
15. Describe the etiology of gastroenteritis.
16. Discuss the pathologic conditions that may result in intestinal obstruction.
17. Explain the difference between a mechanical obstruction and a functional obstruction of the bowel.
18. Distinguish between diverticulosis and diverticulitis.
19. Discuss the screening program for and the treatment of colorectal cancer.
20. Explain the relationship between broad-spectrum antibiotics and pseudomembranous enterocolitis.
21. Explain the preventive measures for *Clostridioides difficile* infection.
22. List the causes of inflammation of the peritoneum.
23. Explain the pathologic symptoms and signs of cirrhosis of the liver.
24. Contrast the causes and preventive measures of hepatitis A and hepatitis C. Explain how health care providers are at special risk for hepatitis B.
25. Name the most important etiologic factor for hepatocellular carcinoma (HCC) and other additional risk factors.
26. Name the most common bloodborne infection in the United States.
27. Describe the clinical picture of an individual with (1) biliary colic and (2) acute pancreatitis.
28. State the prognosis of pancreatic cancer.
29. State the components of a successful weight loss program.
30. Describe the clinical manifestations of malnutrition and malabsorption.
31. Explain the diagnostic criteria for celiac disease.
32. List some ways to lower the risk of food poisoning.
33. Distinguish between the clinical picture of the patient with anorexia and that of the patient with bulimia.

KEY TERMS

adenocarcinoma (**ad**-ih-no-**kar**-sin-**OH**-ma)
anastomosis (ah-**nas**-toh-**MOH**-sis)
antiemetic (**an**-tih-ee-**MET**-ik)
aphthous (**AF**-thus)
ascites (ah-**SIGH**-teez)
cholinergic (**ko**-lin-**ER**-jik)

endoscopy (en-**DOS**-ko-pee)
fistula (**FIS**-tew-lah)
fulminant (**FUL**-mih-nant)
gastroscopy (gas-**TROS**-koh-pee)
gingivitis (jin-jih-**VIE**-tis)
hematemesis (hem-ah-**TEM**-eh-sis)

KEY TERMS—cont'd

hepatomegaly (**hep**-ah-toh-**MEG**-ah-lee)
hypokalemia (**high**-poh-ka-**LEE**-me-ah)
inguinal (**ING**-gwih-nal)
intussusception (in-tah-sus-**SEP**-shun)
periodontitis (**per**-ee-oh-don-**TIE**-tis)
peritonitis (**per**-ih-toh-**NIE**-tis)

proctoscopy (prock-**TAHS**-ko-pee)
pseudomembranous (**soo**-doe-**MEM**-brah-nus)
sigmoidoscopy (**sig**-moy-**DOS**-ko-pee)
temporomandibular (**tem**-poh-roh-man-**DIHB**-you-lar)
varices (**VAR**-ih-seez)

Orderly Function of the Digestive System

The digestive system comprises the alimentary canal, or digestive tract, and the accessory organs of digestion (Fig. 8.1). Each unit, or organ, of the system must be normal in structure and function to regulate the ingestion, digestion, and absorption of nutrients. The alimentary canal processes and transports the products of digestion. The accessory organs, located outside the gastrointestinal (GI) tract, manufacture and secrete endocrine and exocrine enzymes, secretions that are essential to the breakdown, digestion, and absorption of nutrients.

Diseases of the GI tract negatively affect health and threaten life because they interfere with the critical functions of ingestion and digestion of food, absorption of nutrients for metabolism, and elimination of wastes. General categories of

diseases and conditions of the digestive system include erosion of tissue, inflammation, infection, benign and malignant tumors, obstruction, interference with blood or nerve supply, malnutrition, and malabsorption syndromes.

Disorderly Function of the Digestive System

Diseases and Conditions of the Oral Cavity and Jaws

The function of the teeth is mastication (chewing) to break down food into pieces that can be swallowed and digested easily (Fig. 8.2). Hindrance of the chewing function caused

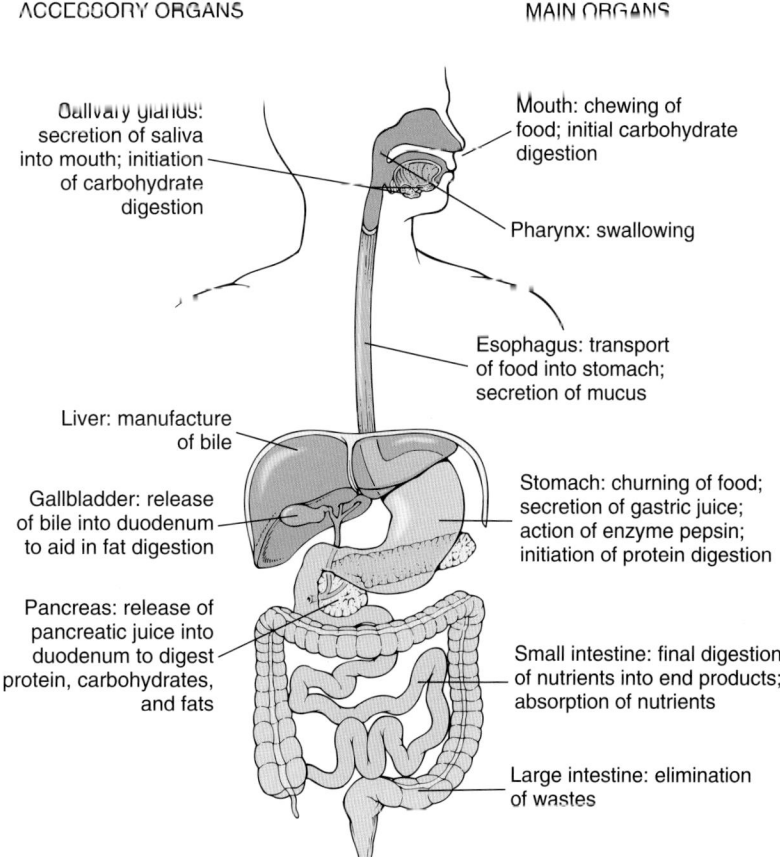

• **Fig. 8.1** Main and accessory organs of the normal digestive system. (Redrawn from Miller M: *Pathophysiology: principles of disease,* Philadelphia, 1983, Saunders.)

U.S. Tooth Numbering

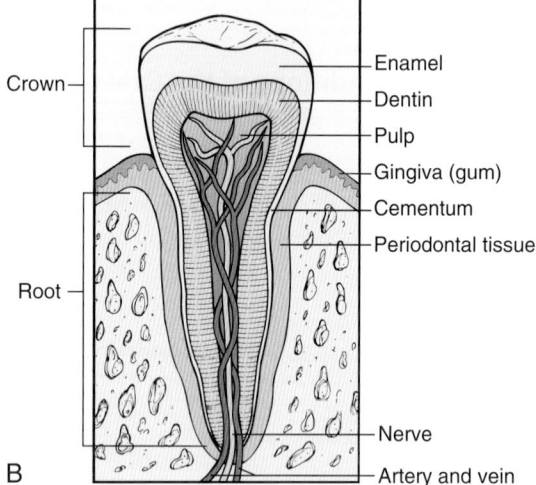

• **Fig. 8.2** (A) Thirty-two permanent teeth. (B) Structure of a tooth.

by decay, infection of the teeth or gums, malocclusion, or missing teeth can interfere with this phase of the digestive process. A decrease in saliva production, called *xerostomia,* can adversely affect the digestive process. Xerostomia may be caused by dehydration, medications, either prescription or over-the-counter (OTC) ones, or less often by an autoimmune condition called *Sjögren disease.* Recent research has identified the interrelationship between oral health and general health. For instance, there can be a connection between oral infections and cardiovascular diseases, respiratory diseases, or diabetes. Periodontal disease (gum disease) and the increase in systemic cross-reactive protein have been recognized as risk factors for cardiovascular disease (arteriosclerosis), diabetes, and pancreatic cancer. An example of the serious nature of gum disease is seen in the reported death of an infant that was directly connected to the bacteria identified in the oral infection of the mother. Most disorders affecting the mouth or the tongue are not this serious.

Most treatments for oral disease are simple and effective. Because malignant tumors are possible, the dentist performs screening examinations for any lump or change in the mouth or on the tongue as part of a routine oral examination. Patients should report any oral lesions (white, red, or blue) or lumps in any part of the mouth that persist for longer than 10 days.

Missing Teeth

Description
Permanent teeth are missing.

ICD-10-CM Code	K08.109 *(Complete loss of teeth, unspecified cause, unspecified class)*
	(K08.101-K08.199 = 25 codes of specificity)

Loss of tooth is coded by causative factors. Refer to the physician's diagnosis and then to the current edition of the ICD-10-CM coding manual to ensure the greatest specificity.

Symptoms and Signs
The loss of permanent teeth, after the loss of primary teeth, can cause serious dental problems later in life (Fig. 8.3). Missing teeth can alter the bite, that is, how the teeth come together (occlusion). Malocclusion eventually leads to jaw pain, called *temporomandibular joint disorder* (see the Temporomandibular Joint Disorder section), if not corrected. Missing teeth can cause bolting (inadequate chewing) of food. Digestive disturbances (i.e., gastritis or constipation) and loss of the nutrient value of food may result. Patients may express cosmetic concerns with tooth loss.

Patient Screening
Schedule an appointment for the patient for an evaluation by the dentist.

Etiology
There are four main causes of missing permanent teeth. The most common is loss resulting from dental decay in all age groups but is most commonly caused by periodontal disease in adults. Tooth loss increases with age or may be a result of

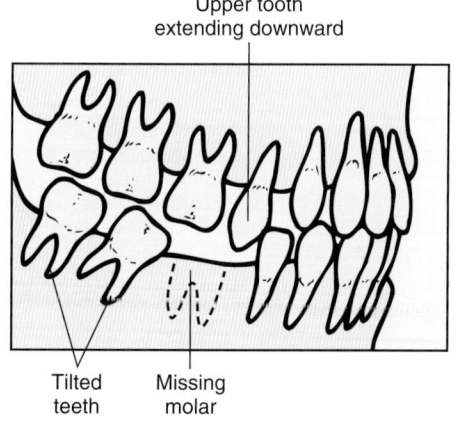

• **Fig. 8.3** Missing molar.

dental injury. Teeth also may be congenitally missing, or they may be impacted and prevented from erupting by the root of an adjacent tooth. Tooth loss may present as a sign of certain rare inherited or systemic diseases.

Diagnosis

Diagnosing missing teeth may be as simple as performing an oral examination and obtaining radiographs to determine whether the tooth is absent or impacted.

Treatment

Treatment is aimed at restoring the occlusion. This is accomplished by placement of a permanent or removable prosthesis (false tooth) with orthodontics or by placing a dental implant.

Prognosis

The prognosis is good when a prosthesis or a dental implant provides replacement.

Prevention

Regular dental hygiene is the only method to prevent tooth decay and tooth loss.

Patient Teaching

Emphasize the importance of complying with the individualized treatment plan. When the patient has a dental appliance in place, teach the proper cleaning technique to prevent tooth decay. Make sure the patient knows what to expect after any surgical procedure or cosmetic dentistry.

Impacted Third Molars

Description

An impacted third molar is malpositioned, thereby preventing normal eruption.

ICD-10-CM Code	K00.6 *(Disturbances in tooth eruption)*
	K01.0 *(Embedded teeth)*
	K01.1 *(Impacted teeth)*

Symptoms and Signs

Third molars, also known as *wisdom teeth,* are the last teeth in the back of the mouth and can become impacted (pressed together) and cause pain. They begin developing between ages 8 and 10 years and emerge or erupt (through the gums) between ages 17 and 21 years. In some people, one or more of these teeth never erupt. There are usually no symptoms until these teeth begin to emerge. Even when wisdom teeth develop normally, they are difficult to clean because of their position at the back of the mouth. Because of this, they decay much more often compared with other teeth, resulting in pain.

Patient Screening

Schedule an initial consultation with the dentist for diagnostic evaluation.

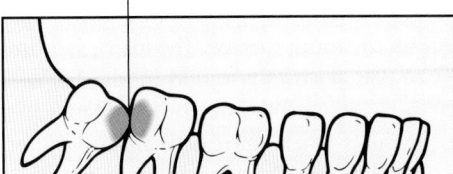

Site of impaction

• **Fig. 8.4** Impacted wisdom tooth.

Etiology

Third molars become impacted when they do not have enough room to erupt because of bone structure or because adjacent teeth block eruption (Fig. 8.4). Sometimes they erupt at an angle, creating a space in which food can become trapped. This can lead to pericoronitis around the tooth, which, in turn, causes pain when biting and a foul taste in the mouth. The gum around the tooth becomes red and swollen.

Diagnosis

Radiographic studies are needed to determine the position of the tooth if it has not erupted completely. An examination also is performed to look for any infection.

Treatment

The dentist is likely to prescribe an antibiotic (penicillin or amoxicillin) to clear up any infection that is present and an analgesic (e.g., acetaminophen, ibuprofen, codeine combinations, or hydrocodone combinations) to relieve pain temporarily. After the infection clears up and pain has lessened, the impacted tooth must be extracted to prevent recurrence of infection.

Prognosis

Treatment of the infection and extraction of the impacted tooth solve the problem.

Prevention

No prevention is known.

Patient Teaching

Emphasize the importance of taking the entire course of antibiotics as prescribed. Explain the procedure of tooth extraction and what to expect after surgery. Inform the patient that swelling often occurs after surgery and that ice compresses will help reduce this swelling.

Dental Caries

Description

Dental caries is considered an infection resulting in erosion of the tooth surface.

| ICD-10-CM Code | K02.9 *(Dental caries, unspecified)* |
| | (K02.51-K02.9 = 8 codes of specificity) |

Symptoms and Signs

Dental decay, also known as *dental caries,* first manifests as white spots on the tooth surface. The major symptom in the early stage of dental caries is a mild toothache, with hypersensitivity to sweets and temperature extremes in foods or beverages. If caries is left untreated, an unpleasant taste in the mouth results from the accumulation of food and bacteria in the cavity area. Eventually the pulp of the gum becomes inflamed, and the pain is persistent. Some patients say they feel a stabbing pain in the jaw. As the tooth continues to decay, an abscess may form (see the Tooth Abscesses section).

Patient Screening

Schedule an appointment for the patient for an immediate dental examination and evaluation.

Etiology

Dental caries occurs when bacteria in the mouth break down the sugars present in foods, converting them into acid plaque. Sugars in foods include sucrose, glucose, and fructose in fruits; lactose in milk products; and breakdown products of simple carbohydrates, such as chips, crackers, and breads. The acid plaque erodes the calcium in the tooth's enamel (demineralization), causing the formation of a cavity (Fig. 8.5). In addition to this plaque in the mouth, other disorders, such as stomach acid from gastroesophageal reflux disease (GERD) or episodes of purging in bulimia, may contribute to tooth decay.

Diagnosis

The dentist examines the patient's teeth for signs of cavity formation and may obtain radiographs to determine the extent of the decay.

Treatment

In early treatment, the dentist removes the diseased portion of the tooth enamel and pulp and fills the cavity with dental amalgam composite material (gold, silver, or porcelain fillings) to prevent further decay and to restore the tooth's size and shape. If the decay has advanced into the pulp, the dentist may perform a root canal procedure. In this procedure, the infected pulp tissue is removed, and then the canals in the roots of the tooth are filled, treated with antibiotics, and sealed. Tooth extraction may be necessary if the tooth is not salvageable or if root canal therapy fails. In this case, a dental implant (an artificial tooth root) may be inserted to support restorations that resemble a tooth or group of teeth (Fig. 8.6).

Prognosis

The prognosis is good with prompt treatment. Dental decay can spread quickly, and the bacteria that cause decay can be transmitted through saliva. When swallowed, the bacteria in saliva enter the bloodstream, and damage to other major organs may occur. When the cavity is allowed to erode and damage the inner pulp of the tooth, infection and tooth abscess can result.

Prevention

Caries may be prevented with good oral hygiene, including brushing, flossing, and using an effective antibacterial mouthwash after eating, and biannual professional cleaning of the teeth. Limiting ingestion of sweets, simple carbohydrates, and between-meal snacks is suggested. Some dentists prescribe the use of oral fluorides. Chewing self-cleaning foods after meals is helpful when tooth brushing is delayed; celery and apples help scour away food scraps and plaque. Dental scalants are plastic coatings, similar to a Teflon coating, and when applied to the surfaces of permanent molars, they are effective in creating a physical barrier to prevent cavities.

Patient Teaching

Demonstrate good brushing, flossing, and rinsing with antibacterial mouthwash techniques. Explain what causes

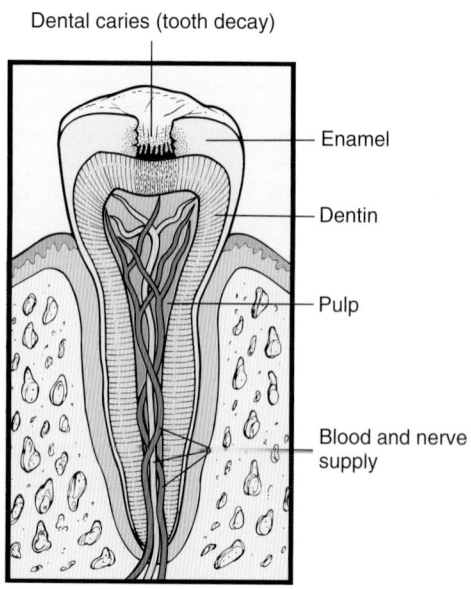

Dental caries (tooth decay)

— Enamel

— Dentin

— Pulp

— Blood and nerve supply

• **Fig. 8.5** Dental caries (tooth decay).

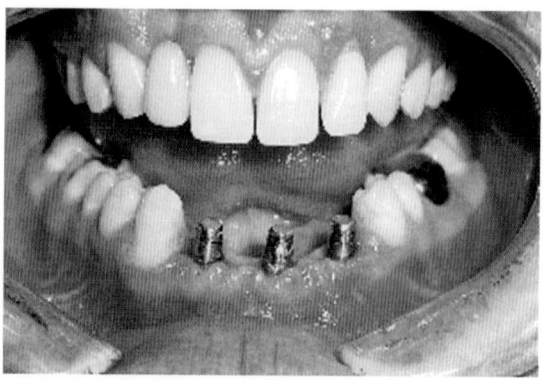

• **Fig. 8.6** Dental implant. (From Christensen GJ: *A consumer's guide to dentistry,* ed 2, St Louis, 2002, Mosby.)

dental caries. Offer nutritional counseling to promote healthy and strong enamel formation and help reduce the number of acid-producing bacteria in the mouth. Professional cleaning of teeth and biannual dental examinations should be strongly recommended.

Discolored Teeth

Description

In this condition, teeth are discolored.

ICD-10-CM Code	K03.7 (Posteruptive color changes of dental hard tissues)

Symptoms and Signs

Symptoms of discolored teeth are obvious, and colors may range from a slight yellow to brown and gray. Some teeth may have brown spots, patches, and dark lines in or on them.

Patient Screening

Schedule an appointment for the patient for a dental consultation.

Etiology

Discoloration of teeth can have many causes. Aging causes slight yellowing of teeth; smoking turns teeth surfaces brown; and a dead tooth often turns gray. Red wine, coffee, tea, and foods such as blueberries can stain teeth. Certain drugs (e.g., tetracyclines) taken in large quantities during childhood can cause the formation of defective, discolored enamel (Fig. 8.7). An antibacterial mouthwash, such as chlorhexidine, can discolor teeth. Severe attacks of pertussis (whooping cough) and measles in children can cause discolored patches to form on teeth. Naturally occurring fluoride, in excessive amounts, can produce white or brown spots in teeth.

Diagnosis

The dentist performs an oral examination. A pertinent history includes recent illnesses, medications, and trauma to teeth. Hereditary factors also are considered.

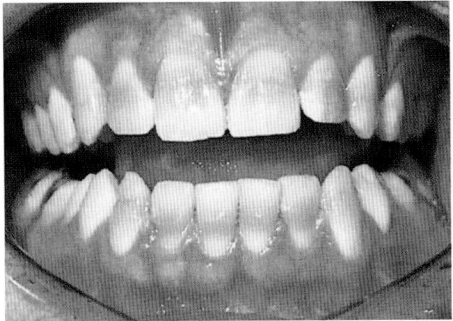

• **Fig. 8.7** Discolored teeth. (From Christensen GJ: A consumer's guide to dentistry, ed 2, St Louis, 2002, Mosby.)

Treatment

The extent of treatment varies, depending on the discoloration being superficial or deep within enamel. Superficial discoloration can be removed or reduced by polishing with a rotary polisher. Deeper discolorations can be treated by dentist-provided bleaching procedures or by capping or crowning by bonding a synthetic veneer to the tooth. Dentists offer treatments for cosmetic whitening of teeth (i.e., application of a whitening gel that is activated by a light source).

Prognosis

Resolution of discoloration is possible with a range of treatments.

Prevention

Dental hygienists suggest avoiding smoking and drinking coffee, tea, or red wine to prevent staining of teeth. Many products on the market claim to whiten teeth and use various forms of peroxide as a bleaching agent. Harsh or abrasive whitening agents should be avoided because they can damage enamel. Intrinsic causes may or may not be preventable.

Patient Teaching

In addition to the preventive measures mentioned previously, the dentist may suggest treatment for deeper discoloration. Currently there are many OTC products (gels, toothpastes, whitening strips, and mouth rinses) on the market that claim to whiten teeth; most of them simply remove stains caused by foods and drinks but have limited effectiveness on deep stains. Some of these products have side effects, including a burning sensation in the gum area. Consultation with a dentist is advised before beginning use of an at-home whitening system. Explain the planned dental procedures to help reduce anxiety.

Gingivitis

Description

Gingivitis is inflammation and swelling of the gums (Fig. 8.8).

ICD-10-CM Code	K05.00 (Acute gingivitis, plaque induced)
	(K05.00-K05.01 = 2 codes of specificity)
	K05.10 (Chronic gingivitis, plaque induced)
	(K05.10-K05.11 = 2 codes of specificity)

Symptoms and Signs

Gums that are normally pale pink and firm become red, soft, and shiny. They bleed easily, even with gentle tooth brushing. The disease can be painless and therefore be discovered after it has progressed. If gingivitis is not treated, it leads to destruction of the gums and bone disease called

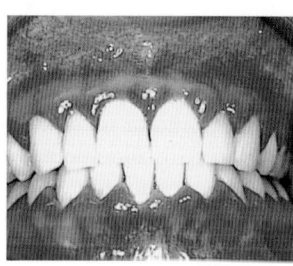

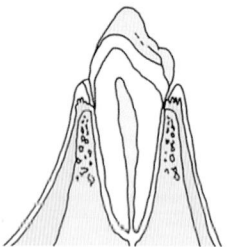

• **Fig. 8.8** Gingivitis. (From Murray PR, et al: *Medical microbiology,* ed 6, Philadelphia, 2009, Mosby.)

periodontitis (see the Periodontitis section). Advanced cases of gingivitis can cause loss of healthy teeth.

Patient Screening

Schedule an appoint for the patient for a dental examination and consultation.

Etiology

Approximately half of U.S. adults have some areas of gingivitis, and it is the second most common cause of toothache. The most common cause of gingivitis is plaque. Plaque is a sticky deposit of mucus, food particles, and bacteria that builds up around the base of teeth as a result of inadequate or incorrect technique when brushing or flossing. As the gums become inflamed and swollen, the plaque causes a pocket to form between gums and teeth, and that space becomes a food trap. Other causes of gingivitis include vitamin deficiencies, glandular disorders, blood diseases, viral infections, and the use of certain medications. Pregnant women and patients with diabetes are particularly susceptible to gingivitis as a result of vascular and hormonal changes.

Diagnosis

If symptoms develop, a dentist should be seen as soon as possible to confirm gingivitis and to begin treatment to prevent complications.

Treatment

Treatment includes removal of plaque and calculus by a professional dental hygienist. In advanced cases of gingivitis, the dentist may prescribe an antibacterial mouthwash, such as chlorhexidine (Periogard), to clear up the infection.

In some cases, a local anesthesia may be used to thoroughly clean teeth and exposed teeth roots, in a procedure called *root planing* and *subgingival curettage.* Oral antibiotics may follow to treat gum infection or abscess. Follow-up

treatment is required for loosened teeth or when there is bone destruction.

Prognosis

It has been estimated that 80% of adults will suffer from some type of gum (periodontal) disease during their lifetime. Identifying and treating underlying causes offers the best outcome.

Prevention

Prophylaxis includes good oral hygiene and removal of plaque at the gum line. Toothbrush trauma caused by brushing teeth incorrectly and excessively should be avoided. Excessive use of abrasives (teeth whitening products) is contraindicated.

Patient Teaching

See the preventive measures listed earlier. Encourage the patient to have regular dental examinations and keep follow-up appointments. Discuss symptoms to report to the dentist if the patient is on antibacterial therapy. Share research findings that support the strong correlation between cardiac disease and plaque and poor dental status in patients.

Periodontitis

Description

Periodontitis, also called *periodontal disease,* is a destructive gum and bone disease around one or more teeth (Fig. 8.9).

ICD-10-CM Code	K05.20 *(Aggressive periodontitis, unspecified)*
	(K05.20-K05.22 = 3 codes of specificity)
	K05.30 *(Chronic periodontitis, unspecified)*
	(K05.30-K05.32 = 3 codes of specificity)

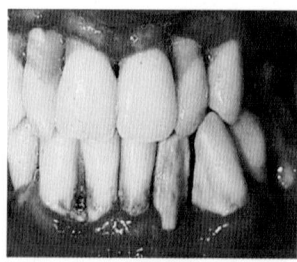

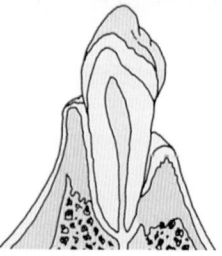

• **Fig. 8.9** Advanced periodontitis. (From Murray PR, et al: *Medical microbiology,* ed 6, Philadelphia, 2009, Mosby.)

Symptoms and Signs

Periodontitis is the end result of gingivitis (see the Gingivitis section) that was treated too late or not at all. The pockets that form between teeth and gums in gingivitis gradually deepen, exposing the root. Plaque develops in this area, causing an unpleasant taste in the mouth and offensive breath (halitosis). As more root is exposed, one or more teeth become extremely sensitive to temperature extremes in foods, and pain may be experienced when chewing. Abscesses can form (see the Tooth Abscesses section), and eventually a tooth or several teeth become loose and possibly fall out.

Patient Screening

Schedule a complete dental examination and consultation immediately.

Etiology

The cause of periodontitis is plaque biofilm and unchecked gingivitis. This commonly results from poor oral hygiene and lack of professional dental periodontal care. Over time, the bacteria in plaque destroy the bone surrounding and supporting teeth. Contributing factors include smoking, certain medications, chemotherapy, diabetes, and human immunodeficiency virus (HIV) infection. Stress, poor nutrition, hormonal medications, and pregnancy may also contribute to periodontitis.

Diagnosis

To determine the stage of the periodontal disease, the dentist measures the depth of the pockets and obtains radiographs. Radiographs reveal the condition of the underlying bone, and this knowledge aids the dentist in deciding how to treat the disease.

Treatment

Conservative treatment includes thorough cleaning of the root surfaces of teeth, a procedure called *scaling and root planing (SRP)* and *curettage*. Multiple daily sessions of brushing and flossing of teeth are required. An oral or local application of a sub-antimicrobial dose of an antibiotic may be prescribed. Periodontal surgery may be required if the pockets have become deep and nonresponsive to more conservative therapy. The procedure, called *respective periodontal surgery*, requires the dentist to trim the gums to reduce the depth of the pockets and to remove any damaged bone. In certain situations, the dentist may graft bone and/or gum tissue to resolve the periodontal condition.

Prognosis

The prognosis varies with the extent of the disease process, the presence of complications, and the effectiveness of treatment.

Prevention

Adherence to a schedule for professional cleaning and examination of teeth by a dentist is of primary importance. Poor oral hygiene, lack of regular professional dental cleaning, smoking, and certain medications are primary contributors to periodontal disease. In some cases, medication and periodontal surgery may prevent tooth loss.

Patient Teaching

Reinforce the education provided by the dentist regarding an ongoing dental care plan. The care plan may include having teeth cleaned every 2 to 4 months to remove/disrupt the causative bacteria and prevent further disease. Emphasize the long-term advantages of early detection and treatment to save teeth, because a history of periodontal disease predisposes the patient to rapid progression of the disease. Education for patients with diabetes should include adherence to periodontal therapy, and good oral hygiene may enhance diabetic control.

Oral Tumors

Description

Oral tumors, or neoplasms, are classified as benign or malignant and localized or invasive.

ICD-10-CM Code	D10.0 *(Benign neoplasm of lip)*

Benign oral tumors have code modifiers according to location. Refer to the physician's diagnosis and then to the current edition of the ICD-10-CM coding manual to ensure the greatest specificity. See oral cancer for coding of malignant oral tumors.

Symptoms and Signs

Tumors can develop anywhere in or on the surface of the mouth, gums, cheeks, or palate but not on teeth. They begin as single, small, pale lumps, in or on the mouth, which may or may not bleed easily and may or may not cause pain. There are two types of tumors: benign (or noncancerous) and malignant (or cancerous). Benign tumors grow slowly over several years, do not metastasize (spread to other areas), and are not usually life-threatening. Malignant tumors are generally not painful until they reach advanced stages (see the Oral Cancer section).

Patient Screening

The lesion(s) or lumps should be evaluated without delay. Patients may describe a lesion as being red, blue, or white. Biopsy of the lesion may be required.

Etiology

The cause of benign and malignant oral tumors is unknown, although certain factors, such as tobacco use, seem to cause development of a tumor into a malignancy.

Diagnosis

An oral surgeon or a physician should be consulted if the patient has a lump, an ulcer, or a color change in or on the surface of the mouth that does not clear up within 10 days. If a tumor is discovered, biopsy is needed to determine whether it is benign or malignant.

Treatment

If the tumor has been determined to be benign, it should be observed periodically by a medical professional to ensure that it has not become malignant. Benign tumors will be assessed and may be excised if they are subject to chronic irritation or interfere with the fit of a denture, implant, crown, and so on. See the Oral Cancer section for a discussion about malignant oral tumors.

Prognosis

Benign tumors are usually curable with excision.

Prevention

Avoid chronic irritation to the lips and the mouth. This includes excessive brushing, tongue probing, and so on. Any mouth lesion that does not heal must be evaluated and treated to avoid potential invasive disease.

Patient Teaching

Educate the patient regarding causes of lesions that result from chronic irritation. Review the course of action prescribed to promote healing.

Malocclusion

Description

Malocclusion describes specific angles of malposition and contact of the maxillary and mandibular teeth.

ICD-10-CM Code	M26.4 *(Malocclusion, unspecified)*

Symptoms and Signs

The relationship of the upper and lower teeth when the mouth is closed is called *occlusion,* or bite; a faulty bite is called *malocclusion* (Fig. 8.10). Signs of malocclusion include protrusion or recession of the jaws and teeth that are turned or twisted out of position because of crowding. The patient may or may not experience some degree of difficulty with mastication or chewing.

Patient Screening

Schedule an appointment for dental examination and consultation. Inform the patient that radiographic studies may be indicated.

Etiology

Malocclusion generally results from genetic factors. It is a rarity to have perfectly aligned teeth. Heredity is not the only cause of malocclusion; crowding can result from the early loss of primary teeth or from oral habits, such as thumb/finger sucking. Thumb/finger sucking often causes orthopedic (skeletal) changes and dental crowding. Airway problems (deviated septae, enlarged tonsils, or allergies) can affect the normal growth and development of the facial skeleton and dentition. Other teeth may shift to fill the space left by this loss of teeth, causing the loss of space where the permanent tooth normally would erupt.

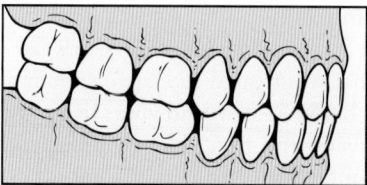
Normal teeth

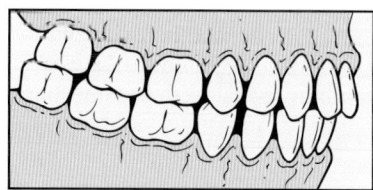
Protruding upper teeth

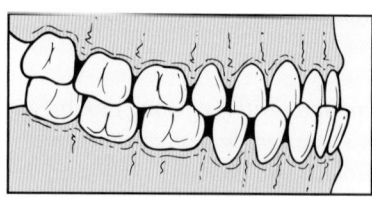
Receding upper teeth

• **Fig. 8.10** Malocclusion.

Diagnosis

A visual examination and radiographic studies clearly identify the malocclusion.

Treatment

Several treatments are used to correct this problem. These include the application of braces for a minor problem, extraction of one or more teeth, or surgical removal of portions of the jaw in situations of protrusion and recession of the jaw. Additional treatment includes combining crowns or bridges to replace the missing teeth.

Prognosis

The prognosis is favorable with treatment.

Prevention

If caused by genetics, there is no prevention. Parents are reminded to discourage thumb/finger sucking, and they are encouraged to seek professional dental advice to curtail the behavior in the child. Airway problems need to be addressed when major skeletal development begins at age 6 to 8 years. Professional dental evaluation can help decrease costly orthodontic/orthopedic treatment in the future.

Patient Teaching

Special care is needed to avoid the development of caries while wearing corrective dental appliances. The patient should practice thorough, regular cleaning of teeth and avoid eating candy and gum. Often use of alternative flossing instruments, such as Waterpik, may be advised to reach tooth areas that are not accessible with a standard brush.

Temporomandibular Joint Disorder

Description

Temporomandibular joint disorder (TMD) is a symptom complex related to inflammation, disease, or dysfunction of the temporomandibular joint (TMJ).

ICD-10-CM Code   M26.60 *(Temporomandibular joint disorder, unspecified)*
    M26.69 *(Other specified disorders of temporomandibular joint)*
    (M26.60-M26.69 = 5 codes of specificity)

Symptoms and Signs

The synovial joints between the condyles of the mandible and the temporal bones of the skull are known as *temporomandibular joints.* When these joints are inflamed or diseased, jaw movement is markedly limited. The patient reports hearing clicking sounds during chewing or experiences severe pain or aching in or around the ears and jaw joints, and the pain is worse with chewing. This pain and limitation of movement can be unilateral but is usually bilateral, with one side markedly more painful than the other. Headache, dizziness, a feeling of pressure, tinnitus, or a draining sensation may be present in one or both ears; deafness may be experienced. Patients often complain of sinus pain, which is, in reality, muscle pain from the superior or deep masseters. Reduced ability to open the jaw not only interferes with chewing but also prevents adequate cleaning of teeth and treatment of cavities. It also may prevent the making of dentures, crowns, or implants because of the inability to take impressions of teeth.

Patient Screening

Significant pain usually prompts a request for medical treatment. Complete medical and dental assessments may be necessary.

Etiology

Temporomandibular disorders result from unbalanced activity of the jaw muscles caused by a number of conditions, including bruxism (grinding of teeth, an action emanating from the central pattern generator in the brain); malocclusion; poorly fitting dentures; rheumatoid, degenerative, or traumatic arthritis; and neoplastic diseases. Emotional stress, with accompanying clenching and grinding of teeth, and habitual gum chewing are also contributing factors.

Diagnosis

The diagnosis of TMD is made through oral examination, patient history, and radiographic studies, including computed tomography (CT) and magnetic resonance imaging (MRI), to analyze the hard and soft tissues of the temporomandibular complex. There may be history of previous trauma to the jaws or fractured facial bones. An assessment for domestic violence or child or elder abuse may be indicated. In the case of a neoplasm, biopsy would rule out malignancy.

Treatment

Treatment is aimed at the cause of the condition or disease. Symptoms of rheumatoid or traumatic arthritis often subside after 3 to 5 days of immobilization of the mandible. In cases where inflammation causes TMD, nonsteroidal antiinflammatory drugs (NSAIDs) often are used to treat the condition. Some patients wear special appliances to prevent them from grinding their teeth. If TMD is caused by jaw misalignment, a plastic bite plate, called a *splint,* may be used to better align the jaw. The splint is worn over teeth and establishes proper alignment, which can eliminate jaw locking, pain, and clicking sensations associated with TMD. Intraarticular injections of hydrocortisone may be needed in more severe cases of rheumatoid or degenerative arthritis. When teeth experience premature contact, the dentist adjusts the occlusion by grinding the surfaces of teeth. More complex dental conditions, such as worn or broken teeth or restorations, may require orthodontic and/or comprehensive restorative dental care. Physical therapy, stress counseling, and the use of muscle relaxants may be prescribed. As a last resort, TMJ arthroscopy, joint restructuring, and joint replacement are considered.

Prognosis

Mild cases respond well to resting of the joint. More complicated chronic cases require extended treatment of the underlying cause.

Prevention

Regular dental checkups can identify the underlying conditions. Treatment of these conditions can prevent the onset of TMD. Assessment for domestic violence and child or elder abuse may reveal physical trauma that can be prevented with appropriate interventions.

Patient Teaching

When the dentist prescribes an appliance, tell the patient what kind of initial discomfort he or she may expect. The patient is encouraged to use the appliance exactly as directed and is urged to report any unusual discomfort during treatment. Referrals appropriate to the cause are made.

Tooth Abscesses

Description

A tooth abscess is a pus-filled sac that develops in the tissue surrounding the base of the root.

ICD-10-CM Code   K04.7 *(Periapical abscess without sinus)*
    (K04.6-K04.7 = 2 codes of specificity)

Symptoms and Signs

An abscessed tooth aches or throbs persistently and can be extremely painful when biting and chewing food. Glands in the neck and face on the affected side may become swollen and tender. Fever also can develop, along with a feeling of general malaise.

Patient Screening

Tooth abscesses require prompt medical attention.

Etiology

An abscess forms when a tooth is decayed or dying or when the tooth structure loss (i.e., from aggressive brushing, traumatic fracture, or acid erosion) exposes the dental nerve to bacteria from the mouth. Severely receding gums, which expose the root, are a risk factor. The dead pulp, along with invading bacteria, can infect the surrounding tissues and the jaws, even after a root canal procedure, and form an abscess.

Diagnosis

If any of the symptoms or signs is present, the patient should see the dentist immediately. Swelling in the neck or face must be treated immediately to prevent spreading of the infection.

Treatment

Antibiotic therapy is prescribed to relieve pain and acute swelling. The definitive treatment is root canal therapy, which entails removal of the infected dental pulp and the cleansing, shaping, and definitive filling of the root canal system of the tooth. Restorative procedures, such as a dental crown or sometimes a filling, are required to seal the root canal system from the oral environment. If a lesion is a longstanding one, is large, or does not heal after a period, an apicectomy may be necessary. In this procedure, the dentist or the oral surgeon makes an incision into the gum and removes the bone that covers the tip of the root and the infected tissue as well. If this fails to clear the infection, the tooth must be extracted.

Prognosis

A positive outcome is likely with early intervention and a favorable response to antibiotic therapy.

Prevention

Prophylaxis includes good oral hygiene and regular dental checkups.

Patient Teaching

Educate patients that neglect of a tooth abscess may cause serious complications resulting from spread of infection to bone. If untreated, this becomes systemic and life-threatening.

Mouth Ulcers

Description

An ulcer in the mouth is a lesion on the mucous membrane, exposing the underlying sensitive tissue.

ICD-10-CM Code	K13.70 (Unspecified lesions of oral mucosa)
	K13.79 (Other lesions of oral mucosa)

Symptoms and Signs

Mouth ulcers (sometimes called *canker sores*) are common and look alike but vary considerably in their causes and degrees of seriousness. The two most common types of ulcers are aphthous ulcers (Fig. 8.11), which occur during stress or illness, and traumatic ulcers, which result from injury and are caused by burns by hot foods, rough dentures, or even toothbrushes. Ulcers appear as pale yellow spots with red borders. Aphthous ulcers usually occur in clusters and last for 3 or 4 days. Traumatic ulcers are usually single and larger and last for a week or longer.

Patient Screening

Ulcers that do not heal within 10 days require a physician's or health care provider's attention. Any mouth ulcer that is not caused by trauma from mechanical devices (braces) or brushing must be assessed irrespective of duration.

Etiology

A viral cause for aphthous ulcers has not been established. Acute ulcerations are usually the result of mechanical trauma (braces, excessive brushing, and so on), viral and bacterial infections, stress (inducement of hormonal changes), illness, or certain medications used in chemotherapy. In rare instances, an ulcer may be the first sign of a tumor in the mouth, anemia, or leukemia.

Diagnosis

If an ulcer does not heal within 10 days or recurs, the patient should consult a medical professional. Blood tests and biopsy of the ulcer are needed to determine the cause. When the ulcer results from trauma, it does not heal until it is diagnosed and treated.

Treatment

Self-treatment of ulcers includes using antiseptic mouthwashes, rinsing with warm salt water, and avoiding spicy or

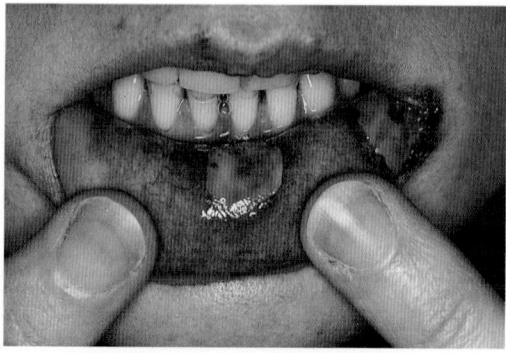

• **Fig. 8.11** Mouth ulcers. (From Stevens A, et al: *Core pathology*, ed 3, London, 2010, Mosby.)

acidic foods and hot foods or drinks. Topical analgesics, such as benzocaine, and soothing agents, such as spirit of camphor, can be used to reduce painful irritation. The medical professional may prescribe a steroid mouthwash and topical or oral antiviral agents to promote healing.

Prognosis

Most ulcers heal spontaneously in less than 10 days.

Prevention

No specific prevention is known, except when the ulcer is attributed to mechanical trauma or improper brushing.

Patient Teaching

Educate the patient regarding the self-help measures listed previously under the Treatment section.

Herpes Simplex (Cold Sores)

Description

Herpes simplex is a contagious, recurrent viral infection that affects the skin and mucous membranes. Herpes type 1 commonly produces cold sores and fever blisters (Fig. 8.12).

ICD-10-CM Code	B00.9 *(Herpes viral infection, unspecified)*

Symptoms and Signs

Herpes simplex (cold sore) blisters can develop on the lips and inside the mouth, producing painful ulcers that last a few hours or days. Exposure to strong sun, wind, stress, nicotine, and stimulants (caffeine and chocolate) are associated with the onset of recurrent oral facial herpes simplex. These ulcers also can form on the gums, causing them to become red and swollen. Tingling and numbness around the mouth precede their appearance. This is called the *prodrome*. Untreated, the prodrome is followed by the appearance of the vesicles (blisters), their rupture and scabbing, and finally healing of the scabs; this pathogenesis can often last 14 days or more. Although most infections are subclinical, constitutional symptoms can occur.

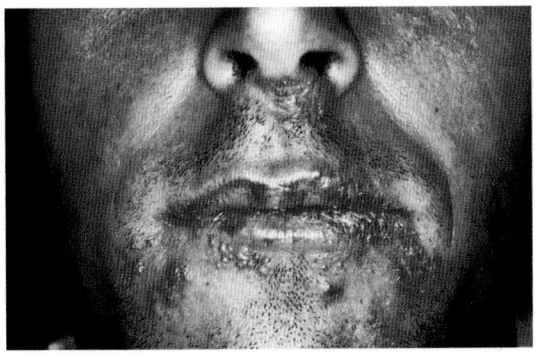

• **Fig. 8.12** Herpes simplex virus type 1 (HSV-1). (From Damjanov I, Linder J: *Pathology: a color atlas,* St Louis, 1999, Mosby.)

Patient Screening

Lesions near the eye are considered more serious. A patient having generalized symptoms, such as fever, anorexia, and lymphadenopathy, should be seen by the physician or health care provider immediately, especially if the patient is pregnant.

Etiology

The vesicles are caused by the herpes simplex virus type 1 (HSV-1) and are common. They tend to recur because the virus can lie dormant. Exposure to sunshine or wind or the presence of another infection, such as a common cold, can reactivate the virus. Once patients develop extraoral and/or intraoral herpes, they can have recurrent attacks throughout their lives. Patients may anticipate an outbreak of herpes with symptoms of the prodrome (burning tingling sensation in the soon-to-be affected area).

Diagnosis

An oral examination is usually sufficient for the diagnosis. Isolating HSV-1 from local lesions can confirm the cause of the infection. The HSV-2 causes a similar lesion in the oral cavity.

Treatment

Currently no cure is known. If the infection is mild, no treatment is necessary, but severe cases require medical attention. Herpes simplex usually does not cause serious risks to health, but rubbing the eyes after touching the ulcer could cause the formation of a herpetic corneal ulcer, and the infection can produce severe illness in an immunocompromised patient. A physician or health care provider may advise using an antiviral ointment or capsules, such as acyclovir or penciclovir, to arrest or shorten the duration of the episode. Immediate attention to the symptoms and use of an antiviral ointment are the most conservative and comfortable measures for the treatment of extraoral herpes. Intraoral herpes benefits from a prescription of an antiviral, such as acyclovir (Zovirax). Comfort measures include resting, taking aspirin, and using an anesthetic mouthwash and a topical cream to relieve the pain and to heal the sores. Creams proven to shorten the duration of herpes sores and speed healing of cold sores are docosanol (Abreva) and Novitra, a homeopathic cream. Both contain particles that bind to the virus and inhibit further spreading. Recently a single-day dosage of antiviral medication (acyclovir, famciclovir, or valacyclovir), begun at the very onset of symptoms, has been proven to shorten the severity of cold sores.

Prognosis

Cold sores usually clear up uneventfully in 7 to 14 days. Lesions tend to recur when reactivated by trauma or stress. Serious complications can result from lesions close to the eye. Secondary bacterial infection of the skin may occur.

Prevention

Early treatment with an antiviral medication controls the outbreak and reduces the risk of transmission. Direct contact with cold sores from associates with the patient should be avoided. Gentle cleansing with antiseptic soap may help prevent spreading of infection or secondary bacterial infection.

Patient Teaching

Recommend that close contact between the patient and his or her partner be avoided. This includes kissing of any part of the body of the infected person, because the virus may remain in saliva after the vesicle has healed. Personal items (cups, eating utensils, towels, razors, and so on) should not be shared between an infected individual and others. Touching the affected vesicles as they appear should be avoided, because a break in the skin of the finger can result in a *whitlow finger* (extremely painful herpetic infection of the finger). When the patient has multiple lesions in the oral cavity, use of anesthetic mouthwashes helps reduce pain, enabling the patient to eat and drink. Avoidance of proper nutrition may result in dehydration or vitamin deficiencies.

Thrush

Description

Thrush is candidiasis of the oral mucosa and involves the mouth, tongue, palate, and gums.

ICD-10-CM Code	B37.0 *(Candidal stomatitis)*
	B37.83 *(Candidal cheilitis)*
	(B37.0-B37.9 = 16 codes of specificity)

Symptoms and Signs

Thrush is a fungal infection of relatively short duration that produces sore, slightly raised, pale-yellow patches in the mouth and sometimes the throat. These lesions cause a burning sensation in the mouth and become painful when rubbed by dentures, toothbrushes, or food when eating; light bleeding may occur. Some patients suffering from severe cases of thrush have the smell of yeast in their breath. Thrush most often develops in young children, in immunodeficient individuals, and in older adults, but it can occur at any age.

Patient Screening

If the patient also complains of fever or other systemic symptoms, he or she should see a health care provider immediately.

Etiology

The fungus *Candida albicans* causes most cases of thrush. Normally present in the mouth in small numbers, the fungus can multiply out of control. This may occur during lowered resistance or as a result of prolonged treatment with antibiotics, which upsets the normal number of protective microbes. Other predisposing factors are cancer chemotherapy, diabetes, or glucocorticoid therapy. It is also very common in patients with removable dental prostheses, such as complete or partial dentures. The infection rarely

becomes systemic or infectious. This same fungus can cause vaginitis.

Diagnosis

Diagnosis is made by the dentist, physician, or health care provider through an oral examination and laboratory analysis of a sample taken from a lesion. Blood tests may rule out a serious underlying disease, such as iron deficiency anemia or early HIV infection.

Treatment

Thrush is treated successfully with an antifungal medication for 14 days. The antifungals used most often are nystatin, an antifungal suspension that is swished and then swallowed, and fluconazole (Diflucan), available as a suspension or an oral tablet. After diagnosis of thrush, patients with removable dental prostheses are advised to soak their prostheses in a cup of water with a few drops of household bleach (5% sodium hypochlorite) for a few hours to disinfect them and to subsequently use an OTC denture cleaner on a daily basis to prevent reinfection.

Prognosis

The infection tends to recur in some patients. In all cases, treatment must begin immediately after a confirmed diagnosis, because thrush can extend into the esophagus, causing esophagitis. Thrush can spread to other parts of the body in those with weakened immune systems.

Prevention

Patients who have had treatment with antibiotics should report any signs of thrush. Those using inhaled corticosteroids should rinse their mouths thoroughly after use to avoid the development of thrush.

Patient Teaching

Palliative care includes a soft diet and the use of a nonirritating mouthwash and a soft toothbrush for oral hygiene. Foods containing sugar or yeast should be limited. Good oral hygiene is encouraged. The patient is advised to quit smoking. See the procedure for disinfection of dental prostheses earlier in the Treatment section.

Necrotizing Periodontal Disease

Description

Necrotizing periodontal disease (formerly called *acute necrotizing ulcerative gingivitis* [trench mouth]) is a common infection affecting gums and the anchoring structure of teeth.

| ICD-10-CM Code | A69.0 *(Necrotizing ulcerative stomatitis)* |
| | A69.1 *(Other Vincent's infections)* |

Symptoms and Signs

Necrotizing periodontal disease is a rare, painful ulceration and disease of the gums, particularly between teeth, and is

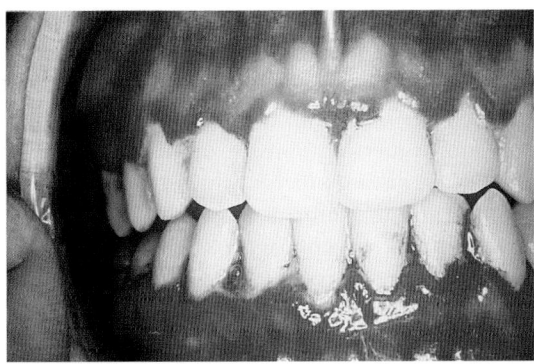

• **Fig. 8.13** Necrotizing periodontal disease. (From Stevens A, et al: *Core pathology*, ed 3, London, 2010, Mosby.)

sometimes called *Vincent angina*. The primary symptom is painful, red, swollen gums with ulcers that bleed. Gums also can appear grayish in areas of decomposing tissue. The patient also may report a metallic taste in the mouth and bad breath (Fig. 8.13). Mild systemic symptoms include fever and enlarged lymph nodes.

Patient Screening

Prompt medical treatment is advised. An oral examination by a dentist or appropriate physician or health care provider is needed as soon as possible.

Etiology

Anaerobic opportunistic bacteria cause necrotizing periodontal disease. It results from poor oral hygiene and bacterial infection secondary to gingivitis (see the Gingivitis section). Nowadays, the infection is most often seen in association with HIV/AIDS, especially in the early stages. Stress, poor nutrition, throat infections, smoking, and serious illnesses, such as leukemia, are also contributing factors. Some cases have been linked to the use of oral contraceptives.

Diagnosis

Throat culture and blood work may be necessary to rule out serious illness.

Treatment

The patient receives antibiotics and hydrogen peroxide mouthwash to relieve pain and inflammation. After the disease has been halted, teeth and gums must be professionally cleaned. A minor surgery on the gums, called *gingivectomy*, may be advised.

Prognosis

With treatment, improvement can be expected within days.

Prevention

Prophylactic professional cleaning of teeth, good oral hygiene, and avoidance of the contributing factors, such as smoking and poor diet, are recommended.

Patient Teaching

Emphasize prevention as described earlier. Explain that particular medications and systemic diseases can aggravate periodontal disease.

Oral Leukoplakia

Description

Leukoplakia is hyperkeratosis or epidermal thickening of the buccal mucosa, palate, or lower lip.

ICD-10-CM Code	K13.21 (*Leukoplakia of oral mucosa, including tongue*)

Symptoms and Signs

Leukoplakia, or white plaque, is thickening and hardening of a part of the mucous membrane in the mouth (Fig. 8.14). It develops over several weeks and can vary in size. At first, the patient is asymptomatic, but as the leukoplakia progresses, the mucous membrane becomes rough, hard, and whitish gray and is sensitive to hot or highly seasoned foods.

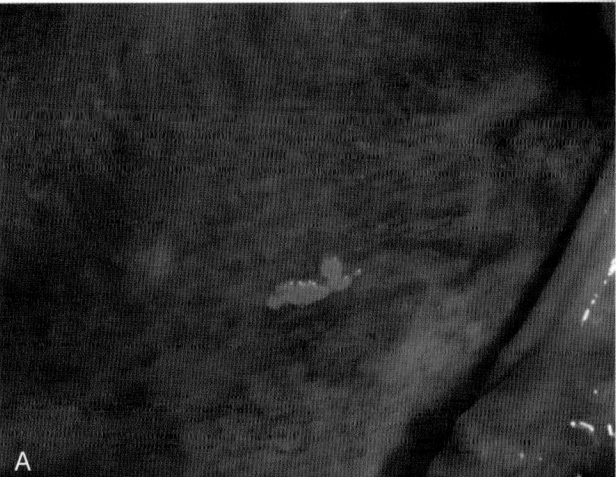

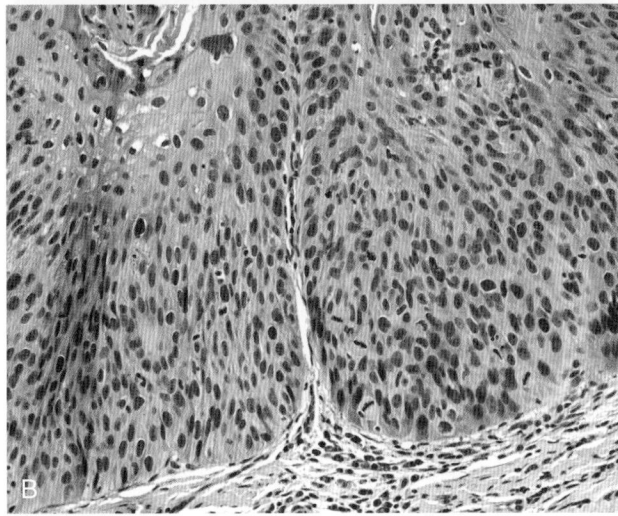

• **Fig. 8.14** Leukoplakia. (From Kumar V, et al: *Robbins basic pathology*, ed 10, Philadelphia, 2018, Saunders.)

Patient Screening

Schedule an appointment for the patient for an oral examination.

Etiology

Leukoplakia may develop at any age, but it is more common in older adults. It usually results from chronic irritation, such as friction caused by habitual cheek biting, dentures, or a rough tooth that rubs an area raw. Leukoplakia also may be a reaction to the heat from tobacco smoke or local irritation from chewing tobacco.

Diagnosis

An oral examination is needed. If the condition has not cleared up in 14 to 21 days, biopsy is advised, because in about 3% of cases, oral leukoplakia progresses to oral cancer.

Treatment

The treatment of leukoplakia consists of eliminating the source of irritation. A rough tooth or denture may be smoothed, and giving up smoking may be advised. These measures are usually all that is needed to correct the condition. Until proven otherwise, the leukoplakia is considered precancerous.

Prognosis

The lesions require monitoring because of the risk of malignant transformation.

Prevention

Although the cause is not always known, the patient is urged to eliminate tobacco and avoid exposure to persistent irritants.

Patient Teaching

Advise patients to avoid common potentiating influences, including consumption of alcohol and tobacco (especially chewing tobacco); ill-fitting dentures; and frequent eating of spicy foods.

Oral Cancer

Description

Oral cancer includes squamous cell carcinoma (SCC) or adenocarcinoma of the lips, cheek mucosa, anterior tongue, floor of the mouth, hard palate, and upper and lower gingivae.

ICD-10-CM Code   C06.9 *(Malignant neoplasm of mouth, unspecified)* (C06.8-C06.9 = 3 codes of specificity)

Refer to the physician's diagnosis and then to the current edition of the ICD-10-CM coding manual for malignant neoplasm of other parts of the mouth to ensure the greatest specificity.

Symptoms and Signs

Oral cancer usually appears as a white, patchy lesion or an oral ulcer that fails to heal. If the cancer is on the lip or the tongue, the ulcer is likely to be associated with pain. However, for most other locations of oral cancer, pain occurs very late in the disease process, which often leads to delay in seeking medical treatment. Associated symptoms may include dysphagia, odynophagia, weight loss, bleeding, or referred pain in the ear or jaw. The patient also may experience loose teeth or dentures.

Patient Screening

Follow office policy for new referrals or oncology follow-up.

Etiology

Greater than 90% of oral cancers are SCCs. The lip is the most common location of oral cancer because it has the risk factor of sun exposure. Those who smoke and drink have 15 times higher incidence of oral cancer compared with those who do not. Use of alcohol and tobacco, especially cigarette smoking and snuff dipping, accounts for up to 80% of cases of oral cancer. The combined effect of alcohol and smoking is multiplicative. Betel nut chewing, a practice common in Southeast Asia and Micronesia, also presents an increased risk, as do infection with human papillomavirus (HPV), poor oral hygiene, and periodontal disease. HPV-16 infection is specifically of concern because of an increase in its prevalence and because it leads to oral cancer. Tobacco use decline is affecting statistics, which are being monitored.

Oral leukoplakia (see Fig. 8.14), a reactive process that presents as a white patch on the oral mucosa, and erythrodysplasia, a red patch on the mucosa, can progress to oral cancer in some individuals, so patients with these lesions require close monitoring.

Diagnosis

Although the patient often notices the oral lesion, he or she often ignores it because the lesion is usually painless. Therefore the diagnosis of oral cancer is most often made in a dental office. The diagnosis is confirmed via fine-needle aspiration biopsy. Staging of oral cancer is performed via contrast-enhanced CT, MRI, or positron emission tomography (PET) to determine the extent of tumor infiltration. The lung, liver, and bone are the most common sites for metastasis, so chest x-ray and measurement of serum alkaline phosphatase and liver function tests are usually performed. Oral tumors are classified and staged according to the TNM classification system proposed by the American Joint Committee on Cancer (AJCC). See Chapter 1 for information about the staging and grading systems used to assess malignant neoplasms.

Treatment

The treatment for oral cancer depends on the stage. Early oral cancers are treated with surgery, with or without radiotherapy, although the use of laser therapy in the excision of early-stage oral cancers has been increasing. Neck dissection may be performed at the time of surgery to detect nodal metastases. Therapeutic irradiation is often employed for advanced tumors. Regular follow-up is needed to evaluate for recurrences after tumor removal. Speech and swallowing rehabilitation may be needed after treatment.

Prognosis

Patients with large tumors or nodal metastases have a worse prognosis compared with patients with small, localized tumors. Because oral cancer often is diagnosed late, the overall expected 5-year survival rate is about 59%. Survival percentages increase in patients who stop smoking.

Prevention

Oral examination to detect premalignant or early malignant lesions should be performed during routine visits to the dentist. Abstinence from tobacco and alcohol is recommended. Immunization with the HPV vaccine decreases the risk of HPV-associated oral cancer. After treatment, close follow-up is needed, because many of these cancers recur.

Patient Teaching

Review information about the treatment plan, and encourage questions. Ensure that the patient understands the plan for control of pain and side effects of any therapeutic intervention. Educate treated patients on the symptoms of recurrences such as hoarseness, pain and lymphadenopathy

Diseases of the Gastrointestinal Tract

The alimentary canal, or GI tract, is a hollow continuous tube that extends from the mouth to the anus. It propels the products of digestion by peristalsis, a coordinated, wavelike muscular motion that forces food along the alimentary canal. It is also the site of the processes of mechanical and chemical breakdown of food. As the food passes through the tract, it is broken down into molecules that can be absorbed through the intestinal wall for distribution to body cells for metabolism via the bloodstream.

Water and electrolytes are absorbed in the proximal colon; waste material is stored in the rectum, and indigestible wastes are voluntarily evacuated through the anus.

Gastroesophageal Reflux Disease

Description

GERD refers to clinical manifestations of regurgitation of stomach and duodenal contents into the esophagus, frequently occurring at night (Fig. 8.15). Mild episodes may be described as heartburn by the patient.

ICD-10-CM Code	K21.9 (Gastroesophageal reflux disease without esophagitis) (K21.0-K21.9 = 2 codes of specificity)

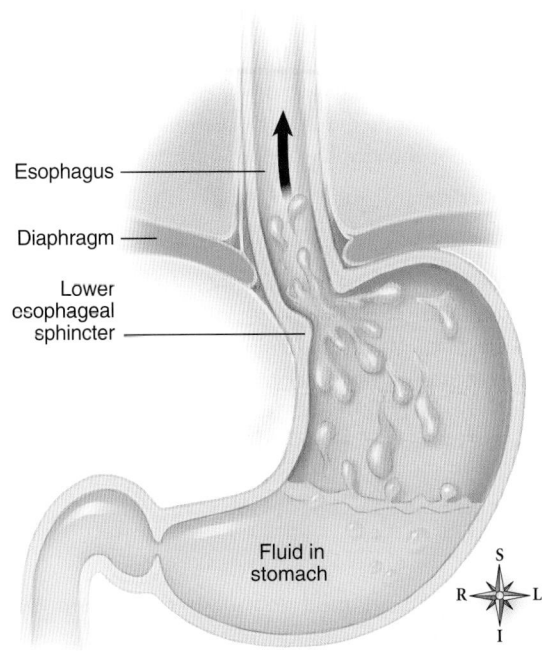

• **Fig. 8.15** Gastroesophageal reflux disease (GERD). (From Patton KT, Thibodeau GA: *The human body in health & disease,* ed 6, Maryland Heights, 2014, Elsevier.)

Symptoms and Signs

The patient typically experiences belching, with a burning sensation in the chest and mouth. A coughing spell and wheezing caused by irritation to the oropharynx or respiratory tree may follow. Vomitus may regurgitate into the mouth. Chronic and frequent GERD may lead to dysphagia and erosive esophagitis with bleeding. Acid gastric fluid (pH < 4) is extremely caustic to the esophageal mucosa and is the major injurious agent in the majority of cases. In some patients, reflux of bile or alkaline pancreatic secretions may be contributory. Tooth enamel may become eroded, leading to caries. Other complications include esophageal stricture caused by scar tissue, ulceration of the mucosa, and pulmonary aspiration. A subtype of GERD is laryngopharyngeal reflux (LPR), which may present as a chronic nonproductive cough, hoarseness, or frequent clearing of the throat.

Patient Screening

The patient may have symptoms that mimic angina pectoris or may report blood in sputum. These are indications for prompt evaluation by the appropriate health care professional.

Etiology

Reflux can result from overeating, pregnancy, or weight gain. GERD that causes pathology frequently is associated with relaxation of the lower esophageal sphincter (LES) or an increase in intraabdominal pressure. Patients with hiatal hernia frequently experience GERD. Certain medications, including theophylline, calcium channel blockers, alendronate, and meperidine, can contribute to GERD. Some foods, coffee, and alcohol can aggravate the condition. Some medications, such as birth control pills, antihistamines, antispasmodics, and some asthma drugs, can reduce the strength of the esophageal sphincter, causing the symptoms of GERD.

Diagnosis

The history and clinical evidence of GERD are most important in establishing a diagnosis. A radiographic test called *Barium swallow* may help diagnose gross changes, such as strictures or ulcerations. Esophagoscopy or esophagogastroduodenoscopy (EGD) is a superior diagnostic method, which may include biopsy of any abnormality or dilation of strictures. Esophageal pH monitoring and scanning tests are other probative methods of diagnosis.

Treatment

When symptoms are mild and of short duration, simple measures to eliminate episodes of reflux may be employed. These include elevating the head of the bed about 6 inches, using multiple pillows to maintain the non-supine position, ingesting a light evening meal no less than 4 hours before bedtime, and using antacids. Weight loss is indicated if the person is obese. Strict limitation or elimination of alcohol ingestion and smoking is recommended. Should these interventions fail, systemic medical management is initiated. Use of an histamine-2 (H_2) receptor antagonist, such as ranitidine or famotidine, or a proton pump inhibitor (PPI; omeprazole, lansoprazole, rabeprazole, or esomeprazole), inhibits acid secretion and allows for healing of the esophagus. Antireflux surgery is used conservatively. Symptomatic complications of chronic GERD are treated as needed.

Prognosis

When simple interventions fail and the condition is chronic, symptoms typically improve with drug therapy. Complications include ulceration and strictures of the esophagus, asthma, and Barrett esophagus, a precancerous condition.

Prevention

Preventive measures are directed at managing the causes that can be controlled.

Patient Teaching

Explain how positional therapy uses gravity to reduce the onset of reflux. Instruct the patient not to recline until 4 hours after eating. List the warning signs of complications, such as dysphagia, odynophagia, pulmonary symptoms, an increase in esophageal burning, bleeding, or unexplained weight loss and dehydration. Explain the importance of follow-up appointments with the physician or health care provider to monitor the treatment plan.

◆◆ ENRICHMENT

Digestive Distress Signals

- Hiccup is an involuntary spasmodic contraction of the diaphragm in which the beginning of an inspiration is suddenly checked by closure of the glottis, resulting in the characteristic sound. It is usually transient.
- *Indigestion* is a term frequently used to denote vague abdominal discomfort after meals. Indigestion and eructation (belching) are common symptoms of upper GI tract disease.
- Heartburn is a sensation of retrosternal warmth or burning occurring in waves and tending to rise upward toward the neck; it may be accompanied by reflux of fluid into the mouth (regurgitation).
- Nausea is an unpleasant sensation in the epigastrium. It often culminates in vomiting.
- Vomiting is the forcible expulsion of the contents of the stomach through the mouth.
- Colic is acute visceral pain caused by spasm, torsion, or obstruction of a hollow organ.
- Flatulence is the presence of extensive amounts of air or gases in the stomach or intestines, leading to distention of the organs.
- Diarrhea is abnormally frequent passage of loose stools.
- Constipation is a condition of infrequent bowel evacuation. It may have functional or organic causes.
- Fecal incontinence is an inability to control defecation.

Esophageal Varices

Description

Esophageal varices are dilated submucosal veins that develop in patients with underlying portal hypertension and may result in serious upper GI bleeding.

ICD-10-CM Code	I85.00 (*Esophageal varices without bleeding*)
	I85.01 (*Esophageal varices with bleeding*)
	(I85.0-I85.11 = 4 codes of specificity)

Symptoms and Signs

The superficial veins lining the esophagus become dilated and twisted at the distal end of the esophagus (Fig. 8.16). In some cases, there may be preceding retching or dyspepsia attributable to alcoholic gastritis or withdrawal. Actual varices do not cause symptoms, such as dyspepsia, dysphagia, or retching. Varices may be asymptomatic until a rupture causes a massive hemorrhage. With rupture, the patient experiences hematemesis or melena, and signs of hypovolemic shock may develop.

Patient Screening

Variceal hemorrhage can be life-threatening and is a medical emergency. If the patient is not already hospitalized, immediate referral to an emergency room is essential.

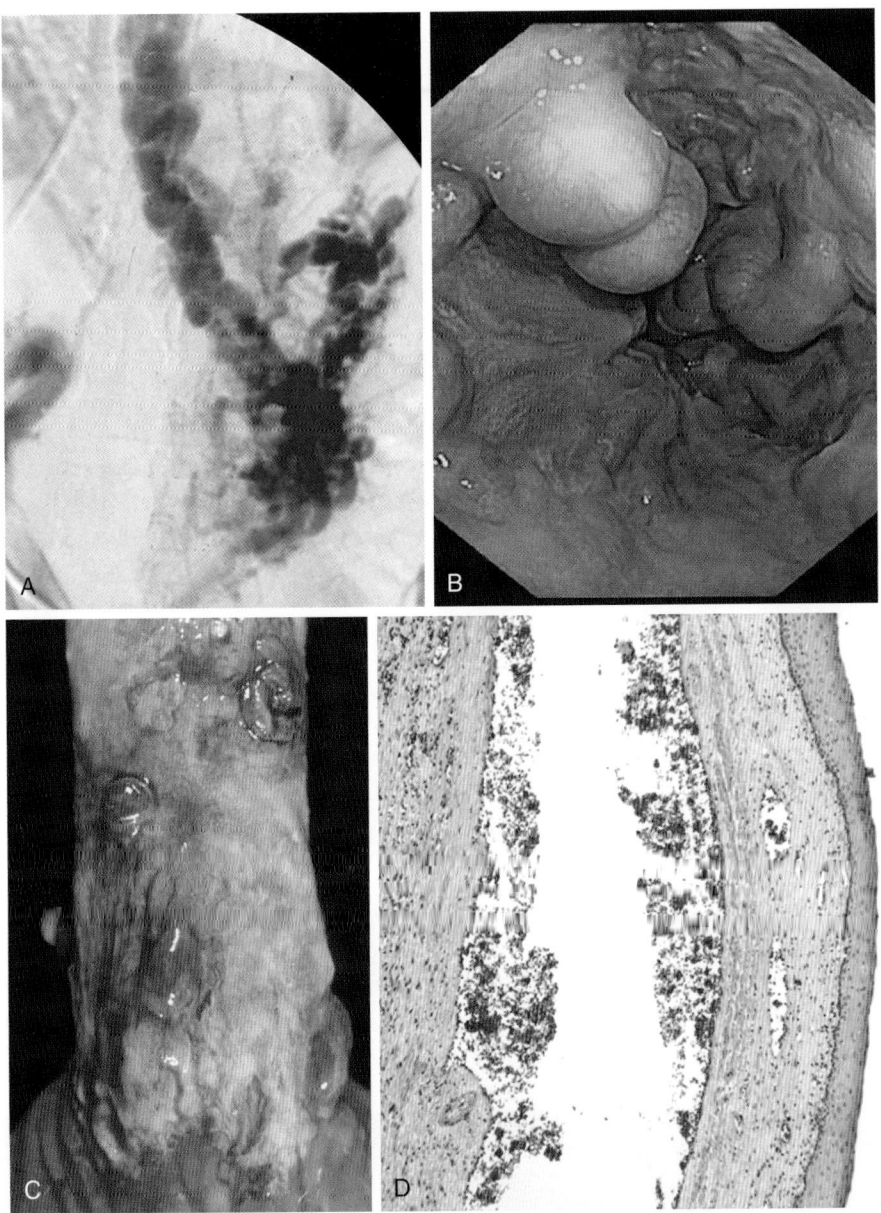

• **Fig. 8.16** Esophageal varices. (From Kumar V, et al: *Robbins basic pathology,* ed 10, Philadelphia, 2018, Saunders.)

Etiology

Varices result from increased pressure within the veins. This pressure develops when the venous return to the liver is impeded. Esophageal varices occur in about two-thirds of all patients with cirrhosis of the liver and are often associated with alcoholic cirrhosis. Esophageal varices are a common complication of cirrhosis of the liver because destruction of hepatic tissue interferes with emptying of the portal vein, resulting in portal hypertension. Although approximately 50% of patients with cirrhosis have esophageal varices, only one-third of patients with varices develop serious bleeding from the varices.

Diagnosis

Diagnosis is based on the clinical picture and a history of hepatic disease, specifically cirrhosis. Radiographic examination is indicated to study any obstruction of blood flow that causes back pressure in the esophageal vessels. Esophageal varices can be noted during endoscopic examination. Patients with cirrhosis are prone to varices and should be screened with endoscopy so that preventive measures can be instituted.

Treatment

The principal treatment of a patient with bleeding esophageal varices is the same as that for any patient with gross GI bleeding: replacing the blood volume and maintaining the fluid and electrolyte balance to restore homeostasis. Interventions to control and prevent recurrences of bleeding include endoscopic sclerotherapy and ligation of bleeding varices. In patients with variceal bleeding that cannot be controlled with pharmacologic or endoscopic therapy, emergency portal decompression may be considered.

Prognosis

Bleeding esophageal varices have a higher morbidity and mortality rate than any other source of upper GI bleeding. The long-term prognosis is somewhat guarded because of the tendency to hemorrhage. Forty percent of patients die during the first episode of massive hemorrhage. Of those who survive, recurrent bleeding frequently occurs within 1 year, with a similar mortality rate for each episode.

Prevention

Esophageal varices are often associated with hepatic disease, which may or may not be preventable.

Patient Teaching

Illustrate how obstruction of blood flow causes back pressure in the esophageal vessels. Teach the patient how to monitor for overt signs of upper GI bleeding. When intervention is required to control bleeding, explain the procedure and its purpose.

Esophagitis

Description

Esophagitis is inflammation and tissue injury of the esophagus.

ICD-10-CM Code	K20.9 *(Esophagitis, unspecified)*
	(K20.0-K20.9 = 3 codes of specificity)

Esophagitis is coded according to types and causes. Refer to the physician's diagnosis and then to the current edition of the ICD-10-CM coding manual to ensure the greatest specificity.

Symptoms and Signs

The main symptom that the patient experiences is burning chest pain (heartburn), which can make the patient believe that he or she is having a heart attack. The onset of pain typically follows eating or drinking. The patient even may have some vomiting of blood (hematemesis).

Corrosive esophagitis is severe inflammation of the esophagus resulting from ingestion of a caustic chemical (alkali or acid) that causes tissue damage (Fig. 8.17). In children, ingestion is usually accidental; in adults, chemical ingestion often is a suicide attempt. The degree of damage to the esophageal tissue ranges from pain and inability to swallow and speak to perforation and even destruction of the esophagus.

Patient Screening

Acute cases caused by ingestion of a caustic chemical require emergency care.

Etiology

The most common cause of esophagitis is reflux of the acid contents of the stomach resulting from a defect of the LES. The stomach acids irritate the esophageal lining and may cause an inflammatory response. Erosive esophagitis may occur after taking antibiotics, such as tetracycline, without drinking adequate amounts of water. Chemical injury may also be a cause. Esophagitis also can appear as a GI manifestation of HIV infection.

Diagnosis

Assessment begins with patient history and radiography of the upper GI tract (esophagoscopy) to confirm diagnosis and determine the extent of inflammation and tissue

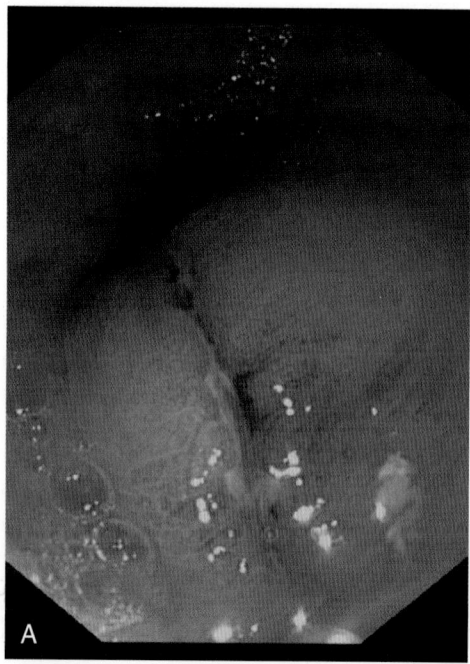 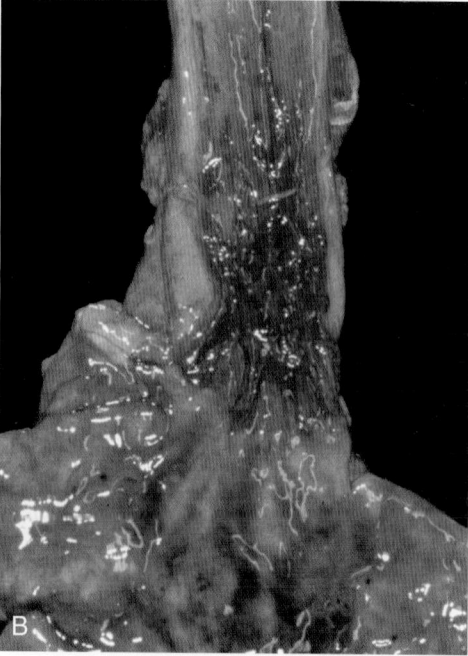

• **Fig. 8.17** Corrosive esophagitis. (Endoscopic image Courtesy Dr. Ira Hanan, The University of Chicago, Chicago, Illinois.)

damage. A history of chemical ingestion and the presence of redness and oropharyngeal burn point to caustic esophagitis.

Treatment

The treatment of esophagitis is determined by etiology. In mild cases of reflux esophagitis, treatment may include a bland diet and a course of antacids. Underlying causes of reflux, such as hiatal hernia, are addressed in the treatment plan. Medications to reduce gastric acid production, such as cimetidine (Tagamet) or omeprazole (Prilosec), are effective. Sucralfate (Carafate) suspension sometimes is prescribed to relieve discomfort and to promote healing. Meals should be small and frequent, and alcohol must be avoided.

Esophageal stricture may require dilation; esophageal perforation requires emergency endoscopic or surgical repair.

Prognosis

The prognosis for esophagitis is good if the patient adheres to treatments prescribed by the health care professional. Complications of chronic or caustic esophagitis include scarring and stricture of the esophagus. Caustic ingestions increase the risk of esophageal cancer throughout the patient's lifetime.

Prevention

There is no known prevention for esophagitis, but avoiding alcohol, spicy foods, and caffeine helps relieve the symptoms.

Patient Teaching

Advise the patient that close monitoring of the condition is required during the treatment and the healing process. Assess the need for psychological counseling when chemical ingestions result from suicide attempts or any nonaccidental causes.

Esophageal Cancer

Description

Esophageal cancer occurs in two main forms. The esophagus is lined for most of its length with squamous epithelium, which can give rise to SCC (Fig. 8.18). Adenocarcinoma may develop in the columnar epithelium near the esophagogastric junction.

ICD-10-CM Code	C15.9 *(Malignant neoplasm of esophagus, unspecified)*
	(C15.3-C15.9 = 5 codes of specificity)

Esophageal cancer is coded according to the site of the lesion. Refer to the physician's diagnosis and then to the current edition of the ICD-10-CM coding manual to ensure the greatest specificity.

Symptoms and Signs

Symptoms may include dysphagia, weight loss, and retrosternal discomfort or a burning sensation. Iron deficiency anemia may result from chronic esophageal blood loss. If the

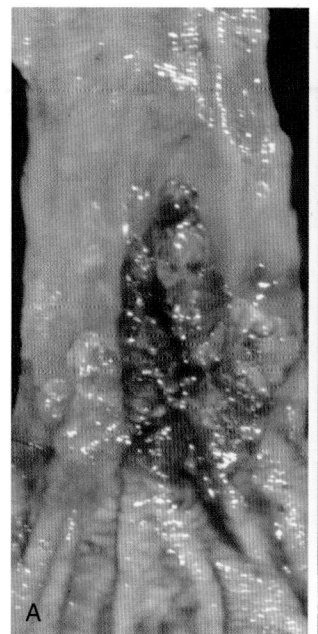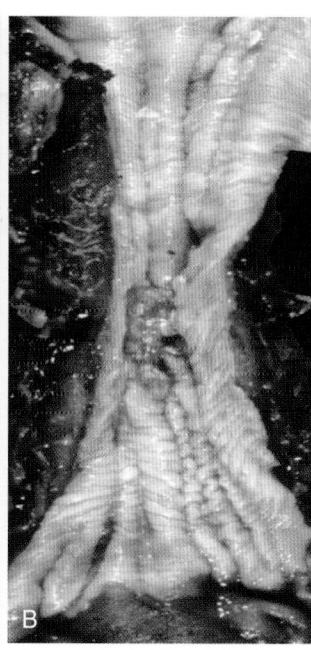

• **Fig. 8.18** Carcinoma of the Esophagus. (A) Esophageal adenocarcinoma. (B) Esophageal squamous cell carcinoma. (From Kumar V, et al: *Robbins basic pathology,* ed 10, Philadelphia, 2018, Saunders.)

tumor involves the laryngeal nerve, hoarseness may result. A tracheoesophageal **fistula** may develop during the late stages of the disease, with coughing or frequent pneumonias occurring when saliva, liquid, or food spills into the lungs.

Patient Screening

A health care professional must be contacted for patient referrals and follow-up appointments.

Etiology

The incidence of SCC of the esophagus varies, with the highest rates being found in Asia, Africa, and Iran. Risk factors for SCC include cigarette smoking, alcohol consumption, betel nut chewing (a practice common in some Asian countries), drinking of very hot beverages (greater than 149°F [65°C]); eating of foods containing N-nitroso compounds (e.g., pickled vegetables); a diet low in fruit and vegetables; a history of head and neck cancer; and underlying esophageal disease, such as achalasia or caustic strictures. Adenocarcinoma predominantly affects Caucasians and males. The major risk factors are Barrett esophagus (see the Enrichment box about Barrett Esophagus) and chronic GERD. The risk of adenocarcinoma is greater in patients who smoke or those who are obese.

Diagnosis

Physicians and other health care providers detect most esophageal cancers during evaluation of symptomatic patients or incidentally during screening of high-risk individuals with endoscopic examination. Among patients who have symptoms suggestive of esophageal cancer, a barium study may be used for the initial assessment. An endoscopic biopsy is necessary to confirm the diagnosis.

Barrett Esophagus

One of the most severe consequences of chronic gastroesophageal reflux disease (GERD) is the replacement of the normal stratified squamous epithelium of the distal esophagus by abnormal columnar epithelium. This condition is known as *Barrett esophagus*. In one sense, it is a protective metaplastic change produced because the columnar epithelium is more resistant to acid damage compared with the original stratified squamous epithelium, but at the same time, this adaptation predisposes the individual to the development of adenocarcinoma of the esophagus and of the proximal stomach.

Barrett esophagus is usually diagnosed during endoscopic examination of middle-aged and older adults (Fig. 8.19). The metaplasia itself causes no symptoms, and the condition is usually discovered when patients are being seen for symptoms of GERD, such as heartburn, regurgitation, and dysphagia. Endoscopic screening of patients with GERD is only recommended if the patient has multiple other risk factors for adenocarcinoma, such as obesity, age greater than 50 years, male gender, or a history of hiatal hernia.

The gene-related changes leading from the development of Barrett esophagus to adenocarcinoma are not completely understood. We do know that before the cells acquire enough DNA damage to become malignant, dysplastic morphologic changes appear. The use of acid-suppressive medications has been shown to slow the progression of dysplasia.

Although no management strategy has been proven to prolong life, there are several options currently in use: treatment of GERD, endoscopic surveillance to detect dysplasia, and treatment of the dysplasia. GERD is usually treated with PPI medications. For patients found to have diffuse low-grade dysplasia on endoscopic examination, the frequency of endoscopic examination often is increased from every 3 to 5 years to every 6 months to 1 year. In patients with high-grade dysplasia, progress to adenocarcinoma is much more common but still varies. Because of this risk, however, the American Gastroenterological Association now recommends endoscopic eradication of the dysplastic tissue by using radiofrequency ablation, photodynamic therapy, or resection.

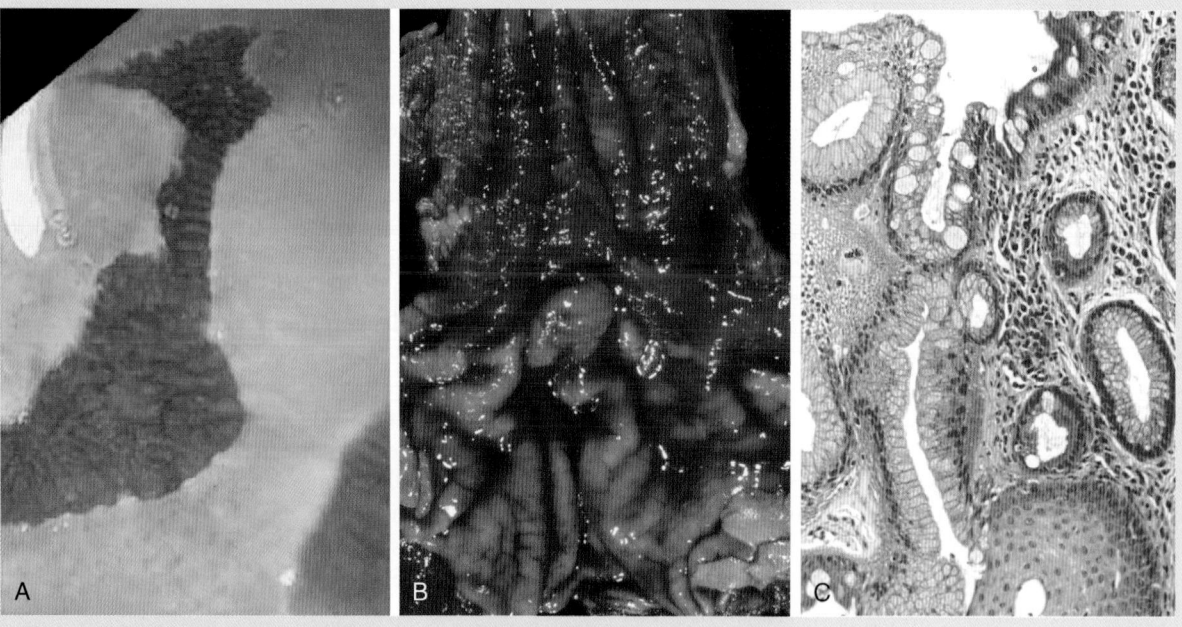

• **Fig. 8.19** Barrett esophagus. (Endoscopic image Courtesy Dr. Ira Hanan, The University of Chicago, Chicago, Illinois.)

After the initial patient evaluation, diagnosis includes assessment of the operative risk and staging. Esophageal tumors are staged according to the TNM classification system proposed by the AJCC. SCCs and adenocarcinomas have different staging groups. Staging involves CT, PET, and endoscopic ultrasonography (EUS) to evaluate for metastatic disease and to determine whether surgical resection of the tumor is a realistic option. The most common sites of metastasis are the lung, liver, bone, and adrenal gland. At times, a diagnostic laparoscopy is required for complete staging. See Chapter 1 for information about the staging and grading systems used to assess malignant neoplasms.

Treatment

Accurate staging is critical to selecting a treatment method. Patients with clinically localized cancer often undergo chemoradiotherapy either before or after surgery. EUS is used to detect recurrence of the disease after successful tumor excision. For patients with advanced, unresectable disease, the therapeutic goal is to maintain the ability to swallow. Nonoperative measures may be used to palliate symptoms. Radiation, with or without chemotherapy, and endoscopic stent placement are used to treat dysphagia by shrinking the tumor and dilating the esophagus, respectively. These methods also reduce the risk of aspiration and weight loss but rarely improve the survival of the patient. There is little doubt that SCC and adenocarcinoma represent different disease processes, but it is unknown whether or how they should be treated differently.

Prognosis

The prognosis is highly associated with the stage but is generally poor because esophageal cancer of both types has a high propensity for metastasis even in the earliest stages. The overall 5-year survival rate is less than 20%.

Prevention

Those with Barrett esophagus usually undergo endoscopics to screen for progression to adenocarcinoma. In addition, the patient should avoid practices associated with increased risk, such as the use of alcohol and tobacco.

Patient Teaching

Assess the patient's comprehension of the diagnosis and the treatment plan. Discuss the possible side effects of radiation, chemotherapy, or surgery, as appropriate. Encourage the patient to ask questions and discuss his or her anxiety. Provide a list of local cancer support groups and other appropriate referrals.

Gastric and Duodenal Peptic Ulcers

Description

Should the protective mucous membrane of the stomach or upper intestinal tract break down, the lining is prone to ulceration. These internal surface lesions can be acute or chronic, clustered or singular, and shallow or deep. Deep sores develop within the deep muscle layer of tissue (Fig. 8.20).

ICD-10-CM Code	K25.9 *(Gastric ulcer, unspecified as acute or chronic, without hemorrhage or perforation)*
	(K25.0-K25.9 = 9 codes of specificity)
	K26.9 *(Duodenal ulcer, unspecified as acute or chronic, without hemorrhage or perforation)*
	(K26.0-K26.9 = 9 codes of specificity)
	K27.9 *(Peptic ulcer, site unspecified, unspecified as acute or chronic, without hemorrhage or perforation)*
	(K27.0-K27.9 = 9 codes of specificity)

Gastric, duodenal, and peptic ulcers are coded according to the pathology involved. Refer to the physician's diagnosis and then to the current edition of the ICD-10-CM coding manual to ensure the greatest specificity.

Symptoms and Signs

When the peptic ulcer occurs in the stomach (gastric ulcer), often the patient is asymptomatic, particularly if it is caused by ingestion of antiinflammatory agents, such as NSAIDs (e.g., ibuprofen [Motrin]). However, the patient may report heartburn or indigestion and epigastric pain that is described as gnawing, dull, aching, or "hungerlike." Some patients experience pain or a feeling of uncomfortable fullness after eating, causing them to avoid eating, and this results in loss of weight and predisposition to dehydration.

The most common type of peptic ulcer is the duodenal ulcer (an ulcer of the first part of the small intestine), which causes symptoms that range from subtle midepigastric pain and heartburn to intense pain in the upper abdomen with nausea and vomiting. The patient may be observed guarding the painful area by clutching the stomach, assuming a crouching position, or sitting with the knees drawn up to the chest. Some patients have reported that frequent eating helps relieve discomfort; attacks of the most intense pain may erupt 2 hours after a meal.

Two-thirds of duodenal ulcers and one-third of gastric ulcers cause nocturnal pain that awakens the patient.

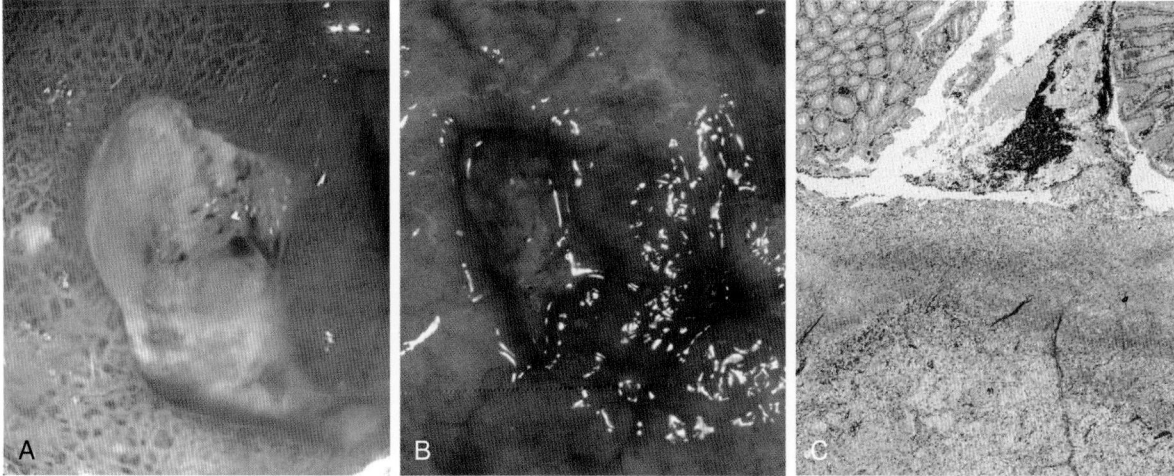

• **Fig. 8.20** Peptic ulcer. (Endoscopic image Courtesy Dr. Ira Hanan, The University of Chicago, Chicago, Illinois.)

If these ulcers bleed internally, occult (hidden) or frank (obvious) blood is found in the vomitus or stool. The situation is more serious if the lesion invades deeply and perforates, causing hemorrhage and leakage of the contents of the stomach or intestine into the abdominal cavity. A change from a patient's typical rhythmic discomfort to constant or radiating pain may indicate penetration or perforation.

Patient Screening

Sudden onset of pain and vomiting with overt signs of bleeding present an urgent need for medical care.

Etiology

Although the cause is not always clear, an area of breakdown of the mucous membrane precipitates ulceration of the epithelial lining of the stomach or the intestine. A crucial causal factor of peptic ulcers is *Helicobacter pylori* infection, which is thought to be the most common worldwide human bacterial infection (Fig. 8.21). When present, it produces inflammation in the mucous membrane of the GI tract. The second most common form of ulcer is related to the use of NSAIDs (e.g., ibuprofen [Motrin]). The less common gastric ulcers follow chronic gastritis, in which the gastric mucosa becomes less able to defend itself against erosion. Some of the known contributing catalysts are the ingestion of gastric irritants; the use of ulcerogenic drugs, such as alcohol, aspirin, and other antiinflammatory agents; smoking; and the presence of a bacterial infection *(H. pylori)*. Gastric ulcers are most common in middle-aged men.

Duodenal ulcers are associated with an increase of acid and gastric juice (pepsin). Predisposing factors include the presence of *H. pylori* infection, drinking alcohol, and use of NSAIDs. In the United States, about 500,000 new cases of peptic ulcer and 4 million ulcer recurrences are diagnosed per year. Ulcers occur five times more commonly in the duodenum. Ulcers occur more commonly in men than in women (1.3 : 1). Although ulcers can occur in any age group, duodenal ulcers most commonly occur in patients 30 to 55 years of age, whereas gastric ulcers are more common in patients 55 to 70 years of age.

Diagnosis

The patient report of an illness can help distinguish between a gastric ulcer and a duodenal ulcer. The diagnosis of a peptic ulcer can be suspected on the basis of the patient's history and physical examination findings. The diagnosis may be confirmed with barium radiography of the upper GI tract to detect abnormal appearance and function, or the ulcer may be visualized through upper GI tract endoscopy (Fig. 8.22). Diagnostic studies are available to identify *H. pylori*. Gastric contents are sometimes collected and analyzed for the level of acidity or the presence of blood in the secretions. The patient's stool also is analyzed for evidence of blood. Blood tests indicating reduced hemoglobin (Hgb) concentration and reduced hematocrit (Hct) may confirm a bleeding ulcer. Biopsy, with microscopic study of the tissue specimen, rules out or confirms the presence of cancer. Serum albumin and transferrin levels may be reduced if the patient has weight loss and malnutrition. Abdominal radiographic studies are performed to investigate the possibility of perforation or other abdominal conditions.

Treatment

The management of peptic ulcers requires rest, medication, changes in the diet, and adjustments in lifestyle, especially for stress reduction. Surgery may be indicated in severe cases. If the etiology is confirmed (e.g., use of an ulcerogenic drug, such as aspirin; NSAIDs; and alcohol), the identified agent must be eliminated. Drug therapy includes

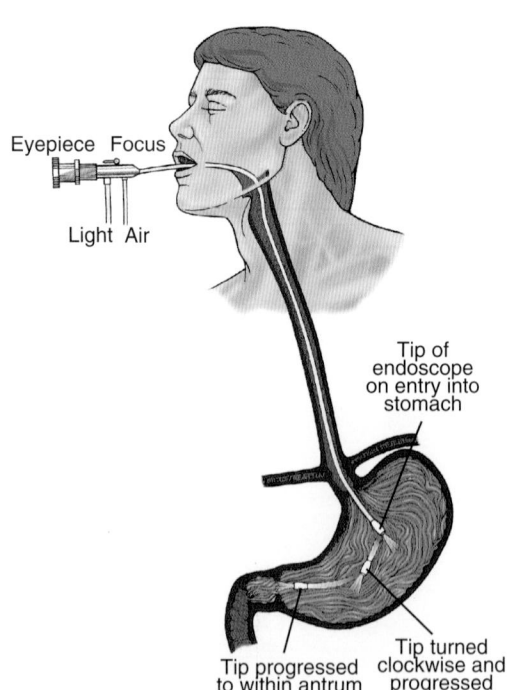

• **Fig. 8.22** Upper gastrointestinal (GI) tract endoscopy is a procedure that allows direct visualization of the interior of upper GI structures resulting in an accurate and sensitive evaluation of mucosal lesions; it is possible to obtain biopsy specimens, to perform superficial operative procedures, or to make an assessment of the course of a disease. The endoscope, a thin flexible tube equipped with a camera and a light source, is inserted through the mouth and guided by a television monitor. (From *Mosby's dictionary of medicine, nursing and health professions,* ed 8, St Louis, 2009, Mosby.)

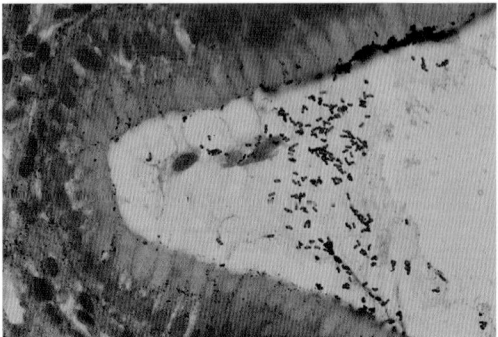

• **Fig. 8.21** *Helicobacter pylori.* (From Cotran R, et al: *Robbins pathologic basis of disease,* ed 6, Philadelphia, 1999, Saunders.)

one or more of the following: H₂ receptor blocking agents to control gastric secretion (e.g., nizatidine [Axid], famotidine [Pepcid], cimetidine [Tagamet], and ranitidine [Zantac]); antacids (e.g., magnesium hydroxide-aluminum hydroxide [Maalox]) to reduce gastric acidity; coating agents (e.g., sucralfate) to protect the mucosa; and PPIs (e.g., omeprazole [Prilosec], esomeprazole [Nexium], pantoprazole [Protonix], and lansoprazole [Prevacid]) to suppress the secretion of gastric acid. When *H. pylori* is identified as the cause, antibiotic therapy, such as clarithromycin (Biaxin) with amoxicillin, combined with a PPI, may be prescribed. Small, frequent meals of soft, bland foods are better tolerated.

All of these measures attempt to relieve symptoms and encourage the healing process. Significant bleeding or perforation of the ulcer calls for more aggressive measures, such as surgical intervention, the administration of intravenous (IV) fluids, and blood replacement.

Prognosis

Peptic ulcers can heal. Patients are instructed to follow the recommended preventive measures even after healing, because peptic ulcer disease tends to recur. Any nonhealing ulcer, and all gastric ulcers should be evaluated via endoscopy to rule out cancer.

Prevention

Avoid alcohol ingestion and smoking. NSAIDs and aspirin must be used appropriately.

Patient Teaching

Refer the patient to a registered dietitian (RD) for nutritional consultation. Have the patient eliminate caffeine, alcohol, smoking, and any other identified irritants. Reinforce the importance of strict adherence to a bland diet high in vitamin K. Instruct the patient to take prescribed analgesics or **antiemetics** 1 hour before meals to help control pain or nausea. Warn the patient to report any signs of hematemesis and any occurrence of black or bloody stools.

Gastritis

Description

Gastritis is inflammation of the lining of the stomach; the acute form is a common disorder.

ICD-10-CM Code	K29.70 *(Gastritis, unspecified, without bleeding)*
	K29.90 *(Gastroduodenitis, unspecified, without bleeding)*
	(K29.00-K29.91 = 18 codes of specificity)

Gastritis is coded according to the pathology involved. Refer to the physician's diagnosis and then to the current edition of the ICD-10-CM coding manual to ensure the greatest specificity.

Symptoms and Signs

The mucosal layer of the stomach normally acts as a physical barrier to protect against injury, inflammation, and erosion. When the stomach lining becomes inflamed, the patient experiences epigastric pain, indigestion, and a feeling of fullness after meals. Other discomforts, such as nausea, belching, and fatty food intolerance, cause the patient to lose his or her appetite. When the gastric mucosa is inflamed and swollen, it can bleed, and blood can be seen and detected in the patient's vomitus and stool. Chronic gastritis is more common in older adults.

Patient Screening

Sudden onset of pain and hematemesis requires emergency medical care.

Etiology

Similar to symptoms of peptic ulcers, the main cause of gastritis is inflammation associated with *H. pylori*. Many agents damage the gastric lining, including common medications, such as aspirin and other antiinflammatory drugs, poisons, alcohol, smoking tobacco or other substances, infectious diseases, stress, and mechanical injury resulting from the swallowing of a foreign object (Fig. 8.23). The repeated ingestion of irritating foods or allergic reaction to foods irritates the gastric mucosa.

Chronic gastritis is associated with peptic ulcer disease and recurring exposure to irritating substances. It can also occur in patients with a history of chronic disease, such as pernicious anemia. A substantial number of patients have idiopathic gastritis. Paradoxically, gastritis also can result from the lack of production of gastric acids, which is sometimes associated with a condition caused by vitamin B₁₂ deficiency called *pernicious anemia.*

Diagnosis

Gastroscopy allows for visualization of the interior of the stomach, and radiography helps rule out other structural abnormalities. Biopsy specimens are obtained to determine the cause and extent of disease. Blood counts and serum tests offer additional findings. Fecal occult blood test results may be positive because of gastric bleeding.

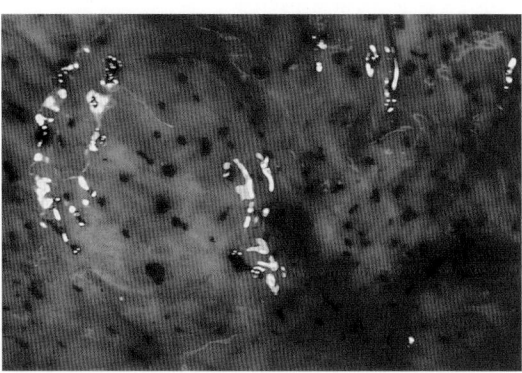

• **Fig. 8.23** Chemical gastritis caused by aspirin. (From Damjanov I, Linder J: *Pathology: a color atlas,* St Louis, 1999, Mosby.)

Treatment

Curing *H. pylori* infection with antibiotic therapy often rapidly resolves superficial gastritis. If any other source of irritation is known, it is eliminated or controlled. Gastric discomfort is relieved with the use of antacids and medications, such as cimetidine (Tagamet), ranitidine hydrochloride (Zantac), famotidine (Pepcid), omeprazole (Prilosec), or pantoprazole (Protonix) to reduce the secretion of gastric acid. If the patient has bleeding, it is monitored and treated with medicines that constrict blood vessels. Antibiotics are given for *H. pylori* infection, and antiemetics are given to help control nausea and vomiting. The patient is given a bland diet as tolerated, with vitamin and mineral supplements as needed. If the patient has vitamin B$_{12}$ deficiency, injections of vitamin B$_{12}$ must be administered each month for an indefinite period.

Prognosis

Acute mild cases of gastritis improve with conservative treatment and elimination of the known irritant. Chronic gastritis is monitored for complications.

Prevention

Preventive measures are the same as those for gastric and duodenal ulcers.

Patient Teaching

It is essential to refer patients to a psychologist for extreme stress resulting from experiencing a serious illness. Teaching the patient about the relationship between gastritis and the contributing lifestyle factors can promote healing and prevent recurrences (see Patient Teaching in the Gastric and Duodenal Peptic Ulcers section).

Gastric Cancer

Description

Gastric cancer occurs in the stomach, the organ located in the upper abdomen that connects the esophagus and the small intestine (Fig. 8.24).

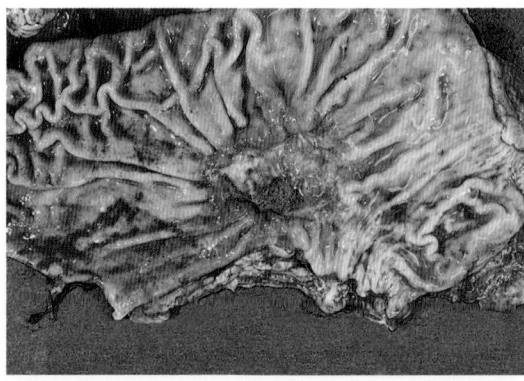

• **Fig. 8.24** Ulcerative gastric carcinoma. (From Cotran R, et al: *Robbins pathologic basis of disease,* ed 6, Philadelphia, 1999, Saunders.)

ICD-10-CM Code   C16.9 *(Malignant neoplasm of stomach, unspecified)*
(C16.0-C16.9 = 9 codes of specificity)

Gastric cancer is coded according to the site of the lesion. Refer to the physician's diagnosis and then to the current edition of the ICD-10-CM coding manual to ensure the greatest specificity.

Symptoms and Signs

The patient with early carcinoma of the stomach is frequently asymptomatic. As the disease progresses, the most common symptoms at initial presentation are weight loss and persistent abdominal pain, although nausea, dysphagia, melena, and anorexia are also seen. Anorexia is present more often with gastric cancer than with ulcers. The most common physical finding is a palpable abdominal mass, which usually indicates advanced disease. Left supraclavicular adenopathy (Virchow node) is commonly found in metastatic disease.

Patient Screening

The patient being treated for gastric cancer may experience a variety of complications resulting from surgery, chemotherapy, or radiation. Symptoms of GI obstruction or malnutrition may be present. Physicians and other health care providers often give priority attention to these patients.

Etiology

Japan has the highest incidence of gastric cancer in the world. *H. pylori* is a known carcinogen and can cause gastric cancer, usually in the distal stomach. Barrett esophagus is the main risk factor for the development of gastric cancer in the proximal stomach. A diet high in salt, smoking, previous gastric surgery, and prior abdominal radiation exposure are known risk factors. There can be a genetic predisposition (e.g., family history of gastric cancer and blood type A). Twenty-five percent of patients have a history of gastric ulcer. A diet rich in fruits and vegetables can be protective.

Diagnosis

When gastric cancer is suspected, upper GI endoscopy with biopsy of any suspicious lesion is used for diagnosis. If biopsy of an ulcer proves it to be benign, follow-up endoscopy is recommended in 8 to 12 weeks to verify healing of the ulcer detected on the initial test. Gastric cancer is staged by using the TNM classification system proposed by the AJCC. Staging is performed on the basis of findings from the physical examination; CT of the chest, abdomen, and pelvis to detect metastases; and EUS to assess the depth of tumor invasion. For patients with significant tumor depth, laparoscopy also may be used to directly visualize the surface of the liver, peritoneum, and local lymph nodes, which are the most likely sites of metastasis. See Chapter 1 for information about the staging and grading systems used to assess malignant neoplasms.

Treatment

The treatment regimen is identified after accurate tumor staging. All patients should be tested for *H. pylori* infection and, if infected, treated with antibiotics. Gastric resection, often followed by combined chemoradiotherapy, offers the best chance of long-term survival for patients with localized disease. Total gastrectomy is performed for lesions of the proximal stomach (upper third), and subtotal gastrectomy with resection of adjacent nodal tissue is usually sufficient for distal gastric cancer. Chemoradiotherapy is often added for more advanced disease. Palliation is an important part of care of patients with gastric cancer because the majority have advanced disease at the time of diagnosis and because of the high rate of recurrence after surgical resection.

Prognosis

The prognosis of gastric cancer has improved only slightly over the last few decades despite surgical advances and a decline in incidence. Most patients will develop metastases at some point during the course of their illness. Advanced, incurable cancer is present in about 50% of patients at initial presentation. Even those who undergo potentially curative surgery have high rates of local and distant recurrences. The overall combined 5-year survival rate is about 20%.

Prevention

The high mortality rate of gastric cancer largely results from the advanced stage of the disease at presentation. Therefore detection at an early stage is very important to improve survival. The cost-effectiveness of screening asymptomatic patients remains controversial, but in Japan, Venezuela, and Chile, this practice has rendered positive outcomes with early detection of gastric cancer. In the United States, with a relatively low incidence of gastric cancer, screening is limited to those who are identified as "high risk" (those with gastric adenomas, pernicious anemia, partial gastrectomy, or familial colon cancer syndromes). These patients should receive screening endoscopy every 1 to 3 years, depending on their underlying conditions. *H. pylori* infection should be eradicated to reduce the risk of progression to gastric cancer.

Patient Teaching

Assess the patient's knowledge of the disease process and the medical management prescribed by the physician, usually an oncologist. Address any related impairment to eating and nutrition. Encourage the patient to ask questions and express any feelings of anxiety. Discuss the side effects of chemotherapy or surgery. Ensure that the patient understands all of the palliative measures provided and the warning signs to report to a physician or health care provider. Provide referrals to cancer support groups.

Acute Appendicitis

Description

Appendicitis is inflammation of the appendix, a narrow pouch that is about 3.5 inches long and extends from the first part of the large intestine (cecum) (Fig. 8.25).

ICD-10-CM Code	K35.2 (*Acute appendicitis with generalized peritonitis*) (K35.2-K38.9 = 12 codes of specificity)

Appendicitis is coded according to the pathology involved. Refer to the physician's diagnosis and then to the current edition of the ICD-10-CM coding manual to ensure the greatest specificity.

Symptoms and Signs

The appendix has no known function in humans. Classic symptoms of appendicitis include abdominal pain that usually starts as vague discomfort around the navel and, within a few hours, localizes in the right lower quadrant. As the condition worsens, the patient becomes nauseated and may vomit, runs a fever, and has diarrhea or constipation.

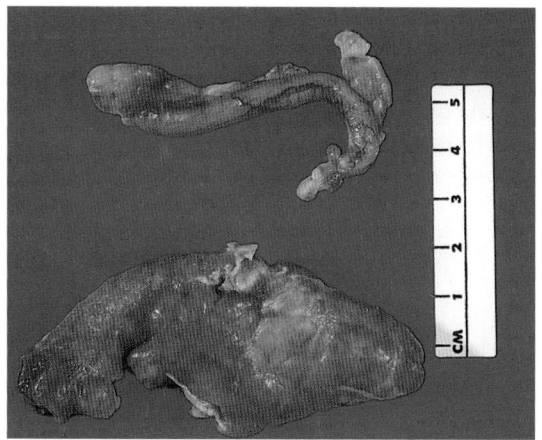
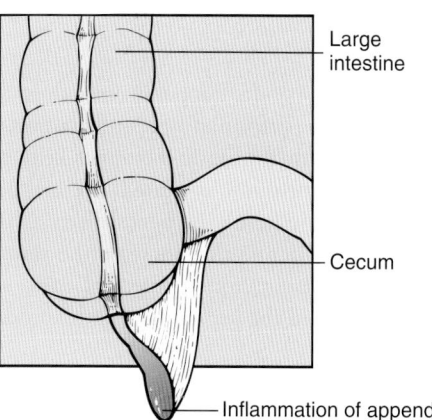

• **Fig. 8.25**   Acute appendicitis. (From Cotran R, et al: *Robbins pathologic basis of disease,* ed 6, Philadelphia, 1999, Saunders.)

Patient Screening

Clinical signs vary but usually follow a sequence, as described previously. A patient with lower abdominal pain, fever, and nausea and vomiting requires immediate medical attention.

Etiology

Obstruction of the narrow appendiceal lumen initiates the clinical illness of acute appendicitis. Obstruction has multiple causes, including lymphoid hyperplasia (related to viral illnesses, including upper respiratory infection, mononucleosis, and gastroenteritis), fecaliths, parasites, foreign bodies, Crohn disease, and primary or metastatic cancer. Whatever the cause, the pathophysiology of the disease is the same. As bacteria multiply, they invade the wall of the appendix, and eventually the circulation to the appendix is compromised. Appendicitis is most common in the 20- to 40-year-old age group.

Diagnosis

The physician or health care provider makes a differential diagnosis to rule out other causes of right lower abdominal pain and acute abdomen. Appendicitis generally can be diagnosed on the basis of physical examination findings and reported symptoms; one significant diagnostic indicator is maximal tenderness of the abdomen at the McBurney point. Rebound tenderness on the opposite side may be a sign of peritoneal irritation. Complete blood count (CBC) and urinalysis are performed and possibly repeated during hospital observation. Laboratory findings indicate an elevation in the white blood cell (WBC) count (leukocytosis). The WBC count is elevated in 80% of all cases of acute appendicitis. Unfortunately, the WBC count is elevated in up to 70% of patients with other causes of right lower abdominal pain. Thus an elevated WBC count has a low predictive value. Serial WBC measurements (over 4–8 hours) in suspected cases may increase the specificity because the WBC count often increases in acute appendicitis. The usual signs and symptoms of appendicitis in older patients are diminished, atypical, or absent and remain unrecognized, leading to a higher rate of perforation.

Treatment

Surgical removal of the appendix (appendectomy) is the indicated treatment and is performed on confirmation of appendicitis. Broad-spectrum antibiotic therapy is initiated before surgery. If appendicitis is left untreated, necrosis and rupture of the appendix can result in peritonitis, a life-threatening complication. Factors that increase the rate of perforation are delayed presentation to medical care, age extremes (the very young and the very old), and the hidden location of the appendix.

Prognosis

Complete recovery is expected with prompt medical and surgical intervention. Laparoscopic appendectomy allows for expedited recovery.

Prevention

No prevention is known, but the appendix may be removed during unrelated abdominal surgery as a prophylactic measure.

Patient Teaching

Local application of heat to the abdomen is contraindicated in the presence of the characteristic clinical symptoms of appendicitis. Postsurgical instructions include deep breathing and early ambulation to prevent complications. Review all postoperative instructions. Encourage the patient to notify the physician or health care provider with any signs of infection at the incision site.

Hiatal Hernia

Description

A hiatal hernia is a defect in the diaphragm that causes a segment of the stomach to slide into the thoracic cavity.

ICD-10-CM Code	K44.9 *(Diaphragmatic hernia without obstruction or gangrene)* (K44.0-K44.9 = 3 codes of specificity)

Symptoms and Signs

Hiatal hernia is the condition in which the upper part of the stomach protrudes through the esophageal opening of the diaphragm and into the thoracic cavity (Fig. 8.26). As a consequence, the LES muscle at the junction of the esophagus and stomach malfunctions, allowing the contents of the stomach to be regurgitated into the esophagus. This esophageal reflux (see the Gastroesophageal Reflux Disease section) can irritate the lining of the esophagus. The patient reports heartburn, which is usually worse when reclining or after a large meal. Symptoms of chest pain and difficulty swallowing may suggest that a large portion of the stomach has slipped into the opening. Respiratory complications can develop as a result of aspiration.

Some hiatal hernias are asymptomatic.

Patient Screening

When patients report heartburn, excessive belching, or distention of the stomach, a routine appointment is scheduled. If the patient has substernal chest pain, dysphagia, or bleeding, he or she should be seen as soon as possible.

> **NOTE**
> Cardiac ischemia may present as chest discomfort, nausea, or belching, which may be mistaken as symptoms of reflux or hiatal hernia.

Etiology

Hiatal hernia, a common condition, can be caused by a congenital defect in the diaphragm or a weakness that develops in the diaphragm, causing protrusion of part of the include a cholinergic agent, which helps control the episodes of reflux by strengthening the LES. Smoking is discouraged because it aggravates heartburn. Because gravity plays a role in hiatal hernia, the patient is advised to avoid lying down for 4 hours after a meal; elevating the head of the bed on blocks also helps.

If these measures fail to provide symptom relief or if the hernia becomes strangulated, surgical repair of the hiatus is the treatment of choice.

Prognosis
Compliance with conservative measures may result in control of symptoms. Should complications occur, antireflux surgical repair may be required.

Prevention
Prevention is not possible when the condition results from congenital weakness or aging.

Patient Teaching
Encourage the patient to follow the conservative measures listed earlier to control symptoms. Suggest ways to manage obesity and avoid any physical exertion that increases intraabdominal pressure.

Abdominal Hernia
Description
Abdominal hernia is the condition in which an organ protrudes through an abnormal opening in the abdominal wall,

ICD-9-CM Code	553.9 *(Unspecified site)*
ICD-10-CM Code	K46.9 *(Unspecified abdominal hernia without obstruction or gangrene)*
	(K46.0-K46.9 = 3 codes of specificity)

Symptoms and Signs
An abdominal hernia results from a weakness in the muscles and membranes of the abdominal wall that allows an organ or part of an organ to break through the wall (herniate) or protrude. This can occur to an individual of either sex and at any age. The signs and symptoms of abdominal hernias vary with the site and the size of the hernia.

The inguinal canal is a common site for hernias. A loop of bowel protrudes into the inguinal canal and, in a male, may progress to fill the scrotal sac (Fig. 8.27A). The patient notices a lump or bulge in the inguinal area and may discover that pressing on the hernia to push it back into the abdomen can reduce it. A sharp pain in the groin is continuous or made worse when standing or straining.

Complaints of severe pain usually indicate the hernia may be trapped or strangulated (see Fig. 8.27B). This means that the blood flow to the herniated organ or bowel has been stopped, and gangrene, a serious condition, can set in. The umbilicus is another common site of herniation (see Fig. 8.27C), as are surgical incisions.

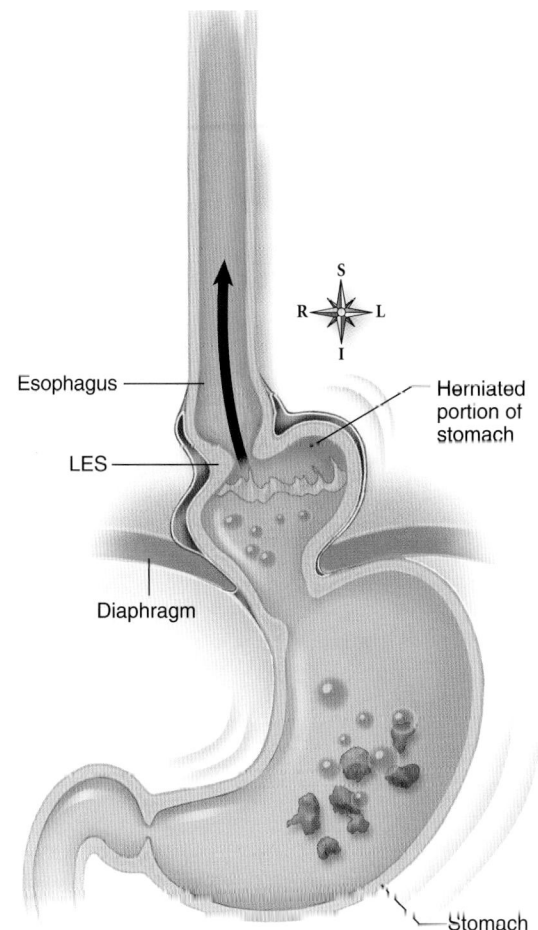

• **Fig. 8.26** Hiatal hernia. (From Patton KT, Thibodeau GA: *The human body in health & disease,* ed 6, Maryland Heights, 2014, Elsevier.)

stomach into the thoracic cavity. The weakening of the muscle can result from obesity, old age, trauma, or intraabdominal pressure; sometimes the exact cause is uncertain.

Diagnosis
Large hiatal hernias may be seen on a chest radiograph. Diagnosis is based on barium radiographic studies of the esophagus and the stomach. Endoscopy confirms the diagnosis and differentiates the condition from other diseases, such as peptic ulcers and malignant tumors. Additional diagnostic studies include measurement of reflux pH and examination of the reflux contents for the presence of blood.

Treatment
Initial treatment identifies the symptoms and prevents complications. This includes dietary modifications (smaller, more frequent meals of bland food). The patient is advised to minimize activities that increase intraabdominal pressure, such as straining and coughing. The obese patient is advised to lose weight.

Antacids (Maalox and Mylanta) and medications that control acid secretions in the stomach, such as H_2 blockers or PPIs (Prevacid or Nexium), are given. Drug therapy may

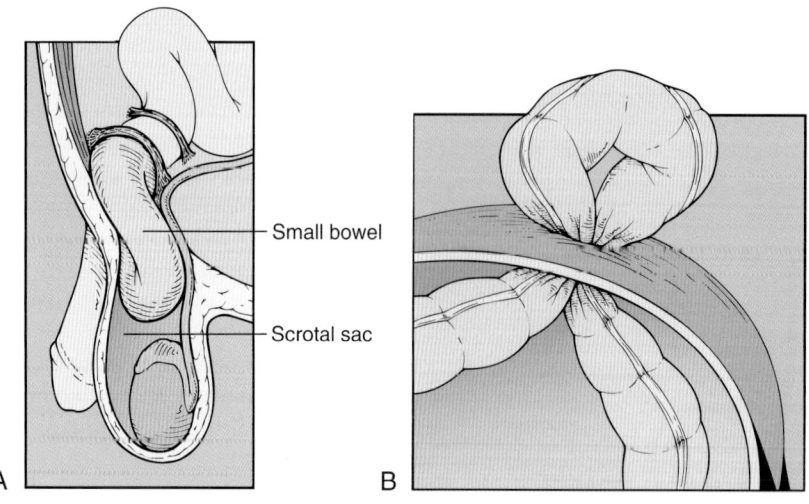

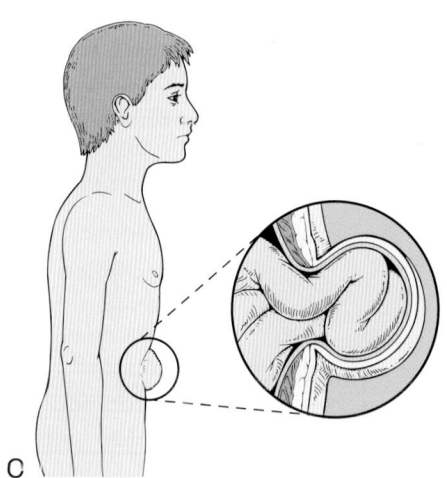

• **Fig. 8.27** Abdominal Hernias. (A) Inguinal hernia. (B) Strangulated hernia. (C) Umbilical hernia.

Patient Screening
Unless the patient complains of severe pain, there is no urgency.

Etiology
An abdominal hernia begins when an abnormal opening develops in a weak area or when a congenital malformation exists in the containing structures of the abdominal cavity. Trauma or increased intraabdominal pressure resulting from heavy lifting or pregnancy also can cause a hernia. A hernia occasionally develops near the weakened site of a previous surgical scar.

Diagnosis
A visible hernia can be assessed by palpation for size, with the patient standing or supine. The physician or health care provider listens for bowel sounds. An inguinal hernia can be detected in the male by asking him to perform the Valsalva maneuver. The medical assessment also might include radiographic studies of the abdomen and WBC count.

Treatment
Therapeutic measures vary with the type of hernia and are dependent on the age and physical condition of the patient. If the hernia is uncomplicated and the hernial sac can be reduced back into the abdominal cavity, the patient can wear a device called a *truss*. If this measure keeps the patient comfortable and there are no signs of strangulation, surgical intervention may be avoided. Surgical repair of the hernia (herniorrhaphy) is the treatment of choice in children and healthy adults.

Prognosis
In uncomplicated cases, the prognosis is good. An incarcerated or strangulated hernia requires prompt surgical repair and a variable postoperative recovery time.

Prevention
When the patient has a known weakness in the abdominal wall, heavy lifting and trauma should be avoided. Coughing may contribute to hernias. Encourage patients to stop smoking.

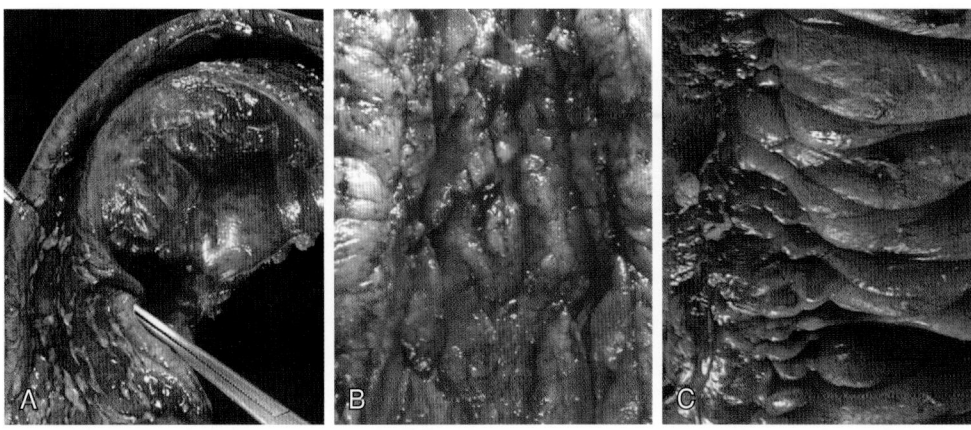

• **Fig. 8.28** Gross pathology of Crohn Disease. (A) Small-intestinal stricture. (B) Linear mucosal ulcers and thickened intestinal wall. (C) Creeping fat. (From Kumar V, et al: *Robbins basic pathology,* ed 10, Philadelphia, 2018, Saunders.)

Patient Teaching

Provide patient education on how to apply a truss, which is a device that is often recommended to reduce a hernia. Discuss any activity restrictions or permissions. When surgical repair (herniorrhaphy) is planned, review the preoperative and postoperative procedures, and discuss the warning signs of complications.

Crohn Disease (Regional Enteritis)

Description

Crohn disease is a chronic inflammatory disorder of the GI tract that affects up to 480,000 persons in the United States. It is also called *regional enteritis.*

ICD-10-CM Code	K50.90 *(Crohn disease, unspecified, without complications)* (K50.00-K50.919 = 28 codes of specificity)

Symptoms and Signs

Crohn disease is a chronic inflammatory disorder of the alimentary canal in which all layers of the bowel wall are edematous and inflamed (Fig. 8.28). Any portion of the GI tract from the mouth to the anus can be affected. Patients with Crohn disease may have chronic diarrhea or crampy, intermittent abdominal pain, often in the right lower quadrant of the abdomen. They also may experience weight loss, malaise, nausea, anorexia, fever, and abdominal fullness. If obstruction develops, patients have symptoms of an acute abdomen. The abdomen is tender and distended, and patients may vomit, and there may be blood in the stools. However, symptoms of Crohn disease are often insidious. Patients may have intermittent symptoms, with varying periods of remission. Over time, symptomatic periods may increase in frequency and severity. If the condition is chronic, signs and symptoms of malnutrition begin to manifest; perianal *fissures* and fistulas usually develop. Complications associated with chronic inflammation include deep ulcerations, symptoms of bowel obstruction, adhesions, and abscesses. Symptoms may mimic those of small intestine bacterial overgrowth (SIBO). In this condition, abdominal pain, bloating, and diarrhea result from an abnormally high level of normal small intestinal bacteria. After treatment, relapse may occur, with symptoms reemerging.

Patient Screening

The acute symptoms of Crohn disease can mimic those of appendicitis and require prompt medical investigation.

Etiology

The cause remains unknown despite major research endeavors. Immunologic factors play a role; autoimmune factors, allergies, and genetic causes also have been investigated.

Diagnosis

Diagnosis is based on symptoms, radiographic studies of the small and large intestines, colonoscopy (Fig. 8.29), and enteroscopy (examination of the small intestine with an endoscope or a swallowed pill-sized camera). Radiographs reveal the diseased segments (strictures) separated by normal bowel in a characteristic distribution called *skip lesions.* Direct examination with endoscopy shows characteristic ulcerations; biopsy confirms the diagnosis. Anemia, leukocytosis, and hypoalbuminemia may be detected in blood tests. Electrolyte abnormalities reflect the severity of diarrhea. CT may help identify abscesses and other complications. The differential diagnosis includes also small bowel obstruction, ulcerative colitis, irritable bowel syndrome (IBS), malabsorption syndromes, infectious or ischemic colitis, neoplasia, hemorrhoids, and diverticular disease.

Treatment

Crohn disease is considered a medically incurable condition. Therapy has two goals: to treat acute disease flareups and to maintain remission. General medical management includes nutritional support and control of symptoms by controlling the inflammation. The patient may require dietary supplements of vitamins, minerals, protein, and

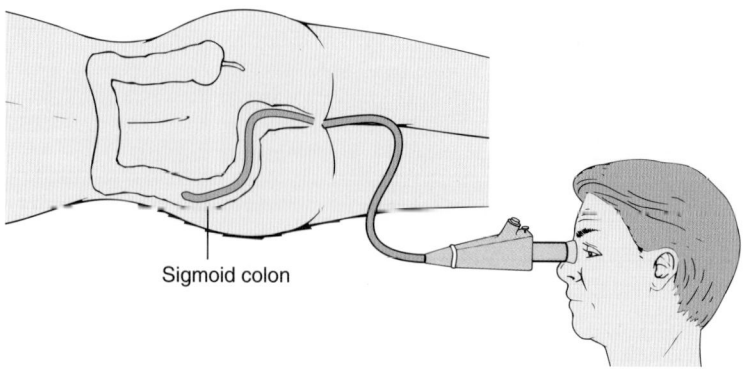

• **Fig. 8.29** Colonoscopy. A lighted fiberoptic endoscope is inserted through the anus to allow direct examination of the colon. This method is useful in differential diagnosis of bowel disease to obtain a biopsy and in minor surgery, such as polypectomy.

calories. In cases of severe and prolonged bouts of diarrhea, IV nutrition may be necessary to avoid dehydration and electrolyte imbalance. Medication therapy is determined by the phase of the disease: acute or chronic. Acute therapy may include antibiotics or steroids. Chronic therapy may include azathioprine, methotrexate, infliximab, adalimumab, certolizumab, or natalizumab. Drug therapy with anticholinergics and narcotic agents relieves cramping and diarrhea, but its use should be limited. If the disease is complicated by infection, the physician prescribes antibiotics. Mesalamine is an effective agent for mild infections. Corticosteroid therapy controls inflammation, but duration of use should be limited because of side effects. Immunosuppressive drugs also are used to decrease underlying inflammation and promote healing. Administration of antibodies to tumor necrosis factor (TNF) is effective and used in moderate to severe cases. When there is blood loss, attempts are made to detect the site of bleeding. If bowel obstruction, uncontrolled GI hemorrhage, or perforation develops, surgery to remove the affected portion of the intestine may be indicated. Abscesses can be drained by placement of a percutaneous catheter. Poorly controlled disease or strictures may require surgical resection.

Prognosis

Crohn disease has a high rate of recurrence and requires continuous treatment. The course of the disease varies. High stress levels cause exacerbations as a result of changes in the body's hormone balance as a reaction to stress. A slightly increased risk for colon cancer exists, possibly because of constant inflammatory injury to the GI tract.

Prevention

Because the cause is uncertain, prevention is directed toward avoiding complications, with careful monitoring of the patient.

Patient Teaching

The clinician is challenged to address the many physical and psychological implications of this type of chronic disease. Teaching includes compliance with medications to prevent progression of the disease; good nutrition; diet that is tolerated; lifestyle modifications; and coping with altered body

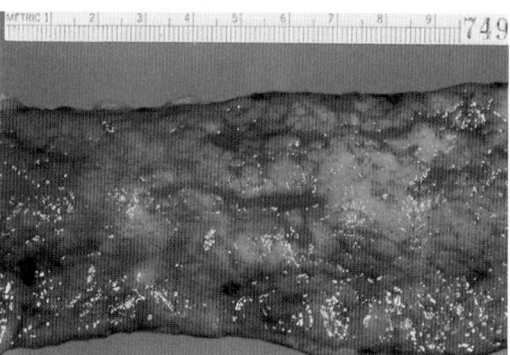

• **Fig. 8.30** Ulcerative colitis. (From Doughty DB, Jackson DB: *Gastrointestinal disorders—Mosby's clinical nursing series,* St Louis, 1993, Mosby.)

image. Educate the patient that signs of intestinal bleeding or a fever associated with increased abdominal tenderness must be reported to the physician. Because this disease is chronic in nature, patients may benefit from counseling, participation in a support group, and physical rest. Low-impact exercise programs also have been shown to improve patients' quality of life.

Ulcerative Colitis

Description

Ulcerative colitis is a chronic inflammatory bowel disease (IBD) affecting the mucosa and submucosa of the rectum and colon (Fig. 8.30).

ICD-10-CM Code	K51.90 *(Ulcerative colitis, unspecified, without complications)* (K51.00-K51.919 = 49 codes of specificity)

Symptoms and Signs

Ulcerative colitis, a common cause of serious bowel disease, does not discriminate for age or gender but usually occurs between ages 15 and 30 years, and less frequently between ages 50 and 70 years. A higher incidence of ulcerative colitis is seen in white people and those of Jewish descent. The symptoms result from a chronic, diffuse, continuous inflammation of the mucosa of the rectum and colon. The patient reports intermittent episodes of bloody diarrhea, abdominal cramping, urgency to defecate, and mucoid stools. As the disease progresses, the stools become looser and more frequent (10–20 per day), with cramping and rectal pressure; the patient also experiences weight loss, fever, and malaise. Some patients report tenesmus, which is mistaken as constipation. The watery stools contain blood, mucus, and pus resulting from mucosal ulceration of the bowel. If the disease is fulminant, major complications result from severe diarrhea, massive bleeding, and perforation.

Patient Screening

The hallmark sign is frequent and bloody diarrhea. A prompt evaluation by a physician or health care provider is warranted.

Etiology

Approximately 20% of people with ulcerative colitis report a family member or relative with ulcerative colitis. The cause is unknown. Current thinking suggests an association with autoimmune response.

Diagnosis

The diagnosis is based on the clinical symptoms, examination of the stool for blood, and laboratory values. Findings could include a reduced Hgb level and leukocytosis. Electrolyte abnormalities may be noted when the diarrhea is severe. Plain film radiographs of the abdomen also are taken. Stool cultures are needed to rule out pathogenic bacteria or parasites. Barium enema studies and colonoscopy are performed to confirm the diagnosis. Colonoscopy with biopsy shows typical inflammatory changes in the mucosa.

Treatment

The patient is encouraged to consume a well-balanced diet devoid of foods that are irritating to the stomach. The diet usually is low in fat and bulk and high in protein, vitamins, and calories. The goal of drug therapy is to induce and maintain remission and to improve the quality of life for people with ulcerative colitis. Anticholinergic drugs and occasionally antidiarrheal agents are prescribed. Mesalamine and sulfasalazine are used for mild to moderate cases. Corticosteroid therapy is used in more severe cases, but the duration is limited because of side effects. Anti-TNF (antibodies to TNF) is effective in severe disease. Surgical removal of the diseased colon is indicated for severe hemorrhage or perforation. Surgery to remove the colon and rectum, known as *proctocolectomy*, is followed by ileostomy or ileoanal anastomosis. The patient is examined annually, because chronic ulcerative colitis is associated with an increased risk of colon cancer.

Prognosis

The severity varies from mild to fulminant disease. The risk for colon cancer increases with the duration of the disease and how much the colon has been damaged. If the entire colon is involved, the risk of cancer may be as much as 32 times the normal rate.

Prevention

As in other types of IBDs, the etiology may be uncertain. The medical approach is to prevent and manage recurrent attacks and complications.

Patient Teaching

A multidisciplinary health care team approach is important to address multiple aspects of care in IBD. During an acute phase, encourage the patient to identify emotional or physical stressors. Discuss the results that the patient can expect from the prescribed regimen of diet, rest, and medication. Advise patients regarding dehydration and GI bleeding. Severe episodes of bleeding or diarrhea require parenteral nutrition. Uncontrolled disease despite maximal medical therapy requires surgical intervention. Referral to IBD support services is useful.

Gastroenteritis

Description

Gastroenteritis is a general term for acute inflammation of the lining of the stomach and intestines.

ICD-10-CM Code	K52.89 *(Other specified noninfective gastroenteritis and colitis)*
	K52.9 *(Noninfective gastroenteritis and colitis, unspecified)*
	(K52.0-K52.9 = 7 codes of specificity)

Symptoms and Signs

The stomach and intestines remain protected from infections and irritations by the presence of normal bacterial flora and acid secretions and by the healthy motility of the GI tract. When these mechanisms fail to rid the body of toxins or large numbers of disease causing bacteria and viruses, the stomach and intestines become filled with the products of inflammation, resulting in gastroenteritis. The patient experiences increased intestinal motility, sometimes with the presence of mucus, pus, and blood in the stool. The body may lose fluids too rapidly, causing dehydration with a disturbance in the body's electrolyte balance.

A common syndrome of gastroenteritis called *traveler's diarrhea* is characterized by varying degrees of anorexia, abdominal cramping, frequent loose stools, and nausea and profuse vomiting. If the infection is severe enough, fever and weakness follow. The same symptoms occur with viral gastroenteritis, which is referred to as *stomach flu*; food or chemical poisoning; allergic reactions to food; and some drug reactions.

Patient Screening

Weakness, dizziness, reduced urine output, and mental confusion are indications of dehydration. A patient who experiences acute vomiting and hematemesis or reports ingestion of a poisonous or corrosive agent should be treated as a medical emergency.

Etiology

Ingestion of disease-causing bacteria or parasites from contaminated food or water is the primary cause of traveler's diarrhea, whereas viral gastroenteritis is the result of a virus. Some bacteria produce toxins in food that cause food poisoning when ingested (see the Food Poisoning section). Ingestion of the poison in certain food (e.g., poisonous mushrooms) or chemicals (e.g., arsenic) causes gastroenteritis. Other causes are chronic ingestion of spicy or irritating food, alcohol, caffeine, aspirin, and antiinflammatory agents. Gastroenteritis may be a complication of acute illness.

Diagnosis

The first important step in identifying the cause is to consider the medical history. Laboratory analysis and culture of the stool reveal the signs and the actual causes of infection or poisoning. The stool is inspected by microscopy for leukocytes, erythrocytes, and ova and parasites (O&P). The clinical evaluation includes blood studies for causative organisms, the presence of antibodies, abnormal blood cell counts, and serum electrolyte values. Endoscopy also may be indicated.

Treatment

The treatment varies with the cause, the severity of the disease, and the age and general health of the patient. Viral and most bacterial gastroenteritis often is self-limiting, although it can become severe and life-threatening. Children, older adults, and the chronically ill are most vulnerable to serious complications from electrolyte imbalance resulting from dehydration.

The goal of treatment is to control symptoms and to maintain a normal fluid and electrolyte balance. Direct management of the cause as diagnosed accomplishes this; the subsequent treatment includes the use of antiemetics, antibiotics, antacids, and either oral or IV rehydration solutions. The patient should rest and eat as tolerated. Antidiarrheal agents should not be used for treatment of traveler's diarrhea because they delay the body's elimination of the offending organisms, thus increasing the duration of symptoms.

Prognosis

Simple gastroenteritis is self-limiting.

Prevention

Education directed at eliminating the cause helps prevent recurrences. Excellent preventive measures for the most common causes of gastroenteritis include frequent and thorough hand washing and avoidance of food that has not been well refrigerated and well cooked.

Patient Teaching

Teach infection control measures. Advise the patient that when traveling, well-cooked foods, rather than raw foods, and purified bottled water should be consumed.

Intestinal Obstruction

Description

Intestinal obstruction is mechanical or functional blockage of the intestines.

ICD-10-CM Code	K56.60 *(Unspecified intestinal obstruction)*
	(K56.60-K56.69 = 2 codes of specificity)

Mechanical obstructions of the intestines are coded according to the nature of the obstruction. Refer to the physician's diagnosis and then to the current edition of the ICD-10-CM coding manual to ensure the greatest specificity.

Symptoms and Signs

Intestinal obstruction occurs when the contents of the intestine cannot move forward because of a partial or complete blockage of the bowel. Although the cause and nature of the obstruction can vary, the patient's discomfort and the signs of blockage are characteristic and include severe pain, nausea, and vomiting, and a bloated and painful abdomen without passage of stool or gas. Symptoms also include an electrolyte imbalance and an elevated WBC count. The bowel sounds can be hyperactive or absent, depending on the nature of the obstruction. This condition is more common in middle-aged and older people.

Patient Screening

The level of intestinal obstruction dictates the severity of the symptoms. A sudden increase in symptoms or an acute onset of symptoms requires urgent medical care.

Etiology

Mechanical blockage of the bowel narrows the normal lumen and prevents the flow of intestinal contents. Mechanical causes of intestinal obstruction are many and include:
- neoplasm (benign or malignant)
- foreign bodies
- fecal impaction
- strictures, from Crohn disease
- compression of the bowel
- volvulus (a twisting of the bowel on itself) (Fig. 8.31)
- intussusception (in which the bowel telescopes into itself; see Fig. 8.31)
- strangulated hernia (see Fig. 8.31)
- adhesions that form tight bands of scar tissue on the bowel (see Fig. 8.31)

In some cases of mechanical obstruction, blood supply to the affected area of intestine is blocked, resulting in tissue death; this leads to the risk of perforation, with spillage of the intestinal contents into the abdominal cavity. This becomes a toxic condition that endangers the patient.

A paralytic condition of the small bowel, called *ileus*, can occur after abdominal surgery, when peristalsis and bowel sounds are absent. Normal peristalsis also can be inhibited by the use of certain medications (e.g., codeine

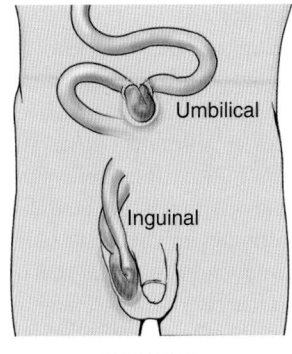

Umbilical

Inguinal

Herniation

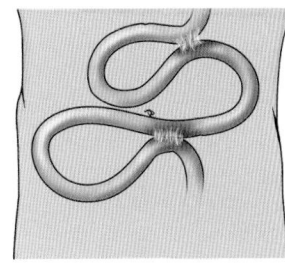

Adhesions

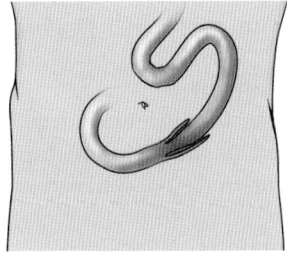

Intussusception

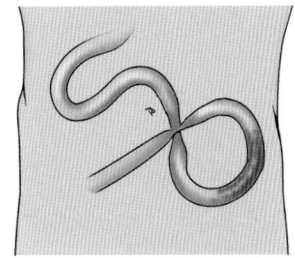

Volvulus

• **Fig. 8.31** Schematic of intestinal obstructions. (From Cotran R, et al: *Robbins pathologic basis of disease,* ed 6, Philadelphia, 1999, Saunders.)

and aluminum-containing antacids) or disease conditions, such as peritonitis. The motility of the bowel often returns spontaneously.

Diagnosis

Radiographic studies of the abdomen with barium or Gastrografin contrast show the point of obstruction of the bowel. CBC shows an elevated WBC count; the patient also has electrolyte imbalances and acid–base disturbances.

Treatment

When the obstruction is mechanical and does not resolve with conservative measures, surgery is performed to remove the cause of blockage. If necessary, the diseased bowel is resected. An ostomy may be needed. A second surgical procedure is often required to reverse the ostomy and rejoin the bowel. When this is not possible, the patient retains a permanent ostomy.

In a nonmechanical or functional obstruction (ileus), the patient is not given anything by mouth and is fed intravenously until peristalsis has returned. A nasogastric tube is inserted to relieve distention and vomiting. Surgery is not usually indicated for functional obstruction. In cases of fecal impaction, manual disimpaction or enemas are used in treatment.

Prognosis

The prognosis generally is good for mechanical obstructive bowel conditions treated promptly. The outcome, however, is guarded with malignant tumors.

Prevention

Screening tests for colorectal cancer permit early detection and treatment of malignant tumors of the colon. Laxative therapy, especially for older adults or bedridden persons, helps prevent fecal impaction.

Patient Teaching

Review the physician's explanations, and discuss any anticipated surgical procedure. Ensure that the patient has a list of signs and symptoms that need to be reported to a doctor, such as any change in bowel habits or sign of GI bleeding. Refer the patient with a colostomy to an ostomy care nurse. Review any diet restrictions, and urge adequate fluid intake. Obtain referrals for home health care, as needed.

Diverticulosis (Diverticular Disease)

Description

Diverticulosis is a progressive condition, common with age, characterized by defects in the muscular wall of the large bowel (Fig. 8.32).

ICD-10-CM Code	K57.30 *(Diverticulosis of large intestine without perforation or abscess without bleeding)*
	K57.31 *(Diverticulosis of large intestine without perforation or abscess with bleeding)*
	(K57.30-K57.93 = 16 codes of specificity)

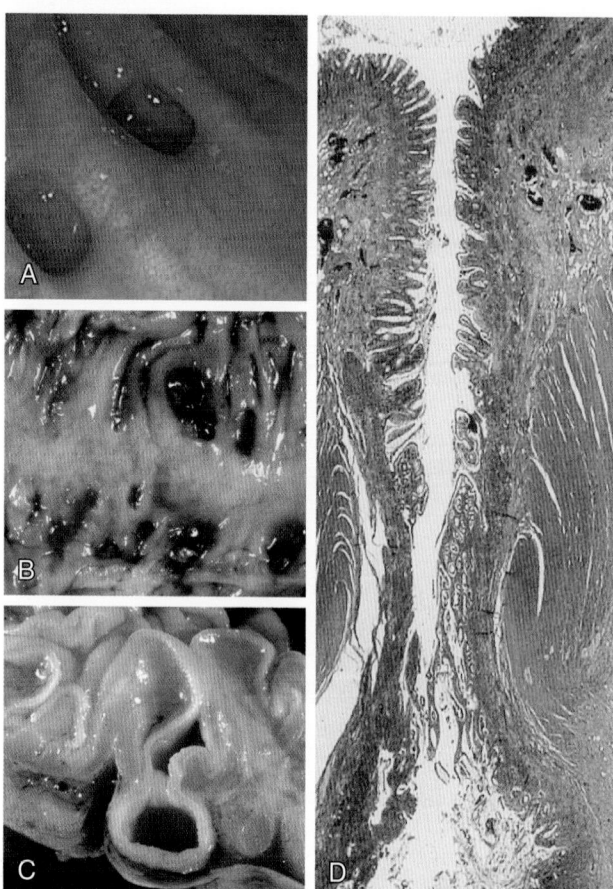

• **Fig. 8.32 Sigmoid Diverticular Disease.** (A) Endoscopic view of two sigmoid diverticula. Compare with B. (B) Gross examination of a resected sigmoid colon shows regularly spaced stool-filled diverticula. (C) Cross-section showing the outpouching of mucosa beneath the muscularis propria. (D) Low-power photomicrograph of a sigmoid diverticulum showing protrusion of the mucosa and submucosa through the muscularis propria. (Endoscopic image Courtesy Dr. Ira Hanan, The University of Chicago, Chicago, Illinois.)

Symptoms and Signs

Diverticulosis is a condition in which outpouches (diverticula) of the mucosa penetrate the weak points in the muscular layer of the large intestine. Colonic diverticula may vary in size, from a few millimeters to several centimeters, and in number, from one to several dozen. Diverticulosis occurs particularly in the distal part of the colon, the sigmoid colon, because intraluminal pressures are higher in this region (see Fig. 8.32). Diverticulosis usually causes no symptoms or inflammation. Occasionally the patient reports nonspecific abdominal distress, such as pain and flatulence, and difficulty in defecation. The patient may experience alternating constipation and diarrhea and even blood in the stool.

Patient Screening

Vague symptoms of intermittent abdominal pain and constipation are typical. Schedule a consultation with the health care provider.

Etiology

The causes are not clear. A diet that contains inadequate roughage and excessive amounts of highly refined food is thought to contribute to diverticulosis. Lack of roughage produces small-caliber, drier stools, which fail to distend the bowel lumen. The small volume of stool causes higher intraluminal pressure during peristalsis and defecation, which, in turn, contributes to the small herniations or pouches through the mucosa of the muscular wall of the intestine. Colonic diverticulosis increases with age, ranging from 5% in those younger than 40 years of age to 30% at age 60 years to greater than 50% in those older than 80 years of age in Western societies.

Diagnosis

Diagnosis is based on the clinical picture and an air-contrast barium enema radiographic study or colonoscopy.

Treatment

A diet that includes adequate fluids and roughage is indicated to produce soft, formed stools daily. Fiber supplements and stool softeners are helpful.

Prognosis

The prognosis is positive unless the condition progresses to diverticulitis.

Prevention

The onset cannot be prevented. Adequate hydration and a high-fiber diet rich in fruits and vegetables help prevent constipation and straining during defecation.

Patient Teaching

Instruct the patient to follow the preventive measures mentioned earlier. Inform the patient to report rectal bleeding or symptoms of colon obstruction to the physician.

Diverticulitis

Description

Diverticulitis is infection of one or more diverticula.

ICD-10-CM Code	K57.32 (*Diverticulitis of large intestine without perforation or abscess without bleeding*)
	K57.33 (*Diverticulitis of large intestine without perforation or abscess with bleeding*)

Symptoms and Signs

When fecal matter becomes trapped in one or more diverticula, inflammation and infection can ensue, causing diverticulitis (see Fig. 8.32C). The patient has abdominal pain or tenderness, usually in the left lower quadrant. The patient may or may not have a fever. A palpable mass may be felt, and the patient reports changes in bowel function. Constipation or loose stools may present. The pain sometimes appears in the right lower quadrant or in the suprapubic area. Blood in the stools indicates small hemorrhages.

Perforation into the abdominal cavity can produce symptoms of peritonitis, intestinal obstruction, and sepsis. Recurrent diverticulitis can cause complications, such as the formation of adhesions, abscesses, and fistulas. Fistula formation may involve the bladder, ureter, vagina, uterus, bowel, and abdominal wall.

Patient Screening

A patient previously diagnosed with diverticulitis can develop acute symptoms that require prompt medical attention. Warning signs may include persistent abdominal pain, fever, and change in bowel habits. Because diverticulitis carries the risk of bowel perforation and peritonitis, the condition may progress to a medical emergency.

Etiology

Diverticulitis, which is not nearly as common as diverticulosis, can develop when one or more diverticula become inflamed and infected. Lack of dietary bulk, inadequate fluid intake, and constipation are thought to contribute. Fecal plugs in the diverticula can predispose patients to infection of the diverticula by colonic bacteria.

Diagnosis

The patient is assessed through history and physical examination with attention to signs of inflammation at the location of the patient's symptoms, usually pain or tenderness. Blood tests may show leukocytosis, low Hgb level, and low Hct. CT will confirm the diagnosis. Colonoscopy or barium enema should not be performed in acute diverticulitis but can be helpful after treatment with antibiotics.

Treatment

Antibiotics may be prescribed for infection. Stool softeners may be indicated, and a liquid diet is often encouraged. If the symptoms are severe or if the bowel is perforated, hospitalization is indicated. Surgical intervention to remove the diseased portion of the colon may be necessary. Small perforations can be treated without surgery with IV antibiotics, nutritional support, and percutaneous drainage if an abscess develops.

Prognosis

In mild cases, the disease is self-limiting. Recovery becomes more complicated when surgery is required or an abscess is present, but the final outcome is usually favorable. Diverticulitis recurs in one-third of patients treated with medical management. Multiple recurrent attacks warrant elective surgical resection, which carries lower morbidity and mortality risks compared with emergency surgery.

Prevention

Regular elimination of soft-formed stools is recommended, especially in a patient with diverticulosis.

Patient Teaching

Explain diverticulosis, the underlying contributing condition. Surgical patients who have had a colon resection need

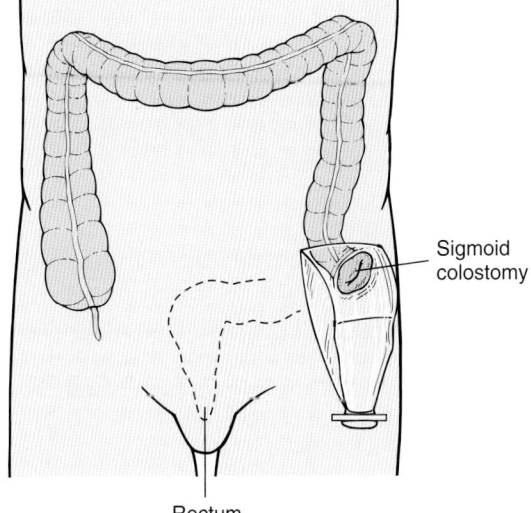

• **Fig. 8.33** Colostomy. Colostomy is a surgical procedure that creates an opening for feces to pass through the abdominal wall. The opening in the colon is brought to the surface of the skin to divert feces into an external pouch worn by the patient. The colostomy may be temporary to promote healing or permanent if the distal bowel has been removed because of malignancy or other disease.

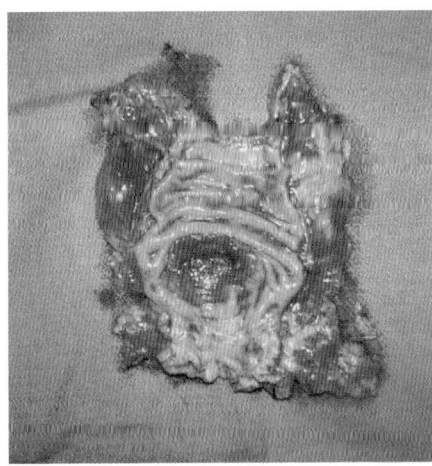

• **Fig. 8.34** Adenocarcinoma of distal rectum. (From Doughty DB, Jackson DB: *Gastrointestinal disorders—Mosby's clinical nursing series,* St Louis, 1993, Mosby.)

to understand the progression to a normal diet and the schedule for antibiotic therapy. Those who have had a colon resection with a diverting colostomy can be referred to an enterostomy nurse for ostomy care and education (Fig. 8.33). Assess for signs of depression after surgery.

Colorectal Cancer

Description

Colorectal cancer is a cancer that arises in any part of the colon or the rectum (Fig. 8.34). According to the 2015 Surveillance Research estimates of the American Cancer Society, it is the third most common site in new cases of cancer and the third most common cause of cancer death (see Chapter 1, Fig. 1.3).

ICD-10-CM Code   C19 *(Malignant neoplasm*
of rectosigmoid junction)
Colorectal cancer is coded according to the site of the
lesion. Refer to the physician's diagnosis and then to
the current edition of the ICD-10-CM coding manual to
ensure the greatest specificity.

Symptoms and Signs

Although symptoms in the early stages are often vague and nonspecific, most patients with colorectal cancer have one or more of the following symptoms at presentation: abdominal pain, change in bowel habits (diarrhea, constipation), bloody stools, weakness, weight loss, or symptoms related to iron deficiency anemia. Colon cancer should be considered in any older patient who develops iron deficiency anemia or stool positive for occult blood. Later symptoms include abdominal distention, pallor, ascites (Fig. 8.35), cachexia, lymphadenopathy, and **hepatomegaly**.

Patient Screening

Follow office policy for referrals and follow-up appointments.

Etiology

The risk of developing colon cancer increases with age. Greater than 90% of cases occur after age 50 years. The rare genetic disorders of familial adenomatous polyposis and hereditary nonpolyposis colorectal cancer predispose affected individuals to the early development of colorectal cancer. Risk factors also include a history of large adenomatous polyps, diabetes mellitus, ulcerative colitis, or Crohn disease; a first-degree relative with colorectal cancer; cigarette smoking; and obesity. Several dietary factors may be protective against colorectal cancer, such as higher intake of fruits and vegetables. Aspirin and NSAIDs may also offer a protective effect. The highest incidences are in Western Europe and North America, possibly because of the higher average dietary fat intake in those living in countries of these regions.

Adenomatous polyps of the colon are the precursor lesion of colorectal cancer. Adenomas are composed of

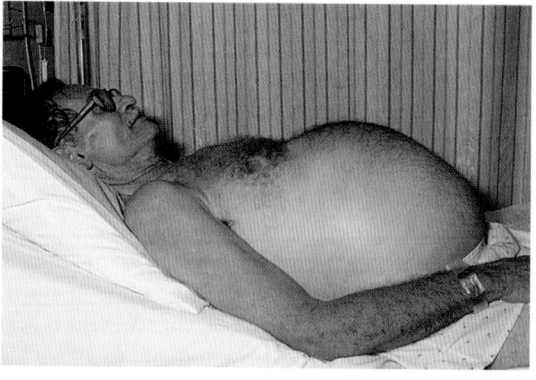

• **Fig. 8.35** Abdominal bloating in ascites. (From Swartz MH: *Textbook of physical diagnosis,* ed 6, Philadelphia, 2010, Saunders.)

dysplastic epithelium that has proliferated to form a mass. Most colorectal carcinomas arise from adenomas over an average time frame of 7 years. Most adenomas, however, do not develop into carcinoma.

Diagnosis

Many early-stage cases of colorectal cancer are detected with prevention screening tests, such as colonoscopy or the fecal occult blood test, along with either a double-contrast barium enema. Colonoscopy is the best test to use in symptomatic patients and for screening because it allows the physician to visualize, sample, and remove lesions throughout the colon. The differential diagnosis of a colonic mass includes many benign and malignant disorders, so histologic evaluation is necessary for the diagnosis of cancer.

Although several staging systems have been proposed for colorectal cancer, physicians now prefer to use the TNM classification system proposed by the AJCC. In the case of colorectal cancer, however, "T" reflects the depth of penetration by the tumor into or through the bowel wall rather than the size of the lesion. Clinical staging is determined through physical examination and CT of the chest, abdomen, and pelvis. For rectal cancers, EUS also may be performed. The level of carcinoembryonic antigen (CEA) can be obtained for postoperative follow-up purposes but should not be used for screening or diagnosis of colorectal cancer. The most common sites for distant metastases are the liver and lungs.

See Chapter 1 for information about the staging and grading systems used to assess malignant neoplasms.

Treatment

Surgical resection of the affected part of the colon or rectum, and any affected lymph nodes, is the mainstay of treatment. A colostomy may be indicated should surgical intervention be unable to reconnect the parts of the colon (see Fig. 8.33). Locally advanced colon cancer is treated with chemotherapy. Radiation therapy can be helpful if the cancer is confined to the rectum. Although treatment for metastatic colorectal cancer is still aimed at palliation of symptoms, advances have been made in the use of chemotherapy that can prolong overall survival. Metastatic colon cancer can also be treated with surgery if the metastatic tumor (usually in the liver) can be removed as well.

Prognosis

The pathologic stage at diagnosis remains the best prognostic indicator. In addition, patients with preoperative serum levels of CEA of greater than 5 ng/mL have a worse prognosis, stage for stage, compared with those with lower levels. Elevated CEA levels that do not become normal after surgery indicate persistent disease. The survival rate for rectal cancer is lower than that for colon cancer.

Prevention

Relatively simple improvements in nutrition and physical activity and the use of available screening procedures may help prevent many cases of colorectal cancer and resulting deaths. A diet high in fruits and vegetables, regular exercise, and maintenance of a healthy weight reduce the risk of colorectal cancer. Screening for colorectal cancer has two functions: It enables the discovery and removal of adenomas to prevent the incidence of cancer, and it detects cancer in the earlier, more curable stages. First, the patient's relative risk of developing colorectal cancer must be determined. A person is considered to be at high risk for colorectal cancer if he or she has hereditary nonpolyposis colon cancer, familial adenomatous polyposis, a previous history of colon cancer or polyps, a history of IBD, or a first-degree relative with colorectal cancer or adenoma. People at average risk for colorectal cancer are urged to start screening at age 50 years with a colonoscopy no less frequently than every 10 years. High-risk patients should start screening by age 40 years or 10 years younger than the earliest colorectal cancer diagnosis in their family, with repeat screening every 5 years. Those with familial cancer syndromes should begin screening in the third decade of life. Patients with a history of colorectal cancer should receive surveillance colonoscopy at 1 year and then every 3 to 5 years to screen for new cancer. Despite the availability and effectiveness of screening, however, only 60% to 70% of adults age 50 years or greater participate in it.

Patient Teaching

Assess the patient's knowledge of the disease process and the medical plan. Encourage the patient to ask questions and discuss any anxiety he or she feels. Answer questions about procedures. Discuss the side effects of surgery, chemotherapy, or intraoperative radiation therapy. Refer the patient to an ostomy nurse for stoma care. Give emotional support, and refer the patient to cancer support groups. Encourage the patient to call the physician or the nurse if complications occur. Inform the patient that family members have increased risk and should undergo screening.

Pseudomembranous Enterocolitis

Description

Pseudomembranous enterocolitis is acute inflammation with a plaquelike necrotic debris and mucus adhered to the damaged superficial mucosa of the small and large intestines.

ICD-10-CM Code	A04.7 (Enterocolitis due to Clostridioides difficile) (A04.0-A04.9 = 10 codes of specificity)

Symptoms and Signs

Enterocolitis, in which bowel mucosa has a membranous appearance, is a disease marked by mild to severe greenish, foul-smelling watery diarrhea (up to 30 stools per day). The patient may have a fever and weakness and report abdominal cramping and tenderness. Some patients experience nausea and vomiting. A patient with severe diarrhea will exhibit signs of dehydration, including dry mouth, light-headedness, and dizziness. The urine is concentrated, and the skin displays decreased *turgor*. Irritation develops around the anal area as a result of the frequent and watery stools; fecal incontinence can be a problem. Blood and mucus in stools may be reported.

Patient Screening

A patient who has been on antibiotics during the preceding 6 weeks, is currently on antibiotics, has a history of long-term use of PPIs, and complains of sudden onset of copious watery diarrhea, abdominal pain, and fever should seek the advice of the physician who prescribed the antibiotics.

Etiology

Pseudomembranous enterocolitis often is related to the use of broad-spectrum antibiotics; the patient either is taking the antibiotics or has been undergoing antibiotic therapy during the previous 6 weeks. Although almost all antibiotics have been implicated, colitis most commonly develops after the use of ampicillin, clindamycin, third-generation cephalosporins, and fluoroquinolones. Antibiotic therapy reduces the body's protective natural intestinal flora (along with the target pathogens) and allows development of a bacterial infection with *Clostridioides difficile*. This organism, a cytotoxic-producing strain of a normal gut organism, produces powerful toxins that cause the bowel wall to become inflamed, ulcerated, and necrotic (Fig. 8.36). The products of inflammation and dead tissue form a coating that is called a *pseudomembrane*. Pseudomembranous enterocolitis is more common in health care facilities, including skilled nursing facilities, where fecal contamination is more likely. Hospitalized patients are most at risk, especially those who are severely ill, malnourished, or receiving chemotherapy. Most infections occur as a result of fecal-oral transmission. Those who have had abdominal surgery and those older than age 65 years of age are more susceptible. Asymptomatic patients with colonization by *C. difficile* can be a source of contamination. Long-term use of PPIs increases risks of *C. difficile* infections.

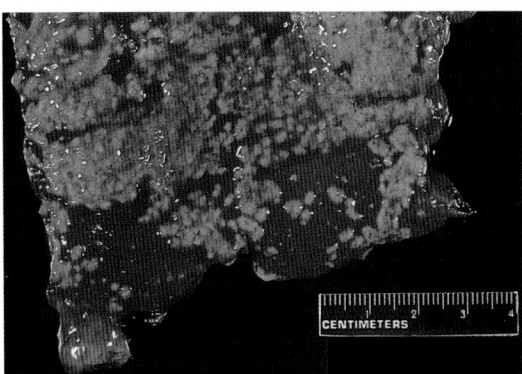

• **Fig. 8.36** Pseudomembranous colitis. (From Kumar V, et al: *Robbins basic pathology,* ed 8, Philadelphia, 2008, Saunders.)

Diagnosis

Pseudomembranous enterocolitis is diagnosed when *C. difficile* toxin is found in the stool or rectal biopsy confirms pseudomembranous enterocolitis. The WBC count is elevated as a result of the immune response to the infection. In severe cases, blood protein (serum albumin) levels are reduced, the serum electrolyte levels are abnormal; abdominal radiographs may show a distended colon.

Treatment

Treatment is initiated by discontinuing the broad-spectrum antibiotic and substituting it with metronidazole or vancomycin to fight the infection. Cholestyramine (Questran) may be given to bind the toxins produced by the causative bacteria. Drugs that slow bowel activity are not recommended because they boost the retention of the toxins, thereby increasing damage to the bowel.

The general management of the patient includes monitoring of the fluid and electrolyte balance, with oral or IV supplement as needed. Surgery is rarely necessary. Careful hand washing with soap and water (not alcohol-based antibacterial sprays or foam), isolation, and decontamination measures are encouraged to prevent cross-infection.

Prognosis

Some cases may require more than one course of autoinfection therapy. Severe infection, although rare, can be life-threatening. With the emergence of a new, more virulent strain of *C. difficile* (BI/NAP1), the numbers of severe infections and fatal complications in hospitals across the United States and Canada have increased. This toxin-gene variant strain (higher toxin production) has been associated with several hospital outbreaks. The 30-day mortality attributed to infection with this strain is 7%, increasing to 14% in older adults.

Prevention

Prevention includes infection control in health care facilities and caution in prescribing broad-spectrum antibiotics to patients who have had abdominal surgery. Complete environmental disinfection of all patient care equipment is challenging because some disinfectants do not kill the highly resistant spores. *C. difficile* bacteria and spores are easily transmitted from infected patients to the hands of health care workers. All health care providers should be educated about the precautions to avoid transmitting *C. difficile* to other patients. Public swimming pools can be a source of *C. difficile;* it is advisable, especially for children and older adults, to avoid swallowing pool water.

Patient Teaching

It is important to note that alcohol-based hand sanitizers are ineffective against *C. difficile.* Thorough hand washing with soap and water is stressed. Additionally, inform the patient with pseudomembranous enterocolitis that drugs that slow peristalsis are contraindicated.

Short Bowel Syndrome

Description

In short bowel syndrome, the small bowel fails to absorb nutrients because of inadequate absorptive surface.

ICD-10-CM Code	K91.2 *(Postsurgical malabsorption, not elsewhere classified)*

Symptoms and Signs

Short bowel syndrome is the result of an insufficient amount of functioning small bowel to absorb the nutrients, fluid, vitamins, and minerals that the body needs. Depending on the amount of missing or damaged bowel, significant signs of malnutrition, including pathologic changes in other organs and body systems, are noted. Because there is insufficient small bowel to digest and absorb food adequately, diarrhea and abnormal stools occur. The patient loses weight and feels weak, tired, and dizzy. As the malnutrition continues, the hair and nails become brittle, and rashes develop.

Patient Screening

Patients may require frequent follow-up appointments with their physician or health care provider after bowel surgery. Nutritional status assessment is a priority.

Etiology

Short bowel syndrome develops when the length of intact or functioning small bowel is altered significantly by disease or surgery. Crohn disease, intestinal infarction, radiation enteritis, volvulus, tumor resection, and trauma are conditions that may cause extensive resection of the small intestine. This loss of functioning small bowel interferes with the digestion and absorption of needed nutrients. The type and degree of malabsorption depend on the length and site of the resection and the degree of adaptation of the remaining bowel.

Diagnosis

The patient history initially may indicate the presence of bowel disease, with or without surgical intervention that has reduced the length or function of part of the small bowel. In short bowel syndrome, the results of blood tests reflect abnormal electrolyte levels, pH disturbance, and anemia. Stool studies show an increased amount of fat.

Treatment

The treatment plan depends on the cause of the syndrome and the particular manifestations of malnutrition. Medical management includes prescription drugs for infection, diarrhea, vitamin and mineral deficiency, and pain, as required. Food supplements are administered orally or intravenously, as needed. Surgery may be performed to correct the underlying condition or to reconstruct the bowel. Postoperative parenteral hyperalimentation is required for weeks or until the remaining gut adapts and becomes functional, at which time oral feeding is gradually introduced.

Prognosis

Many patients recover without difficulties, even with extensive resection, as the remaining bowel adapts to increased nutrient absorption.

Prevention

After surgical resection of the small bowel, the patient is monitored closely for manifestations of malnutrition, dehydration, or weight loss.

Patient Teaching

After surgery, the patient needs nutritional counseling as oral food is gradually reintroduced. Give instructions for controlling diarrhea with the prescribed agents.

Irritable Bowel Syndrome

Description

IBS is a *functional* bowel disorder characterized by chronic abdominal pain or discomfort, bloating, and erratic dysfunction of bowel habits.

ICD-10-CM Code	K58.0 *(Irritable bowel syndrome with diarrhea)*
	K58.9 *(Irritable bowel syndrome without diarrhea)*

Symptoms and Signs

Classic symptoms of IBS include episodes of cramping or aching abdominal pain typically relieved by defecation. A key feature of IBS is a change of bowel habits with predominant diarrhea or constipation, or an alternation between the two. Bloating and abdominal distention are commonly experienced, and the patient may complain of tenesmus (a feeling of incomplete or ineffectual straining). Some patients report gastroesophageal reflux, nausea, and the feeling of a lump in the throat. Patients may express anxiety over the course of the disease and its effect on limiting their lifestyle because of the need for access to bathroom facilities.

Patient Screening

A patient requesting an appointment for recurrent abdominal pain and changes in bowel habits should be seen as soon as possible by a physician or a health care provider.

Etiology

The exact cause of IBS is unknown. The incidence of developing IBS increases after acute GI infection; this may suggest an immune or neuroimmune contribution. Many patients report other chronic pain disorders, such as fibromyalgia, lactose intolerance, back pain, urinary symptoms, anxiety, and depression. Risk factors include age (20–40 years) and a significant female gender predominance. Stressful events may precipitate the onset of symptoms.

Diagnosis

A positive clinical diagnosis of IBS begins with history, physical examination, and tests to exclude organic disease. Typically routine clinical tests yield no abnormalities, and the gross and macroscopic evaluation is often normal. The diagnosis depends largely on physical symptoms based on abnormal GI motility. Diagnosis of IBS involves excluding other conditions with similar symptoms, such as parasitic infections, lactose intolerance, Crohn disease, and other IBDs. Older patients (age > 50 years) with recent onset of symptoms require colonoscopy or a double-contrast barium enema with **sigmoidoscopy**.

Treatment

There is no cure for IBS. There are treatments to relieve and manage symptoms. Patients need reassurance and explanation of the necessary diagnostic testing to rule out certain organic diseases. Because symptoms tend to fluctuate, refinement of the medical treatment may require adjustment of medications based on patient feedback. Medications may include soluble fiber supplements (e.g., psyllium), stool softeners, and laxatives in constipation-dominant IBS (IBS-C); for diarrhea-dominant IBS (IBS-D), an antidiarrheal medication (e.g., loperamide) may provide relief. Ondansetron has been shown to block 5-hydroxytryptamine (5-HT3) receptors in the gut and may also be used. Antispasmodic drugs (dicyclomine and hyoscyamine) for postprandial pain are available. Tricyclic antidepressants are useful for chronic pain for their anticholinergic effects. The probiotic *Bifidobacterium* has been shown to reduce pain and bloating. Nonabsorbed antibiotics have alleviated the symptoms in some patients with IBS-D. There is a newer class of drugs that show promise for patients with IBS-D. A new class of medications, guanylate cyclase-c agonists (Trulance, Linzess, Amitiza), have shown promise for patients with IBS-C.

A multidisciplinary team approach to the treatment plan, including referral for relaxation therapy, cognitive behavioral therapy, or psychotherapy, may be indicated. Dietary modifications may be included.

Prognosis

IBS does not usually lead to more serious conditions, but it can affect the quality of life of the patient. As a chronic illness, it can be a source of fatigue and pain with increased absenteeism and increased medical costs. The prognosis is related to the duration of symptoms with longer duration reducing the chance of improvement. About one-third of patients with IBS become asymptomatic with time. IBS does not affect life expectancy, and prolonged remissions are possible.

Prevention

Because the exact cause is not known, there is no prevention.

Patient Teaching

Patients with IBS can benefit from positive reinforcement that their symptoms are real and not psychosomatic or imaginary. Provide reassurance that IBS is not life-threatening and does not cause cancer. Advise the patient to avoid heavy use of alcohol or caffeinated or decaffeinated products, because these may precipitate or exacerbate symptoms. Stress reduction has been correlated to mitigating symptoms. Inform patients to avoid taking unnecessary medications, because some may aggravate symptoms. Encourage patients to follow specified dietary recommendations and follow the medical therapy prescribed by their health care provider for the best outcome. IBS support group referrals benefit chronic sufferers.

Peritonitis

Description
Peritonitis, inflammation of the peritoneum, can be acute or chronic and local or generalized.

ICD-10-CM Code	K67 (Disorders of peritoneum in
	infectious diseases classified
	elsewhere)

Peritonitis is coded by etiology. Refer to the physician's diagnosis and then to the current edition of the ICD-10-CM coding manual to ensure the greatest specificity.

Symptoms and Signs
The large serous membrane that lines the abdominal cavity and folds over the visceral organs is normally transparent and sterile. When it is irritated or infected, the peritoneum becomes *hyperemic* and edematous as fluid accumulates in the peritoneal space. The inflammatory process of peritonitis has the potential to cause abscesses and adhesions to form in the abdominal cavity (Fig. 8.37).

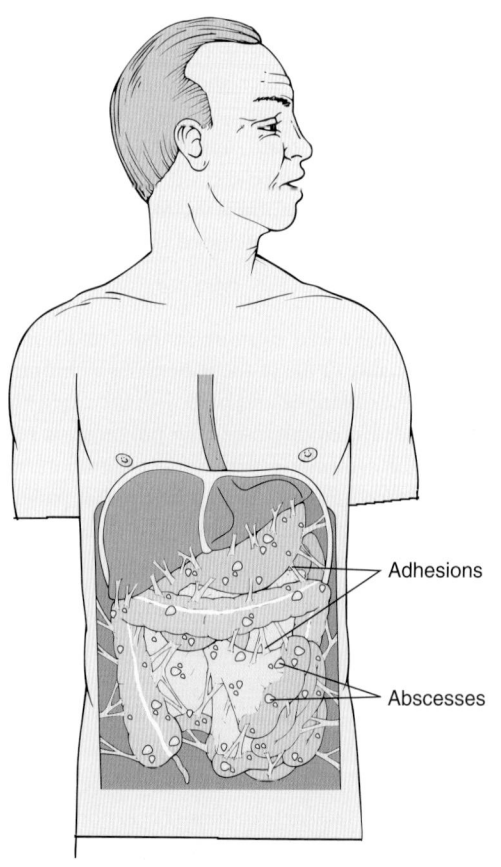

Adhesions

Abscesses

• **Fig. 8.37** Peritonitis.

The patient reports abdominal pain, nausea and vomiting, weakness, and profuse sweating. Abdominal pain may be so severe that the patient may prefer not to move. Symptoms include fever and abdominal tenderness and distention. Occasionally a paralytic ileus is present. Examination of the abdomen reveals tenderness to direct touch and rebound (or percussion), indicating peritoneal inflammation. In a fulminating case of peritonitis, the bacteria or bacterial endotoxins enter the circulation, leading to septicemia, shock, and death.

Patient Screening
A patient having sudden, severe, and diffuse abdominal pain, fever, weakness, nausea, and vomiting requires emergency medical attention.

Etiology
Peritonitis can occur as a primary infection caused by blood-borne organisms or organisms originating in the GI or genital tract. The infection is considered secondary if the source of infection is contamination by GI secretions resulting from a perforation of the GI tract or intraabdominal organs. For example, bacterial invasion could occur after surgery as a result of a breakdown of anastomoses, allowing contaminated intestinal contents to spill into the abdominal cavity. Causes of secondary bacterial peritonitis include appendicitis, diverticulitis, perforated peptic ulcer, and perforated gallbladder. A penetrating wound to the abdomen is another common cause. Systemic lupus erythematosus also can cause bouts of peritonitis as a result of continuous inflammation.

Noninfective secretions (e.g., bile from a ruptured, inflamed gallbladder) can cause aseptic peritonitis resulting from chemical irritation of the membrane. Eventually there is bacterial invasion. The organisms most often involved include *Escherichia coli, Klebsiella pneumoniae, Enterococcus* species, anaerobic streptococci, and *Pseudomonas aeruginosa.*

Diagnosis
Diagnostic findings include an elevated WBC count, abnormal serum electrolyte levels (e.g., altered levels of sodium, potassium, and chloride), and gaseous distention of the bowel evident on radiographic examination of the abdomen. Radiographic studies or CT also may reveal perforation of an abdominal organ evidenced by air in the abdominal cavity. Aspiration of peritoneal fluid shows cloudy peritoneal fluid and allows for a culture and sensitivity study to identify the causative organism.

Treatment
The clinical manifestations of peritonitis must be assessed and the source of the irritation or infection identified. The patient is promptly and aggressively treated with broad-spectrum antibiotics, analgesics, and antiemetics. The patient is not given anything by mouth, and fluid and electrolyte losses are replaced parenterally. If there is a perforation, surgery is required to correct the source of infection and to drain the spilled contents.

Prognosis

Without prompt and aggressive medical intervention, including antibiotics, peritonitis is life-threatening.

Prevention

Many of the underlying causes are not easily predicted.

Patient Teaching

After the patient has been stabilized with medical interventions, emphasize special instructions in writing about activity, medications, surgical wound care, and follow-up visits.

Hemorrhoids

Description

Hemorrhoids are varicose dilations of a vein in the anal canal or the anorectal area.

ICD-10-CM Code	K64.8 *(Other hemorrhoids)*
	(K64.0-K64.9 = 8 codes of specificity)

The codes vary by the location and complications. Refer to the physician's diagnosis and then to the current edition of the ICD-10-CM coding manual to ensure the greatest specificity.

Symptoms and Signs

Hemorrhoids are tumorlike lesions in the anal area caused by dilated veins; hemorrhoids often are painless. When hemorrhoids are symptomatic, the patient experiences rectal pain, itching, protrusion, or bleeding, especially after defecation. The patient also may experience a mucous discharge from the rectum, a sensation of incomplete evacuation, and difficulty cleaning the anal area. A painful anal lump may indicate thrombosis of an external hemorrhoid requiring medical attention.

Patient Screening

The patient reporting frequent, unrelieved urge to defecate, severe constipation, or bright red rectal bleeding needs a consultation with the physician.

Etiology

The veins in the rectal and anal area become varicose, swollen, and tender as a result of blockage. If they are located within the rectum above the junction of skin and rectal mucosa, these swollen and twisted varicosities are considered internal hemorrhoids; varicosities lower in the anal area covered by skin are considered external hemorrhoids (Fig. 8.38). A large, firm subcutaneous lump indicates thrombosis of the external hemorrhoids. Constipation, straining, pregnancy, and any condition that increases pressure on the veins often exacerbate this condition.

Diagnosis

The diagnosis is based on visual inspection of the anal area and **proctoscopy** to visualize internal hemorrhoids of the rectum. The patient's Hgb level and red blood cell (RBC)

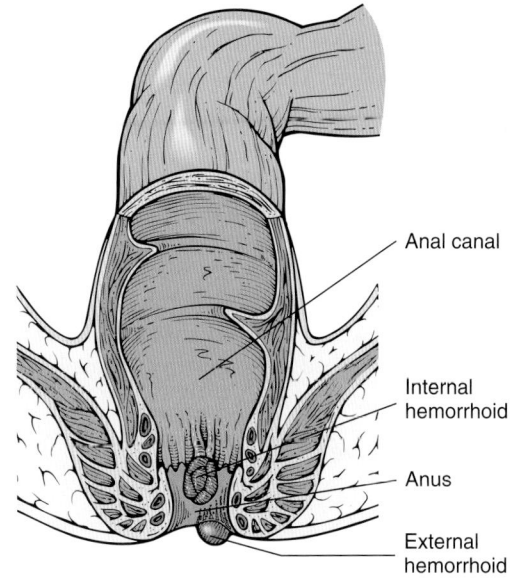

• **Fig. 8.38** Hemorrhoids.

count may be below normal if the patient has experienced significant bleeding.

Treatment

Conservative treatment consists of measures to correct constipation and to prevent straining. Stool softeners and a diet high in fruits, vegetables, and whole-grain cereals are recommended. If the patient is symptomatic, warm sitz baths may be prescribed, along with a topical anesthetic ointment or witch hazel compresses. Products, such as hydrocortisone acetate or pramoxine hydrochloride (ProctoCream-HC), may be applied locally to reduce inflammation. If these measures do not help, sclerotherapy injections may be used to induce scar formation and to reduce prolapse. The hemorrhoids can be destroyed by band ligation or by cryosurgery, a procedure that uses a probe to expose the hemorrhoids to extreme cold. Photocoagulation using an infrared device also is effective. Electrocoagulation and thermocoagulation are other alternatives. When bleeding and other symptoms are severe, hemorrhoidectomy is the best treatment. The newest surgical therapy is called *stapled hemorrhoidectomy.*

Prognosis

The procedures used to treat hemorrhoids produce positive outcomes. Complications are uncommon, and recurrences are unusual.

Prevention

To prevent exacerbation of the condition, the patient should avoid constipation, prolonged sitting at the stool, straining during defecation, and heavy lifting. A high-bulk diet is recommended to promote regular bowel habits.

Patient Teaching

Reinforce the preventive measures listed earlier. Encourage adequate fluid intake. Urge good anal hygiene with gentle wiping after stools along with the other comfort measures listed in the Treatment section. Recommend weight loss for patients who are obese. Give special consideration during pregnancy to minimize discomfort.

Diseases of the Liver, Biliary Tract, and Pancreas

The liver, gallbladder, and pancreas are accessory organs of digestion that introduce digestive hormones and enzymes into the alimentary canal, ensuring that the nutrients critical to life can be absorbed selectively by the small intestines into the bloodstream.

Cirrhosis of the Liver

Description

Cirrhosis of the liver is a chronic degenerative disease that is irreversible. It brings slow deterioration of the liver, resulting in the replacement of normal liver cells with hard, fibrous scar tissue, known as *hobnail liver*.

ICD-10-CM Code	K70.30 *(Alcoholic cirrhosis of liver without ascites)*
	(K70.30-K70.31 = 2 codes of specificity)
	K74.0 *(Hepatic fibrosis)*
	K74.60 *(Unspecified cirrhosis of liver)*
	K74.69 *(Other cirrhosis of liver)*
	(K74.0-K74.69 = 8 codes of specificity)

Symptoms and Signs

Cirrhosis is twice as common in men as in women. As many as 40% of people with cirrhosis of the liver are asymptomatic.

In the early stages of the disease, the symptoms are vague and mild. As the liver is destroyed, the patient experiences loss of appetite and weight, nausea and vomiting, indigestion, abdominal distention (caused by ascites), and edema. The patient tends to bleed and bruise more easily, and frequent nosebleeds are common. The skin appears *jaundiced* and is dry with pruritus. Small, red, spidery marks (spider nevi) may appear on the face and body. Changes in the endocrine system cause testicular atrophy, gynecomastia, and loss of chest hair in the male (Fig. 8.39).

As the cirrhosis advances, memory is impaired, and confusion and drowsiness occur and intensify. If cirrhosis is left untreated, hepatic failure and death eventually follow.

Patient Screening

The medical history determines the urgency to see the physician or health care provider. The following changes in a patient diagnosed with cirrhosis should be reported to the provider immediately: changes in behavior or intellectual function, increased ascites, edema, shortness of breath, or GI bleeding.

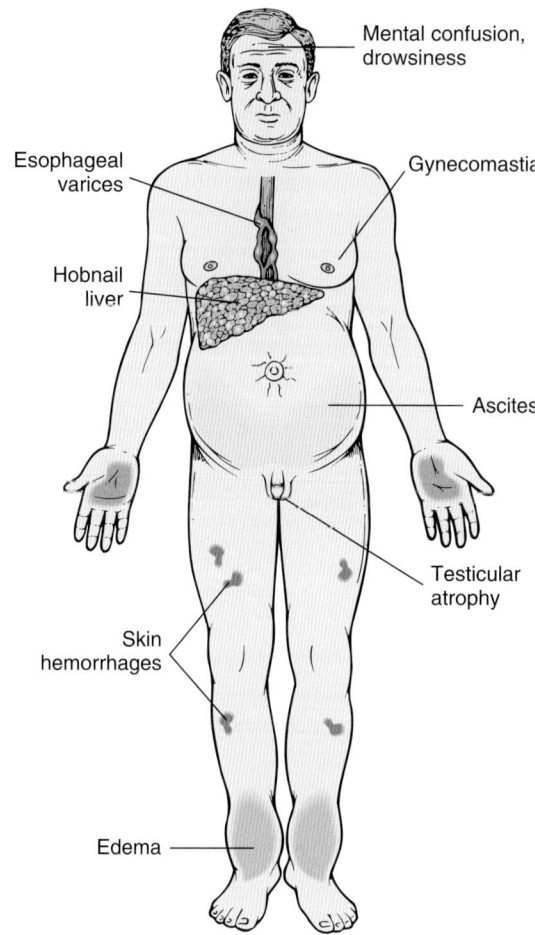

• **Fig. 8.39** Cirrhosis of the liver (in the male).

Etiology

The causes of cirrhosis are many, but the most common cause is chronic alcoholism. Malnutrition, hepatitis (see the Hepatitis B and Hepatitis C sections), parasites, toxic (poisonous) chemicals, and congestive heart failure are other possible causes of this disease. Inherited disorders, such as Wilson disease and *hemochromatosis,* can be predisposing conditions leading to cirrhosis of the liver. Cirrhosis also may be idiopathic.

Diagnosis

On physical examination, the liver appears enlarged, firm to hard; palpable blunt edge; abdominal radiographs show this enlargement. Blood studies may reveal elevated liver enzyme and bilirubin levels. CT, ultrasonography, and needle biopsy of the liver are helpful to determine the type and extent of fibrosis.

Treatment

Treatment is directed at the cause of the disease in an attempt to prevent further damage to the liver. Regardless of the underlying cause, alcohol intake is prohibited. Malnutrition must be prevented, and adequate rest is essential. Vitamin and mineral supplements, along with antacids, are given. Diuretics reduce the excessive fluid (edema) that accumulates in the abdomen (ascites) and ankles. With significant ascites, it is sometimes necessary to drain the accumulated fluid by inserting a large needle into the peritoneal cavity (paracentesis). Paracentesis alleviates the discomfort from all of the fluid causing edema, but it also carries risk of infection. In other cases, fluid accumulates in tissues, and paracentesis is not indicated. When the disease progresses to liver failure, liver transplantation is a viable option.

Prognosis

Some early liver damage can be reversed. Patients with cirrhosis are at risk for the development of hepatocellular carcinoma (HCC). Liver transplantation has greatly improved the outlook for patients who are acceptable candidates and are referred early for evaluation.

Prevention

Early diagnosis of the cause of the patient's abnormal liver function tests and institution of appropriate treatment can prevent progression to cirrhosis.

Drinking alcohol only in moderation is the most effective prevention; about half of all cases result from chronic alcoholism. Chemical toxins, such as arsenic and carbon tetrachloride, should be avoided. Exposure to infections known to damage the liver, such as those that cause hepatitis, must be shunned. Caution must be exercised when taking medications known to be damaging to the liver.

Patient Teaching

Because the cause and progression of symptoms vary, patient teaching is highly customized. Give the patient a written schedule explaining how to take prescribed medications. Advise the patient to inform any other health care professional, including the dentist, about the cirrhotic liver disease because of the resulting reduction in medication tolerance. Explain the importance of a low-sodium, highly nutritious diet, and give the patient a list of food and alcohol restrictions.

Viral Hepatitis

Description

Viral hepatitis is a systemic infection causing symptoms ranging from mild inflammation of the liver to severe involvement with destruction of hepatic cells. Viral hepatitis, a common cause of acute hepatitis, is endemic in much of the world. Most cases are caused by one of several viral agents described by the letters of the alphabet. Some cases lead to chronic viral hepatitis, which is the 10th leading cause of death among adults in the United States. The transmission of the disease varies with the type of virus: Hepatitis A virus (HAV) moves through the fecal-oral route; hepatitis B virus (HBV) and hepatitis C virus (HCV) are bloodborne. Similar symptoms occur with all forms of viral hepatitis. The differential diagnosis is based on the results of laboratory tests. Treatment is symptomatic in acute cases; some chronic cases respond to antiviral agents.

Patient Screening

When the patient complains of an abrupt onset of fatigue, fever, jaundice, malaise, dark urine, and/or yellowing of the sclera of the eyes, prompt medical evaluation is indicated.

> ### ✖ *NOTE*
>
> All universal precautions should be observed when the patient is treated. Administration of hepatitis B vaccine is recommended for health care workers as a means of primary prevention.
> Viral hepatitis is contagious until recovery is complete. Once recovered, the patient is immune to future infection with the same virus.

Symptoms and Signs

Many patients, especially children, are asymptomatic. Clinical manifestations of viral hepatitis can range from mild to chronic or severe. Many cases are self-limiting, with complete recovery. Severe viral hepatitis can be life-threatening when liver function is destroyed and waste products accumulate in blood. Because the liver has many functions, many abnormal findings are possible on blood and urine tests. The specific type of hepatitis can be established through laboratory tests that look for antibody and antigen markers.

Common symptoms in all forms of hepatitis include abrupt onset of headache, anorexia, malaise, fever, nausea, dark urine, and clay-colored stools. Jaundice and yellowing of the sclera of the eyes are evident in most patients. The patient may complain of abdominal discomfort and myalgia. Liver enlargement may be noted during physical examination.

Hepatitis A

Description

Hepatitis A is highly contagious and results in mild acute liver infection. The incubation period varies from 15 to 50 days. Symptoms can be mild to severe. In most cases, the infection is self-limiting, liver function is fully recovered, and lifelong immunity to HAV is conferred. Hepatitis A is the only viral hepatitis causing spiking fevers.

ICD-10-CM Code	B15.9 *(Hepatitis A without hepatic coma)* (B15.0-B15.9 = 2 codes of specificity)

Etiology

The causative virus, HAV, is highly contagious and is transmitted by the fecal-oral route from contaminated food (including shellfish and contaminated raw fruit and vegetables), water, and stools. HAV is present in the stool before symptoms are evident. This form of hepatitis is sometimes known as *epidemic* or *infectious hepatitis* because it frequently occurs at schools, camps, or institutions.

Diagnosis

A hepatitis profile is performed to identify the antibody and antigen markers and thereby establish the causative virus. Liver function studies are used to support the diagnosis. Blood tests show elevated serum levels of alanine aminotransaminase (ALT) and aspartate aminotransaminase (AST), usually found in the liver. The prothrombin time

(PT) is prolonged, and the serum bilirubin level is elevated. Urine tests show bilirubinuria. The presence of antibody to HAV in serum confirms the diagnosis.

Treatment

General medical management includes rest and symptom control. Intramuscular administration of immune globulin is recommended within 2 weeks of exposure. The patient is isolated, and care is taken to prevent cross-infection. Medications to control nausea and pain are given, as needed. Other measures taken while the liver heals are a low-fat, high-carbohydrate diet and restriction of physical activity. Alcohol should be avoided at all costs because of its potential to strain the liver.

Prognosis

In adult patients, the disease can be severe during the acute stage and lasts 4 to 8 weeks. Recovery is usually complete. Chronic hepatitis A does not occur, and there is no carrier state. Clinical illness is more severe in adults; children may not present symptoms.

Prevention

Vaccination against hepatitis A is recommended before travel into areas where hepatitis A is prevalent and where sanitation is poor. The vaccine should be received at least 2 weeks before potential exposure. One dose is sufficient for primary immunization, and a booster dose is given 6 to 12 months later. The duration of immunity has not been established. Vaccination is recommended for anyone with close contact with an infected person.

Prevention includes education about proper sanitation, hand washing, food preparation, and immunizations.

Patient Teaching

Preventive measures and immunization are recommended. The patient should habitually practice proper hand washing, careful food preparation, cooking, and storage. The patient should dispose of fecal matter, including soiled diapers, properly. Person-to-person contamination is common in such places as day care centers, among family members, and spread to customers in eating places. Inform the patient that the virus can be spread until recovery is complete.

Hepatitis B

ICD-10-CM Code	B16.9 (*Acute hepatitis B without delta-agent and without hepatic coma*)
	(B16.0-B16.9 = 4 codes of specificity)
	B19.10 (*Unspecified viral hepatitis B without hepatic coma*)
	(B19.10-B19.11 = 2 codes of specificity)

Symptoms and Signs

The symptoms and signs of hepatitis B, or serum hepatitis, can mimic flu and are similar to those mentioned previously. The onset of hepatitis B is more insidious and the aminotransferase levels are higher than in HAV infection. Liver inflammation causes destruction of liver cells and necrosis. These changes can be detected in abnormal results of liver profile studies.

Etiology

HBV is transmitted primarily through the percutaneous and permucosal routes. When the virus enters the body, it multiplies quickly and destroys liver cells. The mode of transmission includes contact with blood, semen, vaginal secretions, and saliva. Many infections result from sexual contact or blood exchange from the sharing of contaminated needles. Health care providers are at risk of infection from "needlesticks"; therefore all patients must be considered potential sources of infection, and standard precautions must be maintained (see Chapter 3 or Chapter 12 for a list of standard universal precautions). An infected mother can transmit the virus to her infant during birth.

Diagnosis

Patient history indicates both the mode of transmission and source infection. The detection of hepatitis B surface antigen (HBsAg) in blood confirms the diagnosis. When HBsAg is detected in blood for more than 6 months, chronic hepatitis is present. While the hepatitis B antigen is present in blood, the disease is highly transmissible with exposure to blood and body fluids of the infected individual.

Treatment

Some cases are self-limiting; general medical management is the same as that described previously for hepatitis A virus. Oral antiviral therapy may be employed in chronic cases when effective results are long lasting without relapses. Interferon can be effective; younger patients may prefer it because of its shorter duration of therapy. Hepatitis B immune globulin (HBIG) is given to create passive immunity and is given to the exposed, nonimmune individual. Such exposure may occur through needlesticks or sexual relations with an infected person.

Prognosis

Because HBV infection can be acute or chronic, the prognosis varies. Some people become chronic carriers because the virus remains in blood. In most cases, however, the liver heals and regenerates, but this takes time, perhaps several months. Later in life, patients with chronic hepatitis are prone to cirrhosis and cancer of the liver. Some patients may require liver transplantation.

Prevention

Hepatitis B is common enough to cause concern about unvaccinated health care workers. Employers are required by the Occupational Safety and Health Administration (OSHA) to make hepatitis B vaccine available to workers in high-risk occupations, such as staff at hemodialysis centers, physicians, dentists, nurses, physical therapists, and personnel working in clinical and pathology laboratories and blood banks. Initially, hepatitis may not cause symptoms, so it is important that high-risk individuals be screened for the disease. Among the general population, IV drug users, those who have multiple sexual partners, and homosexual or bisexual men are at high risk. Other transmissions of the disease may occur through mother-to-newborn, blood transfusions, nonsterile tools during acupuncture, tattoos, and body piercings. Hepatitis B is not transmitted through casual contact. The vaccine for hepatitis B is recommended for all children and for individuals at high risk for contracting the disease. Cases of HPB must be reported to the appropriate county or state health department.

Patient Teaching

Compliance with medical treatment and follow-up care improve outcome. Safe practices are taught for procedures that involve blood or body fluids to avoid transmission of HBV. High-risk behaviors and high-risk occupations should be discussed, as indicated by the medical history or as needed. Not everyone who is infected with hepatitis is symptomatic, so it can be transmitted unknowingly. This makes awareness of safe practices very important.

Hepatitis C

ICD-10-CM Code   B17.10 (Acute hepatitis C without hepatic coma)
(B17.10-B17.11 = 2 codes of specificity)
B18.2 (Chronic viral hepatitis C)
(B18.2; B19.20-B19.21 = 3 codes of specificity)

Symptoms and Signs

HCV infection, considered a widespread epidemic, is the most common bloodborne infection in the United States. Many of those infected by HCV, often young adults, are asymptomatic and may unknowingly infect others. The incubation period varies from 2 weeks to 6 months. When present, symptoms resemble those of hepatitis A but are typically less severe and sometimes without jaundice. Chronic HCV infection results in gradual, insidious liver disease. Over a period of years, the infection causes necrosis, fibrosis, and cirrhosis of the liver (Fig. 8.40).

Abnormal laboratory findings may include elevated serum levels of liver enzymes and bilirubin, although this evidence is inconclusive without a positive blood test for anti-HCV antibodies. Physical assessment may find liver tenderness and enlargement.

Etiology

Hepatitis C is caused by HCV, which is transmitted via blood and body fluids. Exposure may be traced to blood

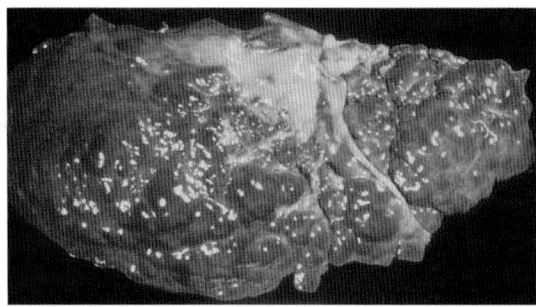

• **Fig. 8.40** Cirrhosis of the liver resulting from hepatitis C. (From Cotran R, et al: *Robbins pathologic basis of disease,* ed 6, Philadelphia, 1999, Saunders.)

transfusions, especially those performed before 1990, when blood bank procedures became rigorous; kidney dialysis; organ transplantations before 1990; or behaviors involving contact with the blood of an infected person. Other risk factors include working in the health care environment, injecting illegal drugs, sexual transmission, or sharing articles of personal hygiene (i.e., razor, dental floss, and toothbrush) with an infected person. When a person infected with HIV becomes infected with HCV, a more rapid progression to end-stage liver disease is likely and may necessitate liver transplantation. In many cases, the source of infection is not discovered.

Diagnosis

A clinical history of possible exposure to HCV accompanied by symptoms of hepatitis may point to the diagnosis. Ultrasonography of the liver may rule out other causes of liver disease. Laboratory findings include elevated serum levels of liver enzymes, elevated serum bilirubin, and bilirubinuria. HCV ribonucleic acid (RNA) serum tests detect circulating virus in the blood. A positive blood test result for the presence of anti-HCV antibodies indicates infection, past or present. Liver biopsy confirms the diagnosis.

Treatment

New medication therapy for hepatitis C has been approved. Sofosbuvir (Sovaldi) is the first treatment believed to cure hepatitis C. It must be used in conjunction with ribavirin or peginterferon and ribavirin. Sofosbuvir may be effective on genotypes 1, 2, and 4 with a 12-week regimen. Genotype 3 may be treated with a 24-week regimen. Sofosbuvir can cause birth defects and death in neonates. It should not be used with certain prescription medications or St. John's wort. Several other similar medications quickly followed, some with significantly fewer side effects and shorter treatment course. They include glecaprevir/pibrentasvir (Mavyret), sofosbuvir/velpatasvir/voxilaprevir (Vosevi), sofosbuvir/velpatasvir (Epclusa), elbasvir/grazoprevir (Zepatier), daclatasvir (Daklinza), and ledipasvir/sofosbuvir (Harvoni).

Standard treatment is typically aimed at control of symptoms and improving long-term liver function. Drug therapy may include gamma globulin, the antiviral agent interferon-α, and ribavirin to reduce inflammation. Glucocorticoids may be given to reduce inflammation. Supportive measures include rest and a well-balanced diet. The increase in HCV infection (particularly when coinfection with HIV is present) has contributed to a high demand for liver transplants in the United States.

Prognosis

Patients may recover completely. Most patients develop chronic hepatitis. In about 20% of the cases, cirrhosis of the liver eventually occurs. As mentioned previously, coinfection with HIV presents a more complicated prognosis. Chronic hepatitis carries an increased risk of liver cancer and may result in patients succumbing to liver failure.

Prevention

Standard universal precautions must be enforced. The risk factors of acute hepatitis C are employment in the health care field, IV drug abuse, intranasal cocaine use, multiple sex partners, a history of sexually transmitted diseases, tattooing and body piercing with contaminated needles, and other factors mentioned previously. There is no vaccine for hepatitis C. HCV can exist in a carrier state, that is, without any active disease or in a low-grade infection. There are more than 2.7 million HCV carriers in the United States. In the case of a known infection, every precaution must be taken to prevent transmission of the virus.

Patient Teaching

The patient is taught the importance of diet and rest during the acute stage of infection by HCV. In the case of known infection, one should emphasize precautions to prevent transmission of the virus. Risk factors should be clearly identified. Patients addicted to alcohol or actively using IV drugs should delay treatment until these addictions are under control. When drug therapy is begun, the patient should be taught the possible side effects. Pregnancy is not contraindicated in HCV-infected women, and breastfeeding is considered safe. Medical follow-up and treatment may be recommended.

Cancer of the Liver

Description

HCC is a primary tumor of the liver that usually arises in the setting of chronic liver disease (Fig. 8.41). Hepatoblastoma is a childhood cancer that arises in an otherwise normal liver.

ICD-10-CM Code	C22.0 *(Liver cell carcinoma)*
	C22.2 *(Hepatoblastoma)*
	C22.7 *(Other specified carcinomas of liver)*
	C22.8 *(Malignant neoplasm of liver, primary, unspecified as to type)*
	(C22.0-C22.9 = 8 codes of specificity)

Symptoms and Signs

Patients who develop HCC often have no symptoms other than those associated with their chronic liver disease. Symptoms of HCC or hepatoblastoma may include upper abdominal pain, weight loss, early satiety, and a palpable abdominal mass. Physical findings may include ascites, hepatomegaly, splenomegaly, and jaundice. Laboratory evaluation may reveal thrombocytopenia, elevated bilirubin, low albumin, and electrolyte abnormalities. Serum alpha-fetoprotein (AFP), a protein secreted by neoplastic liver cells, is usually elevated.

Patient Screening

Schedule prompt appointment, on request, for a patient with a history of cirrhosis.

Etiology

The most important etiologic factor in HCC worldwide is HBV infection. Additional risk factors include hereditary hemochromatosis, cirrhosis resulting from any cause (e.g., hepatitis C and alcoholism), and exposure to aflatoxins (toxins produced by molds that may contaminate food supplies, such as corn, soybeans, and peanuts). The incidence of HCC varies widely with geographic location. It is a major cause of cancer-related death in Africa and Asia. Hepatoblastoma is

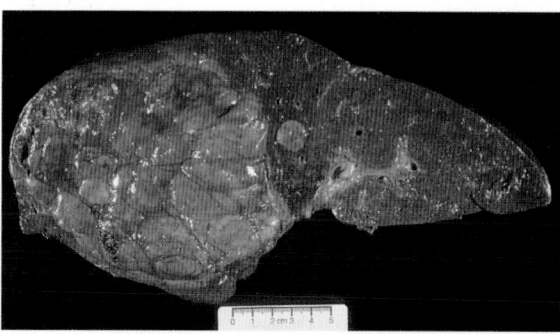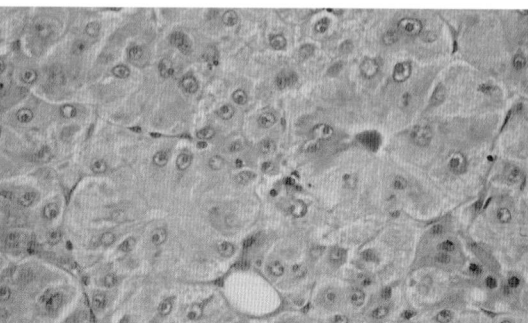

• **Fig. 8.41** Hepatocellular carcinoma (HCC). (From Cotran R, et al: *Robbins pathologic basis of disease,* ed 6, Philadelphia, 1999, Saunders.)

more common in children with a history of prematurity or with certain genetic syndromes, such as Beckwith-Wiedemann syndrome or familial colonic polyposis.

Diagnosis
The diagnosis of HCC should be suspected in a patient with cirrhosis whose condition suddenly deteriorates. An increase in AFP level to greater than 500 g/L (normal value 10–20 g/L) in a high-risk patient is diagnostic of HCC, although any AFP elevation should arouse suspicion. In any patient with an elevated AFP level, ultrasonography, CT, or MRI of the liver is the next diagnostic procedure. Liver biopsy can help make a definitive diagnosis, but it may be risky in patients with cirrhosis. Therefore it is attempted only in these patients when the result will affect disease management. Common sites of metastatic spread include bone, lungs, brain, peritoneum, and adrenal glands. A biopsy is typically necessary for hepatoblastoma diagnosis.

Treatment
Surgical resection (partial hepatectomy) of the liver is the treatment of choice for HCC, but many patients are not eligible because of tumor extent or underlying liver disease. For patients with no extrahepatic spread, liver transplantation is an option. Nonsurgical options for nonmetastatic disease are radiofrequency ablation or percutaneous ethanol injection. In some patients with unresectable disease, systemic therapy with sorafenib has shown benefit. Research into other molecularly targeted therapies for HCC is currently underway. Unlike HCC, hepatoblastoma is often sensitive to chemotherapy. Surgical resection or liver transplantation can be curative.

Prognosis
The most important factors predicting survival are tumor size, severity of underlying liver disease, and presence of metastatic disease. Because HCC often is detected late, the median survival after diagnosis is 6 to 20 months. Patients living in high-incidence regions and those with higher AFP levels often have a worse prognosis. For hepatoblastoma, a low AFP level is also associated with a poor prognosis. The 5-year overall survival for hepatoblastoma is around 70%.

Prevention
Vaccination against the hepatitis B virus could reduce the high rate of HCC worldwide. Other methods of prevention include treatment of viral hepatitis and cessation of alcohol use. Patients with cirrhosis should be screened for HCC with ultrasonography every 6 months. Children with genetic conditions associated with hepatoblastoma should get regular ultrasound screening.

Patient Teaching
The clinical effects of liver cancer present many indications for comprehensive support measures. Explain the need for special diet restrictions and total abstinence from alcohol. The treatment plan will be highly customized, depending on the therapies employed and the stage of the cancer. Give written and oral directions. Preoperative and postoperative instructions may be indicated. Emotional support is of primary importance for the family and the patient.

ENRICHMENT
Nonalcoholic Fatty Liver Disease
There are patients who drink little or no alcohol but are diagnosed with various liver conditions that fall under the diagnosis of nonalcoholic fatty liver disease (NAFLD). Patients with NAFLD have one thing in common: too much fat stored in the cells of the liver. The incidence rates of NAFLD are increasing around the world, and in the United States, this is the most frequently seen form of chronic liver disease. About 25% of the population is affected. Those who have NAFLD are at risk of developing nonalcoholic steatohepatitis (NASH). NASH causes liver inflammation and can advance to cirrhosis of the liver and liver failure. Although the liver damage is similar to that with heavy alcohol use, the etiology is not alcohol use. Obesity is one thing that puts a patient at a higher risk for developing NAFLD and NASH. Patients diagnosed with NAFLD can reverse the process toward scarring and potential liver damage by losing 10% of their body weight in the first year after diagnosis. A healthy diet and moderate approach to losing weight, rather than resorting to extreme measures to change one's entire lifestyle, are more effective. In addition, regular exercise is recommended as part of the treatment protocol.

Cholelithiasis (Gallstones)
Description
Cholelithiasis is a common condition in which there is an abnormal presence of calculi or gallstones that form in the bile.

ICD-10-CM Code	K80.20 (Calculus of gallbladder without cholecystitis without obstruction) (K80.00-K81.9 = 44 codes of specificity)

Symptoms and Signs
The patient with cholelithiasis (gallstones) may be asymptomatic until the bile ducts become obstructed by the stones (Fig. 8.42). Colicky pain, or biliary colic, signals the obstruction of the cystic duct or the common bile duct by one or more stones. The pain is in the epigastric region or the right upper quadrant of the abdomen, often radiating to the right upper back in the area of the scapula. Nausea and vomiting accompany the typically severe pain. The patient may report flatulence and clay-colored stools. If the obstruction is prolonged, jaundice may appear. Laboratory studies may show transient elevations of bilirubin and alkaline phosphate, AST, and ALT.

Patient Screening
Biliary colic begins with sudden severe waves of pain in the upper right quadrant (URQ) of the abdomen that may

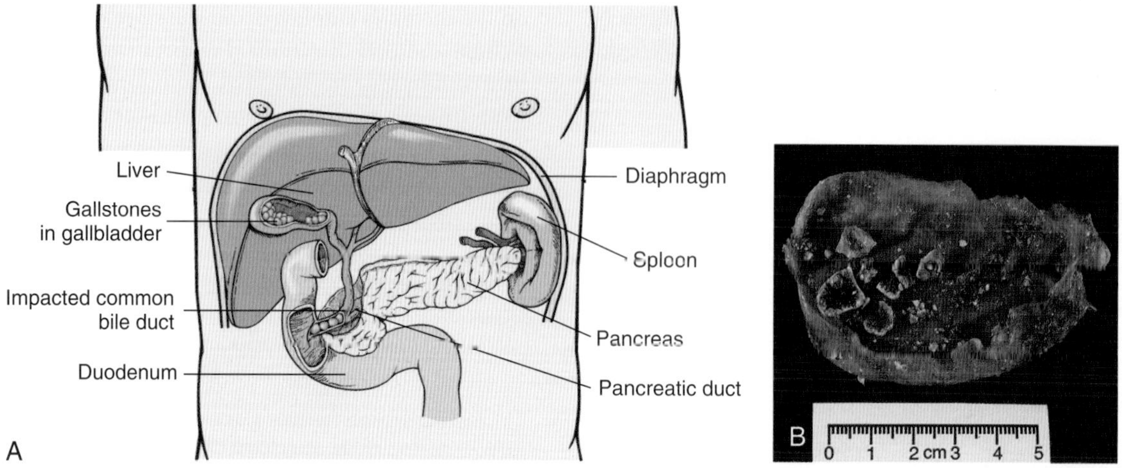

Liver

Gallstones in gallbladder

Impacted common bile duct

Duodenum

A

Diaphragm

Spleen

Pancreas

Pancreatic duct

B

• **Fig. 8.42** (A) Cholelithiasis. (B) Cholesterol gallstones. (From Kumar V, et al: *Robbins basic pathology,* ed 8, Philadelphia, 2008, Saunders.)

radiate to the back; the patient may describe this as "gripping or stabbing pain." Initially, medication for pain is given as soon as possible. The patient should be asked about nausea and vomiting and the presence of jaundice noted.

Etiology

Gallstones form in the gallbladder from insoluble cholesterol and bile salts; they vary in size and number. The reasons they form are not always clear, although they are more common with increasing age, with the high-calorie, high-cholesterol diet associated with obesity, and in the female population. Other risk factors are oral contraceptive use and ileal disease. People with alcoholic cirrhosis or biliary tract infection are also susceptible. The incidence of gallstones is increased in patients with diabetes mellitus.

In the United States, greater than 10% of men and 20% of women have gallstones by age 65 years; the total exceeds 20 million.

Diagnosis

The clinical picture and ultrasonography of the gallbladder and biliary ducts are highly accurate in confirming the presence of cholelithiasis. One can estimate the size and type of stones with some accuracy through test results (Fig. 8.43). The serum bilirubin level is elevated with obstruction of the common bile duct.

Treatment

Asymptomatic gallstones are usually left alone. Fatty intake should be controlled through dietary changes. If the patient experiences recurring pain, surgical removal of the gallbladder (cholecystectomy) is indicated. A surgical procedure called *laparoscopic cholecystectomy* has shortened hospitalization and recovery time. Endoscopic retrograde cholangiopancreatography (ERCP) is used to identify and remove stones in the common bile duct. The use of oral preparations, called *bile acids* (chenodeoxycholic or ursodeoxycholic acid), to dissolve the gallstones may be attempted in some cases, for example, in patients who are

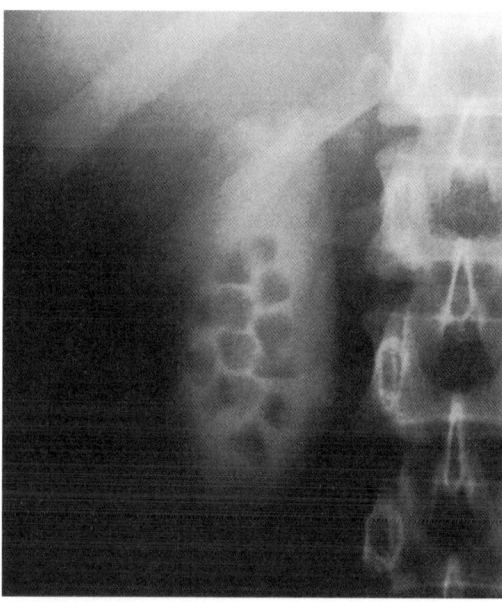

• **Fig. 8.43** Oral cholecystogram. (From Doughty DB, Jackson DB: *Gastrointestinal disorders—Mosby's clinical nursing series,* St Louis, 1993, Mosby.)

too ill to undergo surgery. It is most successful in patients with pure cholesterol gallstones that are less than one-half inch in diameter. It is usually not successful in patients with calcified stones. Another nonsurgical treatment is called *extracorporeal shock wave lithotripsy (ESWL).* This method is considered safe and preserves the function of the gallbladder, but positive results have been limited.

Prognosis

In mild cases, diet modifications may resolve symptoms, but a cholecystectomy provides the best prognosis by eliminating recurrences. In patients with longstanding gallstone disease, chronic cholecystitis can develop. When there is infection, the recovery depends on a good response to antibiotics. Recovery varies with the method of treatment, as mentioned earlier. Nonsurgical interventions require more time to achieve results and have a limited role.

Prevention

A low-fat diet may help prevent attacks of biliary colic. Once the patient becomes symptomatic, surgery is required to prevent the complications of chronic obstruction, including sepsis, stricture of the bile ducts, and pancreatitis.

Patient Teaching

Explain the risk factors, including a high-fat, high-calorie diet; hormone replacement therapy; obesity; diabetes; and liver disease. Emphasize the importance of the low-fat diet and the purpose of the prescribed medication. List the signs and symptoms that may indicate the onset of cholecystitis (see the Cholecystitis section).

Cholecystitis

Description

Cholecystitis is acute or chronic inflammation of the gallbladder, usually associated with obstruction of the cystic duct.

ICD-10-CM Code	K81.2 *(Acute cholecystitis with chronic cholecystitis)*

(K81.0 K81.9 — 4 codes of specificity)

Refer to the physician's diagnosis and then to the current edition of the ICD-10-CM coding manual to ensure the greatest specificity.

Symptoms and Signs

Cholecystitis, or inflammation of the gallbladder, usually is associated with cholelithiasis; infection often follows the inflammation (Fig. 8.44). The condition can become chronic.

The patient experiences acute colicky pain, which localizes in the URQ of the abdomen and becomes more severe when radiating around to the right lower scapular region. In addition, the patient may experience nausea and vomiting, followed by guarding of the URQ muscles and shallow

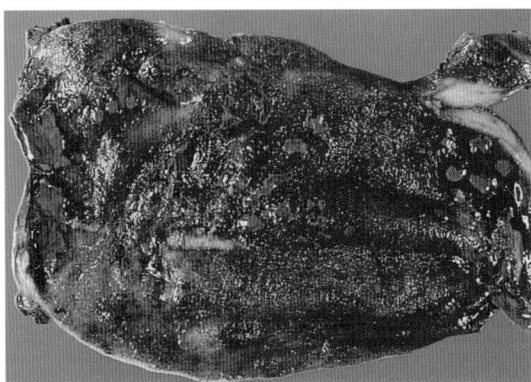

• **Fig. 8.44** Cholecystitis. (From Damjanov I, Linder J: *Pathology: a color atlas,* St Louis, 1999, Mosby.)

respirations. A fever may ensue. Other signs are jaundice, clay-colored stools, dark urine, and pruritus. In some cases, the acutely inflamed gallbladder ruptures, causing peritonitis. Otherwise the cholecystitis may subside spontaneously, and the pain begins to abate in a few days; there is a high likelihood of recurrence unless a cholecystectomy is performed.

Patient Screening

Acute onset of biliary colic with nausea, vomiting, chills, fever, and jaundice requires a prompt medical evaluation.

Etiology

Most cholecystitis results from an obstruction of the gallbladder caused by gallstones. Trauma or other insult to the gallbladder, including infection, occasionally is the cause.

Diagnosis

The diagnosis is based on the clinical picture and ultrasonography of the gallbladder and biliary ducts. Radioisotope gallbladder study (hepatobiliary iminodiacetic acid [HIDA] scan) that indicates a nonvisualized gallbladder points to acute gallbladder disease. Other findings include an elevated WBC count and an increased serum bilirubin level.

Treatment

Treatment in uncomplicated cases consists of dietary modification with elimination of fatty foods. The acutely ill patient with persistent vomiting is given nothing by mouth, and a nasogastric tube might be inserted. IV solution is given to replace fluids and electrolytes. When the patient is stabilized, surgical intervention to remove the gallbladder (cholecystectomy) is indicated. Medical management may include the administration of antibiotics, analgesics, and antiemetics while the patient is awaiting surgery.

Prognosis

Mild and uncomplicated cases have a positive prognosis. Acute complications include gangrene of the gallbladder, gallbladder perforation, emphysematous cholecystitis (secondary infection with a gas-forming organism), and empyema. Chronic cholecystitis has been associated with fibrotic changes and may predispose the patient to adenocarcinoma of the gallbladder.

Prevention

Early medical attention and dietary modifications at onset of symptoms related to inflammation of the gallbladder are the initial attempts to control the stages and complications of chronic gallbladder disease.

Patient Teaching

Explain the relationship between a high-calorie, high-fat diet and the onset of gallstone disease that can, in turn, predispose to inflammation of the gallbladder. If a patient undergoes a cholecystectomy, explain that the liver will continue to produce bile for fat digestion.

Acute and Chronic Pancreatitis

Description

Pancreatitis is acute or chronic inflammation of the pancreas with variable involvement of adjacent and remote organs.

ICD-10-CM Code	K85.9 *(Acute pancreatitis, unspecified)*
	(K85.0-K85.9 = 6 codes of specificity)
	K86.1 *(Other chronic pancreatitis)*
	(K86.0-K86.9 = 6 codes of specificity)

Symptoms and Signs

The pancreas functions as both an endocrine and an exocrine organ (Fig. 8.45). Pancreatitis is inflammation of the pancreas. It can range from a mild and self-limiting disease to chronic and fatal destruction of pancreatic tissue. In pancreatitis, the pancreas becomes inflamed, edematous, hemorrhagic, and necrotic (Fig. 8.46). The patient with acute pancreatitis has a sudden onset of severe abdominal pain that radiates to the back and nausea and vomiting. Epigastric pain is often worsened by walking and lying supine or improved by sitting and leaning forward. In acute pancreatitis, the patient appears acutely ill, diaphoretic, and tachycardic, with shallow, rapid respirations. Blood pressure falls, and body temperature rises. The abdomen is tender mainly in the upper quadrants, most often without guarding and rigidity. Bowel sounds are reduced. Mild jaundice is common. Many local and systemic complications (e.g., pancreatic abscess, necrotizing pancreatitis, and pneumonia) are possible.

Chronic pancreatitis can present a vague clinical picture. The patient may report constant pain in the back, with repeated mild episodes of the symptoms of acute pancreatitis. Anorexia, nausea, vomiting, constipation, flatulence, and weight loss are common. As pancreatic function deteriorates and the organ becomes fibrotic, signs of malabsorption and diabetes mellitus appear. Psychiatric disturbances, including depression and anxiety, have been reported.

Patient Screening

Acute pancreatitis is a life-threatening emergency. Systemic symptoms listed previously require emergency medical intervention.

Etiology

Acute pancreatitis is thought to result from the "escape" of activated pancreatic enzymes from acinar cells (i.e., cells of the tiny lobules of the gland) into surrounding tissues. Several theories have been proposed for the mechanism that initiates acute pancreatitis and that triggers pancreatic autodigestion. Alcoholism, biliary tract disease, trauma, infection, structural anomalies, greatly elevated calcium levels in the blood, hemorrhage, hyperlipidemia, or drugs may cause pancreatitis. Gallstones are often the cause of pancreatitis in the nonalcoholic individual. Less often, the cause is a metabolic or endocrine disorder. Some cases are idiopathic. Smoking may increase the risk of alcoholic and idiopathic pancreatitis.

Diagnosis

The diagnosis is based on the clinical picture, with dramatically elevated serum amylase and lipase levels on the first day of the attack. Serum amylase and lipase levels

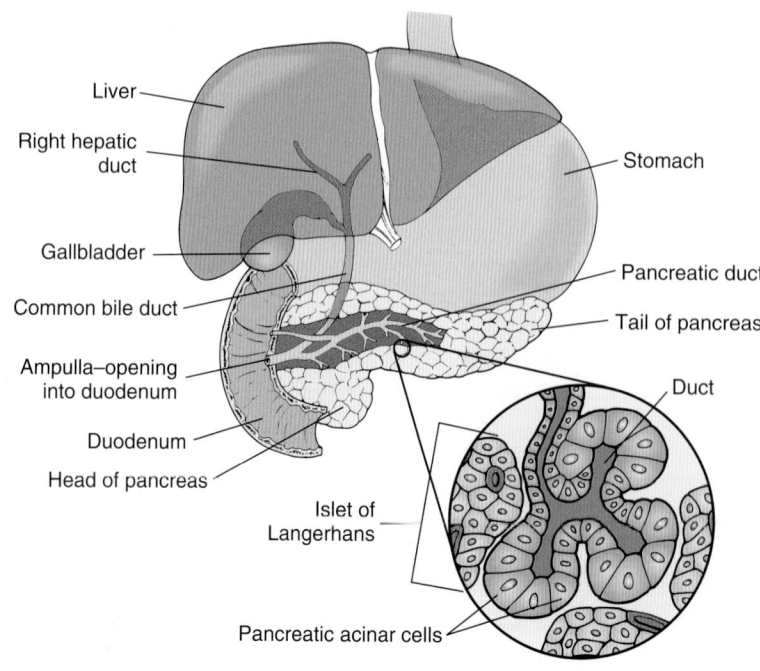

• **Fig. 8.45** Location and structure of the pancreas.

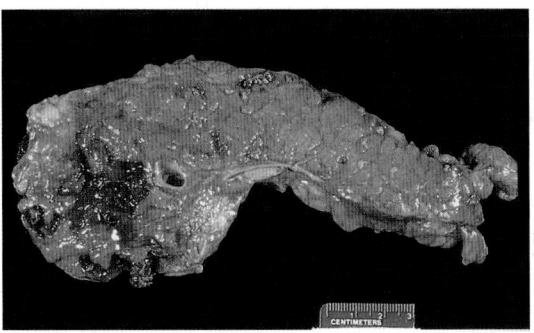

• **Fig. 8.46** Acute pancreatitis. (From Cotran R, et al: *Robbins pathologic basis of disease,* ed 6, Philadelphia, 1999, Saunders.)

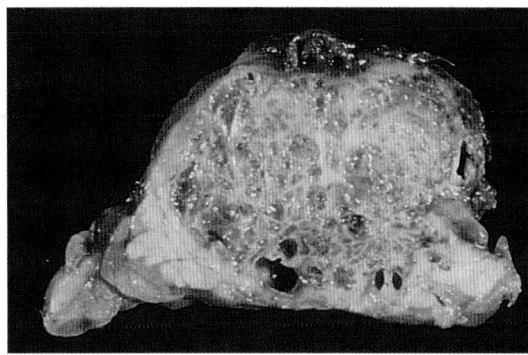

• **Fig. 8.47** Pancreatic cancer. (From Cotran R, et al: *Robbins pathologic basis of disease,* ed 6, Philadelphia, 1999, Saunders.)

usually return to normal by the third day. The WBC count and Hct are usually elevated. Hyperglycemia is commonly present. Radiography and ultrasonography may reveal stones in the biliary tract or dilation of the common bile duct, and the bilirubin level may be elevated. CT, with oral or IV contrast material, identifies pancreatic changes and complications.

Treatment

Most cases are mild without systemic and local complications; treatment includes general supportive care. In contrast, acute pancreatitis may require emergency treatment consisting of IV fluid and electrolyte replacement. The patient is given nothing by mouth, and in some cases, a nasogastric suction tube is introduced with intermittent suction. Pain medication, usually a narcotic, is given per health care provider's order. Laboratory blood values of electrolytes, serum amylase and lipase, Hct, glucose, and serum calcium are monitored. The development of a pancreatic abscess is an indication for prompt percutaneous or surgical drainage.

In chronic pancreatitis, the patient also must be monitored closely for malabsorption, steatorrhea, and impaired glucose tolerance indicating diabetes mellitus. If the underlying cause of pancreatitis is an obstructed pancreatic duct, then surgery may be necessary to remove the obstruction.

Prognosis

In approximately 80% of mild cases, the condition resolves within a week. Severe cases with systemic complications or pancreatic necrosis face a variable outcome. The mortality rate in these cases ranges from 15% to 100%. Half the deaths occur within the first 2 weeks, usually from multiorgan failure. Recurrences are common in alcoholic pancreatitis.

Prevention

Preventive measures are based on the many clinical conditions, medications, and toxins associated with acute pancreatitis.

Patient Teaching

Explain the measures needed to reduce recurrent episodes: forgoing alcohol, if the cause is alcohol related; and carefully managing gallstone disease, including treatment with

cholecystectomy. Teach the warning signs of endocrine and exocrine insufficiency: weight loss, digestive disturbance, and the signs and symptoms of hypoglycemia and hyperglycemia.

Pancreatic Cancer

Description

Cancer of the pancreas is a neoplasm, usually an adenocarcinoma, and occurs more often in the head of the pancreas (Fig. 8.47). Most neoplasms arise from the exocrine cells of the pancreas, whereas 1% to 2% involve the endocrine cells.

ICD-10-CM Code	C25.9 *(Malignant neoplasm of pancreas, unspecified)* (C25.0–C25.9 = 8 codes of specificity)

Symptoms and Signs

Most patients with pancreatic cancer experience abdominal pain, weight loss, or jaundice. Nausea, vomiting, acholic (without bile) stools, and steatorrhea are also common. On examination, the patient may have ascites, abdominal tenderness, or a palpable gallbladder. As pancreatic tissue is infiltrated and destroyed, the patient can experience glucose intolerance, increasing weakness, fatigue, and diarrhea. Laboratory studies may reveal elevated bilirubin and alkaline phosphatase concentrations.

Patient Screening

The patient often reports feeling generally quite ill and experiencing the symptoms listed previously; a prompt appointment is indicated.

Etiology

Cancer of the pancreas is the fourth leading cause of cancer-related deaths in the United States. The peak age of incidence is in the 45- to 60-year-old age group. Risk factors include cigarette smoking, obesity, a history of chronic pancreatitis or diabetes, and a family history of pancreatic cancer. Mutations in the cancer susceptibility genes *BRCA1, BRCA2,* and *STK11* are also associated with an increased risk of pancreatic cancer.

Diagnosis

Because of the retroperitoneal location of the pancreas, carcinoma is difficult to detect. The pancreas is inaccessible to palpation and insensitive to many diagnostic techniques. The diagnosis of pancreatic cancer is typically made radiographically and histologically. The initial study in a patient with suspected pancreatic cancer is either an abdominal ultrasonography or CT. ERCP may be done. Cancer is suggested by dilated bile ducts or a mass in the pancreas. There is a serum tumor marker for pancreatic cancer, CA 19-9. An elevated level suggests the presence of cancer and very high levels correlate with a poor prognosis.

If cancer is suspected or a mass lesion is present, a tissue diagnosis by EUS fine-needle aspiration biopsy of the mass and lymph nodes is necessary to guide treatment. If EUS is not available, a staging laparoscopy may be performed. The patient may be a candidate for surgery if the patient shows no evidence of distant metastases and no involvement of the major vessels. Pancreatic tumors are classified and staged according to the TNM classification system. See Chapter 1 for information about the staging and grading systems used to assess malignant neoplasms.

Treatment

Surgical resection is the only potentially curative treatment for pancreatic cancer. It is a viable option only for patients with disease confined to the pancreas and peripancreatic nodes. Because of late detection of the disease, however, only 15% to 20% of patients are candidates for surgery. For palliative treatment of advanced pancreatic cancer, chemotherapy with or without radiation therapy is the current standard of care. Stents can be placed to relieve bile duct obstruction or gastric outlet obstruction. Control of pain and treatment of depression are also important in the palliation of pancreatic cancer. Weight loss and malabsorption often are treated with pancreatic enzyme replacement. Patients need to be monitored closely after treatment with repeat serum CA 19-9 and CT examinations.

Prognosis

The prognosis is poor even after surgical resection; the 5-year survival rate is about 5% to 25%. The median survival is 8 to 12 months for those with locally advanced, unresectable disease and 3 to 6 months for those with metastatic disease. The tumor can invade adjacent structures, such as the duodenum, stomach, and liver, and death often results from these local effects.

Prevention

Cessation of cigarette smoking is recommended. Although screening programs are available for people at high risk (those with family cancer syndromes or hereditary pancreatitis), experts have not reached a consensus regarding the type and the interval of screening.

Patient Teaching

Give the patient and his or her family both written and verbal instructions, as indicated, about surgery, pain management, and chemotherapy. Allow the time and opportunity for the patient and the family to ask questions and express their feelings and anxiety. Make referrals for home care, hospice care, and social services, as needed.

Disorders of Nutrient Intake and Absorption

Proper nutrition is needed to enable the regulation and function of all processes to ensure that the human body is healthy and has the energy and nutrients to build and repair tissues. Nutritional deficiencies, excesses, or imbalances can affect the body's homeostasis. Any inability of the GI tract to digest or absorb nutrients can cause forms of malnutrition, even with adequate intake of food. Prolonged malnutrition or malabsorption results in anatomic lesions or disease entities.

Malnutrition

Description

Malnutrition is a disorder of nutrition caused by primary deprivation of protein-energy (seen in poverty or self-imposed starvation) or secondary to deficiency diseases (e.g., cancer or diabetes).

ICD-10-CM Code	E46 (Unspecified protein-calorie malnutrition)

Symptoms and Signs

Disturbances in nutrition can result from eating too much or too little food or from having an imbalanced diet. When a body cannot absorb or use food properly, malnutrition will result, even with sufficient nutritional intake. Malnutrition disrupts the body's metabolic processes, disturbing normal physical structure and biologic function.

Malnourishment can cause many specific disease conditions, such as abnormal growth, with physical and intellectual impairment. A human body deprived of adequate nutrition cannot maintain health. The appetite may decrease or increase, resulting in emaciation or obesity. Signs and symptoms of malnutrition include loss of energy, diarrhea, drastic weight change, skin lesions, loss of hair, poor nails, and generalized edema; delayed healing and greasy stools may result from loss of fat. More advanced signs may include muscle wasting (most noticeably in the temporalis and interosseus muscles), enlarged glands, and hepatomegaly. Many abnormal findings of blood and urine tests are possible.

Patient Screening

A patient with a recent, unintended, or unexplainable weight loss of 10 lb or greater should be scheduled for a complete physical examination.

Etiology

Protein-energy malnutrition has been described as two distinct syndromes. Kwashiorkor, caused by a deficiency of protein in the presence of adequate energy, is typically seen in weaning infants at the birth of a sibling in areas where food

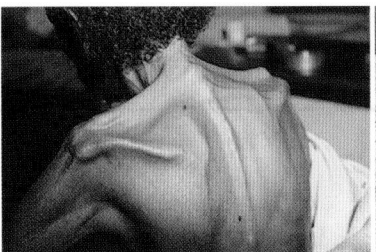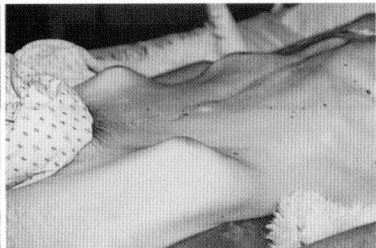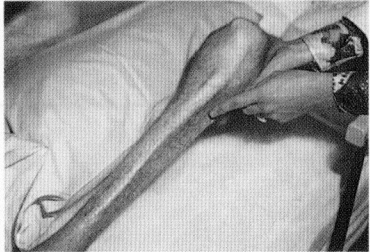

• **Fig. 8.48** Protein-energy malnutrition. (From Morgan SL, Weinsier RL: *Fundamentals of clinical nutrition,* ed 2, St Louis, 1998, Mosby.)

containing protein is insufficiently abundant. Marasmus (extreme malnutrition and emaciation), caused by combined protein and energy deficiency, is most commonly seen where adequate quantities of food are not available (Fig. 8.48).

In industrialized societies, protein-energy malnutrition is most often secondary to other disease. Kwashiorkor-like secondary protein-energy malnutrition occurs primarily in association with increased metabolic acute illnesses, such as trauma, burns, and sepsis. Marasmus-like secondary protein-energy malnutrition typically results from chronic diseases, such as chronic obstructive pulmonary disease (COPD), congestive heart failure, cancer, or AIDS.

In both syndromes, protein-energy malnutrition is caused either by decreased intake of energy and protein, increased nutrient losses, or increased nutrient requirements dictated by the underlying disease. For example, diminished oral intake may result from poor dentition or various GI disorders. Loss of nutrients results from malabsorption and diarrhea and from glycosuria. Nutrient requirements are increased by fever, surgery, neoplasia, and burns.

Diagnosis

Clinical evaluation of the patient includes a complete physical examination with special attention to weight and measurements of body fat and muscle mass. Laboratory diagnostic findings vary, depending on the cause and type of malnutrition. Laboratory tests include blood protein level, CBC, and a 24-hour urine test for urea nitrogen. The tests may show evidence of mineral deficiency, anemia, abnormal protein metabolism, and other changes in metabolism related to malnourishment.

Treatment

The treatment of malnutrition is based on the underlying cause. After the patient's nutritional needs are assessed, nutritional supplements and replacement begin with appropriate oral and IV feedings. Certain pathologic conditions may necessitate feedings through a nasogastric tube. Treatment may include a combination of dietary modifications with appropriate supplements of proteins, vitamins, and minerals. Diarrhea and infections are controlled with medications.

Surgery may be indicated when lesions of the GI tract cause the malnutrition. Patients with eating disorders require special counseling or psychiatric interventions in addition to medical treatment. Vulnerable populations, such as those in poverty or older adults, may require community services that make healthy nutrition available on a daily basis.

Prognosis

The prognosis varies with the nature and severity of malnutrition. Severe cases have a high morbidity and mortality rate. Loss of 35% to 40% of body weight usually results in death.

Prevention

Address the underlying cause to correct nutritional deficiencies, restore weight, and prevent complications.

Patient Teaching

After contributing factors have been identified, one can explain the treatment plan and the goals of therapy. Nutritional status is monitored, and the therapeutic diet is adjusted to allow for the patient's preferences. Address the psychological problems associated with eating disorders by making referrals for counseling and support.

ENRICHMENT

Hypervitaminosis

- Hypervitaminosis is a condition of toxicity resulting from an excess of any vitamin, but especially the fat-soluble vitamins A and D.
- The four fat (lipid)–soluble vitamins A, D, E, and K are stored in fat tissue.
- Symptoms of vitamin A toxicity include irritability, loss of hair, anorexia, enlargement of the liver and spleen, jaundice, skin changes, and psychiatric disorders. Vitamin A excess can be toxic to a developing fetus. Chronic toxicity in infants and children can cause increased pressure in the brain, tinnitus, pruritus, swelling of the optic nerve, and abnormal bone growth.
- Vitamin D is considered highly toxic, especially in infants and children. It can cause calcification of soft tissue, poor appetite, weakness, kidney damage, excessive thirst and urination, and mental changes. Note: The tolerable upper level for adults has been set at 2000 international units (IU; 50 mcg). 4000 IU is the new upper limit recommendation for ages 8 years or greater.
- Very high doses of vitamin E may interfere with the blood-clotting action of vitamin K.
- Vitamin K toxicity is uncommon. Rapid infusion causes dyspnea, flushing, cardiovascular complications, red blood cell (RBC) hemolysis, jaundice, and brain damage.
- Water-soluble vitamin C taken in excess causes nausea, diarrhea, and acidification of urine; niacin (B_3) may cause flushing, hyperglycemia, and liver damage; vitamin B_6 may cause photosensitivity and peripheral nerve damage.
- Overload of nutritional trace elements also produces toxicity.

Facts about Obesity

- Overweight and obesity are identified objectively by the use of the body mass index (BMI). The formula is weight-adjusted for height. For instance, the calculation is weight in pounds, divided by (height in inches)^2 and multiplied by 703. A number greater than 25.0 defines overweight, and a BMI of 30.0 or higher is classified as morbid obesity. A BMI of 40.0 or higher defines extreme obesity.
- In the United States, more than 2 of 3 people are overweight or obese. Adult obesity is an epidemic in the country despite the popularity of fad diets and sugar-free and fat-free products that are presented as the antidotes to overweight and obesity.
- More women are obese compared with men, especially as they age.
- The causes of obesity are complex, but a major correlation has been made with greater energy intake than output.
- Fatness and the regional distribution of fat have a strong genetic component.
- Factors that may contribute to obesity include overeating (sometimes linked to psychological stress or environment), a low rate of energy expenditure, inactivity, and more rarely, endocrine disorders.
- Obesity contributes to severe health problems, such as diabetes mellitus, hypertension, cardiovascular disease, sleep apnea, blood lipid abnormalities, orthopedic problems, and skin problems. Obesity has been associated with metabolic syndrome. Being overweight when younger than 45 years of age is more dangerous.
- Obesity can make a person feel self-conscious and can impair social relationships; overweight people sometimes experience prejudice and discrimination. Obese children are often bullied.
- Treatment goals are (1) to lose as much nonessential fat as possible while minimizing the loss of lean body mass and (2) to maintain a balance between energy intake and energy expenditure.
- Important elements in successful weight loss are active patient self-control; a supportive physician; a reduced-calorie, nutritionally adequate diet; and increased physical activity. Portion control alone has proven to be successful in weight loss.
- Other controversial treatment modalities that have known risks, or lack proven long-term success, include extremely low-calorie diets, anorectic drugs, and surgical procedures. Newer medications given to aid in weight loss include orlistat (Xenical) and rimonabant (Acomplia).
- The study of overweight people is called *bariatrics*. Some bariatric surgery centers are gaining recognition for their favorable outcomes. Bariatric surgery requires a lifetime commitment to lifestyle changes to prevent nutrient deficiencies.
- Many patients have great difficulty maintaining their reduced body weight. Lifestyle changes to include exercise and control of food intake through behavior modification remain important.
- Consultation with a health care provider is recommended before a patient starts on a substantial weight-loss program.

Malabsorption Syndrome

Description

Malabsorption syndrome refers to a group of disorders in which intestinal absorption of dietary nutrients is impaired.

ICD-10-CM Code	K90.9 *(Intestinal malabsorption, unspecified)* (K90.4-K90.9 = 4 codes of specificity)

Symptoms and Signs

A person with malabsorption syndrome has impaired digestion and is unable to absorb fat or certain other components of diet. Symptoms include abdominal discomfort, bloating with gas, chronic diarrhea, and abnormal bowel movements. Stools may appear yellowish gray and may be greasy looking. The stools tend to float because of their high fat content. Over time, untreated malabsorption leads to weight loss, anemia, shortness of breath, and symptoms of vitamin and mineral deficiencies.

Patient Screening

The patient with malabsorption syndrome needs regular appointments for follow-up care until stable.

Etiology

The main cause of malabsorption syndrome is defective mucosal cells in the small intestine. Absorption also is hindered if the intestinal enzymes and chemicals are not properly assisting the digestive process. A diseased pancreas or a blocked pancreatic duct, which deprives the small intestine of amylase and lipase, may cause secondary malabsorption syndrome. Reduced secretion of bile, caused by hepatic disease or a bile duct obstruction, also prevents lipid (fat) digestion. Metabolic or endocrine disorders, such as hyperparathyroidism and diabetes mellitus, are other possible causes of the syndrome. Severe parasitic and worm infestations, more common in developing countries, can cause malabsorption.

Diagnosis

The health care provider usually orders several blood tests to determine the levels of proteins, fats, and minerals in the patient's bloodstream. A laboratory analysis of a stool sample also may be performed. Biopsy of the small bowel may reveal a primary condition responsible for malabsorption.

Treatment

The main task for the physician or health care provider is to discover the underlying cause and to choose the course of treatment. Diet is controlled carefully. A high-protein, high-calorie diet with vitamin and mineral supplements, such as the fat-soluble vitamins A, D, E, and K, which are not being absorbed, aids the recovery.

Prognosis

Improvement can be expected when the underlying causes are identified and successfully treated. When areas of the intestines are damaged or resected, the remaining bowel can adapt to absorb nutrients.

Prevention
Many specific and nonspecific therapies are available for malabsorption.

Patient Teaching
Refer the patient to a dietitian for a nutrient-specific therapeutic diet. Give written instructions about prescribed vitamins and supplements. Instruct the patient to monitor his or her weight and return for follow-up testing for anemia.

Celiac Disease (Gluten Enteropathy)

Description
Celiac disease (celiac sprue), a disease of the small intestine, is characterized by malabsorption, gluten intolerance, and damage to the lining of the intestine.

ICD-10-CM Code	K90.0 (Celiac disease)

Symptoms and Signs
Celiac disease has multisystem effects that can produce serious health problems. Symptoms include weight loss, anorexia, abdominal cramping, diarrhea, flatulence (gas), abdominal distention, intestinal bleeding, weakness, muscle wasting, dermatitis herpetiformis (a characteristic skin rash consisting of pruritic papulovesicles over the extensor surfaces of the extremities and over the trunk, scalp, and neck), and the characteristically large, pale, greasy, foul-smelling stools. The end result of celiac disease is malabsorption and malnutrition.

Patient Screening
Assess the severity of symptoms to determine the patient's level of urgency to be seen by the health care provider.

Etiology
The cause of this disease may be either a toxic or an immunologic reaction to a component of gluten (a protein that is found in wheat and wheat products, barley, and rye). Celiac disease is linked to genetic factors because the occurrence is higher in siblings. Females are affected twice as often as males.

Diagnosis
Celiac disease is often difficult to diagnose and differentiate from other intestinal diseases and disorders. For a positive diagnosis, three criteria are needed: (1) positive serologic testing, (2) biopsy of the small intestine showing changes or destruction in the mucosal lining, and (3) improvement while on a gluten-free diet. In addition to celiac serology, laboratory tests that may be ordered include blood tests for WBC count, platelet count, albumin level, and PT, and the glucose tolerance test. Upper GI and small bowel radiographic series demonstrate the characteristic abnormal patterns of barium passage.

Treatment
The patient must strictly adhere to a lifelong gluten-free diet; eliminating gluten allows the bowel to heal and reverses malabsorption. If the patient does not improve while on the diet, it usually results from noncompliance with a strict gluten-free diet. For a resistant form of celiac disease, known as *refractory sprue,* corticosteroid drugs may be used. Consultation with a skilled dietitian is important to prevent even inadvertent consumption of gluten. Patients with this disease are more prone to abdominal lymphoma and cancer later in life, and they should be examined if GI symptoms develop.

Prognosis
A lifelong gluten-free diet usually leads to gradual recovery. When undiagnosed or improperly treated, there is an increased risk for cancer and malnutrition, especially in children.

Prevention
No prevention for celiac disease is known. Delayed recognition and treatment exposes the affected individuals to long-term complications.

Patient Teaching
Provide education about the disease process. Refer the patient to a dietitian. With regard to grains, the patient should consume corn and rice. All wheat, rye, and barley must be eliminated. Family members should be screened. To help the patient and family members cope with the complex impact this disease has on quality of life, suggest resources, such as the Celiac Disease Foundation and advocacy groups.

Food Poisoning

Description
Food poisoning is an illness resulting from the eating of food that contains bacterial toxins and viral, chemical, or toxic substances. The Centers for Disease Control and Prevention (CDC) estimates that there are up to 33 million cases of food poisoning in the United States each year.

ICD-10-CM Code	A05.9 (Bacterial foodborne intoxication, unspecified)
	(A05.0-A05.9 = 8 codes of specificity)

Symptoms and Signs
The symptoms of food poisoning are determined, in part, by the cause. The onset is sudden, with rumbling stomach sounds, nausea, vomiting, diarrhea with abdominal pain and cramps, malaise, and fever. The symptoms usually disappear within 24 to 48 hours. If an extreme case of food poisoning persists, the situation becomes life-threatening as a result of dehydration and electrolyte imbalances that can affect the cardiac system.

Patient Screening

Screen the patient for severity of symptoms and signs of dehydration, mindful that the very young and the very old are more prone to dehydration. It is appropriate to inquire about skin turgor, dry tongue, sunken eyes, and/or parched lips.

Etiology

True food poisoning includes poisoning from cheese, mushrooms, shellfish, food contaminated by poisonous insecticides, and toxic substances, such as lead and mercury. In addition, poisoning results from eating food that has undergone putrefaction or decomposition and food contaminated with bacteria or their toxins (Table 8.1).

Diagnosis

The patient's history is important to diagnosis and can point to the cause. The physician may perform endoscopy. A stool or blood culture reveals the presence of any parasites or bacteria. The actual contaminated food also may be cultured.

Treatment

Most treatment is symptomatic. Bed rest is beneficial. To prevent or minimize fluid and electrolyte imbalances, nutritional support and fluid replacement are essential. These may have to be given intravenously if the patient becomes dehydrated. The health care provider may prescribe antidiarrheal and antiemetic agents.

TABLE 8.1 Bacterial Causes of Food Poisoning

Organism	Major Food Source(s)	Pathophysiologic Mechanism	
		Toxin in Food	Ingestion of Bacteria
Staphylococcus aureus	Cooked meat, cheese, pasta, cream buns, custard pies	Yes	No
Clostridium perfringens type A	Cooked meat, vegetable soup (prepared in bulk)	No	Yes (bacteria release enterotoxin in intestine)
Clostridium botulinum	Uneviscerated cured fish, preserved or fermented meat, home-preserved vegetables	Yes	No
Salmonella enteritidis/ Salmonella typhimurium	Raw eggs, mayonnaise, incompletely cooked meat and poultry	No	Yes
Salmonella dublin	Raw milk, unpasteurized cheese	No	Yes
Salmonella typhi/ Salmonella paratyphi	Food contamination by infected food handlers	No	Yes
Vibrio cholerae O1	Raw seafood	No	Yes
Vibrio cholerae non-O1	Raw oysters	No	Yes
Vibrio parahaemolyticus	Raw seafood	No	Yes
Vibrio vulnificus	Raw seafood (especially oysters)	No	Yes
Listeria monocytogenes	Soft cheese	No	Yes
Shigella species	Food contamination during preparation	No	Yes
Escherichia coli O157:H7	Ground beef	No	Yes
Campylobacter jejuni/ Campylobacter coli	Incompletely cooked poultry and other meats, raw milk	No	Yes
Bacillus cereus Heat-stable toxin Enterotoxin	Fried rice Meat products	Yes Yes	No No
Yersinia enterocolitica	Pork, raw milk	No	Yes

(From Goldman L, Schafer AI: *Goldman's Cecil medicine*, ed 24, Philadelphia, 2012, Elsevier/Saunders.)

Prognosis

The prognosis for this condition varies with the cause. The prognosis generally is good if the cause has been determined and the treatment has begun. The earlier the diagnosis is made and treatment is begun, the better are the chances for a successful recovery. Many infections are mild and self-limiting.

Prevention

Food poisoning can be prevented by the fastidious practice of infection control techniques as primary prevention. Careful hand washing to prevent oral-fecal transmission of disease-causing organisms is especially important in restaurants, day care centers for children or elders, and health care institutions. Avoid swimming in contaminated water and drinking untreated water. Careful handling of food, eating of well-cooked food, and proper refrigeration of food reduce the risk.

Patient Teaching

Emphasize the preventive measures listed earlier. Patients who are stabilized after a severe episode are given a diet as tolerated and are advised to rest and rehydrate.

Anorexia Nervosa

Description

Anorexia nervosa, an eating disorder, is linked to a psychological disturbance in which hunger is denied by self-imposed starvation, resulting from a distorted body image and a compulsion to be thin (Fig. 8.49).

ICD-10-CM Code   F50.00 (Anorexia nervosa, unspecified)
(F50.00-F50.02 = 3 codes of specificity)
Refer to the current edition of the ICD-10-CM coding manual for exclusions.

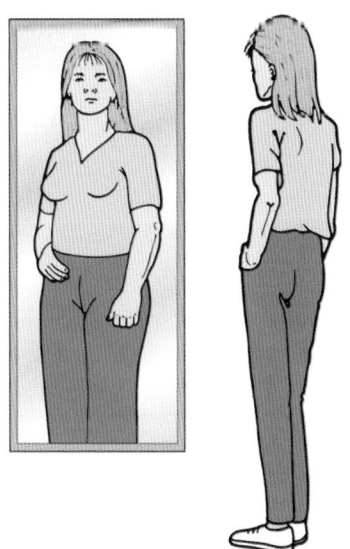

• **Fig. 8.49** Anorexia nervosa. Persons with anorexia overestimate their body width, insisting that they are too fat despite profound weight loss.

Symptoms and Signs

The typical patient with anorexia is a female adolescent who is meticulous, is a high achiever, and refuses food intake; she is preoccupied with obesity and obsesses about her weight. Although she experiences continued weight loss, she does not believe that anything is wrong with it. The patient with anorexia is one of the most difficult to treat. Concerned family members usually are the ones who bring the problem to the health care provider's attention when the girl loses weight and body mass. Other physical signs of malnutrition include thinning hair, poor wound healing, and dental changes. She may have amenorrhea, cold intolerance, constipation, bloating, or abdominal distress. The patient with anorexia usually is hyperactive and overexercises, is hypotensive, and experiences bradycardia and hypothermia. Feelings of sadness, insomnia, and withdrawal from friends and family may occur. Bulimia, which includes purging and binging, may occur concurrently.

Patient Screening

A parent or responsible party may be the first to report concern about a person's weight loss, anorexia, behavioral changes, and malnutrition-related health problems; the patient frequently denies the condition until it is more advanced. Recommend a physical examination and consultation with the physician or health care provider as soon as possible.

Etiology

The etiology is unknown, although it is believed that family and social factors may precipitate the condition. Anorexia nervosa afflicts predominately younger, affluent females, although its prevalence among the male population is rising. The risk among middle-aged women to develop body image dissatisfaction and anorexic behavior is being recognized. Stress hormones are biologic factors, which have been linked to the onset in some people. Current social and cultural factors that promote thinness reinforce anorectic behavior. Many females engaged in some sports, such as cross-country running, track, gymnastics, and swimming, may be encouraged by their coaches to attain a less-than-healthy body weight. This often triggers the anorexic behavior. There may be a genetic predisposition. The patient often is intelligent, has a compulsive personality, and is driven to achieve. Notable depression or anxiety may be present.

Diagnosis

The diagnosis is based on the clinical picture and history: The patient has lost significant weight (at least 15% of total body weight) and may appear emaciated, has intense fear of weight gain, and, if female, has absent or irregular menstruation. Assessment of vital signs may reveal hypotension and bradycardia. The nutritional status and the electrolyte balance are evaluated through laboratory tests, including blood tests, urinalysis, and an electrocardiography. Other organic causes and psychiatric disorders that cause physical wasting are ruled out.

Treatment

The goal of treatment is to promote normal weight and to restore nutrition. A team approach combining medical management, psychotherapy, behavior modification, family counseling, and nutritional counseling works best. The patient often is hospitalized to provide fluid and electrolyte replacement, to remove the patient from the home environment, and to place the patient in a controlled environment. Long-term emotional support is needed, and long-term psychiatric counseling often is indicated to correct any underlying dysfunction. Support groups for eating disorders help many patients.

Prognosis

The outcome is more favorable when the patient seeks help willingly. Without medical intervention, life-threatening complications, such as cardiac arrest, are possible. Recovery is usually slow, and some patients become suicidal. Long-term health complications include anemia, osteoporosis, loss of kidney function, and heart failure. There is a high incidence of recurrence of the disease. Two percent to 6% of patients die as a result of the complications of the disorder, particularly cardiac complications caused by electrolyte deficiencies.

Prevention

Until the causes and risk factors are better understood, there is no certain prevention. Education of coaches regarding the dangers of expecting the female athlete to achieve an unhealthy body weight as a means of excelling is needed. Self-esteem building exercises in school often improve a young female's ability to accept her body image. Because of the high incidence of anorexia in the United States, clinicians suggest prevention programs and media based awareness campaigns are essential. Some health experts suggest that an educational shift from valuing people for body size and shape to valuing people for positive inner qualities and personality is needed.

Patient Teaching

It is of utmost importance for the health care team to build trust and sensitivity in presenting the plan for recovery to the patient. Establish a target weight. Give the patient as much control as possible over his or her preferred food and drink while beginning an adequate diet. Encourage the patient to share her or his struggles in a "safe" setting, such as an eating disorder support group. Discourage obsessive exercise activities.

Bulimia

Description

Bulimia is a behavioral disorder characterized by recurring episodes of binge eating followed by self-induced vomiting or purging, usually in secret. The incidence of binge eating disorders is much lower in men than in women. Like anorexia nervosa, bulimia is predominantly a disorder of young, white, middle- and upper-class women. It is more

difficult to detect than anorexia, and some studies have estimated that the prevalence may be as high as 19% in college-age women.

ICD-10-CM Code	F50.2 *(Bulimia nervosa)*

Symptoms and Signs

The binge-purge eating pattern of bulimia is fueled by a morbid fear of becoming fat. Vomiting can result in poor dentition, pharyngitis, esophagitis, aspiration, and electrolyte abnormalities. Gastric dilatation and pancreatitis have been reported after binges. The patients also abuse laxatives and diuretics by using them excessively. Other signs are compulsive exercise, swollen salivary glands, and broken blood vessels in the eye. These patients, usually females, typically weigh more than patients with anorexia and experience a wide fluctuation in weight. Some report feeling guilty about the binge-purge episodes. Periods of binging may be followed by intervals of self-imposed starvation. Menstruation is usually preserved.

Patient Screening

Be alert to recognize the shame and denial associated with the disease. The patient may admit only to depression and resist medical intervention.

Etiology

Although the etiologic factors are similar to those of anorexia nervosa, the exact cause is uncertain. Psychosocial factors, depression, control issues, and conflict frequently are identified. The patient reports a typical disordered eating pattern with self-induced vomiting; the patient often denies this ritual and keeps it secret. Characteristic perfectionist personality traits are identified, as in anorexia nervosa. The condition is associated with depression and, in some cases, compulsion.

Diagnosis

The diagnostic approach is similar to that for anorexia nervosa. Increased loss of electrolytes and metabolic acidosis are noted on laboratory tests. The patient exhibits a loss of muscle mass, cardiac irregularities, and dehydration. Anger and denial are part of the emotional state. Sudden death can result from **hypokalemia** and resulting cardiac arrhythmias.

Treatment

Treatment is similar to that of anorexia nervosa, with a multidimensional approach, including the administration of antidepressant drugs and participation in a support group. After the patient has discontinued the bulimic behavior, she or he should be taught proper nutrition in the form of a balanced diet.

Prognosis

Treatment may continue for years, because recovery may be a slow process. Although death from bulimia is rare, the long-term psychiatric prognosis in severe bulimia is worse than that in anorexia nervosa.

Prevention
No prevention is known.

Patient Teaching
Encourage the patient's efforts to comply with medical management, psychotherapy, and self-help groups for eating disorders. Describe the risks of abusing laxatives and diuretics. Praise the patient for reaching goals in weight gain and behavior modification.

Motion Sickness

Description
Motion sickness is loss of equilibrium experienced during motion.

ICD-10-CM Code	T75.3XXA (Motion sickness, initial encounter)

Symptoms and Signs
During an episode of motion sickness, the patient experiences nausea and vomiting when riding in a motor vehicle, boat, airplane, or other means of transportation. Air hunger, excessive salivation, pallor, sweating, dizziness, or headache may precede the nausea and vomiting.

Patient Screening
A person susceptible to motion sickness may require medication before an airplane flight, car trip, or boating excursion. Some OTC medications are available.

Etiology
Motion sickness results from a disturbance in the sense of balance. The fluid in the semicircular canals of the ears becomes dislocated because of the motion. In addition, excessive stimulation of the vestibular apparatus in the inner ear is caused by repetitive acceleration and deceleration and by angular and linear motions.

Diagnosis
The diagnosis is based on the clinical picture.

Treatment
Prevention of this condition is easier than treatment. The patient is encouraged to sit in the vehicle in the position that has the least amount of motion and where he or she can see the horizon. The patient is urged to avoid food and liquid before travel. If the patient must eat, only small amounts of food should be eaten. Prophylaxis with dermal patches of scopolamine (Transderm-Scop) often is employed. Dimenhydrinate (Dramamine) is another drug that helps prevent and treat motion sickness.

Prognosis
The prognosis is good with prophylactic medication.

Prevention
Good results can be expected from taking an antiemetic in anticipation of a motion event.

Patient Teaching
Refer to the comments listed previously under the Treatment section. Warn the patient about any possible adverse effects associated with the medication.

Review Challenge

Answer the following questions:
1. What are the accessory organs of digestion and their functions?
2. How does malocclusion lead to complications?
3. What problem may result from untreated gingivitis?
4. How would you describe the symptoms of temporomandibular joint disorder (TMD)?
5. What is the difference between an aphthous mouth ulcer and a "cold sore?"
6. What causes gastroesophageal reflux disease (GERD)? How is it treated?
7. How does *Helicobacter pylori* relate to peptic ulcers and gastritis?
8. What is a serious possible complication of esophageal varices?
9. How are peptic ulcers treated?
10. What is the diagnostic value of (1) endoscopy and (2) colonoscopy?
11. Is pain usually the initial symptom of gastric cancer?
12. What is the diagnostic significance of the McBurney point?
13. What is strangulated hernia?
14. What is the difference between ulcerative colitis and Crohn disease?
15. What is the goal in the treatment of gastroenteritis?
16. What is the difference between functional and mechanical intestinal obstructions? Give an example of each.
17. How would you compare the pathology of diverticulosis with that of diverticulitis?
18. How is colorectal cancer detected?
19. What causes pseudomembranous enterocolitis?
20. If a person has peritonitis, what serious complications may occur?
21. What are the signs and symptoms of cirrhosis of the liver?
22. How do hepatitis A and hepatitis C compare in etiology? What are the preventive measures for each disease?
23. What are the presenting symptoms of a patient with (1) biliary colic and (2) acute pancreatitis?
24. What are the causes of pancreatitis?
25. What are some examples of disorders of nutrition caused by deficiencies and excesses?
26. In what ways do pathogens cause food poisoning?

27. What are three diagnostic criteria for celiac disease?
28. What are the similarities and differences between anorexia nervosa and bulimia?
29. What is the leading cause for liver transplantation in the United States?

30. What is the third most common site of cancer incidence in men and women?
31. What are recommendations for patients diagnosed with nonalcoholic fatty liver disease (NAFLD) and nonalcoholic steatohepatitis (NASH)?

Real-Life Challenge: Cholelithiasis

A 43-year-old woman is experiencing an intermittent colicky type of pain in the upper right quadrant (URQ) of the abdomen, radiating to the right scapular region. The onset was approximately 1 week ago. In the past few days, she has had nausea and vomiting, increasing in the past 24 hours. The pain is more severe today, and the emesis is bile colored. Vital signs are temperature, 99.68°F; pulse, 96 beats per minute; respirations, 26 breaths per minute; and blood pressure, 144/92 mm Hg. Her skin is warm, dry, and slightly jaundiced. The patient is somewhat obese and has been on oral contraceptives for 15 years.

Cholelithiasis is suspected. CT of the gallbladder confirms the presence of stones in the gallbladder and also in the common bile duct. Serum bilirubin is elevated. The patient is scheduled for laparoscopic surgery.

Questions

1. When would a patient with gallstones be asymptomatic?
2. How do gallstones develop?
3. Which type of person would be most likely to have gallstones?
4. Which diagnostic imaging studies would be ordered when gallstones are suspected?

5. Which blood studies would be ordered when gallstones are suspected?
6. What is the usual treatment for asymptomatic gallstones?
7. What is the treatment for symptomatic gallstones?
8. What is the difference between cholelithiasis and cholecystitis?

Real-Life Challenge: Ulcers

A 50-year-old man is experiencing midepigastric pain and heartburn along with nausea and vomiting, with the onset occurring approximately 1 week ago. The patient says that the pain is better after eating and more severe 2 hours after eating. The patient is observed sitting slightly bent over with knees drawn up. Vital signs are temperature, 99.88°F; pulse, 104 beats per minute; respirations, 24 breaths per minute; and blood pressure, 136/88 mm Hg. His skin is warm, dry, and pale. The physician suspects a duodenal ulcer. The abdomen is slightly distended and tender to palpation.

Diagnostic investigation includes hemoglobin (Hgb), hematocrit (Hct), gastric analysis, stool examination for occult blood, upper gastrointestinal (GI) series, and gastroscopy. Drug therapy includes antacid, histamine (H_2) blockers, and an antibiotic. The patient is instructed to adhere to a bland diet, with small and more frequent meals.

Questions

1. What population is most prone to ulcers?
2. Compare gastric, duodenal, and peptic ulcers.
3. Why would symptoms of gastric and duodenal ulcers vary?
4. Discuss theories of the cause of ulcers. Compare theories of ulcerogenic drugs versus bacterial origin.
5. What warnings should be given to patients taking non-steroidal antiinflammatory drugs (NSAIDs)?

6. Explain the complications of perforation.
7. Discuss the various forms of drug therapy available to treat ulcers.
8. What side effects might a patient on H_2 blockers experience?
9. What would a positive guaiac test indicate?

Internet Assignments

1. Explore the American Dental Association website, and report the latest news about the call for early detection of oral cancer. What do the relevant statistics suggest about oral cancer?
2. Visit the website of the National Eating Disorders Association, and report on a relevant headline article. For

example, what is being done to reach preteen children with a positive message about body image to prevent tragic deaths resulting from eating disorders?
3. Research the latest approaches to the treatment of hepatitis C by searching the American Liver Foundation website and related links.

Critical Thinking

1. Discuss the relationship between neglecting oral infections, such as dental decay, gingivitis, or periodontal disease, and the risk of damage to major organs including the heart. What exactly is plaque?

2. Discuss the possible damage to the oral cavity, the larynx, the esophagus, and respiratory tree that can be caused by frequent and chronic gastroesophageal reflux disease (GERD). Explain the interventions a patient can use to help control GERD.

3. Why is it important for a patient to understand how to take a prescription for nonsteroidal antiinflammatory drugs (NSAIDs)?

4. A patient being treated for gastritis benefits from understanding the many agents that damage the gastric lining. Explain them as you would to a patient.

5. The symptoms experienced by a person suffering from irritable bowel syndrome (IBS) can be unpredictable and cause embarrassment with social interaction. How would you address the psychological and emotional concerns of the patient?

6. Discuss the advantages of screening for early detection and prevention of colorectal cancer.

7. Discuss how the distorted body image and self-imposed starvation of a patient with anorexia nervosa affect family members she or he lives with. What are some ways the family may try to reinforce the treatment plan?

8. Discuss the lifestyle changes recommended to lower the risk of oral cancer.

9. What measures can be taken to help prevent food poisoning in day care centers and institutions?

Prepare to discuss Critical Thinking case study exercises for this chapter that are posted on Evolve.

9

Diseases and Conditions of the Respiratory System

CHAPTER OUTLINE

Orderly Function of the Respiratory System, 343

Common Cold/Upper Respiratory Tract Infection, 344

Sinusitis, 346

Pharyngitis, 347

Nasopharyngeal Carcinoma, 348

Laryngitis, 349

Deviated Septum, 350

Nasal Polyps, 350

Anosmia, 351

Epistaxis (Nosebleed), 352

Tumors of the Larynx, 352

Laryngeal Cancer, 353

Hemoptysis, 354

Atelectasis, 355

Pulmonary Embolism, 357

Pneumonia, 358

Influenza, 362

Chronic Obstructive Pulmonary Disease, 365

Pneumothorax, 370

Hemothorax, 371

Flail Chest, 371

Pulmonary Tuberculosis, 372

Infectious Mononucleosis: Epstein-Barr Virus Infection, 373

Adult Respiratory Distress Syndrome, 374

Sarcoidosis, 375

Lung Cancer, 376

LEARNING OBJECTIVES

After studying Chapter 9, you should be able to:

1. Explain the process of respiration.
2. Discuss the causes and medical treatment for (1) the common cold, (2) sinusitis, and (3) pharyngitis.
3. Name the treatment of choice for nasal polyps.
4. Name some systemic disorders that might cause epistaxis.
5. Discuss the prognosis of cancer of the larynx.
6. Define atelectasis and discuss some possible causes.
7. Compare the clinical pictures of (1) a patient with pulmonary embolism and (2) one with pneumonia.
8. List some health hazards of common molds.
9. List some possible causes of pulmonary abscess.
10. Compare Legionnaires disease with Pontiac fever.
11. Explain who is at greatest risk for (1) respiratory syncytial virus (RSV) pneumonia and (2) histoplasmosis.
12. List the groups recommended to receive prophylactic use of influenza vaccines.
13. Recall what the acronym COPD stands for.
14. Contrast the pathologic course of acute bronchitis with that of chronic bronchitis.
15. Compare the pathology involved in bronchiectasis with that of pulmonary emphysema.
16. Name and describe three causes of pneumoconiosis.
17. Describe the presenting symptoms of pleurisy.
18. Explain the difference between pneumothorax and hemothorax.
19. Describe the cause of the instability of the chest wall in a patient with flail chest.
20. Discuss contributing factors to, and concern about, the rising prevalence of pulmonary tuberculosis (TB).
21. Describe the clinical course of infectious mononucleosis.
22. Explain the pathologic changes in the lungs in adult respiratory distress syndrome (ARDS).
23. Explain what determines the prognosis of sarcoidosis.
24. Name the leading cause of cancer deaths worldwide for both men and women.
25. Explain the possible health consequences of smoking tobacco.
26. What are potential health risks for individuals who use tobacco-free nicotine delivery devices, such as electronic cigarettes and atomizers?

KEY TERMS

anosmia (an-**OZ**-me-ah)
anthracosis (an-thrah-**KOE**-sis)
aphonia (ah-**FOE**-nee-ah)
asbestosis (as-beh-**STOH**-sis)
aspiration (as-pih-**RAY**-shun)
circumoral cyanosis (sir-kum-**OH**-ral sigh-an-**OH**-sis)
dysphonia (dis-**FOE**-nee-ah)
epistaxis (**ep**-ih-**STAK**-sis)
exsanguination (eck-**sang**-win-**AY**-shun)
hemoptysis (he-**MOP**-tih-sis)

laryngectomy (lar-in-**JECK**-toh-me)
lymphadenitis (limf-**ad**-eh-**NIGH**-tis)
lymphadenopathy (limf-**ad**-eh-**NOP**-ah-thee)
pneumoconiosis (**nu**-moh-koh-nee-**OH**-sis)
rhonchi (**RONG**-ki)
silicosis (sill-ih-**KO**-sis)
sinusotomy (sigh-nus-**OT**-oh-me)
stridor (**STRY**-dor)
syncytial virus (sin-**SIGH**-shal virus)
tachypnea (**tach**-ip-**NEE**-ah)

Orderly Function of the Respiratory System

The primary functions of the pulmonary system are ventilation and respiration. Respiration maintains life by supplying oxygen to organs, tissues, and cells and by allowing for the removal of carbon dioxide (a waste product of metabolism). This process is made possible by ventilation (the bellows-like action of the chest) and healthy lung tissue that is adequately perfused with blood. Breathing is controlled by the central nervous system (CNS); nerve stimulation of breathing begins in the medulla oblongata and the pons. Pulmonary circulation is composed of pulmonary arteries, which carry deoxygenated venous blood from the heart to the lungs; pulmonary capillaries, in which gas exchange occurs; and pulmonary veins, which return freshly oxygenated blood to the heart for systemic circulation. The lung tissue itself is supplied with oxygen and nutrients by the blood supply that is carried to it by the bronchial arteries.

The lungs, along with the kidneys, have a major metabolic function: the maintenance of acid–base (pH) balance of blood. Lack of oxygen with hypercapnia (increased carbon dioxide in the blood) causes respiratory acidosis; hyperventilation may produce hypocapnia (a decreased amount of carbon dioxide in blood), causing respiratory alkalosis. In both conditions, arterial blood gases are abnormal. The kidneys work to adjust bicarbonate in blood in response to carbon dioxide.

In the lungs, oxygen inhaled from the air is exchanged with carbon dioxide from blood; this process is called *external respiration. Internal respiration* refers to the exchange of gases between blood and tissue cells. Carbon dioxide then is exhaled as a waste product. Inhaled air and exhaled air pass through the respiratory tract, which includes the nose, pharynx, larynx, and trachea (Fig. 9.1).

In the chest, the trachea bifurcates into bronchi. Each bronchus enters a lung, where it further divides into increasingly smaller air passages called *bronchioles.* At the end of each bronchiole is a saclike cavity called an *alveolus.* There are approximately 300 million alveoli in each lung. The vital exchange of carbon dioxide for oxygen takes place through capillaries that lie next to the walls of the alveolus.

A muscular, dome-shaped partition, called the *diaphragm,* attaches to the lower ribs and separates the thoracic cavity from the abdominal cavity. On inspiration, the diaphragm contracts, pulling downward and causing air to be sucked into the lungs. During expiration, the diaphragm relaxes, pushing upward and forcing air out of the lungs (Fig. 9.2). Expansion of the chest cavity and diaphragmatic contraction are active, energy-requiring processes. Exhalation occurs as the stretched chest cavity springs back to its resting state along with the relaxation of the diaphragm. This is a passive process.

A membrane called the *visceral pleura* encases the lungs, and the *parietal pleura* line the inside of the chest or thoracic cavity. The potential space between the visceral and parietal pleura is called the *pleural cavity.* Depending on the body size, approximately 10 to 20 mL of pleural fluid is contained in the space between the pleurae, preventing friction and allowing the pleurae to slide easily on each other. Between the lungs is the mediastinum, where the heart, great vessels, trachea, esophagus, and lymph nodes are located.

Respiratory failure can result from the impairment of alveolar-arterial gas exchange (hypoxia), which results in a decrease of oxygen in blood. Additionally respiratory failure can be caused by the inability to ventilate, which results in an increasing buildup of carbon dioxide. Diseases of the respiratory system result from infection, circulatory disorders, tumors, trauma, immune diseases, congenital defects, CNS damage or diseases, inflammatory disturbances, or environmental conditions.

The chief symptoms indicating respiratory tract disorders that should receive medical attention include:

- chest pain
- dyspnea (difficulty in breathing), shortness of breath
- productive or nonproductive cough that is acute or chronic
- hemoptysis (spitting up blood)
- dysphonia (hoarseness)
- chills

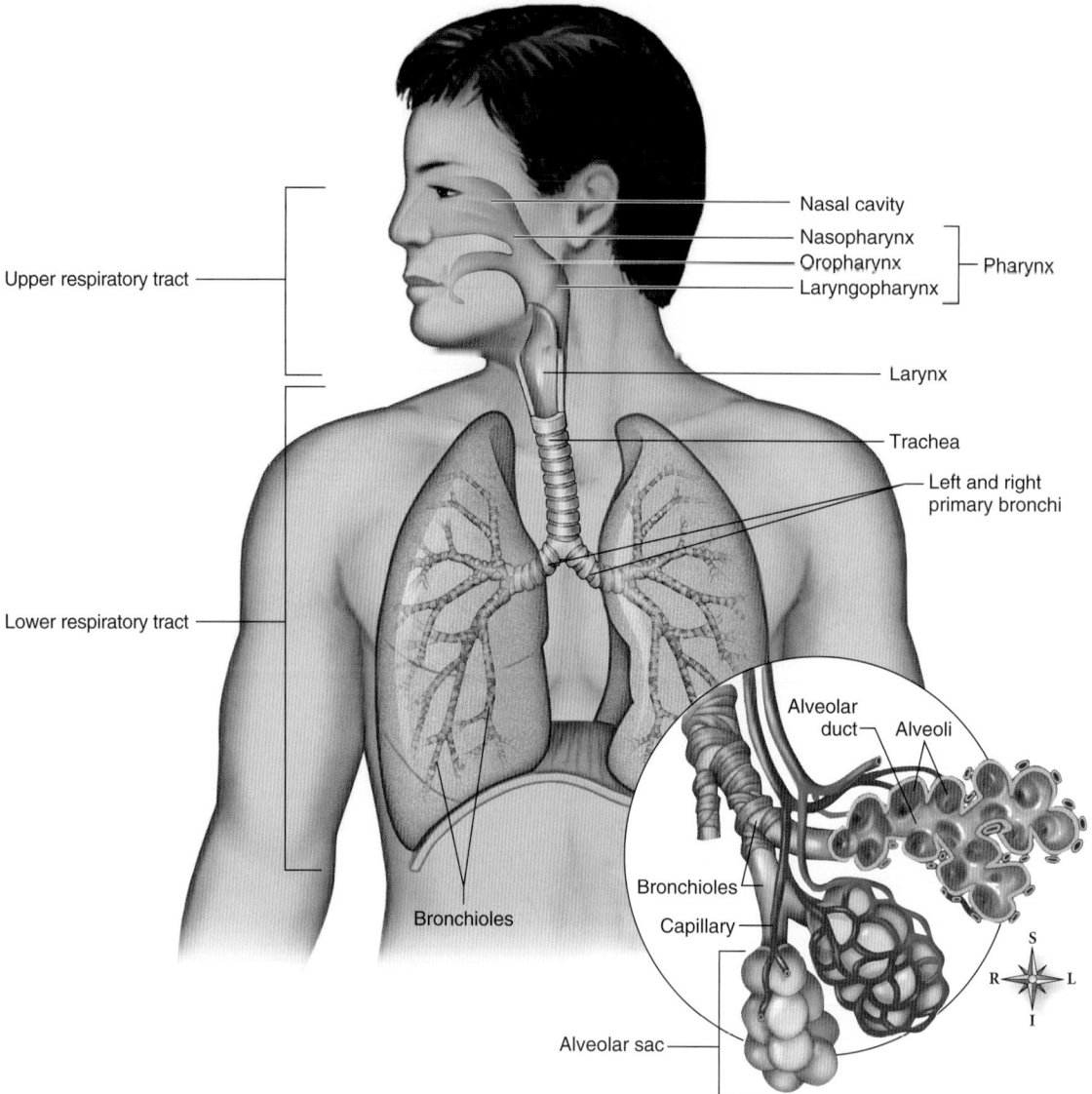

• **Fig. 9.1** Structural plan of the respiratory system. (From Patton KT, Thibodeau GA: *The human body in health & disease,* ed 6, Maryland Heights, 2014, Elsevier.)

- low- or high-grade fever
- wheezing
- fatigue

Common Cold/Upper Respiratory Tract Infection

Description

The common cold, also referred to as an *upper respiratory infection* (URI), is an acute inflammatory process that affects the mucous membrane that lines the upper respiratory tract.

ICD-10-CM Code	J00 (Acute nasopharyngitis [common cold])

Symptoms and Signs

Although the common, or "head," cold is confined to the nose and the pharynx, the same viruses can infect the larynx (see the Laryngitis section) and various areas of the lungs (see the Acute and Chronic Bronchitis section). The suffix *-itis* is added to the anatomic location where most of the inflammation occurs (i.e., pharyngitis, laryngitis, tracheitis, or bronchitis). The symptoms of a cold tend to be subjective and, to some extent, depend on which virus is responsible; the symptoms include nasal congestion and discharge, sneezing, watery eyes, sore throat, hoarseness of the voice, and coughing. When this highly contagious inflammatory process first begins, the nasal discharge is usually clear and thin. In the adult, the symptoms usually abate in 5 to 7 days without antibiotic therapy. In some cases, the cold progresses, and the discharge becomes greenish yellow and thick. Headache, slight fever, and chills often accompany a cold. A high fever and malaise, however, are more likely to be symptoms of influenza (see the Influenza section).

Patient Screening

Symptoms of a cold that are prolonged or accompanied by fever, chest pain, chest congestion, earache, severe headache,

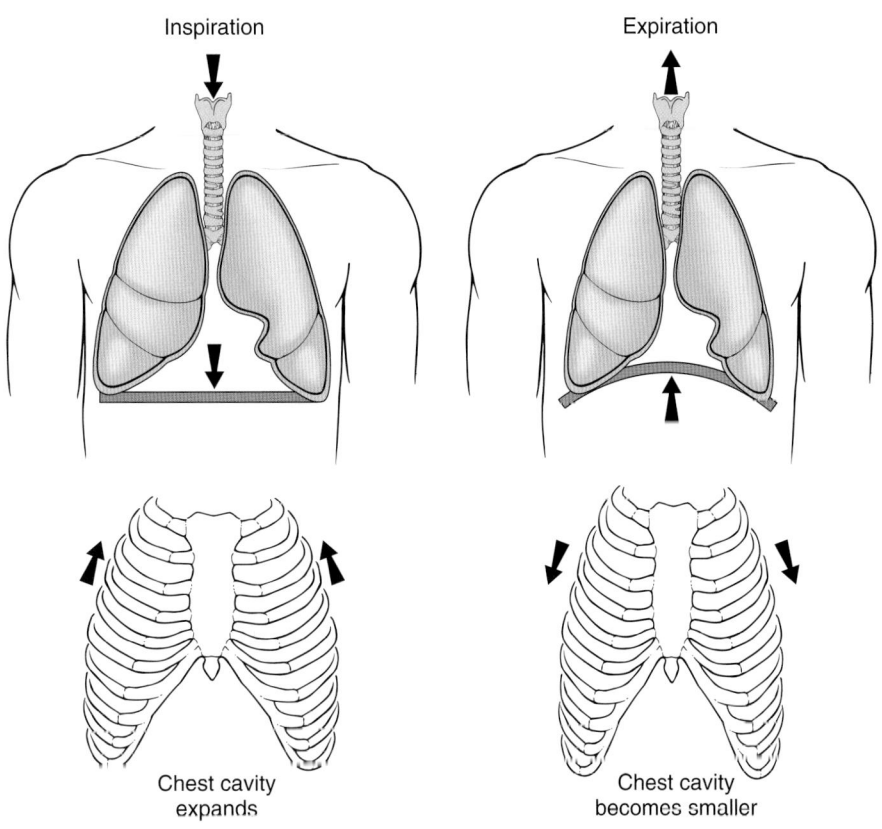

Inspiration

Expiration

Chest cavity
expands

Chest cavity
becomes smaller

• **Fig. 9.2** Diaphragm and chest movement on inspiration and expiration.

stiff neck, decreased urine, or other complications indicate the need for medical care within 24 hours.

Etiology

The common cold is a group of minor illnesses that can be caused by almost 200 different viruses. Cold viruses are not part of normal body flora; thus viruses that cause a cold are passed from one human to another. Colds are frequent diseases and a common cause of absenteeism from work and school. Rhinoviruses cause about one-half of the colds in adults. (Some colds may result from *Mycoplasma* and other atypical organisms that are more like bacteria than viruses. These are also transmitted by airborne respiratory droplets.) Viral infections sometimes are followed by bacterial infections of the pharynx, middle ear (see the Otitis Media section in Chapter 5), sinuses, larynx, or lungs. General poor health, lack of exercise, and poor nutrition predispose a person to the common cold.

Diagnosis

Diagnosis is made from the symptoms described by the patient. To rule out a more serious disease, cultures of the nasal discharge and sputum, along with a complete blood count (CBC), may be needed.

Treatment

An ordinary cold should clear up in 4 or 5 days, and a bacterial infection should resolve in no longer than 7 to 10 days.

Persistent cough or nasal congestion may suggest the presence of another process, such as allergies or asthma. There is no cure for a cold. Resting, drinking plenty of fluids, using a vaporizer, and taking over-the-counter antihistamines, decongestants, cough suppressants, and mild analgesics can give temporary relief of symptoms.

> **NOTE**
> Aspirin is contraindicated in infants and children; acetaminophen is the drug of choice.

Mechanism of Action. *Antihistamines* are drugs that inhibit the action of or inhibit the formation of histamine in the body. Antihistamines help dry up nasal secretions, diminish itchy or watery eyes, and decrease flare-ups of allergic reactions. Antihistamines may cause drowsiness.

Decongestants are drugs that stimulate adrenergic receptors, induce vasoconstriction of blood vessels in the nose, throat, and sinuses. Stimulation of the alpha-adrenergic receptors decreases the swelling of the nasal tissue and reduces mucus formation.

Expectorants (mucolytics) are medications that help dissolve mucus and reduce the viscosity of mucous secretions.

Cough suppressants are medications used to treat or lessen cough. The efficacy of these drugs is questionable. Cough suppressants are no longer recommended for children younger than 6 years of age. The American Academy of

Pediatrics recommends buckwheat honey as a cough suppressant for those age 12 months to 6 years. Honey should not be given to children under 1 year of age.

Antibiotics are of little value in treating viral infections; however, patients with recurring attacks of bronchitis (see the Acute and Chronic Bronchitis section) or frequent middle ear infections may receive some protection against these complications caused by bacteria by taking antibiotics. Some data suggest that taking zinc lozenges may shorten the course of the common cold slightly.

Prognosis

The common cold is usually benign and self-limiting. Patients who are immunocompromised may be more susceptible to developing frequent colds and complications. Possible complications include secondary bacterial infections, as listed previously under the Etiology section.

Prevention

The mechanisms of the transmission of cold viruses are not always clearly defined. In many cases, the mode of transmission is airborne respiratory droplets and hand-to-hand contact, so prevention is difficult.

Patient Teaching

Colds are more common in children than in adults and are a frequent cause of absenteeism. Once infected, children can easily transmit new strains to family members. Frequent, thorough hand washing and isolation during the acute stage of illness are commonsense measures that can help control transmission. Stress to the patient that antibiotics do not cure the common cold. Instruct the patient to avoid overuse of drugs, such as nasal sprays, and to take all medications only as instructed. List the warning signs of complications that should be reported to the health care provider (i.e., shortness of breath, severe headache, chest pain, high fever, and symptoms of dehydration or stiff neck).

Sinusitis

Description

Sinusitis is acute or chronic inflammation of the mucous membranes of the paranasal sinuses.

ICD-10-CM Code	J01.90 (Acute sinusitis, unspecified)
	(J01.90-J01.91 = 2 codes of specificity)
	J32.9 (Chronic sinusitis, unspecified)
	(J32.0-J32.9 = 7 codes of specificity)

Sinusitis is classified by location, type, and extent of pathology. Refer to the physician's diagnosis and then to the current edition of the ICD-10-CM coding manual for greatest specificity.

Symptoms and Signs

The sinuses, which are cavities behind the facial bones that shape the nose, cheeks, and eye sockets, are normally air filled. In sinusitis, the frontal sinuses (located in the forehead above the eyes) and the maxillary sinuses (located under the maxillary bones in the face) are the most commonly involved sinuses (Fig. 9.3). When the frontal sinuses are affected, a headache is common over one or both eyes, especially on waking in the morning. Pain and tenderness, which are felt just above the eyes and usually intensify when bending over, are also common symptoms. Pain in the cheeks and upper teeth is a symptom of sinusitis in the maxillary sinuses. If present, drainage will be a thick, greenish yellow, mucopurulent liquid. The course of acute sinusitis is 3 to 4 weeks.

Patient Screening

Individuals with symptoms of acute sinusitis (fever, sinus congestion, facial tenderness and pain, and severe

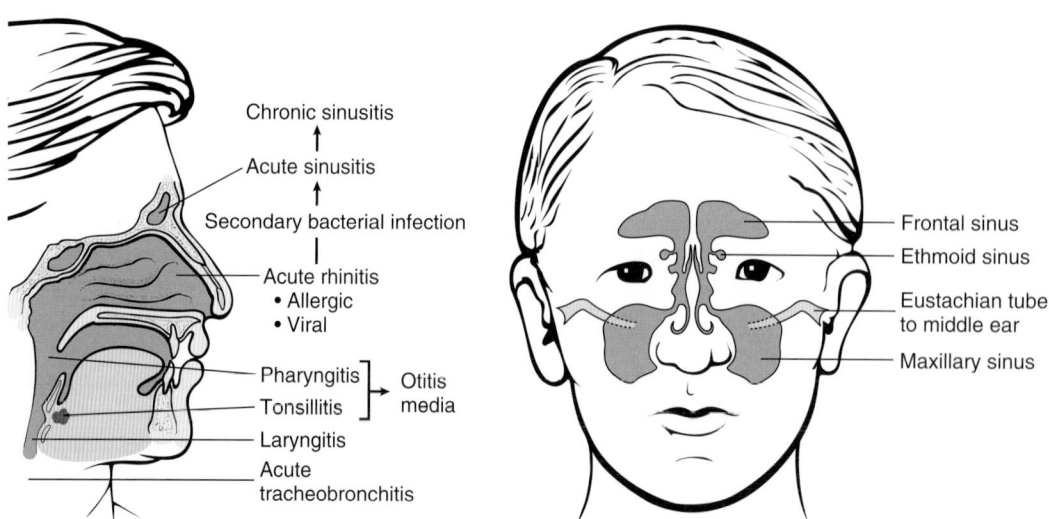

• **Fig. 9.3** Sinusitis. (From Damjanov I: *Pathology for the health-related professions*, ed 4, St Louis, 2011, Saunders/Elsevier.)

headache) are encouraged to seek medical attention as soon as possible.

Etiology

Sinusitis can be caused by viral, fungal, or, more commonly, bacterial infections that travel to the sinuses from the nose, often after the patient has been infected by a common cold. This occurs easily because the mucous membranes that line the nasal cavity extend into and also line the sinuses. One is predisposed to sinusitis by any condition that blocks sinus drainage and ventilation (e.g., a deviated nasal septum or nasal polyps). Sinusitis also may result because of swimming or diving, tooth extractions, tooth abscess, or allergies that affect the nasal passages. The cause of chronic sinusitis may never be determined; however, common variable immunodeficiency disease may be involved (see Chapter 3).

Diagnosis

The diagnosis of sinusitis is made by evaluating the findings from the physical examination, patient history, sinus radiographic studies, computed tomography (CT), and endoscopic sinoscopy. Sinuses that are air filled appear as dark patches on a radiograph, whereas fluid-filled sinuses appear as white areas. Bedside transillumination can suggest the presence of sinusitis. Additionally, a specimen of nasal secretions may be taken for culture to identify or rule out bacterial agents.

Treatment

Treatment of sinusitis can include saline nasal spray, topical steroid nasal sprays, broad-spectrum antibiotics, oral corticosteroids, antihistamines, and decongestants. Decongestants alleviate symptoms by shrinking the swollen mucous membranes and drying up the nasal discharge to expand the airway and ease breathing. Oral and topical corticosteroids decrease the inflammation of the affected area and decrease sensitivity to aggravating stimuli. Oral antibiotics are used if bacterial infection is present and may include amoxicillin, doxycycline, sulfamethoxazole-trimethoprim, or cephalosporins. Other antibiotics may be used depending on the infecting organism. Determination of allergic sinusitis may include allergy testing followed by appropriate desensitization with immunotherapy and corticosteroids. If the inflammation persists, a minor surgery called sinusotomy may be advised by the physician. With the patient under local anesthesia, the physician pierces the maxillary sinus, allowing drainage and relief of pressure. Often the physician instills sterile water into the sinus to flush out any residual material. Analgesics are usually given for pain relief.

Prognosis

The prognosis for uncomplicated acute sinusitis is good. Chronic sinusitis may require more prolonged medical treatment with antibiotics.

Prevention

Management of conditions that predispose an individual to sinusitis may help prevent chronic sinusitis.

Patient Teaching

Use visual aids to explain the function of sinus cavities. Emphasize the importance of complying with the treatment plan and returning for follow-up appointments. List the warning signs of complications, such as chills, fever, facial edema, severe headache, stiff neck, lethargy, or confusion. Prepare the patient for diagnostic testing or surgery by explaining each procedure and what to expect in terms of preparation and postprocedure care.

Pharyngitis

Description

Pharyngitis (sore throat) is acute or chronic inflammation or infection of the pharynx.

| ICD-10-CM Code | J02.9 (Acute pharyngitis, unspecified) |
| | (J02.0-J02.9 = 3 codes of specificity) |

Symptoms and Signs

Pharyngitis may be acute or chronic and often involves inflammation of the tonsils, uvula, and palate. A sore throat with dryness, a burning sensation, or the sensation of a lump in the throat is common. Clinical manifestations vary with the type of pharyngitis. Generally chills, fever, dysphonia, dysphagia, and cervical lymphadenopathy are common. On examination of the throat, the mucosa of the pharynx is found to be red and swollen, with or without tonsillar exudate, depending on the causative organism.

Patient Screening

An individual complaining of a persistent sore throat with systemic symptoms should be seen by a physician within 24 hours. The patient should be advised not to initiate antibiotic therapy before the appointment because this can impede the accuracy of diagnostic testing.

Etiology

The most common cause of pharyngitis is a viral infection; tonsillitis is the most important cause. In children, it is often an extension of streptococcal infection from the tonsils, adenoids, nose, or sinuses. Persistent infection, or chronic pharyngitis, occurs when an infection (respiratory, sinus, or oral disease) spreads to the pharynx and remains. Acute pharyngitis may be secondary to systemic viral infections, such as chickenpox and measles, whereas chronic pharyngitis may accompany other diseases, such as syphilis and tuberculosis (TB). Gonococcal pharyngitis may result from oral-genital sexual activity with an infected partner. Pharyngitis also can be caused by irritation and inflammation without infection. Occasionally inhalation or swallowing of irritating substances, such as tobacco smoke and alcohol, is responsible for trauma to the mucous membranes of the pharynx. Breathing in excessively heated air or chemical irritants and swallowing sharp objects (e.g., a large ice chip or hard candy) also can cause trauma. Seasonal allergies may induce pharyngitis.

Diagnosis

Physical examination usually shows red, swollen mucous membranes. Along with patient history, this is usually sufficient for determining the diagnosis of acute pharyngitis. For chronic pharyngitis, the physician needs to identify and locate the primary source of the infection or irritation. Further examination of the nasopharyngeal area, a CBC, and sinus radiography may be necessary.

Treatment

Home treatment with the use of lozenges, mouthwashes, salt water gargles, an ice collar, and antiinflammatory medication may be helpful in viral infections. When symptoms persist for longer than a few days, a physician should be consulted. Because most cases of pharyngitis are viral in origin, antibiotics are not prescribed. However, acute bacterial infections necessitate systemic administration of antibiotics or sulfonamides. Documented streptococcal pharyngitis is treated with a 7- to 10-day course of antibiotics. Chronic tonsillitis, adenoiditis, and adenoid hypertrophy may be treated with surgical excision. Bed rest and copious amounts of fluids may be advised.

> **NOTE**
>
> Aspirin is not given to children because of the threat of Reye syndrome.

Prognosis

Uncomplicated pharyngitis resolves within a few days. Bacterial causes are cured with appropriate antibiotics. Chronic cases may require eliminating the underlying cause, such as smoking or allergens, before improvement can be achieved. A potential complication of streptococcal pharyngitis is peritonsillar abscess. This is a pocket of infection that occurs behind the tonsil (usually unilateral) and can compromise the airway. This is an emergent issue and needs to be addressed the same day.

Prevention

Prevention measures include maintaining general good health, avoiding infections, evading known irritants, and controlling allergies.

Patient Teaching

Instruct the patient to take the entire course of antibiotic therapy and keep follow-up appointments to ensure complete cure and to prevent complications. Provide a list of comfort measures, such as safe use of analgesics, warm saline gargles, adequate fluid intake, and a soft diet. Advise patients with chronic pharyngitis to stop smoking; refer them to a support group.

> **NOTE**
>
> A more serious condition may appear initially as routine pharyngitis. Ludwig angina involves cellulitis on the floor of the mouth, whereas epiglottitis involves infection of the structure overlying the larynx (voice box). Both are often characterized by fever and severe sore throat. However, drooling, difficulty breathing, and inability to swallow may occur and indicate some compromise to the respiratory tract. *Patients should seek emergency medical attention if these symptoms develop.*

Nasopharyngeal Carcinoma

Description

Nasopharyngeal tumors arise in the area of the pharynx that opens into the nasal cavity anteriorly and the oropharynx inferiorly. They are unique among head and neck cancers in that they are not as strongly linked to tobacco use. Instead they are often linked to dietary intake or Epstein-Barr virus (EBV) infection.

ICD-10-CM Code	C11.9 *(Malignant neoplasm of nasopharynx, unspecified)* (C11.0-C11.9 = 6 codes of specificity)

Symptoms and Signs

Because of the anatomic location of the nasopharyngeal tumor, patients are often asymptomatic during the early stages of the disease. The classic clinical triad of symptoms is neck mass, nasal obstruction with epistaxis, and serous otitis media. Although it is rare to find all three symptoms in a patient, the individual symptoms occur frequently. Other symptoms include headache, hearing loss, tinnitus, pain, and impaired function of the cranial nerves.

Patient Screening

Provide the first available appointment to the individual reporting neck mass or related symptoms.

Etiology

Although nasopharyngeal carcinoma is a rare disease in the United States and Western Europe, several subpopulations do have a relatively high incidence. These include people from southern China, areas around the Mediterranean Sea, Southeast Asia, and the Arctic. It is two to three times more common in males than in females and has peak incidence in persons between ages 10 and 25 years or 50 and 60 years. Several known risk factors in the high-risk areas include consumption of salted fish as a diet standard, foods with high levels of nitrates (e.g., processed meats), and Chinese herbs; infection by EBV; and having a first-degree relative with nasopharyngeal carcinoma. Use of alcohol and tobacco is a risk factor in low-risk areas.

Diagnosis

Diagnosis is made after a full clinical examination of the head and neck and an endoscopic examination of the nasopharynx with biopsy of suspicious lesions. Testing for EBV should also be performed. Staging is determined according to the tumor-node-metastasis (TNM) system, in which T stands for the extent of tumor invasion into adjacent structures and N for lymph node location and size. Magnetic resonance imaging (MRI) of the head and neck, bone scanning, and a CT or positron emission tomography (PET) are used for staging. See Chapter 1 for information about the staging and grading systems used to assess malignant neoplasms.

Treatment

Because of the anatomic constraints of the nasopharynx, surgery is usually not performed. Nasopharyngeal carcinoma commonly is quite radiosensitive, and most patients with early-stage cancer are treated with radiation therapy, with or without adjuvant chemotherapy. Those with recurrent or more advanced carcinomas are generally treated with chemoradiotherapy. Close follow-up is important after completion of therapy to monitor for recurrence.

Prognosis

Because early neoplasms rarely cause symptoms, most patients present with advanced carcinoma, and many already have distant metastases to bones, the lungs, or the liver. If the tumor has extended to involve one of the cranial nerves or has metastasized to the cervical lymph nodes, the prognosis is worse. In addition, the presence of high plasma levels of EBV deoxyribonucleic acid (DNA) at the time of diagnosis or after treatment is correlated with a poorer outcome.

Prevention

It is possible to detect circulating EBV DNA in the serum of affected individuals. However, screening for EBV in first-degree relatives of patients with nasopharyngeal carcinoma is not currently performed, except in southern China, where the disease is most prevalent.

Patient Teaching

Prepare the patient for diagnostic testing by providing information about endoscopy of the nasopharynx and biopsy of any lesion in the nasopharynx. Tell the patient when to expect results. After diagnosis, explain the treatment of choice and the possible side effects. Encourage the patient to ask questions, and defer to the physician for revealing the prognosis. Provide information regarding cancer support groups.

Laryngitis

Description

Inflammation of the larynx (hoarseness), including the vocal cords, is called *laryngitis*.

| ICD-10-CM Code | J04.0 (Acute laryngitis) |

Laryngitis coding includes modifiers that specify causative agents and factors, such as obstruction. Refer to the physician's diagnosis and then to the current edition of the ICD-10-CM coding manual for the appropriate modifiers.

Symptoms and Signs

Because the opening of the larynx is narrow, inflammation of the larynx sometimes interferes with breathing. Symptoms vary with the severity of the inflammation, but the main symptom of laryngitis is hoarseness, which causes aphonia. Fever, malaise, a painful throat, dysphagia, and other symptoms associated with influenza occur in more severe infections.

Patient Screening

Laryngitis associated with recent trauma requires immediate medical attention. A sensation of swelling in the throat, difficulty breathing, and laryngitis indicate a medical emergency. An individual reporting persistent hoarseness and symptoms of infection should be seen in the medical office within 24 hours.

Etiology

The cause of laryngitis can be either viral or bacterial infection, and the condition can be either chronic or acute. URIs, such as the common cold, tonsillitis, pharyngitis, and sinusitis, are the most common causes of inflammation of the larynx. Laryngitis also occurs with bronchitis, pertussis, influenza, pneumonia, measles, mononucleosis, diphtheria, syphilis, and TB. Occasionally laryngitis is caused by irritation without infection. Reflux laryngitis may result from repeated attacks of acid reflux. Inclement weather, tobacco smoking, alcohol consumption, inhalation of irritating materials, and excessive use of the voice are all predisposing factors, especially in the case of chronic laryngitis. Hoarseness can also be caused by benign or malignant lesions of the larynx. In most cases, the pathology is benign, but malignancy must be ruled out.

Diagnosis

Laryngoscopic examination reveals mildly or highly inflamed mucosa, and vocal cord movement may be limited. If no inflammation is present, laryngitis is not the cause of dysphonia, and further diagnostic tests are needed to determine the underlying condition.

Treatment

Treatment of viral laryngitis includes the following palliative measures: absolute voice rest, bed rest in a well-humidified room, liberal fluid intake, no tobacco or alcohol consumption, and the use of lozenges and cough syrup. Improvement should be seen in 4 or 5 days. Antibiotic administration gives good results when laryngitis occurs in conjunction with bacterial infection. Corticosteroids may be used to decrease inflammation when symptoms are more severe. When hoarseness persists for longer than 1 week, the condition may be chronic. Treatment of chronic laryngitis is based on elimination, as much as possible, of the causative factors.

Prognosis

Recovery is generally complete within 1 week.

Prevention

Known irritants that cause laryngitis are avoided or treated, if possible. Infections are difficult to prevent.

Patient Teaching

Explain the importance of resting the voice and taking medications as prescribed, along with drinking plenty of fluids. When the cause of chronic laryngitis has been determined to be irritation from excessive alcohol intake or smoking, provide information on support groups that offer help to those with such addictions, if appropriate.

Deviated Septum

Description

A crooked nasal septum (the cartilage partition between the nostrils) is called a *deviated septum* (Fig. 9.4).

ICD-10-CM Code	J34.2 *(Deviated nasal septum)*

Symptoms and Signs

A deviated septum causes narrowing and obstruction of the air passage, making breathing somewhat difficult. Other than mild breathing problems or a slightly increased tendency to develop sinusitis, no significant symptoms are associated with a deviated septum. The nose can appear normal externally, with the deviation visible only on examination with a nasal speculum.

Patient Screening

Unless the deviation is severe, it may not be noted until found by chance during a routine physical examination. The condition may be of no consequence until aggravated by trauma to the nose. In that case, schedule the first available appointment for evaluation.

Etiology

Congenital anomaly is usually the cause of minor deviation of the septum. Substantial septal deviation is uncommon and is usually the result of trauma to the nose.

Diagnosis

A deviated septum may not be visible without the aid of a nasal speculum. Patient history and the amount of

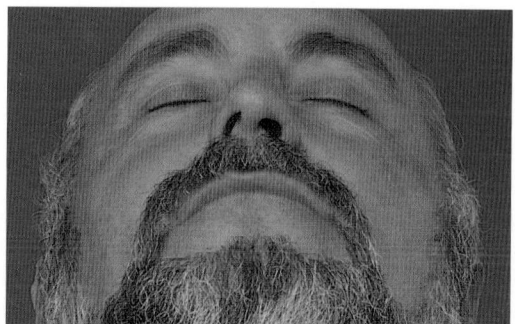

• **Fig. 9.4** Deviated septum. (From Monahan FD, Neighbors M: *Medical-surgical nursing: foundations for clinical practice,* ed 2, Philadelphia, 1998, Saunders.)

obstruction aid the physician in determining the diagnosis and treatment of this condition.

Treatment

Treatment is not usually necessary unless compromise of the air passage is noted. The septum can be straightened surgically to repair a significant obstruction or for cosmetic reasons. Straightening a deviated septum involves removing the cartilage (rhinoplasty or septoplasty). Once removed, the cartilage can be reshaped and repositioned in the nose, if needed, to maintain the nasal structure.

Prognosis

This fairly common condition has a good prognosis.

Prevention

The only possible prevention is avoiding trauma to the nose.

Patient Teaching

If surgical correction is scheduled, tell the patient what to expect after surgery, such as the use of nasal packing to control bleeding and analgesics for pain.

Nasal Polyps

Description

Nasal polyps are benign growths that form as a consequence of distended mucous membranes protruding into the nasal cavity (Fig. 9.5).

ICD-10-CM Code	J33.9 *(Nasal polyp, unspecified)*
	(J33.0-33.9 = 4 codes of specificity)

Nasal polyps are coded by anatomic site and underlying pathology. Refer to the physician's diagnosis and then to the current edition of the ICD-10-CM coding manual for greatest specificity.

Symptoms and Signs

Nasal polyps are not harmful but can become large enough to obstruct the nasal airway, making breathing difficult. Polyps often affect or impair the sense of smell (see the Anosmia section). When polyps obstruct one of the sinuses, symptoms of sinusitis are present (see the Sinusitis section).

Patient Screening

Nasal polyps may be found in the patient exhibiting symptoms of allergic rhinitis and/or sinusitis. The degree of urgency for an appointment is based on severity of symptoms.

Etiology

Polyps are caused by the overproduction of fluid in the cells of the mucous membrane. This overproduction is often the result of a condition called *allergic rhinitis.* Some aspirin-sensitive persons have the triad of nasal polyps, asthma, and urticaria (hives).

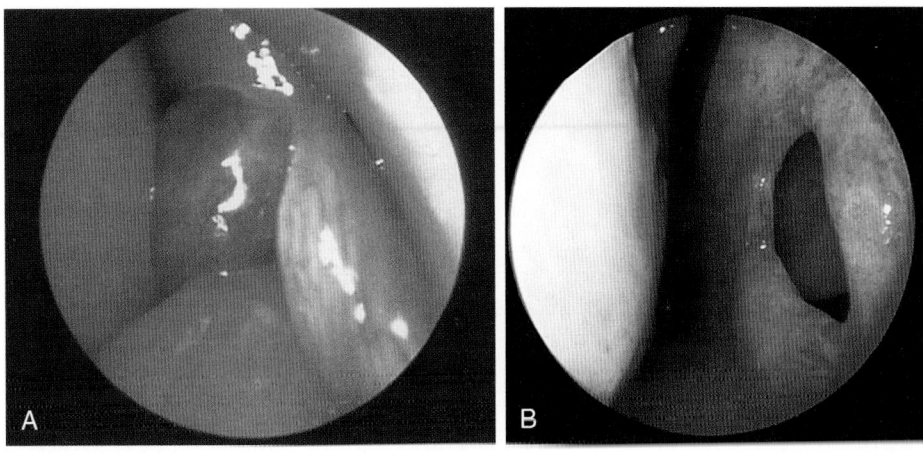

• **Fig. 9.5** Nasal polyps. (From Jarvis C: *Physical examination & health assessment*, ed 5, St Louis, 2008, Saunders.)

Diagnosis

The physician examines the inside of the nose using an instrument called a *nasal speculum.* Polyps appear as pearly gray lumps along the nasal passage.

Treatment

Surgical removal is the treatment of choice; however, considerable relief may be obtained through the injection of a steroid directly into the polyps. This procedure is repeated at 5- to 7-day intervals until relief is obtained. Removal of polyps is a minor procedure necessitating local anesthesia. Rhinoplasty may also be indicated. When the lining of the sinus also must be removed, general anesthesia is used.

Prognosis

The prognosis is good, although nasal polyps tend to recur.

Prevention

No specific preventive measures are known. Management of allergic rhinitis is beneficial.

Patient Teaching

Instructions given to the patient are related to the treatment of choice. When appropriate, explain the relationship of allergic rhinitis to nasal polyps.

Anosmia

Description

Anosmia is the impairment or loss of the sense of smell.

ICD-10-CM Code	R43.0 *(Anosmia)*
	R43.1 *(Parosmia)*
	R43.2 *(Parageusia)*
	(R43.0-R43.9 = 5 codes of specificity)

Symptoms and Signs

The loss of smell that continues without an obvious cause is termed *anosmia.* The ability to taste liquids and food also is impaired or lost.

Patient Screening

The patient complaining of prolonged, unexplained loss of the sense of smell is scheduled for a diagnostic evaluation.

Etiology

A chronic condition, such as nasal polyps and allergic rhinitis, is the most common cause of anosmia. Intranasal swelling accompanying an upper respiratory condition causes temporary anosmia. Sometimes a phobia concerning a particular odor accounts for a psychological basis for anosmia. It may, however, be the result of damage to the olfactory nerves caused by a head injury or, rarely, a symptom of a brain tumor.

Diagnosis

If the physician does not find any physical abnormality on examination or the patient's history does not reveal recent head trauma or an allergic condition, a neurologist may be consulted with regard to diagnostic tests.

Treatment

Treatment is aimed at the cause of the condition. When polyps are found, they are removed. Correction of nerve damage may not be possible. For allergic rhinitis, a series of injections containing increasingly stronger concentrations of the offending allergen is used to desensitize the patient.

Prognosis

Anosmia is often related to a URI and is thus a temporary condition. Other causes, as listed earlier, have a guarded prognosis.

Prevention

No means of prevention other than avoiding head injury is known.

Patient Teaching

Patients may benefit from an explanation of how the olfactory nerve normally functions and how it is affected by the determined cause of anosmia. (Fig. 1.9 illustrates the structure of the olfactory nerve.)

Epistaxis (Nosebleed)

Description

Epistaxis is hemorrhage from the nose.

ICD-10-CM Code   R04.0 (Epistaxis)

Symptoms and Signs

Hemorrhage from the nose, known as *epistaxis,* is a common, sudden emergency. Bleeding usually occurs from only one nostril, and often no apparent explanation for the bleeding is known. Most nosebleeds are seldom a cause for concern. They are unlikely to be a symptom of any other disorders, unless injury has occurred or associated serious systemic conditions are present. With significant blood loss, systemic symptoms will occur, such as vertigo, an increase in pulse, pallor, shortness of breath, and drop in blood pressure. Epistaxis is more common in children than in adults.

Patient Screening

Hemorrhage from the nose that persists for 10 minutes or more after constant pressure is applied is considered severe and requires immediate emergency care. If the patient reports a severe headache at the onset of epistaxis or is experiencing sequential nosebleeds, an immediate appointment should be arranged.

Etiology

Common causes of epistaxis are colds and infections, such as rhinitis, sinusitis, and nasopharyngitis, which can cause crusting that damages the mucous membrane lining the nose or the rupture of tiny vessels in the anterior septum of the nose. Direct trauma to the nose, picking the nose, and the presence of a foreign body are the most common causes of epistaxis. Nasal hemorrhage also has been encountered in relation to many systemic disorders, such as measles, scarlet fever, pertussis, rheumatic fever, hypertension, congestive heart failure, and chronic renal disease. Epistaxis may be the foremost symptom of some blood disorders, such as hemophilia, thrombocytopenia, agranulocytosis, and leukemia. Risk factors include vitamin K deficiency, hypertension, aspirin ingestion, high altitude, and anticoagulant therapy. An infrequent cause of epistaxis is extensive hepatic disease.

Diagnosis

The diagnosis of epistaxis is made on the basis of the patient history regarding the frequency of the nosebleeds, whether an injury has occurred, or whether the symptoms indicate that systemic disease may be present. All medications, dietary supplements, and herbal preparations taken by the patient are noted to identify contributing offenders.

Treatment

First the severity of blood loss is assessed. Mild hemorrhage may be controlled by applying constant direct pressure on either side of the bridge of the nose for 5 to 10 minutes. An internal compression device, such as Rhino Rocket, may be used. Persistent bleeding is treated with local application of epinephrine followed by cauterization with silver nitrate or laser cauterization. If bleeding continues, a posterior nasal packing left in place for 1 to 3 days may be necessary. A mild sclerosing agent also may be injected into a bleeding vessel if it can be visualized by the physician. Additional measures, such as surgical ligation of a bleeding artery, may be necessary if other measures fail.

Prognosis

The prognosis is generally good.

Prevention

Specific treatment of the underlying disease, if present, is of prime importance. Prevention includes instructing patients on how to avoid recurrences.

Patient Teaching

Demonstrate first-aid measures for controlling epistaxis, sitting with the head tilted forward while applying constant local pressure by compressing the side of the nose against the septum. Tell the patient to report repeated or severe nosebleeds immediately to the health care provider. Discuss measures for preventing recurrences.

Tumors of the Larynx

Description

Growths or tumors on the larynx may be benign or malignant.

ICD-10-CM Code   C00 D49
The above general codes represent the broad category of neoplasms that are classified by such diagnostic criteria as malignant or benign, as primary or secondary, or according to site, function, and morphology. Refer to the physician's diagnosis and then to the current edition of the ICD-10-CM coding manual to ensure the greatest specificity of pathology.

Symptoms and Signs

Dysphonia is usually the only symptom of a tumor on the larynx. No influenza-like symptoms occur as with laryngitis (see the Laryngitis section), but when the tumor is malignant, dysphagia may be experienced. In children with tumors, a high-pitched crowing sound, called **stridor**, is present because of the small airways. Hoarseness caused by a benign tumor is usually intermittent, whereas hoarseness caused by cancer is continuous and gradually becomes worse. Neither type of laryngeal tumor is common, but malignant tumors are slightly more common in men than in women.

Patient Screening

Unexplained, persistent hoarseness lasting longer than 2 weeks requires medical evaluation. Other symptoms related to the throat also may be present. The appointment can be made at the first available time or at the patient's first convenience.

Etiology

There are two types of benign tumors: papillomas, which usually appear in multiples, and polyps, which usually appear as single lesions (Fig. 9.6). These tumors are caused by misuse or overuse of the vocal cords, although smoking and acid reflux are contributing factors. Malignant tumors occur more often in those who indulge in heavy tobacco use.

Diagnosis

The physician or otolaryngologist thoroughly examines the larynx and vocal cords. When a tumor or tumors are found, biopsy is done to determine whether a malignancy is present. Cancer of the larynx almost always can be cured if it is diagnosed early.

Treatment

Benign growths, whether papillomas or polyps, may be treated with correction of the vocal strain, management of acid reflux, and smoking cessation. The growths may also be excised under local anesthesia. Malignant tumors, if discovered early, often are treated and cured by radiation therapy. When the cancer has metastasized, laryngectomy may be needed. After a laryngectomy, the patient needs extensive speech therapy to learn a substitute form of speech.

Prognosis

The prognosis depends on the type of tumor.

Prevention

Avoidance of smoking or any chronic irritation of the larynx is recommended.

Patient Teaching

Give the patient preoperative instructions, and encourage the patient to express any concerns about treatment. When laryngectomy is necessary, provide every venue of psychological support available to the family and the patient. Help the patient plan alternative means of communication during speech rehabilitation.

Laryngeal Cancer

Description

Laryngeal cancer describes a neoplasm of the larynx, the part of the respiratory tract between the pharynx and the trachea that houses the vocal cords. It is the most common site for head and neck tumors. Most laryngeal tumors are squamous cell carcinomas.

ICD-10-CM Code	C32.9 *(Malignant neoplasm of larynx, unspecified)* (C32.0-C32.9 = 6 codes of specificity)

The above code is a nonspecific code and may be valid as a principal diagnosis, except for Medicare. Refer to the physician's diagnosis and then to the current edition of the ICD-10-CM coding manual to ensure the greatest specificity.

Symptoms and Signs

If the tumor involves the vocal cord area of the larynx, persistent hoarseness tends to occur early in the disease process and is the most common initial complaint. Hoarseness related to benign causes, such as a vocal cord polyp or nodule caused by chronic irritation or overuse, is usually intermittent, whereas that caused by a malignant neoplasm is continuous and gradually becomes worse over time. Other symptoms may include dysphagia, hemoptysis, chronic cough, referred pain to the ear, and stridor (a high-pitched crowing sound). Airway obstruction also may occur depending on the tumor location. No influenza-like symptoms, as with laryngitis, are present (see the Laryngitis section).

Patient Screening

Unexplained, persistent hoarseness lasting longer than 2 weeks requires medical evaluation. Other symptoms related to the throat also may be present. The appointment can be made at the first available time or at the patient's earliest convenience.

Etiology

The major risk factors for development of laryngeal cancer are smoking and alcohol abuse. The combined effect of

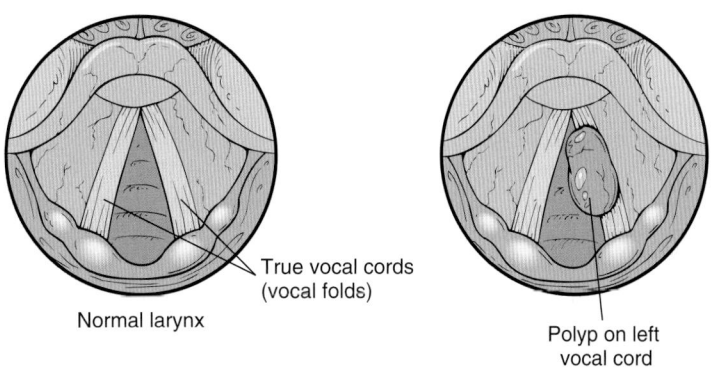

True vocal cords (vocal folds)

Normal larynx

Polyp on left vocal cord

• **Fig. 9.6** Vocal cord polyp.

alcohol and tobacco in causing cancer is multiplicative, with heavy smokers and drinkers having a 200-fold greater risk of developing laryngeal cancer compared with nonsmokers and nondrinkers. Other risk factors include infection with human papillomavirus (HPV)-16 or -18, occupational exposure to carcinogenic agents, such as perchloroethylene (a dry cleaning agent) or asbestos, and having a first-degree relative with laryngeal cancer. Tumors of the larynx have a peak incidence in the sixth and seventh decades of life.

Diagnosis

Laryngeal cancer is often diagnosed at an earlier stage compared with other head and neck cancers because hoarseness usually occurs early in the disease process. Flexible fiberoptic endoscopy allows visualization of the larynx and assessment of vocal cord mobility. The diagnosis of cancer requires biopsy, which is usually done through fine-needle aspiration. Staging is done by using the TNM system. CT or MRI is performed to evaluate the depth and extent of tumor invasion and to look for nodal metastasis. A panendoscopy (laryngoscopy, esophagoscopy, and bronchoscopy) is also generally done to look for other areas of tumor growth, because tobacco and alcohol use often have widespread toxic effects on the aerodigestive tract. PET can be done to look for distant metastases. See Chapter 1 for information about the staging and grading systems used to assess malignant neoplasms.

Treatment

The larynx plays an important role in speech, swallowing, respiration, and protection of the lower airway. Therefore quality-of-life considerations are often incorporated into the treatment plan. For early-stage cancer, often the physician will explain the risks and benefits of surgery and radiation therapy, both of which have similar outcomes, and will let the patient decide on the therapy. Usually the patient will choose the option that preserves voice, that is, radiation. Surgical options include partial laryngectomy, total laryngectomy, and endoscopic laser resection. The choice largely depends on tumor stage. Treatment of later-stage (III and IV) cancer is more difficult. For patients with resectable tumors, treatment usually consists of surgery followed by radiation therapy or radiation alone. Chemoradiotherapy may be tried in patients choosing an organ-sparing approach. For patients who do undergo laryngectomy, follow-up care generally requires the services of a speech therapist for speech therapy and swallowing therapy.

Prognosis

Because of the early manifestation of symptoms, laryngeal cancer is often diagnosed at a stage in which a cure is possible. The most significant prognostic indicator is the status of the cervical lymph nodes. The overall 5-year survival rate ranges from 30% to 90%, depending on the tumor stage at diagnosis. Patients with laryngeal cancer are more likely to develop second primary cancers compared with patients with malignancies outside the head and neck region because of the widespread carcinogenic effects of tobacco and alcohol in the head and neck area. The development of another primary tumor often indicates a worse prognosis.

Prevention

Cessation of smoking and reducing alcohol consumption are highly recommended. Periodic panendoscopy may be used to detect primary cancers occurring after treatment for laryngeal cancer.

Patient Teaching

Encourage the patient to express any concerns about the diagnostic procedures or the course of treatment chosen. Provide every venue of psychological support available to the patient and the family. Give specifics about the postoperative care after laryngectomy, as appropriate. Help the patient plan for alternative means of communication during speech rehabilitation.

Hemoptysis

Description

Hemoptysis is the coughing or spitting up of blood from the respiratory tract.

ICD-10-CM Code	R04.2 *(Hemoptysis)*
	P26.9 *(Pulmonary hemorrhage originating in the perinatal period)*
	(P26.0-P26.9 = 4 codes of specificity)
	A15.0 *(Tuberculosis of lung)*
	A15.7 *(Primary respiratory tuberculosis)*

Symptoms and Signs

Sputum streaked or spotted with blood can be present in minor infections. Hemoptysis can be massive, indicating a serious underlying condition. The patient expectorates bright or dark blood-streaked sputum or dark red clots from the pulmonary or bronchial circulation. Profuse bleeding is present in severe lung infections (i.e., aspergillus infection with angioinvasion), a respiratory malignancy, or erosion of a pulmonary vessel.

Patient Screening

Blood of unknown origin in the sputum is a symptom that requires medical evaluation. If the bleeding is slight and associated with a known respiratory infection, an appointment should be scheduled within 24 hours. Advise the patient experiencing profuse bleeding to seek emergency care, and inform the physician immediately.

Etiology

Trauma, erosion of a vessel, calcification, or tumors can cause bronchial bleeding, as can inflammatory conditions, such as bronchitis or bronchiectasis; chronic infection can result in damaged and irregularly shaped airways. Pulmonary arterial hypertension (often associated with right-sided heart failure) and at times pulmonary venous hypertension (associated with left-sided heart failure) may precipitate bleeding from pulmonary vessels. Additional origins of the bleeding can be fungal infections, pulmonary infarcts, tumors or ulcerations of the larynx or pharynx, and coagulation (clotting) defects.

Diagnosis

Of primary importance is determination of the source of bleeding. This is accomplished by visual examination of the mouth and the nasopharynx; visualization of the larynx, trachea, and bronchi with endoscopy; and inspection of the lung fields with radiographic studies. Pulmonary angiography can be used for diagnosis and therapeutic embolization.

Coagulation studies of blood ascertain whether the problem is caused by a clotting deficiency. The patient is given a purified protein derivative (PPD) skin test to screen for TB. Lung scanning, CT of the chest, and/or pulmonary angiography may be indicated if the previously mentioned investigations are inconclusive.

Treatment

After the location and the cause of the bleeding are determined, the source is treated. When the bleeding is severe, ligation or surgical removal or repair of the involved vessels is indicated. Measures are implemented to prevent asphyxiation by clotted blood in the air passages; to prevent obstruction of the bronchial tree by clots, with resulting lung collapse; and to prevent exsanguination of the patient. If minor bleeding occurs or the cause is uncertain, antibiotics and cough suppressant therapy are often prescribed.

Prognosis

The data may vary; however, in approximately 75% of cases, hemoptysis is not a sign of serious disease. The prognosis is good with treatment but guarded if associated with a serious underlying illness.

Prevention

Hemoptysis is generally considered a symptom, so there is no directed prevention.

Patient Teaching

Steps are taken to allay any fear and anxiety that the patient might be experiencing. Explain the diagnostic procedures and when to expect the results. Reassure the patient that hemoptysis may occur after endoscopy. Reinforce information about the treatment regimen, and encourage the patient to voice any concerns. It is also necessary to advise the patient to seek medical attention on an emergent basis if the amount of hemoptysis increases significantly.

Atelectasis

Description

Atelectasis is an airless or collapsed state of the pulmonary tissue.

| ICD-10-CM Code | J98.11 (Atelectasis) |
| | J98.19 (Other pulmonary collapse) |

Symptoms and Signs

Atelectasis occurs after incomplete expansion of lobules or segments of the lung, with partial or complete collapse of the lung. The condition results in hypoxia, causing the patient to experience dyspnea. When only a small segment of the lung is involved, dyspnea may be the only clinical symptom. When a large area of the pulmonary tissue is involved, the area available for gas exchange is decreased, and the dyspnea becomes severe. Substernal retraction and cyanosis may be seen on physical examination, and diminished breath sounds over the affected area are noted on auscultation. Chest radiographs may indicate a mediastinal shift toward the side of collapse. Additionally the patient experiences anxiety, diaphoresis, and tachycardia. Fever may be present, because collapsed lung tissue is prone to infection. Atelectasis also can occur with incomplete expansion of the lungs at birth.

Patient Screening

The patient experiencing dyspnea requires prompt medical attention for evaluation. Severe dyspnea with or without a history of previous atelectasis is a medical emergency; instruct the patient and the family to call an ambulance. The physician should be notified immediately.

Etiology

Atelectasis is caused by an obstruction in the bronchial tree; this can be a mucous plug, foreign body, or bronchogenic cancer. Compression atelectasis results when a tumor exerts pressure on the lung and does not allow air to enter that part. Inflammatory pulmonary disease can result in accumulation of fluid in the pleural cavity (pleural effusion) and induce atelectasis. Any condition that makes deep breathing difficult can lead to atelectasis (Fig. 9.7). Failure to breathe deeply postoperatively or prolonged inactivity also can induce the collapse of pulmonary tissues. In the newborn, causes include prematurity, hyaline membrane disease, decreased stimulus to breathe, narcotics that cross the placental barrier during labor, and obstruction of the bronchus by a mucous plug. Any condition that decreases the amount of surfactant (a lubricating fluid in the air sacs) can lead to collapse of these air sacs and hence atelectasis.

Diagnosis

Chest radiography, a thorough history, and physical examination play important roles in the diagnosis. CT of the chest may be necessary to detect subtle changes. Breath sounds are diminished over the affected area, and percussion is dull. Bronchoscopy may be indicated to evaluate obstruction by a foreign body or a neoplasm.

Treatment

Because postsurgical patients are at high risk for atelectasis, they are encouraged to ambulate as soon as possible, breathe deeply, and cough periodically; an incentive spirometer is often used to encourage deep breathing. Other therapeutic measures include suctioning of the airway to remove any obstruction, spirometry, and the use of antibiotics to treat accompanying infection. Analgesics are given for chest pain. Surgical drainage of pleural effusion (abnormal fluid accumulation in the intrapleural spaces of the lungs) may be indicated to reduce intrathoracic pressure.

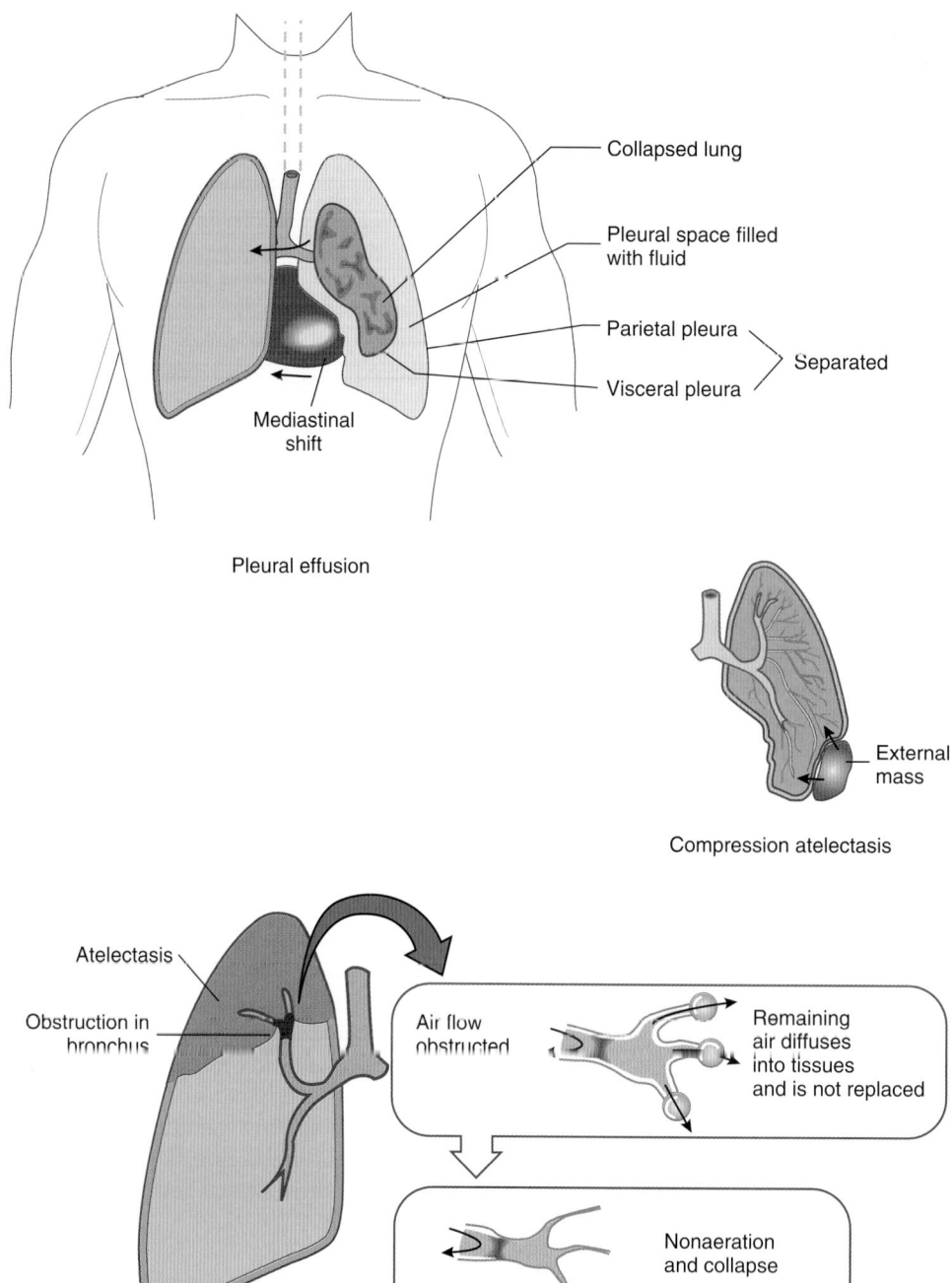

Pleural effusion

Compression atelectasis

Obstructive atelectasis – Absorption atelectasis

• **Fig. 9.7** Atelectasis. (From Gould B: *Pathophysiology for the health professions,* ed 3, Philadelphia, 2006, Saunders.)

Suctioning the trachea of the newborn is indicated to remove mucus and to facilitate a patent airway. Suctioning usually is followed by the administration of oxygen.

Prognosis

The outcome depends on treatment of the primary cause. Mild cases may resolve spontaneously. More severe cases are prone to complications, such as pneumonia. Individuals with obesity, upper abdominal or chest surgery, neuromuscular weakness, or pulmonary disease are at higher risk.

Prevention

Early ambulation and good ventilation therapy, after surgery or for any condition that causes prolonged immobility, are important. Individuals with lung disease are strongly advised not to smoke.

Patient Teaching

Discuss the diagnostic and therapeutic procedures. Use visual aids depicting the respiratory system to explain atelectasis. Explain the importance of postoperative ambulation and ventilation therapy. Tell the patient to seek prompt medical care for respiratory infections.

Pulmonary Embolism

Description
A pulmonary embolism occurs when a blood clot or other material (e.g., foreign body or tumor) lodges in and occludes an artery in the pulmonary circulation (Fig. 9.8).

ICD-10-CM Code	I26.99 *(Other pulmonary embolism without acute cor pulmonale)* (I26.90-I26.99 = 3 codes of specificity)

Symptoms and Signs
The size and location of the embolism, coupled with the general physical condition of the patient, determine the consequences of the interruption of blood supply to the area and the resulting symptoms and signs. The most common symptom of acute pulmonary embolism is the sudden onset of dyspnea and chest pain when the embolism enters the pulmonary circulation and interrupts the blood flow. It should also be mentioned that pulmonary embolism is one of the masqueraders in medicine. It often presents with nonrespiratory symptoms, such as tachycardia. Apprehension is common. The patient with a small, uncomplicated embolism experiences a cough, chest pain, and a low-grade fever. The patient with a more extensive infarction experiences dyspnea, **tachypnea** (with a respiratory rate of at least 20 breaths per minute), chest pain, and occasionally hemoptysis. Massive embolism leads to the sudden onset of cyanosis, shock, and death.

Patient Screening
Pulmonary embolism may have symptoms that mimic a heart attack, with the onset of sudden chest pain and shortness of breath. The patient may be extremely apprehensive.

An ambulance should be called immediately and immediate emergency care sought. The physician should be notified promptly. Individuals with milder symptoms of chest pain, fever, and dyspnea should be given prompt medical attention.

Etiology
Although most emboli are thrombi (blood clots) that have broken loose from a deep vein in the legs or the pelvis, emboli also may be composed of air, fat globules, a small piece of tissue, or a cluster of bacteria. The mass moves through the venous circulation and is pumped by the right side of the heart to the pulmonary circulation, where it becomes lodged in a vessel, usually at a division of an artery where it narrows.

Stasis of blood flow from immobility, injury to a vessel, predisposition to clot formation, thrombophlebitis, cardiovascular disease, smoking, or pulmonary disease increases the risk of embolism formation. In pregnancy, multiple factors predispose individuals to venous thrombosis. Oral contraceptives high in estrogen, diabetes mellitus, and myocardial infarction are considered contributing factors.

Diagnosis
The clinical picture, along with a history of physical immobility or other risk factors, leads to further investigation of respiratory status. Lung scanning and CT angiography of the chest are used to image the pulmonary blood flow. Echocardiography is also used to assess pulmonary artery pressure and right heart function. With the advances in CT technology, pulmonary angiography, once the definitive method for making the diagnosis, is rarely needed now. Auscultation often reveals rales and pleural rub in the area of the embolism. Arterial blood gas determination shows reduced partial pressure of oxygen and carbon dioxide. Studies performed to find residual thrombi in the veins of the lower extremities are helpful because the vast majority of pulmonary emboli originate there.

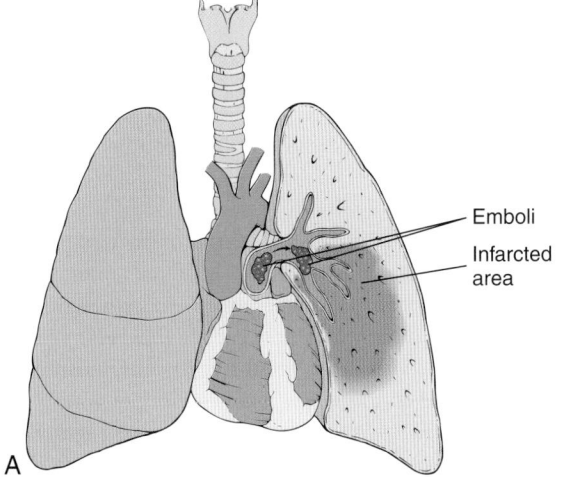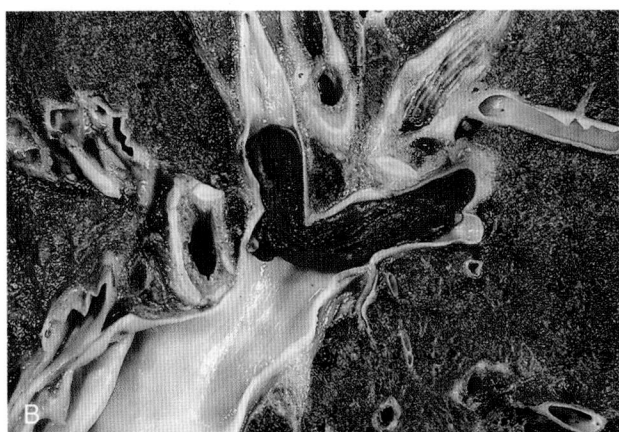

• **Fig. 9.8** Pulmonary embolism. (B, From Kumar V, et al: *Robbins basic pathology,* ed 10, Philadelphia, 2018, Saunders.)

Treatment

Primary treatment is aimed at preventing a potentially fatal episode and maintaining cardiopulmonary integrity and adequate ventilation and perfusion. Oxygen therapy and anticoagulant administration are used to meet these goals. Heparin or its analogues are often used initially in the treatment because therapeutic levels can be obtained quickly. Warfarin, an oral agent, is then used and maintained for weeks to months, depending on the clinical situation. A newer class of drugs has replaced warfarin as the treatment of choice for pulmonary embolism; these include apixaban (Eliquis), rivaroxaban (Xarelto), and dabigatran (Pradaxa). They do not require laboratory tests for monitoring the levels in blood and have fewer drug and food interactions compared with warfarin. Additionally, when there are hemodynamic compromises (shock and right-sided heart failure), thrombolytic drugs sometimes are administered to dissolve a clot, especially when low blood pressure or cardiac arrest occurs.

Prevention is important; most hospitalized patients should be placed on some form of prophylactic therapy.

Early ambulation, low-dose anticoagulant agents, and the use of a variety of stockings, such as thromboembolic deterrent (TED) stockings or sequential stockings that intermittently pump the legs, are employed as preventive measures for patients.

Prognosis

Mild cases can have a positive outcome with treatment. Mortality is high in cases of massive pulmonary embolism.

Prevention

Management of risk factors, such as long-term immobility, can prevent the formation of emboli that can potentially obstruct pulmonary circulation. Postoperative prophylactic measures should be employed. Optimal management of systemic diseases, such as myocardial infarction, thrombophlebitis, and atrial fibrillation, is beneficial.

Patient Teaching

Use visual aids to demonstrate normal pulmonary circulation. Explain anticoagulation therapy and the importance of regular blood monitoring to ensure that therapeutic levels of the anticoagulant are being maintained. Make the patient aware of the side effects that should be reported to the health care provider, such as nosebleeds, blood in the stool, or spontaneous bruising under the skin. Explain the postoperative measures prescribed to prevent venostasis, such as antiembolism stockings.

Pneumonia

Description

Pneumonia is infective inflammation of the lungs.

| ICD-10-CM Code | J18.9 *(Pneumonia, unspecified organism)* |
| | (J12.0-J18.9 = 29 codes of specificity) |

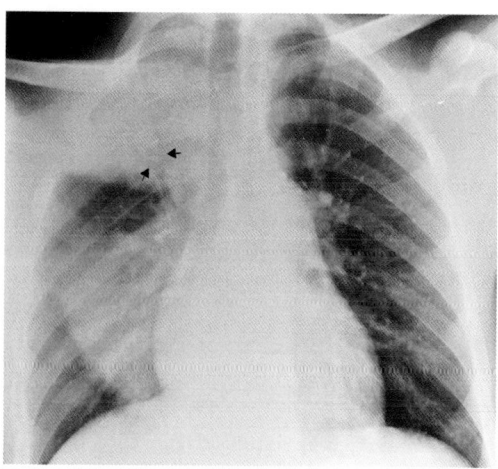

• **Fig. 9.9** Appearance of pneumonia. (From Long BW, Frank ED, Ehrlich RA: *Radiography essentials for limited practice,* ed 4, St Louis, 2013, Elsevier.)

Symptoms and Signs

Pneumonia is not only a condition but also a general term applied to several types of inflammation of the lungs. The inflammation may be either unilateral or bilateral and involve all or only a portion of an infected lung (Fig. 9.9). The symptoms of pneumonia vary. The patient may have a cough, fever, shortness of breath even while at rest, chills, sweating, chest pains, cyanosis, and blood in the sputum. The infant or child exhibits "panting" or shallow, rapid respirations. The larger the area of lung affected, the more severe the symptoms are. How quickly the symptoms develop and which symptoms are most evident vary with the cause.

Aspiration pneumonia results from aspiration of liquids or other material into the tracheobronchial tree. It tends to occur in patients who have serious problems with swallowing; it is commonly seen in older adults, especially those weakened by cancer or those with neurological problems, such as stroke or Parkinson disease.

Patient Screening

Cough, fever, and shortness of breath are symptoms that require a prompt, same-day appointment for medical evaluation. Parents of infants may report that the child exhibits symptoms of a cold with fever and fast respirations. The infant or child should be given top priority for a medical examination by a physician within 2 hours.

Etiology

Pneumonia usually is caused by viral or bacterial infections. Organisms commonly causing bacterial pneumonia are pneumococci, staphylococci, group A hemolytic streptococci, *Haemophilus influenzae* type B, *Klebsiella pneumoniae* types 1 and 2, and other gram-negative organisms. A syndrome referred to as *atypical pneumonia,* previously referred to as *walking pneumonia,* often demonstrates marked abnormalities on the chest radiograph, yet the patient does not appear significantly ill. The organisms most commonly identified with this syndrome include *Legionella, Mycoplasma,* and *Chlamydia.* Viruses, such as adenoviruses, influenza viruses, and respiratory syncytial viruses (RSVs), also can produce pneumonia. It also may be caused by damage to the lungs from inhalation of a poisonous gas, such as chlorine, or by aspiration of foreign matter. The pneumonia can range from a mild complication of URI to a life-threatening illness. Bacterial pneumonia can be community acquired by patients living independently in the community, or it may arise in a hospital setting associated with health care or with use of a ventilator.

Diagnosis

The diagnostic evaluation begins with physical examination, patient history, and chest radiography to evaluate the pulmonary system. Further tests, such as arterial blood gas, bronchoscopy, and sputum and blood cultures, are also done.

Treatment

Treatment is based on the underlying cause of the pneumonia. Organism-specific antibiotics are prescribed for bacterial pneumonia. Penicillin is the drug of choice for pneumococcal pneumonia. Tetracycline drugs, erythromycin, doxycycline, and sulfonamides may be administered. *Mycoplasma* infections may be treated with broad-spectrum antibiotics. Fungal infections require the use of various antifungal medications, whereas viral infections are treated with specific antiviral agents. The use of analgesics, such as aspirin, helps relieve chest pain, and oxygen therapy may be necessary for shortness of breath. Bed rest, increased fluid intake, a high-calorie diet, and postural drainage also prove beneficial.

Prognosis

The prognosis is good for otherwise healthy individuals. Severely or chronically ill patients are more predisposed to pneumonia. Pneumonia is the leading cause of death worldwide and the eighth leading cause of death in the United States.

Prevention

The pneumococcal vaccine is the only way to prevent pneumococcal pneumonia. Vaccines are available for adults, children, and certain groups. Anyone can contact their health care provider to find out if they should be vaccinated to prevent pneumococcal pneumonia.

Antibiotic therapy for URIs determined to be caused by bacteria, such as *Streptococcus* or *Staphylococcus,* can prevent pneumonia. Prophylactic measures against aspiration in patients with stroke or those in an altered state of consciousness are prudent.

Patient Teaching

Instruct the patient to take the full course of antibiotics and other medications as prescribed. Stress the importance of rest, plenty of fluid intake, and coughing to clear secretions. Counsel the patient to avoid smoking, limit alcohol intake, and not to take over-the-counter medications. Tell the patient to seek prompt medical care for signs of respiratory infection in the future, to stay away from persons with infections, and to take seasonal influenza vaccines, if appropriate. Stress the importance of follow-up appointments to determine sufficient resolution of pneumonia.

! ALERT!

Health Hazards of Common Molds

Recent concern about the health hazards of mold infestation in homes and other buildings has made its way into the public health media and medical arena. There are reports that toxic mold inside homes can cause allergic symptoms or unique or rare health conditions, such as pulmonary hemorrhage or memory loss. Reported cases of illnesses from molds, in the indoor and outdoor environment, that contain mycotoxins (poisons produced by fungi) have prompted a plethora of questions from the public about how to identify mold infestation, what action to take, and when to seek medical attention. Listed below are some facts presented to the public by the Centers for Disease Control and Prevention (CDC):

- Molds grow naturally in both the indoor and outdoor environments, especially where there is moisture. A constant supply of moisture is required for its growth.
- Large mold infestations usually can be seen or smelled.
- The hazards presented by molds that contain mycotoxins, such as *Stachybotrys chartarum*, should be considered the same as other common molds.
- Mold exposure does not always present a health problem.
- People with allergies may be more sensitive to molds. Possible allergic symptoms experienced are nasal stuffiness, eye irritation, skin irritation, and/or wheezing. Severe reactions may occur among workers exposed to large amounts of molds in occupational settings.
- Individuals who have decreased immunity, such as those with acquired immunodeficiency syndrome (AIDS) or those with underlying lung disease or chronic diseases, are more susceptible to fungal infections and allergic pneumonitis.
- A commonsense approach that includes routine measures of control should be used for any mold contamination existing inside homes and buildings. Decisions about treatment required for extensive mold infestations of homes or buildings are made individually; sometimes professional cleaning companies and reconstruction are employed.
- In most cases, mold can be removed by a thorough cleaning with commercial products, soap and water, or a bleach solution of no more than 1 cup of bleach in 1 gallon of water. Moldy items are to be discarded.
- All molds should be treated the same with respect to potential health risks and removal.
- Recommendations for preventing mold infestation include ensuring adequate ventilation, using paints with mold inhibitors, cleaning bathrooms with mold-killing products, and promptly removing flooded carpets.
- A physician should be consulted for appropriate medical intervention when symptoms or illnesses are suspected to be the result of exposure to mold.

Modified from the CDC National Center for Environmental Health: Questions and answers on *Stachybotrys chartarum* and other molds, 2010, http://www.cdc.gov/mold/stachy.htm.

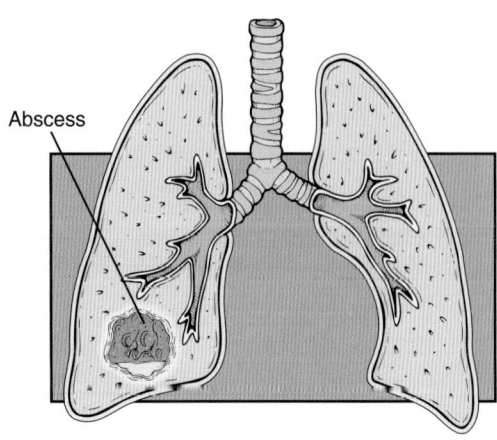

• **Fig. 9.10** Pulmonary abscess.

Pulmonary Abscess

Description

A cavity of contained infectious material in the lung is known as a *pulmonary abscess* (Fig. 9.10).

ICD-10-CM Code	J85.0 *(Gangrene and necrosis of lung)*
	J85.1 *(Abscess of lung with pneumonia)*
	J85.2 *(Abscess of lung without pneumonia)*

Symptoms and Signs

Abscesses are more common in the lower portions of the lungs and in the right lung because of its more vertical bronchus. The main symptoms are alternating chills and fever. Chest pain and a productive cough accompanied by purulent, bloody, or foul-smelling sputum and foul-smelling breath may also be present.

Patient Screening

Fever, bloody and/or foul-smelling sputum, and chest discomfort indicate a serious respiratory infection that requires immediate medical care. The patient may report "a turn for the worse" while under treatment for pneumonia. Generalized fatigue, weight loss, and persistent vacillating fever may be the only symptoms.

Etiology

Lung abscesses are often a complication of pneumonia caused by bacteria. Aspiration of food, a foreign object, bronchial stenosis, or neoplasms may cause pulmonary abscesses to form. A pulmonary abscess also may develop when a septic embolism is carried to the lung via the pulmonary circulation. Background factors include periodontal disease, gingivitis, sinus infection, intravenous drug abuse, and general anesthesia or other causes of reduced levels of consciousness.

Diagnosis

Decreased breath sounds are revealed on chest auscultation. The patient history may indicate recent aspiration. Chest radiography is necessary to locate the site of the affected portion of the lung. Blood and sputum cultures are used to detect the causative organism.

Treatment

The treatment of choice for an abscess is the use of antibiotics for a fairly long duration or until the abscess is gone. Surgical resection of the abscess and a portion of the affected lung may be required if the antibiotic therapy is not successful.

Prognosis

The otherwise healthy individual who responds favorably to treatment has a good prognosis. Prognosis is guarded for the very young, older adults, the immunocompromised, or the chronically ill. A history of aspiration and/or poor dentition carries a higher risk for abscess formation.

Prevention

Precautions should be taken to minimize aspiration. Proper treatment of dental infections and early treatment of pneumonia minimize the risk for bacterial lung abscess. Some individuals (e.g., older patients) benefit from taking the influenza vaccine.

Patient Teaching

Explain to the patient the importance of taking medications exactly as prescribed, especially taking the entire course of antibiotics. Stress the importance of follow-up care until the condition is completely resolved.

Legionellosis (Legionnaires Disease and Pontiac Fever)

Description

Legionellosis is a type of pneumonia caused by the bacterium *Legionella pneumophila*.

ICD-10-CM Code	A48.1 *(Legionnaires' disease)*
	(A48.1-A48.2 = 2 codes of specificity)

Symptoms and Signs

This infection can evolve in two different forms: the more severe legionnaires disease and the milder form, Pontiac fever. Legionnaires disease, an acute respiratory tract infection that produces severe pneumonia-like symptoms or possibly fatal pneumonia, was named after an epidemic outbreak at an American Legion convention in Philadelphia in July 1976. More than 200 people became ill, and 34 died as a result of the disease.

Typical symptoms include general malaise, headache, and cough. These are followed rapidly by the onset of chills, fever, chest pain, dyspnea, myalgia, vomiting, diarrhea, and anorexia. The symptoms often mimic those of pneumonia. The incubation period for Legionnaires disease is 2 to 10 days, usually about 1 week. The symptoms of Pontiac fever are less severe and include a high fever and muscle aches, with duration of 2 to 5 days. The incubation period for Pontiac fever is much shorter than that for Legionnaires disease, and pneumonia does not occur.

Patient Screening

Initially the patient may experience malaise, fatigue, and flulike symptoms that progress to be more severe: headache, chills, high fever, dyspnea, restlessness, confusion, nausea, and vomiting. A prompt medical evaluation should be scheduled. Hospitalization may be required.

Etiology

Both disorders are caused by *L. pneumophila* and are not contagious. These bacteria thrive in warm aquatic environments and are inhaled from contaminated aerosolized water droplets. Air conditioning systems, cooling towers, whirlpool spas, showers, and the hot water plumbing of buildings in which the temperature of the water is between 95°F and 115°F permit the reproduction of the bacterium. Predisposing factors include smoking, physical debilitation, especially among patients with chronic obstructive pulmonary disease (COPD), immunosuppression, and alcoholism. Pontiac fever usually occurs in otherwise healthy individuals.

Diagnosis

Complete physical examination and patient history, along with chest radiographic studies and testing of blood samples, are performed. Laboratory analysis of blood indicates elevated white blood cell (WBC) count, liver enzyme level, and erythrocyte sedimentation rate (ESR). A culture from the sputum to isolate the *Legionella* bacterium is necessary for confirmation of Legionnaires disease. The detection of the presence of bacteria in a urine sample indicates the disease. Evaluating convalescent serum samples to detect antibodies is the best diagnostic tool.

Treatment

Typically antibiotic therapy is initiated before confirmation of the diagnosis is made, because the response to treatment is usually slow. Antibiotics of choice are azithromycin or levofloxacin, except for mild cases, when erythromycin or doxycycline is prescribed. Rifampin may be added when response to the antibiotic is not adequate. Oxygen may be used for the dyspnea; antipyretics, antiemetics, and analgesics are also helpful.

Pontiac fever usually resolves itself in a few days, requiring no specific treatment. Legionellosis occurs worldwide. The National Center for Infectious Diseases monitors the incidence of legionellosis in the United States. Attempts are made to identify the sources of disease transmission, and recommendations for prevention and control measures are made.

Prognosis

Improvement of symptoms occurs in 2 to 4 days with specific antimicrobial therapy and without complications. The prognosis is guarded in severe cases and in the immunocompromised.

Prevention

Prevention can be accomplished by the appropriate design of facilities to prevent stagnant water. The temperature of the water in cooling towers and air conditioning units must be maintained either below 95°F or above 115°F, or it must have adequate chlorination to kill the *Legionella* bacillus. Monitoring of chlorine content of whirlpool baths and spas is a necessary obligation of the owners.

Patient Teaching

Urge the patient to take the entire course of antibiotics as prescribed. Give the patient appropriate instructions regarding hospitalization, when required.

Respiratory Syncytial Virus Pneumonia

Description

RSV pneumonia, an inflammatory and infectious condition of the lungs, is most common in infants, young children, and older adults.

ICD-10-CM Code	J12.1 *(Respiratory syncytial virus pneumonia)*

Symptoms and Signs

RSV causes coldlike symptoms, including nasal congestion, otitis media, and coughing, in the mild upper respiratory tract form of infection. As the virus progresses downward to the lower respiratory tract, the patient experiences fever, malaise, lethargy, more frequent coughing, wheezing, and dyspnea.

Patient Screening

Infants with symptoms of a lower respiratory tract infection require prompt medical attention and close monitoring thereafter until well. Older adults are considered to be at high risk, especially those in nursing homes. In young adults, symptoms consist of nasal discharge, pharyngitis, and low-grade fever.

Etiology

RSV is the causative agent of RSV pneumonia. The greatest occurrence of these annual epidemic infections is during the winter months, December to March, and they most seriously affect children younger than 3 years of age and older adults, especially patients whose respiratory systems already are compromised by underlying disease or predisposing factors. At greatest risk are infants who were premature, have a congenital cardiac defect, or have a preexisting pulmonary disorder. Most people have experienced several RSV URIs in their lifetimes, and most cases of mild RSV infection are self-limiting.

RSV is spread by contact with the secretions of an infected person. Thorough hand washing and the use of disposable tissues for nasal secretions can prevent the spread of this disease.

Diagnosis

Clinical findings, a thorough physical examination, and lavage of the nasal pharynx aid in determining the diagnosis of RSV pneumonia. The secretions obtained from the lavage are examined for the presence of RSV. When grown in a tissue culture, RSV produces giant syncytial cells.

Treatment

Most cases of RSV infection involving the upper respiratory tract are self-limiting. Antipyretics are prescribed for fever, and antibiotics are given for otitis media. When the infection invades the lower respiratory tract of an infant or a young child, treatment may involve inhalation therapy. Inhalation of 3% hypertonic saline is frequently used to treat RSV. Hospitalization may be required for oxygen therapy and hydration.

Prognosis

The prognosis is generally good. Infants are prone to otitis media as a complication.

Prevention

Adults with symptoms of respiratory infection should not handle infants. Strict hand washing is prudent because the virus is transmitted by respiratory secretions. No vaccine is available.

Patient Teaching

Infants are usually hospitalized so that supportive therapy can be provided; thus parents need reassurance and support. Parents are encouraged to hold and interact with the infant. Inform the parents that the head of the crib or bed is elevated to prevent aspiration of secretions and aid respirations.

Histoplasmosis

Description

Histoplasmosis is a fungal disease originating in the lungs and is caused by inhalation of dust containing *Histoplasma capsulatum*.

ICD 10 CM Code	B39.9 *(Histoplasmosis, unspecified)* (B39.0-B39.9 = 7 codes of specificity)

Symptoms and Signs

Histoplasmosis may cause pneumonia or may become systemic. Many patients with histoplasmosis are *asymptomatic* at onset of disease; it is not contagious. As the fungus disseminates throughout the pulmonary tissue, the patient reports dyspnea and loss of energy to the point of incapacitation. The patient becomes febrile. The spleen and lymph nodes become enlarged. In patients with AIDS, histoplasmosis may occur as an opportunistic infection.

Patient Screening

The patient having the above-mentioned symptoms should be seen for medical evaluation within 24 hours.

Etiology

Histoplasmosis is caused by the fungus *H. capsulatum*, which is carried by dust and is inhaled. It is the most common endemic mycosis in the United States. The greatest occurrence of histoplasmosis is in the Midwestern United States. Often the fungus is found in soil contaminated by droppings from birds or bats specific to the area, which may

be a source of the airborne fungus. Infections are associated with disruption of soil, cleaning attics or barns, and tearing down old structures.

> **NOTE**
>
> Blastomycosis (also called *Gilchrist disease*) is a fungal infection caused by inhaling the fungus *Blastomyces dermatitidis*, which grows as a mold in moist soil and wood. It is found in specific endemic areas in North America and has the greatest prevalence in the upper Midwest and southward along the Mississippi and Ohio riverbeds. In the Southwest, coccidioidomycosis is caused by the fungus *Coccidioides immitis*, which produces spores that live in the soil. This is the agent that causes the disease known as San Joaquin Valley fever. The disease is contracted when dry soil is picked up by wind and the spores are breathed in; it is not communicable.

Diagnosis

Diagnosis is made by evaluating the clinical findings, a positive skin test result, blood serologic findings specific for the fungus, or the identification of the fungus in pus, sputum, or tissue specimens. Chest radiographs may be normal or may reveal patchy infiltrates and diffuse opacities.

Treatment

When the disease is self-limiting, no antifungal therapy is necessary. The antifungal drugs, itraconazole, fluconazole, and amphotericin B, are used to treat more severe or progressive disease. In severe cases, corticosteroid use may be beneficial.

Prognosis

Spontaneous recovery is usual. Secondary infections may occur. Reinfection is possible, especially in a setting of high exposure. Small calcifications remain in the lungs after infection. Progressive histoplasmosis can be fatal. Infection confers immunity.

Prevention

It is prudent to teach safety practices to workers in high-risk jobs that expose them to contaminated soil.

Patient Teaching

Review appropriate prevention measures with individuals at risk because of poor health. Advise the patient to avoid contact with soil contaminated with bat or bird droppings. Use available computer-based health education on how to avoid histoplasmosis infection.

Influenza

Description

Influenza is a generalized, highly contagious, acute viral disease that occurs in annual outbreaks.

ICD-10-CM Code	J10.1 *(Influenza due to other influenza virus with other respiratory manifestations)* (J10.0-J10.89 = 9 codes of specificity)

The above codes are nonspecific and may be valid as a principal diagnosis, except for Medicare. Refer to the physician's diagnosis and then to the current edition of the ICD-10-CM coding manual to ensure the greatest specificity.

Symptoms and Signs

Influenza is characterized by inflammation of the upper and lower respiratory tract mucous membranes, a severe protracted cough, fever, headache, sore throat, and generalized malaise. The onset is usually sudden and marked by chills and a feverish feeling. In mild cases, the temperature may reach 101°F to 102°F, and the fever may last for 2 or 3 days. In severe cases, a temperature of 103°F to 104°F is possible, lasting 4 or 5 days. Acute symptoms usually subside rapidly with decreasing fever. The weakness, sweating, and fatigue may continue for a few days to a few weeks; malaise may persist several days before full recovery.

Fever, cough, and other respiratory symptoms persisting for longer than 5 days may indicate a secondary bacterial pneumonia. Possible complications of influenza are bronchitis, sinusitis, otitis media, and cervical lymphadenitis.

Patient Screening

During a known epidemic, the health care provider may give the telephone screener(s) guidelines to address callers with symptoms typical of influenza.

Individuals with severe symptoms or those who are at high risk for complications (i.e., the very young, older adults, or those chronically ill) are given a prompt appointment for close medical monitoring.

Etiology

Known viruses that cause influenza are designated as orthomyxovirus types A, B, and C. However, many mutant strains also reproduce in both humans and animals. Acute uncomplicated influenza with recovery is the most frequently encountered type of this disease. Secondary bacterial pneumonia after influenza most often is caused by hemolytic *Streptococcus, Staphylococcus,* or *Pneumococcus.*

Influenza outbreaks may be sporadic or epidemic. Epidemics occur every 1 to 4 years and spread rapidly because the incubation period is only 1 to 3 days. Transmission is from person to person by inhalation of the virus in airborne mucus discharge. Fatalities can occur in as short a time as 48 hours after the onset of symptoms.

Diagnosis

Clinically, influenza (Fig. 9.11) may be indistinguishable from the common cold. When differentiating influenza from other respiratory tract infections, consideration should be given to the amount of time passed since onset, the presence of an epidemic in the community, and the severity of the patient's symptoms. Frequent recurrences of influenza-like syndromes may make the physician suspect TB (see the Pulmonary Tuberculosis section). A complicating pneumonia may be present if the patient has dyspnea, cyanosis, hemoptysis, or rales in the lungs. The WBC count may indicate leukopenia with relative lymphocytosis. Confirmation of the influenza diagnosis is made by isolation of the virus from nasopharyngeal culture. A sputum culture isolates bacteria in secondary infections.

Treatment

Treatment is symptomatic; vaccines are useless after the disease is established. Bed rest, increased fluid intake, a light diet, and the use of antipyretic and analgesic drugs, when needed, are helpful. Oseltamivir may be used for influenza A or B. All of these agents are only effective if given within the first 48 hours of symptoms, usually when the disease is known to be present in the community. In less severe cases, treatment of respiratory tract symptoms may not be necessary; however, warm salt water gargles, steam inhalation,

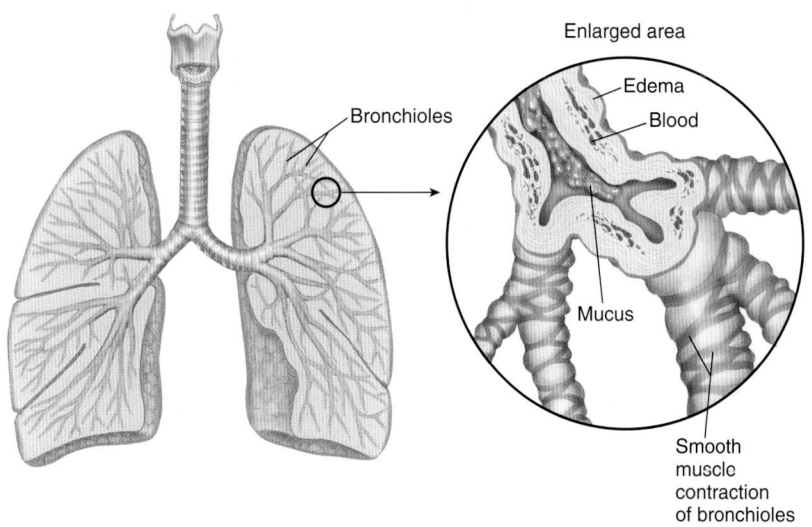

• **Fig. 9.11** Influenza. (From Seidel HM, et al: *Mosby's guide to physical examination,* ed 5, St Louis, 2003, Mosby/Elsevier.)

and the use of cough syrups may be comforting. Antibiotics are effective against bacterial pneumonia and other less serious complications, such as sinusitis, otitis media, and lymphadenitis. *Aspirin should not be used, especially in children, because of its association with Reye syndrome* (see Reye Syndrome in Chapter 2).

Prognosis

Recovery is usually complete; however, complications, such as pneumonia, can occur. Those at highest risk are the very young, older adults, and the chronically ill. Epidemics can cause substantial morbidity, financial loss, and even death. During seasonal influenza, the vast majority of deaths occur in persons 65 years and older.

Prevention

The prophylactic use of vaccines against influenza is effective in reducing the occurrence of the disease, especially in older adults or infirm (Box 9.1). Because immunity from vaccination lasts only 1 year, annual booster doses are needed for optimal protection. After vaccination, about 2 to 4 weeks is required for immunity to develop.

Patient Teaching

Reinforce the use of comfort measures, including antipyretics and analgesics as prescribed. Advise the patient to rest and take adequate fluids. Infection control, such as thorough and frequent hand washing, is prudent to reduce the spread of the virus. Educate individuals at high risk about annual influenza immunizations.

> **NOTE**
>
> Warn parents that aspirin is contraindicated for children because Reye syndrome can result.

◆ ENRICHMENT

Swine-Origin Influenza A Virus (H1N1) Infection (Swine Flu)

The novel influenza A virus (subtype H1N1) is of swine origin (commonly called *swine flu*) and causes a respiratory disease that was first detected in April 2009. H1N1 virus is a highly unusual mix of swine, bird, and human flu viruses. Because this is a relatively new virus, *most people have little or no immunity against it.*

The Centers for Disease Control and Prevention (CDC) has determined that the H1N1 virus is contagious, and in the 2009 epidemic, it spread from human to human in all 50 states in the United States, with cases occurring internationally as well. The disease has spread mostly among children and young adults. Lower rates of hospitalization have been noted in people 65 years of age and older; this is quite different than what is seen with seasonal flu. Like seasonal flu, H1N1 infection in humans can vary in severity from mild to severe.

The symptoms of H1N1 infection in people are similar to the symptoms of regular human flu and include fever, cough, sore throat, body ache, headache, chills, and fatigue. Some people have reported diarrhea and vomiting associated with swine flu. The incubation period is estimated to be 1 to 7 days. Although some experience milder symptoms, in others, symptoms can be severe and even cause death, usually as a result of pneumonia. At this time, in the United States, most people who have become ill with H1N1 and have experienced typical flu symptoms have recovered without requiring medical treatment.

H1N1 virus is susceptible to both oseltamivir (Tamiflu) and zanamivir (Relenza). These drugs are effective for the treatment and/or prevention of infection with swine influenza viruses.

Laboratory diagnostic tests are available for confirmation of H1N1 virus infection, and they include real-time reverse transcription polymerase chain reaction (RT-PCR) and a viral culture. It is wise to stay informed as new information about seasonal flu vaccine guidelines becomes available.

•BOX 9.1   Target Groups for Influenza Immunization

Groups at Increased Risk of Complications (Recommended)

- Persons age 50 years and older
- Residents of nursing homes and other chronic care facilities
- Patients with chronic pulmonary (including asthma) or cardiac disorder
- Patients with chronic metabolic disease (including diabetes), renal dysfunction, hemoglobinopathies, or immunosuppression
- Children and teens receiving long-term aspirin
- Women who will be pregnant during the influenza season
- Children age 6 months to 5 years

Groups in Contact with High-Risk Persons (Recommended)

- Physicians, nurses, and other health care providers
- Employees of nursing homes and chronic care facilities
- Providers of home care to high-risk persons
- Members (including children) of the households of high-risk persons

Other Groups (Encouraged)

- Providers of essential community services (e.g., police, fire)
- International travelers
- Students, dormitory residents
- Anyone wishing to reduce the risk of influenza, young and old alike, when the flu vaccine is not restricted by supply

Modified from Advisory Committee on Immunization Practices, Centers for Disease Control and Prevention: *MMWR* 43(No RR-9):1, 1994. From Bennett JC, Plum F: *Cecil textbook of medicine,* ed 23, Philadelphia, 2008, Saunders.

Chronic Obstructive Pulmonary Disease

COPD is a condition of slow and irreversible progressive airway obstruction. It encompasses several obstructive diseases of the lungs, including chronic bronchitis, bronchiectasis, asthma, emphysema, cystic fibrosis, and pneumoconiosis. Although the mechanism of the obstruction can vary, the consequence is the same; the patient with COPD is unable to ventilate the lungs freely, which results in ineffective exchange of respiratory gases. This causes the patient's normal respiratory response to elevated carbon dioxide levels to become diminished.

Acute and Chronic Bronchitis

Description

Bronchitis is inflammation of the mucous membrane lining the bronchi.

ICD-10-CM Code	J40 (Bronchitis, not specified as acute or chronic)
	J41.8 (Mixed simple and mucopurulent chronic bronchitis)
	(J40-J42 = 5 codes of specificity)

Symptoms and Signs

In acute bronchitis, a deep, persistent, productive cough is the main symptom. The patient has thick, yellow to gray sputum. Other symptoms include shortness of breath, wheezing, a slightly elevated temperature, and pain in the upper chest, which is aggravated by the cough. Acute symptoms subside within a week, but the cough may continue for 2 to 3 weeks. Physical signs within the lungs are few or absent if the bronchitis is uncomplicated. Scattered or occasional rales often are heard on auscultation. There is no clinical or radiologic evidence of pneumonia.

Chronic bronchitis is similar to acute bronchitis, except that the inflammation persists and becomes worse for at least 3 months of the year for 2 consecutive years. Mild forms may exist for many years, with the patient having only a slight cough in the mornings. Then the condition becomes aggravated when the patient contracts acute URIs. Obstructive and asthmatic symptoms and dyspnea appear as the condition progresses. Chest expansion becomes diminished, and scattered rales and wheezing are often heard. In the beginning stages of the disease, flare-ups of chronic bronchitis are likely to occur after the patient has experienced severe colds or influenza. In later stages, even a minor head cold can cause a severe attack. During the final stages, the coughing, shortness of breath, and wheezing occur almost continuously. Prolonged, recurrent attacks cause gradual deterioration of the lungs.

For both acute and chronic bronchitis, the symptoms appear more troublesome during the winter months. Living or working in a cold, damp environment or in a polluted atmosphere can aggravate the condition.

Patient Screening

An individual complaining of a persistent, productive cough is advised to seek medical care if there has been no improvement. When the cough is described as chronic, with purulent sputum, and fever and/or wheezing are present, the patient should be examined by a health care professional within 24 hours. Persons known to have chronic bronchitis should be seen promptly to be examined for suspected infections or sudden worsening of symptoms.

Etiology

Acute bronchitis is part of a general URI. It begins after a common cold or other viral infections of the nasopharynx and pharynx or occurs as a complication of bacterial infections. Recurring attacks in adults may indicate a focus of infection, such as chronic sinusitis (see the Sinusitis section), bronchiectasis (see the Bronchiectasis section), and pneumonia (see the Pneumonia section). In children, hypertrophied tonsils and adenoids may be the source of acute bronchitis. Allergens are also frequently predisposing factors. The same bacteria known to cause pneumonia (as mentioned previously) may be responsible for chronic bronchitis. Progressive and irreversible changes in the bronchi can result from constant irritation from smoking or exposure to industrial pollution or recurrent infections.

Diagnosis

Acute or chronic bronchitis can be suspected on the basis of the patient's symptoms and history. The presence of other diseases or their complications must be ruled out, especially if the symptoms are serious or prolonged. Diagnostic tests include chest radiographic studies, pulmonary function tests, arterial blood gases, and other blood and sputum analyses.

Treatment

Because acute bronchitis usually is caused by a viral infection, no specific treatment is prescribed, except for those measures that will relieve the symptoms. Aspirin may be used to control fever. Increased fluid intake, along with the use of a vaporizer and humidifier, helps clear the nasal passages and bronchi. The physician may prescribe the use of a bronchodilator aerosol inhaler for wheezing and shortness of breath and a cough suppressant if the chest is sore from coughing. If a secondary bacterial infection is suspected, an antibiotic is prescribed.

The treatment of chronic bronchitis is based on the stage of the disease at the time the patient consults professional help. Prompt treatment of acute infections, when they occur, is of primary importance. Low-flow oxygen therapy may be administered, as needed, for hypoxemia. Postural drainage and percussion are techniques used to help loosen and expectorate thick mucus. Aerosolized corticosteroids may be ordered to control inflammation. The patient is advised to give up smoking, to avoid smoke-filled rooms, to stay away from people with colds, and to avoid crowds.

Prognosis

Acute bronchitis resolves completely within a few days; however, a residual cough can remain for 2 to 3 weeks. Chronic bronchitis has a guarded prognosis because it may be progressive and involves airway obstruction and general debilitation.

Prevention

It is important for the patient to avoid the primary causative factors: smoking, chronic exposure to pollutants in the air, and recurrent respiratory infections.

Patient Teaching

For acute bronchitis, advise the patient to rest and take any palliative medications as prescribed. Advise patients with chronic bronchitis not to smoke or expose themselves to known respiratory irritants. Demonstrate methods of chest physiotherapy. Explain the use of home equipment designed for oxygen therapy or inhalation therapy. Make use of manufacturers' website information to demonstrate the use of equipment. Encourage smokers to take advantage of smoking cessation programs available in the community.

Bronchiectasis

Description

Bronchiectasis is the permanent, irreversible dilation or distortion of one or more of the bronchi, resulting from destruction of muscular and elastic portions of the bronchial walls (Fig. 9.12).

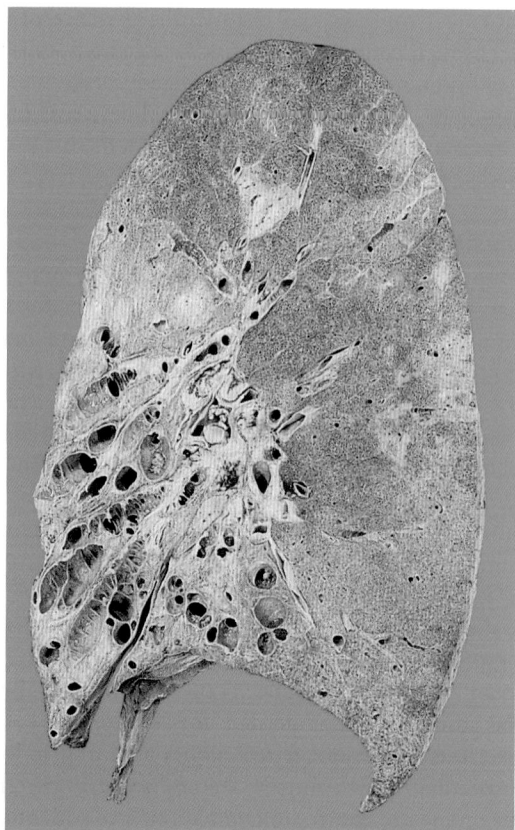

• **Fig. 9.12** Bronchiectasis. (From Cross S: *Underwood's pathology: a clinical approach,* ed 7, Philadelphia, 2019, Elsevier.)

ICD-10-CM Code	J47.9 *(Bronchiectasis, uncomplicated)* (J47.0-J47.9 = 3 codes of specificity)

Symptoms and Signs

Bronchiectasis, a condition that takes many years to develop, is usually bilateral and involves the lower lobes of the lungs. A chronic cough producing large quantities of purulent, foul-smelling sputum is the main symptom of bronchiectasis. Hemoptysis, dyspnea, wheezing, fever, and general malaise develop as the condition progresses. The patient also may experience chronic halitosis.

Patient Screening

Schedule the patient having a chronic, highly productive cough for a clinical examination at his or her earliest convenience.

Etiology

Bronchiectasis may be caused by repeated damage to the bronchial wall caused by recurrent airway infections. It also can result from pneumonia, TB, bronchial obstruction, or inhalation of a corrosive gas. This condition is a common life-threatening complication of cystic fibrosis or other childhood infections, such as measles and pertussis (whooping cough), and also may result from immune deficiency (e.g., hypogammaglobulinemia).

Diagnosis

Initially, when symptoms are vague, determining the diagnosis of bronchiectasis may be difficult. Physical examination, history of symptoms, chest radiography, high-resolution CT of the chest, bronchoscopy, sputum culture, and pulmonary function tests are of the most value in making the diagnosis.

Treatment

Antibiotics and bronchodilators are prescribed, and postural drainage is encouraged. Sputum removal management is very important and can be accomplished with vibratory devices, such as the Acapella or a high-frequency chest compression inflatable vest. Avoiding environmental irritants, such as smoke, fumes, and large amounts of dust, is important. If the patient has a great deal of hemoptysis, surgery to remove the affected part of the lung may be advised.

Prognosis

The prognosis varies with the underlying cause. Serious respiratory and cardiac complications, such as pulmonary hypertension and cor pulmonale (see Chapter 10), develop with advanced bronchiectasis.

Prevention

Childhood immunizations and early treatment of respiratory infections are recommended for prevention, as is avoidance of smoking or exposure to any other respiratory irritants.

Patient Teaching

Provide strong advice to the patient who smokes to cease smoking; offer a referral to a smoking cessation support group. Explain the medical management regimen, and demonstrate how to use home equipment for oxygen therapy and/or inhalation therapy. Teach the patient proper techniques for postural drainage and percussion and how to properly discard secretions. Use demonstration videos or print-on-demand electronic materials to teach the proper technique for postural drainage.

Asthma

Adult-onset asthma manifests for the first time in middle-aged or older individuals, with the usual moderate to severe symptoms of asthma: wheezing, productive cough, and difficulty breathing. During an attack, airway narrowing can be severe and result in airway closure and severe anxiety in the patient. This condition, called *status asthmaticus,* requires emergency hospitalization for treatment. There are many common asthma triggers, and the causes can be intrinsic or extrinsic. Both environmental and genetic factors are important in the etiology of asthma. Medical management includes pharmacologic therapy with antiinflammatory drugs and bronchodilators. Both quick-relief medications and long-term medications are given to treat and prevent asthma attacks. Patient education is crucial for obtaining the maximum benefit from the treatment plan.

See Chapter 2 for a discussion of asthma. See Fig. 9.13 for effects of smoking. See the Alert box on the Health Effects of Exposure to Tobacco Smoke in Chapter 1.

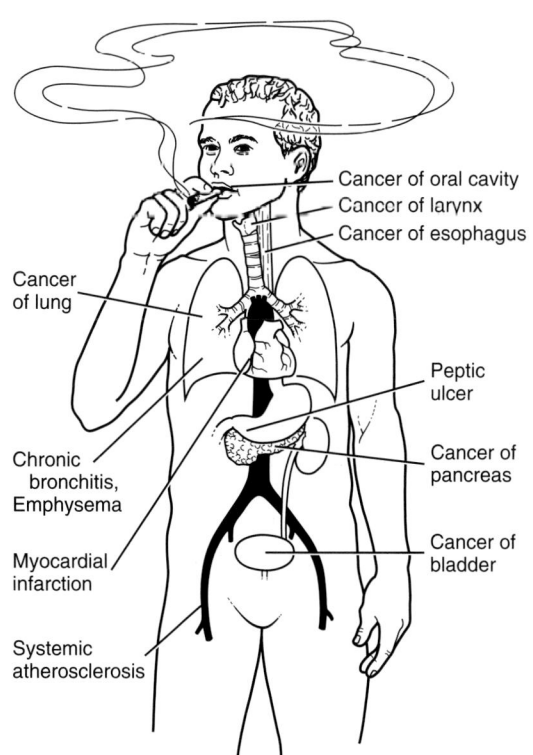

• **Fig. 9.13** Effects of smoking. (From Kumar V, Cotran R, Robbins S: *Robbins basic pathology,* ed 8, Philadelphia, 2008, Saunders.)

Pulmonary Emphysema

Description

Pulmonary emphysema is a chronic obstructive pulmonary disorder characterized by destructive changes in the alveolar walls and irreversible enlargement of alveolar air spaces.

ICD-10-CM Code	J43.9 *(Emphysema, unspecified)*
	(J43.0-J43.9 = 5 codes of specificity)

The above codes are nonspecific codes and may be valid as a principal diagnosis, except for Medicare. Refer to the physician's diagnosis and then to the current edition of the ICD-10-CM coding manuals to ensure the greatest specificity.

Symptoms and Signs

Pulmonary emphysema, a destructive disease of the alveolar septa, interferes with both the breathing process and gas exchange in the lungs. Alveoli become enlarged, which precipitates destruction of the alveolar walls and damage to the adjacent capillary walls. As a result of the decreased area for gas exchange and the trapped air, the patient experiences dyspnea. The onset of symptoms is insidious, with gradually increasing difficulty breathing, dyspnea, tachypnea, and wheezing. Cough can be a minor component or absent in patients with emphysema. Cough, especially productive cough, is more characteristic of chronic bronchitis and asthma. The inability to exhale carbon dioxide in the normal manner requires the patient with emphysema to use accessory muscles to force out air trapped in the alveoli, resulting in the characteristic barrel chest (Fig. 9.14). Shortness of breath and dyspnea increase, and the patient purses the lips to assist in exhaling. As the disease progresses, the patient develops circumoral cyanosis, symptoms of right ventricular heart failure (see Cor Pulmonale in Chapter 10), and digital clubbing.

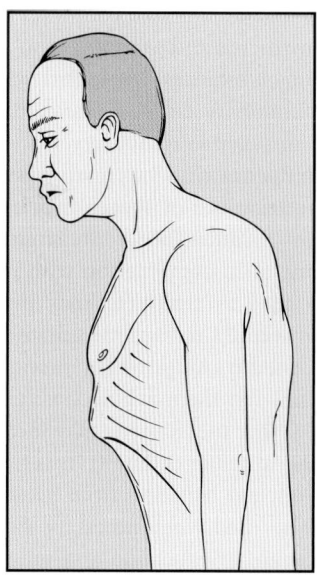

• **Fig. 9.14** Note the barrel chest and bluish discoloration around mouth in a patient with emphysema.

Patient Screening

The patient who complains of an insidious onset of difficulty breathing, wheezing, and/or persistent coughing should be given the first available appointment within 24 hours for clinical evaluation.

Etiology

Although the etiology of pulmonary emphysema is not completely understood, long-term cigarette smoking appears to be a contributing factor. Repeated respiratory tract infections beginning in childhood and continuing throughout adulthood also may contribute to the increased occurrence of the disease. Additionally, irritants, such as ozone, sulfur dioxide, and nitrogen oxides, are thought to play a role in the etiology. The possibility of a familial tendency is supported by the increased frequency of the disease in families who experience an enzyme deficiency (alpha$_1$-antitrypsin).

Diagnosis

Diagnosis is based on a clinical examination and a thorough patient history, which usually shows a prolonged exposure to possible respiratory irritants, especially cigarette smoking. Pulmonary function studies indicate increased tidal volume and residual volume along with decreased vital capacity and expiratory maneuver volumes. Radiographic chest studies show translucent-appearing lungs and a depressed or flattened diaphragm. The patient exhibits tachypnea, tachycardia, hypertension, polycythemia, diminished breath sounds, and wheezing or rhonchi. Anteroposterior chest diameter is increased, producing a typical barrel chest appearance (see Fig. 9.14). Individuals with extensive progressive disease have distended neck veins, hepatomegaly, peripheral edema, clubbed fingers, and cyanosis. Blood gas determinations in the advanced stages indicate decreased arterial oxygen tension and increased carbon dioxide.

Treatment

The patient is instructed and encouraged to avoid the inhalation of irritating substances, particularly cigarette smoke. Patients with pulmonary emphysema should take care to avoid exposure to possible respiratory tract infections and should receive influenza virus vaccination annually. Supplemental low concentrations of oxygen may help as well.

Drug therapy includes beta$_2$-adrenergic sympathomimetic drugs alone or in combination with inhaled corticosteroids. Drugs used in treatment may include albuterol (Ventolin and Proventil), terbutaline sulfate (Brethine), and metaproterenol sulfate (Alupent) for bronchodilation and antispasmodic activity; theophylline (rarely); expectorants; and antibiotics. Other medications may include treatments for gastroesophageal reflux disease (GERD) to prevent tracheal and/or bronchial irritation from gastric reflux. Oxygen therapy is also used when necessary. Pulmonary rehabilitation, a program of education and progressive exercise training, is essential to improve the quality of life in these patients. In some special circumstances, surgery may be an option to improve the serious air trapping seen in severe emphysema.

Prognosis

The prognosis for long-term disease is poor; in the United States, emphysema is the most common cause of death from respiratory disease.

Prevention

Education about the possible health consequences of long-term smoking is imperative. It is helpful for patients to avoid exposure to respiratory irritants and to guard against repeated respiratory infections.

Patient Teaching

Provide strong advice to the patient who smokes to cease smoking; offer a referral to a smoking cessation support group. Explain the medical management regimen, and demonstrate how to use home equipment for oxygen therapy and/or inhalation therapy. Demonstrate appropriate breathing techniques that maximize expiration and ventilation. Have the patient use the appropriate in-house closed-circuit television (CCTV) system, DVDs, or videos to enhance learning of the above teaching. Referral to a pulmonary rehabilitation program can be helpful as well.

Pneumoconiosis

Description

Pneumoconiosis is any disease of the lung caused by long-term mineral dust inhalation.

ICD-10-CM Code	J64 *(Unspecified pneumoconiosis)*

Symptoms and Signs

Pneumoconiosis means presence of dust in the lungs, which results in interstitial lung disease. It refers to a number of occupational diseases that cause progressive, chronic inflammation, fibrosis, and infection in the lungs. The onset of symptoms can be insidious, with dyspnea on exertion being the first symptom. In all types of dust-related disease, a dry cough, which later turns productive and becomes similar to the cough of chronic bronchitis, is typical. The patient may report that increasing effort is required for inspiration. Pulmonary hypertension, tachypnea, general malaise, and recurrent respiratory tract infections are common. Other symptoms may be associated with TB of the lungs (see the Pulmonary Tuberculosis section). Family members are also at risk for pneumoconiosis if constantly exposed to the dust particles in the worker's clothing.

Patient Screening

Persistent cough over a period of weeks or months and dyspnea are symptoms that require clinical evaluation; schedule the first available appointment. Inform the patient to call back for an immediate appointment if signs of infection occur or symptoms worsen.

Etiology

Pneumoconiosis is considered an occupational disease caused by inhaling inorganic dust particles over a prolonged period. It usually takes at least 10 years or longer of continual daily exposure for pneumoconiosis to develop; however, it may take as little as 2 years or as long as 30 years to develop.

Asbestosis is a form of dust disease caused by exposure to asbestos fibers. It is characterized by a slow and progressively diffuse fibrosis of the lungs. Asbestosis is the most commonly occurring type of pneumoconiosis. Asbestos fibers were considered effective in the past as insulation and reinforcing materials.

Another form of pneumoconiosis is anthracosis, also known as *black lung* or *coal miner's lung.* Anthracosis is caused by the accumulation of carbon deposits in the lungs resulting from inhaling smoke or coal dust (Fig. 9.15).

Silicosis, another type of dust disease, affects stone masons and metal grinders and those who work in quarries. Silicosis develops as a result of inhaling silica (quartz) dust and causes a dense fibrosis of the lungs and emphysema with respiratory impairment.

Other workers who are also susceptible to dust diseases are those who work with aluminum, beryllium, iron, cotton, sugar cane, and a number of synthetic fibers.

Diagnosis

A thorough patient history and a complete physical examination are essential for making the diagnosis. Chest radiographic studies, pulmonary function tests, and arterial blood gas determination confirm the diagnosis.

Treatment

The treatment of all pneumoconioses is directed toward relieving symptoms. Typically this includes administration of bronchodilators, oxygen therapy, chest physical therapy to help remove secretions, and the use of short-term corticosteroid drugs. Lung transplantation may be considered in some patients. TB, a common complication, must be treated aggressively. Cessation of smoking is strongly advised.

Prognosis

The damage to lung tissue is irreversible, and infections are common. There is an increased risk for lung cancer, especially in those with asbestosis.

Prevention

Pneumoconiosis is considered an environmental disease, thus dust reduction or cessation of exposure to dust in the work place is essential. Smoking worsens the condition, and embedded asbestos fibers increase the risk of lung cancer.

Patient Teaching

Stress the importance of prompt treatment of infections. Advise the patient to avoid exposure to the offending dust particles. Explain the medication dosage schedule, and demonstrate the proper use of the inhaler and/or home oxygen therapy equipment. Offer referral to a support group for cessation of smoking, if appropriate.

Pleuritis

Description

Pleurisy is inflammation of the membranes surrounding the lungs and lining the pleural cavity (Fig. 9.16).

ICD-10-CM Code	R09.1 *(Pleurisy)*

Symptoms and Signs

The patient reports generally unilateral sharp, needlelike pain, which increases with inspiration and coughing. Additionally, the patient experiences a cough, fever, and chills. Inspirations are shallow, rapid, and restricted. Pain may radiate to the shoulder or the abdomen. The patient may attempt to splint the painful area, especially on inspiration.

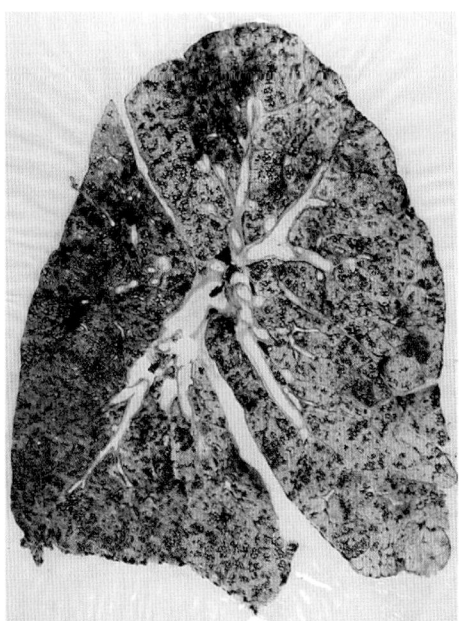

• **Fig. 9.15** Pneumoconiosis. (From Damjanov I, Linder J: *Pathology: a color atlas,* St Louis, 1999, Mosby.)

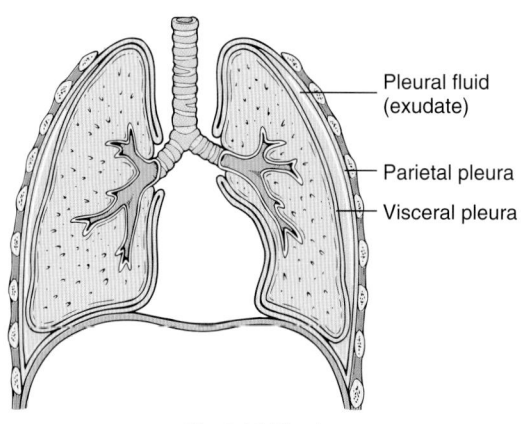

• **Fig. 9.16** Pleurisy.

Patient Screening

Usually significant pain with inspiration prompts the call for medical intervention. Schedule the first available appointment within 24 hours.

Etiology

Pleurisy is usually secondary to other diseases or infections. The inflammation also may result from injury or the presence of a tumor.

Two types of pleurisy exist: wet and dry. When extra pleural fluid (effusion) is present between the two layers of the plural membranes that cover the lungs, the increased volume causes compression of the pulmonary tissue and dyspnea. Dry pleurisy occurs when the pleural fluid decreases in volume, resulting in dryness between the pleura; the layers rub together and become congested and edematous.

Diagnosis

Diagnosis is made from the symptoms, history, and physical examination. A pleural rub can be heard on auscultation of the lungs. Radiography or CT may indicate the presence of pleural effusion and/or underlying pulmonary disease. Thoracostomy may be performed to determine the diagnosis or for therapeutic value.

Treatment

Treatment is directed at the underlying cause. Antibiotic therapy and analgesics to control the pain may be given. Splinting of the chest and deep breathing exercises help promote good ventilation. As mentioned earlier, therapeutic thoracostomy may be performed.

Prognosis

Recovery is usually complete. In some cases, permanent adhesions may restrict lung expansion.

Prevention

No specific prevention is known.

Patient Teaching

Explain to the patient the importance of deep breathing exercises and demonstrate proper splinting for adequate lung expansion. Stress the importance of taking medications as prescribed.

Pneumothorax

Description

Pneumothorax is a collection of air or gas in the pleural cavity that results in a collapsed or partially collapsed lung (Fig. 9.17).

ICD-10-CM Code	J93.9 (Pneumothorax, unspecified)
	(J93.0-J39.9 = 4 codes of specificity)
	P25.1 (Pneumothorax originating in the perinatal period)

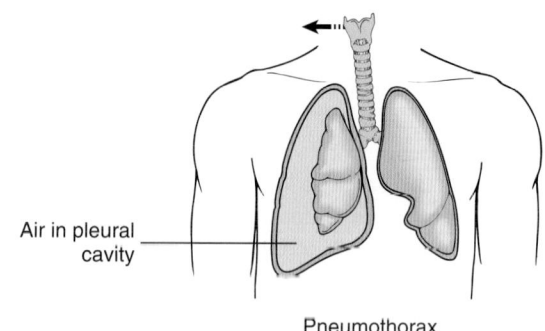

Pneumothorax

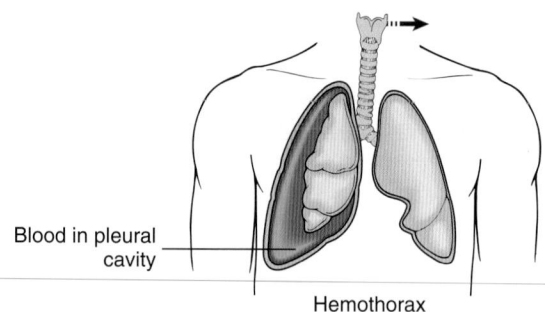

Hemothorax

• **Fig. 9.17** Pneumothorax and hemothorax.

	(P25.1-P25.3 = 3 codes of specificity)
	J95.81 (Post procedural pneumothorax)
	J93.8 (Other pneumothorax)
	(J93.0-J93.9 = 7 codes of specificity)
	S27.0 (Traumatic pneumothorax [7 digits required])

Symptoms and Signs

Collapse of a lung causes severe shortness of breath, sudden and sharp chest pain, falling blood pressure, rapid weak pulse, and shallow and weak respirations. The patient may be cyanotic and appear anxious. Increased air pressure on the affected side causes a mediastinal shift to the unaffected side.

Patient Screening

The patient experiencing the crisis, as described earlier, requires urgent care and immediate transport to the emergency room.

Etiology

Pneumothorax can be spontaneous or traumatic. Spontaneous pneumothorax occurs when an opening occurs on the surface of a lung. Causative factors can be erosion of alveoli from tumor or disease, increased pressure from within the respiratory system (too great a force with artificial ventilation), or a spontaneous tear in the tissue. Traumatic pneumothorax occurs when the integrity of the pleural cavity is breached from outside as the result of trauma, such as a gunshot wound, stab wound, or crushing type of wound to the chest. The object (possibly the patient's own rib) penetrates the chest cavity, allowing air to enter from the atmosphere. Gas or an accumulation of pus in the pleural space generated by microorganisms can result in a pneumothorax.

Diagnosis

Diagnosis is made after evaluating the history, the clinical findings, and radiographic studies. Radiographs will show the air in the pleural cavity, the collapsed portion of the lung, and mediastinal shift. Breath sounds are diminished, and sucking air sounds are heard at the wound site. The patient is in acute distress.

Treatment

The patient is more comfortable in the Fowler or semi-Fowler position and may require oxygen. An occlusive dressing is placed over any sucking wound to seal the portal of entry and to prevent additional air from entering the chest cavity. Thoracostomy is performed to withdraw air from the cavity. A closed drainage system is established if air continues to leak into the pleural space. This allows expansion and healing of the lung.

Prognosis

Recovery depends on the degree of lung collapse, the cause, and prompt medical intervention.

Prevention

No specific measures of prevention are known.

Patient Teaching

Throughout emergency care and after the patient is medically stable, offer support to the individual and family. Encourage patients receiving conservative therapy to rest during a period of close monitoring. Provide teaching about treatments used to expand the lungs to more severe cases or those that result from trauma. Use visuals, such as customized electronically generated patient education material on the anatomy and physiology of the lungs.

Hemothorax

Description

Hemothorax is the accumulation of blood and fluid in the pleural cavity (see Fig. 9.17).

ICD-10-CM Code	J94.2 (Hemothorax)
	P54.8 (Other specified neonatal hemorrhages)
	S27.1 (Traumatic Hemothorax)
	A15.6 (Tuberculous pleurisy)

Symptoms and Signs

The patient experiences symptoms similar to those of a pneumothorax. Signs of hemorrhage include pale and clammy skin, a weak and thready pulse, and falling blood pressure. The patient may experience chest pain, and respirations are labored and shallow or gasping.

Patient Screening

A hemothorax is a life-threatening condition that requires emergency medical care.

Etiology

Blood enters the pleural space as a result of trauma, erosion of a pulmonary vessel, or hematologic disorders. This causes the lung to collapse.

Diagnosis

Breath sounds are diminished or absent on the affected side, as is chest wall movement. Radiographs show blood in the pleural space. Blood tests indicate hemorrhage; arterial blood gas analysis reflects respiratory failure. The patient is in acute distress.

Treatment

The treatment employed is similar to that for a pneumothorax. The lung must be reexpanded, usually by performing thoracostomy, with closed drainage to evacuate blood. The underlying cause, once discovered, is treated, often necessitating surgical intervention to repair the wound. Vital signs are monitored, and blood loss is replaced.

Prognosis

The prognosis for a hemothorax is guarded, depending on the cause and the availability of effective treatment.

Prevention

No specific prevention measures are known.

Patient Teaching

Make every effort to reassure the patient while emergency and diagnostic measures are taking place. Once the patient is stabilized, explain the purpose of therapeutic procedures, such as chest tube drainage and thoracentesis. Use available visual aids to demonstrate the therapeutic procedures.

Flail Chest

Description

Flail chest is a condition of instability in the chest wall caused by multiple rib fractures; the sternum also may be fractured.

ICD-10-CM Code	S22.5XXA (Flail chest, initial encounter for closed fracture)
	S22.5XXB (Flail chest, initial encounter for open fracture)
	S22.5 (Flail chest, 7 digits required)
	(S22.5XXA-S22.5XXS = 6 codes of specificity)

Symptoms and Signs

The patient with flail chest, a double fracture of three or more adjacent ribs, experiences severe pain and dyspnea and is cyanotic and extremely anxious. The segment of the chest involved moves inward during inspiration and outward during expiration; this is termed *paradoxical breathing.*

Patient Screening

Flail chest is a medical emergency and may be a life-threatening condition.

Etiology

Direct trauma to the chest wall that fractures three or more adjacent ribs is the cause of flail chest. This trauma may be from direct compression by a heavy object, a motor vehicle accident (especially injury caused by the steering wheel), a hard fall onto a solid object, or an industrial accident. The paradoxical movement and instability of the chest wall occur when three or more adjacent ribs are broken in two places or break loose from the sternum while also being broken at another site (Fig. 9.18).

Diagnosis

Diagnosis is made by noting history of chest trauma and observing the paradoxical movement of the chest wall. Chest radiography will confirm the diagnosis.

Treatment

First responder emergency care employs measures to stabilize the chest wall until surgical repair is possible. The treatment of flail chest involves allowing the rib fractures to heal while maintaining respiratory integrity. This may entail mechanical ventilation and sedation of the patient with an endotracheal tube in place. Pain medications are administered to keep the patient comfortable. Additionally, supplemental oxygen is administered. Rib fixation can be done to facilitate healing and pain relief.

Prognosis

Emergency medical care and transport to the hospital as soon as possible help achieve a positive outcome. Delayed medical intervention and complications resulting from trauma can worsen the chances for recovery.

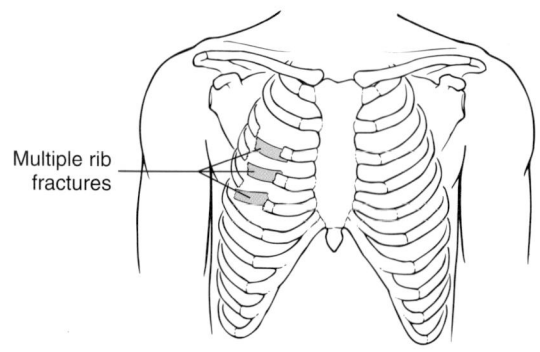

Multiple rib fractures

• **Fig. 9.18** Flail chest.

Prevention

Use of safety measures, such as wearing seat belts that protect the chest from trauma, are prudent.

Patient Teaching

Make every effort to dispel the patient's anxiety during emergency measures to stabilize the chest wall. Continue to advise the patient of all procedures necessary to achieve respiratory integrity.

Pulmonary Tuberculosis

Description

Pulmonary TB is a chronic, acute, or subacute infection of the lungs by *Mycobacterium tuberculosis.*

ICD-10-CM Code	A15.0 *(Tuberculosis of lung [includes: infections due to* Mycobacterium tuberculosis *and* Mycobacterium bovis*])*

Symptoms and Signs

Pulmonary TB, an infectious and inflammatory disease of the lungs, is acquired by inhaling dried droplet nuclei that contain the tubercle bacillus. These droplet nuclei may remain suspended in room air for many hours. The patient with a primary TB infection is often asymptomatic initially. When the infection is secondary, the patient experiences vague symptoms, such as weight loss, reduced appetite, listlessness, vague chest pain, dry cough, loss of energy, and fever. As the disease progresses, the patient has a productive cough with purulent sputum, the appearance of blood streaking or hemoptysis, fever, and night sweats.

Patient Screening

Schedule a prompt appointment for the patient complaining of a persistent cough with blood-tinged or purulent sputum. Constitutional symptoms, such as fatigue, fever, and night sweats, may also exist.

> **NOTE**
>
> All patients having a cluster of symptoms that indicate a serious respiratory infection should be escorted on arrival to the first available examination room. It is prudent to follow strict infection control.

Etiology

The tubercle bacillus *M. tuberculosis* causes TB and is spread by droplet nuclei. The primary lesion usually is located in the lungs. The bacteria can survive in the dried form for months if not exposed to sunlight. Any tissue of the body can be affected; however, the lung is the typical site (Fig. 9.19).

The infection begins with a primary lesion in the lower area of the lung. As the body's defense mechanisms respond to the bacterial invasion, antigens that cause necrosis are

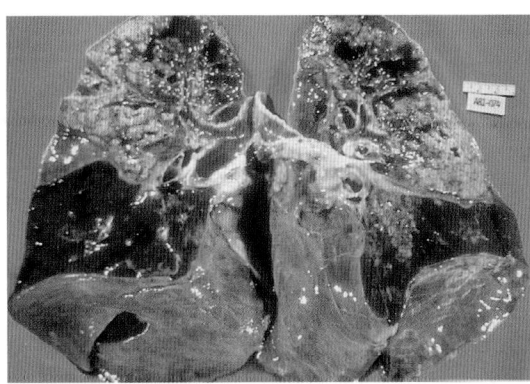

• **Fig. 9.19** Tuberculosis (TB). (From Kumar V, Cotran R, Robbins S: *Robbins basic pathology*, ed 8, Philadelphia, 2008, Saunders.)

produced, and this is followed by fibrosis and calcification of the affected tissue. The infection then may be arrested, and the disease becomes inactive, remaining so for years. If the infection is not arrested, the patient experiences progressive primary TB.

The patient's resistance to secondary TB depends on general health and environment. Malnutrition, poor health, an unsanitary and crowded living environment, and the presence of other illnesses tend to lower resistance to reinfection. The source of a secondary exacerbation of TB can be a reactivation of the previous primary infection or another infection process.

During the period 1982 to 1985, increased immigration and travel from Asia and South and Central America and the AIDS epidemic contributed to an upsurge of TB in the United States. Since then, improved prevention and treatment measures have resulted in a significant drop in the case rate, and TB is no longer considered an epidemic. TB still remains a public health risk. TB remains a leading cause of infectious disease–related adult mortality worldwide.

Diagnosis

The Mantoux test (purified protein derivative [PPD] test) is a standard intradermal test used to detect the presence of tuberculin antibodies. The test result is available in 48 to 72 hours; an induration of 8 to 10 mm indicates sensitivity to the bacillus and is considered a positive result. The positive test result is followed by chest radiographic studies, examination of gastric washings, fiberoptic bronchoscopy, and sputum cultures. The typical walled-off lesions (tubercles) can be seen on chest radiographs. Apical pulmonary infiltrates with cavities are present in patients with TB. Final confirmation is a positive result on culture of the sputum for the tubercle bacillus.

> ### ✗ NOTE
>
> Some individuals who have no symptoms or signs of tuberculosis (TB) can have a positive skin reaction and are said to have latent tuberculosis infection (LTBI). Most do not progress to active disease and are not considered infectious.

Treatment

Persons with communicable TB must be either treated or quarantined; new cases must be reported to the local health department. Concern has been raised recently over the increasing prevalence of drug-resistant TB and the resulting progression to complications.

Treatment is dependent on whether the TB is latent or active. Latent TB is generally treated with isoniazid (INH). Therapy can last upward of 6 to 9 months. Active TB consists of drug therapy with use of multiple antituberculosis agents. INH is administered with rifampin, ethambutol, or pyrazinamide. Drug-resistant TB is treated more aggressively with various combinations of medications.

Prognosis

Early and complete treatment affords an excellent prognosis. Drug therapy may continue for several months to a year. The prognosis is not as good for individuals infected with strains that are drug resistant. Risk factors exist for reactivation of infection.

Prevention

Bacillus Calmette-Guérin (BCG) vaccination has not been proven effective in preventing TB. All those who come in contact with infected patients are advised to have the tuberculin skin test, chest radiography, and prophylactic treatment with INH.

Patient Teaching

TB is considered infectious and is reportable to the local public health department; therefore, thorough, consistent hand washing techniques and respiratory precautions must be practiced. Patient and family education about sources of contagion and transmission is indicated. A nutritious diet and sanitary living conditions are important for recovery. Provide information on adverse drug effects to report to the health care provider. Stress the importance of regular follow-up care. Inform the caregiver and/or family members that the disease is no longer infectious when the sputum test result is negative. The final culture result can take up to 6 weeks.

Infectious Mononucleosis: Epstein-Barr Virus Infection

Description

Infectious mononucleosis, also known as *glandular fever*, is an acute herpesvirus infection.

ICD-10-CM Code	B27.90 (*Infectious mononucleosis, unspecified without complication*) (B27.90-B27.99 = 4 codes of specificity)

Symptoms and Signs

The two main symptoms of this infection are lymphadenopathy and fever that typically peaks in the afternoon.

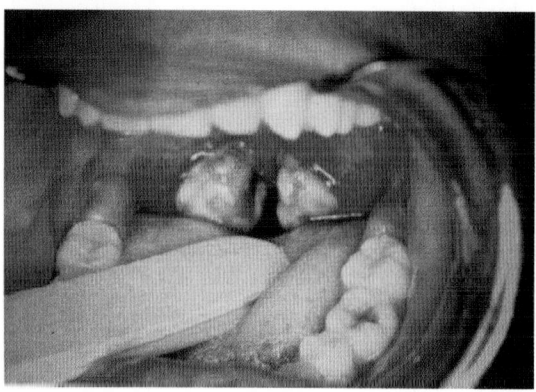

• **Fig. 9.20** Tonsils coated with debris during infection of mononucleosis. (From Sigler B: *Ear, nose, and throat disorders—Mosby's clinical nursing series,* St Louis, 1994, Mosby.)

Initially, symptoms are vague. They include general malaise, anorexia, and chills. As the infection progresses, symptoms include sore throat, fever, headache, fatigue, and cervical and generalized lymphadenopathy; the tonsils may appear coated with debris (Fig. 9.20). The syndrome causes mild transient hepatitis and atypical lymphocytosis. The incubation period ranges from 5 to 15 days. This disease affects primarily adolescents and young adults. Infection is rare after age 35 years.

Patient Screening

Schedule a prompt appointment for a patient (likely to be a teenager or a young adult) complaining of fever, sore throat, fatigue, and swollen glands.

Etiology

Mononucleosis is caused by EBV, a herpesvirus. The virus is carried in the saliva of previously infected individuals and may be transmitted through the oral pharyngeal route (e.g., during kissing), through blood transfusions, or organ donation. After it is inside the body, the virus infects a type of WBC found in lymph, blood, and connective tissue. EBV infection is not highly contagious but is lifelong. The virus is shed asymptomatically in oropharyngeal secretions.

Diagnosis

Thorough patient history and physical examination are essential to rule out hepatitis and other lymphomatous disorders, such as leukemia, Hodgkin lymphoma, and lymphosarcoma. Two procedures of prime diagnostic importance are blood smear examination and immunologic study of blood serum. Laboratory tests include the infectious mononucleosis blood screening test, antinuclear antibody (ANA), total serum bilirubin, liver function tests, and EBV serology.

Treatment

Treatment is based almost entirely on symptoms. During the acute phase of fever and malaise, bed rest should be enforced. Fluid intake should be forced orally, or with high fever, intravenous fluids are given, if needed. Antipyretic medications, such as acetaminophen, are needed when the temperature becomes high (103°F in adults and 104°F in children).

Prevention

Prevention is difficult because infectious mononucleosis can be transmitted by infected people before they have developed any symptoms. Carriers exist among the general population. No vaccine is available.

Prognosis

Barring complications, recovery is complete within 3 to 4 months. Infection confers permanent immunity.

Patient Teaching

Stress the importance of bed rest to prevent serious complications affecting the liver or the spleen. A soft, bland diet is often better tolerated. Advise the patient and the caregiver that although the disease is not highly infectious, strep throat also may be present; it is prudent to practice infection control during the recovery period. Another important patient teaching point is to report any abdominal pain immediately to their health care provider. Although rare, spontaneous splenic rupture may occur and is a medical emergency. Reassurance is beneficial, because recovery can be slow.

Adult Respiratory Distress Syndrome

Description

Adult respiratory distress syndrome (ARDS) is a type of acute lung injury, characterized by severe pulmonary congestion, acute respiratory distress, and hypoxemia.

ICD-10-CM Code	J95.3 *(Chronic pulmonary insufficiency following surgery)*

Symptoms and Signs

The sudden onset of severe hypoxemia, progressive hypercapnia, and acidosis in the patient who recently has experienced trauma, septicemia, shock, or insult to the lungs or the rest of the body is termed *adult respiratory distress syndrome,* or *shock lung.* The lungs are hemorrhagic, wet, boggy, congested, and unable to diffuse oxygen; atelectasis results. The onset of symptoms is usually 24 to 48 hours after a medical or surgical insult to the body. Primary symptoms include sudden and severe dyspnea with rapid and shallow respirations. Inspiratory intercostal and suprasternal retractions are noted, along with cyanosis or mottled skin. During the Vietnam War, this condition was referred to as *Da Nang lung.* No improvement in the respiratory status is noted with the administration of supplemental oxygen. Rales, rhonchi, and wheezes may be present.

Patient Screening

The sudden onset of respiratory distress is a medical emergency. The patient is directed to call an ambulance for immediate transport to an emergency care facility. The physician is notified.

Etiology

ARDS is considered secondary to some agent of insult that precipitates increased capillary permeability in the lungs, pulmonary edema, and resulting respiratory failure. Injury to the cells activates the leukocytes and platelets in the capillaries to release products that cause additional injury. The alveoli fill with exudate 12 to 48 hours after the insult. The fluid-filled alveoli tend to collapse at the end of expiration, leaving less pulmonary tissue available for gas exchange. Consequently, low pulmonary compliance, pulmonary hypertension, decreased functional residual capacity, and hypoxemia result.

Diagnosis

Patients with ARDS have an underlying cause, such as pneumonia, fulminating sepsis, aspiration of gastric contents, hypovolemic shock, a near-drowning episode, fat embolism, or cardiopulmonary bypass. Most patients appear to be doing well just before they experience dyspnea, and arterial blood gas determinations indicate reduced perfusion and increased pH. Chest radiographs show diffuse bilateral alveolar infiltration with a normal cardiac silhouette.

Treatment

No cure for ARDS is known; therefore the patient receives supportive care only. Efforts are made to correct the underlying cause of ARDS. Treatment of hypoxemia can be complicated, because changes in the lung tissue leave less pulmonary tissue available for gas exchange, thereby causing inadequate perfusion. Oxygenation may be accomplished by establishing an airway, administering humidified oxygen, and suctioning the air passages, as necessary. Protective lung ventilation strategy is important to pamper the lung. For instance, instead of ventilating with 10 mL/kg ideal body weight, it is prudent to lower the tidal volume at 6 mL/kg ideal body weight; this has been shown to reduce mortality.

When ventilation cannot be maintained, mechanical ventilation is attempted with the addition of positive end-expiratory pressure (PEEP). Nutritional status and cautious hydration are maintained intravenously. The patient is observed for signs of renal failure and superinfection; intervention is undertaken, if necessary. Arterial blood gases, blood pressure, and urine output are monitored.

Prognosis

Prognosis is guarded, depending on the cause. Many individuals (60%–75%) do recover, with no permanent lung damage.

Prevention

The onset of ARDS is generally unpredictable and therefore cannot be prevented.

Patient Teaching

Patients with ARDS are admitted to a hospital, usually in an intensive care unit, where they can receive constant monitoring, reassurance, and meticulous care.

Sarcoidosis

Description

Sarcoidosis is a multisystem granulomatous (small lesions of inflamed cells) disorder most commonly detected in the lungs.

ICD-10-CM Code	D86.9 (Sarcoidosis, unspecified)
	(D86.0-D86.9 = 13 codes of specificity)

Symptoms and Signs

Patients may have no complaints or mild to severe symptoms, depending on the site of the lesions and the degree of involvement. In pulmonary sarcoidosis, patients may have a dry cough, shortness of breath, or mild chest pain resulting from loss of lung volume and abnormal lung stiffness. Other symptoms are fatigue, fever, weight loss, swollen ankles, and joint pain. Organ-specific symptoms can occur in chronic, multisystem cases. The typical epithelioid lesions can also affect the skin, eyes, musculoskeletal system, and other internal organs.

Granulomas in the lungs are often found incidentally when chest radiography or CT is performed for some other reason. Lesions may also be found in the walls of the bronchioles, the alveoli, and the lymph nodes of the chest.

Patient Screening

In most cases, the disease is insidious and can have a range of symptoms. Acute onset or worsening of respiratory symptoms always requires immediate attention by a physician. Follow office policy for a possible referral to a pulmonary specialist.

Etiology

The exact cause is not clear. The disorder is thought to be a malfunction of the immune system or caused by a virus. Some scientists suspect exposure to toxins in the environment or other insult can be a trigger. Although the disease is found throughout the world, in the United States, it occurs more commonly in young adults between the ages 20 and 40 years and in African Americans. Genetic factors are suspected.

Diagnosis

Sarcoidosis can be difficult to detect. Sometimes symptoms and signs are uncovered through a complete medical evaluation, which includes history, physical examination, and chest radiography. Laboratory tests and pulmonary function studies are also helpful. Biopsy of the affected tissue, when possible, is essential to confirm the diagnosis.

Treatment

In many cases, sarcoidosis resolves spontaneously; at stage 1, spontaneous resolution is greater than 90% within 1 year. Treatment is not necessarily indicated when there are no symptoms or mild symptoms, regardless of radiologic abnormalities. Corticosteroid therapy, such as prednisone, helps relieve severe symptoms. The immunosuppressant drug methotrexate is also used to treat widespread disease, such as disfiguring skin lesions, and cardiac or CNS involvement. A few newer treatments are available as well. These include infliximab, an intravenously administered antibody, and adalimumab, an immunosuppressant.

Prognosis

Serious disability is rare with sarcoidosis, and most people can live normally. The prognosis varies for people with pulmonary sarcoidosis if the lungs become scarred and fibrotic or if other organ damage exists. Relapses can occur after cessation of immunosuppressive drugs. The disease is rarely fatal.

Prevention

Because the cause remains uncertain, there is no known prevention.

Patient Teaching

Review the doctor's instructions, including the medication schedule and possible side effects, such as insomnia and irritability. Advise the patient not to smoke. Explain the importance of follow-up visits with the doctor to monitor the treatment. Patients experiencing the disabling effects of sarcoidosis can benefit from support groups.

Lung Cancer

Description

Lung cancer is the most common cause of cancer-related deaths worldwide among both men and women, accounting for almost 30% of all such deaths. It is usually caused by repeated carcinogenic irritation to the bronchial epithelium, leading to increased rates of cell division (Fig. 9.21).

ICD-10-CM Code	C34.0 *(Malignant neoplasm of main bronchus)* (C34.0-C34.92 = 16 codes of specificity)

The above code is a nonspecific code and may be valid as a principal diagnosis, except for Medicare. Refer to the physician's diagnosis and then to the current edition of the ICD-10-CM coding manual to ensure the greatest specificity of pathology and any appropriate modifiers.

Symptoms and Signs

The most common symptom is cough with or without sputum production. Because many patients diagnosed with lung cancer have coexisting COPD with a chronic cough, it is important to note any changes in the character of the cough. Other symptoms may include dyspnea, hemoptysis, chest pain (usually dull, intermittent pain on the side of the tumor), and weight loss. The brain is a common site for metastasis for some types of lung cancer. Symptoms of brain metastasis include headache, weakness, change in mental status, and seizures. Other common sites of metastasis are the liver, bone, and brain. Sometimes lung cancer is discovered in an asymptomatic patient with an abnormal chest radiograph.

Patient Screening

A patient complaining of a chronic cough, chest pain, or dyspnea is scheduled for medical evaluation at the first available appointment.

Etiology

Lung cancers are subdivided into two main types by histology: non-small cell lung cancer (NSCLC) and small cell lung cancer (SCLC). The distinction is important because it relates to staging, treatment, and prognosis. SCLCs account for about 10% to 15% of all lung cancers. Most of

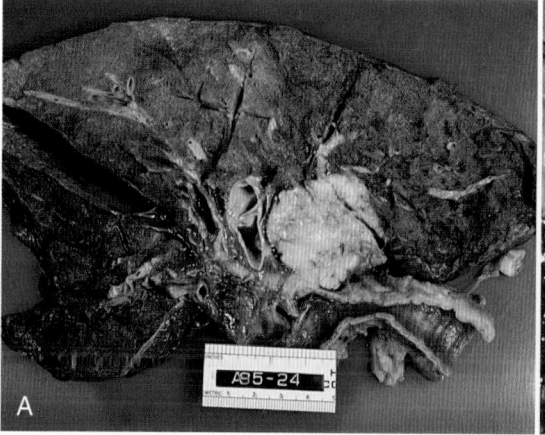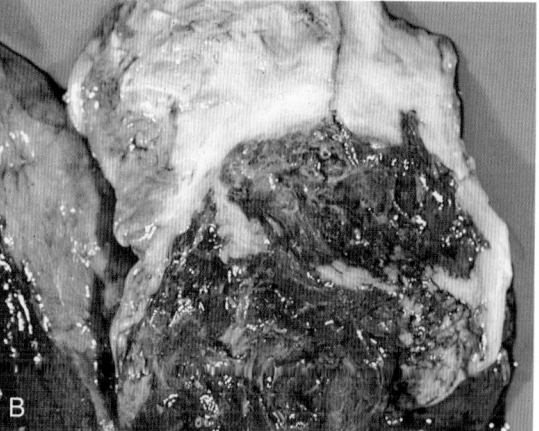

• **Fig. 9.21** Examples of lung carcinomas. (A) Centrally located tumor attached to bronchus. (B) Mesothelioma on pleural surface. (From Damjanov I: *Pathology for the health-related professions,* ed 4, St Louis, 2011, Saunders.)

the remainder are NSCLCs. SCLC occurs almost exclusively in smokers, has a rapid growth rate, and metastasizes early in the disease process.

The primary risk factor for development of lung cancer is cigarette smoking. Smoking has been shown to be responsible for 90% of lung cancers, and smokers are 10 to 30 times more likely to develop lung cancer compared with nonsmokers. A smoker's risk for developing lung cancer is proportional to the total lifetime smoking of cigarettes. The risk does decrease after cessation of smoking, but it remains higher than that in individuals who have never smoked. Other factors that increase the risk of lung cancer include exposure to secondhand smoke, asbestos, radon, arsenic, air pollution, and radiation therapy for other types of cancer.

Diagnosis

Many patients are symptomatic at the time of diagnosis, although some may be diagnosed incidentally by a chest radiograph (Fig. 9.22). A tissue biopsy specimen is required for a definitive diagnosis. It can be obtained through bronchoscopy, mediastinoscopy, or CT-guided fine-needle aspiration. CT of the chest, abdomen, and head and bone scanning are done to look for metastases. Laboratory tests are done to check for abnormalities caused by metastatic disease (Fig. 9.23). Testing is also done to look for specific biomarkers, such as gene mutations in epidermal growth factor receptor (EGFR) or anaplastic lymphoma kinase (ALK), which may affect the treatment choice. SCLC and NSCLC are staged differently. NSCLC is staged by using

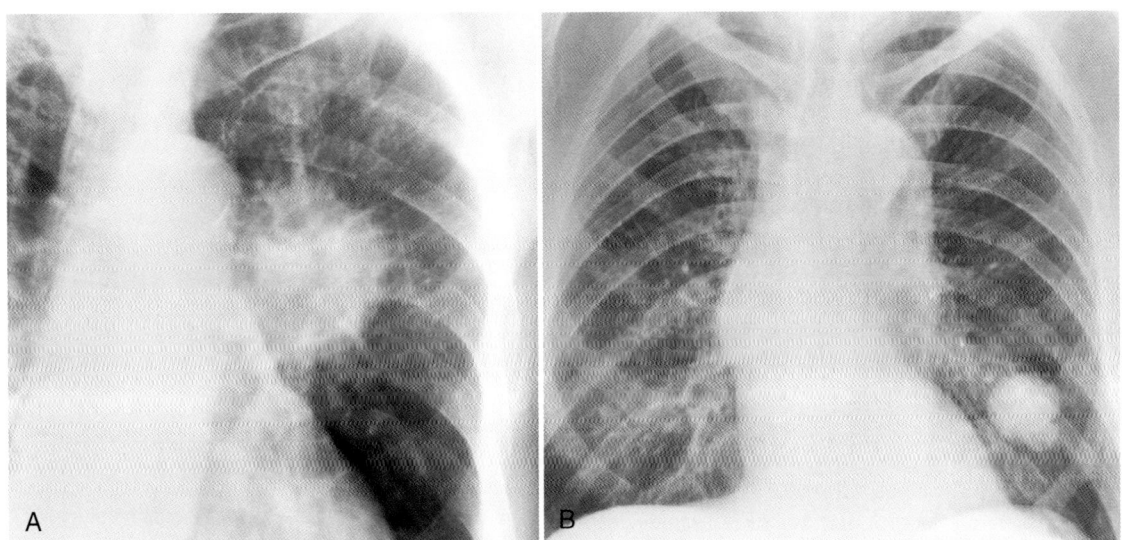

• **Fig. 9.22** Examples of neoplastic lung disease. (From Long BW, Frank ED, Ehrlich RA: *Radiography essentials for limited practice*, ed 4, St Louis, 2013, Elsevier.)

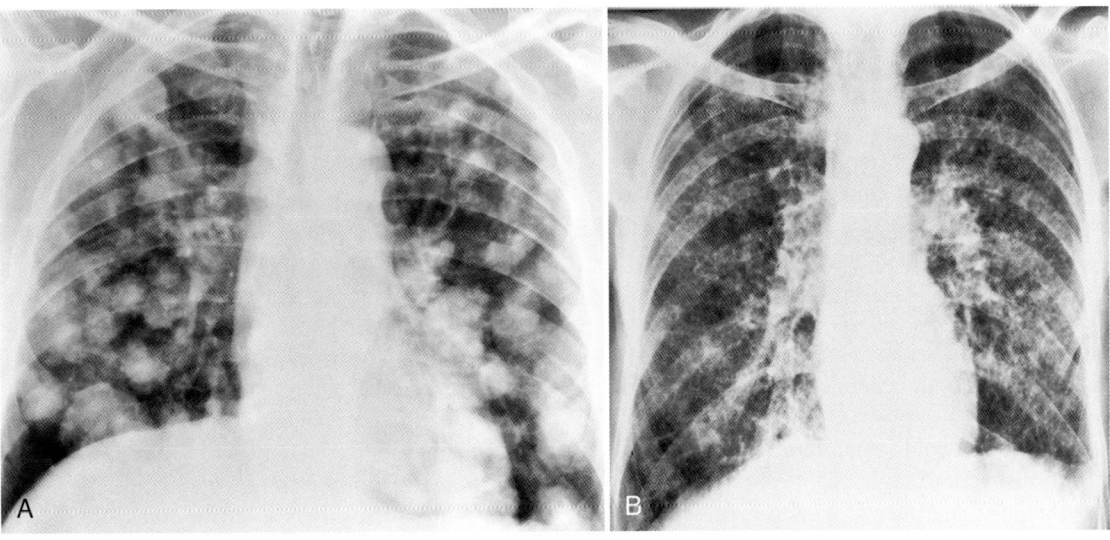

• **Fig. 9.23** Metastatic lung disease. Hematogenous (spread via blood) metastases are well-defined lesions scattered throughout the lungs. (From Long BW, Frank ED, Ehrlich RA: *Radiography essentials for limited practice*, ed 4, St Louis, 2013, Elsevier.)

the TNM system. SCLC staging involves distinguishing between disease that is confined to one side of the chest ("limited") and disease that has spread to encompass the other lung or other parts of the body ("extensive"). See Chapter 1 for information about the staging and grading systems used to assess malignant neoplasms.

Treatment

Treatment decisions are based on the type of tumor (small cell or non-small cell) and the stage of the tumor. For early-stage NSCLC, surgical resection, with or without radiation or chemotherapy, is the preferred option and offers the best chances for survival. Surgery usually involves lobectomy, which is removal of the portion of the lung affected by the tumor, or pneumonectomy, which is removal of the entire affected lung. Later-stage NSCLC is generally not treatable by surgical resection alone. A combined modality approach is used, including chemotherapy, radiotherapy, surgery, and/or palliative therapy for symptom control. Because SCLC often metastasizes early in the disease process, it is usually treated by using systemic chemotherapy along with radiation therapy rather than surgery, even in the limited disease stage.

There have been many recent advances in the use of targeted therapy or immunotherapy in the treatment of lung cancer. For example, patients with EGFR mutations may respond well to treatment with EGFR tyrosine kinase inhibitors. Much research is currently being done in this field, and many clinical trials are underway.

Prognosis

The prognosis for patients with lung cancer is generally poor. The 5-year survival rate for all stages and types combined is just 15%. Some factors that have been shown to affect the prognosis are the stage at the time of diagnosis, the histologic tumor type, the degree of differentiation of the tumor, the presence or absence of symptoms at diagnosis, and the presence and degree of weight loss.

Prevention

The U.S. Preventative Services Task Force now recommends lung cancer screening for high-risk individuals with an annual low-dose chest CT. *High risk* is defined as people age 55 to 80 years with at least a smoking history of 30 packs per year and who are current smokers or have quit within the past 15 years. Screening should be discontinued if

greater than 15 years have elapsed since smoking cessation or if there is limited life expectancy.

The importance of smoking cessation cannot be stressed enough, and reducing exposure to secondhand smoke is recommended. It is important to emphasize the benefits of smoking cessation even to patients who already have lung cancer, especially those with limited SCLC disease. If patients survive their lung cancer, relapse is much more likely in patients who continue to smoke.

Patient Teaching

Explain the diagnostic procedures, their purposes, and when to expect results. Encourage the patient to express concerns and offer to supply answers to any specific questions. After diagnosis, the patient benefits from explanation and clarification of the treatment regimen through verbal and written instructions. Offer referral to community support groups and information agencies, such as the American Cancer Society and the American Lung Association. Provide information on smoking cessation programs, when appropriate. Stress the importance of follow-up care. See the Alert box on Health Effects of Exposure to Tobacco Smoke in Chapter 1.

◆ ENRICHMENT

Vaping and Electronic Cigarettes

Electronic cigarettes (e-cigarettes) deliver nicotine through a device and are used by people of all ages. According to the Centers for Disease Control and Prevention (CDC), e-cigarettes are sometimes called *e-cigs, vapes, e-hookahs, vape pens,* and *electronic nicotine delivery systems (ENDS).* Some e-cigarettes look like regular cigarettes, cigars, or pipes. Some look like USB (Universal Serial Bus) flash drives, pens, and other everyday items.

Vaping has become quite common, particularly among teenagers and young individuals. The use of nicotine while the brain is still developing, which occurs into the mid-20s, can cause problems with brain development and function. The liquid used in e-cigarettes and vape devices can also contain other harmful substances. The battery-operated devices used for this type of nicotine delivery heat the liquid substance that contains nicotine and produce an aerosol that is inhaled. Users of e-cigarettes and parents need to be aware of the risks of this habit. Long-term effects of vaping during the teenage period or young adulthood are still being studied.

Review Challenge

Answer the following questions:

1. What are the physical and chemical dynamics of normal respiration?
2. Why is the common cold so common?
3. How is sinusitis treated?
4. What are the possible causes of nasal polyps?
5. How is severe epistaxis treated?
6. What is the prognosis for malignant tumors of the larynx?
7. What are some causes of and risk factors for (1) atelectasis and (2) pulmonary embolism?
8. What determines the treatment of pneumonia?
9. Why does the patient with pulmonary abscess exhibit foul-smelling sputum?
10. Where does the causative organism of Legionnaires disease thrive?

11. What is the profile of individuals vulnerable to respiratory syncytial virus (RSV) pneumonia?
12. How is histoplasmosis contracted?
13. Who would benefit from influenza immunization?
14. Why is influenza considered a serious infection?
15. What does the abbreviation *COPD* refer to?
16. How is chronic bronchitis associated with other pulmonary conditions?
17. Are emphysema and bronchiectasis reversible? What are some causes of both conditions?
18. Why is pneumoconiosis considered an occupational disease?
19. What is the treatment for a hemothorax and a pneumothorax?
20. Why is pulmonary tuberculosis (TB) more prevalent and difficult to treat today?
21. How would you describe the pathology in a patient with adult respiratory distress syndrome (ARDS)?
22. What steps are recommended to prevent lung cancer?
23. What effect may electronic cigarettes have on the brain?

Real-Life Challenge: Sinusitis

A 45-year-old man is experiencing a headache over both eyes on awakening. The patient says he also experiences pain above the eyes when bending over. Tenderness above the eyes in the frontal area of the forehead and also in both cheeks is noted on palpation. A thick greenish-yellow mucous drainage is present. Sinus radiographs show cloudiness in the region of the maxillary and frontal sinuses.

Vital signs are temperature, 99.88°F; pulse, 90 beats per minute; respirations, 26 breaths per minute; and blood pressure, 136/88 mm Hg. Mouth breathing is noted.

Questions

1. Compare the symptoms and signs of sinusitis and those of an upper respiratory tract infection (URI).
2. What are the causes of sinusitis?
3. Discuss the correlation between allergies and sinusitis.
4. What drug therapy might be prescribed for the treatment of sinusitis?
5. What is the principle behind the use of decongestants for sinusitis?
6. How would air-filled sinuses appear on radiographs?

Real-Life Challenge: Acute Bronchitis

A 39-year-old woman is experiencing a deep cough that produces thick, yellow sputum. She is complaining of shortness of breath and pain in the upper chest. Audible wheezing is heard without a stethoscope. Vital signs are temperature, 100.28°F; pulse, 102 beats per minute; respirations, 32 breaths per minute; and blood pressure, 134/88 mm Hg. Auscultation of the chest confirms the presence of bilateral wheezing and scattered rales.

The patient has a history of an upper respiratory tract infection (URI) 2 weeks before the onset of coughing 3 days ago. Her husband is a cigarette smoker. Diagnostic studies ordered include chest radiography, pulmonary studies, sputum analysis, complete blood count (CBC), and erythrocyte sedimentation rate (ESR). The patient is diagnosed with acute bacterial bronchitis.

Questions

1. Why would it be safe for the patient to take aspirin to control fever?
2. Why would increased fluid intake be recommended?
3. Which treatment would be recommended to relieve wheezing?
4. Which treatment would be recommended to relieve coughing?
5. Compare the symptoms and signs of chronic bronchitis with those of acute bronchitis.
6. Compare the etiology of chronic bronchitis versus acute bronchitis.
7. How significant is the exposure to primary or secondary smoke to patients with acute or chronic bronchitis?
8. What is this patient's risk for developing chronic bronchitis?

Real-Life Challenge: Epistaxis

A 60-year-old woman has called the office stating that she is experiencing a severe nosebleed. She says her nose started bleeding last night and has been bleeding off and on since then. The blood is bright red and seems to be coming from the left side of her nose. On questioning, she reports that she has a few periods of feeling lightheaded. She is advised to apply pressure to the left nostril and to sit down. The physician is not in the office. The patient's son is with her and is able to transport her to an emergency facility. She is instructed to take along her current medication. After talking with her son, you suggest that he take his mother to a nearby facility. You also tell him that you will call the facility ahead to expect her arrival.

Questions

1. On looking at the patient's chart, you see that she is taking Plavix. Why is that important?
2. Should you also advise the son to assist her to his vehicle?
3. Will the emergency facility inquire about her health status?
4. What might be significant about her medical history?
5. What is the significance of the patient feeling lightheaded?
6. Which treatment protocols do you anticipate the patient to receive at the facility?
7. What would you do if the son were not with the patient?

Internet Assignments

1. Research the American Lung Association website (www.lung.org) for an update on a respiratory condition of your interest.
2. Visit the American Lung Association website. Search for "Work" and report on some of the work-related illnesses.
3. Explore the National Institute of Allergies and Infectious Diseases (NIAID) website at https://www.niaid.nih.gov. Search for "asthma," and answer the following questions:
   a. Why is the study of asthma a priority for NIAID?
   b. How is NIAID addressing this critical topic?
4. Perform an Internet search on "vaping statistics," and report on your findings on teenagers and their use of electronic delivery devices.

Critical Thinking

1. Discuss how smoking affects the tissues and structures of the respiratory system.
2. Cancer of the lung and bronchus is the number one cause of cancer-related death. What help is available to those who want to stop smoking?
3. How would you respond to a person choking in a restaurant and obviously unable to dislodge the obstruction? Demonstrate the Heimlich maneuver. What if that person is a child? How would you adjust the procedure?
4. How would you come to the aid of a person experiencing a severe nosebleed (epistaxis)? When should emergency treatment be obtained?
5. Explore how chronic respiratory diseases can present a daily challenge to keep the patient's airway open, to allow for ventilation and respiration. What are some ways anxiety enters into each day of the patient's life?
6. Compensation for lung disease may require the patient to regularly take medication, breathing treatments, and perhaps even different levels of oxygen therapy. In some cases, tracheostomy and an intermittent positive-pressure breathing (IPPB) machine may be used to improve ventilation of the lungs. How can these interventions change a person's life, depending on age and occupation?
7. What makes sputum removal management vitally important for the patient with bronchiectasis?
8. How would you respond to a person who suddenly complains of shortness of breath and chest pain? What possible pathologic conditions come to mind?

Prepare to discuss Critical Thinking case study exercises for this chapter that are posted on Evolve.

10

Diseases and Conditions of the Circulatory System

CHAPTER OUTLINE

Orderly Function of the Circulatory System, 382

Cardiovascular Diseases, 383

Lymphatic and Blood Disorders, 385

Coronary Artery Disease, 385

Myocardial Infarction, 390

Cardiac Arrest, 392

Hypertensive Heart Disease, 394

Congestive Heart Failure, 396

Cor Pulmonale, 398

Pulmonary Edema, 400

Cardiomyopathy, 400

Pericarditis, 402

Myocarditis, 403

Endocarditis, 404

Rheumatic Fever, 405

Valvular Heart Disease, 408

Arrhythmias, 410

Shock, 414

Cardiac Tamponade, 417

Vascular Conditions, 417

Aneurysms, 422

Blood Dyscrasias, 427

Leukemias, 432

Lymphatic Diseases, 436

Transfusion Incompatibility Reaction, 442

Clotting Disorders, 443

LEARNING OBJECTIVES

After studying Chapter 10, you should be able to:

1. Discuss the anatomy and physiology of the heart.
2. Name the common presenting symptoms in patients with cardiovascular disease.
3. Describe the pathology of coronary artery disease (CAD).
4. Name the contributing factors for CAD.
5. Explain what causes the pain of angina pectoris.
6. Explain the difference between angina pectoris and myocardial infarction (MI).
7. Describe the treatment of MI and cardiac arrest.
8. Name and describe the symptoms of the most prevalent cardiovascular disorder in the United States.
9. Explain what happens when the pumping action of the heart fails.
10. Compare left-sided heart failure with right-sided heart failure.
11. Name some causes of cardiomyopathy.
12. Distinguish among pericarditis, myocarditis, and endocarditis.
13. Explain why rheumatic fever is considered a systemic disease.
14. Recall the cardiac manifestations of rheumatic heart disease.
15. Explain the pathophysiology of valvular heart disease.
16. Name the causes of cardiac arrhythmias.
17. Discuss treatment options for cardiac arrhythmias.
18. Describe the signs and symptoms of shock.
19. Discuss cardiac tamponade.
20. Explain the possible consequences of emboli.
21. Compare arteriosclerosis with atherosclerosis.
22. Describe *aneurysm* and explain how it is diagnosed.
23. Explain the treatment for (1) thrombophlebitis and (2) varicose veins.
24. Describe the vascular pathology of Raynaud disease.
25. Define *anemia* and list the presenting symptoms.
26. Describe how anemias are classified and give some examples.
27. State the causes of agranulocytosis.
28. Describe the typical symptoms in all types of leukemias.
29. Distinguish between lymphedema and lymphangitis.
30. Explain the diagnostic significance of Reed-Sternberg cells in lymphoma.
31. Name the signs and symptoms of transfusion incompatibility reaction.
32. Explain the cause of classic hemophilia.
33. Describe disseminated intravascular coagulation.

KEY TERMS

agglutination (ah-**glue**-tih-**NAY**-shun)
aggregation (**ag**-reh-**GAY**-shun)
angioplasty (**AN**-jee-oh-**plas**-tee)
arteriosclerosis (ar-**tee**-ree-oh-skleh-**ROW**-sis)
asystole (a-**SIS**-toh-lee)
atherosclerosis (**ath**-er-oh-skleh-**ROW**-sis)
bradycardia (brady-**KAR**-dee-ah)
bruit (**BREW**-ee)
cardiomegaly (**car**-dee-oh-**MEG**-ah-lee)
cardiomyopathy (**car**-dee-oh-my-**OP**-ah-thee)
cellulitis (sell-u-**LIE**-tis)
dyscrasia (dis-**CRAY**-zee-ah)
ecchymosis (ech-ih-MO-sis)
embolism (**EM**-boh-lizm)
hematopoiesis (**hem**-ah-toh-poy-**EE**-sis)

hemolytic (**hem**-oh-**LIT**-ik)
hypovolemia (**high**-poh-voh-**LEE**-mee-ah)
hypoxia (high-**POX**-see-ah)
ischemia (is-**KEY**-mee-ah)
orthopnea (**or**-**THOP**-nee-ah)
perfusion (per-**FYOU**-zhun)
petechiae (pee-**TEE**-kee-ee)
phlebotomy (phleh-**BOT**-oh-mee)
plaque (**PLACK**)
purpura (**PUR**-pu-rah)
syncope (**SIN**-ko-pee)
tachycardia (**tack**-ee-**CAR**-dee-ah)
tamponade (**tam**-pon-**ADE**)
thrombus (**THROM**-bus)

Orderly Function of the Circulatory System

Circulation of blood to the organs and tissues of the body is the primary function of the circulatory system. The heart is at the center of the circulatory system (Figs. 10.1 and 10.2). Its steady beating pumps about 5 quarts of blood through a complete vascular circuit of the body every minute in an adult; this is called the *cardiac cycle.* This circuit comprises a network of vessels: the arteries, veins, and capillaries (Fig. 10.3).

The heart consists of two side-by-side pumps, each divided into two chambers: two upper chambers called *atria*

and two lower chambers called *ventricles.* As venous blood returns to the heart from the body, it enters the right atrium, passes through the tricuspid valve, and, with atrial contraction, enters the right ventricle. Heart valves prevent blood from flowing backward. From the right ventricle, blood is pumped through the pulmonary valve and, with ventricular contraction, into the pulmonary arteries and on to the lungs. In the lungs, carbon dioxide is removed from and oxygen is added to blood. Freshly oxygenated blood then returns to the heart via the pulmonary veins. Blood enters the left atrium, moves through the mitral (bicuspid) valve with atrial

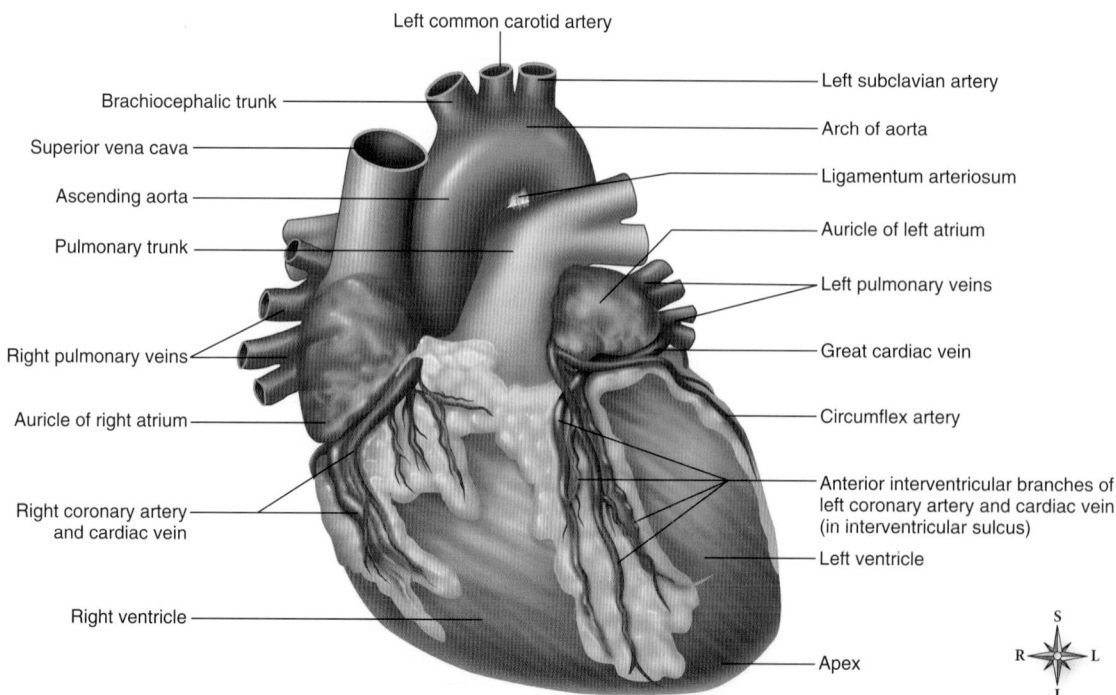

• **Fig. 10.1** The heart and great vessels, anterior view. (From Patton KT, Thibodeau GA: *Anatomy and physiology,* ed 9, St Louis, 2016, Mosby.)

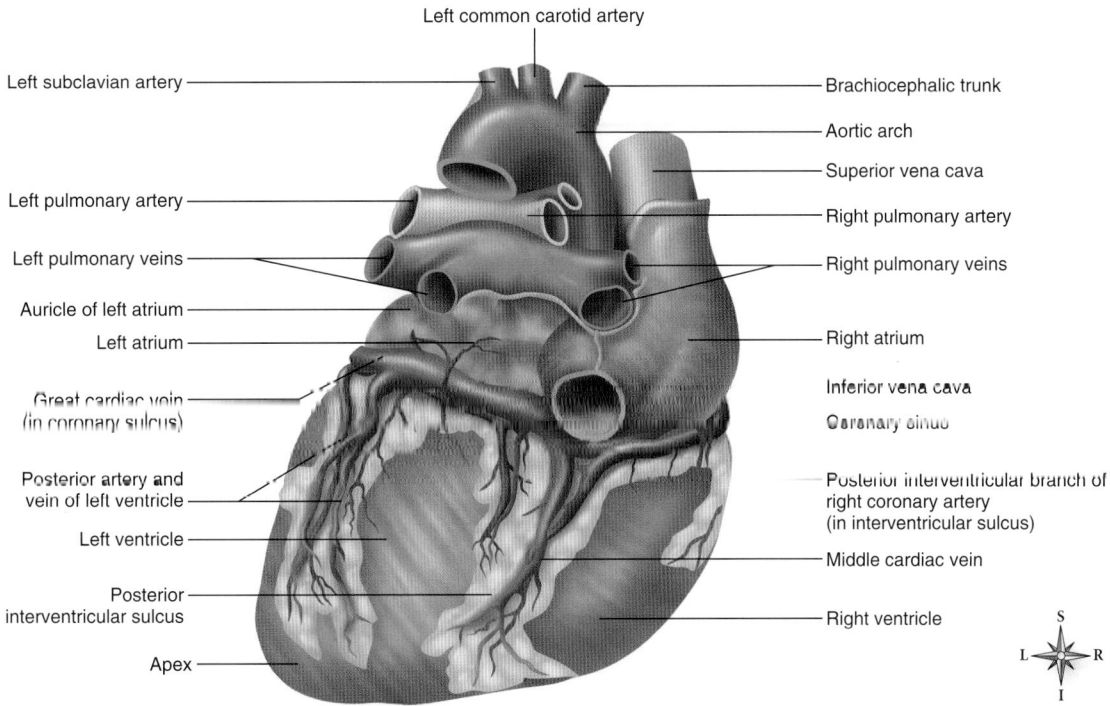

• **Fig. 10.2** The heart and great vessels, posterior view. (From Patton KT, Thibodeau GA: *Anatomy and physiology,* ed 9, St Louis, 2016, Mosby.)

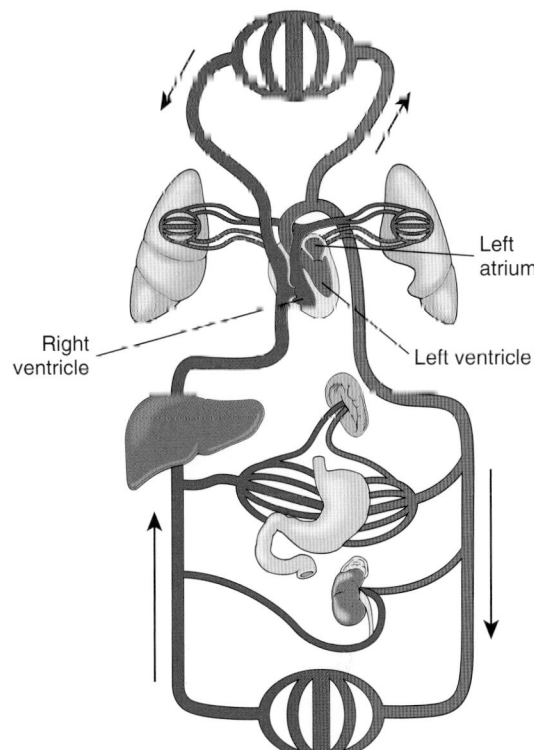

• **Fig. 10.3** Circulation through the body.

contraction, and enters the left ventricle. As the left ventricle contracts, blood is forced through the aortic valve, into the aorta, and on to the rest of the body (see Figs. 10.3, 10.4). This process is called the *cardiac cycle* (Fig. 10.5). Refer to Chapter 2 for a description of fetal circulation.

The heart is enclosed by the double-layered pericardium which is composed of an inner serous layer (visceral pericardium, or epicardium) and an outer fibrous layer (parietal pericardium). Between these layers in the pericardial cavity is a small amount of serous fluid that reduces friction during cardiac movements. Cardiac muscle tissue, or myocardium, is composed of striated muscle cells that can contract rhythmically on their own and characteristically are both voluntary and involuntary responses. Inside the cavities of the heart is a smooth serous lining called *endocardium* (Fig. 10.6). The conduction system of the heart coordinates the contraction and relaxation (cardiac cycle) of the heart by initiating impulses and distributing the impulses throughout the myocardium. Coronary arteries and a network of vessels continuously supply cardiac muscle tissue with oxygen (Fig. 10.7).

Cardiovascular Diseases

There are many and varied disorders of the heart and circulatory system. In some disorders, the rhythm of the heartbeat becomes irregular, may enter **tachycardia** (become abnormally fast), or may enter **bradycardia** (become abnormally slow). Disorders of cardiac rhythm are called *arrhythmias* or *dysrhythmias.*

Almost one-quarter of all deaths in the United States are attributed to heart disease, according to the Centers for Disease Control and Prevention (CDC). Most of these deaths are caused by coronary artery disease (CAD) and hypertension. Cardiovascular disorders, such as angina pectoris, myocardial infarction (MI), congestive heart failure (CHF),

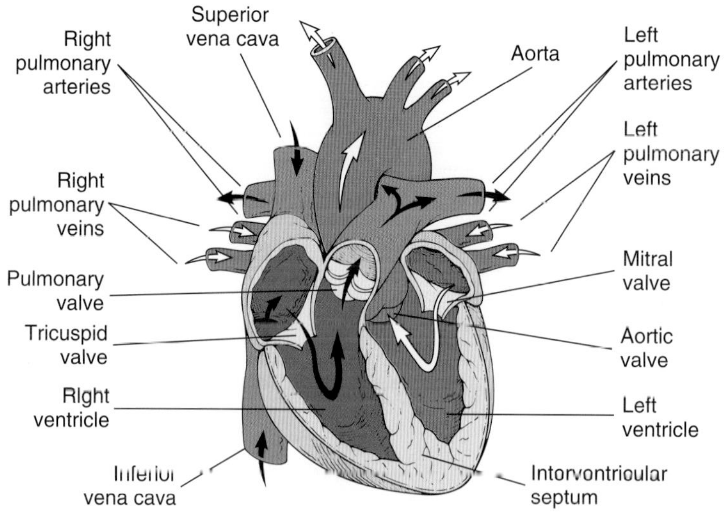

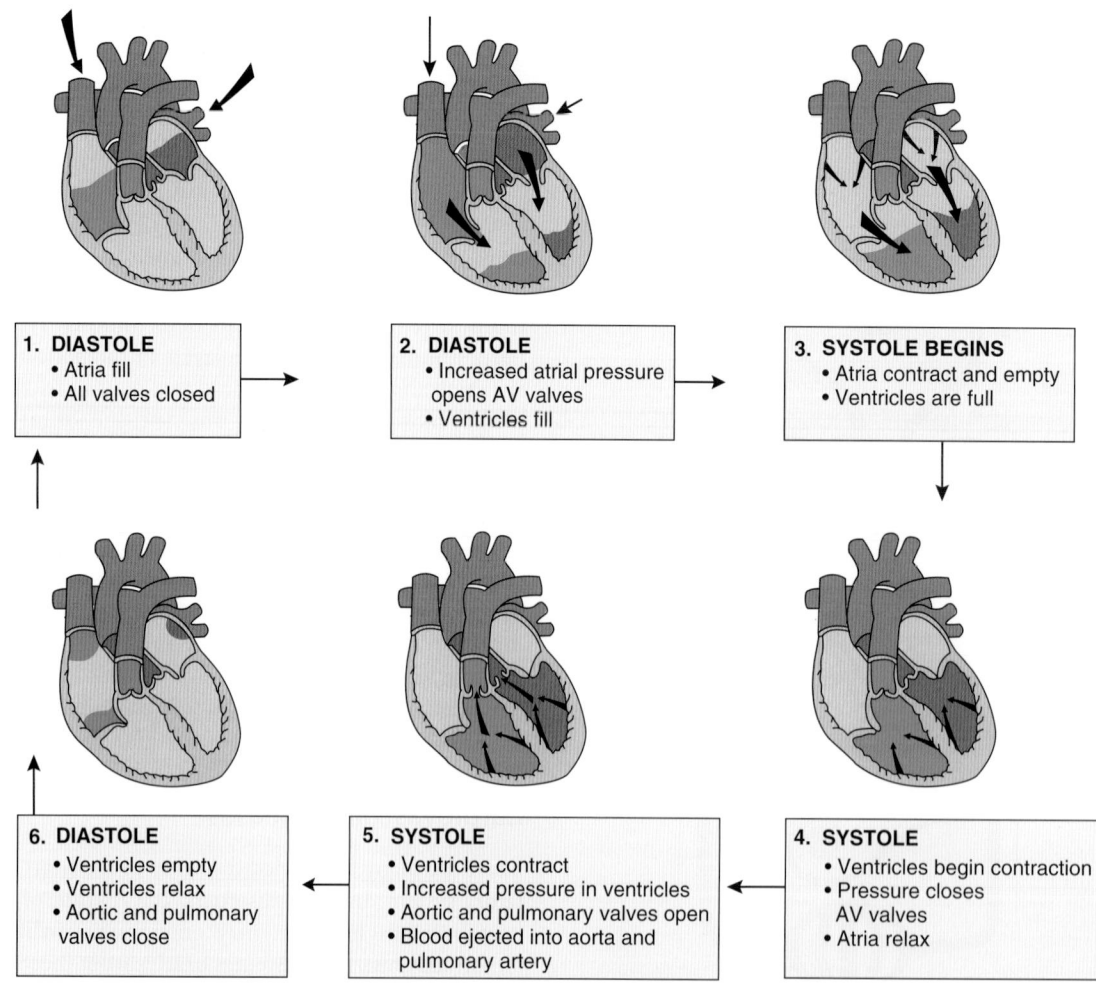

• **Fig. 10.4** Circulation through the heart.

• **Fig. 10.5** Cardiac cycle. *AV,* Atrioventricular valves (both tricuspid and mitral). (From Gould B: *Pathophysiology for the health professions,* ed 3, Philadelphia, 2006, Saunders/Elsevier.)

cardiac arrest, shock, and cardiac **tamponade** also can result in death. Other diseases of the cardiovascular system include rheumatic fever, pericarditis, myocarditis, endocarditis, thromboangiitis obliterans (Buerger disease), Raynaud disease, and vascular (blood vessel) diseases.

Important presenting symptoms that tend to recur in patients with cardiovascular disease and need further investigation include:

• chest pain
• dyspnea (difficulty in breathing) on exertion

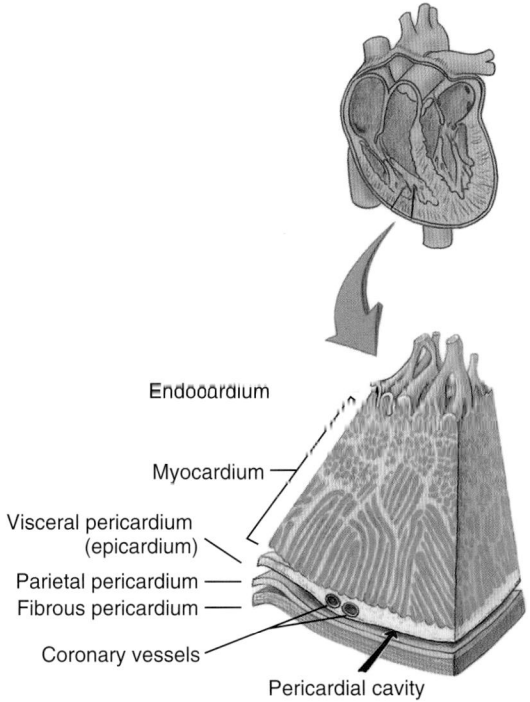

Endocardium

Myocardium

Visceral pericardium
(epicardium)

Parietal pericardium

Fibrous pericardium

Coronary vessels

Pericardial cavity

• **Fig. 10.6** Layers of the heart wall. (From Applegate EJ: *The anatomy and physiology learning system,* ed 4, Philadelphia, 2011, Saunders/Elsevier.)

- tachypnea (rapid breathing)
- palpitations (rapid fluttering of the heart)
- cyanosis (slight blue color)
- edema
- fatigue
- syncope (fainting)

Lymphatic and Blood Disorders

See disorders under discussion of specific diseases.

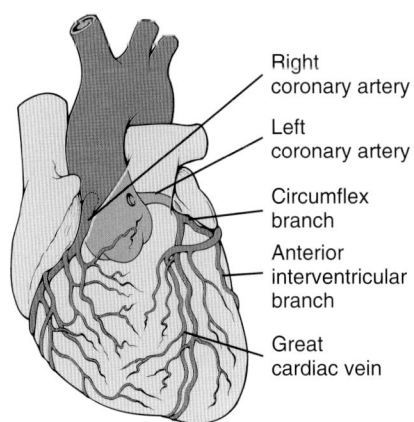

Right
coronary artery

Left
coronary artery

Circumflex
branch

Anterior
interventricular
branch

Great
cardiac vein

Coronary Artery Disease

Description

CAD is a condition involving the arteries supplying the myocardium (heart muscle) (see Fig. 10.7). The arteries become narrowed because of atherosclerotic deposits over time, causing temporary cardiac ischemia and eventually MI (or heart attack).

ICD-10-CM Code	I25.10 *(Atherosclerotic heart disease of native coronary artery without angina pectoris)*
	(I25.10-I25.119 – 5 codes of specificity)

Codes for coronary vascular disease are classified by location and type. Refer to the physician's diagnosis and then to the current edition of the ICD-10-CM coding manual to ensure the greatest specificity.

Symptoms and Signs

Patients are asymptomatic initially, with the first symptom being the pain of angina pectoris (see the Angina Pectoris section). In advanced disease, the severe pain of MI is described as burning, squeezing, crushing, and radiating to the arm, neck, or jaw (see the Myocardial Infarction section) and results from diminished blood flow and lower oxygen saturation. Nausea, vomiting, and weakness also can be experienced. Changes are often, but not always, recognized on the patient's electrocardiogram. Many patients may be asymptomatic until an MI or sudden death event; this is why noninvasive screening of high risk patients is imperative.

Patient Screening

Severe chest pain of sudden onset, with or without previous diagnosis of angina, is considered to be a cardiac event and

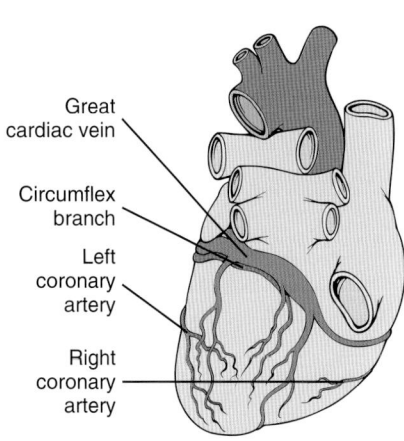

Great
cardiac vein

Circumflex
branch

Left
coronary
artery

Right
coronary
artery

• **Fig. 10.7** Coronary arteries.

has the potential for being catastrophic; therefore the patient should immediately be entered into the emergency medical system.

Etiology

Deposits of fat-containing substances, called plaque, in the lumen (opening) of the coronary arteries result in atherosclerosis and subsequent narrowing of the lumen of the arteries (Fig. 10.8). The myocardium must have an adequate blood supply to function. The coronary arteries supply the cardiac muscle with blood but become constricted by atherosclerosis (Fig. 10.9).

Arteriosclerosis, commonly called *hardening of the arteries*, is associated with older adults and patients with diabetes. The arteries eventually lose elasticity and become hard and narrow, resulting in cardiac ischemia. The cells in the

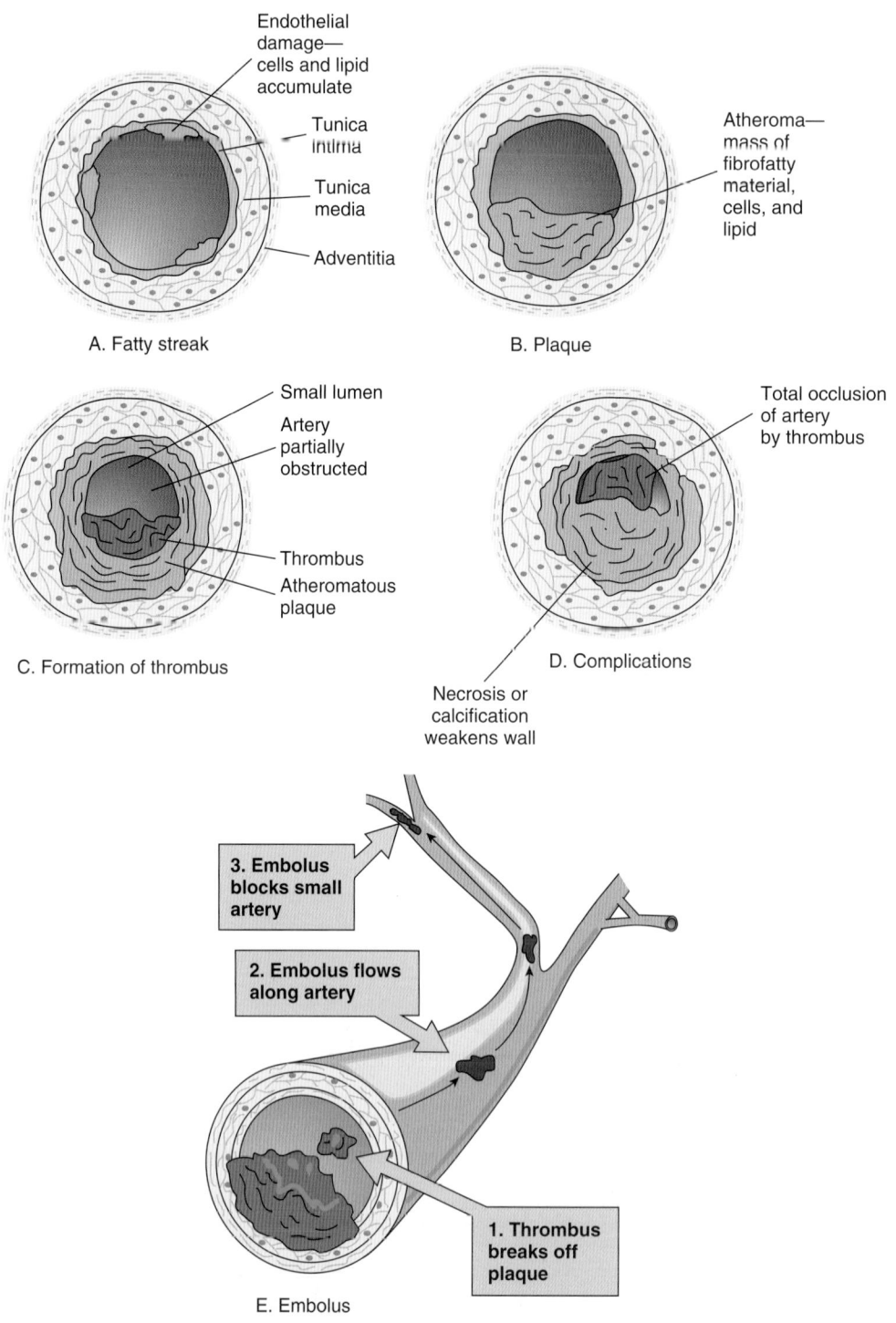

• **Fig. 10.8** Development of an atheroma leading to arterial occlusion. (From Gould B: *Pathophysiology for the health professions*, ed 3, Philadelphia, 2006, Saunders/Elsevier.)

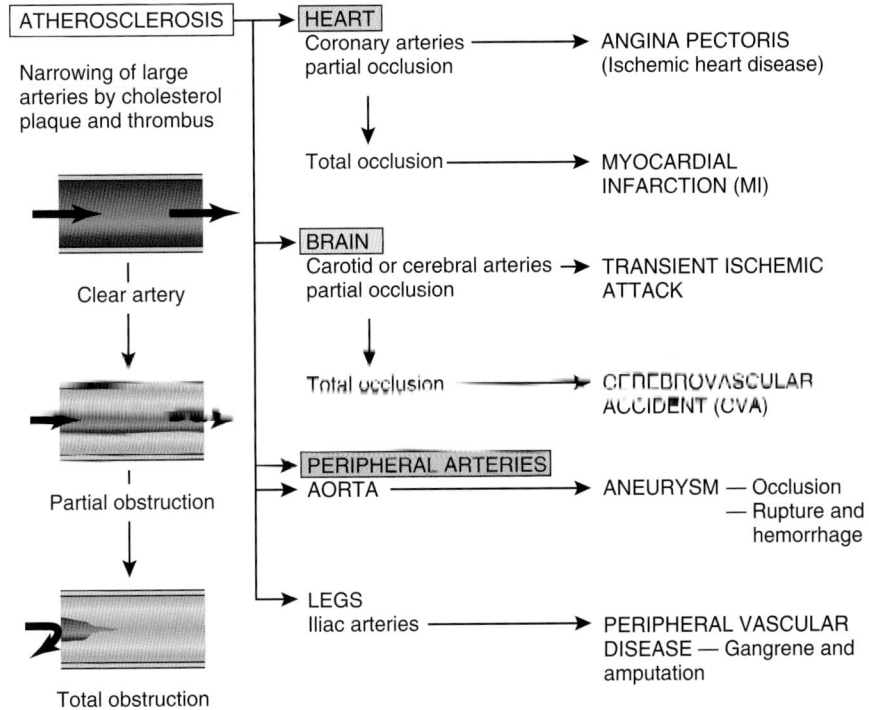

• **Fig. 10.9** Possible consequences of atherosclerosis. (From Gould B: *Pathophysiology for the health professions*, ed 3, Philadelphia, 2006, Saunders/Elsevier.)

myocardium gradually weaken and die. Replacement scar tissue forms, interfering with the heart's ability to pump, resulting in heart failure.

People at higher risk for CAD are those who have a genetic predisposition to the disease, those older than 40 years of age, men (slightly more than women), postmenopausal women, and Caucasians. Other factors contributing to increased risk of the disease include a history of smoking; residence in an urban society; the presence of hypertension, diabetes, or obesity; and a history of elevated serum cholesterol or reduced serum high-density lipoprotein (HDL) levels. Lack of exercise (a sedentary lifestyle) and stress are additional risk factors.

Diagnosis

The patient usually does not experience chest pain from atherosclerosis until the coronary arteries are about 75% occluded. Collateral circulation often develops to supply the tissue with needed oxygen and nutrients (Fig. 10.10). Electrocardiography (ECG) shows ischemia (caused by lack of blood supply) and possibly arrhythmias. Treadmill testing, thallium or Cardiolite scanning, computed tomography (CT), stress echocardiography, cardiac catheterization, and angiography are other tools of cardiac status evaluation used to detect insufficient oxygen supply and to confirm the diagnosis. Electron beam computerized testing, a noninvasive assessment for identifying calcium buildup in arteries, is another means of risk evaluation.

Treatment

Treatment consists of measures to restore adequate blood flow to the myocardium. Vasodilators and other types of medicines are prescribed. Angioplasty with a balloon or stenting is attempted in some instances to open the constricted arteries (Fig. 10.11). Claims of reduction of the plaque buildup with hypolipidemic drugs are being confirmed in some cases. First-line drug therapy for the prevention of CAD may include angiotensin-converting enzyme (ACE) inhibitors, angiotensin receptor blockers (ARBs), calcium channel blockers (CCBs), thiazide diuretics, or vasodilators. Beta blockers and anticoagulants are used to prevent blood clots from breaking off and lodging in the cerebral arteries. When the blockage is severe or does not respond to drug therapy or angioplasty, coronary artery bypass surgery (CABG) may be indicated to restore circulation to the affected myocardium (Fig. 10.12).

Experimental gene therapy uses injections of deoxyribonucleic acid (DNA) directly into cardiac muscle to stimulate new growth of blood vessels; this is still at a very preliminary stage.

Prognosis

The prognosis varies, depending on patient response to the treatment, whether drug therapy, angioplasty, or CABG. An additional factor affecting the prognosis of smokers is the effect of smoking on the coronary arteries and whether the patient ceases smoking.

Prevention

Measures to prevent CAD include a diet that is low in salt, fat, and cholesterol, in addition to exercise. Patients are encouraged to reduce stress and, if they smoke, to stop or reduce smoking.

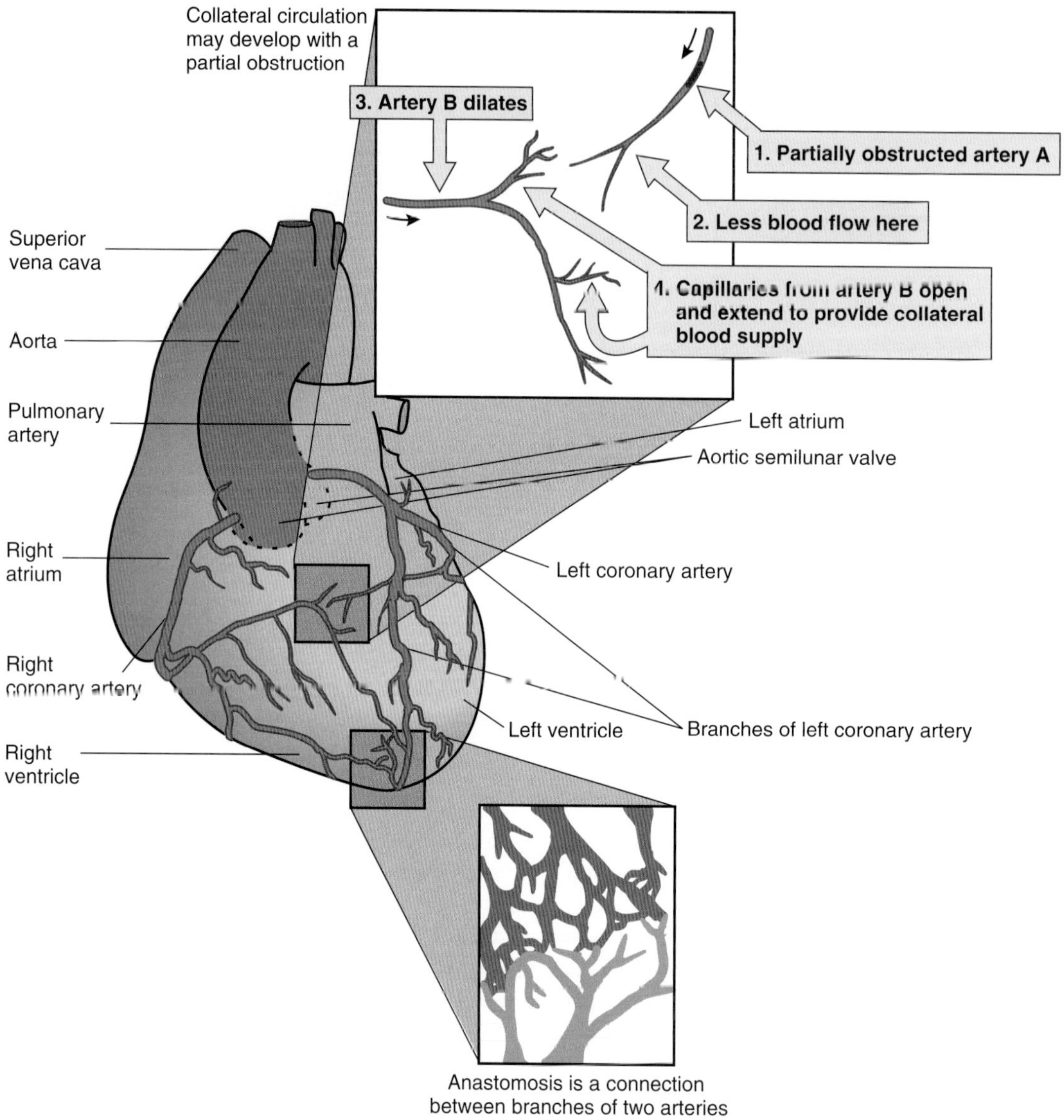

Collateral circulation may develop with a partial obstruction

3. Artery B dilates

1. Partially obstructed artery A

2. Less blood flow here

4. Capillaries from artery B open and extend to provide collateral blood supply

Superior vena cava

Aorta

Pulmonary artery

Right atrium

Right coronary artery

Right ventricle

Left atrium

Aortic semilunar valve

Left coronary artery

Left ventricle

Branches of left coronary artery

Anastomosis is a connection between branches of two arteries

• **Fig. 10.10** Collateral circulation of the heart. (From Gould B: *Pathophysiology for the health professions,* ed 3, Philadelphia, 2006, Saunders/Elsevier.)

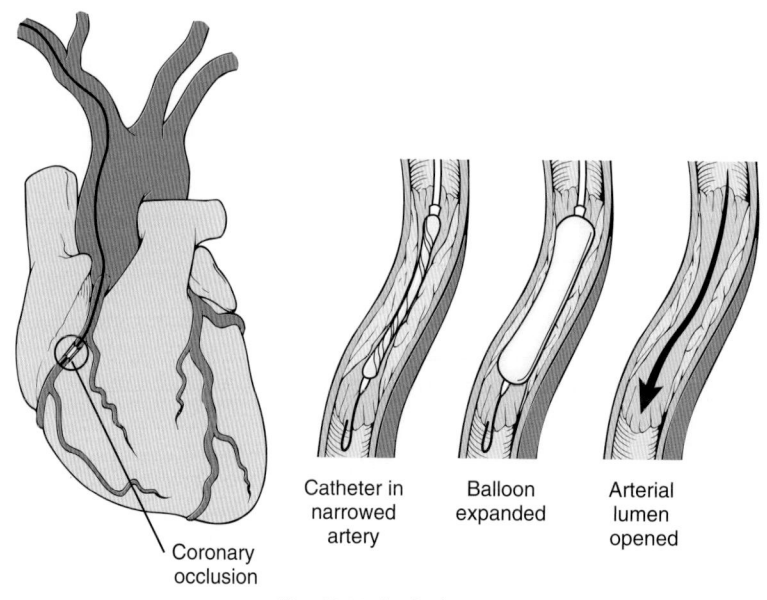

Coronary occlusion

Catheter in narrowed artery

Balloon expanded

Arterial lumen opened

• **Fig. 10.11** Angioplasty.

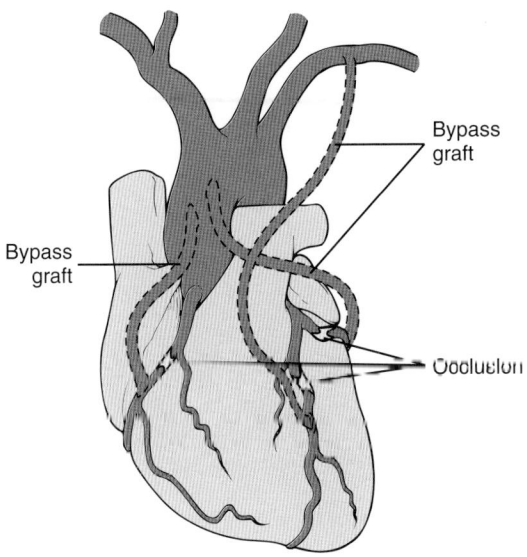

• **Fig. 10.12** Coronary artery bypass.

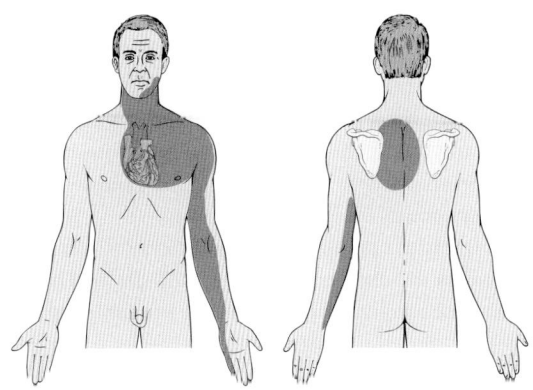

• **Fig. 10.13** Common sites of pain in angina pectoris.

Patient Teaching

Give patients information about symptoms of impending MI, and encourage them to seek immediate emergency medical care at the first sign of any related symptoms. Offer printed information to all patients about the prevention or control of CAD, and emphasize the importance of a low-fat diet, weight control, exercise, and smoking cessation. Encourage follow-up cholesterol blood tests.

Angina Pectoris

Description

Angina pectoris, which is chest pain caused by ischemia during or shortly after exertion, is the result of reduced oxygen supply to the myocardium.

> ICD 10-CM Code   I20.8 (Other forms of angina pectoris)
> I20.9 (Angina pectoris, unspecified)
> (I20.0-I20.9 = 4 codes of specificity)
> Codes for angina pectoris are classified by type. Refer to the physician's diagnosis and then to the current edition of the ICD-10-CM coding manual to ensure the greatest specificity.

Symptoms and Signs

The patient experiences sudden onset of left-sided chest pain during or shortly after exertion. The pain may radiate to the left arm or back (Fig. 10.13). The patient also may experience dyspnea. The pain usually is relieved by ceasing the strenuous activity and placing nitroglycerin tablets sublingually or using nitroglycerin spray also sublingually (under the tongue). Blood pressure may increase during the attack, and arrhythmias may occur.

Patient Screening

Patients experiencing symptoms of angina for the first time require immediate assessment. The sudden onset of chest pain could represent a life-threatening condition, and acute MI must be ruled out. Those who have been diagnosed with angina pectoris and in whom cessation of activity and use of vasodilating medications does not provide relief from the pain within 20 minutes require immediate medical intervention through the emergency medical system.

Etiology

Atherosclerosis causes narrowing of the coronary arteries, compromising the blood flow to the myocardium. Exertion requires increased blood flow to supply more oxygen, but the vessels cannot supply it. Spasms of the coronary arteries also may be a causative factor. Severe prolonged tachycardia, anemia, and respiratory disease also can cause cardiac ischemia.

Diagnosis

The patient history reveals a previous exertional chest pain. ECG performed during the anginal episode may show ischemia; it is important to realize that a normal result on ECG does not preclude the diagnosis of angina. Other diagnostic measures, such as those described for CAD, are performed.

Treatment

Treatment consists of cessation of the strenuous activity and placing of nitroglycerin tablets under the tongue. Transdermal nitroglycerin helps prevent angina. When angina persists after treatment or for longer than 20 minutes, immediate medical attention is indicated.

Prognosis

The prognosis varies, depending on the extent of the arterial involvement. When patients can stop the pain by ceasing strenuous activities and using vasodilating medications, the angina usually will diminish or disappear. The patient's ability to modify his or her lifestyle may improve the prognosis.

Prevention

Preventive measures are similar to those recommended for CAD. Recommendations focus on lifestyle modification, including appropriate exercise; a diet low in fat, cholesterol, and salt; control of hypertension; weight loss; and smoking cessation. Patients are encouraged to reduce stress.

Patient Teaching

Give patients and their families dietary information and suggestions for menu planning within the appropriate diet. Emphasize the importance of compliance with prescribed drug therapy. Help the patient and the family locate and contact community services and support groups.

Patients should be instructed to carry the nitroglycerin tablets with them at all times. Additionally, patients and their families should be instructed that the tablets should not be exposed to light or air and that the tablets should be kept in the original light-resistant bottle with a cap that can be tightened.

Myocardial Infarction

Description

MI is death of myocardial tissue caused by the development of ischemia.

ICD-10-CM Code	I21.0 *(fifth digit required) (ST elevation [STEMI] myocardial infarction of anterior wall)*
	(I21.01-I21.4 = 9 codes of specificity)

Acute myocardial infarction has many codes according to episode and location. The code can include a fifth-digit subclassification according to episode. Codes for location are as follows:

ICD-10-CM Code	I21.09 *(ST elevation [STEMI] myocardial infarction involving other coronary artery of anterior wall)*
	I21.19 *(ST elevation [STEMI] myocardial infarction involving other coronary artery of inferior wall)*
	I21.11 *(ST elevation [STEMI] myocardial infarction involving right coronary artery)*
	I21.29 *(ST elevation [STEMI] myocardial infarction involving other sites)*
	I21.4 *(Non-ST elevation [NSTEMI] myocardial infarction)*
	I21.3 *(ST elevation [STEMI] myocardial infarction of unspecified site)*

Note: The physician must designate the area of the infarction before a code is applied to the episode. Refer to the physician's diagnosis and then to the current edition of the ICD-10-CM coding manual to ensure the greatest specificity.

Symptoms and Signs

Occlusion of a coronary artery resulting in ischemia and infarct (death) of the myocardium causes sudden, severe substernal or left-sided chest pain (Fig. 10.14). The pain

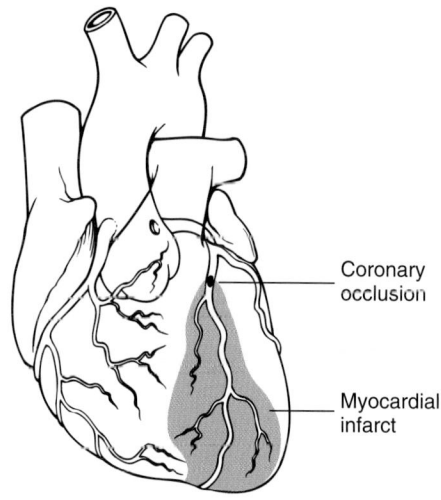

• **Fig. 10.14** Myocardial infarction (MI).

may be crushing, causing a feeling of massive constriction of the chest, may be burning, or may just be a vague discomfort. This pain may radiate to the left or right arm, back, or jaw and is not relieved by rest or the administration of nitroglycerin. Irregular heartbeat, dyspnea, and diaphoresis often accompany the pain, and the patient usually exhibits denial and experiences severe anxiety, sometimes with the feeling of impending doom (Fig. 10.15). Some may experience nausea and diaphoresis. MI occasionally is clinically silent, especially in patients with diabetes.

Patient Screening

Early and immediate intervention improves the chances for survival and minimizes irreversible injury to the myocardium. Recent recommendations include calling 911 for entry into the emergency medical system and chewing one 5-grain/325-mg aspirin tablet. Emergency intervention must be initiated immediately to control pain, stabilize heart rhythm, and minimize damage to the heart muscle. Most deaths caused by MI result from primary ventricular fibrillation. Thus immediate ECG monitoring and possible defibrillation are of primary concern. The American Heart Association (AHA) and the American Red Cross currently recommend defibrillation training for all certified first responders. The latest technology in automated external defibrillators (AEDs) affords auditory instructions to the rescuer, making the use safe for the victim and the rescuer.

Etiology

MI results from insufficient oxygen supply, as occurs when a coronary artery is occluded by atherosclerotic plaque, **thrombus**, or myocardial muscle spasm (Fig. 10.16). The pain is caused by ischemia, and if ischemia is not reversed within about 6 hours, the cardiac muscle dies. Coronary thrombosis is the most common cause of MI.

Diagnosis

The diagnosis includes a thorough history, ECG, chest radiographic studies, and laboratory tests for cardiac enzyme

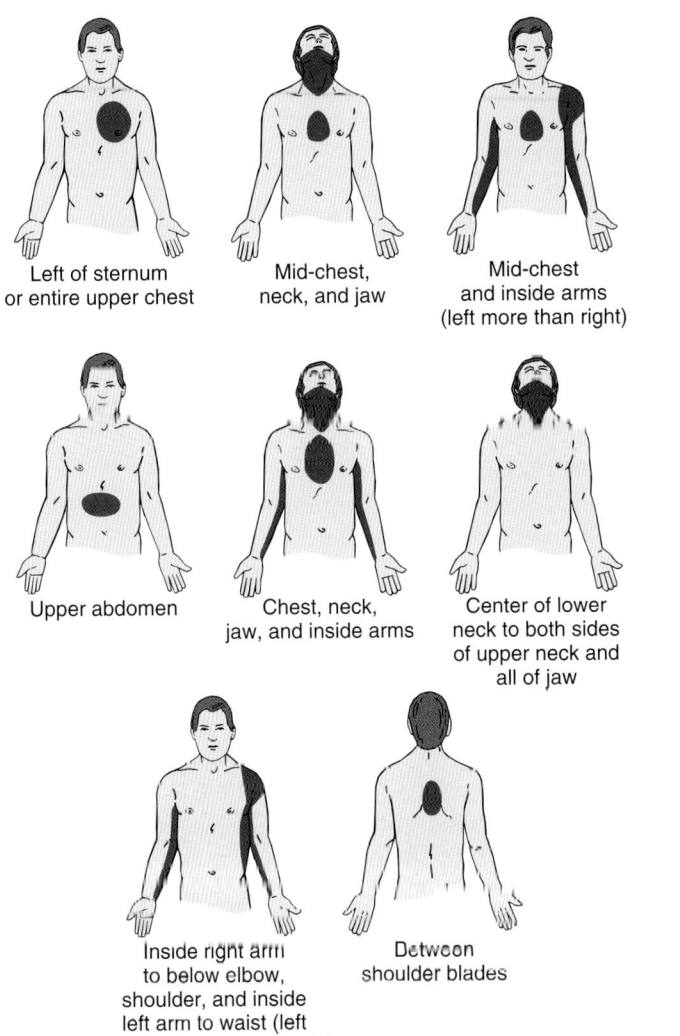

• **Fig. 10.15** Locations of pain from myocardial infarction (MI). (From *Mosby's dictionary of medicine, nursing and health professions,* ed 7, St Louis, 2010, Mosby/Elsevier.)

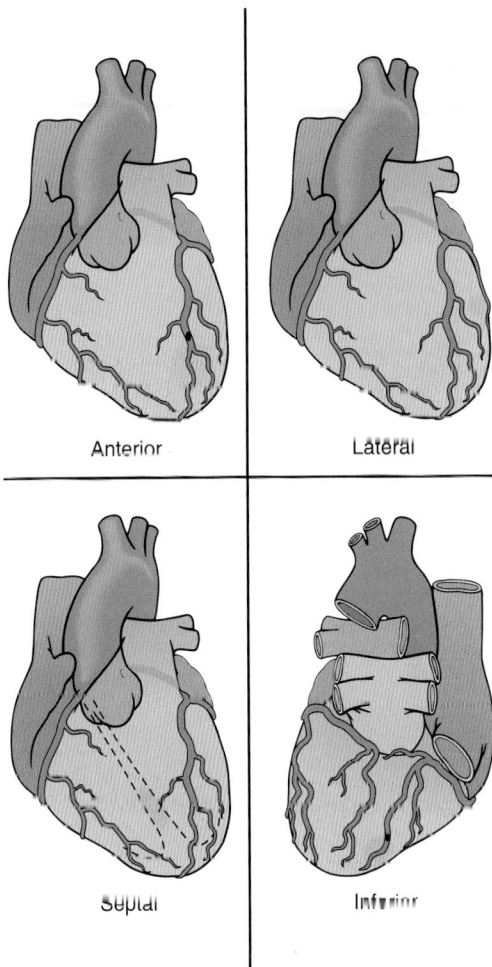

• **Fig. 10.16** Common locations of myocardial infarction (MI). (From Lewis SM, Heitkemper MM, Dirksen SR: *Medical-surgical nursing: assessment and management of clinical problems,* ed 6, St Louis, 2004, Mosby/Elsevier.)

levels. Changes in enzyme levels indicate the death of cardiac tissue and include (1) creatine phosphokinase (CPK) and troponin, which are elevated in the first 6 to 24 hours after MI; (2) lactate dehydrogenase (LDH), which peaks at 48 hours after MI; and (3) aspartate aminotransferase (AST). When elevated levels of these enzymes are detected, a study of cardiac isoenzymes is ordered to confirm the diagnosis. ECG changes in the P-R and QRS complexes and in the ST segment correspond to the ischemic areas. Diagnostic confirmation is assisted by elevated cardiac enzyme levels and altered isoenzyme levels identified through blood tests.

Treatment

Oxygen is administered, and morphine is given for pain. Aspirin is given as soon as possible to reduce the risk of additional damage to the heart and cardiac tissue caused by ischemia. Vasodilation is attempted by administering nitroglycerin drip. Lidocaine or amiodarone given by an intravenous (IV) drip, after a loading bolus, helps control arrhythmias. Thrombolytic drugs, including tissue plasminogen activator (tPA),

streptokinase, or alteplase (Activase) may be administered as soon as possible after the diagnosis, unless there are contraindications. Within the 6-hour window before permanent damage occurs, an attempt may be made to open the occlusion and to restore blood flow to the area through angioplasty, the administration of thrombolytic drugs, or CABG (Fig. 10.17). Currently, the standard of care is to try to emergently open the artery with a stent (Fig. 10.18), preferably within 60 to 90 minutes of the patient's arrival at the hospital; this has been demonstrated to more effectively decrease heart damage compared with IV thrombolytic drugs.

Prognosis

The prognosis of MI is determined by immediate defibrillation for ventricular fibrillation. Late mortality depends on the extent of damage to the heart muscle and the occurrence of complications. In most cases, late cardiac death is sudden, caused by the onset of fatal arrhythmia.

Prevention

Preventive measures are similar to those recommended for CAD. Recommendations focus on lifestyle modification,

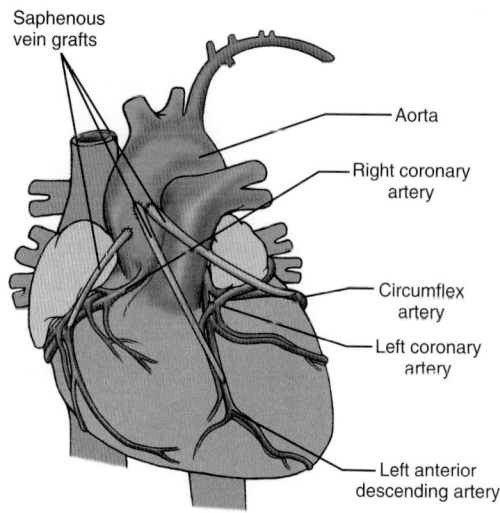

• **Fig. 10.17** Coronary bypass graft. (From *Mosby's dictionary of medicine, nursing and health professions,* ed 7, St Louis, 2010, Mosby/Elsevier.)

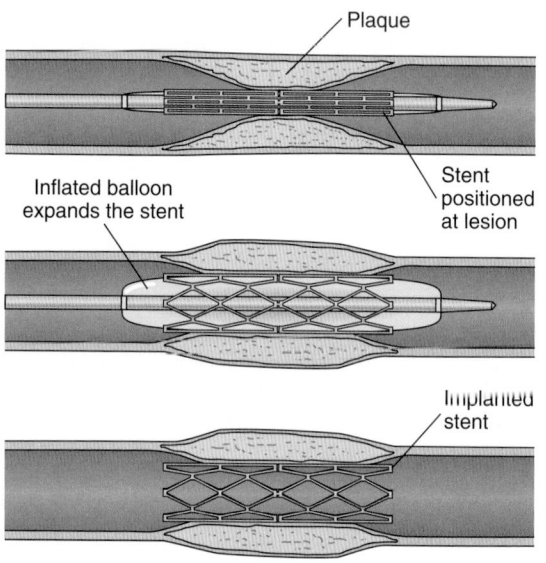

• **Fig. 10.18** Coronary artery stent. (From *Mosby's dictionary of medicine, nursing and health professions,* ed 7, St Louis, 2010, Mosby/Elsevier.)

including appropriate exercise; a diet low in fat, cholesterol, and salt; control of hypertension; weight loss; and smoking cessation. Patients are encouraged to reduce stress. Those surviving MI are urged to take a daily aspirin dose and a beta-blocker or ACE inhibitor for life. Lipid-lowering medications are also recommended.

Patient Teaching
Give patients and their families dietary information and suggestions for menu planning within the appropriate diet. Emphasize the importance of compliance with prescribed drug therapy and cardiac rehabilitation. Help the patient and the family find and contact community services and support groups.

Cardiac Arrest

Description
Cardiac arrest is the sudden, unexpected cessation of cardiac activity.

ICD-10-CM Code	I46.9 *(Cardiac arrest, cause unspecified)*
	(I46.2-I46.9 – 3 codes of specificity)

Symptoms and Signs
The patient is unresponsive, with no respiratory effort and no palpable pulse.

Patient Screening
Cardiac arrest is a true life-threatening emergency. Immediate intervention with instantaneous initiation of cardiopulmonary resuscitation (CPR) and defibrillation by means of an AED may successfully restore contraction of the heart (Fig. 10.19). The AHA or American Red Cross protocol for caregivers in the field requires immediate contact of the emergency medical system by calling 911. Inpatient facilities use the "Code Blue" message to alert personnel.

Etiology
Cardiac arrest results from anoxia (absence of oxygen to the tissue) or interruption of electrical stimuli to the heart. It can be caused by respiratory arrest, arrhythmia, or MI. Electrocution, drowning, severe trauma, massive hemorrhage, or drug overdose also can cause cardiac arrest.

Diagnosis
The diagnosis is based on the absence of respiratory effort and lack of palpable pulse. ECG shows ventricular fibrillation or **asystole**.

Treatment
CPR must be instituted within 4 to 6 minutes of the cardiac arrest. Until recently, cardiac defibrillation was only attempted by personnel trained in advanced life support. AEDs are now available for use by anyone who witnesses

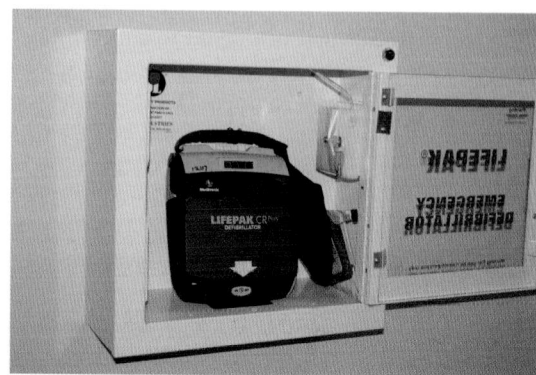

• **Fig. 10.19** Photo of an automated external defibrillator (AED). (Courtesy David Frazier, 2011, in cooperation with St Johns County Sheriff's Office, St Augustine, FL.)

someone experiencing cardiac arrest. The latest technology implemented in these devices talks the rescuer through the defibrillation process (see Fig. 10.19). The rescuer should be familiar with the device he or she is attempting to use. Ambulance or other medical personnel administer cardiac drugs, including epinephrine (Adrenalin) and isoproterenol (Isuprel) or dobutamine to stimulate the heart. Antiarrhythmic drugs, including lidocaine and amiodarone, also may be administered.

Prognosis

The prognosis varies, depending on the length of time the individual has been in cardiac arrest. The earlier CPR and defibrillation are instituted, the greater is the possibility for survival. Within 1 to 2 minutes after cessation of cardiac activity, respiratory efforts cease. At 4 to 6 minutes after the cessation of cardiac activity, brain cells begin to die. At 10 minutes after cardiac activity has ceased with no intervention, the brain dies, and death is inevitable. Many public venues and emergency vehicles now have portable defibrillators to facilitate more rapid resumption of cardiac function.

Successful resuscitation depends on immediate and complete intervention. Other factors that affect the final outcome of the event include the general health and age of the patient and the cause of the arrest. Successful interventions in cold water near drowning and electrical shock have been recorded.

Prevention

Prevention of the catastrophic event of cardiac arrest is difficult. However, as in CAD and MI, the same lifestyle modifications can reduce risk. One cannot predict near-drowning or electrical shock accidents, but the prudent individual will try to avoid situations that carry this risk. Recently in high risk patients with a history of abnormal heart rhythms or weak cardiac muscle, the implanting of defibrillators has been shown to decrease the risk of sudden cardiac death.

Patient Teaching

Encourage all possible candidates for CPR training to become certified. Help families of patients who do not survive cardiac arrest to find and contact support groups in the community. Emphasize safety guidelines to prevent drowning and electrical shock.

Encourage survivors of cardiac arrest to comply with the prescribed regimen of activities and drug therapy. Survivors also may need help in finding and contacting support groups for survivors of cardiac arrest.

Broken Heart Syndrome (Takotsubo Cardiomyopathy)

Description

Broken heart syndrome can occur when the heart's pumping function is abnormal. This can result when there is a temporary problem in a single area or region of the heart.

ICD-10-CM Diagnosis Code I51.81 (Takotsubo syndrome)

! ALERT!

The American Heart Association (AHA) has updated its protocol for cardiopulmonary resuscitation (CPR) of an adult cardiac arrest victim. On observing an individual in what is suspected as cardiac arrest, the first step is to call 911 for help and activate the emergency medical service (EMS) system. The patient should be checked for breathing. The next step is to immediately start giving 30 rapid deep chest compressions (30 in 18 seconds), and the airway should be opened. The rescuer may now give two rapid rescue breaths followed by resumption of rapid chest compressions. The traditional ABCs of CPR are now referred to as *CAB* (compressions, airway, and breathing). See the Enrichment box about Therapeutic Hypothermia.

Courtesy George L. Schiffman, MD, FCCP, Mission Internal Medical Group, Mission Viejo, CA, and AHA updated protocol for postarrest treatment.

♦ ENRICHMENT

Therapeutic Hypothermia

After cardiac arrest and in spite of cardiopulmonary resuscitation (CPR), patients often have a bad outcome, either death or severe brain damage. However, there are many reports of people who fell into lakes in cold climates being resuscitated after some time and returning to a normal life. Recent studies have shown that cooling a select group of patients immediately after cardiac arrest can improve the neurologic outcome and quite possibly decrease mortality. This is referred to as *therapeutic hypothermia*. Patients whose mental status remains impaired are rapidly cooled to 91°F (32°C–33°C) immediately after cardiac arrest. This can be performed using a variety of devices, some as simple as cooling blankets and ice to something as complex as cardiopulmonary bypass. This procedure can be quite uncomfortable for patients because the body fights to maintain normal temperature, primarily by shivering. Therefore patients are heavily sedated and maintained on mechanical ventilation. Patients must be monitored quite closely for shifts in many of their electrolytes and the possibility of seizures. The procedure is continued for 18 to 24 hours. Then the process of rewarming is begun. This is perhaps the most critical time of this therapy. Rapid rewarming can be disastrous, so rewarming must be performed with the utmost care. Several sophisticated devices have been developed to slowly rewarm patients by less than 1° an hour (e.g., external devices, such as the Artic Sun; or internal devices, such as the InnerCool catheter). As this therapy is used more commonly, the mortality rate of cardiac arrest will be reduced, and better neurologic outcomes are likely to result.

Courtesy George L. Schiffman, MD, FCCP, Mission Internal Medical Group, Mission Viejo, CA.

Symptoms and Signs

The individual experiences chest pain and shortness of breath. This may occur after a stressful event or even an exciting event, such as a surprise party or a lottery winning. Examples of stressful events are divorce or job loss. Although the cause is unclear, it is believed that a sudden surge of stress hormones may be responsible.

Patient Screening

When a patient or a family member reports that the patient is experiencing sudden onset of chest pain and shortness of breath, instruct the individual to call 911 for emergency assistance.

Etiology

Although the cause is unclear, it is believed that a surge of stress hormones may be responsible. The event usually is preceded by a powerful emotional or physical incident. Examples include death of a loved one; domestic abuse; certain drugs; surprises; physical stressors, including asthma; and motor vehicle accidents. The left ventricle temporarily enlarges and does not pump properly. The remaining portion of the heart pumps normally or with more forceful contractions.

Diagnosis

The arteries are not obstructed. Blood flow may be reduced. Chest x-ray may or may not show an abnormal size or shape of the heart. ECG is performed, and echocardiography may also be performed. ECG may show changes from normal rhythm. Echocardiography may show an enlarged left ventricle. Coronary angiography is performed to rule out arterial blockages. The lungs will be evaluated for pulmonary edema. Blood pressure is monitored. Blood tests do not show indications of a heart attack.

Treatment

Treatment is the same as that for a coronary obstruction until it is ruled out. Usually the patient will remain in the hospital for a few days until magnetic resonance imaging (MRI) rules it out. The patient may be put on medications to reduce the workload of the heart. Medications may include beta-blockers, ACE inhibitors, and/or diuretics.

Prognosis

Many patients will recover within a month.

Prevention

The only prevention would be avoidance of stressful situations. Availability of support during a severe event is helpful.

Patient Teaching

Being supportive to those who are dealing with a stressful situation may help prevent the reaction.

Hypertensive Heart Disease

Hypertensive heart disease is the result of chronically elevated pressure throughout the vascular system. Atherosclerosis, arteriosclerosis, renal disease, and any condition that creates increased vascular pressure cause the heart to work harder as it pumps against the increased resistance.

Essential Hypertension

Description

Essential, or primary, hypertension, a condition of abnormally high blood pressure in the arterial system, has an insidious onset, with the patient exhibiting few, if any, symptoms until permanent damage has occurred.

ICD-10-CM Code	I10 (Essential [primary] hypertension)

Essential hypertension is listed in several ways under hypertensive heart disease. Other mentions of hypertension are listed under hypertensive heart disease, hypertensive renal disease, hypertensive heart and renal disease, and secondary hypertension. Refer to the physician's diagnosis and then to the current edition of the ICD-10-CM coding manual to ensure the greatest specificity.

Symptoms and Signs

The patient may experience headaches, epistaxis, lightheadedness, or syncope, although there usually are no symptoms. The hypertension generally is detected when blood pressure is taken during a physical examination or a screening process. Hypertension is more common with increased age in all groups. If hypertension is accompanied by hyperlipidemia, it may lead to atherosclerosis.

Patient Screening

Many patients with essential hypertension have no indication of the condition. They may seek an appointment for a headache and should be scheduled for the next available appointment. Others may have had a blood pressure reading at a recent health screening or other event and have been advised to see their physician to report the elevated reading. For these patients also, the next available appointment should be scheduled, preferably on the day of or the day after the call. Likewise for patients with a history of essential hypertension requesting an appointment for any hypertension-related symptoms, an appointment should be scheduled the same day or the next day.

Etiology

The etiology is unknown, but many factors are thought to contribute to the condition. Stress is considered a major factor in hypertension. Age, heredity, smoking, obesity, sedentary lifestyle, poor dietary habits, and hyperactive personality or type A personality are possible causative factors in essential hypertension (Fig. 10.20).

Diagnosis

Elevated blood pressure readings are the first indication of hypertension. A systolic reading of greater than 140 mm Hg and a diastolic reading of greater than 90 mm Hg indicate hypertension. Patients with systolic readings of 120 to 139 and diastolic readings of 80 to 89 mm Hg are prehypertensive. The diagnosis is based on a series of blood pressure readings in which elevated values are obtained several

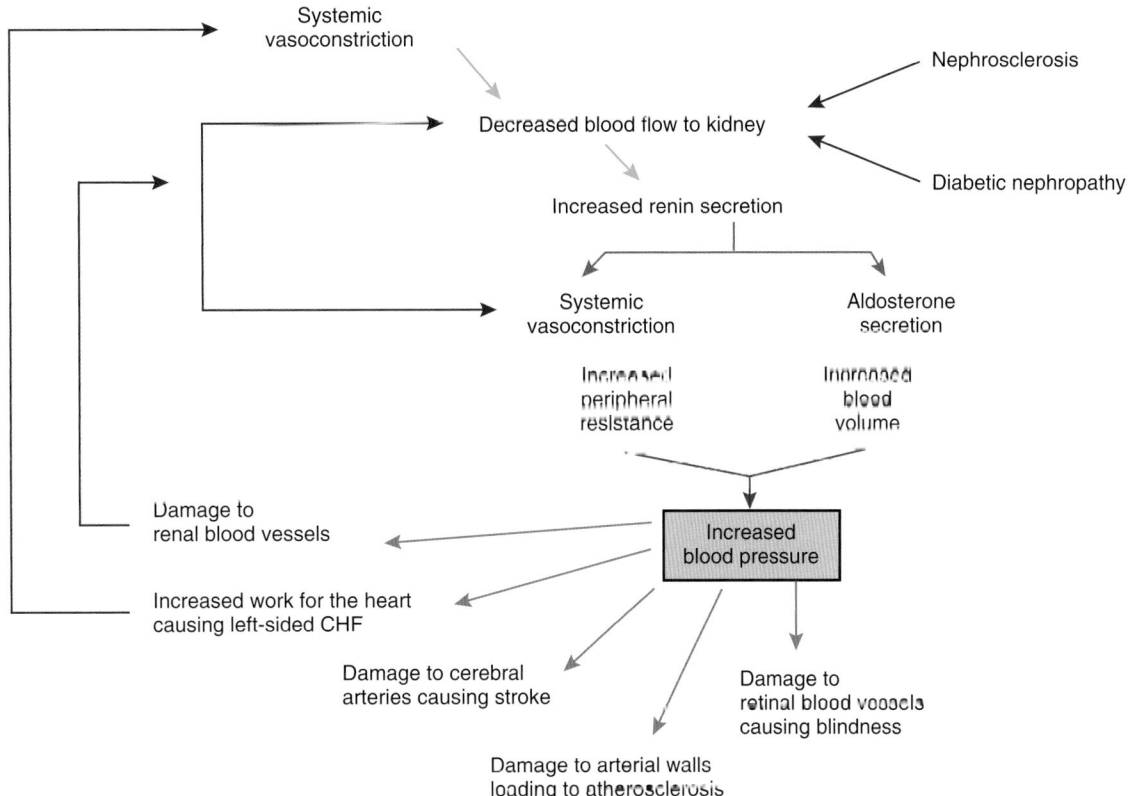

• **Fig. 10.20** Development of hypertension. (From Gould B: *Pathophysiology for the health professions,* ed 3, Philadelphia, 2006, Saunders/Elsevier.)

tumor. A careful, complete medical history, physical examination, and laboratory evaluation should be performed before diagnosis is confirmed and therapy is initiated.

Treatment

Drug therapy used in the treatment of hypertension includes diuretics (to reduce circulating blood volume), ACE inhibitors (to produce vasodilation and to increase renal blood flow), ARBs, vasodilators (to dilate vessels), and CCBs (to slow the heartbeat, to reduce conduction irritability, and to dilate vessels). These drugs may be prescribed singly or in combination. Additional modes of therapy include limitation of sodium intake, dietary management, weight reduction, exercise, reduction of stressful situations, and cessation of smoking.

Prognosis

The prognosis varies, depending on the patient's response to prescribed drug therapy and lifestyle modifications. A reduction of blood pressure by as little as 5% may decrease the risk of stroke by 30% or greater.

Prevention

Because the etiology is unknown, one cannot always prevent essential hypertension. The patient may be able to alter contributing factors by reducing stress levels, reducing sodium intake, controlling weight, exercising, and stopping smoking. Altering the individual's underlying personality, which plays a part in the condition, is difficult.

Patient Teaching

Teaching the patient that this condition is not cured but only controlled by drug therapy is essential. Education reinforces the need to monitor the blood pressure on a regular basis and the need to continue drug therapy for life. When available, use computer-based health education to teach patients about home monitoring of blood pressure.

Malignant Hypertension

Description

Malignant hypertension, a life-threatening condition, is a severe form of hypertension.

ICD-10-CM Code	I10 *(Essential [primary] hypertension)*

Malignant hypertension is listed in several ways under hypertensive heart disease. Other mentions of malignant hypertension are listed under hypertensive heart disease, hypertensive renal disease, hypertensive heart and renal disease, and secondary hypertension. Refer to the physician's diagnosis and then to the current edition of the ICD-10-CM coding manual to ensure the greatest specificity of pathology.

Symptoms and Signs

Severe headache, blurred vision, and dyspnea are symptoms that suggest the condition. The onset of symptoms may be sudden.

Patient Screening

As with essential hypertension, many people with malignant hypertension are unaware of the condition. Some may report having been advised to contact their doctor for an elevated blood pressure reading. Others may complain of a severe headache. Previously diagnosed patients with essential hypertension may complain of the sudden onset of a severe headache, blurred vision, and dyspnea. These patients are at risk for a cerebrovascular accident (CVA) and require prompt assessment and intervention.

Etiology

The etiology of this severe form of essential hypertension is unknown, although extreme stress is thought to be a contributing factor.

Diagnosis

Notable blood pressure elevation is considered malignant hypertension. In severe cases, the systolic pressure reading may be greater than 200 mm Hg and the diastolic pressure reading greater than 120 mm Hg.

Treatment

Aggressive intervention is indicated in severe malignant hypertension. IV vasodilators, such as diazoxide (Hyperstat) and sodium nitroprusside (Nipride), should be administered. After the condition is under control, blood pressure should be monitored on a regular basis and drug therapy continued for life.

Prognosis

The prognosis varies, depending on the patient's response to drug therapy. These patients are at risk for a CVA, or stroke, and irreversible renal damage. When drug therapy is unsuccessful, the patient is likely to succumb to the condition after a CVA.

Prevention

With the etiology being unknown, preventing this condition is difficult. Those who have been diagnosed with hypertension, however, should comply with drug therapy and reduce their stress. The preventive measures suggested for essential hypertension also apply to malignant hypertension. If high blood pressure happens quickly and results in some type of organ damage, then it is referred to as *malignant hypertension.*

Patient Teaching

Emphasize the importance of complying with drug therapy to patients and their families. Encourage patients to modify lifestyles to reduce stress in their lives. Give patients and their families dietary information about low-fat, low-cholesterol, and low-sodium diets and blood pressure management. Educate overweight patients about the importance of weight reduction and exercise. Encourage discussion concerning the dangers of malignant hypertension.

Congestive Heart Failure

Description

CHF is the acute or chronic inability of the heart to pump enough blood throughout the body to meet the demands of homeostasis.

ICD-10-CM Code	I50.9 *(Heart failure, unspecified)*
	(I50.1-I50.9 = 14 codes of specificity)

Refer to the physician's diagnosis and then to the current edition of the ICD-10-CM coding manual to ensure the greatest specificity.

Symptoms and Signs

CHF usually has an insidious onset, with the patient experiencing gradually increasing dyspnea. Cardiac and respiratory rates increase, and the patient becomes anxious. As the condition progresses, the neck veins distend, and edema is noted in the ankles. When the right side of the heart fails, the liver and spleen enlarge, and peripheral edema is more prominent. Left-sided CHF causes increased pulmonary congestion and more pronounced respiratory difficulties (Fig. 10.21).

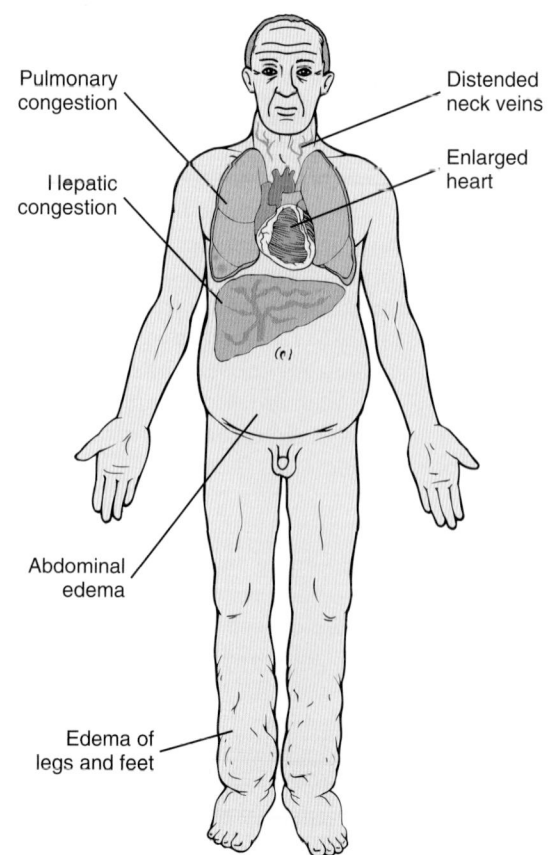

• **Fig. 10.21** Signs of congestive heart failure (CHF).

Patient Screening

Patients reporting unexplained chest discomfort, shortness of breath, or swelling of limbs require prompt medical assessment.

Etiology

Underlying conditions can compromise the pumping action of the heart, resulting in heart failure and inadequate perfusion. A common cause of acute CHF is MI (Fig. 10.22). Some causes of chronic CHF are hypertension, CAD, chronic obstructive pulmonary disease (COPD),

cardiac valve damage, arrhythmias (dysrhythmias), and cardiomyopathy.

Diagnosis

The diagnosis is made after a thorough history and physical examination. Breath sounds are diminished, and radiographs indicate the presence of fluid in the lungs (Fig. 10.23). ECG is used to discover the underlying causes. Echocardiography helps evaluate cardiac chamber size, ventricular function, and disease of the myocardium,

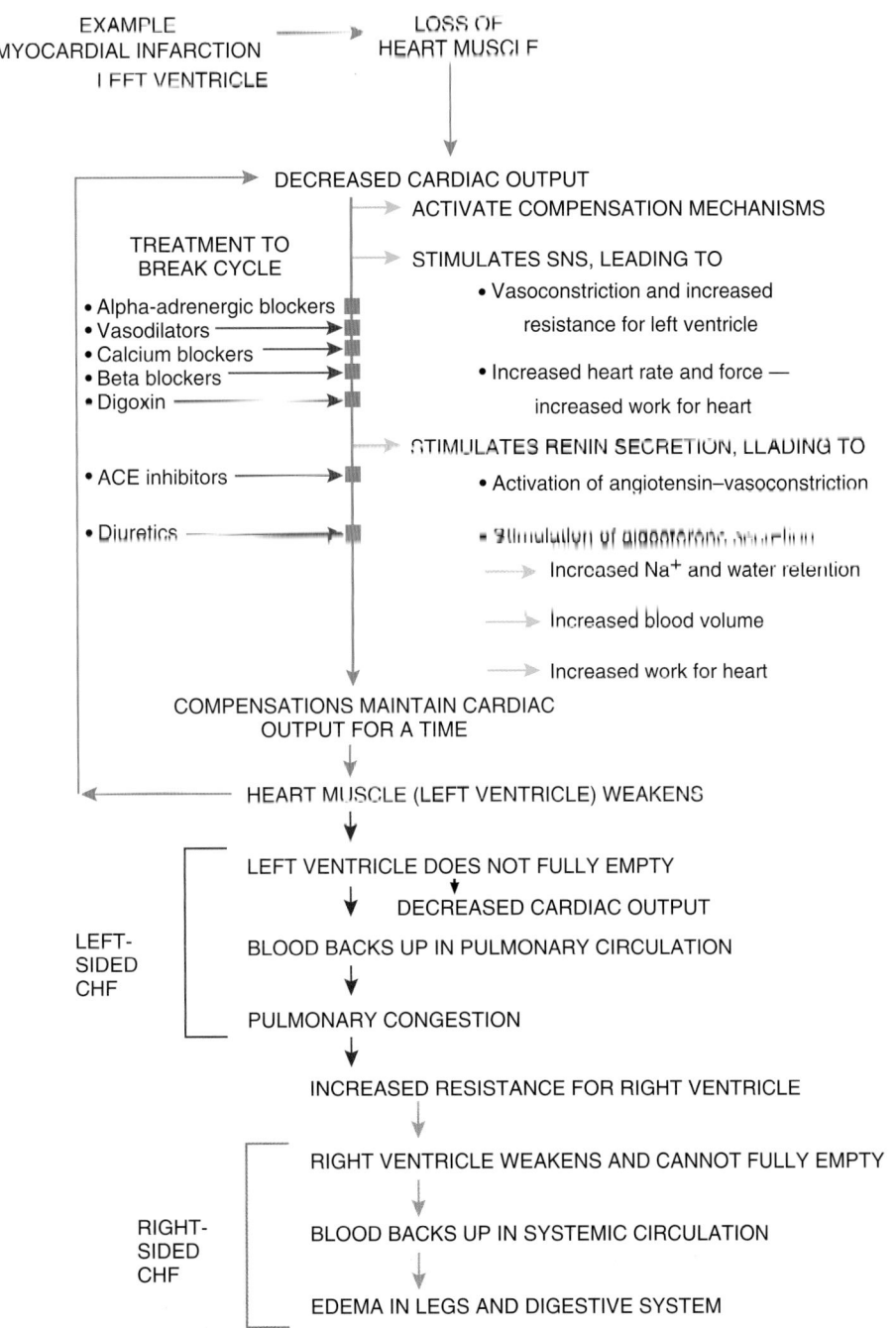

• **Fig. 10.22** Course of congestive heart failure (CHF). *ACE,* Angiotensin-converting enzyme; *CHF,* congestive heart failure; *SNS,* sympathetic nervous system. (From Gould B: *Pathophysiology for the health professions,* ed 3, Philadelphia, 2006, Saunders/Elsevier.)

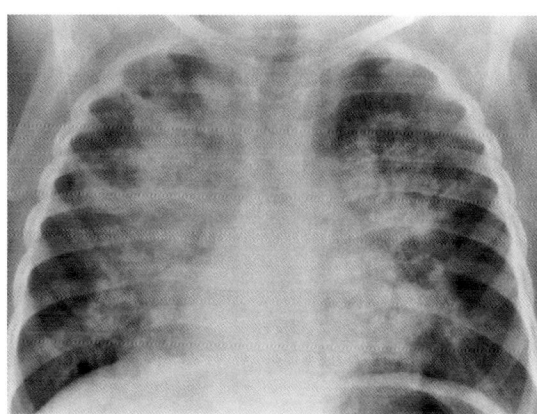

• **Fig. 10.23** Radiograph: Congestive heart failure (CHF). (From Long BW, Frank ED, Ehrlich RA: *Radiography essentials for limited practice*, ed 4, St Louis, 2013, Elsevier.)

valves, cardiac structures (walls, septum, and papillary muscles), and pericardium (the covering of the heart) (Fig. 10.24). Catheterization can be used to monitor the pressures in the circulation.

Treatment

Treatment is directed at reducing the workload of the heart and increasing its efficiency. ACE inhibitors and ARBs recently were approved for use in the treatment of CHF, mainly to increase blood flow. Diuretics help reduce the volume of fluid in the body, and vasodilators help reduce vascular pressure. Aldosterone antagonists (eplerenone or spironolactone) may be used in combination with other drug therapies. Digoxin may also be prescribed in specific cases to strengthen and slow the heartbeat. Intake of fluid and sodium is restricted. Some patients with severe CHF may require special pacemakers, defibrillators, or, in extreme cases, heart transplantation.

Prognosis

The prognosis varies. Acute CHF usually responds well to medical interventions and therefore has a positive outcome. The patient with chronic CHF is vulnerable to major organ impairment and resulting complications.

Prevention

Public education about the contributors to heart health and control of blood pressure continue to produce positive statistical results, especially in the male population. Early medical intervention for CHF is important to prevent multiple organ complications.

Patient Teaching

A primary goal is promoting good patient compliance with the medical treatment plan. Explain that many patients experience quick alleviation of symptoms when they take medications as prescribed, follow dietary instructions, and modify activities to allow required rest and to avoid fatigue. The use of diuretics requires patients to monitor their weight on a daily basis.

Cor Pulmonale

Description

Cor pulmonale, also known as *right-sided heart disease,* results in enlargement of the right ventricle as a sequela of primary lung disease.

ICD-10-CM Code	I27.81 *(Cor pulmonale [chronic])*
	I27.9 *(Pulmonary heart disease, unspecified)*
	(I27.0-I27.9 = 7 codes of specificity)

Symptoms and Signs

Cor pulmonale causes the patient to experience dyspnea, distended neck veins, and edema of the extremities. The liver is enlarged and tender.

Patient Screening

Patients reporting unexplained chest discomfort, shortness of breath, or swelling of limbs require prompt medical assessment.

Etiology

Right-sided heart failure is an outcome of acute or chronic pulmonary disease and pulmonary hypertension. The diseased pulmonary blood vessels impair the flow of blood to pulmonary tissue. The increased pulmonary blood pressure increases the workload of the right side of the heart, causing the right ventricle to hypertrophy and thus to become less effective in pumping blood to the lungs. Chronic conditions causing cor pulmonale include emphysema and fibrotic pulmonary lesions, and the primary acute causative factor is pulmonary emboli. Chronic hypoxemia stimulates bone marrow in an adaptive response to produce an increased number of red blood cells (RBCs) to carry additional oxygen. This condition of abnormally high levels of RBCs (polycythemia) increases the viscosity of blood.

Diagnosis

The diagnosis is based on a history of pulmonary disease and hypoxia. The patient's respiratory status and cardiac status are assessed for neck vein distention and peripheral edema. Chest radiographic studies and echocardiography reveal pulmonary congestion and right-sided heart enlargement, and ECG frequently shows arrhythmias. If polycythemia is present, the RBC count is elevated.

Treatment

Treatment entails relieving the causative factors in the pulmonary system and reducing hypoxemia. Bronchodilators are administered. Supplemental oxygen provides additional comfort to the patient. Bed rest is encouraged, and digitalis preparations are administered to strengthen and slow the heartbeat. Diuretics are prescribed when edema is present. Anticoagulants are given to avoid the

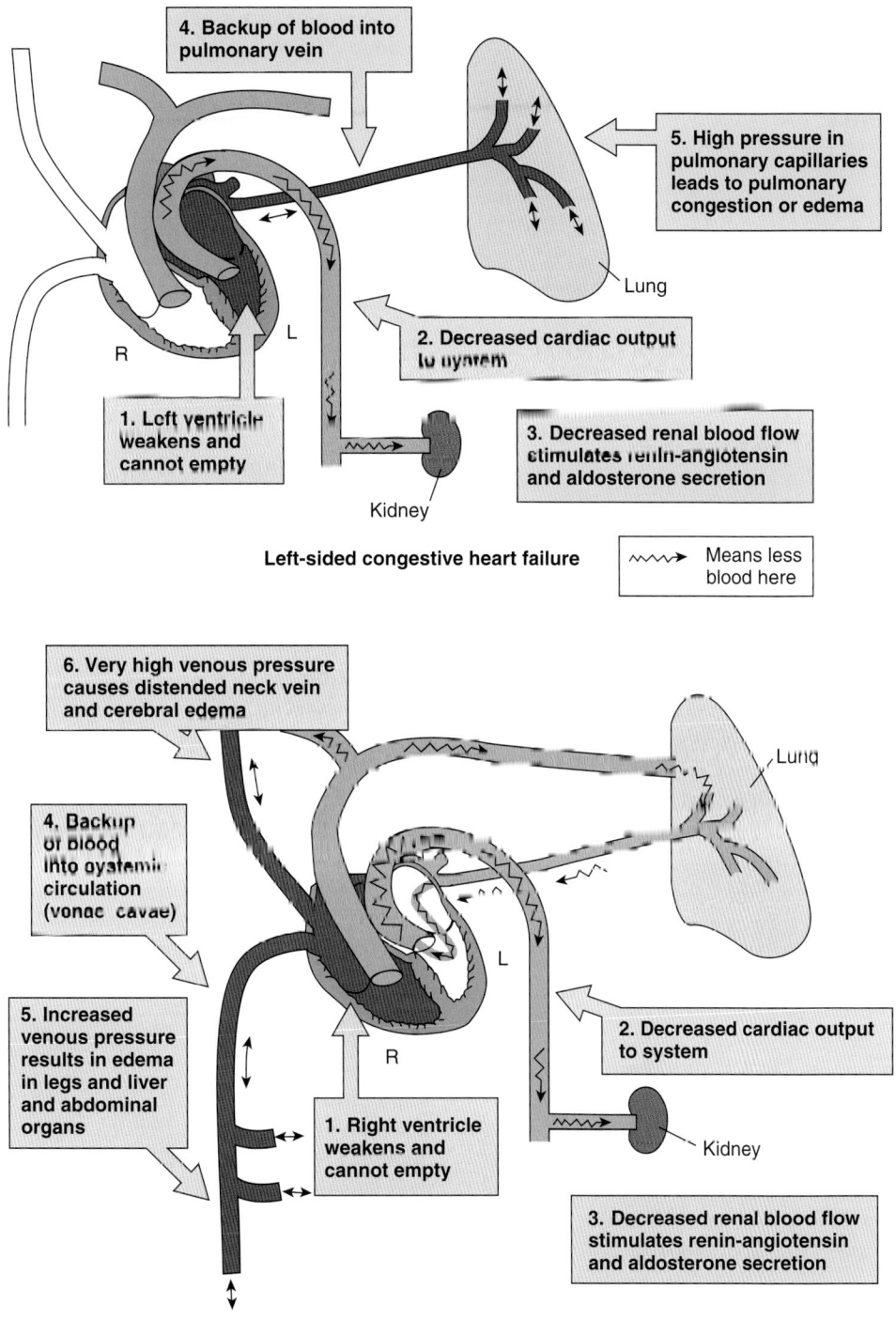

• Fig. 10.24 Effects of congestive heart failure (CHF). (From Gould B: *Pathophysiology for the health professions,* ed 2, Philadelphia, 2002, Saunders/Elsevier.)

risk of thromboembolisms. **Phlebotomy**, surgical puncture of a vein to withdraw blood, may be used when polycythemia is a problem. A low-salt diet is encouraged.

Prognosis

The outcome depends on the patient's response to treatment of the many possible disorders that predispose to cor pulmonale.

Prevention

No direct prevention of this condition is known. Many of the predisposing factors have no preventive measures to be taken.

Patient Teaching

Emphasize the instructions given by the physician. Explain the dosage schedule, and encourage compliance with drug therapy. Give patients information on possible side effects. Advise patients to report any adverse effects of medications.

Pulmonary Edema

Description

Pulmonary edema is a condition of fluid shift into the extravascular spaces of the lungs.

ICD-10-CM Code	J81.0 (Acute pulmonary edema)
	(J81.0-J81.1 = 2 codes of specificity)
	I50.1 (Left ventricular failure)
	J18.2 (Hypostatic pneumonia, unspecified organism)
	(J18.0-J18.9 = 5 codes of specificity)
	J81.1 (Chronic pulmonary edema)

Refer to the physician's diagnosis and then to the current edition of the ICD-10-CM coding manual to ensure the greatest specificity.

Symptoms and Signs

Pulmonary edema causes patients to experience dyspnea and coughing; orthopnea, a condition in which breathing becomes easier in the upright standing or sitting position; increased cardiac and respiratory rates; and often bloody, frothy sputum. Blood pressure may fall, and the skin becomes cold and clammy. The symptoms often occur at night after the patient lies down.

Patient Screening

Patients complaining of shortness of breath, typically when lying down, should be instructed to seek emergency care.

Etiology

Pulmonary edema is caused by left-sided heart failure, mitral valve disease, pulmonary embolus, systemic hypertension, arrhythmias, and renal failure. Head trauma, drug overdose, and exposure to high altitudes are other causes. Excessive fluid accumulates in the pulmonary tissue and air spaces of the lungs. The pulmonary circulation is overloaded with an excessive volume of blood (Fig. 10.25).

Diagnosis

The clinical picture of dyspnea, orthopnea, and bloody, frothy sputum leads to further investigation. Breath sounds are diminished, with the presence of rales, rhonchi, and wheezing. Arterial blood gas measurement shows reduced oxygen saturation, increased carbon dioxide retention, increased bicarbonate levels, and decreased pH of the blood. Chest radiographs show increased opacity of the pulmonary tissue, an enlarged heart, and prominent pulmonary vessels.

Treatment

The patient is placed in the Fowler position (sitting), and oxygen therapy is administered. Drug therapy includes diuretics to improve fluid excretion; IV vasodilators, such as nitroglycerine or nitroprusside; morphine sulfate to induce venous dilation; and beta$_2$-adrenergic drugs to dilate the bronchioles and to control bronchial spasms. Severe cases may require mechanical ventilation.

Prognosis

Pulmonary edema is a life-threatening condition and is considered a medical emergency. The prognosis varies, depending on the severity of the pulmonary edema and the patient's response to intervention.

Prevention

Certain causes are controlled by prevention of heart disease and avoidance of risk factors, such as drug overdose.

Patient Teaching

Encourage compliance with drug therapy and follow-up care. Patients taking diuretics are instructed about the importance of monitoring weight on a daily basis.

Cardiomyopathy

Description

Cardiomyopathy is a noninflammatory disease of the cardiac muscle resulting in enlargement of the myocardium and ventricular dysfunction. Refer to Chapter 2 for a discussion about hypertrophic cardiomyopathy.

ICD-10-CM Code	I42.3 (Endomyocardial [eosinophilic] disease)

Cardiomyopathy is coded according to type. Refer to the physician's diagnosis and then to the current edition of the ICD-10-CM coding manual to ensure the greatest specificity.

Symptoms and Signs

Cardiomyopathy causes the patient to experience symptoms of CHF, including dyspnea, fatigue, tachycardia, palpitations, and occasionally chest pain. Peripheral edema and hepatic congestion also may be present. Syncope and cardiac murmurs may occur. The symptoms and signs vary with the type and cause of this condition.

Patient Screening

Patients reporting dyspnea, fatigue, tachycardia, palpitations, and occasional chest pain require prompt assessment by a physician.

Etiology

Primary causes are mostly unknown. Cardiomyopathies are divided into three groups: dilated, hypertrophic, and restrictive. Dilated cardiomyopathy can be the result of chronic alcoholism, an autoimmune process, or viral infections. Regardless of the cause, dilated cardiomyopathies result in diffuse degeneration of the myocardial fibers. This is followed by a decrease in contractile effort.

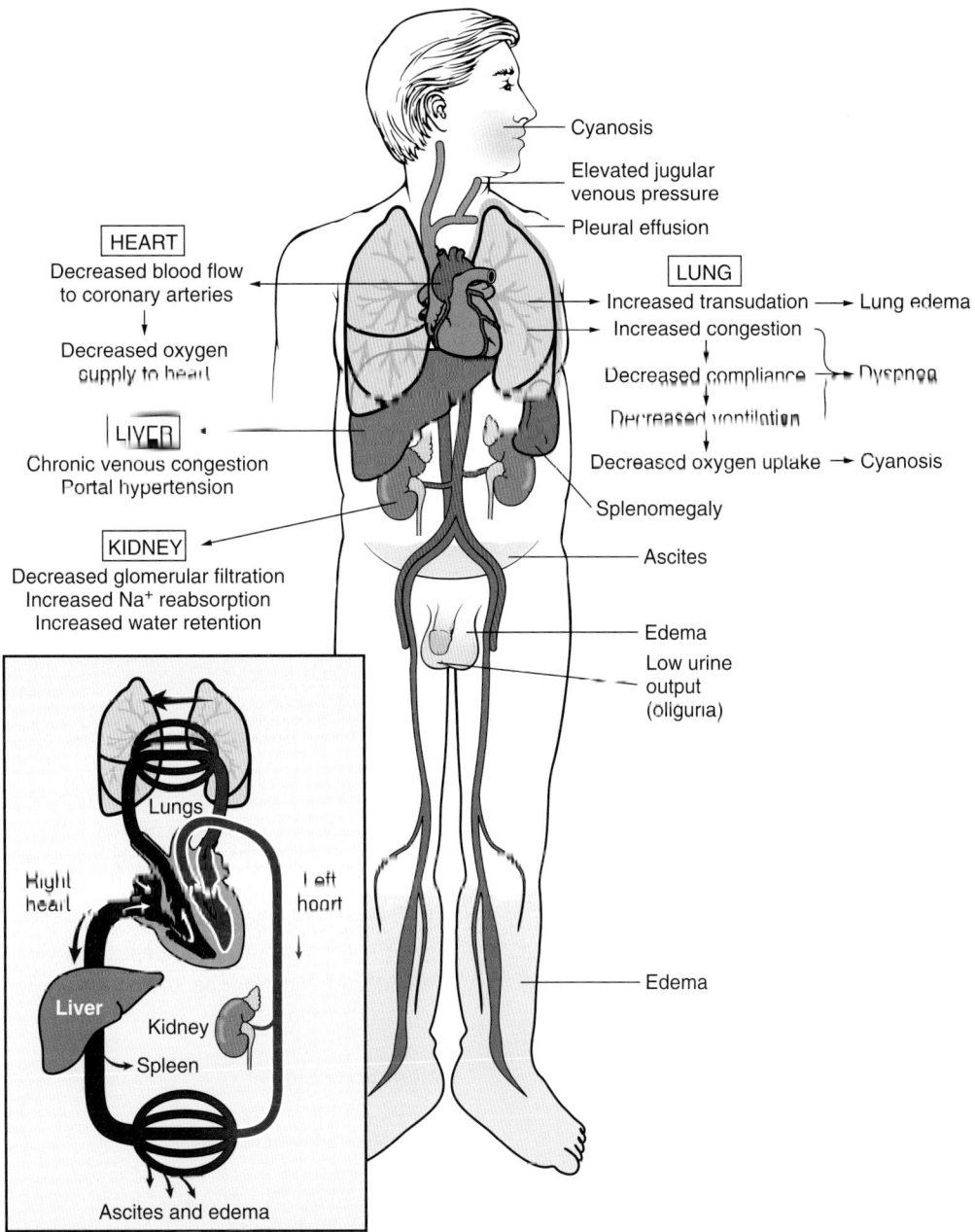

HEART
Decreased blood flow
to coronary arteries
↓
Decreased oxygen
supply to heart

LIVER
Chronic venous congestion
Portal hypertension

KIDNEY
Decreased glomerular filtration
Increased Na⁺ reabsorption
Increased water retention

Cyanosis

Elevated jugular
venous pressure

Pleural effusion

LUNG
Increased transudation → Lung edema
Increased congestion
↓
Decreased compliance → Dyspnea
↓
Decreased ventilation
↓
Decreased oxygen uptake → Cyanosis

Splenomegaly

Ascites

Edema

Low urine
output
(oliguria)

Edema

Lungs

Right
heart

Left
heart

Liver

Kidney

→ Spleen

Ascites and edema

• **Fig. 10.25** Chronic passive congestion. Left heart failure leads to pulmonary edema. Right ventricular failure causes peripheral edema that is most prominent in the lower extremities. (From Damjanov I: *Pathology for the health-related professions,* ed 4, St Louis, 2011, Saunders/Elsevier.)

Hypertrophic cardiomyopathies are thought to be genetic and are considered idiopathic. The left ventricular wall hypertrophies, as does the interventricular septum, resulting in a small and elongated left ventricle and possible obstruction of the aortic valve.

Restrictive cardiomyopathy is a rare condition occurring when any infiltrative process of the heart causes fibrosis and thickening of the myocardium resulting in the walls of the ventricles becoming stiffened.

The walls are usually normal in size or only slightly thickened. The stiff muscle that does not relax normally results in the chamber not filling properly with blood. Thus it is harder for the ventricles to fill with adequate blood. The rigidity of the walls does not permit the ventricular muscles to pump correctly, resulting in reduced amounts of blood being pumped from the ventricles. The inability of the heart to pump blood properly may lead to heart failure.

Diagnosis

The diagnosis includes a thorough patient history and a complete physical examination. Cardiomegaly at various stages is present, along with assorted cardiac murmurs. Chest radiographs confirm the presence of cardiomegaly, and ECG reveals rate and rhythm abnormalities. Echocardiography and cardiac catheterization may help identify the type of cardiomyopathy and the extent of the condition. Biopsy may be required.

Treatment

Treatment is determined by the type of cardiomyopathy. Therapy for dilated cardiomyopathies is aimed at appropriate control of the CHF by means of the measures previously described for the treatment of CHF. Antiarrhythmic agents, digitalis, and anticoagulant drugs are prescribed. Activities are limited, with some patients restricted to bed rest. Treatment of hypertrophic cardiomyopathies also is aimed at reducing the workload of the heart. Beta-adrenergic blockers, such as propranolol hydrochloride (Inderal), reduce myocardial contractility, heart rate, and conductivity, thus preventing arrhythmias. CCBs are prescribed to help reduce blood pressure and relax the heart muscle. ACE inhibitors are used to help relax blood vessels and reduce the heart's workload. Treatment of restrictive cardiomyopathies also includes reducing the workload of the heart. The changes in the cardiac muscle caused by the infiltrates are irreversible, making the prognosis poor for these patients.

Prognosis

Medication improves the survival of these patients. Some conditions can be fatal, with the only hope for survival being offered by heart transplantation.

Prevention

In many cases, these conditions are idiopathic. Prevention is nonspecific, depending on the original underlying causative factor.

Patient Teaching

Focus on improving the patient's compliance with the medical treatment plan. Encourage patients to avoid alcohol and to limit salt intake. Provide information about support groups for people living with chronic disease.

Pericarditis

Description

Pericarditis is an acute or chronic inflammation of the pericardium (serosa), the sac enclosing and protecting the heart (Fig. 10.26).

ICD-10-CM Code	I31.9 *(Disease of pericardium, unspecified)*
	(I30.0-I32 = 12 codes of specificity)

Pericarditis is coded by type. Refer to the physician's diagnosis and then to the current edition of the ICD-10-CM coding manual to ensure the greatest specificity.

Symptoms and Signs

The space between the outer parietal layer of pericardium and the inner visceral layer of epicardium (heart wall) normally is filled with a small amount of thin, lubricating serous fluid (see Fig. 10.6). When blood or inflammatory exudate is released into the pericardial sac, or pericardial

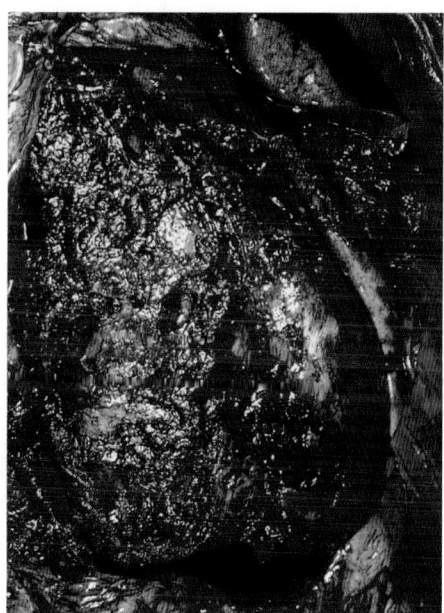

• **Fig. 10.26** Pericarditis. (From Damjanov I: *Pathology for the health professions,* ed 5, St Louis, 2017, Elsevier.)

space, friction and irritation between the layers result in pericarditis. Associated manifestations include fever, malaise, chest pain that fluctuates with inspiration or heartbeat, dyspnea, and chills. The patient may feel anxious and report a "pounding heart." A detectable friction rub, or grating sound, in phase with the heartbeat can be heard on auscultation with a stethoscope. Tachycardia may be present. Pericarditis can occur in different forms. It can be a benign or isolated process or can be secondary to infection elsewhere in the body, so the clinical signs vary.

Patient Screening

Patients complaining of chest pain are advised to seek immediate medical attention.

Etiology

Pericarditis is idiopathic or a consequence of inflammation or infection elsewhere in the body. Other causative agents are viruses, bacteria (producing a suppurative pericarditis), trauma, rheumatic fever, and malignant neoplastic disease. The condition may occur secondary to MI. Acute inflammation of the pericardium can cause adhesions (scarring) to form between the pericardium and the heart, or it can cause a loss of elasticity, producing constrictive pericarditis. Conversely, chronic pericarditis can incite fibrous calcification of the visceral membrane, which comes in direct contact with the myocardium. A scarred and rigid pericardium interferes with the heart's ability to contract normally, with a subsequent drop in cardiac output (Fig. 10.27).

Diagnosis

Blood studies may lead to the identification of a causative organism. They also may reveal elevated white blood cell (WBC) count, erythrocyte sedimentation rate (ESR), and

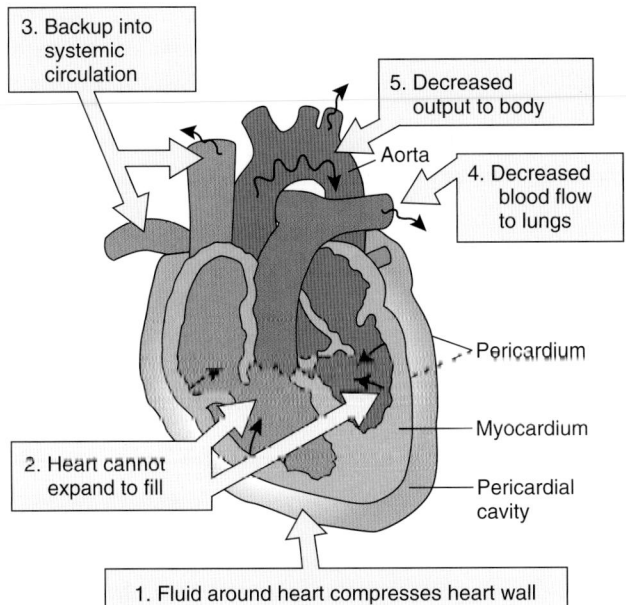

3. Backup into systemic circulation

5. Decreased output to body

Aorta

4. Decreased blood flow to lungs

Pericardium

Myocardium

2. Heart cannot expand to fill

Pericardial cavity

1. Fluid around heart compresses heart wall

• **Fig. 10.27** Effects of pericardial effusion. (From Gould B: *Pathophysiology for the health professions,* ed 3, Philadelphia, 2006, Saunders/Elsevier.)

cardiac enzyme levels. Changes are noted on ECG. Echocardiography may confirm the presence of pericardial fluid and reveal a thickened pericardium. In constrictive pericarditis, cardiac catheterization shows elevated pressures in the cardiac chambers.

Treatment

Treatment is directed at managing the underlying systemic disease and at reducing inflammation and pain. Therapy for infectious pericarditis requires treatment with antibiotic drugs and possibly surgical drainage or aspiration. Complete bed rest and the administration of analgesics, antipyretics, and nonsteroidal antiinflammatory drugs (NSAIDs) are prescribed. Corticosteroids may be prescribed.

Prognosis

Acute pericarditis usually resolves with complete recovery. Extensive adhesions or calcification resulting from chronic pericarditis may necessitate resection of the pericardium.

Prevention

Prompt treatment of infections is a preventive measure for pericarditis.

Patient Teaching

Encourage the patient to seek prompt treatment for infections. Emphasize the importance of completing the antibiotic regimen.

Myocarditis

Description

Myocarditis is inflammation of the muscular walls of the heart.

ICD-10-CM Code   I51.4 *(Myocarditis, unspecified)*

Symptoms and Signs

Myocarditis involves damage to the myocardium by pathogenic invasion or toxic insult. The condition may be acute or chronic, may involve a small part of the myocardium or be diffuse and can occur at any age. The patient may report palpitations, fatigue, and dyspnea. Physical examination may reveal fever, arrhythmia, and tenderness in the chest.

Patient Screening

Patients complaining of dyspnea and palpitations are advised to seek immediate medical attention.

Etiology

Myocarditis is frequently a viral, bacterial, fungal, or protozoal infection or a complication of other diseases, such as influenza, diphtheria, mumps, and, most significantly, rheumatic fever; it is occasionally idiopathic. It also may be associated with MI. Exposure to certain toxic agents through lithium use, chronic use of cocaine, chronic alcoholism, radiation, and chemical poisoning can cause inflammation of the myocardium. In addition, it may be a complication of a collagen disease.

Diagnosis

Diagnostic findings may include an elevated WBC count, increased ESR, elevated cardiac enzyme levels, ventricular enlargement noted on chest radiographs, and an abnormal ECG reading. Myocardial biopsy confirms the inflammation of cardiac muscle tissue and may identify the cause.

Treatment

When infection is the underlying cause, appropriate antiinfective agents are given. The patient is advised to rest and to reduce the heart's workload. Medications, such as quinidine procainamide, digoxin, and diuretics, may be required to stabilize arrhythmia. Analgesics, antiinflammatory agents, ACE inhibitors, and oxygen are also prescribed.

Prognosis

The prognosis for complete recovery is favorable unless the condition is chronic and causes damage to the cardiac muscle.

Prevention

Depending on the underlying cause, prevention is not always possible. In some cases, early treatment of infections with a complete course of antimicrobial agents can prevent the onset of myocarditis.

Patient Teaching

Emphasize the importance of rest and close monitoring by the physician through follow-up appointments during the recovery process. Give the patient a list of the complications that should be reported to the physician, such as difficulty breathing, weakness, and accumulation of fluid in the extremities.

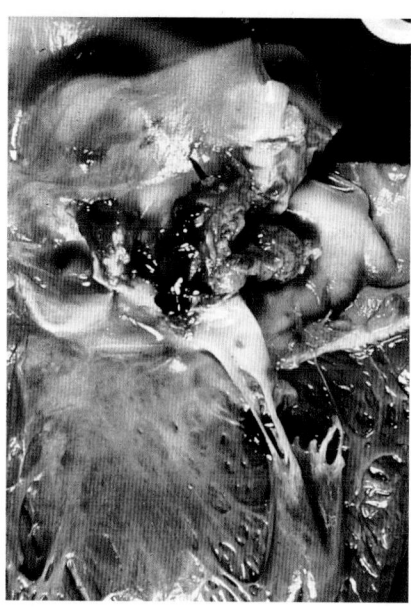

• **Fig. 10.28** Bacterial endocarditis. The valves are covered with extensive vegetations. (From Damjanov I: *Pathology for the health professions*, ed 5, St Louis, 2017, Elsevier.)

Endocarditis

Description
Endocarditis is inflammation of the lining and the valves of the heart (Fig. 10.28).

| ICD-10-CM Code | I38 (Endocarditis, valve unspecified) |

Endocarditis is coded by type and site. Refer to the physician's diagnosis and then to the current edition of the ICD-10-CM coding manual to ensure the greatest specificity.

Symptoms and Signs
Endocarditis is usually secondary to infection elsewhere in the body (Fig. 10.29), the result of preexisting heart disease, or the consequence of an abnormal immunologic reaction. The patient may have vague to pronounced symptoms of infection, including fever, chills, night sweats, weakness, anorexia, and fatigue.

The condition is characterized by vegetative growths on the cardiac valves that may be released into the bloodstream in the form of emboli. These emboli can lodge in vessels and cause symptoms of ischemia. The sites of ischemia may be the heart, lungs, kidneys, brain, or extremities. Dysfunction of the valves, which may not close effectively, disrupts or obstructs blood flow through the chambers of the heart; this dysfunction of the valves usually produces a cardiac murmur heard on auscultation. Serious obstruction or regurgitation of blood flow through the heart affects the pumping effectiveness of the heart and causes complications.

Patient Screening
A patient complaining of persistent fatigue, night sweats, and/or fever requires prompt assessment by a physician.

Etiology
Bacteremia, or the presence of infectious agents in the bloodstream, can lead to endocarditis. Common infecting organisms include *Staphylococcus aureus,* group A beta-hemolytic streptococci, and *Escherichia coli.* IV drug users are at high risk for fungal endocarditis. Patients with damaged cardiac valves as a result of rheumatic disease are more prone to endocarditis. Septic emboli from endocarditis can be carried by the arterial circulation and then embed in major organs, resulting in infarcts and new places of bacterial infections (Fig. 10.30).

Diagnosis
A complete blood count (CBC) may indicate leukocytosis, and an elevated ESR may be present. Blood cultures may reveal the causative organism. Echocardiography shows valve involvement with vegetation or abscesses. ECG may indicate arrhythmia and conduction defects.

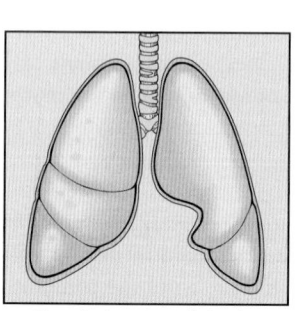
Respiratory tract infection

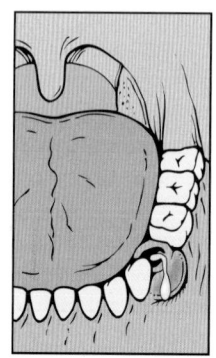
Dental infection

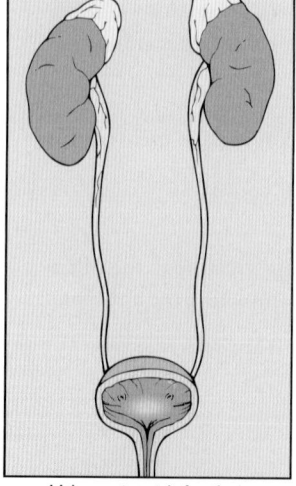
Urinary tract infection

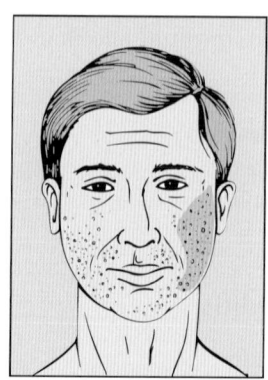
Skin infection

• **Fig. 10.29** Causative factors in endocarditis.

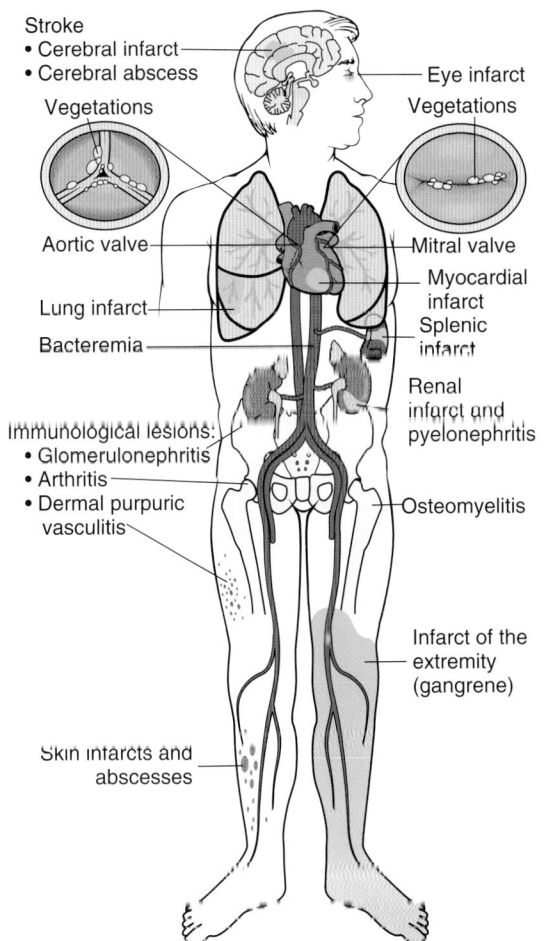

• **Fig. 10.30** Septic emboli from endocarditis are carried by the arterial circulation and may lodge in major organs, causing infarcts and new sites of bacterial infection. (From Damjanov I: *Pathology for the health professions,* ed 5, St Louis, 2017, Elsevier.)

Treatment

Identification of the causative organism dictates the antiinfective therapy (usually IV antibiotics), which continues for several weeks. Other medications include antipyretics, anticoagulants, and drugs indicated to treat any complications. Bed rest is recommended during the acute phase. Damaged cardiac valves may need surgical repair or replacement.

Prognosis

Early diagnosis and treatment with antibiotics usually brings complete recovery. Untreated patients can have a poor prognosis.

Prevention

After recovery, the patient must understand the importance of taking prophylactic antibiotics before dental work, childbirth, or any invasive procedures associated with transient bacteremia.

New guidelines established in 2007 by the AHA no longer recommend antibiotics for many routine dental procedures. Prophylaxis is recommended for dental procedures that involve manipulation of the gingival tissue or the periapical region of teeth or perforation of the oral mucosa. (This may include routine cleaning, extraction, biopsy, suture removal, and so on.) Current guidelines should always be checked for updates.

Patient Teaching

Instruct the patient to take the full course of antibiotics and to obtain plenty of rest.

Rheumatic Fever

Description

Rheumatic fever is a systemic inflammatory and autoimmune disease involving the joints and the cardiac tissue.

> ICD-10-CM Code   I00 *(Rheumatic fever without heart involvement)*
> *Rheumatic fever is coded according to mention of heart involvement. Refer to the physician's diagnosis and then to the current edition of the ICD-10-CM coding manual to ensure the greatest specificity of pathology.*

Symptoms and Signs

Rheumatic fever follows a sore throat caused by group A beta-hemolytic *Streptococcus.* The patient, usually a child, experiences a fever and polyarthritis, including joint pain, edema, redness, and limited range of motion. Joints frequently involved include the finger, knee, and ankle joints, with transient inflammation in these joints. In addition, the patient experiences carditis, cardiac murmurs, cardiomegaly, and even CHF. Other symptoms include weakness, malaise, anorexia, weight loss, a rash on the trunk, abdominal pain, and the development of small nodules on the tendon sheaths in the knees, knuckles, and elbows. The symptoms occur 1 to 5 weeks after the upper respiratory tract infection.

Patient Screening

Patients with vague symptoms of fatigue, joint pain, and fever after an episode of upper respiratory infection and sore throat require prompt assessment by a physician.

Etiology

After a sore throat caused by group A beta-hemolytic *Streptococcus,* antibodies against the bacteria develop and cross-react with normal tissue. This autoimmune disease causes the antibodies to attack the body's own cells and to initiate an inflammatory reaction. The antibodies migrate to the endocardium and the mitral and sometimes the aortic valves, where vegetations form on the tissue. The carditis usually follows the joint pain and fever by a week and can affect all layers of the heart (Fig. 10.31).

Diagnosis

The history of an upper respiratory tract infection in the preceding few weeks suggests rheumatic fever. No single diagnostic feature identifies the condition. The presence of

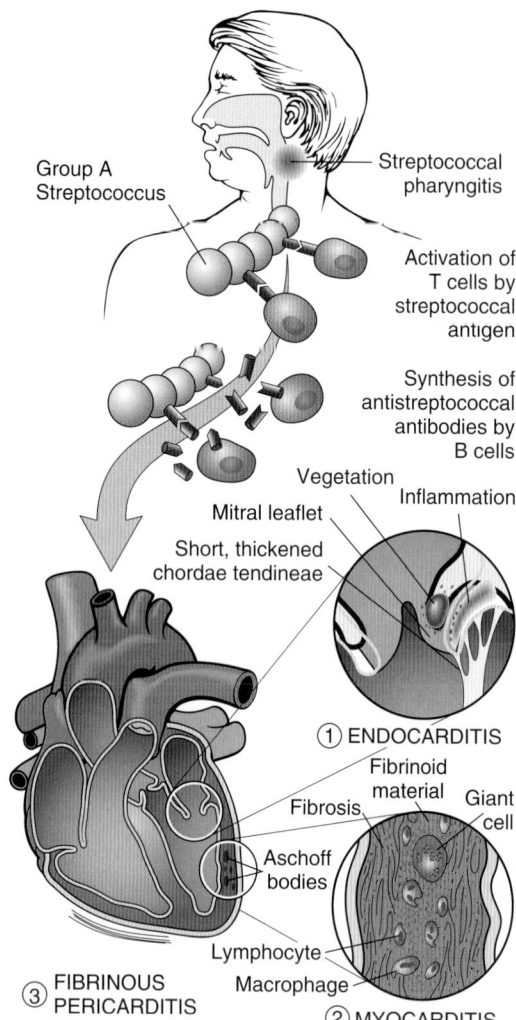

Group A Streptococcus

Streptococcal pharyngitis

Activation of T cells by streptococcal antigen

Synthesis of antistreptococcal antibodies by B cells

Vegetation

Inflammation

Mitral leaflet

Short, thickened chordae tendineae

① ENDOCARDITIS

Fibrinoid material

Fibrosis

Giant cell

Aschoff bodies

Lymphocyte

Macrophage

③ FIBRINOUS PERICARDITIS

② MYOCARDITIS

• **Fig. 10.31** Pathogenesis of rheumatic fever. After infection (with strep throat), an immune response elicited by the streptococci acts on the heart and several other organs, most notably the joints, skin, and central nervous system (CNS). In the heart, it causes endocarditis, myocarditis, and pericarditis. (From Damjanov I: *Pathology for the health professions,* ed 5, St Louis, 2017, Elsevier.)

The completion of the full course of antibiotic therapy is essential. Pediatric autoimmune neuropsychiatric disorders associated with streptococcal infections (PANDAS; an obsessive compulsive disorder) can be the result of untreated or undertreated beta-hemolytic streptococcal infections.

Prognosis
The prognosis is good with treatment.

Prevention
Prevention is through prophylactic administration of antibiotics after a strep throat has been diagnosed.

Patient Teaching
Emphasize the importance of completing the full course of the antibiotic therapy. Reassure the parents of the child with rheumatic fever that recovery usually occurs after medical treatment. Encourage the parents of a child with strep throat to seek medical attention, including beta-hemolytic strep screening.

Rheumatic Heart Disease
Description
Rheumatic heart disease refers to cardiac manifestations that occur after rheumatic fever.

ICD-10-CM Code	I01.0 *(Acute rheumatic pericarditis)*
	(I01.0-I01.9 = 5 codes of specificity)

Rheumatic heart disease is coded according to type and tissue involvement. Refer to the physician's diagnosis and then to the current edition of the ICD-10-CM coding manual to ensure the greatest specificity of pathology.

Symptoms and Signs
Acute endocarditis, which leads to chronic cardiac involvement, includes valvular damage because vegetations cause stenosis of the valves, particularly the mitral and aortic valves (Fig. 10.32). Rheumatic heart disease causes dyspnea, tachycardia, edema, a nonproductive cough, and cardiac murmurs.

Patient Screening
Patients with vague symptoms of fatigue, joint pain, and fever after an episode of upper respiratory infection and sore throat require prompt assessment by a physician.

Etiology
After rheumatic fever, the vegetations may become enlarged or the valves may become scarred, causing stenosis of the openings. The frequency of rheumatic heart disease is decreasing as a result of prompt diagnosis and aggressive antibiotic treatment of streptococcal pharyngitis (strep throat). Patients who experienced rheumatic fever and rheumatic

carditis and polyarthritis adds to the evidence for the disease. The streptococcal antibody level, antistreptolysin O titer, is elevated in a series of tests. Increases in cardiac enzyme levels, WBC count, and ESR aid in the diagnosis.

Treatment
After the diagnosis of streptococcal pharyngitis (strep throat), which precedes rheumatic fever, treatment with a complete course of antibiotics prevents the onset of the fever and subsequent rheumatic heart disease. The administration of antibiotics (penicillin) is necessary to eradicate the streptococcal infection. Antipyretics are given for fever, and antiinflammatory agents are given for relief of the arthritic symptoms. Bed rest is indicated, as is prophylactic administration of antibiotics.

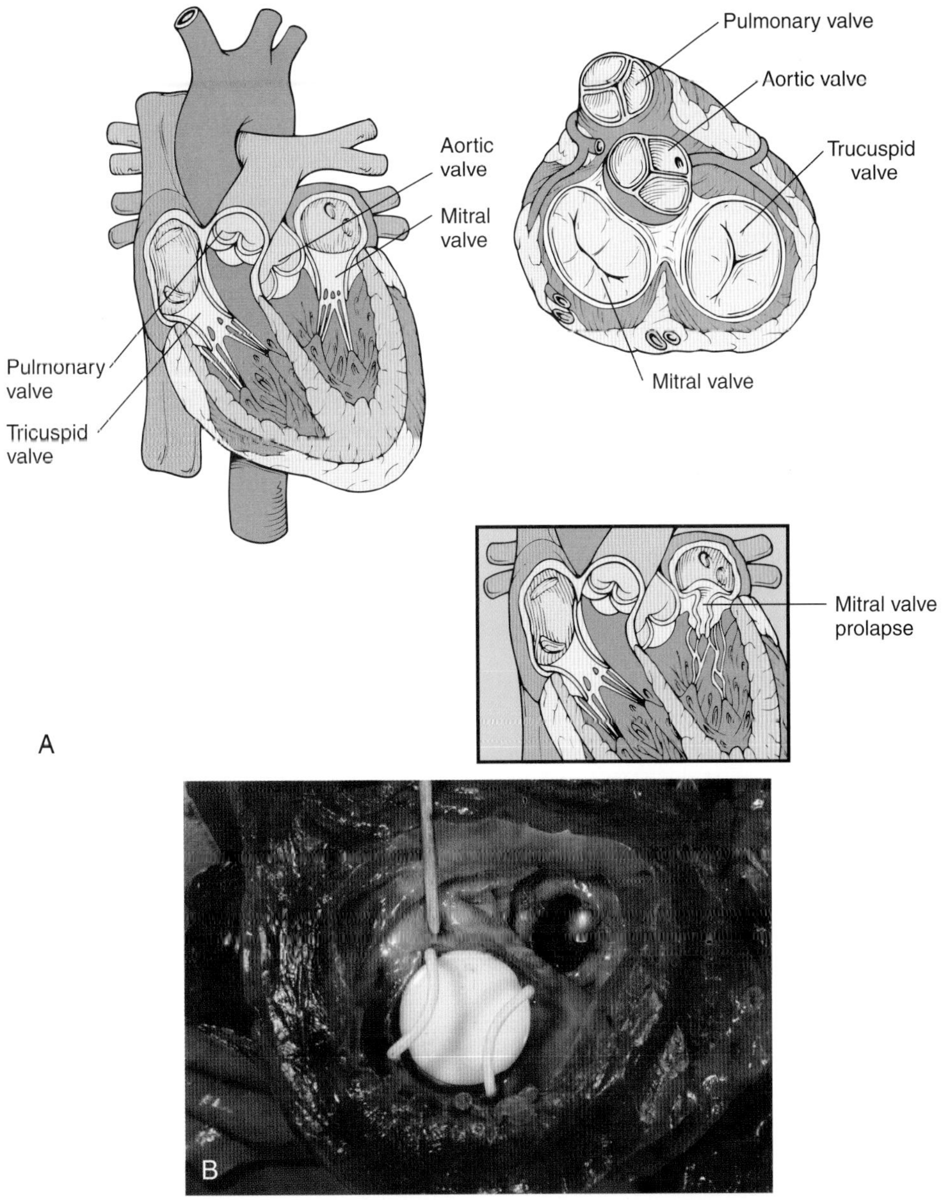

Pulmonary valve

Aortic valve

Aortic valve

Mitral valve

Pulmonary valve

Tricuspid valve

Trucuspid valve

Mitral valve

Mitral valve prolapse

A

B

• **Fig. 10.32** (A) Cardiac valves. (B) Artificial valve. (B, From Damjanov I: *Pathology for the health professions,* ed 5, St Louis, 2017, Elsevier.)

heart disease before the advent of penicillin may have damaged cardiac valves (Fig. 10.33).

Diagnosis

The diagnosis is based on the history of rheumatic fever and cardiac murmurs. Echocardiography shows vegetations or resulting damage to the valves.

Treatment

Treatment is aimed at reducing stenosis of the valves and preventing further damage. Surgery to relieve stenosis or to replace the valve may be necessary. Good dental hygiene is important to prevent gingival infection, which would cause further bloodborne infection and damage the valves. Prophylactic antibiotics are given to the patient before any dental procedures.

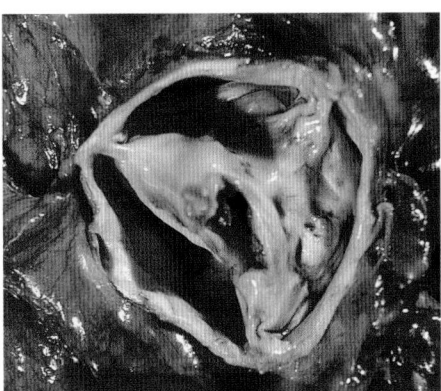

• **Fig. 10.33** Chronic rheumatic endocarditis of the aortic valve. The valves are deformed, and the orifice is stenosed. (From Damjanov I, Linder J: *Pathology: a color atlas,* St Louis, 1999, Mosby/Elsevier.)

Prognosis

The prognosis varies, depending on the extent of damage to the valves. Recurrences are likely. Valve replacement may result in a better outlook.

Prevention

The prevention is prophylactic administration of antibiotics for a diagnosed episode of strep throat.

Patient Teaching

Emphasize the importance of completing the full course of antibiotic therapy. PANDAS (an obsessive compulsive disorder) can be the result of untreated or undertreated beta-hemolytic streptococcal infections.

Encourage the parents of a child with a sore throat to seek medical attention, including beta-hemolytic strep screening. Give information on incision care to patients who have had valve replacement surgery. Encourage the patient to comply with prescribed rehabilitation therapy and activity level.

Valvular Heart Disease

Valvular heart disease is an acquired or congenital disorder that can involve any of the four valves of the heart (see Fig. 10.32). This condition can occur in the form of either insufficiency or stenosis. Insufficiency, the failure of the valves to close completely, allows blood to be forced back into the previous chamber as the heart contracts. This exerts added pressure on that chamber and increases the heart's workload. Stenosis, the hardening of the cusps of the valves that prevents complete opening of the valves, impedes the blood flow into the next chamber (Fig. 10.34). The mitral valve is involved most often. The diagnosis of valvular heart disease requires ECG, chest radiographic studies, echocardiography, and cardiac catheterization. Treatment entails administration of digitalis or quinidine for arrhythmias and antibiotic prophylaxis.

Mitral Stenosis

Description

Mitral stenosis is a hardening of the cusps of the mitral valve that prevents complete and normal opening of the valve for the passage of blood from the left atrium into the left ventricle.

ICD-10-CM Code	I05.0 (Rheumatic mitral stenosis)

Symptoms and Signs

The mitral, or bicuspid, valve lies between the left atrium and the left ventricle. Mitral stenosis causes patients to have exertional dyspnea and fatigue. In addition, they may experience cough and palpitations, followed by hemoptysis. In severe cases, patients may become cyanotic.

Patient Screening

Patients reporting exertional dyspnea and fatigue that may be accompanied by palpitations require prompt assessment by a physician.

NORMAL VALVE

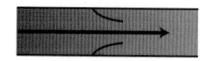 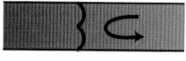

Blood flows freely forward   No backflow of blood

STENOSIS

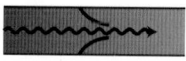 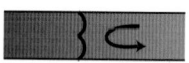

Less blood flows through narrowed opening   No backflow of blood

INCOMPETENT VALVE

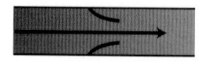 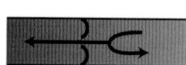

Blood flows freely forward   Blood regurgitates backward through "leaky" valve

EFFECT OF AORTIC STENOSIS

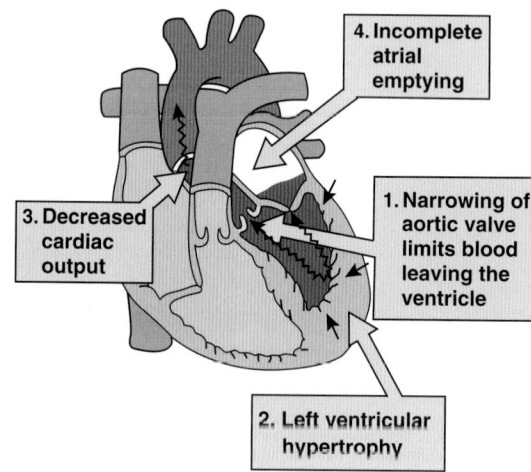

4. Incomplete atrial emptying

1. Narrowing of aortic valve limits blood leaving the ventricle

3. Decreased cardiac output

2. Left ventricular hypertrophy

• **Fig. 10.34** Effects of heart valve defects. (From Gould B: *Pathophysiology for the health professions,* ed 3, Philadelphia, 2006, Saunders/Elsevier.)

Etiology

Rheumatic heart disease is the cause of most cases of mitral stenosis. Group A beta-hemolytic *Streptococcus* stimulates antibody production, and the antibodies often attack the body tissues in an autoimmune response.

Diagnosis

The onset of symptoms of mitral stenosis may be insidious or acute. A cardiac murmur, including a diastolic murmur, is heard. Echocardiography confirms diagnostic suspicions.

Treatment

Limitation of sodium intake, along with the administration of diuretics, helps reduce the workload on the heart. Anticoagulants prevent the formation of thrombi. If atrial fibrillation results from stenosis, digoxin often is given to slow the rapid heart rate. Surgical intervention in the form of a commissurotomy may be needed to free up the valve and to allow adequate blood flow; this can also be done nonsurgically with balloon valvuloplasty. Valve replacement is a final option.

Prognosis
The prognosis improves with corrective intervention.

Prevention
Prevention of rheumatic fever and subsequent rheumatic heart disease is a major factor in preventing mitral stenosis.

Patient Teaching
When possible, use visual aids to demonstrate the effect valvular disease has on blood circulation through the heart. Explain the medical regimen and how medications can improve the condition. Explain the procedure for surgical reconstruction of the valve, if appropriate.

Mitral Insufficiency
Description
In mitral valve insufficiency, the mitral valve fails to close completely and allows blood from the left ventricle to flow back into the left atrium.

ICD-10-CM Code	I05.1 (Rheumatic mitral insufficiency)
	I05.2 (Rheumatic mitral stenosis with insufficiency)
	(I05.0-I05.9 = 5 codes of specificity)

Symptoms and Signs
The patient with mitral insufficiency experiences dyspnea and fatigue. A heart murmur can be heard as blood leaks back into the left atrium as a result of the valve's failure to close completely.

Patient Screening
Patients with mitral insufficiency often call reporting that they are simply very tired and having some difficulty breathing. Anyone complaining of difficulty breathing requires prompt assessment by a physician. For those complaining of generalized fatigue, the next available appointment should be scheduled.

Etiology
The valve may fail to close because of scar tissue resulting from inflammation and vegetations (a consequence of endocarditis), rheumatic fever, mitral valve prolapse (MVP), CAD, or MI or from cardiac dilation.

Diagnosis
The diagnosis is based on a thorough patient history, especially a history of sore throat or rheumatic fever. Physical examination reveals a murmur, and echocardiography discloses the insufficiency. The cardiac status also is assessed with ECG, chest radiography, and cardiac catheterization.

Treatment
Treatment includes bed rest, oxygen therapy, and administration of antibiotics for any infectious process. When severe, surgical repair or replacement of the valve may be necessary.

Prognosis
The prognosis generally is good, but the condition can lead to CHF.

Prevention
Preventing rheumatic fever and the resulting scarring of the mitral valve helps prevent mitral insufficiency.

Patient Teaching
When possible, use visual aids to demonstrate the effect valvular disease has on blood circulation through the heart. Explain the medical regimen and how medications can improve the condition. Explain the procedure for surgical reconstruction of the valve, if appropriate.

Mitral Valve Prolapse
Description
MVP, usually a benign condition, occurs when one or more of the cusps of the mitral valve protrude back into the left atrium during ventricular contraction.

ICD-10-CM Code	I34.0 (Nonrheumatic mitral [valve] insufficiency)
	I34.8 (Other nonrheumatic mitral valve disorders)
	(I34.0-I34.9 = 5 codes of specificity)

Symptoms and Signs
MVP, usually a benign condition, occurs when the valve cusps do not close completely (see Fig. 10.32). Most patients are asymptomatic, and the condition usually is discovered during a routine examination. The few patients who experience symptoms report chest pain, dyspnea, dizziness, fatigue, and syncope. These patients may experience severe anxiety. This fairly common condition can affect all age groups.

Patient Screening
Most individuals with MVP are unaware of any problem. The condition is usually diagnosed incidentally during physical examination. Those who report chest pain require prompt assessment by a physician.

Etiology
Abnormally long or short chordae tendineae may be the cause of the valve's inability to close properly. Malfunctioning papillary muscles may increase the severity of the condition. Regurgitation of blood occurs during left ventricular systole and results in the rushing, gurgling cardiac murmur characteristic of the prolapse.

Diagnosis
The typical click-murmur syndrome is heard on auscultation of the heart. Echocardiography confirms the failure of the valve to close. The premature ventricular contractions (PVCs) that are detected on ECG are not considered harmful and are not an indication of insult to the myocardium.

Treatment

Treatment generally is not required for asymptomatic patients. Those who experience discomfort and anxiety often are treated with beta-blockers, and they are advised to avoid caffeine, smoking, and large, heavy meals.

Prognosis

The prognosis is good.

Prevention

No prevention is known for this condition.

Patient Teaching

Reassure patients that this is usually a benign condition. Emphasize the importance of avoiding caffeine and big meals. The AHA no longer recommends routine antibiotics before dental procedures or other surgical procedures for patients with only MVP, unless they have had bacterial endocarditis in the past.

Arrhythmias

Description

Cardiac arrhythmias are any deviation from the normal heartbeat, that is, the normal sinus rhythm. They are often called *irregular heartbeats.*

ICD-10-CM Code	I47.1 *(Supraventricular tachycardia)*
	(I47.1-I47.9 = 3 codes of specificity)

Arrhythmias or dysrhythmias are coded by type and point of origin. Refer to the physician's diagnosis and then to the current edition of the ICD-10-CM coding manual to ensure the greatest specificity.

Symptoms and Signs

Arrhythmias result when there is interference with the conduction system of the heart, resulting in an abnormality of the heartbeat. Symptoms include palpitations, rapid heartbeat (tachycardia), skipped heartbeats, slow heart rate (bradycardia), syncope, and fatigue.

Patient Screening

Patients who report feeling abnormal heartbeats, usually as missed beats, palpitation, or rapid heartbeats, require prompt assessment by a physician.

Etiology

Arrhythmias can arise from disturbances in the normal conduction system of the heart, including the pacemaker (the sinoatrial [SA] node), the atrioventricular (AV) node, the bundle branches, and the Purkinje fibers (Fig. 10.35). Ischemia and drugs cause many arrhythmias. Failure of the SA node may be responsible. Table 10.1 lists the causes of arrhythmias. Heart block occurs when the impulses from the SA node become slow or irregular at or below the AV node.

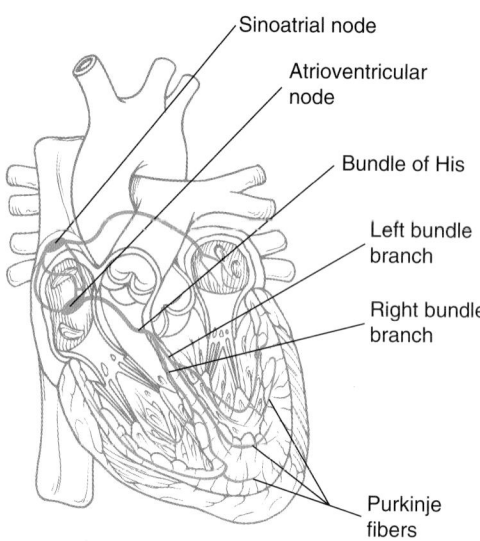

• **Fig. 10.35** Conduction system of the heart.

Diagnosis

The diagnosis is made with the use of 12-lead ECG. Various arrhythmias are evident to the physician. Echocardiography may help confirm a particular arrhythmia (Fig. 10.36). The patient may wear a Holter monitor (ambulatory ECG) to capture any arrhythmic event.

Treatment

Treatment depends on the cause (see Table 10.1). Drug-induced arrhythmias usually resolve with cessation of the drug administration. Anticoagulants, especially warfarin (Coumadin), are given to prevent thromboembolism. Ischemia should respond to oxygen administration and increased blood flow to the tissue. If the arrhythmia is unstable, cardioversion may be performed by electric shock to the heart to restore normal heart rhythm. This mild shock interrupts the arrhythmia pattern by resetting the heart's rhythm and may enable the patient's heart to be normal enough to allow discontinuation of antiarrhythmic medications. Occasionally the heart rhythm does not stabilize, and the arrhythmia can be fatal. Some arrhythmias can be treated with cardiac ablation (radiofrequency ablation) techniques with catheters. Bradycardic heart rates may be treated by the insertion of a pacemaker to maintain a rate at or greater than 60 beats per minute. Implantable cardioverter-defibrillators (ICDs) may be used for those with tachycardic heart rates or ventricular arrhythmias. Refer to Table 10.1 for pacemaker application, ICD application, and ablation procedures. Refer to the Enrichment box about Pacemakers and Implantable Cardioverter-Defibrillators and the Enrichment box about Cardiac Ablation procedures for additional information. Common terms for ablation include *cardiac catheter ablation, radiofrequency ablation, cardiac ablation,* or simply *ablation.*

Prognosis

The prognosis varies, depending on the type and cause of the arrhythmia.

TABLE 10.1   Arrhythmias

Types	Symptoms and Signs	Etiology	Diagnosis	Treatment
Normal sinus rhythm	Rate of 60–100 bpm, regular, P wave uniform	Impulse originates in SA node, conduction normal	Normal	None indicated
Sinus tachycardia	Rate >100 bpm, regular, P wave uniform	Rapid impulse originates in SA node, conduction normal	Rapid rate	Beta-blockers, CCBs; may be candidate for ICD
Sinus bradycardia	Rate < 60 bpm, regular, P wave uniform	Slow impulse originates in SA node, conduction normal	Slow rate	Atropine
Premature atrial contraction	Rate depends on underlying rhythm, usually normal P wave, different morphology from other P waves	Irritable atrium, single ectopic beat that arises prematurely, conduction through ventricle normal	Irregular heartbeat, diagnosis with ECG	Treatment usually unnecessary; if needed, antiarrhythmic drugs
Atrial tachycardia	Rate of 150–250 bpm, rhythm normal, sudden onset	Irritable atrium, firing at rapid rates, normal conduction	Rapid rate with atrial and ventricular rates identical, diagnosis with ECG	Reflex vagal stimulation, CCBs (verapamil), cardioversion; may be candidate for ICD or ablation
Atrial fibrillation	Atrial rate > 350 bpm, ventricular rate < 100 bpm (controlled) or > 100 bpm (rapid ventricular response)	Atrial ectopic foci discharging at too rapid and chaotic rate for muscles to respond and contract, resulting in quivering of atrium; AV node blocks some impulses and ventricle responds irregularly	ECG shows no P waves, grossly irregular ventricular rate	IV verapamil; if unsuccessful, procainamide; if unsuccessful, cardioversion; may be candidate for ICD or ablation
First-degree heart block	Rate depends on rate of underlying rhythm, P-R interval > 0.20 second	Delay at AV node, impulse eventually conducted	ECG shows P-R interval > 0.20 second	Atropine, if unsuccessful, artificial pacemaker insertion
Second-degree heart block, Wenckebach heart block	Intermittent block with progressively longer delay in conduction until one beat is blocked; atrial rate normal, ventricular rate slower than normal, rhythm irregular	SA node initiates impulse, conduction through AV node is blocked intermittently	ECG shows normal P waves, some P waves not followed by QRS complex; P-R interval progressively longer, followed by block of impulse	Mild forms, no treatment; severe, insertion of artificial pacemaker
Classic second-degree heart block	Ventricular rate slow (½, ⅓, or ¼ of atrial rate)—rhythm, regular; P waves normal, QRS complex dropped every second, third, or fourth beat	SA node initiates impulse, conduction through AV node is blocked	ECG shows P waves present, QRS complex blocked every second, third, or fourth impulse	Artificial pacemaker is inserted
Third-degree heart block	Atrial rate normal, ventricular rate 20–40 or 40–60 bpm; no relationship between P wave and QRS complex	SA node initiates impulse, which is completely blocked from conduction, causing atria and ventricles to beat independently	ECG shows P waves and QRS complexes with no relationship to each other, rhythms are regular but independent of each other	Insertion of artificial pacemaker is necessary
Premature ventricular contraction (single focus)	Single ectopic beat, arising from ventricle, followed by compensatory pause	Ectopic beat originates in irritable ventricle	ECG shows a wide, bizarre QRS complex > 0.12 second usually followed by a compensatory pause	Usually no treatment if < 6/min and single focus; may be candidate for ICD or ablation

Continued

TABLE 10.1 Arrhythmias—cont'd

Types	Symptoms and Signs	Etiology	Diagnosis	Treatment
Multifocal arrhythmia • Coupling, two in a row • Bigeminy, every other beat • Trigeminy, every third beat • Quadrigeminy, every fourth beat	Rate dependent on underlying rhythm; rhythm regular or irregular; P wave absent before ectopic beat	Same as single focus (above)	Same as single focus (above)	Same as single focus (above); may be candidate for ICD or ablation
Ventricular tachycardia	Rate of 150–250 bpm, rhythm usually regular; focus of pacemaker normally single, patient experiences palpitations, dyspnea, and anxiety followed by chest pain	Four or more consecutive PVCs at a rapid rate caused by advanced irritability of myocardium, indicating ventricular command of heart rate	ECG shows runs of four or more PVCs, P wave buried in QRS complex	Often forerunner of ventricular fibrillation; immediate intervention necessary—IV lidocaine; if unsuccessful, follow by cardioversion; procainamide or bretylium may be used; this is a candidate for ICD or ablation
Ventricular fibrillation (a lethal arrhythmia)	Patient loses consciousness immediately after onset; no peripheral pulses palpable, no heart sounds, no blood pressure	Ventricular fibers twitch rather than contract, reason unknown	Pulseless, unconscious patient; ECG shows rapid, repetitive, chaotic waves originating in ventricle	Recognize and terminate rhythm; precordial shock (defibrillation); survivors become candidates for ICD or ablation

AV, Atrioventricular; *bpm*, beats per minute; *CCB*, calcium channel blocker; *ECG*, electrocardiography; *ICD*, implantable cardioverter-defibrillator; *IV*, intravenous; *PVCs*, premature ventricular contractions; *SA*, sinoatrial.

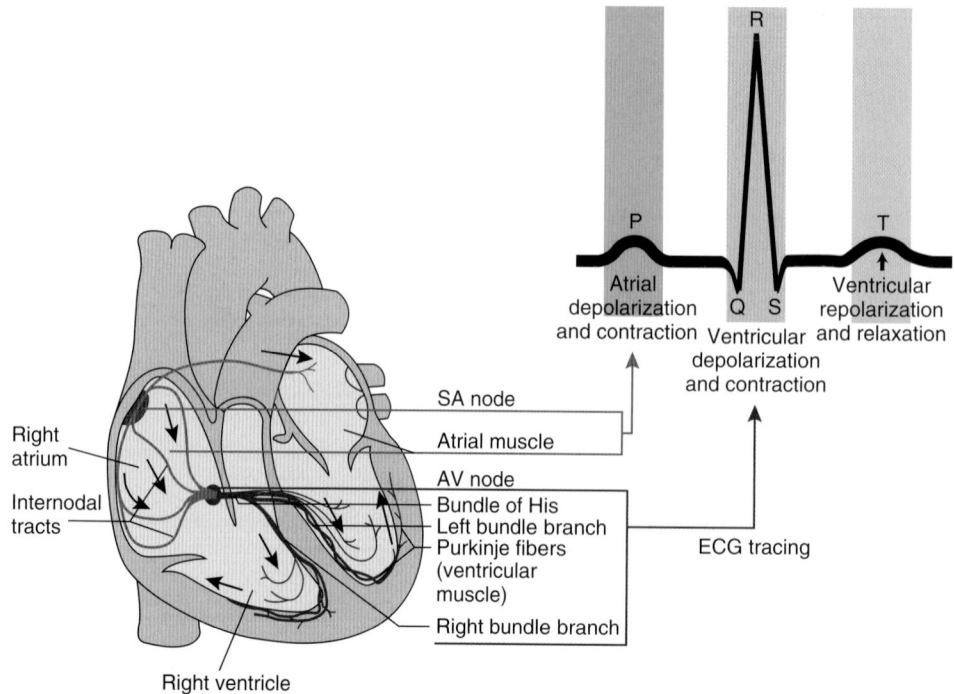

• **Fig. 10.36** Conduction system in the heart and the relationship to the electrocardiogram. *AV*, Atrioventricular; *SA*, sinoatrial. (From Gould B: *Pathophysiology for the health professions*, ed 3, Philadelphia, 2006, Saunders/Elsevier.)

Prevention

Preventing drug-induced arrhythmias requires stopping use of the offending drug substances. Avoiding the identified causative activities helps prevent certain arrhythmias. There is no prevention for certain types of arrhythmias.

Patient Teaching

Give patients information about the causes of arrhythmias. Emphasize the importance of complying with prescribed drug therapy. Encourage patients to comply with the scheduled appointments. Emphasize the symptoms that require prompt medical intervention.

❖ ENRICHMENT

Pacemakers and Implantable Cardioverter-Defibrillators

Implantable electronic cardiac assist devices have extended the lives of those with cardiac arrhythmias. At the present time, there are two programmable devices that can be surgically implanted for regulation of heart rate and for correcting arrhythmias. In an emergent situation, a temporary pacemaker may be used until a permanent pacemaker or an implantable cardioverter-defibrillator (ICD) can be implanted.

Assisting the heart's natural pacemaker, the sinoatrial (SA) node, and, when necessary, the rest of the impulse conduction system, artificial pacemakers can be external (a temporary intervention) or implanted. These devices are used to treat arrhythmias, heart block, and sick sinus syndrome. ICDs are implanted when ventricular tachycardia has the potential to become irregular and unstable, progressing to ventricular fibrillation and even to cardiac arrest.

The artificial pacemaker helps relieve symptoms of heart rhythm bradycardic disturbances. As the normal heart rate and rhythm are restored, circulation of blood returns to normal and symptoms of dizziness, shortness of breath, and fatigue typical of bradycardia usually are abated. The pacemaker also provides treatment for sick sinus syndrome.

ICDs are used to treat tachyarrhythmias, rapid heartbeats that usually result from heart diseases, including coronary artery disease (CAD), myocardial infarction (MI), and cardiomyopathy. The rapid rates originating in the ventricle result in the chambers of the heart not filling adequately, resulting in less blood reaching the brain; pounding heart; and faintness or dizziness. When this rhythm becomes irregular and unstable, the ventricle beats in a disorganized manner, resulting in no blood being pumped out of the heart. This is very rapidly followed by cardiac arrest. The ICD contains an internal defibrillator that will automatically pace or shock the heart out of the dangerous or lethal rhythm. An additional feature of the ICD is that it also is responsive to slow heart rates and at the interpretation of bradycardia, the ICD will act as a pacemaker.

Pacemakers and ICDs are small electronic battery-powered units that are implanted usually just under the skin of either side of the chest wall. The lead that transmits impulses from the pacemaker or ICD to the wall of the heart is threaded through the subclavian vein, the superior vena cava, into the right atrium of the heart, where it is attached to the wall of the right atrium. When a block of impulses exists, as in heart block, a dual-chamber pacemaker with two lead wires is implanted. The second lead is threaded along with the first into the right atrium, then into the right ventricle, where it is attached to the wall of that chamber.

The single-chamber pacemaker sends impulses to initiate the heartbeat in the atrium. When there is a block, either at or below the atrioventricular (AV) node, the second lead will transmit impulses to stimulate the contraction of the right ventricle. Most pacemakers have a rate-responsive feature to adjust the rate of pacing according to the activity of the individual's body. Sensors in the unit monitor changes in the body and adjust the rate according to the body's need for adequate perfusion. The leads for the ICD run through the right chambers of the heart and end in the apex of the right ventricle.

Pacemakers and ICDs contain small microprocessors, batteries, and electronic circuitry. Both store the history of the heart's and the device's activities, which are retrieved at the pacemaker clinic. This information is reviewed by the physician, and any changes may be made to the settings of the devices. Regular pacemaker checks are conducted according to an established schedule. A programming head is placed over the pacemaker. Electrocardiography (ECG) leads remain on the arms and chest, allowing the clinician to view information collected and stored in the recording device in the pacemaker. The computers in the office make a recording of the activity since the last check. Current pacemaker settings are viewed and reset if required. The condition of the battery is checked, including predicted end-of-service date or estimated battery life. Precautions are necessary for patients with implanted pacemakers and ICDs. Electromagnetic fields are to be avoided because they can interfere with the settings of the units. At the present time, MRI are not recommended in patients with ICDs. However, new technology has emerged with MRI-compatible pacemakers and lead systems. Individuals with the devices should avoid magnetic or electronic security scanning and identify themselves (using a pacemaker identification card) as individuals with implantable pacemakers and request a "patdown" or hand-held screening. Cellular phones may present a problem when held within 6 inches of the unit. Therefore individuals with implantable cardiac assist devices should always keep the phone on the ear on the opposite side of the implant site. Other precautions include avoiding arc welding with the cables draped over the neck, not working with a demagnetizer, and not using a gas-powered chainsaw. All of these activities may create an electromagnetic field that can disturb the settings of the unit.

It is important that the patient and the family receive instructions on pacemaker or ICD restrictions. These devices have allowed many with cardiac arrhythmias to live normal lives.

ⓘ ALERT!

Caution During Procedures That Use Electrical Activity

Individuals with pacemakers and/or implantable cardioverter-defibrillators (ICDs) should inform all health care providers that they have these devices. Any procedure that uses electrical activity may cause the devices to fail. Pacemakers interpret the electrical activity as the heart beats and will stop pacing. The impact of the electrical activity depends on its duration and its proximity to the pacemaker. The defibrillator will interpret the electrical activity as ventricular fibrillation and shock the individual.

Any procedure involving electrical activity should be performed in an outpatient setting at a hospital-type setting, where a special magnet can be placed over the device. The magnet prevents the electrical activity from reaching the device.

Cardiac Ablation

Patients with abnormal heart rhythms may be candidates for cardiac ablation. Drug therapy is usually attempted to correct the arrhythmia. When there is little or no response, cardiac ablation may be attempted.

Cardiac ablation is a nonsurgical procedure that uses catheters inserted into the chambers of the heart to administer energy to destroy the small amount of tissue that causes electrical rhythm disturbances in the cardiac conduction system.

The procedure is performed by an electrophysiologist after he or she completes "mapping" of the heart's electrical system. The electrophysiologist watches the procedure with the aid of fluoroscopy, inserting an electrode catheter usually through a vein (sometimes an artery) and threading it into the heart chambers. The electrode catheters sense the electrical activity in various areas of the heart and measure the speed of the impulses. Should it be necessary during the procedure,

the electrodes can pace the heart (cause it to beat). This study, using several electrode catheters, helps isolate where the aberrant pathway is located.

The ablating catheter is introduced into the heart close to where the abnormal electrical pathway is located. Radiofrequency energy is passed through the catheter, causing the tip of the catheter to heat up. The area of the heart containing the abnormal pathway is destroyed. A scar that cannot conduct the electrical impulse results, and the abnormal pathway can no longer cause the arrhythmia.

Ablation is used to treat both atrial and ventricular tachycardias. The idea is to obliterate the focus that is firing too rapidly and prevent the impulse from spreading through the heart. Other common terms for this procedure are *cardiac catheter ablation*, *radiofrequency ablation*, *cardiac ablation*, or simply *ablation*.

Shock

Description
Shock is the collapse of the cardiovascular system, including vasodilation and fluid shift, accompanied by inefficient cardiac output.

ICD-10-CM Code	R57.9 *(Shock, unspecified)*
	R57.0 *(Cardiogenic shock)*
	R57.1 *(Hypovolemic shock)*
	R57.8 *(Other shock)*

Refer to the physician's diagnosis and then to the current edition of the ICD-10-CM coding manual to ensure the greatest specificity.

Symptoms and Signs
Shock causes inadequate perfusion of organs and tissues. The patient has pale, cold, and clammy skin; rapid, weak, and thready pulse; rapid breathing; and altered level of consciousness. Blood pressure drops, and the patient may be anxious, irritable, or restless and often expresses a feeling of impending doom. The patient may experience dizziness, extreme thirst, and profuse sweating. In late stages, the pupils dilate, the eyes become dull and lusterless, and the patient experiences shaking and trembling.

Patient Screening
Shock is a life-threatening condition requiring the patient's immediate entry into the emergency medical system. The caller should be assisted to contact the EMS.

Etiology
This life-threatening emergency can be caused by anaphylaxis, hemorrhage, sepsis, respiratory distress, heart failure, neurologic failure, emotional catastrophe, or severe metabolic insult. Regardless of the cause, the amount of blood that is effectively circulating in the body is reduced. The

final effect is that vital organs (heart, brain, lungs, and kidneys) do not receive sufficient oxygen and nutrients to sustain life. Rapid blood loss or significant fluid loss with subsequent **hypovolemia** precipitates shock. Failure of the heart to pump adequately is another cause of shock. Vascular collapse with subsequent massive dilation or constriction of the vessels can cause blood to pool away from vital areas. Insufficient oxygen supply to the circulating system can generate shock (Fig. 10.37).

Diagnosis
The clinical picture, along with a history of a precipitating event, leads to the diagnosis of shock resulting from inadequate cellular perfusion. Altered level of consciousness and respiratory distress suggest shock. Immediate intervention is needed to halt the progression of the condition.

Treatment
Because of the severity and rapid progression of the condition, aggressive intervention is undertaken at the earliest possible opportunity. The CABs (compressions, airway, and breathing) of emergency care require maintaining an open airway and establishing ventilation to supply vital organs with oxygen. Any visible bleeding is controlled, and surgical intervention may be needed to halt internal bleeding. The patient should be placed in the supine position, with feet and legs elevated, and should be kept warm but not overheated. If the patient is not in an inpatient facility, contacting the EMS for immediate transport to an emergency facility is indicated. Vital signs are monitored, and volume replacement is instituted with IV fluids. Supplemental oxygen is administered, when available.

Prognosis
Immediate assessment and intervention improve the prognosis for complete or near-complete recovery. When the condition is not addressed promptly, shock may become

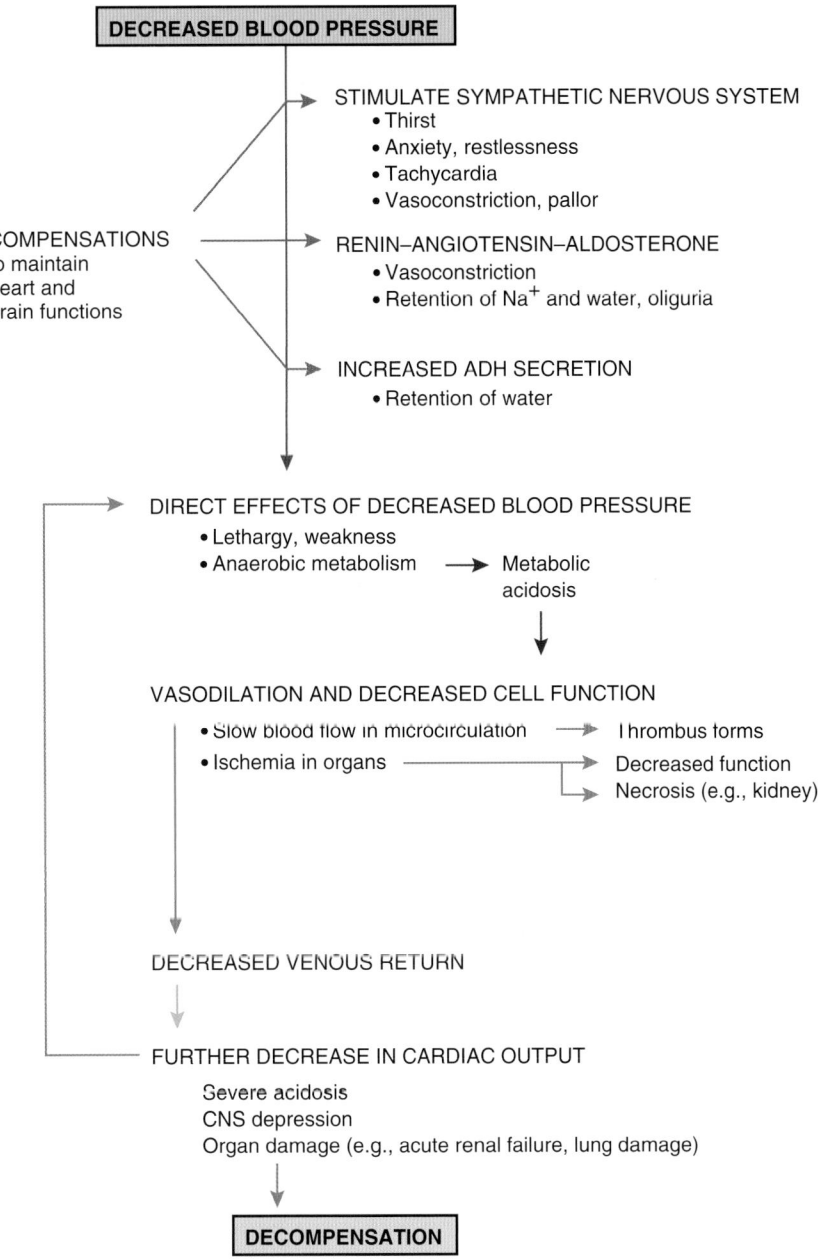

• **Fig. 10.37** Progress of shock. *ADH,* Antidiuretic hormone; *CNS,* central nervous system. (From Gould B: *Pathophysiology for the health professions,* ed 3, Philadelphia, 2006, Saunders/Elsevier.)

unstoppable, and the consequences may be irreversible, resulting in a fatal outcome.

Prevention

Most occurrences of shock are not preventable. Immediate intervention helps prevent rapid progression of the condition to a fatal outcome.

Patient Teaching

Give patients and their family members information about causes and emergency intervention measures for patients with known allergic reactions. Encourage community education in first aid and CPR to help reduce the damaging outcomes of shock.

Cardiogenic Shock

Description

Cardiogenic shock is the inadequate output of blood by the heart.

ICD-10-CM Code	R57.0 *(Cardiogenic shock)*

Symptoms and Signs

In cardiogenic shock (shock resulting from inadequate cardiac output), the myocardium fails to pump effectively. The patient exhibits the previously mentioned symptoms and signs of shock. The event usually is preceded by MI or severe heart failure, certain arrhythmias, or acute valve failure.

Patient Screening

These patients have a life-threatening condition. They should be entered promptly into the emergency medical system.

Etiology

Any insult that disturbs the heart's ability to pump blood can cause cardiogenic shock. MI, severe heart failure, certain arrhythmias, or valve failure can lead to cardiogenic shock (Fig. 10.38).

Diagnosis

The clinical picture and a history of a major cardiac insult lead to the suspicion of cardiogenic shock. ECG is another diagnostic tool, as are chest radiographic studies. A hypotensive state that continues to worsen also indicates the diagnosis.

Treatment

Treatment consists of general measures for shock, along with the administration of medications that increase

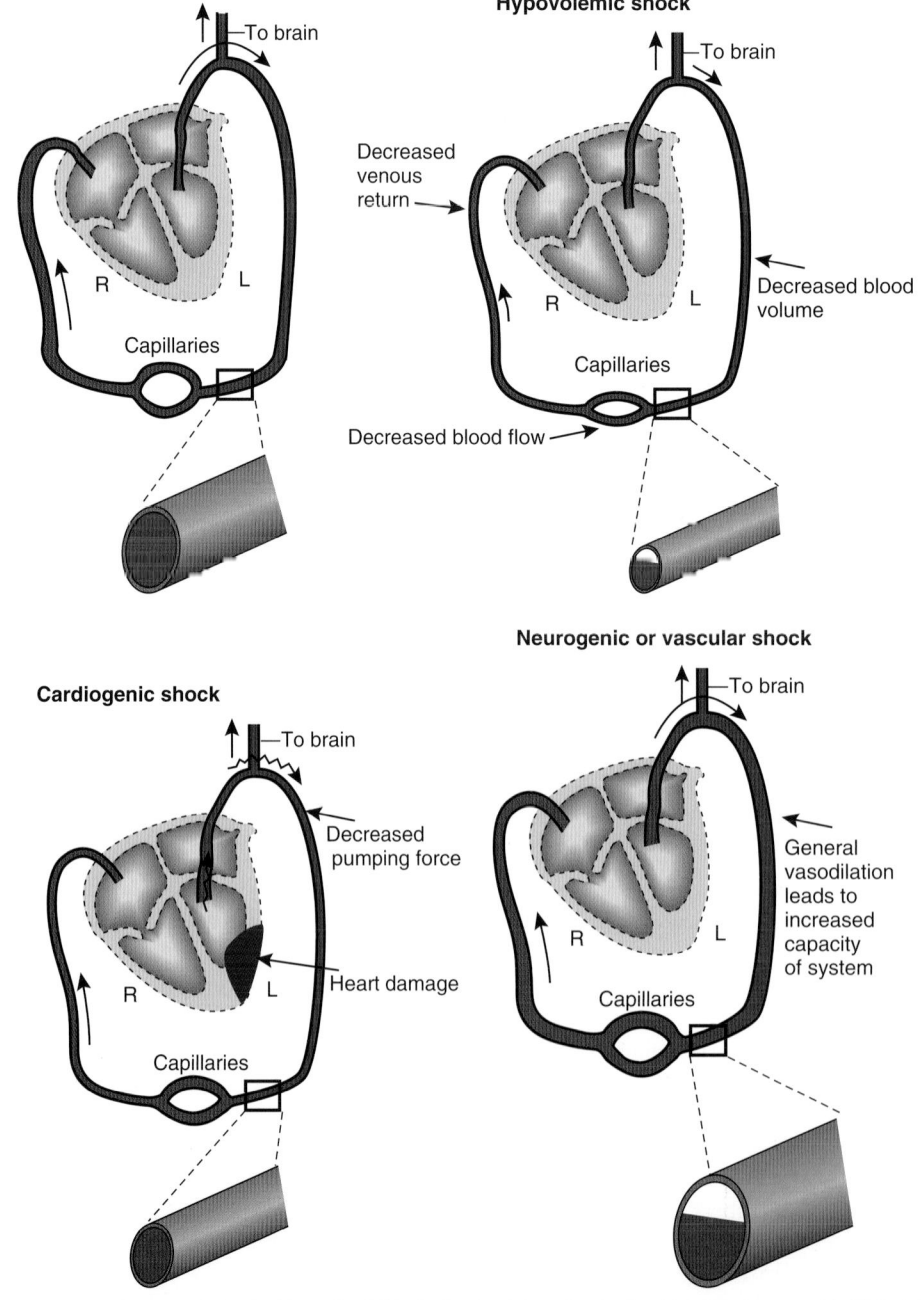

• **Fig. 10.38** Causes of shock. (From Gould B: *Pathophysiology for the health professions,* ed 3, Philadelphia, 2006, Saunders/Elsevier.)

the efficiency of the myocardium and/or affect the blood vessels. Blood supply to vital organs must be improved, and the oxygen demands of myocardial tissue must be reduced. Blood volume assessment determines whether drugs are given to dilate or constrict cardiac vessels. Sometimes an intraaortic balloon pump may be inserted.

Prognosis
The prognosis varies but, in many cases, is poor.

Prevention
Prevention, in most cases, is unlikely. An important factor in preventing a fatal outcome is immediate assessment and intervention when symptoms and signs are identified.

Patient Teaching
Emphasize the importance of immediate emergency intervention when symptoms are detected. Promote community awareness of the benefits of first aid and CPR training in increasing survival rates in the community.

Cardiac Tamponade

Description
Cardiac tamponade is the compression of the heart muscle and restriction of heart movement caused by blood or fluid trapped in the pericardial sac. It may be called *cardiac compression.*

ICD-10 CM Code	I31.4 *(Cardiac tamponade)*

Symptoms and Signs
Cardiac tamponade occurs when a coronary, epicardial, or pericardial vessel breaks and blood is trapped in the pericardial sac. In addition, the myocardium may rupture, also sending blood into the pericardial sac. The blood constricts the heart, thus restricting heart movement, and less blood can enter the heart chambers per beat. The patient with cardiac tamponade experiences sudden severe dyspnea and rapidly falling blood pressure. The pulse becomes weak, thready, and rapid. The patient is in shock and becomes cyanotic above the nipple line. The level of consciousness falls.

Patient Screening
These patients have a life-threatening condition and should be entered promptly into the emergency medical system.

Etiology
Cardiac tamponade may result from an insult to the integrity of a vessel in the pericardium, allowing blood to fill the pericardial space. The pressure of the blood causes the heart to beat inappropriately, leading to cardiac arrest. Cardiac tamponade may also occur in patients with certain cancers, chronic kidney failure, and other medical conditions, such as hypothyroidism or lupus.

Diagnosis
The diagnosis is based on the clinical picture and a history of a traumatic event. Heart sounds become muffled or distant, but breath sounds remain normal.

Treatment
Treatment consists of inserting a needle into the pericardial space and withdrawing the offending blood. Surgery usually is indicated to repair the leak.

Prognosis
The prognosis varies, depending on the causative factor, the success of the intervention, and the health status of the patient. Surgical repair usually has a positive outcome.

Prevention
Because of the etiology of this condition, prevention usually is not possible.

Patient Teaching
Give the patient and the family information about the mechanism and results of the insult. Explain care of the incision and emphasize the importance of following postoperative orders.

If available, provide the patient and family with some form of computer-based health education about postoperative care.

Vascular Conditions

The vascular system, a closed transport system composed of arteries, arterioles, capillaries, venules, and veins, is responsible for supplying tissues with blood containing oxygen and nutrients. This system also conveys waste products and carbon dioxide to the appropriate organs for excretion. Arteries carry blood away from the heart (Fig. 10.39A), veins transport blood back to the heart (see Fig. 10.39B), and capillaries are the point of exchange at the cellular level (see Fig. 10.39C).

Blood vessel walls, other than one-cell-walled capillaries, are composed of three layers: the tunica intima, the tunica media, and the tunica externa (Fig. 10.40). The lining of the vessel lumen, the tunica intima, is composed of smooth, thin endothelium, allowing minimal friction with the flowing blood. The middle portion, the tunica media, is composed of smooth muscle and elastic tissue that are under the control of the sympathetic nervous system. This innervation allows constriction or dilation of the vessel walls and changes in blood pressure. Connective tissue composes the outermost layer, the tunica externa, creating support and protection for the vessels.

Arterial walls are much thicker than venous walls. The tunica media is heavier in arteries to compensate for the stronger blood pressure under which the arteries must function. Veins, with their lower blood pressure, contain valves to prevent backflow and to assist the return of blood to the heart (Fig. 10.41).

Vascular conditions include emboli, arteriosclerosis, atherosclerosis, aneurysms, phlebitis, thrombophlebitis, varicose veins, thromboangiitis obliterans (Buerger disease), and Raynaud disease.

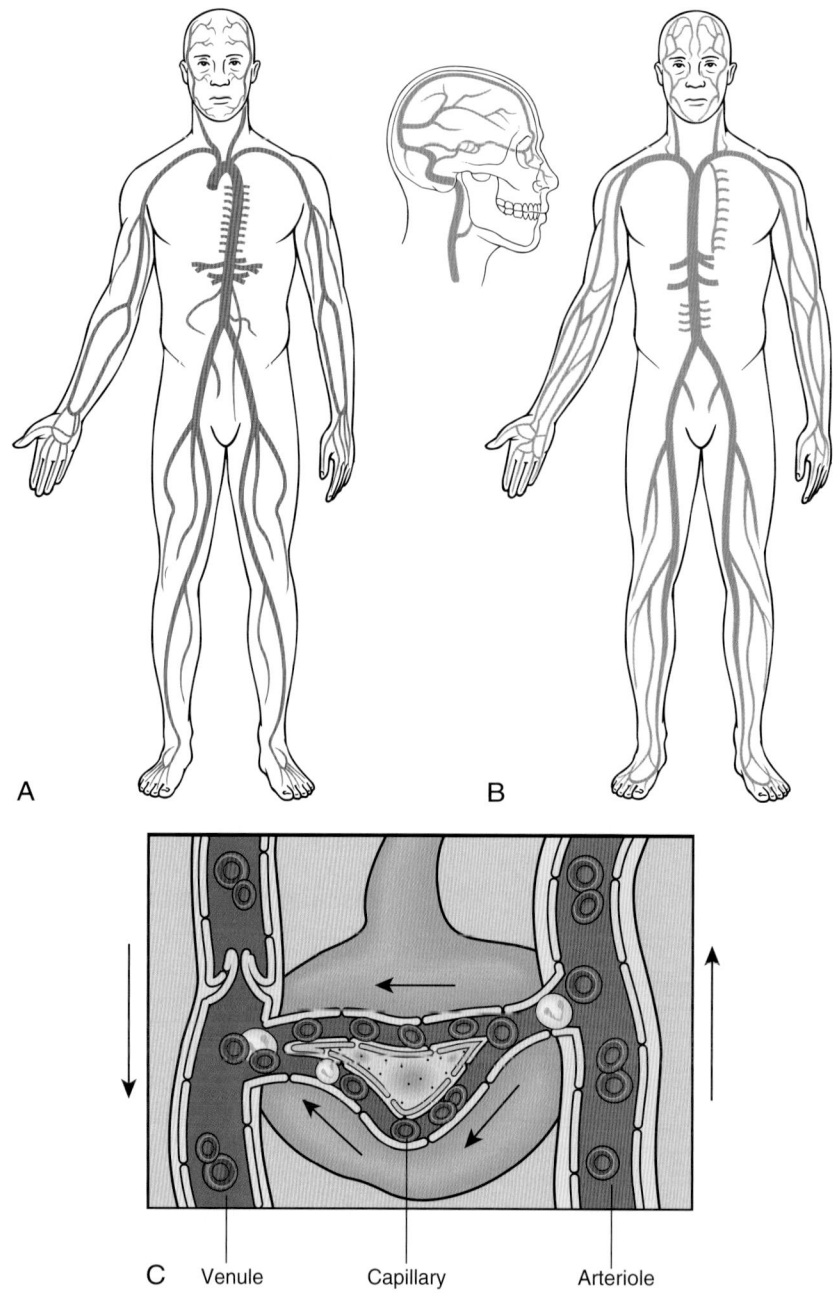

A

B

C   Venule   Capillary   Arteriole

• **Fig. 10.39** Vascular system. (A) Arteries. (B) Veins. (C) Capillary exchange.

Emboli

Description

Emboli are clots of aggregated material (usually blood). They can lodge in a blood vessel and inhibit the blood flow.

ICD-10-CM Code   I74.0 *(Embolism and thrombosis of abdominal aorta)*
(I74.0-I75.89 = 20 codes of specificity)

Emboli are coded according to location of involvement in the arterial system. Refer to the physician's diagnosis for the location of arterial involvement and then to the current edition of the ICD-10-CM coding manual to ensure the greatest specificity.

Symptoms and Signs

Symptoms of emboli depend on the location of the occluded vessel and the magnitude of the area of tissue served by the vessel. The initial symptom is severe pain in the area of the embolus. Emboli lodging in arteries of the extremities cause the area to become pale, numb, and cold to the touch. In addition, arterial pulses are absent below the occlusion if it is arterial. When a large artery is involved, the patient also experiences nausea, vomiting, fainting, and eventually shock. Pulmonary obstructions are discussed in Chapter 9. Cerebral obstructions and CVAs are discussed in Chapter 13.

Patient Screening

A patient reporting severe pain in an extremity that is accompanied by paleness, numbness, and coolness in the area

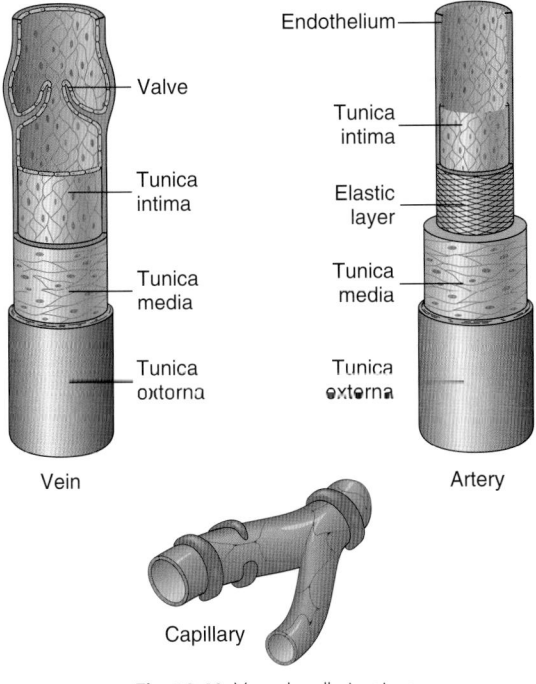

• **Fig. 10.40** Vessel wall structure.

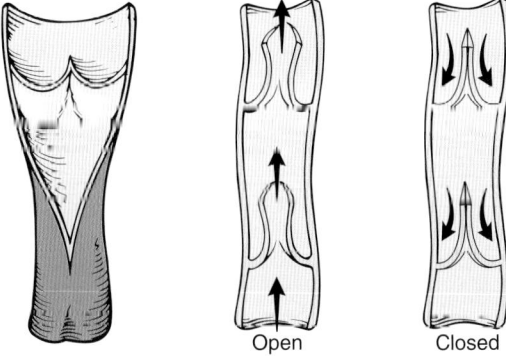

• **Fig. 10.41** Venous valves.

requires prompt assessment by a physician. In addition, those experiencing nausea, vomiting, fainting, and shock are in an emergency state and require immediate entry into the emergency medical system.

Etiology

Emboli are usually blood clots, but the offending embolus also may be composed of air bubbles, fat globules, bacterial clumps, or pieces of tissue, including placenta. The most common offender is a venous thrombus, a blood clot that has formed in the deep veins of the legs as a result of venous stasis (Figs. 10.42, 10.43, and 10.44). A portion of the thrombus breaks loose from the clot and travels through the venous system until it becomes lodged in a vessel that is too narrow to allow passage, often in the lungs. Cardiac arrhythmias also can cause thrombi to form in the heart. Those that travel from the left ventricle can enter the coronary arteries, resulting in MI, or can enter the carotid and cerebral arteries, compromising blood supply and resulting in CVAs.

Diagnosis

The clinical picture and a history of bed rest, physical inactivity, heart failure, arrhythmias, and any condition that has put pressure on or decreased flow in the veins of the legs or pelvis alert the physician to the possibility of an embolus. Pain in the calf of the leg in a patient who has any of the aforementioned predispositions is another clue.

Treatment

Treatment depends on the area of involvement. Treatment of pulmonary embolism (see Chapter 9), MI, and CVA (see Chapter 13) is aggressive and immediate to ensure patient survival. The treatment of a patient with an arterial embolus in an extremity is also aggressive and immediate to prevent the death of tissue and eventual gangrene. Blood flow is reestablished to the affected part by lowering the limb, wrapping it to maintain warmth to the area, and treating any constriction of blood vessels. Heparin or enoxaparin (Lovenox) are administered to prevent further clot formation, and antispasmodic drugs are given for vascular spasms. If this therapy is not successful, surgical intervention may be indicated to remove the obstruction and to restore circulation. In another option, a thrombolytic drug (e.g., urokinase, tPA, tenecteplase, alteplase, reteplase, or streptokinase) can be administered via a central catheter directly into the spot of the coronary embolism to break down the emboli. Apixaban (Eliquis) is prescribed for patients diagnosed with atrial fibrillation, which is an irregular heartbeat.

Prognosis

The prognosis varies, depending on the location of the emboli. When the embolus is in an extremity, aggressive treatment and surgical intervention usually are successful.

Prevention

Preventing the formation of deep vein thrombosis (DVT) during periods of immobilization or reduced physical activity is essential.

Patient Teaching

Encourage those who will be traveling and sitting for long periods to get up and walk every hour for a few minutes. If that is not possible, suggest exercises that stimulate contraction of the calf muscles.

Arteriosclerosis

Description

Arteriosclerosis is a group of diseases characterized by hardening of the arteries. Arteriosclerosis has three forms: atherosclerosis, Mönckeberg arteriosclerosis, and arteriolosclerosis. Atherosclerosis occurs when plaques of fatty deposits form within the arterial tunica intima. Mönckeberg arteriosclerosis, medial calcific sclerosis, involves the arterial tunica media; there is destruction of muscle and elastic fibers along with calcium deposits. Arteriolosclerosis occurs when the walls of the arterioles thicken, resulting in loss of elasticity and contractility.

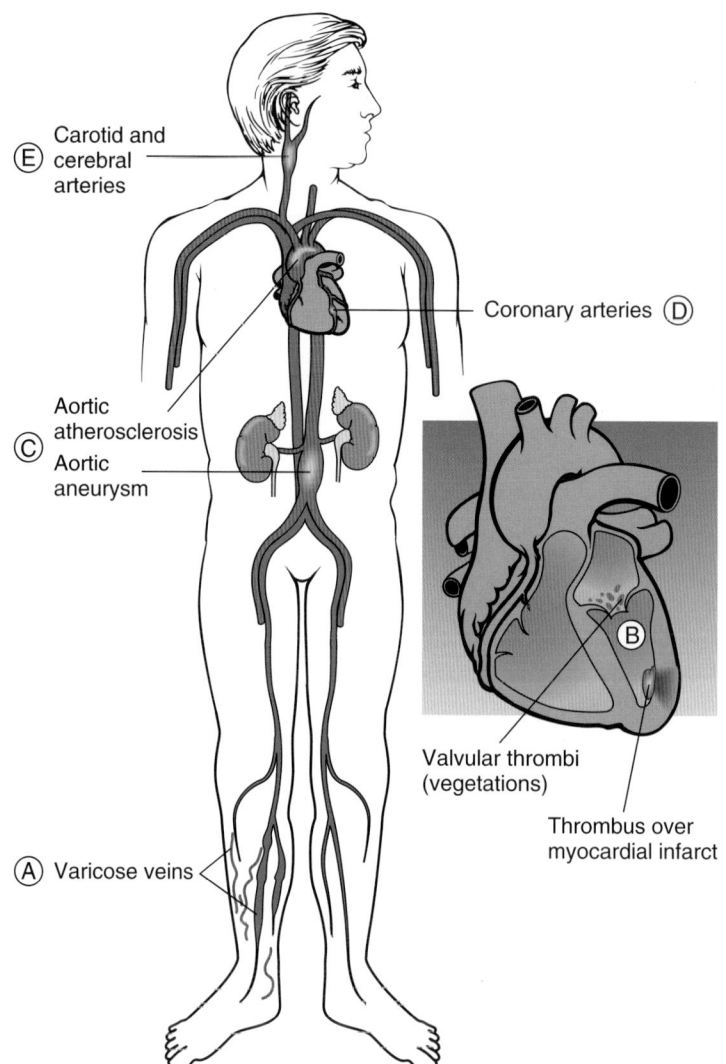

• **Fig. 10.42** Common sites of thrombus formation. (From Damjanov I: *Pathology for the health-related professions,* ed 4, St Louis, 2011, Saunders/Elsevier.)

Atherosclerosis

Description
Atherosclerosis, thickening and hardening of the arteries, occurs when plaques of cholesterol and lipids form in the arterial tunica intima.

> ICD-10-CM Code 170.0 *(Atherosclerosis of aorta)*
> *Atherosclerosis is coded according to the site. Refer to the physician's diagnosis and then to the current edition of the ICD-10-CM coding manual to ensure the greatest specificity.*

Symptoms and Signs
Atherosclerosis is responsible for most MIs and cerebral infarctions. The patient with atherosclerosis often is asymptomatic. The first symptoms may be angina pectoris, dizziness, elevated blood pressure, and shortness of breath.

Patient Screening
Patients reporting symptoms of angina pectoris, dizziness, elevated blood pressure, and shortness of breath require prompt assessment by a physician. Those who are asymptomatic may report just not feeling well; after careful questioning, an appointment should be scheduled as soon as possible or the patient referred to a facility where he or she can be seen quickly.

Etiology
The etiology of atherosclerosis is multifactorial and complicated, but there are risk factors that appear to increase the risk of development of the condition. Heredity seems to increase the occurrence, as do a sedentary lifestyle, a diet rich in lipids and cholesterol-producing foods, cigarette smoking, diabetes mellitus, hypertension, and obesity. The lipids and cholesterol in blood form thick, stiff, and hardened lesions in the medium- and large-size arteries. The lesions are eccentric and eventually expand to occlude the artery (Fig. 10.45). A fatty streak forms in the arterial wall and migrates to the tunica intima. Plaque forms and thickens the arterial wall. A sequela is an ulcer, crack, or fissure in the plaque, where platelets can aggregate and form a

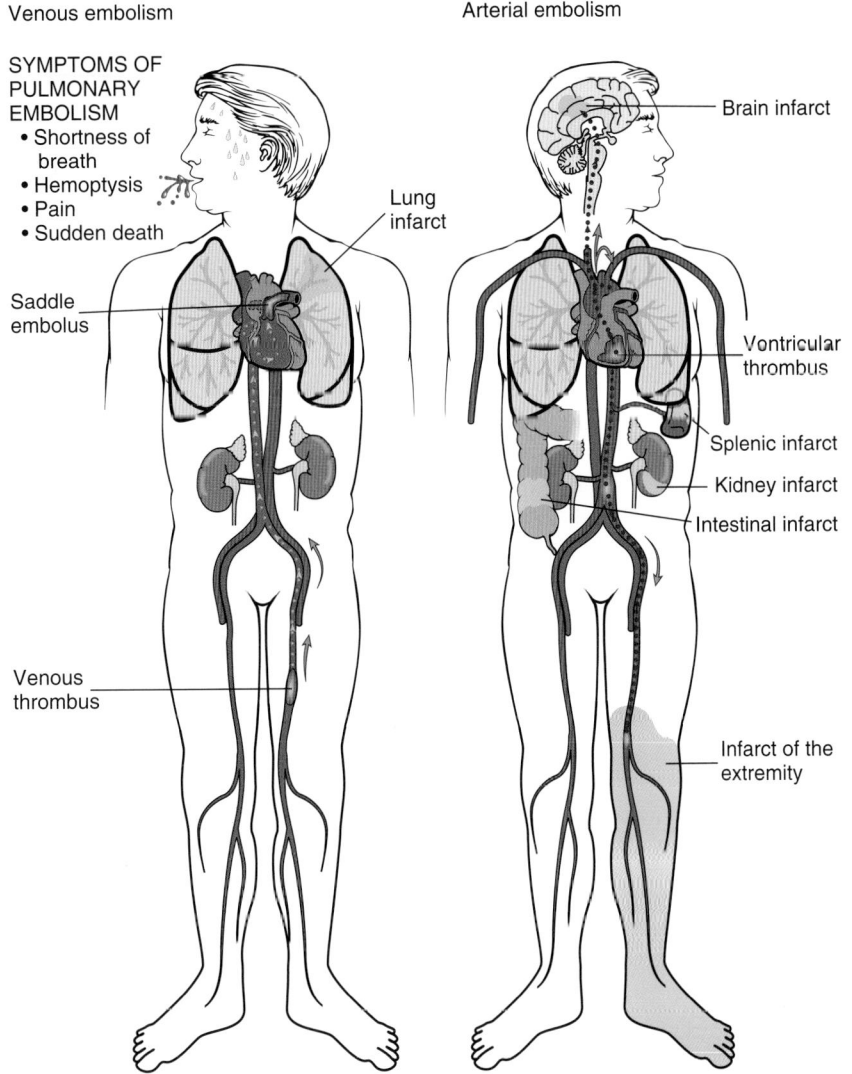

• **Fig. 10.43** Venous and arterial emboli. (From Damjanov I: *Pathology for the health-related professions,* ed 4, St Louis, 2011, Saunders/Elsevier.)

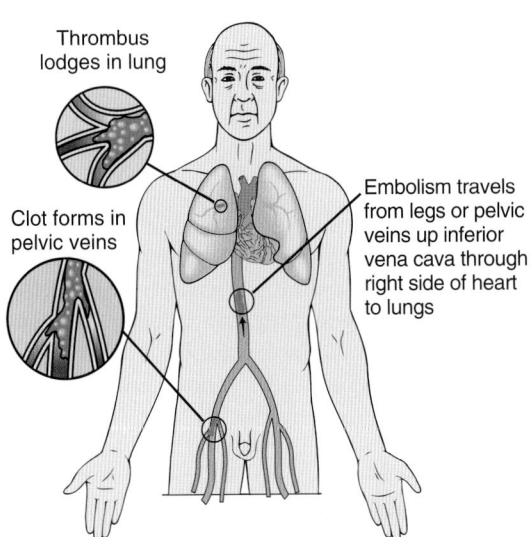

• **Fig. 10.44** Venous thrombosis.

thrombus. Ischemia results from reduced blood supply to the dependent tissue, with resulting pain. Infarct occurs with advanced occlusion of the artery and is followed by tissue necrosis.

Diagnosis

The diagnosis often is made during a routine physical examination or screening process. Blood studies indicate elevated cholesterol, triglyceride, and lipid levels. Hypertension may be noted. Doppler studies of major vessels show reduced blood flow.

Treatment

Treatment consists of dietary changes to reduce saturated fats and foods high in cholesterol and lipids. Cigarette smokers are encouraged to stop smoking. Hypertension and diabetes mellitus are treated and controlled. Hyperlipidemic drugs, such as lovastatin, simvastatin, pravastatin, rosuvastatin, or atorvastatin, are prescribed.

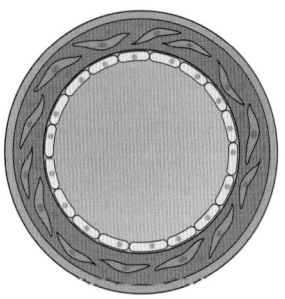
Normal arterial
lumen

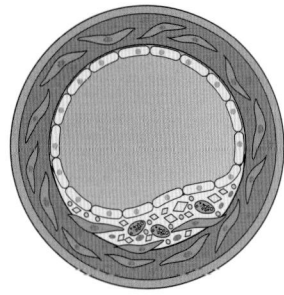
Atherosclerotic
plaque deposit

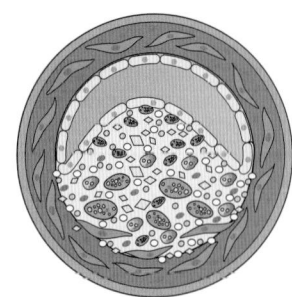
Advanced arterial
atherosclerotic
disease

• **Fig. 10.45** Atherosclerosis.

Recent additions to the recommended drug therapy include a niacin and lovastatin combination (Advicor) and ezetimibe (Zetia), a drug that inhibits the absorption of cholesterol in the intestine. Other therapies include cholestyramine, colesevelam, colestipol, or omega-3 ethyl esters. Research is being conducted to confirm claims that hyperlipidemic drug therapy can bring about regression of the condition and actually reverse the plaque buildup.

Prognosis

The prognosis varies, depending on the patient's compliance with prescribed drug therapy, exercise, and dietary changes. With good compliance, it is possible to prevent progression of the disease.

Prevention

Prevention is important, as is education about risk factors and changes in lifestyle.

Patient Teaching

Emphasize the importance of following dietary and exercise recommendations. If the patient has diabetes, explain the need to keep blood glucose levels within the normal range. Inform smokers of the dangers that smoking poses to their health. Give details about agencies that offer patients additional information about the condition and support groups in the community.

Aneurysms

Description

An aneurysm is a weakening and resulting local dilation of the wall of an artery (Fig. 10.46).

ICD-10-CM Code	I72.9 (Aneurysm of unspecified site) (I72.0-I72.9 = 7 codes of specificity)

Aneurysms are coded according to site and type. Refer to the physician's diagnosis for site and type of aneurysm and then to the current edition of the ICD-10-CM coding manual to ensure the greatest specificity.

Symptoms and Signs

The onset of the symptoms of an aneurysm may be either insidious or sudden and acute. Symptoms depend on the location and size of the aneurysm and the extent of the dilation. Abdominal aortic aneurysm is the most common form. An asymptomatic aneurysm of the aorta often is discovered during a routine physical examination when the abdomen is being palpated or as the result of an abdominal radiographic study conducted for another reason. As the aortic aneurysm enlarges, the patient may experience abdominal or back pain, and a pulsating mass is observed in the abdomen. A complication of any aneurysm is leakage from the wall of the artery or sudden rupture of the weak area. When this occurs, the patient exhibits symptoms and signs of hemorrhagic shock. Signs of rupture of a cerebral aneurysm mimic those of a CVA, with unilateral neurologic deficits being noted.

Patient Screening

Patients reporting a pulsating mass in the abdomen require prompt physician assessment. Those with symptoms of impending or evolving rupture require immediate entry into the emergency medical system.

Etiology

A common cause of aneurysms is buildup of atherosclerotic plaque that weakens the vessel wall. Trauma, infection or inflammation, and congenital tendencies are additional causative factors.

Diagnosis

The aortic mass is noted in the midabdomen, and pulsation is observed. A **bruit** heard on auscultation is another sign of the arterial dilation. Cerebral aneurysms usually are discovered when they rupture with catastrophic consequences. Radiographic studies, ultrasonography, CT, and MRI all help confirm the diagnosis. A ruptured aneurysm precipitates symptoms and signs of shock.

Treatment

Treatment depends on the size, location, and likelihood of rupture of the defect. Most diagnosed aortic aneurysms should be treated with surgical repair before they leak or

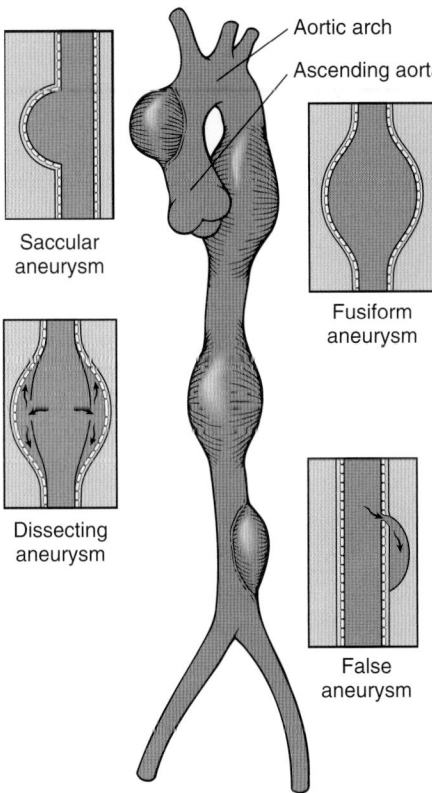

Aortic arch
Ascending aorta

Saccular aneurysm

Fusiform aneurysm

Dissecting aneurysm

False aneurysm

• **Fig. 10.46** Types of aortic aneurysms.

rupture. A newer form of treatment with catheter based stent grafts is now available for many patients as an alternative to surgery. After the integrity of the aortic wall has been breached, immediate surgical intervention is required to repair the rupture, usually with a synthetic graft, to ensure patient survival. Watchful waiting often is employed when the aneurysm itself is small or is located in a small vessel.

Prognosis
The prognosis varies, depending on the location and extent of the aneurysm. Surgical intervention before rupture or severe leakage of the vessel creates a better prognosis than when the aneurysm has ruptured or is leaking large amounts of blood. The speed of emergency intervention also affects the prognosis.

Prevention
Prevention is not possible because the condition is the result of many uncontrollable factors.

Patient Teaching
Instruct those who have had surgery about postoperative care of the incision. Encourage compliance with any prescribed drug therapy, dietary modifications, and exercise regimens.

Phlebitis
Description
Phlebitis, inflammation of a vein, occurs most often in the lower legs, but any vein, including the cranial veins, may be affected.

ICD-10-CM Code	I80.9 *(Phlebitis and thrombophlebitis of unspecified site)*

Phlebitis is coded by site. Refer to the physician's diagnosis for location of phlebitis and then to the current edition of the ICD-10-CM coding manual to ensure the greatest specificity.

Symptoms and Signs
Superficial vein involvement results in pain and tenderness in the affected area, which become more severe as the condition progresses. Swelling, redness, and warmth are noted, followed by the development of a tender, cordlike mass under the skin.

Deep venous inflammation affects the tunica intima, resulting in the formation of clots (thrombophlebitis).

Patient Screening
Patients reporting swelling, redness, warmth, and pain in a limb require prompt assessment by a physician.

Etiology
The cause is uncertain, and the condition may occur for no apparent reason. Possible causes include venous stasis, obesity, blood disorders, injury, and surgery.

Diagnosis
The clinical picture and history of a preceding event help establish the diagnosis.

Treatment
Treatment of superficial phlebitis is symptomatic, with analgesics given for pain. Caution must be taken not to massage the affected tender area, because this manipulation may stimulate the formation of clots or the release of formed clots as emboli.

Prognosis
The prognosis is usually good with treatment.

Prevention
Because the cause is uncertain, prevention is not possible.

Patient Teaching
Warn patients and family members about not massaging the affected area.

Thrombophlebitis
Description
Thrombophlebitis is the result of inflammation of a vein with the formation of a thrombus on the vessel wall.

ICD-10-CM Code	I80.00 *(Phlebitis and thrombophlebitis of superficial vessels of unspecified lower extremity)*

(I80.00-I80.9 = 31 codes of specificity)

Thrombophlebitis is coded by site. Refer to the physician's diagnosis for location of phlebitis and then to the current edition of the ICD-10-CM coding manual to ensure the greatest specificity of pathology.

Symptoms and Signs

Thrombophlebitis causes interference in the blood flow, resulting in edema. As with phlebitis, the patient experiences pain, swelling, heaviness, and warmth in the affected area, along with chills and fever. The involved area is tender to palpation.

Patient Screening

Patients reporting swelling, redness, warmth, and pain in a limb require prompt assessment by a physician.

Etiology

Venous stasis, blood disorders that cause a hypercoagulable state, and injury to the venous wall play important roles in the occurrence of thrombophlebitis. The deep venous inflammation in phlebitis affects the tunica intima, resulting in the formation of clots (thrombophlebitis).

Diagnosis

The clinical picture of gross edema in one leg resulting in a measurable difference in the circumference of the legs suggests thrombophlebitis. The affected area is tender to palpation. Imaging of the vessel with radiographic venography and ultrasonography confirms the diagnosis.

Treatment

Immediate intervention is necessary. The affected part is immobilized to prevent the thrombus from spreading and dislodging to become an embolus. Heparin is administered to prevent the clot from enlarging, and antibiotics are given to prevent infection.

Prognosis

Prompt intervention usually leads to a positive outcome. The condition usually resolves, and no further treatment is indicated. If the condition does not resolve, surgical intervention may be needed to ligate the affected vessel. Collateral circulation develops. As with emboli, preventing DVT during periods of immobilization or reduced physical activity is essential.

Prevention

Prevention of thrombophlebitis includes implementing activities that encourage movement of legs during long periods of sitting, as on long flights or automobile trips. If the individual is unable to walk around during this time, he or she must exercise the leg muscles regularly to encourage blood to flow back to the heart and to prevent the formation of blood clots. Individuals who will be sitting for extended periods are encouraged to drink plenty of fluids to prevent dehydration.

Women using oral contraceptives are encouraged not to smoke while taking the medications because smoking increases the risk of formation of blood clots that may become thrombi.

Patient Teaching

Encourage those who will be traveling and sitting for long periods to get up and walk every hour for a few minutes. If this is not possible for the individual, suggest exercises that stimulate contraction of the calf muscles. Emphasize the importance of immediate attention should the person experience a recurrence of the symptoms.

Varicose Veins

Description

Varicose veins are swollen, tortuous, and knotted veins that usually occur in the lower legs (Fig. 10.47).

ICD-10-CM Code   I83.009 (*Varicose veins of unspecified lower extremity with ulcer of unspecified site*)
I83.019 (*Varicose veins of right lower extremity with ulcer of unspecified site*)
I83.029 (*Varicose veins of left lower extremity with ulcer of unspecified site*)
(I83.001-I83.93 = 57 codes of specificity)

Varicose veins are coded by type. Refer to the physician's diagnosis for specific site and then to the current edition of the ICD-10-CM coding manual to ensure the greatest specificity.

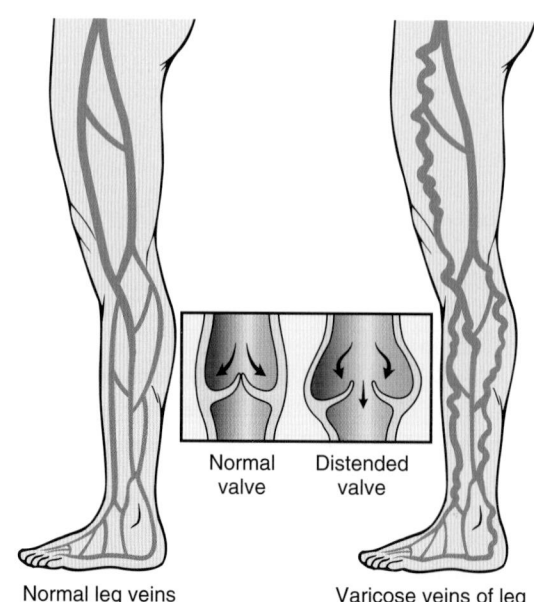

Normal valve   Distended valve

Normal leg veins   Varicose veins of leg

• **Fig. 10.47** Varicose veins.

Symptoms and Signs

Symptoms of varicose veins develop gradually, beginning with a feeling of fatigue in the legs, which is followed by a continuous dull ache. Leg cramps may be experienced at night, and the ankles may swell. As the condition progresses, the veins thicken and feel hard to the touch. The pain worsens and can have a dull or stabbing quality.

Patient Screening

These patients usually are not in acute distress, and the next available appointment can be scheduled for them. Should they report swelling accompanied by pain and redness in the area, prompt assessment by a physician is recommended.

Etiology

Varicose veins have no clearly identifiable cause. However, defective or absent valves may be suspected. Prolonged standing or sitting causes pressure on the valves in the superficial veins of the lower legs. Normal movement of the legs causes the muscles to contract and relax, thus "milking" the blood upward. When the person stands or sits for extended periods, gravity pushes blood downward, with resulting pressure on the valves. Without the normal muscular contractions, the venous walls distend, reaching a point at which they and the valves are no longer competent. Stasis of blood follows, causing swelling of the veins. The enlarging uterus during pregnancy increases pressure on the leg veins and pelvic veins, compromising the free flow of venous blood.

Diagnosis

The presence of the twisted, swollen, knotted veins of the lower legs on clinical inspection and a history of prolonged standing, prolonged sitting, or pregnancy are usually all that is needed to make the diagnosis. Advanced varicosities cause the skin around the affected areas to take on a brown discoloration.

Treatment

Rest periods throughout the day, with the patient lying down and elevating the feet higher than the heart, afford relief in mild cases. Engaging in exercise and submerging the legs in warm water increases the flow of blood. The patient may wear support or compression stockings that promote the return flow of blood. Compression stockings apply different amounts of compression to increase blood flow from the lower extremities back to the heart. Low-compression stockings provide less than 20 mm Hg of pressure to the leg. Medium-compression stockings provide 20 to 30 mm Hg of pressure to the leg. There are also stockings that provide 30 mm Hg or higher pressure. Individuals who have to stand for long periods are instructed to move the legs at frequent intervals to stimulate the muscular milking of the veins.

Painful, twisted, and swollen veins that have progressed beyond treatment with rest and exercise usually require surgical intervention in the form of ligation and stripping of veins or injection of sclerosing solutions that harden and eventually atrophy the affected veins. Collateral circulation develops to augment the return of blood to the heart. Some patients have incompetent valves in their veins that do not function accurately or have varicose veins. This causes venous distention and leg swelling, in addition to pain. This can be treated by destroying the incompetent veins through an endovenous laser ablation procedure. The vein is identified by using ultrasonography, and then injections of an anesthetic and a tissue protecting agent are made near the vein through the entire length of the leg. Then a small incision is made, a catheter is inserted into the vein, and sections of the vein are heated to destroy it. The catheter is advanced until the entire vein is destroyed.

Prognosis

Treatment with venous ligation or injection of sclerosing solutions usually affords relief for the symptoms and resolution of the condition.

Prevention

Wearing support stockings and moving the legs during long periods of standing help prevent this condition. Some individuals, however, may be predisposed to the condition, especially during pregnancy. Weight loss to relieve abdominal pressure also helps. Support hosiery can be worn on a routine basis.

Patient Teaching

Give patients information about preventing stasis of blood flow in the legs. Give information on the care of postoperative incisions.

Thromboangiitis Obliterans (Buerger Disease)

Description

Thromboangiitis obliterans (Buerger disease) is inflammation of the peripheral arteries and veins of the extremities, along with clot formation (Fig. 10.48).

| ICD-10-CM Code | I73.1 (Thromboangiitis Obliterans [Buerger's Disease]) |

Symptoms and Signs

The patient experiences intense pain in the affected area, usually the legs or the instep of the foot, which is aggravated by exercise and relieved by rest. If the condition is not resolved and circulation to the affected area is not restored, atrophy, ulcers, and even gangrene can develop.

Patient Screening

When patients, especially men, report intense limb pain that is aggravated by exercise and relieved by rest, usually the next available appointment is scheduled for them. Those complaining of breakdown of skin tissue require prompt assessment by a physician.

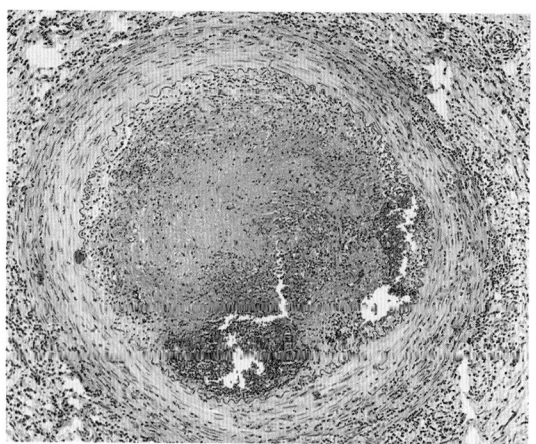

• **Fig. 10.48** Thromboangiitis obliterans (Buerger disease). The lumen is occluded by a thrombus containing two abscesses. The vessel wall is infiltrated by leukocytes. (From Kumar V, Cotran R, Robbins S: *Robbins basic pathology*, ed 8, Philadelphia, 2008, Saunders/Elsevier.)

Etiology

The primary cause of Buerger disease is long-term smoking of tobacco. Inflammation and the resulting clot formation in the vessels continue to advance until the entire vessel is obliterated and circulation to the area is completely compromised. The ischemic tissue dies, and gangrene follows. This condition affects primarily men, most often those of Jewish descent.

Diagnosis

The diagnosis follows reports of intense pain, usually in the legs or the instep. Arteriography and other studies, such as an ultrasonography, identify the site of the clot or the obliteration. Ulcers on the skin are another indication of the disease and its severity. The history of long-term smoking of tobacco products suggests the diagnosis.

Treatment

The first step in treatment is immediate and complete cessation of smoking. This often reduces inflammation and restores partial circulation to the area. Several medications, including prasugrel or clopidogrel, may improve circulation. Buerger-Allen exercises also help improve circulation to the area. In these exercises, the patient elevates the legs by 45 to 90 degrees until the skin blanches and then lowers the legs to the level below the rest of the body until the skin reddens. The patient then rests in the supine position. If these steps do not restore circulation, surgical intervention to establish detours or to bore a pathway through the clot itself may be necessary. Amputation of gangrenous tissue is imperative.

Prognosis

No cure is known for this condition, but cessation of smoking alleviates the symptoms. Surgical intervention may help. When the above-mentioned treatments fail, amputation may be necessary.

Prevention

Because the primary cause is smoking of tobacco products, prevention requires smoking cessation.

Patient Teaching

Give information about the care of foot injuries and instructions on avoiding constrictions around the affected limb.

Raynaud Disease

Description

Raynaud disease is a vasospastic condition of the fingers, hands, or feet. It causes pain, numbness, and sometimes discoloration in these areas.

ICD-10-CM Code	I73.00 *(Raynaud's syndrome without gangrene)*
	(I73.00-I73.01 = 2 codes of specificity)

Symptoms and Signs

This bilateral condition is precipitated by cold and causes white discoloration (blanching), followed by blue discoloration as venous blood remains, and finally red or purple discoloration when circulation is restored. The attacks occasionally are triggered by stressful events. Raynaud disease is much more common in women than in men. The primary disorder is called *Raynaud disease;* when it is secondary to another disease, it is called *Raynaud phenomenon.* In severe cases, the digits may ulcerate and become very painful. In most cases, the prognosis is good.

Patient Screening

Those who have been diagnosed usually know they need to warm the area gently. Those experiencing the condition for the first time and experiencing severe pain require prompt intervention.

Etiology

The small peripheral arteries and arterioles supplying the fingers, hands, and feet go into a spasm and constrict, compromising the circulation to these appendages. The spasm follows exposure to cold or possibly results from a stressful event. The episode usually resolves spontaneously after the application of warmth. The condition also is made worse by smoking tobacco.

Diagnosis

The diagnosis is based on the clinical picture and a history of numbness and paleness of the areas. Normal arterial pulses are present. The condition most often affects women between puberty and age 40 years, especially those who smoke. In severe cases, the compromise in circulation can lead to tissue necrosis and even amputation.

Treatment

Treatment of the episode involves the application of warmth to the affected areas. Patients are encouraged to stop smoking, to avoid exposure to cold, and to avoid stressful situations that bring on the attacks. Drug therapy to dilate the vessels and to increase the blood flow includes vasodilators, alpha-adrenergic blockers, and CCBs. The side effects of these drugs may limit their use in treating the condition.

Prognosis
The painful event resolves with application of warmth to the affected area. The condition will continue to recur, however, with exposure to cold and if the individual continues to smoke.

Prevention
Preventing the attacks requires avoiding exposure to cold and wearing gloves and heavy socks and shoes for protection from extreme cold. Cessation of smoking also helps prevent recurrences of the condition.

Patient Teaching
Give patients information about the effect of smoking on their blood vessels. Encourage them to avoid direct skin exposure to extreme cold and to wear gloves, heavy socks, and warm shoes to protect the fingers, hands, feet, and toes.

Blood Dyscrasias

Blood is composed of formed elements, RBCs (erythrocytes), WBCs (leukocytes), platelets (thrombocytes), and a liquid portion (plasma). Blood is responsible for transporting vital elements, including oxygen, nutrients, and hormones, to the body cells. It also plays a part in the removal of waste products, in the inflammatory response, and in the function of the immune system. In addition, blood helps maintain homeostasis, acid–base and fluid balance, and body temperature.

Blood is synthesized by the hematopoietic system in bone marrow (myeloid) and the lymphoid tissue found in the lymph nodes, spleen, thymus, bone marrow, and gastrointestinal (GI) tract (Fig. 10.49). The reticuloendothelial system is found in the spleen, liver, lymph nodes, and bone marrow. It is responsible for removing worn-out blood cells from the bloodstream and breaking down blood cell components for recycling or elimination from the body.

Stem cells in bone marrow form blast cells, including erythroblasts (rubriblasts), which eventually become erythrocytes, and myeloblasts, which eventually become leukocytes (Fig. 10.50)

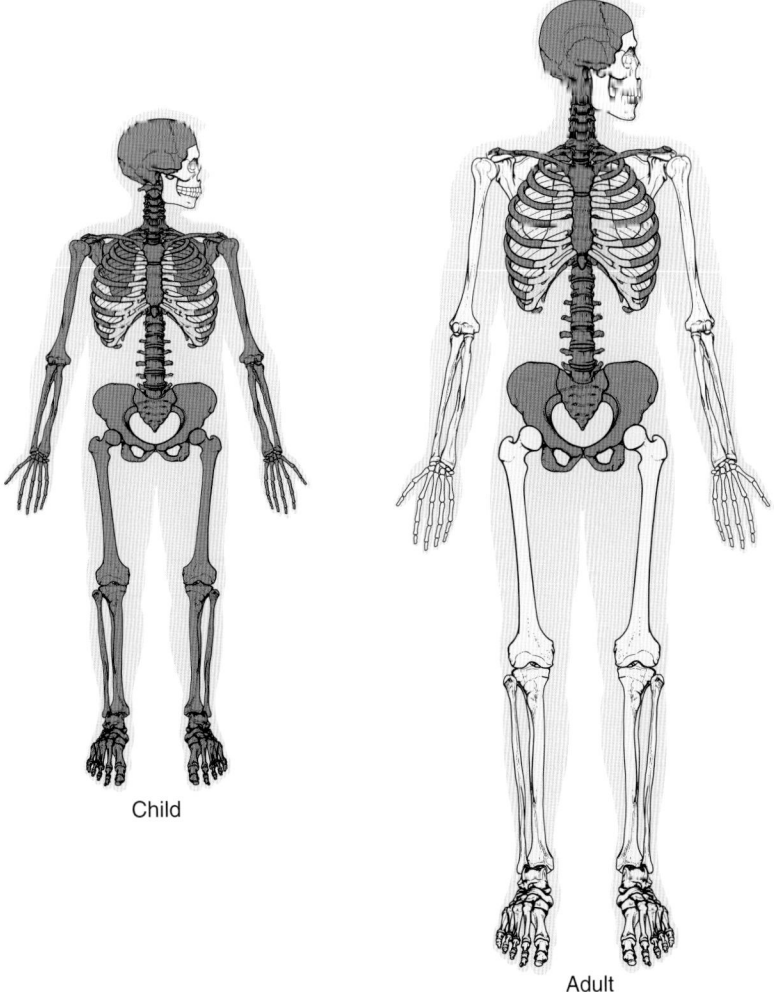

Child

Adult

• **Fig. 10.49** Sites of blood cell formation.

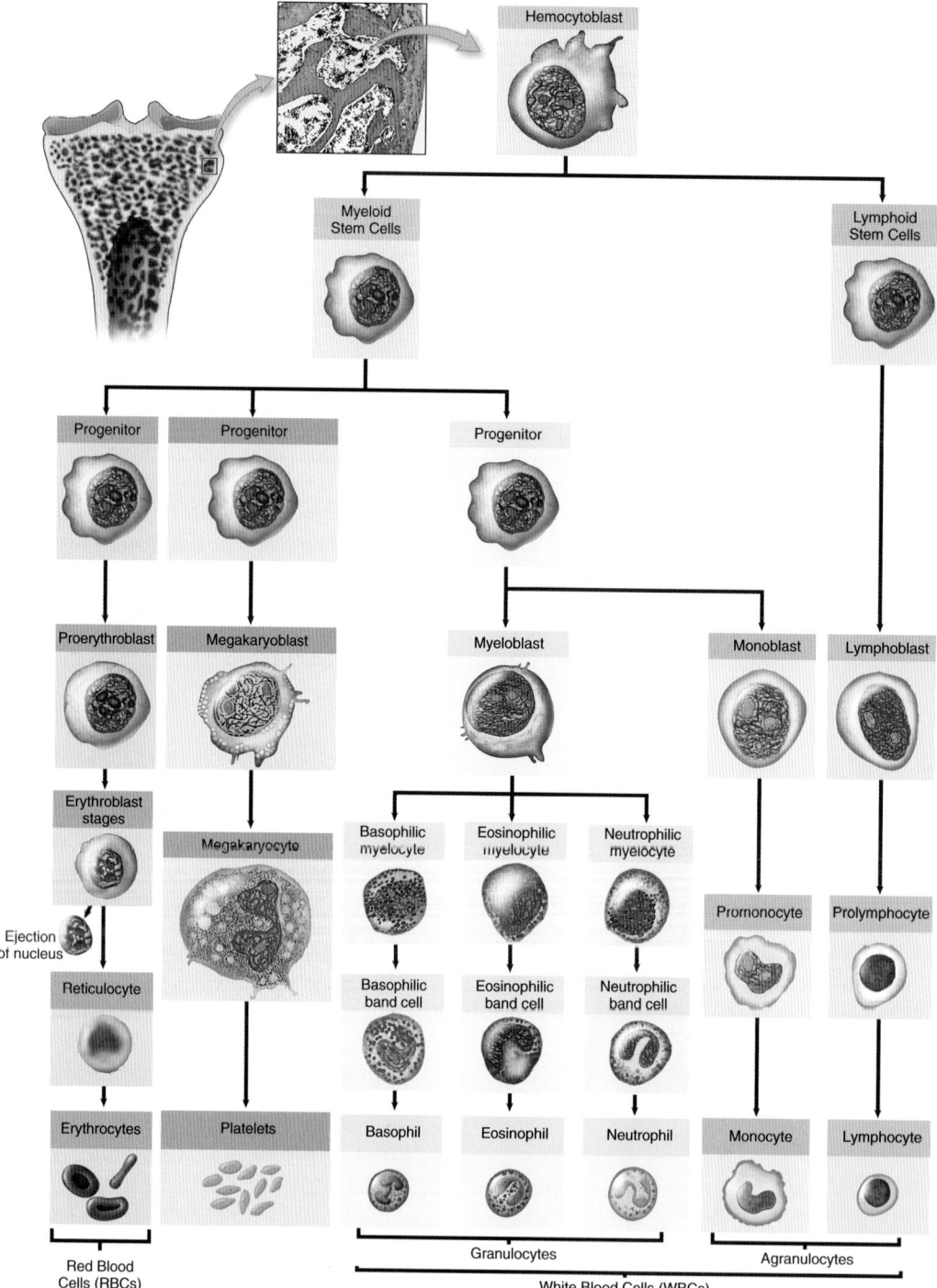

• **Fig. 10.50** Formation of blood cells. (From Patton KT, Thibodeau GA: *Anatomy and physiology,* ed 9, St Louis, 2016, Mosby.)

Deviation or malfunctioning in this system results in various blood **dyscrasias**, either because of impairment in the formation of the blood components or because of unusual destruction of cells. Dyscrasias involving erythrocytes and platelets are anemia, thrombocytosis, thrombocytopenia, and polycythemia. Leukocyte dyscrasias include leukemia, lymphoma, and leukopenia. Bleeding and clotting problems arise from alterations affecting thrombocytes and plasma-clotting factors. Normal values of blood components are measured by performing specific laboratory tests.

Anemias

Description

Anemia is defined as a condition in which there is a reduction in the quantity of either RBCs or hemoglobin in a measured volume of blood, reducing the blood's ability to carry oxygen to cells.

Depending on the severity of anemia, one or many symptoms, including pallor, fatigue, dizziness, shortness of breath, and irregular heartbeats, may occur. Treatment varies, depending on the cause. Several possible causes are acute or chronic blood loss, impaired production of RBCs (including aplastic anemia, iron deficiency anemia, anemias of chronic disease, or megaloblastic anemia), inherited or acquired hemolytic conditions, anorexia nervosa, and hemolytic-hemoglobin disorders. Hemoglobin in RBCs is necessary to transport oxygen to all cells, and any condition that reduces the amount of hemoglobin results in anemia. Iron and other components are needed to synthesize hemoglobin.

Types of anemias include iron deficiency, folic acid deficiency, pernicious, aplastic, sickle cell, hemorrhagic, and hemolytic anemias.

Important presenting symptoms that tend to recur in patients with anemia and need further investigation include:
- fatigue
- dyspnea (difficulty breathing)
- headache
- loss of appetite
- heartburn
- edema, especially of the ankles
- numbness and tingling sensations
- syncope (fainting)
- pallor

ICD-10-CM Code   D50.0 *(Iron deficiency anemia secondary to blood loss [chronic])*
    D51.0 *(Vitamin B$_{12}$ deficiency anemia due to intrinsic factor deficiency)*
    D58.0 *(Hereditary spherocytosis)*
    D59.0-D59.1 *(Autoimmune hemolytic anemia)*
    D64.0-D64.3 *(Sideroblastic anemia)*
    D66 *(Hereditary factor VIII deficiency)*
    D69.0 *(Allergic purpura)*
    D70.9 *(Neutropenia, unspecified)*
    D75.1 *(Secondary polycythemia)*

Anemias are coded by type. Refer to the physician's diagnosis for specific type of anemia and then to the current edition of the ICD-10-CM coding manual to ensure the greatest specificity of pathology.

Symptoms and Signs

Irrespective of the cause, patients with anemia experience fatigue. Most appear pale. As the disease progresses, the symptoms become more pronounced, and the patient may experience dyspnea, tachycardia, and pounding of the heart. Pallor is noted on the palmar surface of the hands and in the nail beds, the conjunctiva, and the mucous membranes of the mouth.

Patient Screening

Anemias often are diagnosed incidentally during a physical examination or during evaluation for other disorders. The individual reporting dyspnea, tachycardia, and a pounding heart requires prompt assessment by a physician. For those reporting they are pale and "just plain tired," the next available appointment should be scheduled.

Etiology

Anemias are classified by the color of the RBC as hypochromic, normochromic, or hyperchromic (spherocytosis), and by size as microcytic, normocytic, or macrocytic (Fig. 10.51). Anemias also are classified by causative factor, as previously mentioned.

Iron deficiency anemia may be secondary to blood loss through hemorrhage; a slow insidious bleed, such as bleeding hemorrhoids, and even heavy menstrual flow or because of insufficient intake of dietary iron.

Folic acid deficiency anemia results when insufficient amounts of folic acid are available for DNA synthesis, thus preventing maturation of blood cells. This can be the consequence of a dietary deficiency and is clinically similar to pernicious anemia.

Pernicious anemia is considered a macrocytic anemia, in which immature RBCs are larger than normal. The hemoglobin volume is reduced, with subsequent reduction in oxygen-carrying capacity. This anemia is considered the result of an autoimmune response and is discussed in Chapter 3.

Autoimmune hemolytic anemia also is considered an autoimmune response and is discussed in Chapter 3.

Aplastic anemia results from an insult to the hematopoietic cells (stem cells) in bone marrow. **Erythrocyte, leukocyte,** and thrombocyte production is reduced because of exposure to myelotoxins, such as benzene, alkylating agents, antimetabolites, certain drugs and insecticides, and radiation.

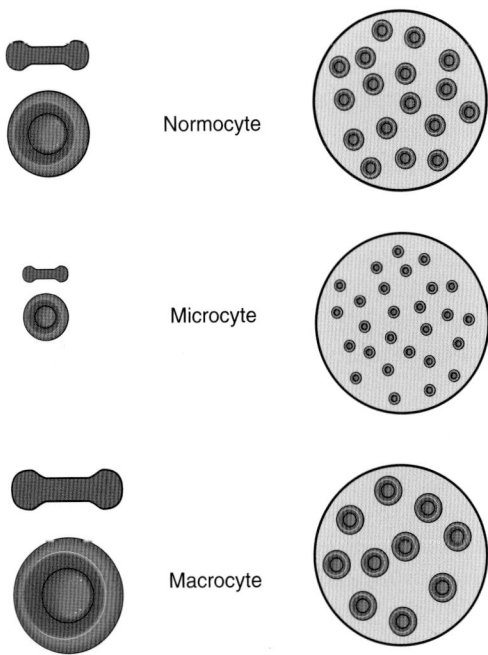

• **Fig. 10.51** Sizes of erythrocytes.

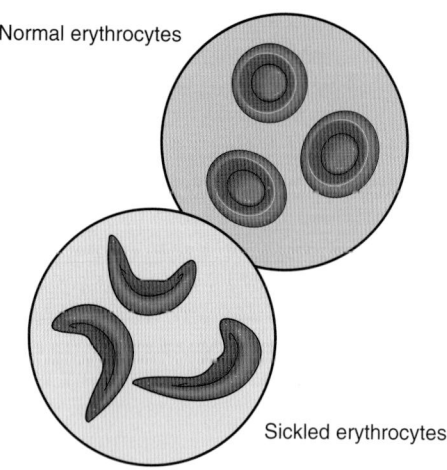

Normal erythrocytes

Sickled erythrocytes

• **Fig. 10.52** Sickled erythrocytes.

Sickle cell anemia is a chronic hereditary hemolytic form of anemia, diagnosed most frequently in the African American population, and the Hispanic American population. A person may also have the sickle cell trait. The true number of people living with sickle cell anemia is unknown. Research includes projects to identify people living with the disease, in order to understand the impact on the individual, and to find treatments to improve health. The presence of hemoglobin S along with hemoglobin A is noted in erythrocytes, causing them to acquire a sickle or elongated shape on deoxygenation (Fig. 10.52). These rigid, misshapen cells obstruct capillary flow and lead to tissue hypoxia and further sickling; this, in turn, causes further obstruction and eventually infarction. When the sickling causes obstruction in the blood flow, the individual experiences severe pain. When the sickled cells are reoxygenated, they resume the natural round disk shape of normal erythrocytes. In addition, hemoglobin S has reduced oxygen-carrying capacity.

Hemorrhagic anemia results from a large decline in blood volume (hypovolemia) in a short time.

Hemolytic anemia is caused by abnormal destruction of RBCs. Heredity plays a role in some hemolytic anemias, but exposure to chemical toxins and certain bacterial toxins or autoimmunity also may be the cause.

Diagnosis
Blood studies show reduced RBC numbers, reduced hemoglobin levels and hematocrit, and changes in the morphology of the corpuscles (Table 10.2). Bone marrow studies may be ordered to detect any aberrations.

Treatment
Treatment is directed at the cause of anemia. Dietary or supplemental iron administration is beneficial in iron deficiency anemia. If anemia is the result of a slow insidious bleed, the underlying cause must be found and treated. Folic acid replacement is indicated in folic acid deficiency anemia. Vitamin B_{12} injections are the treatment of choice for pernicious anemia. The causative factor must be uncovered in hemolytic and aplastic anemias and, if possible, eliminated. No cure is known for sickle cell anemia, so treatment is

symptomatic. Rest, increased fluid intake, and the administration of analgesics are helpful. When the condition is exacerbated, the patient requires hospitalization for oxygen administration, IV therapy, the use of narcotic analgesics, and transfusion of packed RBCs. In all forms of anemia, blood replacement may be needed when other measures fail to restore the RBC numbers and hemoglobin levels.

Prognosis
The prognosis varies, depending on the cause and type of anemia and the patient's response to prescribed therapy.

Prevention
Prevention depends on the type and cause of anemia. Most types of anemia are not preventable. Proper nutrition may play a role in preventing anemia caused by low iron intake.

Patient Teaching
Give patients information about proper nutrition. Emphasize the importance of complying with the prescribed drug therapy.

Agranulocytosis
Description
Agranulocytosis (also called *neutropenia*) is a blood dyscrasia in which leukocyte levels become extremely low.

ICD-10-CM Code D70.9 *(Neutropenia, unspecified)* (D70.0-D70.9 = 7 codes of specificity)

Symptoms and Signs
The onset of this condition can be rapid. The patient experiences severe fatigue and weakness, followed by a sore throat, ulcerations on the oral mucosa, dysphagia, elevated body temperature, weak and rapid pulse, and chills.

Patient Screening
Patients reporting severe fatigue and weakness, followed by a sore throat, ulcerations on the oral mucosa, dysphagia, an elevated body temperature, weak and rapid pulse, and chills, require prompt assessment by a physician.

Etiology
Agranulocytosis usually is caused by drug toxicity or hypersensitivity. For example, cancer chemotherapy with chemotoxic agents can be a cause. Benzene is another chemical agent that causes neutropenia. Agranulocytosis, or neutropenia, is an acute insult to the body's immune system and drastically reduces the body's response to bacterial infection. The infectious agents usually invade the body through the oral or pharyngeal mucosa and often are already present but are no longer held in check by the now-absent granulocytes. Patients occasionally are sensitive to a particular drug, such as chlorpromazine, propylthiouracil, phenytoin, chloramphenicol, and phenylbutazone. Agranulocytosis also can accompany aplastic or megaloblastic anemia, tuberculosis, uremia, or malaria. This condition occurs most often in the female population.

TABLE 10.2   **Blood Values in Anemia**

	Red Blood Cell (per mm³)	Hemoglobin (g/dL)	Hematocrit (%)	Mean Corpuscular Volume (per mm³)	Mean Corpuscular Hemoglobin (pg)	Mean Corpuscular Hemoglobin Concentration (g/dL)	White Blood Cell (per mm³)	Reticulocyte Count (per mm³)	Platelet Count (per mm³)
Normal	Male: 4.7–6.1; female: 4.2–5.4	Male: 14–18; female: 12–16	Male: 42–52; female: 37–47	80–90	27–31	32–36	5000–10,000	0.5–2	150,000–400,000
Acute hemorrhagic anemia	Initial increase, latent decrease	Initial decrease, latent decrease	Normal initially; latent decrease	Increase	Decrease	Normal	Increase	Increase	Decrease
Chronic hemorrhagic anemia	Decrease	Decrease	Decrease	Slight decrease	Slight decrease	Slight decrease	Normal	Decrease	Normal
Iron deficiency anemia	Decrease	Decrease	Decrease	Decrease	Decrease	Decrease	Normal	Decrease	Normal to increase
Aplastic anemia	Gross decrease	Gross decrease	Gross decrease	Moderate decrease	Gross decrease	Gross decrease	Gross decrease	Decrease	Gross decrease
Pernicious anemia	Decrease	Gross decrease	Gross decrease	Increase	Increase	Increase	Slight decrease	Decrease	Slight decrease
Folic acid deficiency anemia	Decrease	Gross decrease	Gross decrease	Increase	Increase	Increase	Slight decrease	Decrease	Slight decrease
Sickle cell anemia	Decrease	Decrease	Decrease	Decrease	Normal	Normal	Increase	Increase	Normal
Hemolytic anemia	Decrease	Decrease	Decrease	Increase	Slight decrease	Normal	Normal	Increase	Normal to increase

Diagnosis

Blood studies show leukopenia, with a substantial decrease in the number of polymorphonuclear cells. Bone marrow studies reveal a lack of granulocytes, and the developing WBCs are not mature and are reduced in number. History may reveal exposure to the offending infectious agents; blood, urine, and oral cultures may be positive for bacteria; and toxins may be present.

Treatment

The primary thrust of treatment is to eliminate any offending microorganism through aggressive antimicrobial therapy. Cultures are repeated several times and are monitored for the growth of microbes. If the cause of the toxicity is identified as a drug or chemical, exposure to the toxic agent must be halted. Aggressive therapy is indicated because the condition can be fatal within a week if left untreated.

Prognosis

The prognosis varies, depending on the etiology of the condition. Cessation of exposure to a toxic substance often results in improvement. As previously mentioned, in some cases, this condition, if left untreated, may be fatal within a week.

Prevention

Prevention involves avoiding the toxic substance after it has been identified. Prevention is not always possible.

Patient Teaching

Give the patient information about exposure to the toxic substance. Help the patient and the family find information about exposure to hazardous materials.

Polycythemia

Description

Polycythemia (polycythemia vera) is an abnormal increase in the amount of hemoglobin, the RBC count, or the hematocrit, causing an absolute increase in the RBC mass.

ICD-10-CM Code	D45 (Polycythemia vera)

Symptoms and Signs

Symptoms of polycythemia are related to the increased RBC mass and include headaches, dyspnea, irritability, mental sluggishness, dizziness, syncope, night sweats, and weight loss. Circulatory stagnation, thrombus, and increased blood viscosity may be noted. Splenomegaly, clubbing of fingers, and cyanosis may be observed.

Patient Screening

Patients reporting headaches, dyspnea, irritability, mental sluggishness, dizziness, syncope, night sweats, and weight loss require prompt assessment. Schedule an appointment as soon as possible. If a prompt appointment is not possible, refer the patient to a facility where assessment can be performed quickly.

Etiology

It is not known why a sustained increase in the hematopoiesis of bone marrow causes absolute, or primary, polycythemia. Relative polycythemia results when plasma volume is reduced by dehydration, plasma loss, fluid and electrolyte imbalances, or burns. Reduced oxygen supply to the tissues results in compensation by the body as it manufactures additional hemoglobin to carry additional oxygen. The body uses this compensatory process when patients have chronic pulmonary and cardiac diseases or live at high altitudes, where the oxygen concentration is reduced.

Diagnosis

An abnormal increase in RBC numbers, hemoglobin levels, and hematocrit suggests the condition. Leukocyte and thrombocyte counts also are elevated, and the spleen may be enlarged. The clinical picture aids in the diagnosis. Evaluation of the total RBC mass is also diagnostic.

Treatment

Periodic phlebotomy is employed to reduce the blood volume. Myelosuppressive drugs and radiation also improve the blood count. Relative polycythemia usually subsides when the causative factors are eliminated.

Prognosis

Periodic phlebotomies help reduce the RBC count and hematocrit. This treatment is a required lifelong protocol for many patients. In some cases, the condition will resolve, as previously mentioned.

Prevention

With no known etiology, no prevention is possible.

Patient Teaching

Emphasize the importance of routine blood cell counts and the need for continued phlebotomy. Encourage patients to keep routine appointments.

Thrombocytopenia

Idiopathic thrombocytopenic purpura is considered an autoimmune response. This dyscrasia involves a reduction in the clotting capability of blood and is discussed in Chapter 3.

Leukemias

Leukemias are malignant neoplasms of the blood-forming organs (bone marrow, spleen, and lymph nodes) and produce an abnormal, uncontrolled, clonal proliferation of one specific type of blood cell in the lymphoid or myeloid cell lines. The large number of leukemic cells leads to bone marrow overcrowding, resulting in the reduced production and function of normal blood cells. The reduced numbers of functional neutrophils, erythrocytes, and platelets result in frequent infections, anemia, and clotting problems.

Leukemias are classified by cell type and degree of differentiation of the neoplastic cells. In acute leukemias, immature-appearing, large hematopoietic cells (blasts) are present. In chronic leukemias, the cells are more mature appearing yet hypofunctional. Acute disease has a rapid progression and can be quickly fatal (with a natural history of 1 to 5 months), whereas chronic leukemias have a slower progression that is measured in years rather than months. Common types of leukemia include acute lymphocytic leukemia (ALL), chronic lymphocytic leukemia (CLL), acute myelogenous leukemia (AML), and chronic myelogenous leukemia (CML).

Acute Lymphocytic Leukemia

Description

ALL is characterized by overproduction of immature lymphoid cells (lymphoblasts) in bone marrow and lymph nodes. It is generally classified into two subtypes, depending on the type of cells affected: B-cell ALL or T-cell ALL.

ICD-10-CM Code	C91.00 (Acute lymphoblastic leukemia not having achieved remission) (C91.00-C91.02 = 3 codes of specificity)

Refer to the physician's diagnosis for specific type of lymphoid leukemia and then to the current edition of the ICD-10-CM coding manual to ensure the greatest specificity of pathology.

Symptoms and Signs

The patient appears pale and may report bone pain, weight loss, sore throat, fatigue, fever, night sweats, and weakness. There is a tendency toward increased bruising and bleeding. As the leukemic cells infiltrate the spleen, liver, lymph nodes, and nervous system, they interfere with the normal functioning of these organs. Lymphadenopathy and splenomegaly are common at presentation. Symptoms of central nervous system (CNS) involvement include headache, blurred vision, nausea, vomiting, and cranial nerve palsies. A mediastinal mass can be found in many patients with the T-cell ALL.

Patient Screening

Patients complaining of bone pain, weight loss, fatigue, night sweats, weakness, persistent fevers, a tendency toward increased bruising and bleeding, recurrent infections, headache, blurred vision, and/or cranial nerve palsies require prompt assessment by a physician.

Etiology

ALL accounts for 20% of adult leukemias and is the most common childhood leukemia. Childhood ALL is covered in more detail in Chapter 2. The exact cause is unknown. Prolonged exposure to radiation, certain chemicals and drugs, smoking, viruses, and genetic factors (certain chromosomal abnormalities) are considered contributing factors.

Diagnosis

Peripheral blood smear analysis shows increased numbers of immature lymphocytes and reduced numbers of erythrocytes and platelets. Microscopic examination of a bone marrow aspiration or biopsy specimen is necessary for definitive diagnosis. Blast cells should make up greater than 25% of all nucleated cells in bone marrow to diagnose ALL. Cerebrospinal fluid (CSF) should be withdrawn and examined for leukemic cells. Karyotyping is performed to look for any abnormalities that may help determine prognosis and treatment options.

Treatment

Treatment regimens for ALL involve aggressive chemotherapy for 2 to 3 years, consisting of three phases: induction, consolidation, and maintenance. Because CNS invasion is common in ALL, the CNS is treated with intrathecally administered chemotherapy even if blasts are not noted in CSF. Those with the Philadelphia chromosome are often treated with tyrosine inhibitors. Hematopoietic stem cell transplantation (HSCT) is an option for patients who have relapsed or for adults with poor prognostic features.

Prognosis

The overall 5-year survival rate is 78% to 85%, with children generally having a better prognosis than adults. Adults often have cytogenetic abnormalities that carry a worse prognosis than the ones found in children. In addition, children often can tolerate relatively higher doses of the drugs currently used to treat ALL than adults can. Poor prognostic indicators include age less than 1 year, CNS invasion, presence of the Philadelphia chromosome or other adverse abnormalities, and failure to achieve remission after induction therapy is completed.

Prevention

No prevention methods are known for ALL.

Patient Teaching

Give patients and parents of affected children information about chemotherapy. Help them find and contact community support groups.

Chronic Lymphocytic Leukemia

Description

CLL is a neoplasm that involves lymphocytes. It is a slowly progressing disease that results in the accumulation of mature-appearing, but hypofunctional, lymphocytes.

ICD-10-CM Code	C91.10 (Chronic lymphocytic leukemia of B-cell type not having achieved remission) (C91.10-C91.12 = 3 codes of specificity)

Refer to the physician's diagnosis for specific type of lymphoid leukemia and then to the current edition of the ICD-10-CM coding manual to ensure the greatest specificity of pathology.

Symptoms and Signs

Patients often have no symptoms when a routine CBC reveals lymphocytosis, thrombocytopenia, or anemia. Symptoms may include weight loss, fever, night sweats, extreme fatigue, splenomegaly, hepatomegaly, and painless swelling of cervical, supraclavicular, or axillary lymph nodes that spontaneously waxes and wanes. Patients are susceptible to frequent viral and fungal infections.

Patient Screening

Patients complaining of weight loss, fever, night sweats, extreme fatigue, and noticeable swelling of the cervical, supraclavicular, or axillary lymph nodes require prompt assessment by a physician.

Etiology

CLL is the most common leukemia in adults. The median age at diagnosis is 70 years, and there is a male predominance. Having a first-degree relative with CLL increases the risk for CLL.

Diagnosis

Nearly 95% of cases are discovered incidentally during routine blood work. Peripheral blood smear analysis, with or without bone marrow studies, is performed and reveals an increased number of mature-appearing lymphocytes. In most cases of CLL, the absolute lymphocyte count is greater than 5000/µL and the bone marrow is hypercellular, with lymphocytes accounting for greater than 30% of all nucleated cells. Because CLL most often involves B lymphocytes, screening for the presence of certain B-cell markers is performed. Karyotyping and testing for certain genetic mutations are performed.

Many staging systems for CLL have been proposed, but the Rai system is the most commonly used one in the United States. The stage of the disease is important in determining the appropriate treatment and the prognosis. The Rai system stratifies patients into risk groups according to their symptoms and assigns average survival times to those groups. Patients usually move through the risk groups during the course of their disease:

- Stage 0: Patients have lymphocytosis and bone marrow infiltration of greater than 30% blasts. Median survival time is 12 years.
- Stage I: Patients have lymphadenopathy. Median survival time is 9 years.
- Stage II: Patients have splenomegaly and/or hepatomegaly. Median survival time is 6 years.
- Stage III: Patients have anemia. Median survival time is 1 year.
- Stage IV: Patients have thrombocytopenia. Median survival time is 1 year.

Treatment

Treatment often is withheld until the patient is symptomatic and has evidence of hemolytic anemia, painful lymphadenopathy, symptomatic organomegaly, cytopenia, prolonged fever, chills, or weight loss. CLL is usually treated with chemotherapy. Radiation therapy can be used to reduce the symptoms caused by lymphadenopathy and splenomegaly. Other therapies include the use of monoclonal antibodies directed against B-lymphocyte surface antigens; these agents include rituximab (Rituxan) (directed against CD20) or alemtuzumab (Campath) (directed against CD52). Other medication therapies may include chlorambucil, pentostatin, prednisone, or cladribine; transplantation is generally not an option for patients with CLL, although the newly developed nonmyeloablative transplants show promise as a potential treatment for CLL.

Prognosis

CLL has a variable natural course. Survival times from diagnosis range from 2 to 20 years. The overall 5-year survival rate is 73%. Poor prognostic indicators are low platelet count and low hemoglobin level at the time of diagnosis. Certain genetic aberrations have prognostic implications as well. For example, the high-risk TP53 corresponds to a 5-year overall survival rate of 51%, whereas the low-risk del13q14 carries a 5-year survival rate of 87%. During the initial asymptomatic phase, patients often can maintain their normal lifestyle, but performance levels during the terminal phase are poor, and frequent causes of death include systemic infection, bleeding, and cachexia.

Prevention

No methods for prevention of CLL are known.

Patient Teaching

Give patients and parents of affected children information about chemotherapy. Help them find and contact community support groups.

Acute Myelogenous Leukemia

Description

AML (also known as *acute myeloid, myelocytic,* or *granulocytic leukemia*) is a rapidly progressive neoplasm of cells committed to the myeloid line of development. Leukemic cells accumulate in bone marrow, peripheral blood, and other tissues.

ICD-10-CM Code	C92.00 *(Acute myeloblastic leukemia, not having achieved remission)*
	(C92.00-C92.02 = 3 codes of specificity)
	C92.40 *(Acute promyelocytic leukemia, not having achieved remission)*
	(C92.40-C92.42 = 3 codes of specificity)
	C92.50 *(Acute myelomonocytic leukemia, not having achieved remission)*

(C92.50–92.52 = 3 codes of specificity)

Refer to the physician's diagnosis for specific type of myeloid leukemia and then to the current edition of the ICD-10-CM coding manual to ensure the greatest specificity of pathology.

Symptoms and Signs

A rapid accumulation of myeloblasts (myeloid precursors) leads to pancytopenia and the resulting symptoms of anemia, easy bleeding and bruising, and increased risk of infection. Bleeding symptoms include gingival bleeding, epistaxis, and menorrhagia. Weight loss, fatigue, and pallor are common. Lymphadenopathy and organomegaly are rare.

Etiology

AML accounts for 80% of acute adult leukemia and 20% of childhood leukemia. Risk factors include a positive family history for AML or other leukemias; prior therapeutic treatment with ionizing radiation; prior aggressive chemotherapy treatment for Hodgkin disease, non-Hodgkin lymphoma (NHL), ovarian cancer, or breast cancer; chronic exposure to benzene (a toxic liquid found in gasoline, rubber cement, and cleaning solvents); and cigarette smoking. In about 10% to 15% of AML cases, the leukemia is treatment related (i.e., prior radiation or chemotherapy). Many cases of AML occurred among Japanese survivors of the atomic bomb attack in 1945 and the Chernobyl nuclear power plant in Russia in 1986.

Diagnosis

The diagnosis is suggested by the clinical picture and the results of peripheral blood smear analysis. Half the patients have an Auer rod (abnormal lysosomal granules) visible inside the leukemic cell (Fig. 10.53). The presence of an Auer rod is diagnostic of AML. Bone marrow aspiration and biopsy are needed for definitive diagnosis. Bone marrow usually is hypercellular, with greater than 20% myeloblasts. After diagnosis, morphologic classification and cytogenetic analysis must be performed to determine the treatment

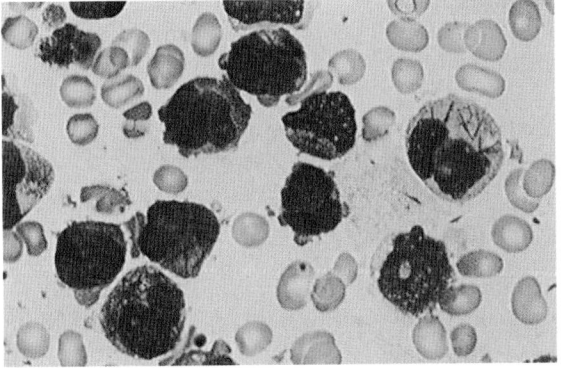

• **Fig. 10.53** Auer rod cells. (From Wiernik, et al: *Neoplastic diseases of the blood,* ed 3, New York, 1996, Churchill Livingstone.)

selection. In addition, molecular studies are done to look for specific genetic mutations that affect treatment choice and prognosis. For the classification of AML based on morphologic cell type, the World Health Organization (WHO) classification scheme is used.

Treatment

Routine laboratory testing (e.g., CBC, liver function tests, and coagulation studies), chest radiography, ECG, and herpes simplex virus (HSV) and cytomegalovirus (CMV) serology are requested to identify potential complications of therapy. Chemotherapy is the first approach to treating AML. Usually cytarabine and daunorubicin are given to induce remission. HSCT during the first remission is recommended in high-risk cases. Complete remission is defined as having normal peripheral blood cell counts and less than 5% blasts in bone marrow.

Acute promyelocytic leukemia (APL) is a form of AML that is distinct from other subtypes. It is characterized by a translocation between the long arms of chromosomes 15 and 17, t(15;17), creating a fusion gene, *PML/RAR-a.* The gene product impairs differentiation and apoptosis of promyelocytes. The impairment can be overcome by administration of all-trans retinoic acid (ATRA), a derivative of vitamin A, often in conjunction with cytotoxic chemotherapy and arsenic trioxide. The patient should be monitored for signs of disseminated intravascular coagulation (DIC) and differentiation syndrome (e.g., fever, peripheral edema, respiratory distress, and renal and hepatic dysfunction).

Prognosis

The overall 5-year survival rate for AML is highly dependent on the prognostic indicators. The 5-year survival rate for patients who are 20 years of age or older is approximately 24%. Patients who are younger than 20 years of age have a 5-year survival rate of 67%. Adverse prognostic indicators are advanced age, history of a prior hematologic disorder, and poor performance status at diagnosis. Some cytogenetic abnormalities, such as the translocations t(8;21) and t(15;17), have a more favorable prognosis. The t(15;17) translocation is considered favorable because of the excellent treatment response of APL to ATRA and chemotherapy.

Prevention

No methods of preventing AML are known.

Patient Teaching

Give patients and parents of affected children information about chemotherapy. Help them find and contact community support groups.

Chronic Myelogenous Leukemia

Description

CML (also known as *chronic myeloid* or *myelocytic leukemia*) is a slowly progressing neoplasm that arises in a hematopoietic stem cell or early progenitor cell, resulting in an excess of mature-appearing but hypofunctional neutrophils.

ICD-10-CM Code   C92.10 (Chronic myeloid leukemia, BCR/ABL-positive, not having achieved remission)
(C92.10-C92.22 = 6 codes of specificity)

Refer to the physician's diagnosis for specific type of myeloid leukemia and then to the current edition of the ICD-10-CM coding manual to ensure the greatest specificity of pathology.

Symptoms and Signs

The disease has a triphasic course: a chronic phase, an accelerated phase, and a blast crisis. Most patients are diagnosed in the chronic phase, where abnormal proliferation of WBCs has begun. These patients are usually asymptomatic at the time of diagnosis, with the disease being suspected on the basis of abnormalities, such as leukocytosis and thrombocytosis, on routine blood tests. Splenomegaly is common, but the symptoms are mild. In the accelerated phase, leukocytosis increases, and neutrophil differentiation becomes further impaired. The patient may experience bone pain, fever, night sweats, and other systemic symptoms. The blast crisis resembles AML and is defined by the presence of 30% or greater blasts in the peripheral blood or bone marrow. Symptoms worsen, and new chromosomal abnormalities are acquired. CML progresses to blast crisis an average of 3 to 5 years after diagnosis and 3 to 18 months after initiation of the accelerated phase. The average survival after blast crisis is 3 months.

Etiology

CML accounts for about 15% of leukemia cases in adults, and the average age of diagnosis is 64 years. CML is almost invariably associated with an abnormal chromosome 22, the Philadelphia chromosome.

Diagnosis

The diagnosis is suggested by the clinical picture and blood and bone marrow studies. CBC reveals anemia, leukocytosis, and thrombocytosis. Bone marrow biopsy shows hyperplasia, but the cells appear more mature than the leukemic cells in AML. Definitive diagnosis requires demonstrating the presence of the Philadelphia chromosome or the *BCR/ABL* fusion gene product with cytogenetic analysis, fluorescence in situ hybridization (FISH), or polymerase chain reaction (PCR). The presence of the Philadelphia chromosome distinguishes CML from other disorders that may resemble CML clinically.

Treatment

Cure can only be achieved via HSCT (see the Enrichment box about Hematopoietic Stem Cell Transplantation). However, HSCT is not a viable option for all patients. Initial treatment is with drugs that specifically inhibit the

BCR/ABL tyrosine kinase, known as *tyrosine kinase inhibitors* (TKIs). Their use is aimed at achieving long-term control of the disease, although they do not cure the disease. With TKIs, many patients can obtain complete remission, which can be sustained for years. *Complete remission* is defined as ablation of the Philadelphia chromosome and its gene product.

Prognosis

The overall 5-year survival rate has increased in the past few years. Indicators of poorer prognosis include large spleen size, older age of the patient, higher percentage of blast cells, and a platelet count greater than 700,000/μL.

Prevention

No methods are known to prevent CML.

Patient Teaching

Give patients and parents of affected children information about chemotherapy. Help them find and contact community support groups.

Lymphatic Diseases

The lymphatic system is composed of lymphatic vessels, lymphatic tissue (lymph nodes, tonsils, thymus, and spleen), and lymph. The lymphatic vessels originate at the capillary level and, along with the venous system, progress to empty into the right and left subclavian veins (Fig. 10.54). This system has no pump. Lymph nodes, collections of lymphatic tissue, filter foreign material (e.g., bacteria and viruses) from the lymphatic circulation (Fig. 10.55). Lymphocytes are produced mainly in the lymph nodes as part of the body's defense mechanism. The lymphatic vessels are thin walled, and the larger vessels contain valves. As in the case of the venous system, the muscles exert intermittent pressure on the vessels, causing the lymph to flow by a milking action. Smooth muscle in the vessel wall contracts to aid the return of lymph to the cardiovascular system. Swollen lymph nodes or glands may indicate trapping of microbes during an infectious process.

Lymphedema

Description

Lymphedema is an abnormal collection of lymph, usually in the extremities.

ICD-10-CM Code   I89.0 (Lymphedema, not elsewhere classified)
I97.2 (Postmastectomy lymphedema syndrome)

Symptoms and Signs

Lymphedema results in swelling of the extremities. Most patients experience no pain, although in severe cases, lymphedema can cause pain and limit movement. The affected extremity becomes swollen and grossly distended (Fig. 10.56).

Hematopoietic Stem Cell Transplantation

Many patients with leukemias and lymphomas cannot be cured with conventional chemotherapy treatments alone. The very large doses of chemotherapy or radiation that would be required to fully destroy all the neoplastic cells in patients with relapsed disease or disease refractory to conventional treatment make people very sick and destroy bone marrow. Few people are able to withstand this severe treatment.

Hematopoietic stem cell transplantation (HSCT), also known as *bone marrow transplantation* (BMT), was developed to treat such patients. In the traditional BMT protocol, the patient first receives high-dose chemotherapy and/or radiation therapy to eradicate all malignant cells in the body and to suppress the body's immune system so that it is less likely to attack the donor marrow. Next stem cells obtained from a donor's bone marrow are infused into the recipient. The stem cells find their way into the marrow space of the recipient and restore marrow functioning in 2 to 4 weeks.

A newer method of HSCT has been developed in recent years. Studies have shown that stem cells may be harvested directly from the donor's peripheral blood after hematopoietic growth factors have been administered to the donor to mobilize stem cells from bone marrow to the bloodstream. The stem cells are collected by using a pheresis machine and then infused into the recipient. These peripheral blood cells can restore neutrophil and platelet production several days faster than stem cells derived from bone marrow. Therefore this peripheral blood stem cell transplantation is preferred over the traditional HSCT for many patients.

An investigational approach called *nonmyeloablative transplantation,* or "mini transplantation," has shown some promise in treating older adults and those who are unable to tolerate the high initial doses of chemotherapy in conventional BMT. It uses mild chemotherapy and low-dose radiation before transplantation of the donor stem cells. The donor cells gradually replace the host marrow and kill neoplastic cells by an immunologic "graft versus tumor" effect.

All of these transplantations carry the risk of severe infections and bleeding, serious damage to vital organs caused by the initial chemotherapy and radiation therapy, and graft rejection by the host's cells. Graft-versus-host disease (GVHD), an immunologic reaction in which the donor T lymphocytes see host tissues, especially the skin, liver, and GI tract, as foreign and attack it, is not uncommon. Relapse may also occur and is seen most often in patients with ALL and CML who received transplantations during blast crisis.

Definitions of some terms commonly used in conjunction with BMT are:

- *Autologous transplantation:* Transplantation in which the patient serves as his or her own donor for stem cells.
- *Allogeneic transplantation:* Transplantation in which the donor is human leukocyte antigen (HLA) identical to the patient (usually a sibling).
- *Haploidentical transplantation:* Transplantation in which the donor is a relative only half-matched to the recipient (usually a parent).
- *HLA type:* The identity of the leukocyte surface antigens, the HLAs, is determined for the patient and donor to define the degree of compatibility. The closer the match is, the lower is the risk of transplantation-related complications.
- *Syngeneic transplantation:* Transplantation in which the patient's identical twin serves as the stem cell donor.
- *Unrelated donor/mismatched transplantation:* Transplantation in which the donor does not match all of the key HLA antigens. This type of transplantation is associated with the greatest risk of complications.

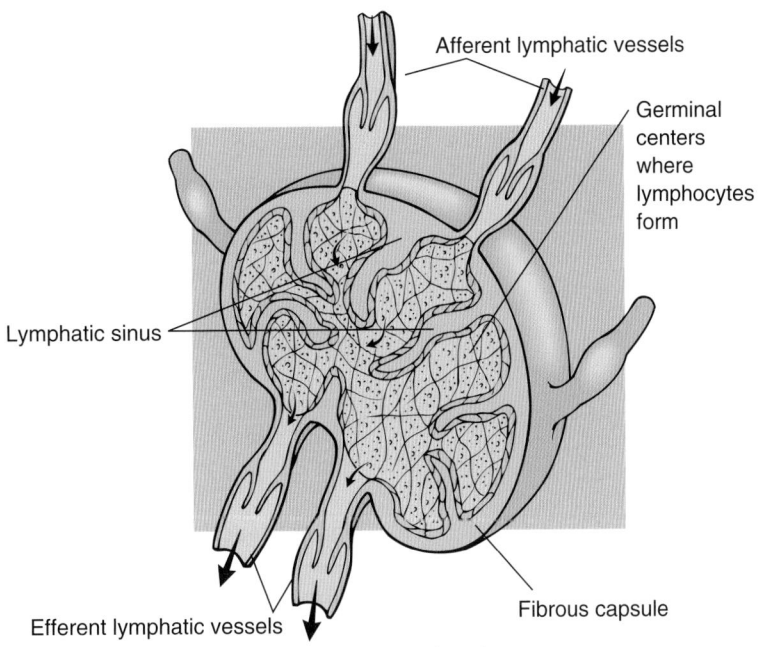

Afferent lymphatic vessels

Germinal centers where lymphocytes form

Lymphatic sinus

Efferent lymphatic vessels

Fibrous capsule

• **Fig. 10.54** Lymph node.

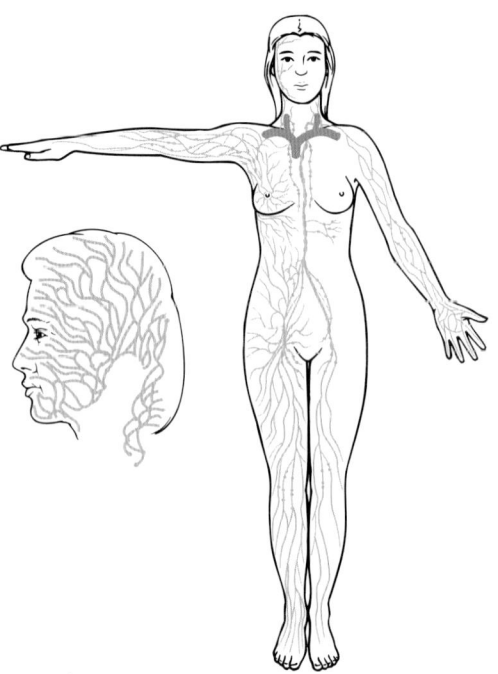

• **Fig. 10.55** Lymphatic system.

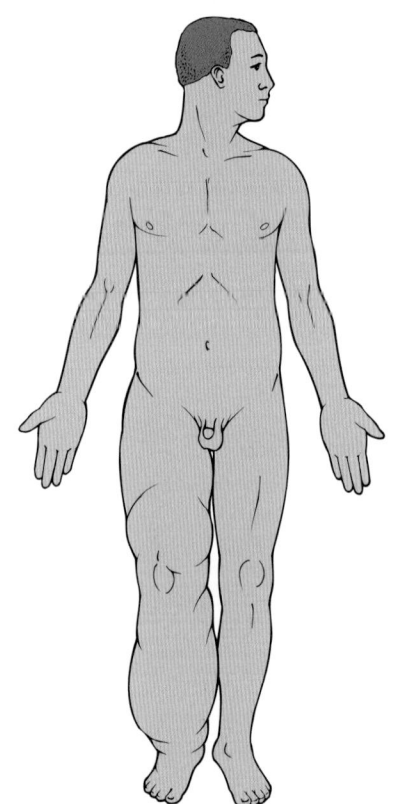

• **Fig. 10.56** Lymphedema.

Patient Screening

Patients reporting unilateral limb swelling require prompt assessment. Schedule an appointment for these patients to be seen as soon as possible, or refer them to a facility where they can be assessed quickly.

Etiology

The obstruction of the lymph vessel or node may be inflammatory or mechanical. If lymphedema is left untreated, the connective tissues lose their elasticity, and the edema becomes permanent. The lymphatic circulation may be compromised by an infection, neoplasm, or thrombus. Allergic reactions also may be implicated, along with trauma or surgery involving the affected part. Tight clothing that constricts the lymphatic vessels can cause temporary lymphedema. Removing the constriction usually resolves the swelling. Women who have had mastectomies may experience lymphedema in the adjacent arm. Prolonged lymphedema rarely is associated with the development of lymphosarcoma (a cancer).

Diagnosis

Painless swelling in an extremity suggests lymphedema. Imaging procedures, including lymphangiography and radioactive isotope studies, are means of confirming the diagnosis and ascertaining the site of obstruction.

Treatment

Treatment is aimed at reducing the swelling. The affected limb is elevated to a level above the heart to encourage drainage of the lymph. Elastic bandages or stockings are applied when the affected part is elevated to compress the area, also encouraging lymph drainage. Diuretics may be administered to reduce fluid volume. Surgical intervention may be attempted to relieve a mechanical obstruction. Antibiotics may be administered if infection is present.

Prognosis

The prognosis varies, depending on the cause of the lymphedema and the patient's response to therapeutic intervention. When conservative measures fail to reduce the swelling, surgical intervention to remove the cause of the obstruction usually has a positive outcome. When lymphedema is left untreated, the connective tissues can lose their elasticity, resulting in the edema becoming permanent.

Lymphedema is not in itself life threatening, but it carries a danger that uncontrolled infection can develop in the affected tissue. The essentially stagnant interstitial fluids are a breeding ground for infections and their resulting toxins (poisons). Local defenses are overwhelmed, and the normal systemic defense system is not activated.

Prevention

Many cases are not preventable. Wearing of tight clothing that can restrict lymphatic flow should be discouraged.

Patient Teaching

Give patients information about the preventable causes of lymphedema. Encourage postmastectomy patients to follow the prescribed rehabilitation exercises that help reduce the incidence of lymphedema.

Lymphangitis

Description
Lymphangitis is an inflammation of the lymph vessels.

ICD-10-CM Code I89.1 *(Lymphangitis)*
(I89.0-I89.9 = 4 codes of specificity)

Symptoms and Signs
Lymphangitis usually manifests as a red streak at the site of entry of the infective organism. The redness extends to the regional lymph node, which is swollen and tender. Cellulitis may develop in surrounding tissue. Manifestations of generalized infection, including fever, chills, and malaise, are present.

Patient Screening
Patients reporting fever, chills, and generalized malaise, accompanied by tenderness and redness in the region of a lymph node, require prompt assessment by a physician.

Etiology
Bacterial invasion into the lymph vessels at the site of local trauma or ulceration is a frequent cause of lymphangitis. Occasionally no portal of entry is detectable. The bacteria travel to the regional lymph nodes and stimulate inflammation.

Diagnosis
Visual inspection of the involved area and observance of typical systemic manifestations of bacterial invasion are usually sufficient for diagnosis. Blood studies indicate leukocytosis. Final confirmation is made by cultures of the infected tissue.

Treatment
Treatment includes administration of systemic antibiotics. The affected area is elevated and rested, and warm, wet dressings are applied locally. Surgical drainage of purulent material is indicated.

Prognosis
The prognosis varies, depending on the amount of tissue involved and the nature of the causative organism. The patient's response to antibiotics also plays a role in recovery. Surgical intervention usually contributes to a more positive outcome.

Prevention
This condition usually cannot be prevented. Good hand washing always helps prevent any infectious process.

Patient Teaching
Give patients information about postoperative care of incision sites. Emphasize the importance of complying with and completing any prescribed antibiotic therapy.

Lymphoma

Lymphomas are malignant neoplasms that arise from uncontrolled proliferation of the cellular components of the lymph system. The dysfunctional cells may be B cells, T cells, or, rarely, both. The neoplastic lymphocytes are migratory and can be found not only in the lymph structures but also in the bloodstream, bone marrow, and, later in the disease, non-lymph organs (e.g., liver or lung). Lymphomas are divided into two main categories: Hodgkin lymphoma and other types that are grouped as NHL.

Treatment selection is determined by the cell type and the stage of the disease. Both kinds of lymphoma are staged by using the Ann Arbor-Cotswolds staging system, which considers the neoplastic involvement of lymph structures (lymph nodes, spleen, and thymus), extranodal tumor sites, and the presence or absence of the systemic "B" symptoms of lymphoma (unexplained weight loss of greater than 10% of body weight in the past 6 months, persistent or recurrent fevers with temperatures greater than 38°C during the previous month, and recurrent, drenching night sweats during the previous month).

- Stage I: A single lymph structure or region is involved.
- Stage II: Two or more lymph structures are involved, with the involvement being on the same side of the diaphragm.
- Stage III: Lymph regions on both sides of the diaphragm are involved.
- Stage IV: There is widespread involvement of extranodal tissue above and below the diaphragm.

Each stage designation carries either an "A" or a "B" after the stage number, indicating whether any of the "B" symptoms are absent (A) or present (B).

Hodgkin Lymphoma

Description
Hodgkin disease (also called *Hodgkin lymphoma*) is a cancer of the body's lymphatic system, in which the involved cells proliferate and interfere with normal functioning by collecting in masses in various parts of the body. Tumors arise in the tissue of the lymph nodes and spread to other lymph nodes, the spleen, the liver, and bone marrow.

ICD-10-CM Code C81.90 *(Hodgkin lymphoma, unspecified, unspecified site)*
C81.99 *(Hodgkin lymphoma, unspecified, extranodal and solid organ sites)*
(C81.00-C81.99 = 70 codes of specificity)

Hodgkin disease is coded by type. Refer to the physician's diagnosis and then to the current edition of the ICD-10-CM coding manual to ensure the greatest specificity of pathology.

Symptoms and Signs
The initial symptoms of Hodgkin lymphoma are painless enlargement of the lymph nodes in the neck or the

mediastinum, fatigue, and pruritus (Fig. 10.57). As the disease progresses, the patient may experience the systemic B symptoms, such as fever, night sweats, and weight loss. Hodgkin disease is differentiated from other lymphomas by the presence in the lymphatic tissue of a Reed-Sternberg cell, a large cell with two or more mirror-image nuclei, each with a single nucleolus (Fig. 10.58).

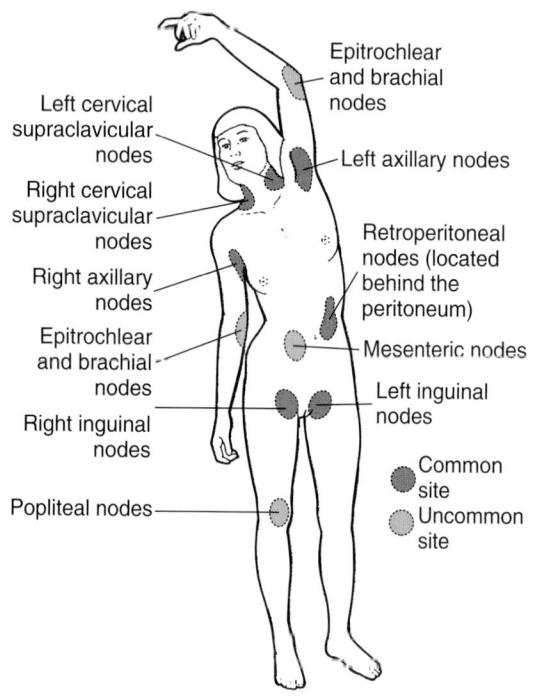

• **Fig. 10.57** Lymph node sites for Hodgkin disease. (From Huether SE, McCance KL: *Understanding pathophysiology*, ed 4, St Louis, 2008, Mosby/Elsevier.)

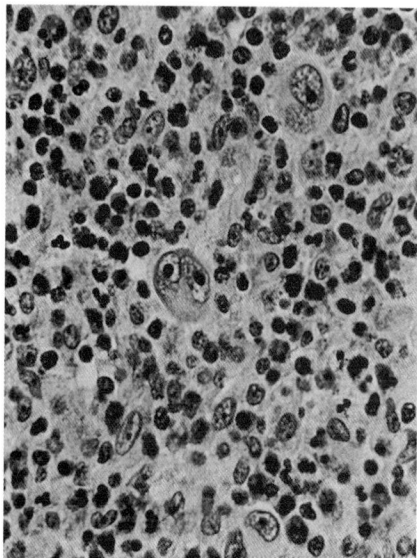

• **Fig. 10.58** Reed-Sternberg cell. (From Wiernik, et al: *Neoplastic diseases of the blood*, ed 3, New York, 1996, Churchill Livingstone.)

Patient Screening

For patients reporting a painless enlargement of cervical lymph nodes, fatigue, and pruritus, an appointment should be scheduled as soon as possible. When the complaints include fever, night sweats, and weight loss, prompt assessment by a physician is required.

Etiology

Hodgkin disease is the most curable type of lymphoma. Young adults 15 to 40 years of age and those older than age 55 years are diagnosed more frequently than at other ages. Risk factors for the development of Hodgkin disease include previous history of malignancy, prior treatment with chemotherapy or radiation therapy, family history of Hodgkin disease or other lymphomas, immunosuppression, and exposure to Epstein-Barr virus (EBV) or similar viruses. Those of male gender have a higher incidence.

Diagnosis

A history of painless lymphadenopathy and the typical symptoms of Hodgkin disease lead to excisional lymph node biopsy for definitive diagnosis. The node biopsy shows the presence of Reed-Sternberg cells. Immunophenotyping of the tissue for certain markers is very helpful in making the diagnosis. Blood studies indicate mild normochromic, normocytic anemia; neutrophilic leukocytosis; lymphopenia; and eosinophilia. The ESR is elevated, as is the serum alkaline phosphatase level. Bone marrow biopsy is performed only on select patients and may show abnormal cells. CT scans of the chest, abdomen, and pelvis help evaluate the extent of disease. Liver and kidney function tests are performed.

Treatment

Combined chemoradiotherapy is preferred for patients in stages I and II and some patients in stage III. Patients in stage IIIB and stage IV often are treated with chemotherapy alone. The preferred regimen is ABVD (doxorubicin, bleomycin, vinblastine, dacarbazine) therapy. Other medication therapies may include chlorambucil, pentostatin, prednisone, or cladribine. Relapses usually are treated with additional chemotherapy. HSCT may be used to treat patients with multiple relapses.

Prognosis

Hodgkin lymphoma is one of the most treatable forms of cancer and can be cured. The overall 5-year survival rate approaches 90%. Death may result from Hodgkin lymphoma itself or from secondary cancers or cardiovascular disease, side effects of treatment that often are not apparent until years after therapy. Important indicators of poor prognosis include the presence of B symptoms, low serum albumin and hemoglobin levels, male gender, age greater than 45 years, anemia, leukocytosis, and a high ESR.

Prevention

No ways of preventing Hodgkin lymphoma are known.

Patient Teaching

Give patients information about chemotherapy and radiation therapy. Help them find and contact community support groups.

Non-Hodgkin Lymphoma

Description

NHL describes a number of heterogeneous neoplasms of the lymphoid cells that exhibit a wide variety of clinical signs and symptoms, ranging from a slow, indolent growth to rapidly fatal progression. Some can be cured with appropriate treatment, but for others, treatment does not prolong survival.

ICD-10-CM Code	C85.80 (Other specified types of non-Hodgkin lymphoma, unspecified site) C85.89 (Other specified types of non-Hodgkin lymphoma, extranodal and solid organ sites) (C85.10-C85.99 = 40 codes of specificity)

Symptoms and Signs

As with Hodgkin lymphoma, symptoms include painless lymphadenopathy, fatigue, pruritus, bone pain, and GI symptoms. Other lymphatic tissue, such as tonsils and adenoids, may be enlarged, and the patient can experience B symptoms, such as fever, night sweats, and weight loss.

Patient Screening

As with Hodgkin lymphoma, patients reporting a painless enlargement of the cervical lymph nodes, fatigue, and pruritus should be scheduled as soon as possible. When the complaints include fever, night sweats, and weight loss, prompt assessment by a physician is required.

Etiology

The incidence of NHL reaches a peak in preadolescence, then drops in incidence, and increases again with increasing age. Risk factors include personal or family history of prior malignancy; previous treatment with radiation therapy, immunotherapy, or chemotherapy; infection with human immunodeficiency virus (HIV), human T-cell lymphotropic virus (HTLV), EBV, or hepatitis C virus; immunosuppression, and connective tissue disorders, such as lupus and rheumatoid arthritis. GI lymphoma may be seen in patients with Crohn disease, celiac disease, and *Helicobacter pylori*-associated chronic gastritis.

NHL is grouped into three main categories based on how aggressively each neoplasm in the group behaves. The indolent lymphomas represent 35% to 40% of NHLs. The most common subtypes are follicular lymphoma (grades I and II behave as indolent; grade III behaves as aggressive), small lymphocytic lymphoma, mantle cell lymphoma, and marginal zone lymphoma. They may arise from any B-cell, T-cell, or natural killer (NK)-cell line. Aggressive lymphomas

represent 50% of NHLs. The most common subtypes are diffuse large B-cell lymphoma and peripheral T-cell lymphoma. Highly aggressive lymphomas are rarer, representing 5% of all NHLs. These include Burkitt lymphoma (thought to be caused, in part, by EBV) and adult T-cell lymphoma (caused by HTLV).

Diagnosis

Patient evaluation must include determination of the histologic subtype, the extent of disease, and the performance status of the patient, because treatment and prognosis greatly depend on this information. All potentially involved lymphoid sites should be physically examined. Excisional biopsy of an intact, involved lymph node is necessary for accurate histopathologic identification of the disease. Immunologic, cytogenetic, and molecular studies may be performed to further aid in therapeutic decisions and in the determination of the prognosis. Bone marrow aspiration and biopsy are performed to determine the extent of disease. If bone marrow is involved, the patient is placed at stage IV. Laboratory tests after diagnosis generally include CBC, peripheral blood smear analysis, and studies of kidney and liver functions. Chest radiography and CT of the abdomen, chest, and pelvis are performed to determine the extent of disease. PET is a useful adjunct. GI endoscopy may detect GI involvement (seen in 10%–60% of patients). MRI of the CNS may be performed if neurologic signs are present.

Treatment

The treatment plan for indolent lymphoma usually involves watchful waiting until the symptoms necessitate starting chemotherapy or local radiation for palliation, as indolent lymphomas are generally not curable with conventional therapies. The more aggressive lymphomas have a rapid progression but may be cured with appropriate treatment. They are treated with CHOP (cyclophosphamide, doxorubicin, vincristine, and prednisone) chemotherapy with or without rituximab and with or without radiation therapy. Relapses may be treated with high-dose chemotherapy followed by HSCT or with chemotherapy alone. Patients are also at increased risk for the development of secondary malignancies and should have periodic follow-up after treatment.

Prognosis

The 5-year overall survival rate is 69%. Histopathology is the most important prognostic indicator, followed by patient age, presence of extranodal disease, presence of B symptoms, and stage at the time of diagnosis. The indolent lymphomas generally are associated with a survival measured in years even if left untreated. However, they generally are not curable with treatment. In contrast, the aggressive lymphomas are curable but are rapidly fatal if left untreated or if unresponsive to therapy.

Prevention

No methods of prevention of NHL are known.

Patient Teaching

Give patients information about chemotherapy and radiation therapy. Help them find and contact community support groups.

Transfusion Incompatibility Reaction

Description

Transfusion incompatibility results when the blood or blood product transfused has antibodies to the recipient's RBCs or the recipient has antibodies to the donor's RBCs.

ICD-10-CM Code	T80.30X(A)(D)(S) *(ABO incompatibility reaction due to transfusion of blood or blood products, unspecified)*
	T80.40X(A)(D)(S) *(Rh incompatibility reaction due to transfusion of blood or blood products, unspecified)*
	T80.92X(A)(D)(S) *(Unspecified transfusion reaction)*

Symptoms and Signs

This hypersensitivity reaction can range from mild to fatal. Most severe transfusion reactions are incompatibility related and are characterized by hemolysis or agglutination. Other forms include bacterial, allergic, and circulatory-overload transfusion reactions. The severity of the reaction depends on the amount of incompatible blood that is transfused and prior transfusion reactions of the patient.

The patient who has incompatibility reaction and is receiving a blood transfusion experiences chills, fever, and tachycardia. The patient with a more severe reaction has severe back pain, vomiting, diarrhea, hives or rash, a substernal tightness, and dyspnea. The patient becomes hypotensive and progresses to a state of circulatory collapse. As the condition worsens, there is bleeding from the puncture site, blood in urine, and eventually renal failure.

The most frequent transfusion reaction is associated with WBCs or WBC remnants in donor blood. It is febrile and short lived, ceasing when the transfusion is halted, and there is no hemolysis or allergic response.

The patient experiencing an allergic reaction exhibits hives and itching and possibly bronchial spasms and anaphylaxis.

Patient Screening

Patients receiving blood transfusions will be in a clinic or hospital environment. The trained professionals observing the patient will immediately institute intervention and care to reverse or modify the reaction. Those who have survived a reaction and their family members may request additional information about the reaction. Schedule an appointment as soon as possible for the discussion. Family members may be included in the discussion as long as the Health Insurance Portability and Accountability Act (HIPAA) guidelines are followed.

Etiology

ABO- and Rh-incompatible blood and antigens that screening does not reveal cause an antigen-antibody reaction that produces hemolysis (destruction of RBCs) or agglutination (clumping of RBCs that obstructs the flow of blood through capillaries). Histamine and serotonin are released from mast cells and platelets. DIC usually is triggered (see the Disseminated Intravascular Coagulation section) with resulting coagulation problems (Fig. 10.59).

Diagnosis

Any sign of chills, fever, hives, back pain, or dyspnea during the transfusion alerts the health care professional attending

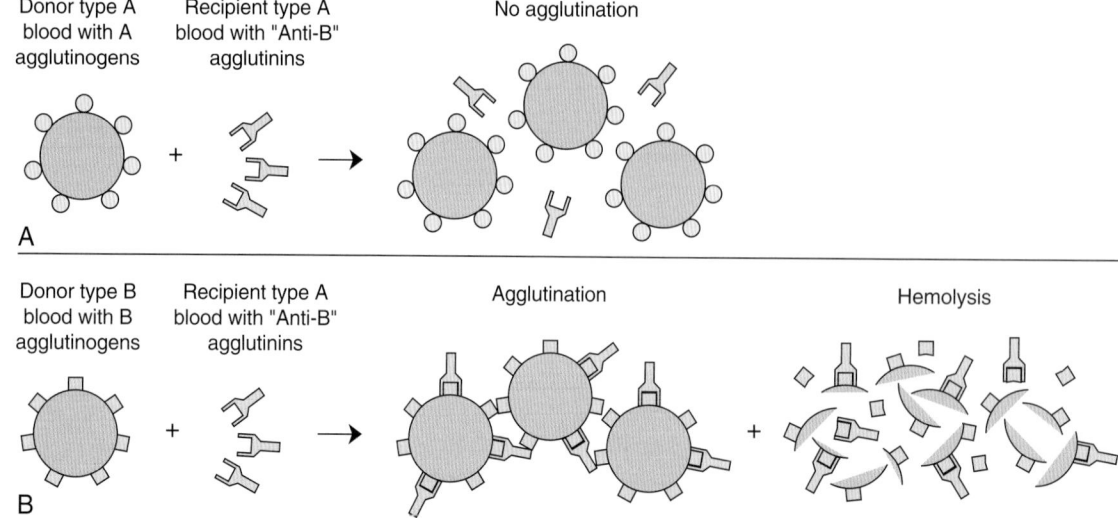

• **Fig. 10.59** Illustration showing agglutination of red blood cells (RBCs) during blood transfusion incompatibility reaction. (From Applegate E: *The anatomy and physiology learning system,* ed 4, St Louis, 2011, Saunders/Elsevier.)

the patient to a possible reaction. Blood and urine specimens are examined, along with the used blood, to confirm the incompatibility and the presence of hemolysis or activated coagulation.

Treatment

Transfusion protocol mandates that a set of baseline patient vital signs be taken before the start of a transfusion. During the first 15 minutes, the patient is observed closely, and assessment of vital signs is repeated. This monitoring of vital signs and observation of the patient continues at designated intervals until the procedure is completed. At the first indication of any symptoms or signs of reaction, the blood transfusion is stopped immediately. Blood and urine samples are obtained from the patient and sent to the laboratory, along with the remaining untransfused blood. Mild reactions are treated with antihistamines, and anaphylaxis is treated aggressively according to institutional protocol.

Prognosis

The prognosis varies, depending on the amount of blood infused, the cause of the reaction, and the speed of the intervention.

Prevention

Prevention is the best form of treatment. Careful typing and crossmatching of the blood product is mandatory. Two attendants must compare the patient's information with that on the blood bag and the physician's orders before starting the transfusion.

Patient Teaching

Instruct the patient to report any untoward symptoms or unusual sensations during the transfusion process immediately, especially early in the transfusion.

Clotting Disorders

Classic Hemophilia
Description
Classic hemophilia is a hereditary bleeding disorder resulting from deficiency of clotting factors.

ICD-10-CM Code   D66 (Hereditary factor VIII deficiency)

Symptoms and Signs
The condition can be mild, moderate, or severe. Any unusually prolonged bleeding episode, easy bruising, hematomas, or excessive nosebleeds in a male child suggest hemophilia. The first sign of hemophilia may be ecchymosis at birth or bleeding resulting from circumcision. Joint swelling and pain suggest bleeding in the joints.

Patient Screening
When parents report that a male infant, toddler, or child has experienced unexplained prolonged bleeding, noticeable hematomas, easy bruising, and/or excessive nosebleeds,

the physician should promptly assess the child. The condition often is diagnosed during the neonatal period of hospitalization. These parents may request an appointment to learn about the disorder. Schedule the next available appointment for the patient as soon as possible.

Etiology
An X-linked genetic disorder in males, hemophilia is transmitted by the asymptomatic carrier mother to her son. Factor VIII, a clotting factor in the intrinsic clotting cascade, is functionally inactive. Any minor trauma can initiate the bleeding episode (Fig. 10.60).

Diagnosis
The diagnosis is based on the clinical picture and a thorough history. Clotting studies indicate normal platelet count, bleeding time, and prothrombin time (PT); prolonged partial thromboplastin time (PTT); and a factor VIII assay of 0% to 30%.

Treatment
Hemophilia cannot be cured, but treatment prevents crippling deformities. Concentrated factor VIII (antihemophilic factor [AHF]) is administered to stop the bleeding. Transfusions of whole blood may be necessary. Patients are encouraged to avoid situations that initiate bleeding episodes. There are documented cases of HIV infection resulting from transfusion of contaminated or infected blood products before 1987; thereafter, blood supplies began to be treated to prevent viral transmission.

Prognosis
No cure for hemophilia is known. Transfusions of blood or blood products may be a lifelong intervention. Bloodborne infections may complicate the condition and place the patient at higher risk for other disease entities.

Prevention
No prevention is known for this condition. Genetic counseling may help explore the probability of the disorder being transferred to offspring.

Patient Teaching
Give parents information about X-linked genetic disorders.

Disseminated Intravascular Coagulation
Description
DIC is a condition of simultaneous hemorrhage and thrombosis. It is a syndrome occurring secondary to other diseases or dramatic events.

ICD-10-CM Code   D65 (Disseminated intravascular coagulation [defibrination syndrome])
Refer to the physician's diagnosis and then to the current edition of the ICD-10-CM coding manual to ensure the greatest specificity of pathology.

Lupus Anticoagulant

The patient with lupus anticoagulant (LA) usually does not have lupus erythematosus; however, some may progress to the disease with joint pain, dermatologic problems, or renal involvement. Therefore, the lupus portion of the name is often considered a misnomer. The anticoagulant portion of the name is also a misnomer because the condition actually does not involve anticoagulant activity but has that of a coagulant with formation of clots.

Many individuals with LA are asymptomatic. Symptoms that may occur are abnormal bleeding of nose or gums, atypical bruising, abnormal menstrual cycles, multiple miscarriages, blood clots in the legs (DVT) or in the lungs (pulmonary embolism), strokes, and heart attacks.

Blood tests for the anticoagulant antibody are performed. When a positive result is obtained, the tests are repeated. Some individuals with positive test results do not require any treatment. Others require ongoing treatment with anticoagulant medications, including heparin or warfarin (Coumadin). Some may be instructed to take aspirin. Many require anticoagulant drug therapy along with routine blood tests for their lifetime. These individuals are at risk for blood clots that may lead to pulmonary embolism, stroke, or heart attack.

Symptoms and Signs

Oozing of blood from needle puncture sites, mucous membranes, or incisions may be noted, as may bleeding in the form of purpura, wound hematomas, or petechiae. Hematemesis, hematuria, and bloody stools may be present. The patient is weak, reports headaches, and experiences air

hunger and tachycardia. DIC follows a major event, such as obstetric complications, septicemia, trauma, burns, hypothermia, and extensive tissue destruction.

Patient Screening

Most of these individuals are usually in an inpatient facility, and immediate intervention is indicated. If they suffer the condition at home after a major precipitating event, they must be entered into the emergency medical system for prompt assessment. When family members request an appointment for information after the event, an appointment should be scheduled as soon as possible, according to the HIPAA guidelines.

Etiology

Thrombin activates the production of fibrin, causing clots to form where they are not needed (i.e., in the microcirculation). The thrombin also causes platelet aggregation, forming more clots. In addition, the fibrinolytic system is activated by the presence of thrombin in plasma; thrombin causes excessive fibrinolysis and additional bleeding. Predisposing factors include hypotension, hypoxemia, acidosis, and stasis of capillary blood. Any of these factors may be the result of the aforementioned major precipitating events (Fig. 10.61).

Diagnosis

The diagnosis is based on the clinical picture; a thorough history, including a probable precipitating event; and laboratory studies. Platelet count and fibrinogen levels are reduced, whereas PT is prolonged.

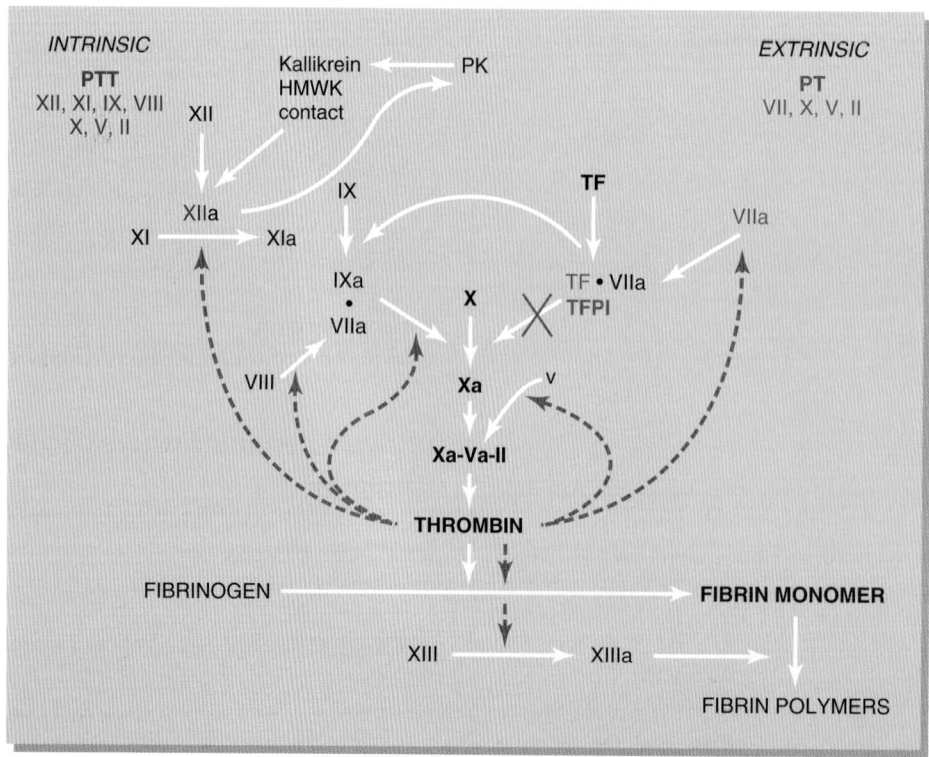

• **Fig. 10.60** Illustration of clotting cascade where factor VIII is inactive. (Andreoli TE, et al: *Andreoli and Carpenter's Cecil essentials of medicine,* ed 8, Philadelphia, 2010, Saunders/Elsevier.)

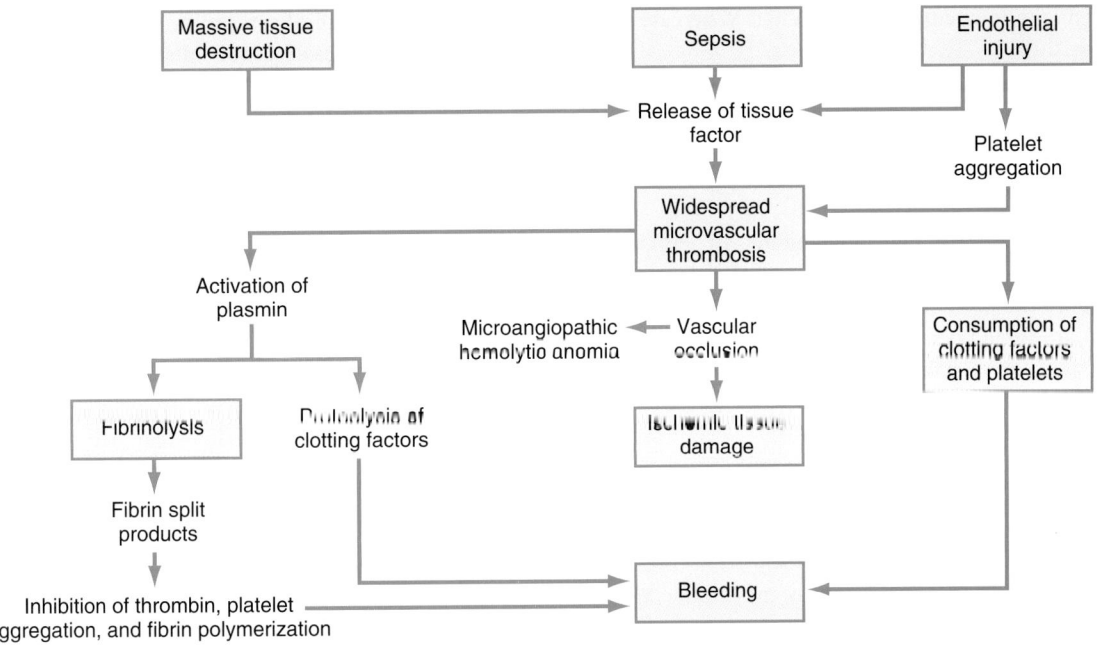

• **Fig. 10.61** Pathophysiology of disseminated intravascular coagulation (DIC). (From Kumar V, Cotran R, Robbins S: *Robbins basic pathology,* ed 8, Philadelphia, 2008, Saunders/Elsevier.)

Treatment

Administration of IV heparin inhibits the formation of additional microthrombi and prevents the aggregation of platelets. Platelet replacement and plasma-clotting factors are administered when serious hemorrhage is present. The condition is life threatening and often fatal.

Prognosis

The prognosis is guarded.

Prevention

Because this condition is a sequela to a major systemic insult, prevention is unlikely.

Patient Teaching

If the patient survives the event, teaching may include an explanation of the incident. Help family members find and contact support groups in the community.

Review Challenge

Answer the following questions:

1. What are the common symptoms of cardiovascular disease?
2. How would you describe the pathology in coronary artery disease (CAD)?
3. How is the patient likely to describe the pain in angina pectoris?
4. How do the symptoms of myocardial infarction (MI) differ from those of angina pectoris?
5. List and discuss possible stress factors contributing to onset of broken heart syndrome.
6. Why is angioplasty used for MI?
7. What conditions can cause cardiac arrest? What is the time frame in which cardiopulmonary resuscitation (CPR) may be successfully initiated?
8. What are the diagnostic criteria for essential hypertension?
9. What happens when the pumping action of the heart is inadequate? How can congestive heart failure (CHF) be treated?
10. Which conditions may lead to cor pulmonale?
11. How is pulmonary edema treated?
12. What does cardiomyopathy refer to, and how is it treated?
13. How does endocarditis affect the cardiac valves?
14. Discuss the importance of completing drug regimen for an infection caused by beta-hemolytic *Streptococcus*.
15. Why is rheumatic fever described as a systemic disease? What infection often precedes it?
16. What is the relationship between rheumatic fever and valvular heart disease?
17. What are the sources of cardiac arrhythmias? How are they diagnosed?
18. What are some of the treatment options for cardiac arrhythmias?
19. Why is shock considered a life-threatening emergency? What are the signs and symptoms?
20. What is cardiac tamponade?
21. What is the relationship between venous thrombosis and pulmonary emboli?
22. What is the difference between arteriosclerosis and atherosclerosis? Why are both conditions a health threat?

23. How might an aneurysm be detected? When are they a serious threat?
24. What is the relationship of phlebitis to thrombophlebitis? Why should the clinician avoid massaging the affected area?
25. What medical intervention is available for severe varicose veins?
26. Which conditions may precipitate an episode of Raynaud disease?
27. What are the presenting symptoms of anemia?
28. What are some possible causes of anemia?
29. How are the following anemias differentiated: aplastic, sickle cell, hemolytic, iron-deficiency, hemorrhagic, and pernicious?
30. What are some usual causes of agranulocytosis?
31. What are typical symptoms in all types of leukemia?
32. Which leukemia is considered more a disease of later life?
33. How does lymphedema differ from lymphangitis?
34. Which lymphoma is characterized by the presence of Reed-Sternberg cells in lymphatic tissue?
35. Discuss the recently identified possible cause of Non-Hodgkin lymphoma (NHL).
36. What symptoms does a patient experience with a transfusion incompatibility reaction?
37. How is classic hemophilia treated?
38. Referring to the American Heart Association's website, list the American Heart Association (AHA)-recommended dietary guidelines for a healthy diet that is suggested as a weapon to fight cardiovascular disease.

Real-Life Challenge: Essential Hypertension

A 46-year-old man reports intermittent headaches and lightheadedness for about 3 months. In the past 2 weeks, he has had several episodes of epistaxis. Vital signs are temperature, 98.6°F; pulse, 106 beats per minute; respirations, 20 breaths per minute; and blood pressure, 168/98 mm Hg. His weight is 265 lb, and his height is 5 feet, 11 inches.

Patient history reveals that he has a highly stressful job requiring extensive travel with overnight stays. He regards himself as a high achiever. His family history reveals that his father died at age 53 years as a result of a CVA and that his mother, age 69 years, has congestive heart failure (CHF) and hypertension. His brother has a history of

hypertension, and his two sisters are alive and well. The patient has been smoking one pack of cigarettes a day for the past 30 years.

The patient is advised to stop smoking or at least reduce the number of cigarettes smoked per day. In addition, he is advised to begin a weight-reduction and exercise program and to reduce his sodium intake. He is also told that he should avoid stressful situations, if possible. Medications ordered are a beta-blocker, atenolol, and an ACE inhibitor, ramipril. The patient is instructed to return in 1 week for reevaluation. Essential hypertension is a suspected diagnosis.

Questions

1. What factors contribute to the symptoms and signs of essential hypertension that this patient is experiencing?
2. Why would his onset of symptoms be considered insidious?
3. Why could the diagnosis of essential hypertension not be confirmed on the initial encounter?
4. Why might a diuretic be ordered?
5. What is the significance of the family history?
6. What is the action of calcium channel blockers (CCBs) in the treatment of essential hypertension?
7. If essential hypertension is not controlled, what complications may evolve from the condition?
8. How important was the symptom of epistaxis in the diagnosis?

Real-Life Challenge: Anemia

A 32-year-old woman reports feeling tired all the time, having an excessively fast heartbeat, having difficulty catching her breath, and experiencing some lightheadedness. She appears quite pale. Vital signs are: temperature, 98.4°F; pulse, 118 beats per minute; respirations, 26 breaths per minute; and blood pressure, 100/69 mm Hg.

The patient is married, has three children ages 7 years, 4 years, and 6 months, and is employed outside the home. She says she can barely get out of bed in the morning and make it through the day. She has had four episodes of

syncope in the past week. Menstrual periods have been regular but heavy. She denies experiencing any observable blood in her urine or stools. CBC with differential is ordered. The RBC count is below normal and normocytic; hemoglobin is 9, hematocrit is 27, and WBC and platelet counts are normal. The patient is diagnosed with iron deficiency anemia and encouraged to rest and to increase her dietary intake of red meat, liver, and egg yolks. Supplementary iron is prescribed in the form of ferrous sulfate tablets, and the patient is instructed to return to the office in 1 week for follow-up.

Questions

1. What might have been the cause of the iron deficiency anemia in this patient?
2. What causes RBCs to be microcytic? Macrocytic?
3. What is the importance of the absence of blood in the stool and urine?
4. What might be the connection with the previous pregnancy?
5. What type of food in addition to the red meat, liver, and egg yolks would help increase the hemoglobin?
6. What might blood tests show if this was sickle cell anemia?
7. Compare hemolytic anemia with iron deficiency anemia.
8. As the hemoglobin improves, what changes might be expected in the vital signs?

Real-Life Challenge: Abdominal Aortic Aneurysms

A 75-year-old female patient with diabetes was diagnosed with two small abdominal aortic aneurysms. She also had a history of elevated blood pressure, 150/90 mm Hg. Lisinopril had been prescribed to maintain an acceptable level. The physician had suggested that the course of treatment could be watchful waiting. A surgeon had been consulted, and after reviewing laboratory values and CT scans of the abdomen and abdominal aorta, the surgeon recommended not pursuing a surgical course at the time of the tests.

Follow-up appointments every 3 months were scheduled. The first 3-month examination revealed no significant change. The second 3-month examination showed that the aneurysm had started to increase in size. The course of watchful waiting was to continue. The patient was instructed to monitor her blood pressure closely and not to lift anything heavier than 10 pounds. Additionally she was advised not to stretch or reach out.

The surgeon preferred to schedule a procedure to install a stent into the abdominal aorta. The patient began to experience severe muscle spasms in the muscles of the lower legs. She also was unsure about the proposed procedure and asked what would happen if she did not have the procedure.

Questions

1. What might be the cause of the aneurysms?
2. Why is controlling blood pressure important?
3. Why would the surgeon want to adopt a wait-and-see approach at first?
4. What is the significance of cramping in the legs?
5. Why would the patient be instructed not to lift or stretch?
6. What would be the outcome if the aneurysm began to leak?
7. What would be the chances of survival if the aneurysm ruptured?

Internet Assignments

1. Research by the American Heart Association (AHA) has suggested treatment interventions for congestive heart failure (CHF). In particular, research and list drug interventions and patient teaching about administration of these drugs.
2. Research by the AHA has suggested treatment interventions for cardiac arrhythmias. Use the arrhythmia chart in the chapter to identify the arrhythmias that are considered potentially lethal arrhythmias. Record your findings from the website about treatment interventions.
3. Research the incidence of hypertension at the AHA website. Record the ages and genders of patients and the seriousness of their conditions. Verify and record any drug therapy suggested.
4. Research the incidence of hemophilia in the U.S. population in the past 10 years at the National Hemophilia Association website. Also research suggested drug treatments and their side effects.

Critical Thinking

1. As a review of the anatomy of the heart, list the four chambers and the four valves.
2. Identify the structures of the conduction system.
3. After reviewing the American Heart Association (AHA) website, discuss the AHA Healthy Heart Recommendations.
4. Locate automated external defibrillators (AEDs) in your educational or work facility, and describe how you would use an AED. Discuss situations when you would use an AED.
5. List and discuss the dangers of malignant hypertension.
6. Discuss the importance of compliance with the prescribed drug regimen in the treatment of hypertension and malignant hypertension.
7. Referring to Fig. 10.22, review the course of congestive heart failure (CHF), and attempt to indicate (where possible) interventions that may offer some relief to the patient with the condition.
8. Discuss the feelings that patients may experience as CHF progresses and there is increasing difficulty breathing.

9. How would you explain the differences between cor pulmonale and CHF?

10. Discuss the feelings of patients experiencing dyspnea.

11. A patient is experiencing the symptoms of cardiomyopathy. Discuss his or her response to dyspnea, fatigue, tachycardia, palpitations, and occasional chest pain.

12. What infectious processes in the body might be the cause of pericarditis?

13. Discuss causative agents, including infections in the body that may be the cause of myocarditis and/or endocarditis.

14. Discuss the psychological effects of an asymptomatic patient being diagnosed with mitral valve prolapse.

15. Explain what you think arrhythmias might feel like, including both atrial and ventricular types.

16. Research and report on interventions for mitral stenosis.

17. Explain the importance of diagnosis and treatment for strep throat.

18. What is the importance of completing the antibiotic regimen prescribed for treatment of strep throat?

19. Patients with pacemakers usually have to wait until the battery reaches the "end of service" before the battery or pacemaker can be replaced. Discuss the psychological aspects of waiting for the "end of service" message to be obtained.

20. Explain some of the precautionary measures that might be taken by travelers or those with sedentary lifestyles to avoid developing a thrombus in the legs.

21. Discuss the psychological effects of an individual being diagnosed with an abdominal aortic aneurysm when a "watch and wait" attitude versus surgical intervention is chosen by the health care provider. Research various methods of treatment, and then discuss treatment options.

22. List the components that make up blood.

23. List various types of anemias, and identify their causes.

24. Discuss the effects of diagnosis of leukemia on the patient and his or her family, workplace, and community.

25. What might be the psychological effects of postmastectomy lymphedema?

26. Discuss hematopoietic stem cell transplantation (HSCT).

Prepare to discuss Critical Thinking case study exercises for this chapter that are posted on Evolve.

11

Diseases and Conditions of the Urinary System

CHAPTER OUTLINE

Orderly Function of the Urinary System, 450

Disorderly Function of the Urinary System, 451

Acute Glomerulonephritis, 451

Chronic Glomerulonephritis, 454

Nephrotic Syndrome (Nephrosis), 458

Acute Renal Failure, 459

Chronic Kidney Disease, 460

Pyelonephritis, 461

Hydronephrosis, 463

Renal Calculi, 465

Infectious Cystitis and Urethritis, 466

Diabetic Nephropathy, 468

Polycystic Kidney Disease, 468

Neurogenic Bladder, 469

Stress Incontinence, 470

Renal Cell Carcinoma, 472

Bladder Tumors, 473

LEARNING OBJECTIVES

After studying Chapter 11, you should be able to:

1. Explain the structure and function of the normal urinary system.
2. Explain how pathologic conditions of the urinary system threaten homeostasis and result in illness.
3. Explain the diagnostic value of urinalysis.
4. Relate the symptoms and signs of acute glomerulonephritis.
5. Describe how immune mechanisms are suspected to be a causative factor of acute and chronic glomerulonephritis (CGN).
6. Distinguish between hemodialysis and peritoneal dialysis.
7. Identify the hallmark sign of nephrosis.
8. List some nephrotoxic agents.
9. Explain why acute renal failure (ARF) is considered a clinical emergency.
10. Discuss treatment measures for prolonging life of the patient with chronic renal failure (CRF).
11. Identify the etiology and diagnosis of pyelonephritis.
12. Describe hydronephrosis.
13. Describe the common symptoms of renal calculi and list the possible complications.
14. List causes of infectious cystitis and urethritis.
15. Describe diabetic nephropathy.
16. Describe the polycystic kidney and discuss the treatment options.
17. Discuss urinary catheterization.
18. Contrast neurogenic bladder with stress incontinence.
19. List and describe symptoms of renal cell and bladder carcinoma.
20. Identify those most at risk for renal cell carcinoma (RCC) and bladder tumors.

KEY TERMS

azotemia (**ah**-zoh-**TEE**-me-ah)
catheterization (**kath**-eh-ter-eye-**ZAY**-shun)
creatinine (kree-**AT**-in-in)
cystoscopy (sis-**TOSS**-ko-pee)
dialysate (dye-**AHL**-ih-sate)
glomeruli (gloh-**MER**-you-lye)
glomerulonephritis (gloh-**mer**-you-low-neh-**FRY**-tis)
glomerulosclerosis (gloh-**mer**-you-low-sklee-**ROW**-sis)
hemodialysis (**he**-moh-dye-**AHL**-ih-sis)

hydronephrosis (**high**-droh-neff-**ROW**-sis)
immunosuppressive (**im**-you-noh-sue-**PRESS**-ihv)
lithotripsy (**LITH**-oh-**trip**-see)
nephrectomy (neh-**FRECK**-toh-me)
nephropathy (neh-**FROP**-ah-thee)
nephrotoxic (**neff**-row-**TOCKS**-ick)
oliguria (ohl-ih-**GOO**-rhee-ah)
peritoneal dialysis (**per**-ih-toe-**NEE**-al dye-**AHL**-ih-sis)
pyelonephritis (**pye**-eh-low-neh-**FRY**-tis)

Orderly Function of the Urinary System

The urinary system is responsible for producing, storing, and excreting urine; these processes prevent the body from becoming toxic. The kidneys facilitate reabsorption of necessary nutrients, water, and electrolytes. Cleansing blood of the waste products of metabolism and regulating the water, salts, and acids in body fluids ensure the body's homeostasis. Regulation of the volume of water in the body is an essential function of the urinary system. The urinary system includes the kidneys, which manufacture urine and play a role in the regulation of systemic blood pressure and the accessory structures. The ureters transport urine, and the bladder stores urine until it is excreted voluntarily through the urethra. The organs and accessory structures of the urinary system consist of two kidneys, two ureters, the urinary bladder, and the urethra (Fig. 11.1).

Each kidney (Fig. 11.2) is composed of about 1 million microstructures called *nephrons* (Fig. 11.3). The nephrons, the units of function in the kidney, are responsible for filtration, reabsorption, and secretion of urine. Fig. 11.4 depicts the formation of urine. Urine is transported from the nephron to the renal pelvis and then to the ureters. The kidney has many other functions, including the secretion of rennin, a hormone that raises blood pressure, and erythropoietin, which acts as a stimulus for red blood cell (RBC) production. It also has a role in the activation of vitamin D.

Nephrons are composed of the glomerulus, Bowman capsule, the proximal convoluted tubule, the loop of Henle, the distal convoluted tubule, and the collecting duct.

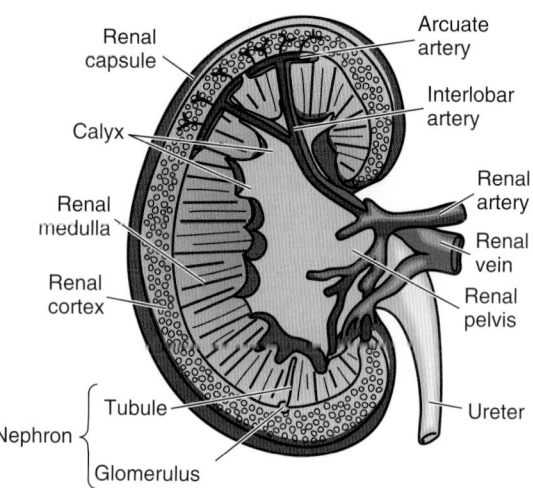

• **Fig. 11.2** Anatomy of the kidney. (From Gould B: *Pathophysiology for the health professions,* ed 4, Philadelphia, 2011, Saunders/Elsevier.)

Each kidney, as a primary organ of the urinary system, processes blood to form urine, which contains waste products to be eliminated from the body (see Fig. 11.2). The bean-shaped organs, about the size of a fist, are located in the back retroperitoneally to the abdominal cavity and lateral to the spinal column. Each kidney is separated into three areas or regions: the cortex, the medulla, and the renal pelvis.

Blood enters the kidneys by way of the renal arteries through the hilum. Refer to Figs. 11.1 and 11.2 for blood supply to and from the kidneys. The arteries divide again and again into smaller arteries that ultimately enter the nephrons. Blood leaves the kidneys by way of the renal veins.

Urine leaves the kidneys by way of two long, slender tubes, the ureters, which enter the lower part of the urinary bladder. Peristalsis in the muscular walls of the ureters moves urine into the urinary bladder, where it is temporarily stored until it is passed from the body by way of the urethra. Urine is voluntarily excreted from the bladder by way of the urethra in a process called *urination* or *micturition*. The urethra is a tubular structure that extends from the base of the urinary bladder to the urinary meatus (urethral orifice) on the external surface of the body (see Fig. 11.1).

Infection, scarring, toxic necrosis, or trauma of the urinary tract can result in disturbances of renal function, and this allows urea (the nitrogenous waste of metabolism in urine) or extracellular fluid and electrolytes to accumulate in blood. Congenital or acquired structural defects and tumors cause obstructive diseases of the urinary system. Other important diseases of the urinary tract are immunologic disorders, circulatory disturbances, cystic disease, and metabolic disorders (e.g., diabetes mellitus).

The function of the urinary system often is evaluated by performing urinalysis (Table 11.1) and blood tests (Table 11.2). Normal results demonstrate proper filtration, absorption, elimination of metabolic waste, and precise

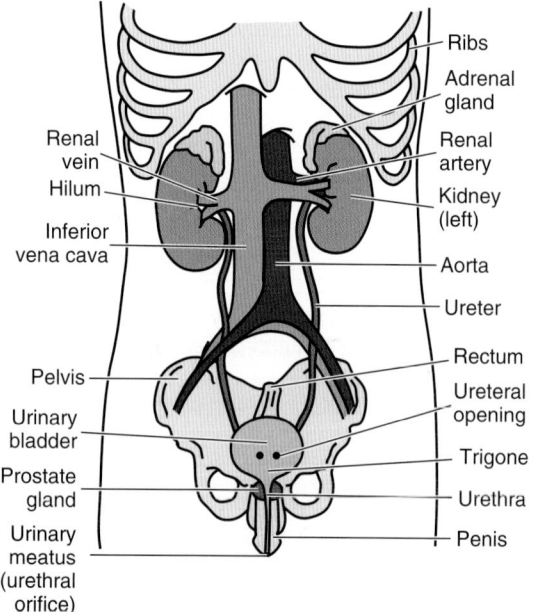

• **Fig. 11.1** Gross anatomy of the urinary system (male). (From Gould B: *Pathophysiology for the health professions,* ed 4, Philadelphia, 2011, Saunders/Elsevier.)

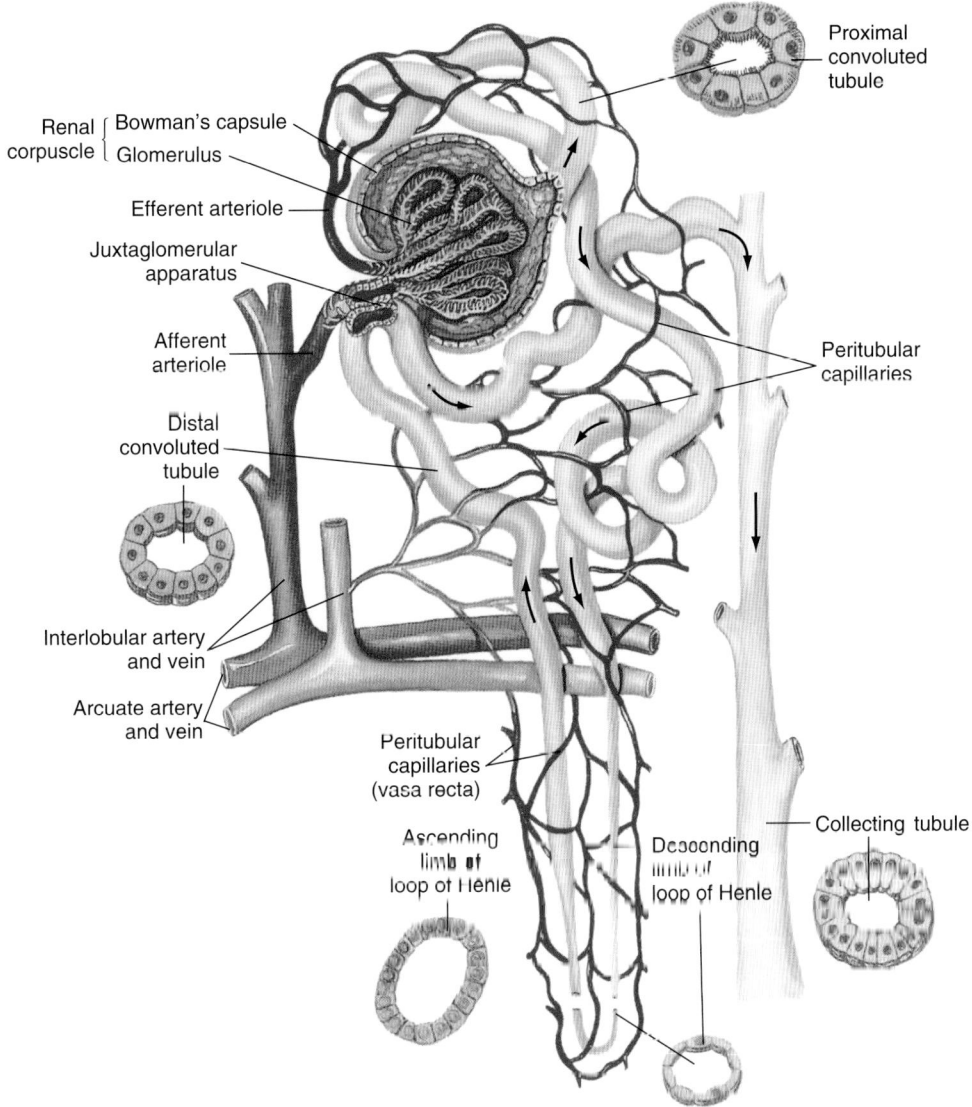

Renal corpuscle { Bowman's capsule / Glomerulus

Efferent arteriole

Juxtaglomerular apparatus

Afferent arteriole

Distal convoluted tubule

Interlobular artery and vein

Arcuate artery and vein

Peritubular capillaries (vasa recta)

Ascending limb of loop of Henle

Descending limb of loop of Henle

Collecting tubule

Proximal convoluted tubule

Peritubular capillaries

• **Fig. 11.3** The nephron. (From Patton KT, Thibodeau GA: *Mosby's handbook of anatomy and physiology,* ed 6, St Louis, 2014, Mosby/Elsevier, p. 536.)

fluid and electrolyte balance. Other tests for urinary tract disorders include culture and sensitivity tests to determine appropriate antibiotic therapy, radiologic tests that visualize structural and functional abnormalities, cystoscopy (see Enrichment box on page 464), and biopsy of lesions.

Usually symptoms of urinary diseases reflect an accumulation of waste products in blood and cause electrolyte imbalances in the body. Common symptoms include the following:

- nausea
- loss of appetite
- fever
- headache and body ache
- flank or low back pain
- bloody urine (hematuria)
- edema
- decreased urinary output
- hypertension
- pruritus

Disorderly Function of the Urinary System

Acute Glomerulonephritis

Description

Acute glomerulonephritis is inflammation and swelling of the glomeruli (see Fig. 11.3) of the kidneys. It can be a primary disease of the kidney or may develop secondary to a systemic disease. This condition usually follows a streptococcal bacterial infection of the throat or skin.

ICD-10-CM Code	N00.3 *(Acute nephritic syndrome with diffuse mesangial proliferative glomerulonephritis)* (N00.0-N00.5 = 6 codes of specificity)

Acute glomerulonephritis is coded according to sites and types of lesions. Refer to the physician's diagnosis for site and type of lesion and to the current edition of the ICD-10-CM coding manual.

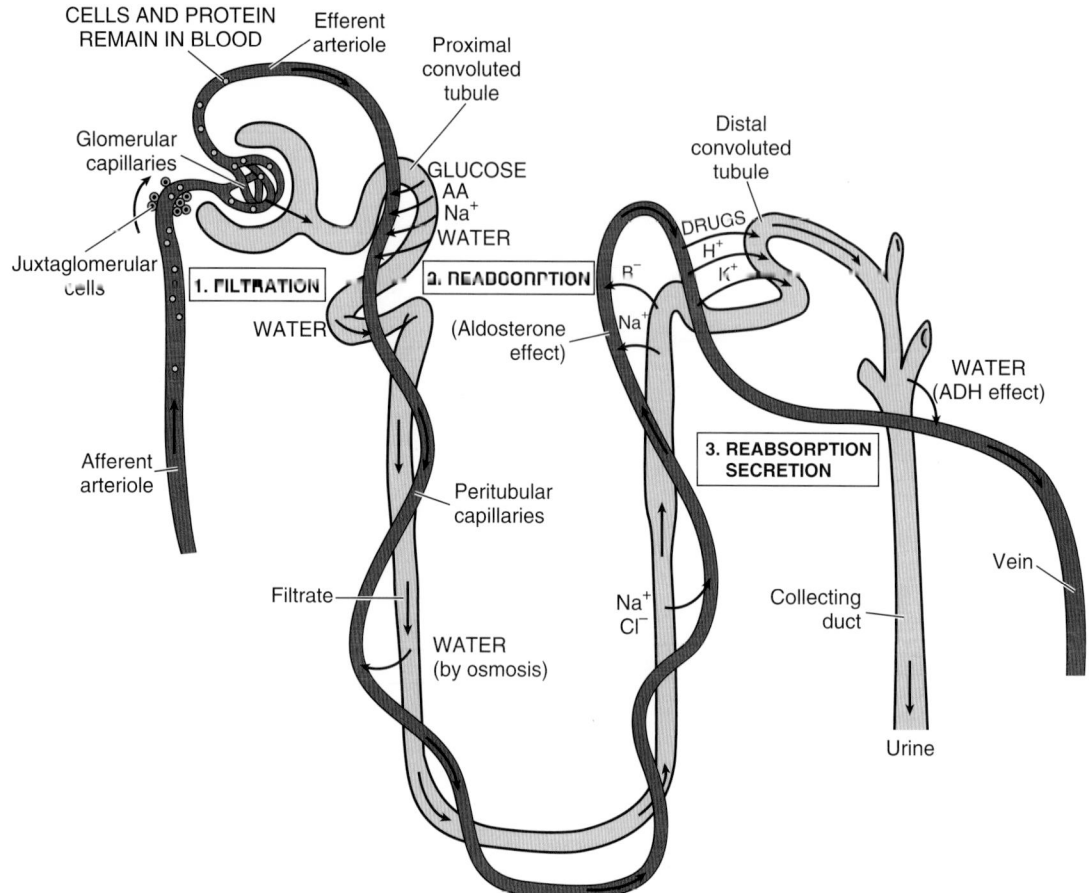

• **Fig. 11.4** Formation of urine. *AA,* Amino acids; *B⁻,* bicarbonate ions; *Cl⁻,* chloride ions; *H⁺,* hydrogen ions; *K⁺,* potassium ions; *Na⁺,* sodium ions. (From Gould B: *Pathophysiology for the health professions,* ed 4, Philadelphia, 2011, Saunders/Elsevier.)

Symptoms and Signs

Acute glomerulonephritis is marked by proteinuria (protein in urine), edema, and decreased urine volume. Hematuria can range from insignificant to a sudden onset of urine that is grossly bloody (gross hematuria). Urine may appear dark or may be described as coffee colored. Occurring most often in children and adolescents, this disease process usually occurs 1 to 2 weeks after a streptococcal infection (poststreptococcal glomerulonephritis). Hypertension related to altered renal function and fluid retention is possible and is accompanied by headaches, visual disturbances, malaise, anorexia, and a low-grade fever. Flank or back pain develops as a result of swelling of the kidney tissue.

Patient Screening

Patients complaining of bloody urine that is accompanied by edema, headache, and flank or pelvic pain require prompt medical attention.

Etiology

This condition usually occurs after an infection caused by group A beta-hemolytic *Streptococcus.* It also can be idiopathic or may result from an immune reaction that causes circulating antigen-antibody complexes to become trapped within the network of capillaries of a glomerulus. In some cases, the antigen is endogenous (arising from within) as an accompaniment of tumors. The injury to the glomeruli results in a decrease in the rate of filtration of blood and consequently retention of water and salts in the body. Fig. 11.5 is a schematic representation of changes occurring in the nephron with acute poststreptococcal glomerulonephritis.

Diagnosis

Diagnosis is made on the basis of clinical findings, clinical history, and urinalysis results. Urine shows gross blood and the presence of RBCs, white blood cells (WBCs), renal tubular cells, and casts. Proteinuria may be present because of the increased permeability of the glomerular membrane. Blood tests show elevated blood urea nitrogen (BUN), hypoalbuminemia, and an elevated erythrocyte sedimentation rate (ESR). Kidney, ureters, and bladder (KUB) radiography and ultrasonography may reveal bilateral enlargement of the kidneys. Renal biopsy may help confirm the diagnosis (Fig. 11.6).

TABLE 11.1 Routine Urinalysis*

	Normal	Abnormal	Pathology
Characteristics			
Color and clarity	Pale to darker yellow and clear	Very pale Cloudy, milky, WBCs Hematuria, RBCs, reddish to reddish brown	Excessive water Pus, UTI Bleeding in infection, calculi, or cancer
Odor	Aromatic	Foul Fruity Foul	Cystitis Diabetes mellitus UTI
Chemical nature	pH is generally slightly acidic, 6.5	Alkaline	Infections cause ammonia to form
Specific gravity	1.003–1.030—reflects amount of waste, minerals, and solids in urine	Higher—causes precipitation of solutes Lower—polyuria	Kidney stones, diabetes mellitus Diabetes insipidus
Constituent Compounds			
Protein	None or small amount	Albuminuria	Nephritis, renal failure, infection
Glucose	None	Glycosuria	Faulty carbohydrate metabolism, as in diabetes mellitus
Ketone bodies	None	Ketonuria	Diabetic acidosis
Bile and bilirubin	None	Bilirubinuria	Hepatic or gallbladder disease
Casts	None or small number of hyaline casts	Urinary casts composed of RBCs or WBCs, fat, or pus	Nephritis, renal diseases, inflammation, metal poisoning
Nitrogenous wastes	Ammonia, creatinine, urea, and uric acid	Azoturia, creatinine, and urea clearance tests disproportionate to normal BUN/creatinine ratio	Hepatic disease, renal disease
Crystals	None to trace	Acidic urine, alkaline urine, hypercalcemia, metabolism error	Not significant unless the crystals are large (stones); certain types interpreted by physician
Fat droplets	None	Lipiduria	Nephrosis

*Routine urinalysis is a physical, chemical, and microscopic examination of urine for abnormal elements that may help estimate renal function and provide clues of systemic disease. This table includes some important characteristics and elements screened for in basic urinalysis. Other normal constituents of urine that are studied routinely for diagnosis include calcium, urea, uric acid, creatinine, sodium chloride, hormones, potassium, magnesium, phosphates, and sulfates.
BUN, Blood urea nitrogen; *RBC,* red blood cell; *UTI,* urinary tract infection; *WBC,* white blood cell.

TABLE 11.2 Some Renal Diagnostic Tests

Test	Designed to Evaluate
Clearance test	Rate of glomerular filtration
Concentration and dilution tests	Functional capacity of renal tubular cells to adaptively retain and/or eliminate water
Serum creatinine and BUN	Capacity to eliminate end products of protein metabolism
Protein in urine	Permeability of glomerular membrane

BUN, Blood urea nitrogen.

Treatment
No specialized therapy is available for the poststreptococcal type of glomerulonephritis other than antibiotic therapy, if infection is still present, and rest. Diuretics help control edema and hypertension. Sodium intake is restricted to prevent circulatory overload and convulsions. Occasionally corticosteroids are used if an immune reaction is the suspected cause. Patients should be instructed to consult their provider before taking any over-the-counter (OTC) medications, especially nonsteroidal antiinflammatory drugs (NSAIDs), because these agents can worsen the renal function.

Prognosis
Most cases resolve within 2 weeks, and the patient experiences spontaneous recovery.

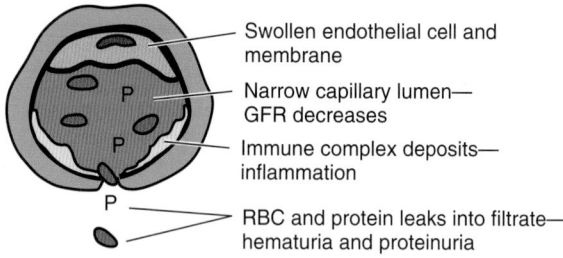

Normal Glomerulus

- Endothelial cell
- Capillary open—blood flow

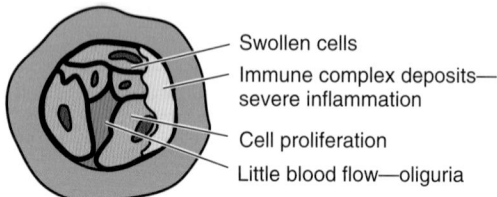

Mild Glomerulonephritis

- Swollen endothelial cell and membrane
- Narrow capillary lumen— GFR decreases
- Immune complex deposits— inflammation
- RBC and protein leaks into filtrate— hematuria and proteinuria

Severe Glomerulonephritis

- Swollen cells
- Immune complex deposits— severe inflammation
- Cell proliferation
- Little blood flow—oliguria

• **Fig. 11.5** Schematic representation of changes occurring in the nephron with acute poststreptococcal glomerulonephritis. *GFR,* Glomerular filtration rate; *P,* protein, *RBC,* red blood cell. (From Gould B: *Pathophysiology for the health professions,* ed 4, Philadelphia, 2011, Saunders/Elsevier.)

Prevention

Prevention depends on the cause of the condition. Streptococcal infections require medical intervention with antibiotics.

Patient Teaching

Explain the underlying cause to patients and their families. Patients are instructed to complete the course of medications as prescribed, especially antibiotics. During the acute stage, bed rest should be instituted along with sodium intake restriction. It is helpful to review the symptoms being reported to the physician. These symptoms include weight gain, decreased urinary output, changes in urine color, and an increase in blood pressure. Pregnant women with a history of acute glomerulonephritis require frequent medical evaluation. Provide the patient with visual aids depicting the urinary system and its functions.

Chronic Glomerulonephritis

Description

Chronic glomerulonephritis (CGN) is a slowly progressive, noninfectious disease that can lead to irreversible renal damage and renal failure. As an advanced stage of many kidney disorders, CGN results in inflammation, followed by progressive destruction of the glomeruli. This progressive destruction causes a reduction in the glomerular filtration rate (GFR), with resulting retention of uremic poisons.

ICD-10-CM Code	N03.2 *(Chronic nephritic syndrome with diffuse membranous glomerulonephritis)*

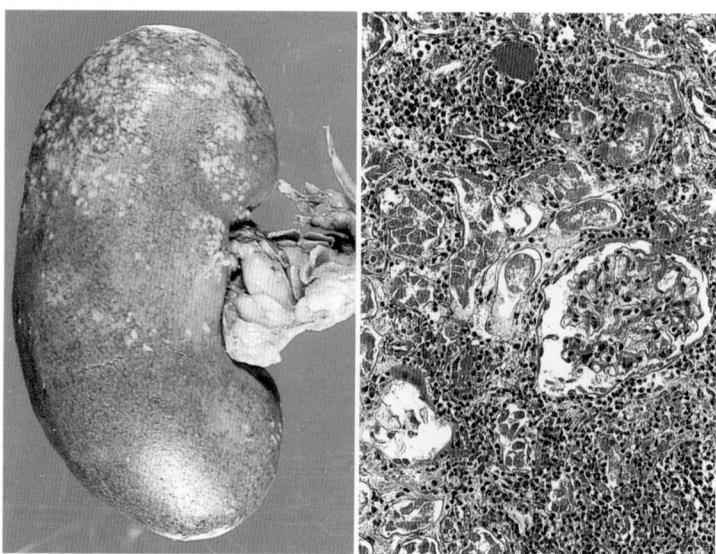

• **Fig. 11.6** Acute pyelonephritis. (From Stevens A, et al: *Core pathology,* ed 3, London, 2010, Mosby/Elsevier.)

(N03.0-N03.5 = 6 codes
of specificity)

*Chronic glomerulonephritis is coded according to sites
and types of lesions. Refer to the physician's diagnosis
for site and type of lesion and to the current edition of
the ICD-10-CM coding manual.*

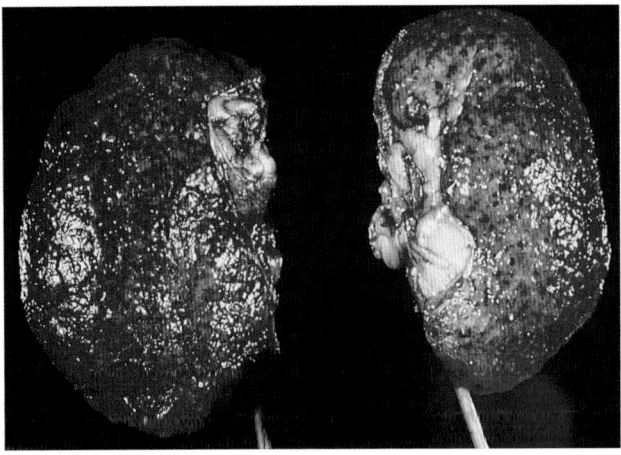

• **Fig. 11.7** End-stage glomerulonephritis. (From Damjanov I: *Pathology for the health professions,* St Louis, 2017, Elsevier.)

Symptoms and Signs

At first, CGN is *asymptomatic;* then subclinical progression of the disease leads to hypertension, hematuria, proteinuria, oliguria, and edema. In the later stages, with increasing renal failure, hypertension becomes severe, and azotemia develops. When the kidneys fail to remove urea from blood (called *azotemia*), the body compensates by attempting to excrete urea through the sweat glands. Tiny crystals of urea appear on the skin; this condition is termed *uremic frost.* The patient experiences fatigue, malaise, nausea, vomiting, pruritus, and dyspnea.

Patient Screening

Patients with CGN have probably been diagnosed already, and routine follow-up visits may have been scheduled. New patients may be referrals and will require an appointment as soon as possible. An appointment should be scheduled as soon as possible for any patient complaining of hematuria. Often hypertension symptoms, along with malaise and edema, are reported and indicate the need for prompt attention.

Etiology

Immune mechanisms are suspected to be a major cause of CGN; antigen-antibody complexes lodge in the glomerular capsular membrane, triggering an inflammatory response and glomerular injury. Primary renal disorders and multisystem diseases, such as systemic lupus erythematosus, are other possible causes.

Diagnosis

The diagnostic studies used to detect CGN are the same as those used for acute glomerulonephritis: urinalysis, blood tests, radiographic studies, ultrasonography, and renal biopsy. The findings include signs of advanced renal insufficiency, rising BUN and serum creatinine levels, and grossly abnormal findings on urinalysis. Renal biopsy and the use of sophisticated tools, such as electron microscopy and immunofluorescence, are valuable in determining the optimal treatment and the prognosis.

Treatment

The goals of treatment are to control edema, treat hypertension, and prevent congestive heart failure and uremia. The patient is given supportive measures for comfort. Medical treatment includes the administration of antihypertensives,

diuretics, and antibiotics if urinary tract infection (UTI) develops. Protein, salt (sodium [Na$^+$] and phosphate), and fluid intake may be limited in the diet. Angiotensin-converting enzyme (ACE) inhibitors are often used to aid in the reduction of excess protein in urine. Guidance should be given to the patient to check with the health care provider before taking any OTC medications, especially NSAIDs, because these medications can further worsen renal function. The patient may require dialysis (see Fig. 11.8) or may be a candidate for kidney transplantation.

Prognosis

Prognosis varies, depending on the extent of destruction of the kidneys and the patient's response to therapy. Eventually CGN will lead to end-stage renal disease (ESRD; Fig. 11.7). Dialysis may help the patient until kidney transplantation can be performed.

Prevention

Prompt treatment of acute glomerulonephritis, diabetes, and hypertension can help in the prevention of CGN.

Patient Teaching

Stress the importance of compliance with treatment regimens to reduce hypertension and on the importance of prompt attention to infections. When dialysis is necessary, encourage the patient and the family to seek out support groups and available community resources. Advise patients to take diuretics in the morning to avoid disruption of sleep at night. Offer visual aids, including videos when available, to explain the anatomy and function of the urinary system.

❖ **ENRICHMENT**

Dialysis and Kidney Transplantation

In the United States, end-stage renal disease (ESRD) develops, on average, in 1.3 in 10,000 people each year. In renal failure, the kidneys no longer can process blood and form urine. Therapy should begin before the development of ultimately fatal uremic symptoms. Dialysis or kidney transplantation, if successful, offer rehabilitation and extended life to patients with ESRD.

Dialysis

Dialysis filters out unwanted elements from blood by diffusion across a semipermeable membrane; the healthy kidneys usually remove these wastes. Thus the proper fluid, electrolyte, and acid–base balances are maintained in the body. Two methods used to perform blood dialysis are hemodialysis and peritoneal dialysis (Fig. 11.8). Although these procedures do not cure renal failure, many patients' conditions stabilize after 10 to 15 years of treatment.

Hemodialysis

Hemodialysis can take place in the patient's home or at a hospital. It removes impurities or wastes from the patient's blood by using an artificial kidney (hemodialyzer). Access to the bloodstream is created surgically in the arm, leg, or subclavian vein with an internal fistula, which allows blood to pass from the patient's body to the semipermeable membrane in the machine. The cleansed blood then returns to the patient in a procedure that takes 3 to 4 hours. The patient usually receives two or three sessions a week.

Peritoneal Dialysis

Peritoneal dialysis is carried out in the patient's own body with the use of a dialysate solution and the peritoneal membrane to filter out harmful toxins and excessive fluid. The clean dialyzing fluid passes into the peritoneal cavity through a permanent indwelling peritoneal catheter, and wastes diffuse across the peritoneal membrane into the fluid. The contaminated fluid then is drained and replaced with fresh fluid.

- Continuous ambulatory peritoneal dialysis (CAPD) takes place without a machine by allowing the solution to drain by gravity into a dialysis bag worn around the waist. This procedure takes about 15 minutes and is repeated three to four times a day and once at night.
- Continuous cycling peritoneal dialysis (CCPD) takes place while the patient sleeps, with the use of a cycling machine.
- Intermittent peritoneal dialysis (IPD) takes several hours, is performed three to five times a week, and usually is done in a clinic.
- See Fig. 11.8C.

Continuous Renal Replacement Therapy

This type of dialysis, also called *hemofiltration,* is performed in the hospital setting. This takes place typically in the intensive care unit for patients in acute renal failure (ARF). CRRT dialysis takes place 12 to 24 hours each day, every day.

Kidney Transplantation

Kidney transplantation is the surgical placement of a donor kidney into a patient with irreversible renal failure. Used synergistically with clinical dialysis, kidney transplantation is one of medicine's success stories. Kidney transplantation leads the field of organ replacement, with many patients being on waiting lists. Immunosuppressive agents are used to prevent or treat rejection syndrome. Sophisticated evaluation of the donor and the recipient to find a good match for human leukocyte antigen (HLA) offers the best chances for a good prognosis. More than 21,000 kidney transplantations were performed in the year 2018. Current research is exploring the option of splitting of the kidney prior to transplantation so that two patients can benefit from one kidney. This is, however, very rare in current practice.

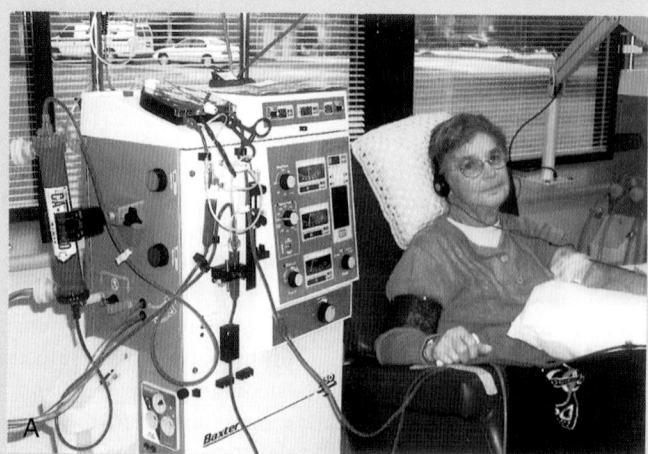

• **Fig. 11.8** Dialysis. (A) Hemodialysis.

Dialysis and Kidney Transplantation

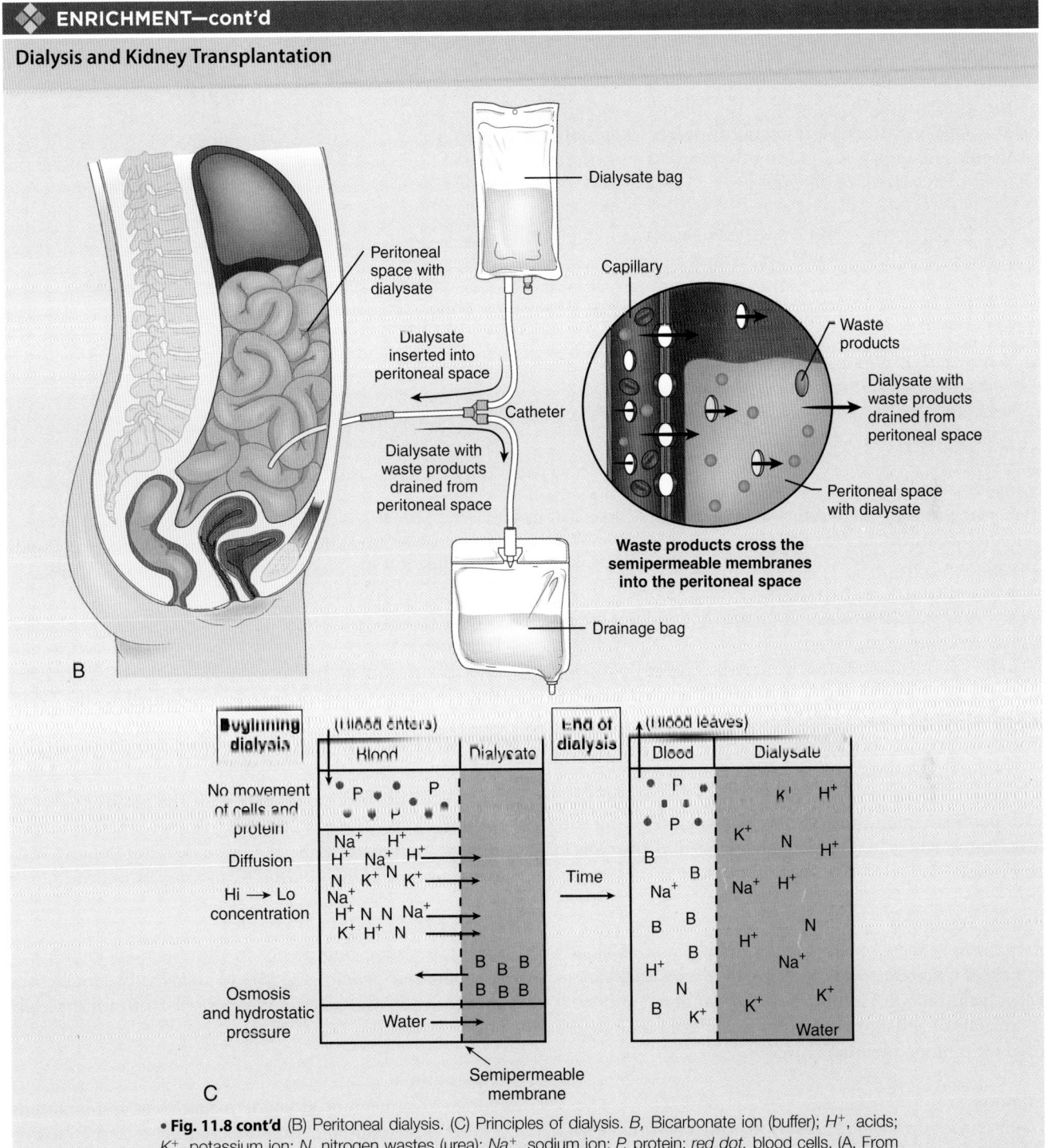

• **Fig. 11.8 cont'd** (B) Peritoneal dialysis. (C) Principles of dialysis. *B,* Bicarbonate ion (buffer); *H⁺,* acids; *K⁺,* potassium ion; *N,* nitrogen wastes (urea); *Na⁺,* sodium ion; *P,* protein; *red dot,* blood cells. (A, From Ignatavicius D: *Medical-surgical nursing: patient-centered collaborative care,* ed 6, St Louis, Saunders. B, From Proctor D, et al: *Kinn's the medical assistant,* ed 13, St Louis, 2017, Elsevier. C, From Gould B: *Pathophysiology for the health professions,* ed 3, Philadelphia, 2005, Saunders/Elsevier.)

Nephrotic Syndrome (Nephrosis)

Description

Nephrotic syndrome, a disease of the basement membrane of the glomerulus, is secondary to a number of renal diseases and a variety of systemic disorders. Nephrotic syndrome encompasses a group of symptoms sometimes referred to as *protein-losing kidney.*

| ICD-10-CM Code | N04.4 (Nephrotic syndrome with diffuse endocapillary proliferative glomerulonephritis) |
| | (N04.0-N04.5 = 6 codes of specificity) |

Nephrotic syndrome is coded according to sites and types of lesions. Refer to the physician's diagnosis for site and type of lesion and to the current edition of the ICD-10-CM coding manual.

Symptoms and Signs

The patient with nephrotic syndrome loses excessive amounts of protein, mainly albumin, in urine (proteinuria). The excessive loss of protein in urine results in depressed plasma protein levels (hypoalbuminemia). Glomerular filtration becomes diminished, and water and sodium are retained, resulting in edema and hypertension. The syndrome includes microscopic or gross hematuria. Plasma lipid levels are elevated, but the reason for this is not understood. Sloughed-off fat bodies can be found in urine. These patients are especially susceptible to infections.

Nephrotic syndrome causes the patient to feel lethargic and depressed, with loss of appetite. He or she appears pale, with puffiness around the eyes, swollen ankles (pitting edema), and weight gain. Skin irritation related to edema may be present.

Patient Screening

As previously mentioned, patients complaining of bloody urine that is accompanied by edema, headache, and flank or pelvic pain require prompt medical attention. Additional complaints of lethargy and sudden weight gain indicate the need for prompt attention as well.

Etiology

Nephrotic syndrome is caused by increased permeability of the glomerulus, indicating renal damage. This condition may occur after an attack of glomerulonephritis, or it may be the result of exposure to certain toxins or drugs, pregnancy, or kidney transplantation (Box 11.1). Metabolic diseases, such as diabetes mellitus; certain infections; and allergic reactions are conditions that may lead to nephrotic syndrome.

Diagnosis

Diagnosis is based on the clinical findings and the presence of gross proteinuria and lipiduria (the presence of fatty casts) in a 24-hour urine specimen. Abnormal blood study

---

• BOX 11.1   Nephrotoxic Agents

Solvents
  Carbon tetrachloride
  Methanol
  Ethylene glycol
Heavy metals
  Lead
  Arsenic
  Mercury
Pesticides
Antibiotics
  Kanamycin
  Gentamicin
  Polymyxin B
  Amphotericin B
  Colistin
  Neomycin
  Phenazopyridine

Nonsteroidal antiinflammatory
  drugs
Iodinated radiographic
  contrast media
Antineoplastic agents
Miscellaneous compounds
  Acetaminophen
  Amphetamines
  Heroin
  Silicon
  Cyclosporine
  Poisonous mushrooms

Modified from Monahan F, et al: *Phipps' medical-surgical nursing, health and illness perspectives,* ed 8, St Louis, 2007, Mosby.

---

serum values, including hypoalbuminemia and hyperlipidemia, support the diagnosis. If a renal tumor is suspected, renal biopsy with histologic study is indicated.

Treatment

Effective treatment begins by addressing the underlying cause. Dietary intake of protein is adjusted to the GFR. Diuretics and decreased sodium intake help control edema. The use of ACE inhibitors is helpful in treating hypertension and usually reduces protein loss. A course of corticosteroids, such as prednisone, may have the positive effect of controlling proteinuria in some patients. Urine output must be monitored. If the condition does not improve with treatment, nephrotic syndrome can progress to ESRD.

Prognosis

Prognosis varies, depending on the extent of kidney destruction and patient response to therapy. Eventually nephrotic syndrome that is nonresponsive to treatment leads to ESRD.

Prevention

Prompt treatment of glomerulonephritis is important to prevent this condition. Avoiding exposure to certain toxins or drugs helps prevent nephrotic syndrome, as does prompt treatment after exposure to these toxins (see Box 11.1). Monitoring kidney function in pregnant women and of any patients with metabolic diseases (e.g., diabetes mellitus), certain infections, and allergic reactions may assist the physician in detecting malfunction early on, and thus treatment can be instituted early on.

Patient Teaching

Advise patients and their families to contact the physician immediately if any exacerbation of symptoms is noted. Encourage patients to remain active, to exercise, and to practice good skin care. Additionally encourage them to seek out support groups and resource agencies in the community. Refer patients to a dietitian for instruction on planning a high-protein, low-sodium diet as prescribed. Offer visual aids, including videos when available, to explain the anatomy and function of the urinary system.

Acute Renal Failure

Description
ARF also known as acute kidney injury (AKI) is a very sudden and severe reduction in renal function, which usually occurs quickly, in a matter of a few days. This is a common clinical emergency because nitrogenous waste products begin to accumulate in blood quickly, thereby causing an acute uremic episode.

ICD-10-CM Code	N17 *(Acute kidney failure)*
	(N17.0-N17.9 = 5 codes of specificity)

Acute renal failure is coded according to sites and types of lesions. Refer to the physician's diagnosis for site and type of lesion and to the current edition of the ICD-10-CM coding manual.

Symptoms and Signs
Initially symptoms of AKI include oliguria, gastrointestinal disturbances, headache, drowsiness, and other alterations in the level of consciousness. A host of other symptoms can occur, depending on the underlying cause, the degree of impairment, and BUN levels.

Patient Screening
In many instances, patients with AKI are already under a physician's care or may even be receiving treatment as inpatients when initial symptoms occur. If not, anyone reporting sudden onset of these symptoms requires prompt attention. Follow office protocol as to scheduling an immediate appointment in the office or referring the individual to an emergency facility for observation and treatment.

Etiology
The causes of AKI are classified as those that result in diminished blood flow to the kidneys (e.g., circulatory shock or heart failure), those that involve intrarenal damage or disease (e.g., glomerulonephritis), and those that result from mechanical obstruction of urine flow. Of special concern is intrarenal damage, which can be prevented by control of exposure to substances known to be **nephrotoxic**, including drugs, insecticides, organic solvents, and cleaning agents (see Box 11.1). Whatever the cause, sudden renal dysfunction disrupts other body systems and, if left untreated, can lead to death. Certain antibiotics (i.e., gentamicin and streptomycin) can cause AKI in patients who have predisposing factors (i.e., existing kidney problems and old age) (Fig. 11.9).

Diagnosis
Blood tests and urinalysis reveal many abnormal findings associated with oliguria and the retention of nitrogenous wastes. BUN, serum creatinine, and potassium levels are elevated in blood. Other diagnostic studies include renal ultrasonography, radiography (computed tomography [CT] or magnetic resonance imaging [MRI]), and intravenous pyelography (IVP). Monitoring of balanced fluid intake and output also is important in determining kidney function.

Treatment
Determining the cause of AKI, if possible, is crucial in the course of medical management to reduce the risk of permanent kidney damage. However, the ultimate goal is to reverse the decreased renal perfusion. All body systems are monitored and supported, as needed, through the uremic crisis. The patient may be evaluated for dialysis. Fluid intake and output are balanced to prevent overload. It is important to carefully manage nutritional support to ensure that protein is being replaced in the right proportions to prevent metabolic acidosis. Initiating a high-carbohydrate/low-protein diet will accomplish this. Sodium and potassium intakes are controlled as well. Drug therapy may include antihypertensives, diuretics, intravenous (IV) fluids, and antiinfective agents because infection is a common complication in AKI.

Prognosis
In many cases, with prompt treatment AKI is reversible, and recovery is rapid and complete. Prognosis varies, depending on the cause and patient response to treatment. Regardless of the cause, sudden renal dysfunction disrupts other body systems and, if left untreated, can lead to death.

Prevention
Prevention methods vary, depending on the causative factors. Promptly treating circulatory shock or heart failure and identifying conditions involving intrarenal damage or disease and those that result from mechanical obstruction of urine flow help prevent AKI. Additionally, controlling exposure to substances known to be nephrotoxic, including drugs, insecticides, organic solvents, and cleaning agents, helps prevent ARF.

Patient Teaching
Encourage patients who have recovered from AKI to be cognizant of the causative factors and to be aware of possible sources of toxins. Warn them of signs and symptoms of renal failure, such as decreased urine output, weight gain, muscle weakness, palpitations, shortness of breath, and excessive bruising. Instruct them to immediately report such symptoms to the physician. Additional instructions on eating a modified diet as tolerated, good skin care and oral hygiene, and a review of the prescribed diet should be given. Assist those who have residual effects of AKI to seek out community resource agencies and support groups. Generate print-on-demand electronic materials, when possible, as teaching tools.

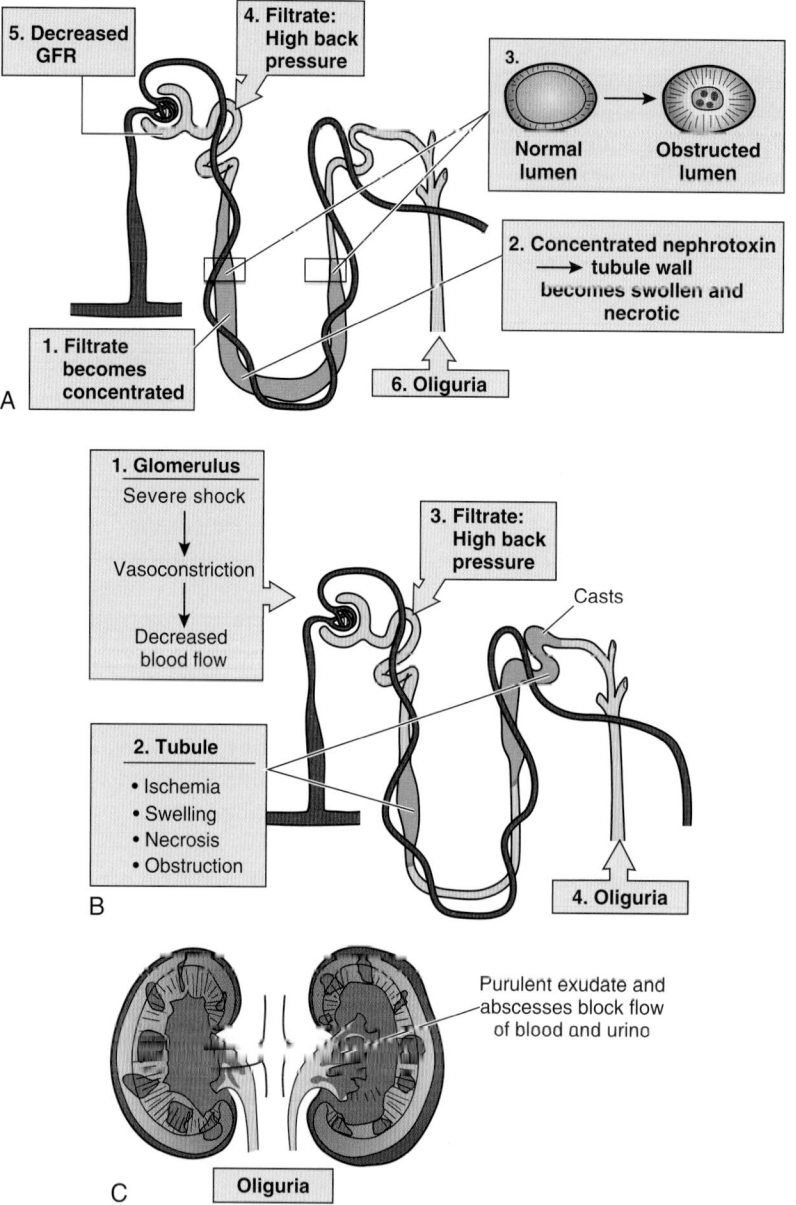

• **Fig. 11.9** Causes of acute renal failure (ARF). (A) Nephrotoxins. (B) Ischemia. (C) Pyelonephritis. *GFR,* Glomerular filtration rate. (From VanMeter: *Gould's pathophysiology for the health professions,* ed 5, St. Louis, 2015, Saunders.)

Chronic Kidney Disease

Description

Chronic kidney disease (CKD) results from the gradual and progressive loss of nephrons, with irreversible loss of renal function and gradual onset of uremia. The systemic effects eventually can manifest in any and all body systems.

ICD-10-CM Code	N18 *(Chronic kidney disease)* (N18.1–18.9 = 7 codes of specificity)

Referral to the current edition of the ICD-10-CM coding manual is recommended to identify the manifestations of this disorder.

Symptoms and Signs

The patient with CKD may feel weak, tired, and lethargic. Hypertension and edema result from retention of fluids in the body as the condition progresses. As uremic syndrome worsens, many other symptoms and signs are generated: arrhythmias, muscle weakness, dyspnea, metabolic acidosis, ulceration of the gastrointestinal mucosa, and hair and skin changes.

Patient Screening

Patients with CRF probably have been diagnosed already, and routine follow-up visits may have been scheduled. New patients may be referrals and require scheduling of appointments as soon as possible. Any patient complaining of hematuria requires prompt attention. Often hypertension symptoms, along with malaise and edema, are the reported symptoms, which indicate the need for prompt attention.

Etiology

There are numerous causes of CRF CKD, including primary diseases or infections of the kidneys, such as glomerulonephritis, pyelonephritis, and polycystic kidneys. Often CRF CKD is the end stage of chronic renal diseases or of chronic obstruction of the outflow of urine.

Diagnosis

Blood studies show elevated BUN, serum creatinine, and potassium levels, along with decreased hemoglobin and hematocrit levels. Urinalysis is grossly abnormal, with excessive protein, glucose, leukocytes, and casts. The 24-hour urine volume is greatly decreased. Diagnostic studies include KUB radiography, renal ultrasonography, kidney scanning, IVP, and renal arteriography.

Treatment

The underlying cause, if known, must be treated. The patient is evaluated for dialysis or kidney transplantation to prolong life. Diet and nutritional modifications help control protein and sodium intakes to reduce the work of the diseased kidneys. Fluid intake and output are monitored and regulated. Drug therapy includes administration of diuretics, antihypertensives, antiinfective agents, and anti emetics. Nausea, vomiting, and loss of appetite may be alleviated by a change in diet that includes more carbohydrate and fat calories and fewer protein calories. Severe anemia can occur with CKD, and often, administration of erythropoietin, a protein that stimulates bone marrow, can help form new RBCs. Bone degeneration also can result from CKD, and calcitriol, a form of vitamin D, can be given to prevent bones from weakening. The patient is given supportive care and kept as comfortable as possible. Numerous complications may occur, so the prognosis is uncertain.

Prognosis

The prognosis for CKD varies, depending on the etiology. No total cure for this condition is known. Preventing complications and providing supportive care are important.

Prevention

Prevention varies, depending on the causative factors. Promptly treating AKI and recognizing and treating the cause of intrarenal damage or diseases that result from mechanical obstruction of urine flow will help prevent further damage. Additionally, controlling exposure to substances known to be nephrotoxic, including drugs, insecticides, organic solvents, and cleaning agents, can help prevent AKI and subsequent chronic failure.

Patient Teaching

Provide a list of support groups, and encourage patients and their families to seek out support groups and resource agencies in the community. Help them become aware of sources of possible toxic exposures that contribute to renal disease. Generate print-on-demand electronic materials, when possible, as teaching tools. Advise patients to consult their provider before taking any OTC medications, especially NSAIDs.

Pyelonephritis

Description

Pyelonephritis, the most common type of renal disease, is inflammation of the renal pelvis and connective tissues of one or both kidneys.

> ICD-10-CM Code   N12 (Tubulo-interstitial nephritis, not specified as acute or chronic)
> N10 (Acute tubulo-interstitial nephritis)
> N11.0-N11.9 (Chronic obstructive tubulo-interstitial nephritis)
>
> *Pyelonephritis is coded according to site and type of lesion. Refer to the physician's diagnosis for site and type of lesion and to the current edition of the ICD-10-CM coding manual.*

Symptoms and Signs

Pyelonephritis usually is caused by infection, pregnancy, or renal calculi. Pus collects in the renal pelvis, with the formation of abscesses. The patient experiences rapid onset of fever, chills, nausea and vomiting, and flank (lumbar) pain. This usually is preceded by a UTI with urinary frequency or urgency and dysuria. The patient may report a foul odor to the urine with hematuria and pyuria. Tenderness is noted in the suprapubic region, the abdomen becomes rigid, and palpation may reveal tender, enlarged kidneys. Urinalysis results show abnormal constituents, including urinary casts, nitrites, and leukocytes.

Patient Screening

Patients complaining of bloody or foul-smelling urine, accompanied by fever, chills, nausea, vomiting, and pelvic and flank pain, require prompt medical attention.

Etiology

Bacteria that ascend from the lower urinary tract to the kidneys usually cause pyelonephritis; it is less commonly caused by hematogenous or lymphatic spread of bacteria. Obstruction and stasis of urine by renal calculi (kidney stones), tumors, and benign prostatic hypertrophy predispose the kidneys to infection. Stasis of urine allows invading bacteria, usually *Escherichia coli,* to cause the infectious process. Women are more at risk because sexual activity or poor perineal hygiene can introduce bacterial contamination into the urinary tract. Catheterization or diagnostic procedures, such as endoscopic (cystoscopic) examination,

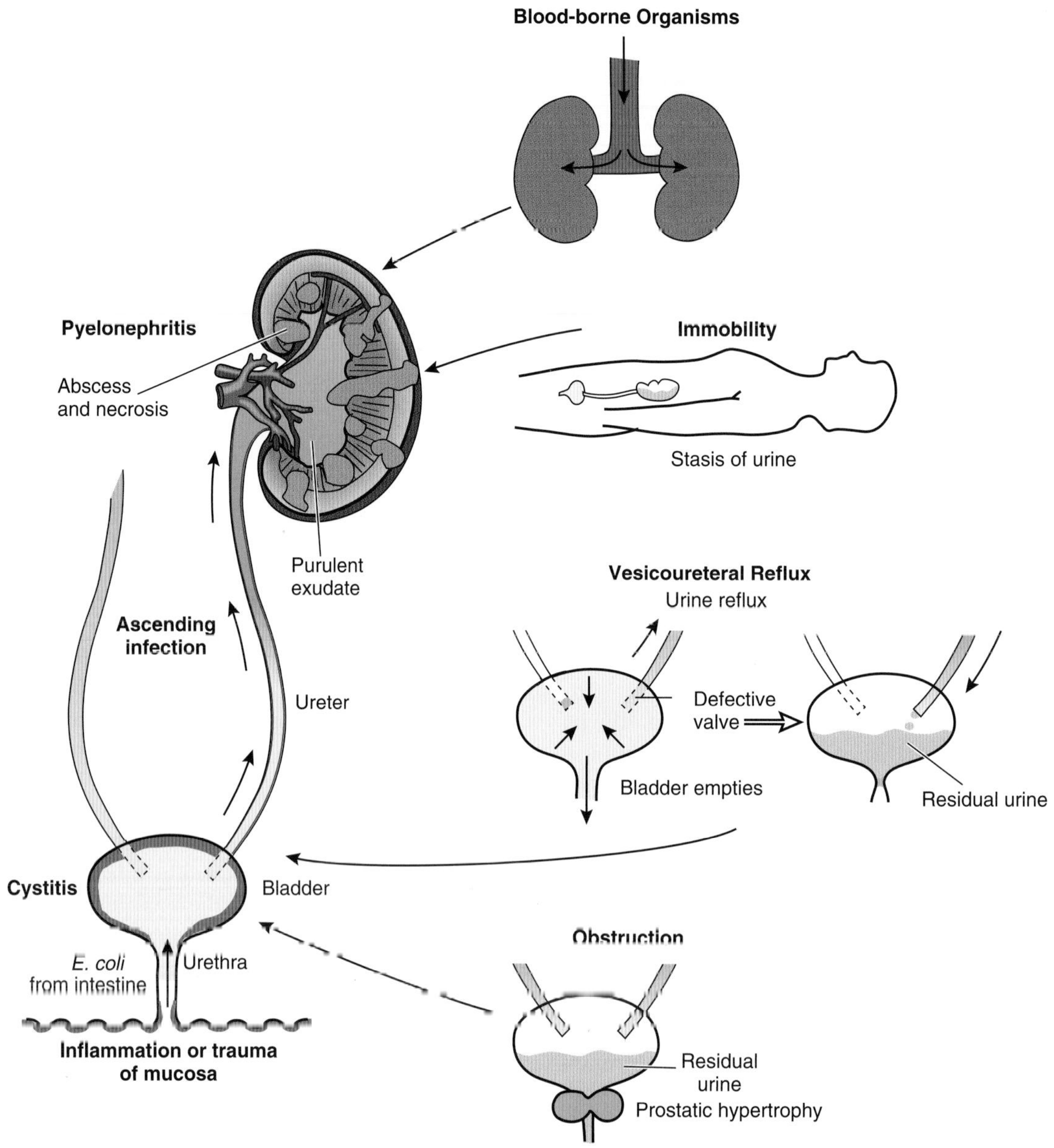

Blood-borne Organisms

• **Fig. 11.10** Causes of infection in the urinary tract. (From Gould B: *Pathophysiology for the health professions,* ed 4, Philadelphia, 2011, Saunders/Elsevier.)

can directly introduce organisms into the urinary bladder. The infection then moves upward in the urinary tract (ascending infection) to one or both kidneys (Fig. 11.10).

Diagnosis

The diagnosis is made by assessing the clinical findings and through urinalysis of a clean-catch urine specimen that shows increased WBCs and RBCs and the presence of bacteria, pus, protein, and casts. Blood culture and urine culture can identify the causative organism. Radiographic studies reveal kidneys that appear swollen or enlarged.

Treatment

The treatment of choice consists of IV or oral antibiotics, usually penicillin fluoroquinolones or cephalosporins, given for a full course of 7 to 14 days. At the present time, common antibiotic treatment is a 10- to 14-day regimen of fluoroquinolones (Cipro, Levaquin). Fluoroquinolones are no longer the drugs of choice because of the increased resistance patterns and adverse side effects related to this class of antibiotics or second- or third-generation cephalosporins also given for 7 to 10 days. Increased fluid intake to dilute urine, along with bed rest, is urged. Unless patients are at high risk for UTIs, they respond well to treatment without recurrences. When pyelonephritis recurs, certain tests (e.g., IVP and/or a renal ultrasonography) need to be performed to determine whether a renal abnormality (e.g., vesicoureteral reflux) is present. In more complicated cases, surgery may be indicated to relieve an obstruction or to correct an anomaly.

Prognosis

Early detection and prompt treatment usually result in a good outcome. However, untreated and recurrent pyelonephritis may be the cause of hypertension, bacteremia, and chronic pyelonephritis, leading to permanent kidney damage.

Prevention

Prevention includes drinking eight glasses of water a day. Those who have a history of pyelonephritis are advised to void frequently. Proper use of toilet tissue when wiping is important in the prevention of infection.

Patient Teaching

Advise women to void (urinate) after engaging in sexual intercourse. Also, patients who begin to experience symptoms should increase their fluid intake, especially of water. Women should be encouraged to wipe the perineum from the front to the back to avoid spreading fecal matter from the rectum to the urethral meatus. Give the patient visual aids that explain the location and function of the urinary system.

Hydronephrosis

Description

Hydronephrosis is abnormal dilation of the renal pelvis caused by pressure from urine that cannot flow past an obstruction in the urinary tract (Figs. 11.11 and 11.12).

ICD-10-CM Code	N13.3 *(Other and unspecified hydronephrosis)*
	(N13.30-N13.39 = 2 codes of specificity)

Symptoms and Signs

When the obstruction is severe and prolonged, fibrotic changes and loss of function of the involved nephrons occurs. Hydronephrosis is usually a chronic condition, with destruction of the kidneys that transpires without pain or symptoms. Its detection often is incidental, occurring during radiographic examination or ultrasonography of the abdomen. A vague backache and diminished urine output might be the only symptoms that the patient can identify. If an infection accompanies the condition, the patient may experience fever, chills, hematuria, and pyuria, and the kidney may be palpable.

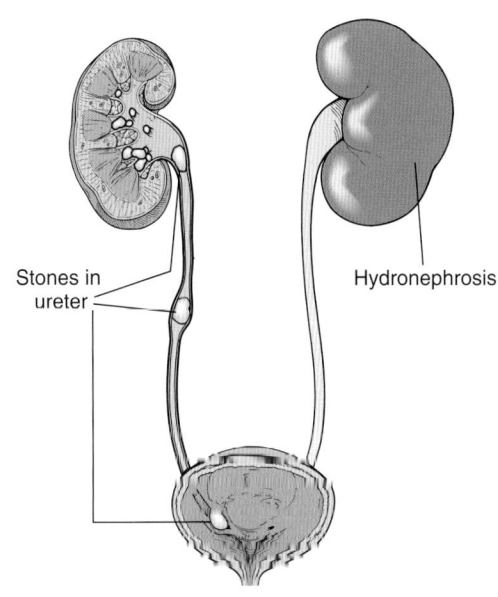

• **Fig. 11.12** Renal calculi.

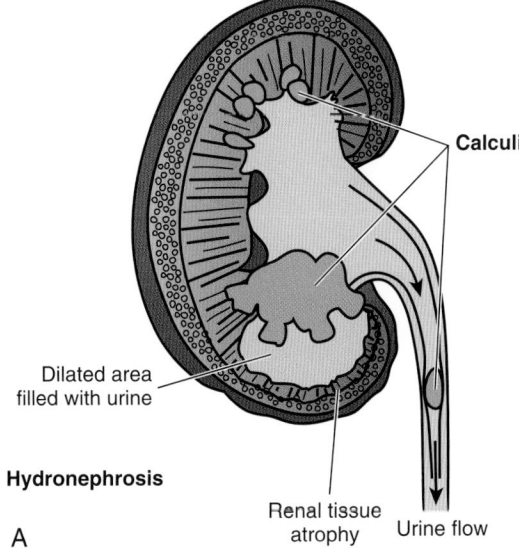

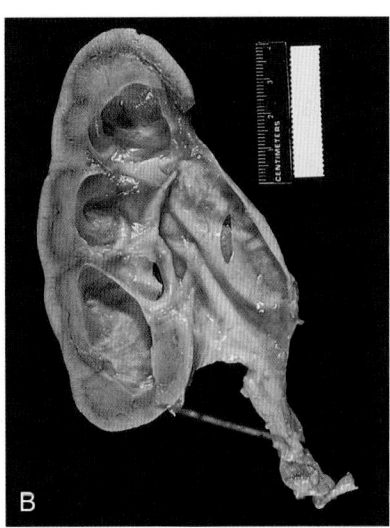

• **Fig. 11.11** (A) Renal calculi and hydronephrosis. (B) Hydronephrosis with dilation of the renal pelvis and calyces and atrophy of renal tissue. (A, From Gould B: *Pathophysiology for the health professions,* ed 4, Philadelphia, 2011, Saunders/Elsevier. B, From Cotran RS, Kumar V, Collins T: *Robbins pathologic basis of disease,* ed 6, Philadelphia, 1999, Saunders/Elsevier.)

Patient Screening

Many patients with hydronephrosis are asymptomatic for some time and request an appointment only when they begin to feel sick. A history of kidney stones or other possible obstruction of the ureter may be mentioned by the patient making an appointment request. As with many other kidney disorders, prompt medical attention is required for these patients.

Etiology

Dilation of the renal pelvis is caused by buildup of pressure in the kidneys because of an obstruction. The cause of the obstruction could be renal calculi, tumors, inflammation caused by infections, prostatic hyperplasia (enlargement), bladder tumors, or congenital abnormalities. During pregnancy, the enlarged uterus can cause hydronephrosis.

Diagnosis

The first indication of hydronephrosis is usually the result of investigation of other abdominal structures. Follow-up contrast studies of the ureters and the kidneys need to be done. Retrograde pyelography is necessary. Cystoscopy to rule out an obstruction by a tumor of the bladder or prostate is helpful (Fig. 11.13).

Treatment

The treatment of hydronephrosis depends on the underlying cause of the obstruction and the duration of the condition. When obstruction is discovered early, the source can be identified and removed by surgical intervention. Concurrent infection necessitates antibiotic therapy. When surgical intervention is not an option and/or the obstruction cannot be relieved, a nephrostomy tube may be inserted.

Prognosis

Once the obstruction causing the hydronephrosis has been resolved, the kidneys may return to normal function. However, when the condition has been present for an extended period, permanent damage may result. Prolonged hydronephrosis may cause permanent damage.

Prevention

Preventing kidney stones and the subsequent obstruction of urine flow they can cause also helps prevent hydronephrosis. As previously mentioned, urine and blood chemistry measurements and stone analysis provide clues that can help determine which preventive measures are likely to prevent recurring kidney stone formation. Additionally, modification of diet, increased exercise, and adequate fluid intake minimize the chance of stone formation. Prompt treatment of an enlarged prostate may prevent obstructions and the resulting hydronephrosis.

Patient Teaching

Encourage patients to follow the suggested diet and fluid regimen to prevent kidney stones. If a nephrostomy tube is in place, care instructions may be necessary.

◆ ENRICHMENT

Cystoscopy

Cystoscopy allows direct examination and treatment of the urinary bladder (see Fig. 11.13). A cystoscope is inserted through the urethra; this instrument has its own lighting system, a viewing scope, and a passage for catheters and surgical devices. Cystoscopy is used to obtain biopsy specimens for diagnosis and to remove stones or tumors.

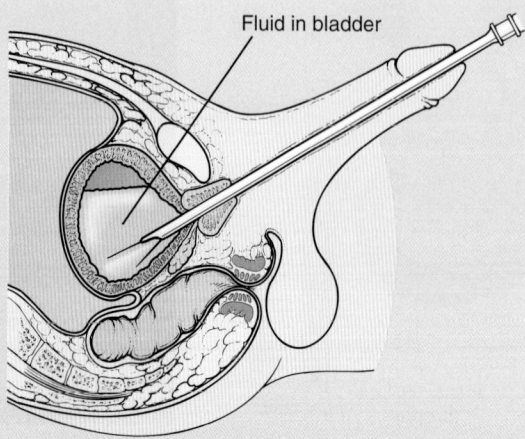

Fluid in bladder

• **Fig. 11.13** Cystoscopy. (From *Mosby's dictionary of medicine, nursing & health professions*, ed 8, St Louis, 2013, Mosby.)

Renal Calculi

Description

Renal calculi are stones in the kidney or elsewhere in the urinary tract formed by the concentration of various mineral salts (see Figs. 11.11 to 11.13).

ICD-10-CM Code   N20 (Calculus of kidney and
                           ureter)
                      (N20.0-N21.9 = 8 codes of
                           specificity)

Renal calculi are coded according to location. Refer to the physician's diagnosis for location of the calculus and to the current edition of the ICD-10-CM coding manual.

Symptoms and Signs

Kidney stones can be solitary or multiple and vary in size. A larger stone formed in the shape of the renal pelvis is known as a *staghorn calculus* (Fig. 11.14). Small stones can be passed spontaneously, unnoticed. The patient's symptoms vary, depending on the degree of obstruction. If infection or blockage caused by the calculi is present, the patient experiences sudden severe pain in the flank area, known as *renal colic,* with urinary urgency and other urinary symptoms. Other symptoms include nausea and vomiting, hematuria, fever, chills, and abdominal distention. Blood in urine can be the result of trauma caused by the presence of small stones, which may be gravel-like in consistency, or larger stones, such as staghorn calculi. Hydronephrosis can develop if urine is prevented from flowing past the calculi.

Patient Screening

Pain caused by a kidney stone should be considered an emergency situation. If these patients cannot be seen in the office as soon as possible, they should be referred to an emergency care facility where they can receive analgesic intervention. The patient experiencing sudden onset of severe flank pain and pelvic pressure and pain that is accompanied by nausea and vomiting requires immediate observation and treatment.

Etiology

Often the cause of calculi is unknown, although a hereditary tendency for development of certain types of stones has been noted. Kidney stones are formed when there is an excessive amount of calcium or uric acid present in urine. Men are more prone to kidney stones compared with women, and the occurrence rate increases from age 30 years up to and including the 50s. Calculi form when sources of crystals are found in urine, along with the absence of crystalline inhibitors, and urine is supersaturated with poorly soluble substances.

Risk factors include prolonged dehydration, prolonged immobilization, infection, urinary stasis from obstruction, long-term ingestion of certain medications, and metabolic factors, such as hyperparathyroidism and gout. (Gout is discussed in Chapter 7.)

Diagnosis

The diagnosis of renal calculi is made on the basis of the family history, clinical findings, urinalysis, KUB radiographic studies, intravenous urography, renal ultrasonography, and CT. The patient is encouraged to strain the urine

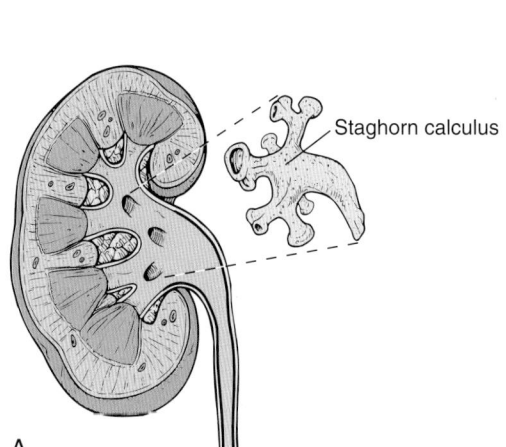
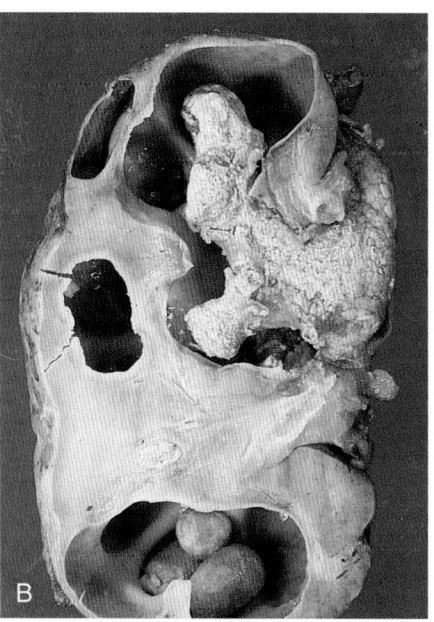

• **Fig. 11.14** Staghorn calculi. (B, From Stevens A, et al: *Core pathology,* ed 3, London, 2010, Mosby/Elsevier.)

to capture any stones that are passed during urination so that the stones can be analyzed in the laboratory. The possible existence of metabolic disorders can be investigated by using blood and urine tests.

Treatment

The goals of medical care are to remove the calculi, treat pain and infection, and resolve the causative factors. These measures should prevent permanent kidney damage and recurrence of calculi.

The treatment begins with analgesic therapy and hydration during the initial evaluation. Sometimes an alpha blocker, such as Flomax, may be prescribed. These work by relaxing the muscles of the bladder, allowing the stone to pass. The location and size of the calculi indicate the course of treatment. Small calculi (< 5 mm) may be treated with just observation and fluid hydration in the hope that the stones will pass spontaneously. Large calculi can be removed by any of several surgical procedures. Attempts are made to crush stones that are (1) too large to pass down the ureter, (2) lodged in the pelvis of the kidney, or (3) trapped in the proximal portion of the ureter. Extracorporeal shock wave lithotripsy (ESWL) is a procedure that breaks apart (crushes) the stones, thus allowing the small particles to be flushed out of the body naturally.

A surgical procedure using an ureteroscope to capture the stone in a basket and remove it is attempted for stones trapped in the distal aspect of a ureter. If the attempt to capture the stone is unsuccessful, electrohydraulic lithotripsy (EHL) or laser lithotripsy is used to attempt to break the stone apart into small particles that can be flushed out of the system. This procedure usually is done with the patient under general anesthesia and with the aid of fluoroscopy. After removal of the calculus, the ureter is visualized via the ureteroscope, and often the pelvis of the kidney also is inspected for any scarring, damage, or residual stone fragments. A stent that extends into the urinary bladder is placed in the pelvis of the kidney as a means of preventing edema and spasms of the ureter and subsequent occlusion of the ureter. The stent is removed in 2 to 5 days.

Stones in the urinary bladder often pass spontaneously. When this does not happen, an attempt to remove bladder stones is done during cystoscopy. When the previously mentioned procedures are unsuccessful in removing the calculi, surgical intervention in the form of percutaneous nephrolithotomy may be indicated to remove the stones before permanent damage is caused. A small incision is made into the kidney, and the stone is shattered by using ultrasound or EHL. Rarely, when the aforementioned procedures are unsuccessful, surgical incision of the kidney is performed to remove the stones.

Depending on the chemical composition, some kidney stones can be dissolved or prevented from forming. Often the patient may pass small or microscopic stones naturally and without pain. The patient is encouraged to drink 8 to 12 glasses of water a day and may be given diuretics to prevent urinary stasis. Patients are encouraged to strain their

urine to catch any stones or particles of stones that may be passed spontaneously. In that way, analysis of the calculi composition is made possible, which can help direct the preventive measures.

Prognosis

Prognosis is good after successful removal or spontaneous passage of the stones. However, additional stone formation is possible.

Prevention

Urine and blood chemistry measurements and stone analysis provide clues as to which preventive measures are likely to help. Prevention includes modification of diet, increased exercise, and adequate fluid intake to minimize the risk of stone formation in the future.

Patient Teaching

Encourage patients to strain their urine for stones, making sure they have an appropriate strainer to use. Instruct them in the proper way of straining urine. Encourage intake of at least eight glasses of water a day. Explain the risk factors, such as UTI, stasis of urine, prolonged dehydration, prolonged immobilization, and long-term ingestion of certain medications. Patients should avoid food high in oxalates, purine, and phosphorus (Box 11.2). Referral to a dietitian for advice on dietary control is helpful. Some physicians prefer limiting the intake of calcium, whereas others place no restrictions on calcium intake.

Infectious Cystitis and Urethritis

Description

Cystitis, inflammation of the urinary bladder, and urethritis, inflammation of the urethra, are two common forms of lower UTI.

• BOX 11.2 Food Containing Oxalates, Purines, and Phosphorus

Containing Oxalates
Chocolate
Coffee
Cola
Nuts
Red beets
Spinach
Strawberries
Tea
Wheat bran

Containing Purines
Anchovies
Beer
Brain
Gravies
Herring

Kidney
Liver
Mackerel
Sardines
Shellfish
Sweetbreads

Containing Phosphorus
Beef
Cheese
Cottage cheese
Dairy products
Ice cream
Liver
Milk
Other meats

ICD-10-CM Code   N30.90 *(Cystitis, unspecified*
without hematuria)
N30.91 *(Cystitis, unspecified*
with hematuria)
(N30.00-N30.91 = 14 codes of
specificity)
N34.1 *(Nonspecific urethritis)*
N34.2 *(Other urethritis)*
(N34.0-N34.3 = 4 codes of
specificity)

Cystitis and urethritis are coded according to type of infectious process. Refer to the physician's diagnosis for type of infectious process and to the current edition of the ICD-10-CM coding manual.

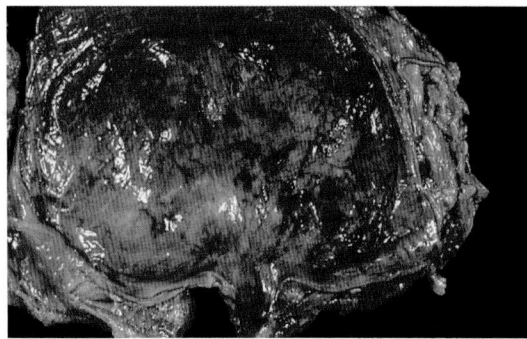

• **Fig. 11.15** Acute cystitis. The mucosa of the bladder is red and swollen. (From Damjanov I: *Pathology for the health professions,* St Louis, 2017, Elsevier.)

Symptoms and Signs

The inflammation and infection cause the patient to experience urinary urgency and frequency, dysuria, and possibly even incontinence. Patients often complain of pressure in the pelvis. Additionally, patients may have pain in the pelvic region and low back, spasm of the bladder, fever and chills, and a burning sensation with urination. The color of the urine may be dark yellow, or pink or red if blood is present.

Patient Screening

Patients experiencing pelvic and low back pain accompanied by fever and chills, along with the classic symptoms of frequency and urgency, require prompt attention. Advise them that they will need to provide a urine specimen on arrival at the office.

Etiology

The usual cause of cystitis and urethritis is an ascending bacterial invasion of the urinary tract. The most common causative microorganism is *E. coli,* followed by the *Klebsiella, Enterobacter, Proteus,* and *Pseudomonas* species. Sexually transmitted diseases can cause cystitis and urethritis. Other causes of these conditions are viruses, fungi, parasites, and inflammation caused by chemotherapy or radiation. Lesions can develop in the bladder secondary to inflammation, thereby intensifying the symptoms.

Diagnosis

The diagnosis is determined by evaluating the clinical findings, urinalysis of a clean-catch urine specimen, urine culture, and cystoscopy. Urinalysis shows dark yellow, pink, or red urine with abnormal urinary sediment and possibly blood and pus. Microscopic examination of the urine specimen shows RBCs (occult blood), increased numbers of epithelial cells or leukocytes, bacteria, and nitrites. Urine may have a foul odor. The urine culture grows the causative agent for identification. Cystoscopy shows a reddened, inflamed bladder wall (Fig. 11.15). Tenderness in the suprapubic region and pain in the lower back may be elicited on palpation.

Treatment

Treatment consists of organism-specific antibiotic or urinary antiseptic therapy, such as amoxicillin (Amoxil), trimethoprim-sulfamethoxazole (Bactrim DS, Septra DS), ciprofloxacin (Cipro), and levofloxacin (Levaquin). The use of fluoroquinolones has fallen out of favor for uncomplicated urinary tract infections because of increased resistance and drug class adverse effects. Penicillin derivatives are used to treat complicated cystitis, which tends to recur often. Treatment is a minimum 3 to 5 days of medication for uncomplicated infections and 7 to 10 days for recurring infections. Antibiotics used to treat UTIs in women may affect the normal vaginal flora, causing yeast infections. Phenazopyridine (Pyridium), a urinary analgesic, also can be given to decrease dysuria, or painful urination. Increased fluid intake is encouraged, as is regular, complete evacuation of the bladder.

Prognosis

Most lower UTIs respond well to antibiotic drug therapy.

Prevention

Prevention includes drinking eight glasses of water a day. Those who have a history of lower UTIs are advised to void frequently. Proper use of toilet tissue when wiping is important in preventing infection. Women with frequent cystitis and urethritis are advised to use prophylactic antibiotic therapy (i.e., nitrofurantoin [Macrobid]) either consistently or directly after intercourse. Postmenopausal women with frequent UTIs are often placed on vaginal estrogen therapy, as new research indicates that the loss of estrogen's effects on perineal tissue is a causative factor in the development of UTIs.

Patient Teaching

Advise women to void (urinate) after engaging in sexual intercourse. Also, patients who begin to experience symptoms should increase their fluid intake, especially of water. Women should be encouraged to wipe the perineum from the front to the back to avoid spreading fecal matter from the rectum to the urinary meatus. Many patients need to be taught the proper procedure for performing a clean-catch midstream sample. Provide the patient visual aids that explain the location and function of the urinary system.

Diabetic Nephropathy

Description

Diabetic nephropathy refers to the renal changes resulting from diabetes mellitus, a systemic endocrine disease caused by failure of the pancreas to release enough insulin into the body (see Diabetes Mellitus in Chapter 4). These changes, called glomerulosclerosis, can be expected to occur eventually in all patients with insulin-dependent (type I) diabetes, which increases their morbidity and mortality. Additionally, many patients with non–insulin-dependent (type II) diabetes also can develop this kidney disorder.

ICD-10-CM Code	E11.29 (Type 2 diabetes mellitus with other diabetic kidney complication)

(E11.21-E11.29 = 3 codes of specificity)
N08 (Glomerular disorders in diseases classified elsewhere)

It is important to code diabetes with renal manifestations first and then list the nephrotic syndrome.

Symptoms and Signs

Clinical manifestations, once they begin, include urinary retention, hypertension, nausea, and protein in urine. UTI and pyelonephritis are common complications. Although nephropathy is more likely to develop in those afflicted by insulin-dependent diabetes mellitus, all patients with diabetes whose blood glucose levels and blood pressure are not controlled are at risk for this irreversible disorder.

Patient Screening

Those diagnosed with diabetes usually are scheduled for routine assessments. Patients with diabetes who report urinary tract symptoms require prompt assessment.

Etiology

Diabetic glomerulosclerosis is a complication of diabetes mellitus; lesions of the glomeruli eventually cause the filtration rate to decrease. Insufficient control of blood glucose levels and blood pressure in the patient with diabetes may hasten the deterioration of renal function.

Diagnosis

Blood tests reveal an elevated BUN level and an increase in cholesterol level. Urinalysis shows protein and pus in urine. Urinary microalbumin signals the presence of urinary albumin, an indication of nephropathy. Hypertension is another factor to be noted. The diagnosis is confirmed by radiographic studies of the kidneys and renal biopsy.

Treatment

In patients with diabetes, susceptibility to renal failure varies, so the treatment plan must be individualized. Medical control of diabetes and blood pressure is important, as is prompt treatment of infection. Drug intervention includes an ACE inhibitor for blood pressure control and prolongation of proper kidney function. Fluid intake and output should be balanced; diuretics may be prescribed, if needed. For patients with diabetes, a modified low-protein and low-fat diet may be recommended. Dialysis or evaluation for kidney transplantation may be part of the long-term management of ESRD.

Prognosis

The prognosis varies, depending on the stage at which intervention begins. Early detection and treatment lead to the best outcome. There is no known cure for diabetic nephropathy. When blood glucose and blood pressure are not kept under control, the outcome becomes bleaker. ESRD is the final outcome. Kidney transplantation is the final option for treatment.

Prevention

Close monitoring of both blood glucose levels and blood pressure, with appropriate treatment intervention, is helpful for all patients with diabetes. Monitoring urine microalbumin is recommended yearly for all patients with diabetes. The sooner these are brought under control, the better is the outcome.

Patient Teaching

Make patients with diabetes aware of the importance of maintaining blood glucose at appropriate levels. Also advise them about the importance of monitoring blood pressure and keeping it at acceptable levels. Compliance with prescribed drug therapy is important.

Polycystic Kidney Disease

Description

Polycystic kidney disease is a slowly progressive and irreversible disorder in which normal renal tissue is replaced by multiple grapelike cysts (Fig. 11.16). The condition is bilateral, with cysts forming from dilated nephrons and collecting ducts. Eventually the kidneys become grossly enlarged, with compression of surrounding tissue leading to impaired renal function and renal failure.

ICD-10-CM Code	Q61.3 (Polycystic kidney, unspecified)

(Q61.1-Q61.3 = 4 codes of specificity)
Q61.2 (Polycystic kidney, adult type)
Q61.19 (Other polycystic kidney, infantile type)

Symptoms and Signs

As the kidneys become dilated, they are palpable on physical examination. The patient experiences lumbar pain, abdominal pain and tenderness, hematuria, and systemic hypertension and is more prone to renal infections and

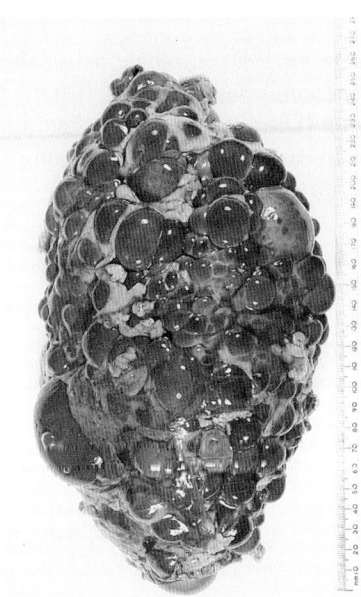

• **Fig. 11.16** Adult polycystic disease. (From Stevens A, et al: *Core pathology,* ed 3, London, 2010, Mosby/Elsevier.)

renal calculi. These patients usually experience chronic high blood pressure and kidney infections.

Patient Screening

Patients complaining of bloody urine accompanied by edema, headache, and flank or pelvic pain, require prompt medical attention.

Etiology

Polycystic kidney disease is inherited but may not manifest until adolescence or adulthood. It is not clearly understood why the cysts form. Acquired cystic kidney disease (noninherited) is a sequela of long-term kidney disease and/or long-term dialysis. Autosomal recessive polycystic kidney disease appears in infants and children and progresses rapidly to ESRD and death. Autosomal dominant polycystic kidney disease usually has its onset during the middle-age years.

Diagnosis

The diagnosis is made by evaluating the clinical findings and the results of renal function tests, such as urinalysis, which shows microscopic blood, proteinuria, and pus. Radiography, abdominal CT, abdominal MRI, and IVP show enlarged kidneys with irregular outlines and a spidery appearance throughout.

Treatment

Because polycystic disease cannot be cured, treatment of this ESRD consists of dialysis and kidney transplantation. The kidneys may have to be surgically removed if the patient has intractable pain, renal stones, or persistent infections. Management of UTIs is necessary, as is management of hypertension.

Prognosis

At the present time, no cure for polycystic disease is known.

Prevention

The majority of cases are inherited; therefore there is no prevention of inherited polycystic kidney disease. Acquired polycystic kidney disease, as a sequela to long-term kidney disease and/or dialysis, also has no means of prevention.

Patient Teaching

Suggest to patients and their families that they seek out community resources for those with kidney disease. Encourage them to locate support groups and possibly interact with those families that are dealing with a similar situation. Be prepared to answer questions about the disease process and outcomes. Advise patients that emptying the bladder regularly is helpful in preventing UTIs. Also remind them to monitor urinary output, blood pressure, and weight and to take frequent rest breaks and to avoid fatigue.

Neurogenic Bladder

Description

Neurogenic bladder is a dysfunction of the urinary bladder that consists of difficulty in emptying the bladder or urinary incontinence.

ICD-10-CM Code   N31.9 (Neuromuscular dysfunction
of bladder, unspecified)
(N31.0-N31.9 = 5 codes of
specificity)

Symptoms and Signs

Symptoms and signs of neurogenic bladder may vary, depending on the cause of the condition. The kidneys may have to be surgically removed if the patient has intractable pain, renal stones, or persistent infections. Some patients with sensory-related problems experience hesitancy and decreased volume of the urinary stream. Others may experience urinary retention resulting from decreased or absent stimuli to void. If the condition is the result of motor paralysis, the patient has the sensation of a full bladder but is unable to initiate the stream to empty. The patient with uninhibited neurogenic bladder is not able to control the voiding pattern and is persistently incontinent of small amounts of urine. In reflex neurogenic bladder, normal sensation is absent, with uncontrolled bladder contractions occurring, which results in spontaneous voiding of spurts of urine. With autonomous neurogenic bladder, all sensations and contraction capabilities are absent, resulting in inability to void without applying pressure to the suprapubic area (Valsalva and Credé maneuvers).

Patient Screening

In most circumstances, inability to empty the bladder and urinary incontinence are stressful for the patient. Prompt assessment should be considered.

Etiology

An insult to the brain, the spinal cord, or the nerves supplying the lower urinary tract, whether by trauma or a disease process, may result in the inability to empty the bladder or to maintain continence. Damage may be caused by cerebrovascular accident, spinal cord trauma, tumors, neuropathies, herniated lumbar disks, poliomyelitis, spinal cord lesions, or myelomeningocele.

Diagnosis

The diagnosis is based on a history of trauma or a disease process, the clinical findings, and the results of urodynamic studies that assess bladder function. Urine flow rate may be evaluated by an uroflowmeter, a device for continuous recording of urine flow in milliliters per second.

Treatment

The treatment is directed toward prevention of UTIs and attempts to restore some normalcy in function. Providing the means for storing urine and bladder emptying are of primary importance. Catheterization, whether intermittent or indwelling, is necessary to help the patient maintain an acceptable quality of life (Fig. 11.17). Drug therapy with parasympathomimetic agents may be indicated in some cases. Surgery and the use of external collection devices are other alternatives. Possible complications include hydronephrosis and renal failure.

Prognosis

Usually no cure for the neurologic defect that caused the bladder dysfunction is possible. Drug therapy may be helpful. Oxybutynin (Ditropan XL) and tolterodine (Detrol A) are both used in cases of urinary urge incontinence caused by muscle spasms of the bladder.

Prevention

Prevention varies, depending on the cause.

Patient Teaching

Patients may require instructions for self-catheterization or other techniques for emptying the bladder. Assist patients and their families in finding community resources available to them. Provide the names and phone numbers of support groups, and encourage patients to contact these groups. Use customized electronically generated educational materials, when available, to reinforce the treatment plan.

Stress Incontinence

Description

Stress incontinence is the uncontrollable leakage of urine from the urinary bladder during physical exertion or actions that stress the pelvic muscles, such as laughing, sneezing, coughing, lifting, stretching, or running.

❖ ENRICHMENT

Urinary Catheterization

Urinary catheterization involves the insertion of a catheter into the urinary bladder through the urethra for withdrawal of urine and for irrigation of the bladder with a therapeutic solution (see Fig. 11.17). Strict sterile technique is necessary to prevent cystitis. Urinary catheterization is indicated to empty the bladder before surgery, to obtain a sterile urine specimen, to relieve urinary retention, and to treat incontinence (an indwelling catheter is attached to a drainage bag).

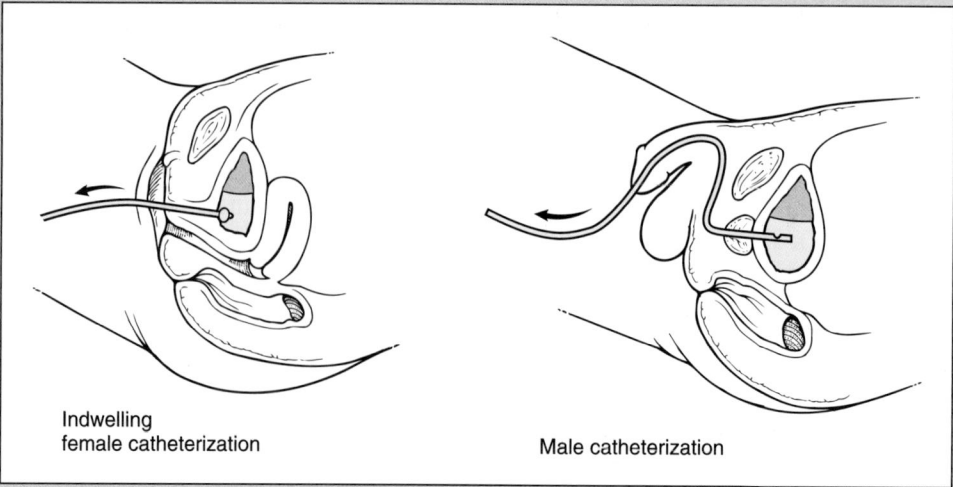

Indwelling female catheterization

Male catheterization

• **Fig. 11.17** Urinary catheterization.

ICD-10-CM Code   N39.3 *(Stress incontinence*
[female] [male])
N39.46 *(Mixed incontinence)*
Referral to the current edition of the ICD-10-CM coding
manual is recommended to confirm the appropriate
code.

Symptoms and Signs

Stress incontinence is a symptom, a sign, and a diagnosis. It occurs when increased abdominal pressure forces urine through the bladder sphincter. The patient (usually female) experiences leakage of urine on coughing, sneezing, laughing, lifting, or running, without feeling prior urgency. The patient is unable to control the leakage during physical exertion.

Patient Screening

Although not a urologic emergency, stress incontinence can seem like an emergency for the individual experiencing it. Therefore the patient should be scheduled for an appointment as soon as possible.

Etiology

Weakening of the pelvic floor muscles and the urethral structure causes this embarrassing disorder. Trauma to the area resulting from childbirth is the most common cause. Pressure from an existing pregnancy also may be the cause. The hormonal changes of aging and menopause make the condition more common in older women. Certain medications and obesity can precipitate the disorder.

Diagnosis

The symptoms clearly point to the diagnosis. Endoscopy and voiding cystourethrography (VCUG) reveal abnormal bladder position, with leakage provoked by coughing or straining, urodynamics.

Treatment

The treatment consists of exercises (Kegel exercises, or pelvic floor muscle tightening), estrogen replacement (most effective when estrogen cream is inserted vaginally), drug therapy, surgical repair, or collagen injections. Drug therapy may include tolterodine (Detrol), darifenacin (Enablex), trospium (Sanctura), or solifenacin (VESIcare).

Prognosis

Prognosis varies, depending on the etiology.

Prevention

Strengthening pelvic and perineal muscles is helpful. Some women experience stress incontinence as a result of the aging process and normal reduction in the amounts of estrogen produced in their bodies. Medications can control the symptoms in some women; for others, there is no prevention.

Patient Teaching

Provide information on Kegel exercises and other exercises to strengthen pelvic and perineal muscles. Discuss diet and fluid intake modifications. Assist with locating community resources or other agencies, and provide relevant information. Suggest locating support groups.

 ENRICHMENT

Urinary Incontinence

Normally, as the bladder distends with urine, a reflex is stimulated to initiate voluntary urination (micturition); the sphincters of the bladder and the pelvic diaphragm relax, the bladder muscles contract, and the bladder empties. Urinary incontinence is partial or total loss of voluntary control of the bladder with inability to retain urine. The causes vary, from muscle or sphincter impairment to nerve damage or structural abnormalities.

This condition is very prevalent in older adults, commonly because of overactivity of the bladder musculature, resulting in urgency and incontinence with an inappropriately small volume of urine. Incontinence sometimes is experienced temporarily after the stretching of muscles during childbirth. Children may experience a form termed *enuresis,* or bedwetting. Older women may experience "stress incontinence" resulting from postmenopausal changes in the pelvic musculature that allow intraabdominal pressure to surpass intraurethral pressure. Other types of overactive bladder, or frequency and urge incontinence, are the subject of much-noted current research. Neurologic damage, such as brain damage or spinal cord injury, may result in permanent incontinence.

Incontinence is treated or managed according to the degree, the type, and the cause. Antispasmodic agents, adult diapers, "bladder training," estrogen therapy for women, and pelvic muscle exercises are some of the therapeutic measures that may be tried. Chronic indwelling catheters are avoided in the management of incontinence because of the risk of infection.

ENRICHMENT

Overactive Bladder

A common bladder problem in today's society is overactive bladder. Individuals with this condition experience urinary urgency or strong, sudden urges to urinate. This sudden, uncomfortable urge to urinate may occur during daytime hours or awaken the individual from sleep. The uncontrollable urge (urge incontinence) can result in urinary incontinence with the accidental loss or leakage of small amounts of urine. Frequency of urination may also be a symptom of overactive bladder.

Additionally, overactive bladder may present social, occupational, and psychosocial problems. The individual with overactive bladder symptoms can never be sure when the symptoms will occur and may not be able to accommodate the urge to urinate. Some of these individuals are afraid to leave the safety of the nearness of their own lavatory or opt for bulky undergarment padding and absorbent protection when they go out in public.

Under normal circumstances, the bladder muscle transmits impulses to the brain indicating it is full and needs to be emptied. Overactive bladder muscles transmit false signals to the brain before the bladder is full, resulting in the strong urge to urinate, even to the point of leakage of urine or incontinence.

Continued

Overactive Bladder

The individual has options in treating this condition, including rehabilitation of pelvic muscles, learning behavior therapies to regain control of the bladder, and drug therapy. Rehabilitation of pelvic muscles and biofeedback trains the sphincter and may not produce the rapid effect that some individuals desire; therefore they decide to try to eliminate or at least lessen the problem with drug therapy.

Drug therapy involves treatment with three different medications. Estrogen may be helpful for postmenopausal women in combination with other drug therapy concepts; however, some may be reluctant to include estrogen in their therapy because of current information about estrogen replacement increasing the risk of cancer. Drugs available for therapy include tolterodine, oxybutynin, solifenacin, trospium, and darifenacin. These medications help alleviate the condition by relaxing the smooth muscle of the bladder and reducing the number of muscle spasms. Patients should be advised that anticholinergic side effects may occur with these medications (e.g., dry mouth, blurred vision, and so on). The patient and her or his physician should discuss the benefits and side effects of each drug before deciding which is best in the patient's situation.

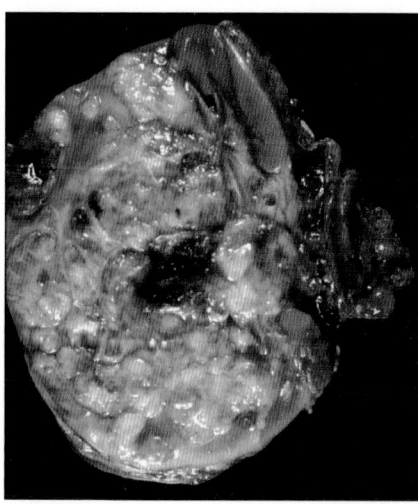

• **Fig. 11.18** Wilms tumor. (From Damjanov I: *Pathology for the health professions,* St Louis, 2017, Elsevier.)

Renal Cell Carcinoma

Description

Renal cancer is a condition in which one or more malignant tumors develop in one or both kidneys. The most common primary tumor of the kidney occurs in the renal cortex and is termed *renal cell carcinoma* (RCC). Less common tumors include Wilms tumor, a congenital renal tumor of childhood, and cancer of the renal pelvis (Fig. 11.18).

ICD-10-CM Code	C64.9 *(Malignant neoplasm of unspecified kidney, except renal pelvis)*
	(C64.1-C65.9 = 6 codes of specificity)

Referral to the current edition of the ICD-10-CM coding manual is recommended to determine appropriate code according to the site and type of the carcinoma.

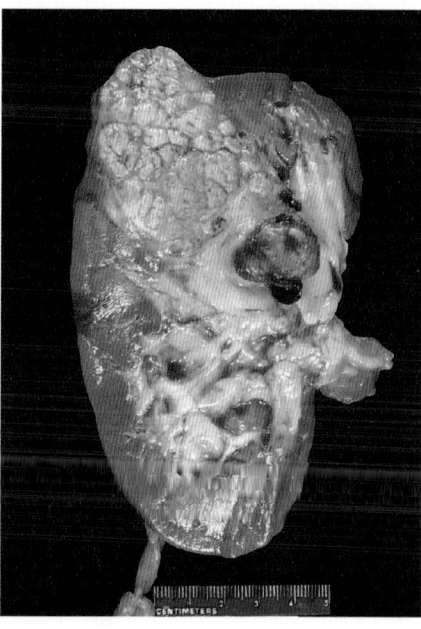

• **Fig. 11.19** Renal cell carcinoma (RCC). Typical cross-section of yellowish, spherical neoplasm in one pole of the kidney. Note the tumor in the dilated, thrombosed renal vein. (From Kumar V, Cotran R, Robbins S: *Robbins basic pathology,* ed 8, Philadelphia, 2008, Saunders/Elsevier.)

Symptoms and Signs

The classic triad of symptoms of RCC is hematuria, abdominal mass, and flank pain. Less than 10% of patients have all three findings, however, and those that do are likely to have advanced disease. Other less common signs and symptoms are weight loss, anemia, fever, hepatic dysfunction, and hypercalcemia. Many patients with RCC experience no symptoms until the disease is advanced.

Patient Screening

Patients experiencing hematuria require prompt assessment, as do those reporting an abdominal mass and/or flank pain.

Etiology

Around 95% of cases of RCC are sporadic, but some familial forms are known. The most common is a component of the von Hippel-Lindau (VHL) syndrome. Patients with this disorder are predisposed to the development of multiple bilateral renal cysts and carcinomas and tumors in other locations (Fig. 11.19). Risk factors for sporadic RCC are smoking, obesity, hypertension, patients with acquired cystic kidney disease undergoing dialysis, and prolonged exposure to chemicals, such as asbestos and cadmium. RCC is more common in men, and the incidence varies geographically, with the highest rates found in the Czech Republic and North America.

Diagnosis

Increasing numbers of RCCs are being detected incidentally on radiologic examinations done for some other unrelated disease. Procedures used to diagnose suspected neoplasms are abdominal CT or abdominal ultrasonography. Once a diagnosis is made, the clinician must look for metastasis by using CT of the abdomen and chest; MRI, in some cases; and bone scanning. Biopsy or tumor resection is then done for histologic confirmation of the diagnosis and to guide therapy. The TNM (tumor–node–metastasis) system developed by the American Joint Committee on Cancer (AJCC) is used for staging. (Refer to Chapter 1 for information on staging of neoplasms.)

Treatment

The treatment of choice for RCC is surgical removal. Depending on the stage, the patient can be treated with partial nephrectomy (for small tumors < 5 cm) or radical nephrectomy. Metastatic RCC is usually resistant to surgical treatment and to radiation or chemotherapy. Drug therapy may include everolimus, temsirolimus, sorafenib, sunitinib, or axitinib. Immunotherapy may also be used with interferon, interleukin-2, or molecularly targeted therapy, such as tyrosine kinase inhibitors.

Prognosis

The single most important determinant of prognosis is the pathologic stage at diagnosis. This is usually determined by histologic evaluation of the resected tumor by a pathologist. High levels of lactate dehydrogenase and serum calcium and low hemoglobin levels are poor prognostic indicators. The overall 5-year survival rate varies greatly, with early-stage tumors having a 5-year survival of greater than 90% and metastatic tumors having a less than 10% survival rate at 5 years.

Prevention

Screening of asymptomatic individuals is not recommended. However, individuals at high risk (those with VHL syndrome, history of kidney irradiation, ESRD and 3 to 5 years on dialysis, or a strong family history of RCC) should undergo periodic screening with abdominal ultrasonography, CT, or MRI to detect early disease. Cessation of smoking and maintenance of a healthy weight are recommended.

Patient Teaching

Encourage patients to seek out support groups and resource agencies in the community. Encourage regular checkups for other family members when a family history of cancer is known.

Bladder Tumors

Description

Bladder neoplasms usually involve the transitional epithelium (urothelium) that lines the surface of the bladder. The urothelium also lines the entire urinary tract from the

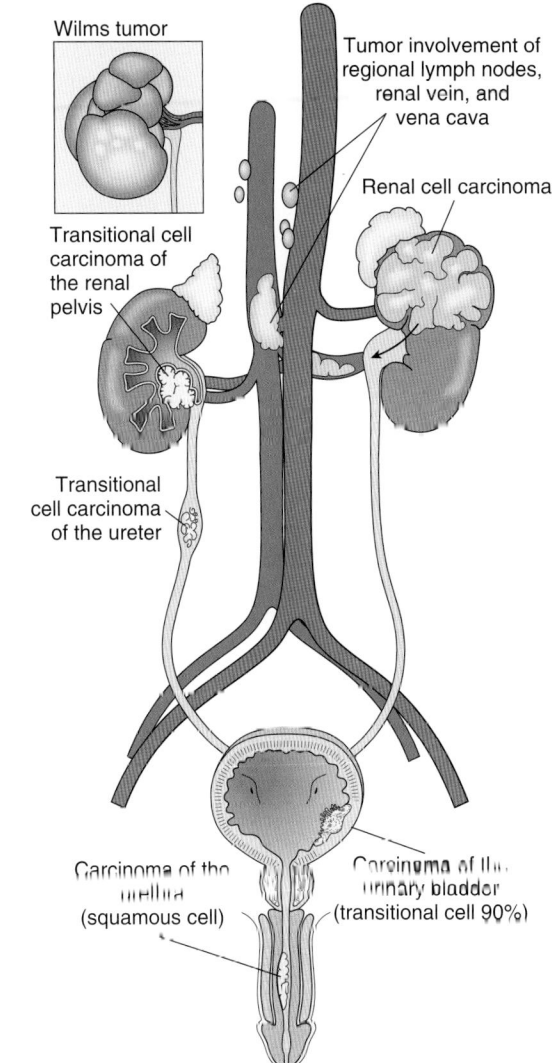

• **Fig. 11.20** Neoplasms of the urinary tract. (From Damjanov I: *Pathology for the health-related professions,* ed 4, St Louis, 2012, Saunders/Elsevier.)

renal pelvis to the prostatic urethra. Although the bladder is the most common site for a tumor to occur, they can develop at any site in the urothelium-lined urinary tract (Fig. 11.20).

ICD-10-CM Code	D49.4 *(Neoplasm of unspecified behavior of bladder)*
	C67.9 *(Malignant neoplasm of bladder, unspecified)*
	(C67.0-C67.9 = 10 codes of specificity)

As with other carcinomas, refer to the physician's diagnosis for specific type and site of carcinoma and to the current edition of the ICD-10-CM coding manual for appropriate code.

Symptoms and Signs

The most common symptom of a bladder tumor is gross, intermittent, painless hematuria. Pain in the flank or suprapubic area may occur as the carcinoma becomes locally advanced or metastatic. Voiding symptoms (e.g., dysuria, urgency, and increased frequency) are sometimes experienced. Symptoms of advanced disease include fatigue, weight loss, and anorexia.

Patient Screening

Patients reporting gross, intermittent, and painless hematuria along with dysuria, urgency, and increased frequency should be assessed as quickly as possible.

Etiology

Environmental exposures are thought to account for most cases of bladder cancer because the surface epithelium is exposed to potential carcinogens excreted in urine (Fig. 11.21). Several risk factors are known: occupational exposure to aniline dyes or diesel exhaust, cigarette smoking, and a history of frequent bladder infections or prior bladder cancer. Human papillomavirus (HPV) infection is associated with an increased risk of bladder cancer. Greater than 80% of cases are diagnosed in patients older than 60 years of age.

Diagnosis

The presence of otherwise unexplained hematuria in a person older than 40 years of age denotes cancer in the urinary tract until proven otherwise. Full urologic evaluation of the entire urinary tract is indicated. This consists of cystoscopy, urinary cytology (examination of transitional cells in the patient's voided urine), and IVP, renal ultrasonography, and/or CT. A biopsy sample can be taken of suspicious lesions during cystoscopy. Once the diagnosis is known, ultrasonography, CT, or MRI may be used to evaluate for extravesical extension and metastatic disease. Tests are being developed to detect biomarkers in urine that can be used to diagnose bladder cancer. The most commonly used staging system is the TNM system proposed by the AJCC, in which T indicates the degree of invasion of the bladder wall. Accurate staging is necessary to direct treatment and predict prognosis.

Treatment

The treatment of bladder cancer has three main goals: (1) to eradicate the disease, (2) to prevent recurrence, and (3) to prevent the development of invasive disease. The standard initial treatment is tumor resection via transurethral resection of the bladder tumor (TURBT). This procedure involves a complete cystoscopic resection of any visible tumors and selected biopsies of bladder mucosa. Despite a complete TURBT, however, up to 80% of tumors will recur within 12 months. For noninvasive carcinoma, post-TURBT follow-up includes urine cytology and cystoscopy at 3- to 6-month intervals for 3 to 5 years. Recurrent tumors are removed by using TURBT. If the patient is at high risk for recurrence, bacillus Calmette-Guérin (BCG) is administered into the bladder. BCG, a mycobacterium modified to a less pathologic state, induces a local immune reaction that suppresses tumor growth. Cystectomy is indicated for patients with many recurrences and resistance to this intravesical therapy.

Invasive carcinoma confined to the bladder is treated with either radical cystectomy or partial cystectomy and adjuvant chemoradiotherapy. For patients with metastatic carcinoma, multidrug chemotherapy may result in tumor shrinkage and moderately increased survival, but it does not result in a cure.

Prognosis

Stage is the most important independent prognostic indicator for disease progression and overall survival. Once invasion outside the bladder or nodal disease is detected, outcomes without systemic therapy are poor. However, recurrence is a more common problem than progression. Lower-grade, well-differentiated tumors have a slower growth rate and a better prognosis.

Prevention

Screening for bladder cancer in asymptomatic individuals is not recommended. Efforts should be made to reduce occupational exposures and to cease cigarette smoking.

Patient Teaching

Encourage patients to seek out support groups and resource agencies in the community. Encourage regular checkups for other family members when a family history of cancer is noted.

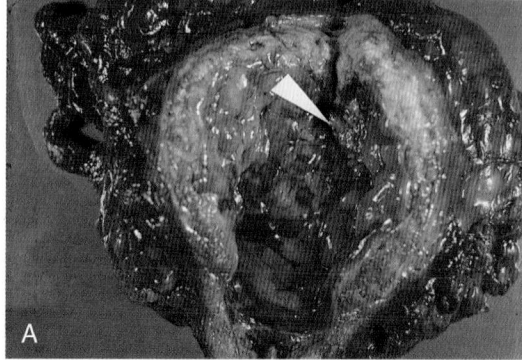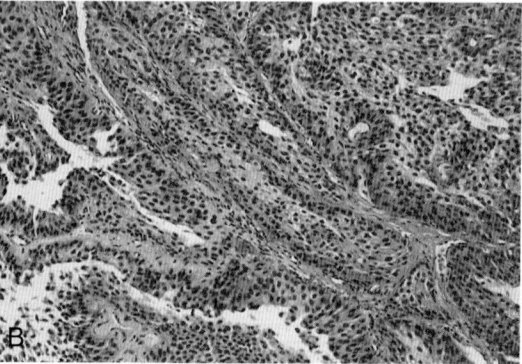

• **Fig. 11.21** Bladder cancer. (A) Gross appearance of an intraluminal mass *(arrow)*. (B) Histologic examination reveals that the mass is a papillary transitional cell carcinoma. (From Damjanov I: *Pathology for the health-related professions,* ed 4, St Louis, 2012, Saunders/Elsevier.)

Review Challenge

Answer the following questions:

1. How does the urinary system work specifically to maintain homeostasis?
2. What are some of the common symptoms of urinary system diseases?
3. Identify the unit of function of the kidney.
4. What are the etiologic factors of acute glomerulonephritis? For chronic glomerulonephritis (CGN)?
5. List some of the goals for the treatment of CGN?
6. What are some examples of abnormal findings in urinalysis?
7. Which individuals may require dialysis? Kidney transplantation?
8. What are possible treatment options for end-stage renal disease (ESRD)?
9. What are the classic clinical symptoms and signs of nephrosis? What causes nephrosis?
10. List some nephrotic agents.
11. Why is acute kidney injury (AKI) considered a clinical emergency?
12. Discuss the difference between acute renal failure (ARF) and chronic renal failure (CRF).
13. When is renal failure irreversible?
14. How would a patient with pyelonephritis describe his or her symptoms?
15. How might organisms be introduced into the urinary tract and cause pyelonephritis?
16. Which condition is a complication of urinary tract obstruction? What are some causes of urinary tract obstruction?
17. What are the risk factors for renal calculi?
18. What are the etiologic sources of infectious cystitis and urethritis?
19. How does diabetes mellitus contribute to diabetic nephropathy?
20. How would you describe the polycystic kidney?
21. How would you compare the pathology of neurogenic bladder with that of stress incontinence?
22. When may catheterization be indicated?
23. Describe overactive bladder.
24. What is the treatment and prognosis for renal cell carcinoma (RCC)? For bladder tumors?
25. Why should children who are being toilet trained be taught to wipe from front to back?

Real-Life Challenge: Cystitis

A 35-year-old woman reports pain in the pelvic region and lower back, frequency and urgency of urination, and burning on urination. The onset of symptoms was about 4 hours before the office visit.

Vital signs are temperature, 100.5°F; pulse, 96 beats per minute; respirations, 18 breaths per minute; and blood pressure, 130/88 mm Hg. A clean-catch urine specimen is obtained, and it is pink in color and has a foul odor. The urine specimen is sent to the laboratory for urinalysis and culture and sensitivity testing. Physical examination reveals tenderness over the bladder. Microscopic examination of the specimen reveals blood, pus, leukocytes, and bacteria.

A diagnosis of cystitis is made, and trimethoprim-sulfamethoxazole (Bactrim DS) is prescribed. The patient is encouraged to force fluids and is instructed to call the office the next day to report her progress.

Questions

1. What is another term for cystitis?
2. What additional symptoms might a patient with cystitis exhibit?
3. What is the usual cause of cystitis?
4. Why is a urinalysis important in diagnosing cystitis?
5. Why would the patient's urine have a foul odor?
6. Why would culture and sensitivity testing be important in the treatment of cystitis?
7. What alternative drug therapy is available to treat cystitis?
8. Why would the patient be encouraged to force fluids?

Real-Life Challenge: Renal Calculus

The wife of a 42-year-old man called the office stating that within the last hour her husband had a sudden onset of severe pain on his left side and back. He also has experienced nausea and vomiting. Questioning revealed the pain to be located in the left flank area and quite severe. The wife also reported that the pain radiated down toward her husband's scrotum and that he was experiencing pressure in the perineal area and frequent urge to urinate. A renal calculus was suspected, and the patient's wife was advised to transport him to an emergency facility.

Vital signs were temperature, 99.6°F; pulse, 96 beats per minute; respirations, 20 breaths per minute; and blood pressure, 124/88 mm Hg. A urine specimen was obtained, and the dipstick indicated blood in urine. The abdomen was slightly distended, the left flank area exhibited tenderness on palpation, and tenderness was noted over the bladder. A renal calculus was suspected, and kidney, ureters, and bladder (KUB) radiography, intravenous pyelography (IVP), and ultrasonography of the kidneys were ordered. An intravenous (IV) line was started, and the patient was given 2 mg of morphine sulfate IV push.

KUB radiography revealed a suspicious area 8 cm distal to the origin of the left ureter. IVP confirmed the presence of a 3.5-mm calculus distal to the ureteral origin. Renal ultrasonography indicated hydronephrosis of the left kidney. The patient was admitted for observation and for pain management.

Questions

1. What causes renal calculi to form?
2. Why would patients' symptoms vary?
3. What would be the significant symptom or symptoms leading to suspicion of renal calculi?
4. What is renal colic?
5. Which conditions cause blood in urine?
6. What is the cause of hydronephrosis?
7. Why would the patient be instructed to strain all urine?
8. What are the treatment options for the patient with renal calculi?
9. Why is IV morphine administered?

Internet Assignments

1. Research the incidence and treatment of urinary incontinence at the websites of the National Kidney Foundation and the American Urological Association. Compare information found on both sites.
2. Research the incidence, types of stones, and treatment of renal calculi at the websites of the National Kidney Foundation and the American Urological Association. Compare information found on both sites.
3. Research transplant donations, by both live and cadaver donors, at the websites of the National Kidney Foundation and the American Urological Association. Include information about the expenses associated with transplantation, including possible third-party payment for the procedure.

Critical Thinking

1. Discuss the importance of drinking eight glasses of water daily.
2. List causes of obstructive diseases of the urinary system, and identify congenital or acquired structural defects and tumors, obstructive diseases of the urinary system, immunologic disorders, circulatory disturbances, cystic disease, and metabolic disorders (e.g., diabetes mellitus).
3. Discuss the importance of good perineal hygiene and emptying the bladder as a preventive measure with a female patient recently diagnosed with pyelonephritis.
4. The patient who has been diagnosed with chronic glomerulonephritis (CGN) requires patient teaching about the progression and prognosis of the condition. Describe how you would approach the topic, because the outcome of this condition is not a positive one. List some teaching aids that could be used to make the explanation more understandable to the patient. Include the essentials of proper nutrition.
5. Discuss with the patient and the family their response to the diagnosis of CGN, and explain that eventually the condition will lead to end-stage renal disease (ESRD) and that dialysis may help the patient until kidney transplantation can be performed.
6. The patient with ESRD may require special funding for treatment. Encourage the patient and the family to begin locating types of assistance that are available to patients with ESRD.
7. List the renal conditions that ultimately may cause ESRD even if aggressively treated.
8. Identify some patients with diabetes, and discuss with them renal complications caused by the diabetes.
9. Explain the importance of straining urine to capture the kidney stone, "gravel," or sand that has been voided after a kidney stone attack. Once an analysis is made, emphasize the need for following dietary restrictions in the prevention of future kidney stones.
10. Stress incontinence creates many difficulties, including emotional and appearance-related issues. Discuss with patients and their families the embarrassment issues and the products available to help deal with the situation.

Prepare to discuss Critical Thinking case study exercises for this chapter that are posted on Evolve.

12

Diseases and Conditions of the Reproductive System

CHAPTER OUTLINE

The Normally Functioning Reproductive Systems, 478

Abnormally Functioning Reproductive Systems, 480

    Sexually Transmitted Diseases, 480

    Sexual Dysfunction, 487

    Contraception/Birth Control, 490

Male Reproductive Diseases, 491

Female Reproductive Diseases, 498

Conditions and Complications of Pregnancy, 514

Diseases of the Breast, 526

LEARNING OBJECTIVES

After studying Chapter 12, you should be able to:

1. Identify risk factors for sexually transmitted diseases (STDs).
2. Discuss male latex condoms and sexually transmitted diseases.
3. Explain what a silent STD is and give an example.
4. Name the complications of untreated gonorrhea.
5. Explain why women with genital herpes are advised to have regular Papanicolaou (Pap) smears.
6. Explain why the human papillomavirus (HPV) vaccine is recommended for girls and young women and, more recently, for men.
7. Describe the stages of untreated syphilis.
8. Explain why hepatitis B is classified as an STD.
9. List the possible causes of sexual dysfunction in men and women.
10. Name drugs that can contribute to impotence.
11. Discuss the possible causes of male and female infertility.
12. Explain how varicocele may contribute to male infertility.
13. Recall the best prevention of epididymitis.
14. Explain why torsion of the testicle is considered a medical emergency.
15. List some likely symptoms experienced by a male with benign prostatic hyperplasia (BPH).
16. Explain the value of prostate-specific antigen (PSA) as a screening test.
17. Discuss the medical interventions for prostatic cancer.
18. Name the common first sign of testicular cancer.
19. Define mittelschmerz.
20. Explain what causes the dysmenorrhea associated with endometriosis.
21. Discuss the importance of early diagnosis and prompt treatment of pelvic inflammatory disease (PID).
22. Explain the etiology of toxic shock syndrome (TSS).
23. Name the hormones that regulate the menstrual cycle.
24. Discuss the advantages and possible risks of hormone replacement therapy for the postmenopausal woman.
25. Explain how uterine prolapse, cystocele, and rectocele may be corrected surgically.
26. List the risk factors for cervical cancer.
27. Name the leading cause of deaths attributed to gynecologic malignancies.
28. Name a condition considered a complication of pregnancy.
29. Discuss possible causes of spontaneous abortion (miscarriage).
30. List some possible causes of ectopic pregnancy.
31. Explain how a pregnant woman is monitored for preeclampsia.
32. Describe abruptio placentae.
33. Name some problems associated with multiple pregnancy.
34. List the factors that place women at higher risk for breast cancer.

KEY TERMS

amenorrhea (ah-**men**-o-**REE**-ah)
autoinoculation (**aw**-toh-in-**ock**-u-**LAY**-shun)
chancre (**SHANG**-ker)
colporrhaphy (kol-**POUR**-ah-fee)
curettage (**ku**-reh-**TAHZH**)
dysmenorrhea (**dis**-men-oh-**REE**-ah)

dyspareunia (**dis**-pah-**RUE**-nee-ah)
dysuria (dis-**YOU**-ree-ah)
genitourinary (**jen**-ih-toe-**YU**-rih-nar-ee)
hysterosalpingography (**hiss**-ter-oh-**sal**-pin-**GOG**-rah-fee)
laparoscopy (lap-ar-**OS**-ko-pee)
leiomyoma (**lye**-o-my-**OH**-ma)

KEY TERMS—cont'd

menorrhagia (**men**-oh-**RAY**-jee-ah)
metrorrhagia (**met**-roh-**RAY**-jee-ah)
orchitis (or-**KYE**-tis)
pessary (**PESS**-ah-ree)
prolapse (pro-**LAPS**)
prostatectomy (**pros**-tah-**TECK**-toh-me)

psychosexual (**sigh**-ko-**SEKS**-you-al)
salpingo-oophorectomy (sal-**ping**-go-oh-ouf-oh-**RECK**-toh-me)
septicemia (sep-tih-**SEE**-me-ah)
ultrasonography (uhl-tra-son-**OGG**-rah-fee)
urethritis (**you**-ree-**THRYE**-tis)
varicocele (**VAR**-ih-ko-seel)

The Normally Functioning Reproductive Systems

The reproductive process in humans is sexual and involves the union of two sex cells: one male and one female. In early embryonic development, the sex organs are not differentiated, and therefore gender is difficult to identify. As the fetus develops, male or female definition becomes evident. The organs of the reproductive system usually are classified into two groups: the gonads (testes and ovaries), which produce germ cells and hormones, and the series of ducts necessary for the transportation of the germ cells.

The male reproductive system functions to transfer the sperm cells to the female for fertilization of the ovum. The testes produce the sperm and the hormones necessary for the development and maintenance of the secondary sex characteristics. The sperm is transported through the series of ducts beginning with the epididymis, the ductus deferens, and the ejaculatory ducts. The seminal vesicles, the prostate gland, the bulbourethral glands, and the penis are accessory organs that help propel the sperm on its journey to meet the egg (Fig. 12.1).

The female reproductive system nourishes and enables the development of the fertilized ovum. The ovaries (which contain the woman's lifetime supply of eggs) produce and release the egg and the hormones necessary for the development of secondary sex characteristics and the maintenance of a pregnancy. The ductal system for transport, nourishment, and growth of the fertilized ovum includes the fallopian tubes and the uterus. Other principal parts of

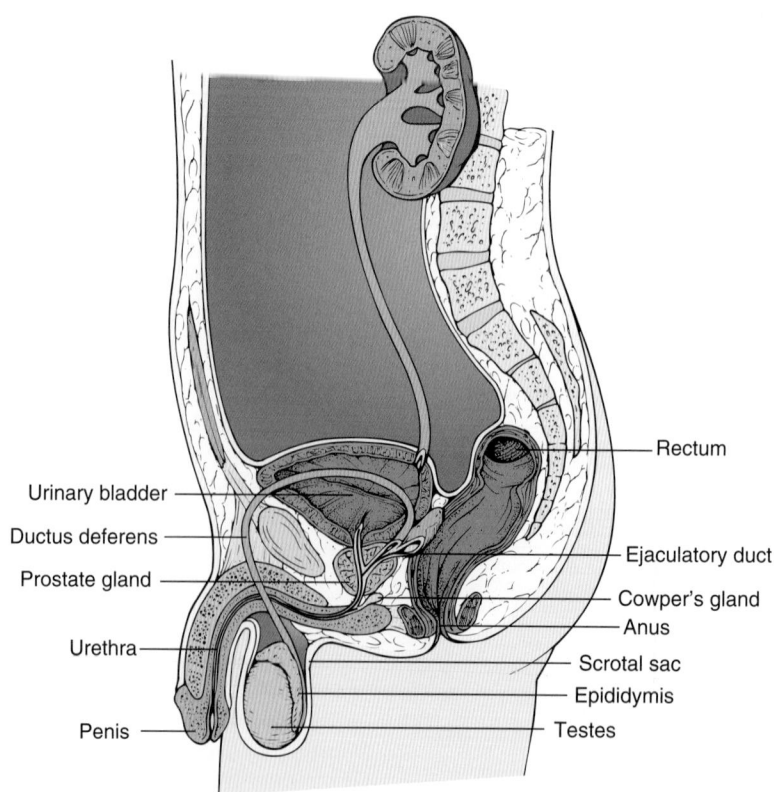

• **Fig. 12.1** Normal male reproductive system.

the female reproductive system include the cervix, the vagina, and the external genitalia (Fig. 12.2).

The breasts are accessory organs of reproduction and are the two milk-producing glands (Fig. 12.3). When a woman is pregnant, the breast tissue is stimulated by both ovarian and placental hormones to prepare for lactation. After delivery, lactating hormones further stimulate the breast tissue to produce and release milk to nourish the infant.

The process of reproduction requires that the sperm fertilize the egg. After release from the ovary, the egg progresses down the fallopian tube. In a typical pregnancy, the egg is met in the fallopian tube by the sperm. After the sperm fertilizes the egg, the zygote continues to travel down the fallopian tube to the uterus, where it eventually attaches to the uterine lining (endometrium) to be nourished and to grow. The placenta forms within the uterine wall and provides a mechanism for the exchange of nourishment and waste products between the mother and the developing fetus. A normal gestational period is 38 weeks after conception, or 40 completed weeks after the start of the last menstrual period, at which time the birth process may begin with labor and subsequent delivery of the infant.

The anterior pituitary gland produces gonadotropic hormones that cause the ovaries to produce estrogen and progesterone, which regulate the menstrual cycle. During menstruation, the endometrium (the disintegrated endometrial cells along with secretions and blood cells) is shed via the vagina. This is followed by the next cycle of ovarian production of estrogen, produced from maturing ovarian follicles, which eventually release the mature ovum during ovulation. The corpus luteum then develops after release of the ovum, and progesterone is secreted into the bloodstream to stabilize the growth of the endometrium to prepare for implantation of the fertilized ovum. If pregnancy does not occur, the endometrium again is shed through menses in anticipation of the next cycle and a possible pregnancy.

Both the male and female reproductive systems are vulnerable to many diseases, including sexually transmitted diseases (STDs), malignancies, benign growths, and chemical imbalances. Abnormal function of the reproductive system sometimes results from functional, structural, dietary, or emotional causes. Complications often develop during pregnancy, some severe and some merely aggravating. This chapter explores the most common disease entities, conditions, and complications of both male and female reproductive systems.

🅐 ALERT!

Risk Factors for Sexually Transmitted Diseases

- Sex with someone whose sexual history one does not know
- Starting sexual activity at an early age
- Drug use with sharing of needles
- Sex with multiple partners
- Sexual intimacy with someone who has been diagnosed with a sexually transmitted disease (STD) or one who is being treated for an STD
- Exposure with skin-to-skin contact in the presence of any open lesion, such as a chancre or a wart
- Use of alcohol or other drugs that may cloud one's judgment about a sexual encounter
- Hemophilia
- Men having sex with men (MSM)
- Transfusion of blood or blood products
- Babies being carried by a human immunodeficiency virus (HIV)-positive mother
- Breast-fed infants of an HIV positive mother
- Lack of education or concern about risky sexual behavior
- Lack of education about the human papillomavirus (HPV) vaccines now on the market to prevent cervical cancer and less common genital cancers

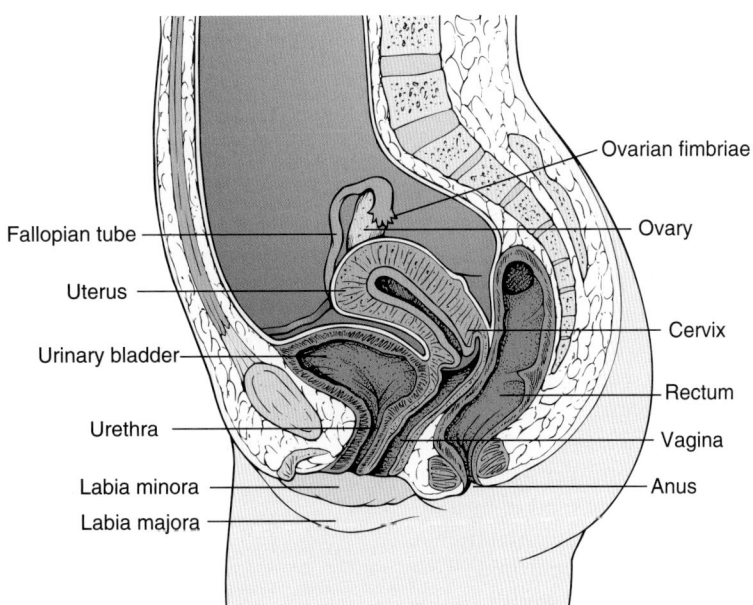

• **Fig. 12.2** Normal female reproductive system.

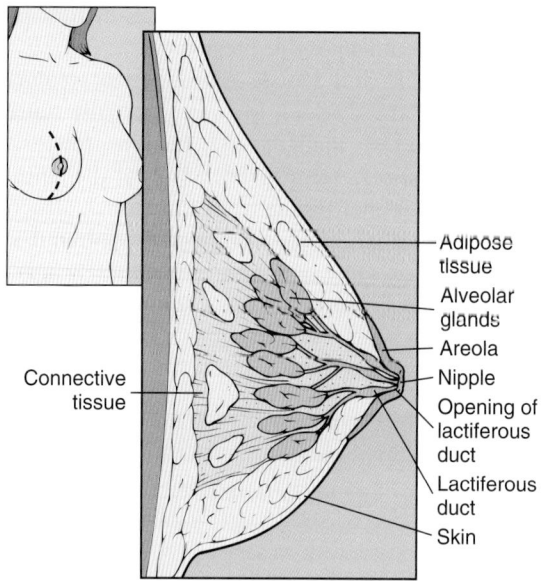

• **Fig. 12.3** Normal female breast.

Abnormally Functioning Reproductive Systems

Sexually Transmitted Diseases

More than 20 infectious diseases are spread by sexual contact, some of which are incurable and all of which can damage health or even threaten life. STDs, formerly called *venereal diseases,* are among the most common contagious diseases in the United States; they remain a major public health problem. The incidence of STDs is increasing among women and among men having sex with men (MSM). In some cases, STDs are asymptomatic and are spread by individuals unaware that they are infected. Many cases are not reported. These diseases represent a "silent epidemic." Untreated STDs can lead to serious long-term health consequences, especially for young women and adolescent girls.

No one is immune, and one can have more than one STD at a time. Recurrent infections are common. The infections are transmitted from one person to another through body fluids, such as blood, semen, and vaginal secretions during vaginal, anal, or oral sex; some are spread by direct contact with infected skin or for example, in the case of pubic lice, are transmitted by clothing, bedding, or infected hairs during coitus. Most STDs are treatable, but there is no cure for viral STDs, such as herpes and human immunodeficiency virus (HIV). Among the many concerns about STDs is the possible transmission by an infected mother to a fetus or a newborn, sometimes with dire consequences to the baby. All pregnant women in the United States should be tested for HIV infection as early in the pregnancy as possible.

STD rates in the United States are among the highest in the world and are growing; syphilis is rising in the United States for the first time in many years. The majority of reported syphilis cases in the United States continue to be among MSM. Recent statistics show one in four teenagers get STDs. Attempts to control this rampant public health problem are focusing on research, education, and prevention campaigns. Prevention messages point out high-risk sexual behavior patterns and lifestyles and warn of possible predisposing health problems. Requirements for reporting STDs vary from state to state. However, several STDs that, when diagnosed, must be reported to state health departments and the Centers for Disease Control and Prevention (CDC) for statistical purposes are chlamydia, gonorrhea, syphilis, chancroid, HIV infection, acquired immunodeficiency syndrome (AIDS), and hepatitis B. See Chapter 8 for a discussion of hepatitis B.

Chlamydia

Description

Chlamydia, the most commonly reported notifiable STD in the United States, causes urethritis in men and urethritis and cervicitis in women.

ICD-10-CM Code	A74.9 *(Chlamydial infection, unspecified)*
	(A74.0-A74.9 = 4 codes of specificity)

Symptoms and Signs

Chlamydia sometimes is called the *silent STD* because it often has no symptoms, and thus it is sexually transmitted unknowingly. A high percentage of women have no symptoms before dangerous complications start. In contrast, 75% of men have symptoms 1 to 3 weeks after exposure. Chlamydia is a major cause of female sterility and a leading cause of pelvic inflammatory disease (PID). According to the Centers for Disease Control and Prevention (CDC), chlamydia is the most commonly reported STD in the United States.

Early female symptoms include dysuria, an odorless, yellow vaginal discharge with a burning sensation, itching, abdominal pain, and dyspareunia. Infected men experience a thin, watery discharge from the penis, with a burning sensation and itching, and a burning sensation when urinating, the latter caused by urethritis. The scrotum may be swollen, and the patient may be feverish. The inguinal lymph nodes often are enlarged in both genders. A small transient lesion and skin irritation may be noticed. Newborns can acquire chlamydia from the infected mother during birth, resulting in conjunctivitis, blindness, arthritis, or overwhelming infection.

Patient Screening

Symptoms usually start 1 or 2 weeks after exposure; they are likely to be mild, such as burning sensation during urination and genital discharge in both men and women. An early appointment should be scheduled to confirm the diagnosis and begin treatment.

Etiology

Chlamydia trachomatis, an intracellular bacterium, is the cause of chlamydia and usually is transmitted through sexual contact. The site of primary infection is usually around the genitals, but it can be oral or anal, depending on sexual practice. The organism can be found in the cervix, throat, or rectum and can be transmitted unknowingly. More cases are now becoming prevalent among adolescents and young adults.

Diagnosis

Testing for chlamydia is most often done by using a deoxyribonucleic acid (DNA) probe test, a test based on DNA detection.

Treatment

Antibiotic therapy is given to both partners, beginning with a single injection, and/or followed by a course of oral antibiotics, such as azithromycin, erythromycin, or a 7-day regimen of doxycycline. More severe cases may require hospitalization and treatment with intravenous (IV) antibiotics. Prompt treatment can cure the infection and prevent complications, such as PID and problematic pregnancy. Follow-up testing is recommended.

Prognosis

Chlamydial infection can be cured with a complete course of antibiotics when taken as directed, even after symptoms subside. Long-term consequences of untreated chlamydia are more serious for women who are prone to PID, which can result in infertility; they are also more likely to become infected by HIV, if exposed. Chlamydia left untreated in men can cause epididymitis, which may lead to infertility.

Prevention

Use standard precautions when caring for a patient with chlamydial infection. Infected patients should inform their sexual contacts of the infection. See the risk factors for STDs. All states require reporting of cases of chlamydia to the public health department. The CDC recommends annual chlamydia screening for sexually active women under age 26 years and for older women with multiple sex partners. Urine tests for chlamydia in men can help reduce the transmission of disease to women. In addition to compromising reproductive health in women, infection with chlamydia facilitates transmission of HIV infection. Use of a protective barrier during sexual activity can help prevent transmission of chlamydial infection.

Patient Teaching

Emphasize the importance of taking the complete course of antibiotic therapy as prescribed. Recommend that patients abstain from intercourse until both partners are cured. Inform patients that meticulous personal hygiene and frequent hand washing are necessary to prevent spreading the infection to the eyes.

Gonorrhea

Description

Gonorrhea, the second most commonly reported notifiable disease in the United States, is a sexually transmitted infection (STI) of the genitourinary tract.

ICD-10-CM Code	A54.00 *(Gonococcal infection of lower genitourinary tract, unspecified)*
	(A54.00-A54.29 = 11 codes of specificity)

Symptoms and Signs

Gonorrhea, also a common infection of the genitourinary tract, causes symptoms and complications similar to those of chlamydia in male and female patients. A purulent discharge from the male or female genitourinary tract and dysuria are often present but can vary in severity. Up to 50% of men and women are asymptomatic in the early stages of infection, so they may unknowingly continue to spread the infection, making transmission difficult to control. The disease also can infect the eyes and throat or become systemic.

Patient Screening

Men develop symptoms, if any, after an incubation period of 3 to 6 days. Symptoms in men vary but may include discharge from the penis, pain or burning with urination, and testicular pain or edema. Women may experience vaginal discharge, heavier menstrual periods, pain in the lower abdomen, dysuria, and urinary frequency. Early treatment is indicated, because untreated gonorrhea can spread among sexual partners.

Etiology

Infection with the common bacterium *Neisseria gonorrhoeae* usually results from sexual transmission. After a decrease in cases, in 2017, the number of cases diagnosed was the highest since the year 2001. Gonorrhea can be transmitted via vaginal, anal, or oral intercourse with an infected individual. Because transmission is also possible during birth, newborns must be protected from eye infections that can lead to blindness (Fig. 12.4). Therefore, prophylactic erythromycin salve is administered routinely at birth.

Diagnosis

Laboratory cultures from the infected site (cervix, rectum, or throat) of infectious body secretions and microscopic examination of exudate with a Gram stain are performed to identify the *N. gonorrhoeae* organism. A DNA-probe technique called *polymerase chain reaction (PCR)* identifies the genetic material of the bacterium.

Treatment

Curative treatment is recommended for the infected individual and any sexual partners as well. Throughout the

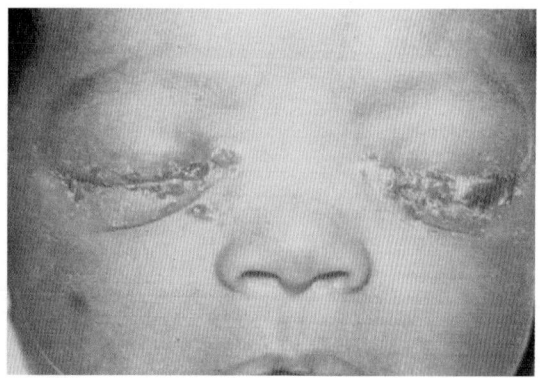

• **Fig. 12.4** Gonorrhea ophthalmia. (From Grimes D: *Infectious diseases—Mosby's clinical nursing series*, St Louis, 1994, Mosby.)

years, gonorrhea has become more difficult to treat because of antibiotic-resistant strains. In 2015, the CDC began recommending that health care providers prescribe a single shot of ceftriaxone accompanied by an oral dose of azithromycin to those diagnosed with gonorrhea. Azithromycin was added to help delay the development of resistance to ceftriaxone. After the antibiotic therapy, follow-up culture studies are ordered to ensure a complete cure, because some strains are becoming increasingly antibiotic resistant. Neglecting treatment of a gonococcal infection can lead to complications, including PID, septicemia, infertility, and septic arthritis. Salpingitis (inflammation or infection of the fallopian tube) is the most common complication of gonorrhea.

Prognosis

With early and complete treatment, the prognosis is excellent, even when there are complications. The presence of gonorrhea infection makes an individual more likely to acquire HIV infection, if exposed.

Prevention

Standard precautions are used when providing care to a patient with gonorrhea. All cases must be reported to the local public health department. Routine instillation of erythromycin or 1% silver nitrate drops into the eyes of newborns is practiced. Abstinence from sexual contact is maintained until treatment is complete and follow-up culture results are negative.

Patient Teaching

Emphasize the importance of complying with a complete treatment plan and follow-up testing to ensure a cure. Inform the patient of the risk factors (see the Alert box about Risk Factors for Sexually Transmitted Diseases). Common bacterium *N. gonorrhoeae* requires specific conditions for growth and reproduction. It is not transmitted from toilet seats or door handles. The organism can exist in the back of the throat (as a result of oral sex), in the genitals, and in the rectum.

Trichomoniasis

Description

Trichomoniasis is a protozoal infection of the lower genitourinary tract; the infection is usually vaginal in females and urethral in males.

ICD-10-CM Code	A59.9 *(Trichomoniasis, unspecified)*
	(A59.00-A59.9 = 7 codes of specificity)

The above code may be valid as a principal diagnosis. Refer to the physician's diagnosis and then to the current edition of the ICD-10-CM coding manual to ensure the greatest specificity of pathology.

Symptoms and Signs

Trichomoniasis is common among people who are sexually active. Most infected men and women, however, are asymptomatic. This contributes to the spread of the unrecognized infection and delays in treatment.

The initial symptoms for male and female patients may include urethritis with dysuria and itching. In addition, women may notice a profuse, frothy, greenish yellow, odorous discharge from the vagina and vulvar irritation. In women, characteristic "strawberry cervix" may be observable on colposcopy. A thin, whitish discharge from the penis may be noted by men. In either case, the discharge may subside without treatment, but the infection remains and can become chronic.

Patient Screening

Discomfort associated with the irritating discharge usually prompts a request for an appointment for examination.

Etiology

Trichomoniasis is a protozoal infection caused by *Trichomonas vaginalis* and usually is transmitted through sexual contact. The incubation period is 5 to 28 days.

Diagnosis

A wet preparation of vaginal secretions from women or discharge from the urethra in men is studied for the microorganism *T. vaginalis*. Urinalysis also may reveal the organism. The cervix is examined for the presence of small hemorrhages with a strawberry-like appearance.

Treatment

If the laboratory culture result is positive, antiprotozoal drugs are given. Metronidazole or tinidazole may be given as a single dose or as a multiday treatment. *Patients are cautioned never to consume products containing alcohol while taking these medications.*

Prognosis

The prognosis is good if both partners receive medical treatment, including a follow-up examination that ensures that the infection is cured completely. Failure to treat both partners causes reinfection, called "ping-pong" vaginitis. An increased risk for HIV transmission has been noted. Pregnant women with trichomoniasis can experience complications.

Prevention

Because this disease is transmitted primarily through sexual contact, prevention requires avoiding sex with someone whose sexual history one does not know. Latex condoms may help prevent the spread of trichomoniasis.

Patient Teaching

Advise the patient that consumption of alcohol is contraindicated while taking metronidazole or tinidazole. See the information in the Prevention and Prognosis sections.

Genital Herpes

Description

Genital herpes is an incurable, recurrent infection of the skin of the genital area, with ulcerations spread through direct skin-to-skin contact, causing painful genital sores similar to cold sores (Fig. 12.5).

ICD 10 OM Code — A60.9 (Anogenital herpesviral infection, unspecified) (A60.00–A60.9 = 8 codes of specificity)

Genital herpes is coded according to the site of the lesion(s). Refer to the physician's diagnosis and then to the current edition of the ICD-10-CM coding manual to ensure the greatest specificity of pathology.

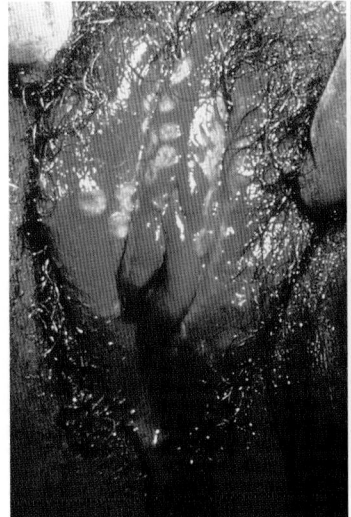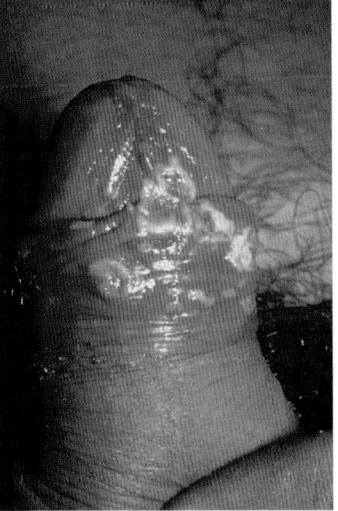

• **Fig. 12.5** Genital herpes in the female *(left)* and the male *(right)*. (From Behrman RE, Kliegman RM, Arvin AM: *Slide set, Nelson textbook of pediatrics,* ed 15, Philadelphia, 1996, Saunders.)

Symptoms and Signs

Genital herpes is caused by herpes simplex virus type 2 (HSV-2), and less frequently by HSV-1, and is a recurrent, incurable viral disease. A large percentage of infections is subclinical, so the initial episode may go unnoticed. More often, one or more blisterlike lesions are noted somewhere on the genitals or around the anus. The painful ulcers and blisters usually occur 2 to 30 days after sexual contact with an infected person. Often the first episode is accompanied by systemic influenza symptoms, swollen glands, fever, headache, and painful urination. The condition is infectious when sores are present, but some people without symptoms, called *shedders*, can transmit the virus. Herpetic lesions occur more often in women than in men, and the infection tends to be more severe in women. Subsequent outbreaks ("breakouts") can occur for months or years, because the virus hides in the nervous system and lies dormant between flare-ups.

Patient Screening

Systemic symptoms may be present during the acute stage. When fever, headache, muscle aches, and swollen glands are present, an appointment for the individual is scheduled promptly for investigative medical evaluation.

Etiology

More than one in six adults between the ages 14 and 49 years are infected with the highly contagious HSV-2; it usually is transmitted sexually via virus-infected body fluids during skin-to-skin contact. Cross-infection may result from oral-genital or anal sex, and the infection is permanent. Genital herpes can also be caused by HSV-1, especially in the younger population.

The presence of open lesions increases the risk of contracting AIDS during sexual acts between persons infected with HSV-2 and those who are positive for HIV infection.

Diagnosis

The presence of the characteristic lesions on the male or female genitalia is noted during physical examination. An antigen test or tissue culture laboratory techniques can identify HSV-2. PCR and a rapid fluorescent test are also used to identify HSV-2.

Treatment

There is no cure, but prescription drugs that reduce the duration and frequency of outbreaks are currently available. These drugs include acyclovir (Zovirax), famciclovir (Famvir), and valacyclovir (Valtrex). In some cases, the person's own immunity makes the episodes less severe. The presence of sores in the genital area and fear of transmitting or acquiring herpes contribute to emotional stress and social embarrassment. In addition, women with genital herpes must be monitored more carefully for cervical cancer. A Papanicolaou (Pap) smear every 6 months is recommended. Finally, a cesarean section may be indicated, because the virus is dangerous to the newborn.

Prognosis

Recurrent herpes usually has prodromal symptoms, such as tingling, itching, or burning 1 to 5 days before the lesion(s) appear. Recurrent episodes are common but tend to be milder and often are triggered by fatigue and stress. Generally, the infection poses no serious problems for healthy adults.

Prevention

The only absolute prevention is by practicing sexual abstinence and mutual monogamy. During an outbreak of symptoms, kissing should be avoided. Condoms do not necessarily provide a complete barrier against skin-to-skin contact. After years of research, attempts to develop a vaccine have been disappointing. There is no effective vaccine for prevention of herpes.

> **NOTE**
>
> Unprotected exposure of health care workers to oral and genital secretions when providing care to patients with HSV infection can result in an intensely painful infection of fingers called *herpetic whitlow*. This is usually caused by autoinoculation or other direct contact between HSV and a break in the skin, such as a torn cuticle.

Patient Teaching

Counsel the patient about the preventive measures and the prognosis, as mentioned previously. Recommend frequent and thorough hand washing; the infection could spread to the eyes and other areas of the skin. Provide the patient with educational material on how to cope with the disease. Address any concerns about how the disease affects personal relationships. Advise the patient to inform anyone they have sex with about their genital herpes. Inform the patient the virus can be shed even while he or she is asymptomatic; thus any sexual partners can be at risk even at this time.

Genital Warts (Condylomata Acuminata)

Description

Condyloma acuminatum is a genital infection that causes raised cauliflower-like growths in or near the vagina or rectum or along the penis (Fig. 12.6). It has become one of the most common STIs in the world.

ICD-10-CM Code	A63.0 *(Anogenital [venereal] warts)*
	(A63.0-A64 = 3 codes of specificity)

Symptoms and Signs

These genital warts are usually painless, and many women have no obvious symptoms. Sometimes the lesions may cause itching or burning. These contagious lesions appear several weeks to several months after direct skin-to-skin contact during sexual intercourse with an infected person. The discomfort experienced varies, depending on the size, number, and location of the warts (see Fig. 12.6).

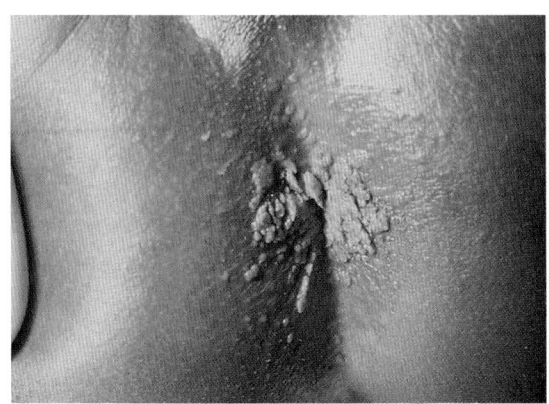

• **Fig. 12.6** Genital warts. (From Behrman RE, Kliegman RM, Arvin AM; Olide sel, Nelson Textbook of pediatrics, ed 15, Philadelphia, 1996, Saunders.)

Patient Screening
Schedule the male or female patient for a pelvic examination.

Etiology
Human papillomavirus (HPV), which is highly contagious, is the cause of genital warts and usually is transmitted sexually. It has a prolonged incubation period of 1 to 6 months. HPV infects epithelial cells. Risk factors for acquiring persistent infection with HPV are early age at initiation of sexual activity and having multiple sexual partners. Coinfection with HIV causes a further increase in the risk for HPV-related cancer.

Many types of HPV have been identified by scientists. The same types of HPV that infect the genital areas can infect the mouth and the throat. Some are low-risk types, whereas the high-risk types can cause cancer.

Diagnosis
Genital warts can be identified by their appearance, but biopsy sometimes is suggested to rule out carcinoma. The wart must be differentiated from a syphilitic lesion. Identification of the genetic material (DNA) of the virus confirms HPV infection.

Treatment
Up to 30% of genital warts go away without treatment, but the underlying virus is never completely eliminated. The treatment is chemical or surgical removal of the warts, but recurrence is common. Topical drug therapy to remove the warts includes a keratolytic agent, such as podofilox and trichloroacetic acid. Imiquimod (Aldara), an antiviral cream, is indicated for the treatment of external genital and perianal warts or condyloma acuminata in patients age 12 years. This is widely used to stop new genital warts from forming. Surgical procedures for wart removal include cryosurgery, which involves the freezing and removal of affected tissue. Electrodesiccation is a process that uses a laser to remove larger warts and is also very effective. Some genital warts go away without treatment.

Studies have shown that women with genital HPV infection are at greater risk for cervical cancer. Because the warts spread more rapidly during pregnancy, a cesarean section may be necessary if the warts occlude the birth canal.

Prognosis
Genital warts have no complications, but the disease tends to recur. Recurrence of symptoms is possible even after treatment. Pregnancy promotes the growth and spread of the lesions.

Prevention
Sexual contact with an infected individual and with someone whose sexual history one does not know should be avoided. The long incubation period introduces an added risk of infecting others or of contracting the disease.

A vaccine to help prevent HPV infection is recommended. (see the Enrichment box about Human Papillomavirus Vaccine and Cervical Cancer).

◆ ENRICHMENT

Human Papillomavirus Vaccine and Cervical Cancer

There are many types of human papillomavirus (HPV), some of which are known to cause cancers of the cervix, anus, vagina, vulva, and penis. HPV infection is most often associated with cervical cancer. Although an invasive neoplasm will not develop in most people infected with HPV, it is important to reduce the risk of infection. The virus may be spread not only via unprotected intercourse but also through close physical contact with an infected area of the body and probably through digital/anal, oral/anal, and digital/vaginal contact as well. Using barrier contraception and limiting the number of sexual partners are recommended to reduce risk of infection. No antiviral drugs currently are available to treat HPV infection. Those who are infected should know the risk of cancer and should follow up periodically with their physician to monitor for premalignant neoplastic changes.

Although the use of annual Pap smear tests to screen for cervical cancer has drastically reduced the number of deaths from cervical cancer in developed countries, cervical cancer remains a leading cause of cancer-related death in countries without these programs. The HPV vaccine is given to prevent the most common types of HPV that can lead to these cancers. This vaccine was approved by the U.S. Food and Drug Administration (FDA) and is recommended by the Centers for Disease Control and Prevention (CDC) for both female and male patients. The vaccine is usually administered at age 11 to 12 years but may be administered as early as age 9 years. Those receiving the injection at age 11 to 12 years, should receive two doses of the vaccine, with the second vaccine 6 to 12 months after the initial dose.

Patients who start the vaccination at age 15 years or later should receive a three-dose series. The second dose is administered 1 to 2 months after the initial vaccination, and the third dose is administered 6 months after the first vaccination. It is important to remember that although the HPV vaccine is a major advance in the prevention of cervical cancer, it will not replace the need for other preventive strategies, such as annual screening with Pap smear tests for early detection of abnormal cells.

Patient Teaching

Counseling about all aspects of prevention and transmission of genital warts is important.

Syphilis

Description

Syphilis is a chronic, systemic STI that has four stages.

ICD-10-CM Code	A51.0 *(Primary genital syphilis)*
	(A51.0-A52.09 = 24 codes of specificity)
	A51.49 *(Other secondary syphilitic conditions)*
	A53.0 *(Latent syphilis, unspecified as early or late)*
	(A53.0-A53.9 = 2 codes of specificity)

Refer to the physician's diagnosis and then to the current edition of the ICD-10-CM coding manual to ensure the greatest specificity of pathology.

Symptoms and Signs

Syphilis begins with the presence of a painless, but highly contagious, local lesion, called a chancre on the male or female genitalia (Fig. 12.7). Without early treatment during the primary stage, it becomes a systemic, chronic disease that can involve any organ or tissue. In 1 to 2 months, when the primary lesion heals, the causative organism (the spirochete *Treponema pallidum*) has disseminated throughout the body and multiplied, producing lesions wherever the organisms are most prevalent, including the skin, lymph nodes, cardiovascular system, brain, and spinal cord.

The disease continues to be contagious during the second stage, when there is systemic manifestation. This stage can present many symptoms, including fever, headaches, aching

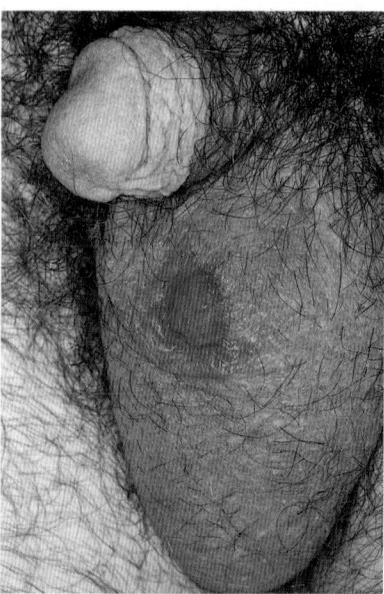

• **Fig. 12.7** Chancre of primary syphilis. (From Kumar V, et al: Robbins basic pathology, ed 10, St. Louis, 2018, Elsevier.)

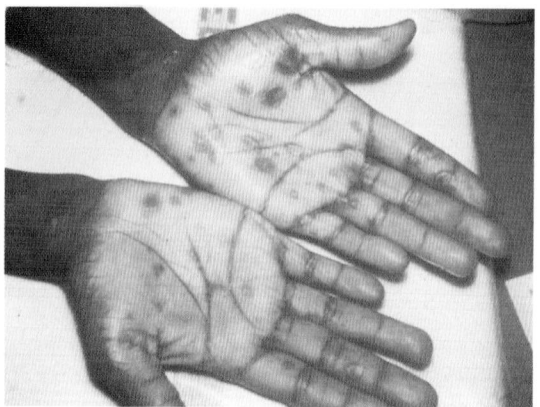

• **Fig. 12.8** Secondary syphilis. (From Grimes D: *Infectious diseases— Mosby's clinical nursing series,* St Louis, 1994, Mosby.)

of joints, mouth sores, and rashes on the palms of the hands and soles of the feet (Fig. 12.8). The third stage is a latent period, lasting from 1 to 40 years, during which the infection is generally subclinical or asymptomatic. In the last stage, the lesions, called *gummas,* have invaded body organs and systems, causing widespread damage to the point of being debilitating and life threatening.

When a fetus is infected, the child may die in utero or be born with congenital syphilis and multiple abnormalities.

Patient Screening

It is important to treat syphilis in the early stage.

> **NOTE**
> For the first time in many years, syphilis is on the rise in the United States, especially among men

Etiology

Syphilis is caused by infection with the spirochete *T. pallidum* through sexual contact or other direct contact with infected lesions or infected body fluids. It is highly contagious when a chancre is present (see Fig. 12.7). During 2014 and 2015, rising rates of syphilis were reported among both women and men. Congenital transmission can occur during pregnancy.

Diagnosis

Standard screening tests are the Venereal Disease Research Laboratory (VDRL) test and the rapid plasminogen reagent (RPR) test. A smear taken from the primary lesion is examined microscopically for *T. pallidum.* Antibodies can be detected in the patient's serum. Further testing confirms the diagnosis and provides a titer to monitor response to treatment. Worldwide, the diagnosis of syphilis requires concurrent HIV testing as well.

Treatment

Syphilis can be easily cured in its early stages with a course of antibiotic therapy by using penicillin G. If the patient is allergic to penicillin, other antibiotics are used, such as doxycycline, azithromycin, and ceftriaxone. The disease is best treated in the primary and secondary stages, before it causes irreversible damage to the body. Patients are monitored with follow-up blood tests for the presence of *T. pallidum* for up to a year.

Prognosis

Treatment can cure syphilis. Untreated syphilis progresses to long-term severe systemic complications. Syphilis facilitates the spread of HIV infection.

Prevention

Health care providers should practice standard precautions while providing care to patients with syphilis. Sexual contact with an infected individual and contact with body fluids should be avoided. Syphilis can be transmitted in the first few years of the latent stage and in the first two stages. When in doubt, a VDRL test should be performed to detect infection. See the list of risk factors for STDs. Syphilis cases are reportable to the local department of health.

Patient Teaching

Emphasize the importance of finishing the course of medication, even if symptoms are alleviated. Urge the patient to inform his or her sexual partners about the infection so that they can seek treatment, if needed. Instruct the patient to avoid all risk factors for STDs.

Chancroid

Description

Chancroid, also called *soft chancre*, is a bacterial infection of the genitalia that causes a necrotizing ulceration and lymphadenopathy.

ICD-10-CM Code	A57 (Chancroid)

Symptoms and Signs

The shallow and painless lesion appears on the skin or mucous membrane, at the site of entry, 7 to 10 days after sexual contact with an infected person (Fig. 12.9). Tender, superlative inguinal adenopathy is noted on physical examination. The ulcer usually deepens and becomes purulent and can be spread to other areas of the body via autoinoculation.

Patient Screening

The presence of a lesion on or near the genitalia usually prompts a request for an appointment for an examination.

Etiology

The causative agent of chancroid is the bacterium *Haemophilus ducreyi*.

Diagnosis

The diagnosis is based on the clinical appearance of the lesions. In the laboratory, Gram staining of smears of the

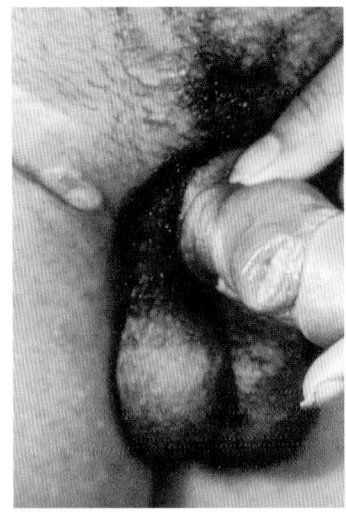

• **Fig. 12.9** Chancroid: Male. (From Grimes D: *Infectious diseases—Mosby's clinical nursing series,* St Louis, 1994, Mosby.)

exudate is performed to confirm the cause of infection. The presence of syphilis or HSV infection is ruled out.

Treatment

The patient usually responds well to antibiotic therapy (i.e., azithromycin, clarithromycin, or ceftriaxone). The lesions sometimes must be drained surgically. Good personal hygiene is advised. The patient is told to keep the infected areas clean and dry and to refrain from sexual contact during the entire time of treatment.

Prognosis

Antibiotic therapy is usually curative. Severe infection may cause scarring.

Prevention

No vaccine is available. Use of a condom helps prevent the spread of infection. Chancroid is a reportable STD.

Patient Teaching

All regular sexual partners should be examined and treated, if needed. Serologic testing for HIV is recommended for patients treated for chancroid.

Hepatitis B

See Chapter 8 for a discussion about hepatitis B.

Sexual Dysfunction

The most common male and female sexual dysfunctions are discussed briefly. Sexual health and proper sexual functioning are important to human beings for the pleasure they provide, for the intimacy they nurture in a relationship, and for reproduction. To fulfill these purposes, the individuals must be free from organic disease and psychosexual disorders.

Ideally the human sexual response cycle progresses from a state of desire or arousal, through orgasm, to resolution or a feeling of well-being and relaxation. This cycle depends on a balance and interplay among physical, mental, and emotional factors.

Erectile Dysfunction/Impotence

Description

Erectile dysfunction (ED)/impotence is a consistent or recurrent inability to achieve or maintain penile erection.

ICD-10-CM Code	N52 *(Male erectile dysfunction)*
	N52.0 *(Vasculogenic erectile dysfunction)*
	N52.01 *(Erectile dysfunction due to arterial insufficiency)*
	N52.02 *(Corporo-venous occlusive erectile dysfunction)*
	N52.03 *(Combined arterial insufficiency and corporo-venous occlusive erectile dysfunction)*
	N52.1 *(Erectile dysfunction due to diseases classified elsewhere)*
	N52.2 *(Drug-induced erectile dysfunction)*
	N52.3 *(Postsurgical erectile dysfunction)*
	N52.31 *(Erectile dysfunction following radical prostatectomy)*
	N52.32 *(Erectile dysfunction following radical cystectomy)*
	N52.33 *(Erectile dysfunction following urethral surgery)*
	N52.34 *(Erectile dysfunction following simple prostatectomy)*
	N52.39 *(Other postsurgical erectile dysfunction)*
	N52.8 *(Other male erectile dysfunction)*
	N52.9 *(Male erectile dysfunction, unspecified)*

Impotence is coded by specific disorders. Refer to the physician's diagnosis and then to the current edition of the ICD-10-CM coding manual to ensure the greatest specificity of pathology.

Symptoms and Signs

ED/impotence is the inability of a man to perform in sexual intercourse, usually because he is unable to attain or maintain an erection of the penis sufficient for satisfactory sexual activity. It is the most common male sexual disorder, affecting most men at some time during their lives. The condition can be temporary or may become chronic.

Patient Screening

A complete physical examination or a private consultation may be scheduled.

Etiology

Sexual arousal causes the arteries in the penis to relax and dilate, thus allowing an increased blood flow to the penis. The expansion and hardening of the penis causes a compression of the veins carrying blood away from the penis, resulting in an erection. Anything that impedes the nerve response or that alters the necessary pattern of blood flow results in failure to achieve an erection.

Many physical or medical conditions can play a significant role in ED. Medical conditions affecting the blood vessels and restricting blood flow to the penis include diabetes mellitus, hypertension, heart disease, obesity, smoking, and hypercholesterolemia. Neurologic elements (e.g., nerve insult resulting from prostate surgery and spinal cord, pelvic, or perineal trauma) may interrupt the impulse transmission between the central nervous system and the penis. Medications prescribed to treat hypertension and depression can cause ED as a side effect. Other common offenders are alcohol, recreational drugs, antihistamines, and diuretics.

ED/impotence may also have a psychosocial basis that is not directly related to the mechanical functioning of the penis. The most common contributing factors include depression and stress.

Diagnosis

A medical history and physical examination to reveal any underlying medical causative factors are necessary. The history should include patient and family history of diabetes mellitus or other endocrine disorders, hypertension, heart disease, cerebral vascular accidents, spinal cord injuries, and vascular or renal disease; any surgery or trauma to the pelvic area; medications that the patient currently is taking or previously has taken; lifestyle, including smoking habits and alcohol consumption; stress levels; and relationship with the sexual partner. Laboratory tests to rule out organic disease help the physician make the diagnosis. Measurement of the testosterone level in blood is helpful, especially if the patient indicates low sexual desire.

Treatment

The treatment may first require management of underlying medical disorders or changing/discontinuing current medications. Testosterone therapy is used for men with androgen deficiency. Other courses of remedies, such as programs for substance abuse or psychological counseling, are more complex and time consuming. Interventions, such as psychoanalysis, discussion, behavioral modification, and sensate exercises, are aimed at restoring the patient's ability to complete the entire sexual response cycle. Other approaches include penile implants, external vacuum devices, and penile injection therapy.

A more recent approach is oral drug therapy with medication, such as sildenafil citrate (Viagra), vardenafil (Levitra), and tadalafil (Cialis). During sexual stimulation, nitric oxide is released in the corpus cavernosum, initiating an enzymatic cascade, ultimately resulting in relaxation of the smooth muscle of the corpus cavernosum and an inflow of blood. This class of medication (phosphodiesterase-5 [PDE5] inhibitors) increases the effect of nitrous oxide, consequently helping the man to have an erection satisfactory for desired sexual activity. Sexual stimulation is needed for these drugs, taken at the recommended dosage, to assist with achieving an erection; they have no effect in the absence of sexual stimulation. See the Alert box about Precautions Concerning Sildenafil Citrate (Viagra), Vardenafil (Levitra), and Tadalafil (Cialis).

ⓘ ALERT!

Precautions Concerning Sildenafil Citrate (Viagra), Vardenafil (Levitra), and Tadalafil (Cialis)

Men who have underlying cardiovascular disease and are advised against sexual activity should not take sildenafil, vardenafil, or tadalafil. In addition, men who have had a heart attack, stroke, or life-threatening arrhythmia in the past 6 months also are warned not to take these drugs, which are classified as phosphodiesterase-5 (PDE5) inhibitors. This class of medication is also contraindicated in patients taking nitrites, both regularly and intermittently, because the combination of the two drugs may lead to severe hypotension.

Other preexisting conditions that may preclude the use of these medications are hypotension, hypertension, unstable angina, liver or kidney impairment, retinitis pigmentosa, or any anatomic deformity of the penis.

Side effects, in order of likelihood of occurrence, may include headache, stomach pain, flushing, nosebleeds, or mild temporary vision changes, including color perception changes and blurred vision. Men are advised to take the smallest possible dose to achieve an erection. In addition, a prolonged erection (lasting longer than 4 hours) is an indication to notify the physician.

Any male experiencing chest pain or other serious side effects after taking these medications should seek immediate emergency medical assistance and should advise emergency personnel of the use of these drugs (sildenafil, vardenafil, or tadalafil). Concurrent use of any form of nitrate drug therapy or short-acting nitrate drug to treat the chest pain may cause life-threatening hypotension.

Prognosis

The prognosis varies greatly, depending on the cause. Effective therapy is available in many cases. The prevalence increases with advancing age.

✗ NOTE

There is growing evidence linking erectile dysfunction (ED) to the eventual onset of the clinical manifestation of coronary artery disease.

Prevention

Impotence is usually secondary to one of many diseases and conditions.

Patient Teaching

If the cause is psychogenic, refer the patient to counseling. Direct other patient teaching toward treating the organic cause.

Male and Female Infertility

Description

Infertility may be defined as the involuntary inability to conceive.

ICD-10-CM Code	N46.9 *(Male infertility, unspecified)*
	(N46.8-N46.9 = 2 codes of specificity)
	N97.9 *(Female infertility, unspecified)*
	(N97.0-N97.9 = 5 codes of specificity)

Symptoms and Signs

With regular, unprotected intercourse, about 90% of couples conceive within 1 year. The inability of a couple to conceive can originate from female factors, male factors, or both. In about 40% of cases, the male causes the infertility; in another 40% of cases, various female factors are found to be the cause, with less than 10% of cases remaining unexplained.

Patient Screening

A complete medical evaluation should be schedules for both partners.

Etiology

The causes of infertility in men may be subdivided into different categories. The most common cause, in about 40% to 50% of infertile men, is idiopathic, meaning that there is no identifiable disorder of sperm number, function, or morphology. Testicular dysfunction, including congenital disorders of the testes, certain developmental disorders, chromosomal abnormalities, and varicoceles, is the next most prevalent cause, resulting in 30% to 40% of infertility cases. The two final categories are disorders of sperm transport and diseases of the hypothalamus or the pituitary gland. Environmental factors, such as certain drugs, radiation, smoking, or pollutants, can also be implicating factors in infertility.

In a woman, in order of prevalence, the causes include:
- ovulatory dysfunction or failure to ovulate
- endometriosis
- scar tissue from infection, ectopic pregnancy, or surgery
- blocked fallopian tubes, caused by PID from STDs
- congenital structural or chromosomal disorders
- tumors
- antisperm antibodies in the female vaginal secretions
- medications that compromise fertility
- psychological distress

Diagnosis

After a physical examination and an interview of both partners, specific testing procedures are chosen. The cause of infertility sometimes is identified quickly and easily. If not, the clinical observation and therapeutic approaches can be time consuming and expensive.

In men, a complete history, with special attention to childhood diseases, is followed by a thorough physical examination for any structural abnormalities. As part of the history, it is pertinent to inquire about any personal or familial genetic or endocrine disorders. Semen analysis is essential and, if relevant, possibly chromosome and testosterone testing. A full semen analysis involves more than just checking to see if sperm are present.

In women, ovulatory function is established by charting of the menstrual cycle. Hormone levels are studied through blood tests. The fallopian tubes and uterine cavity are visualized through hysterosalpingography to determine tubal patency. In some cases, laparoscopy may be necessary to rule out endometriosis or chronic infection.

Treatment

Each treatment plan is unique, depending on the problems that are identified in the medical and psychological evaluations. Unless the condition is untreatable, the course of action to achieve pregnancy may include treatment of infection, surgery to remove blockage, the use of fertility drugs (e.g., follicle stimulating hormone [Follistim]); intrauterine insemination (IUI); or in vitro fertilization (IVF). Many other new assisted reproductive technologies are offered by clinicians specializing in infertility treatment.

Prognosis

Many couples who seek treatment for infertility do achieve pregnancy. Some have untreatable causes, or in some, it may take as long as 3 years to achieve pregnancy.

Prevention

When possible, preventing the causative factors that lead to sterility is preferable. Methods of preventing male infertility include maintaining good overall health to reduce obesity and cardiovascular disease, regular physical examinations, and protection of the testicles during sports. Early and complete treatment of any STD is important for men and women.

Patient Teaching

Much of the patient teaching involves answering questions about the complexity of the medical evaluation and the selected therapeutic approach.

Contraception/Birth Control

Many visits in the medical office are to inquire about contraception methods, also known as *birth control.* There are multiple options available, with each being chosen over another based on the personal preference of the patient, effectiveness, and benefits or risks. Birth control can be considered temporary or permanent. Some permanent methods are reversible, whereas others are not. The patient should be educated on the various methods available and on the benefits and risks of use. Barrier methods of contraception are effective against STDs, such as HIV infection. Nonbarrier methods are used to prevent pregnancy, but they do not to protect against STDs.

Sterilization is a permanent option of birth control for either partner. Female sterilization consist of tubal ligation, commonly referred to as *tying the tubes.* This procedure is accomplished when the physician cuts and closes the fallopian tubes. Sperm are unable to reach the egg for fertilization. Tubal ligation is performed in an outpatient surgical center or a hospital. Immediate sterilization results. Hysterectomy, the removal of the uterus, is another method of permanent sterilization.

Vasectomy is the method for permanent sterilization of a male patient. Vasectomy involves cutting the vas deferens so that sperm cannot travel to the female during intercourse. Both vas deferens are cauterized or sutured shut. After a vasectomy, the patient should have a post-vasectomy sperm count to ensure that the procedure was successful and no sperm are able to reach the partner.

Other methods of contraception are reversible. Intrauterine devices (IUDs); barriers; and fertility awareness-based, hormonal, and lactation amenorrhea are all methods of reversible birth control. Emergency postcoital contraception is also an option if intercourse has taken place without use of contraception.

Currently two categories of IUDs are acceptable. (1) An IUD is placed into the uterus to prevent pregnancy. These IUDs are small, shaped like the letter T (copper T IUD system) and inserted through the cervix. (2) The levonorgestrel intrauterine device (LNG IUD) is another type of IUD system that releases progestin daily, thus preventing pregnancy. The copper T IUD system works by triggering the immune system to prevent pregnancy. This IUD has to be removed after a certain number of years (e.g., it can be left in place for up to 10 years) or if pregnancy should occur while the IUD is in the uterus. The LNG IUD should be removed after 5 years.

Barrier methods of contraception create a barrier that prevents sperm from entering the cervix. The diaphragm (cervical cap) and contraceptive sponge are placed next to the cervix in the vagina before sexual intercourse. Condoms that are now available for male and female partners also provide barrier protection. Spermicide is used with any of these methods, and all instructions for use should be followed with each method.

Fertility awareness-based contraception methods can be used by women who are cognizant of their menstrual cycles. The fertility pattern includes which days of the month a woman cannot get pregnant, or days she is not likely to get pregnant, and which days are considered fertile days, or days when conception can take place.

Hormonal Methods

Hormonal methods of birth control are also popular among women. Implants, progesterone injections, progesterone pills, combined oral contraceptives (containing both progesterone and estrogen), patches, and vaginal rings are all methods indicated for prevention of pregnancy.

Implants are placed under the skin. The progesterone in the small, thin rod is released over 3 years and then can be replaced. Progesterone injections are administered every 3 months. Birth control pills are dispensed in 21- or 28-day packages. The combined form contains both estrogen and progesterone. The pill containing only progesterone is prescribed for women who cannot take estrogen. Patches containing estrogen are placed on the buttocks or on the upper body. The patches have an adhesive material and are changed every week for 3 weeks. The fourth week is patch free. Patches cannot be placed on the breast area. Patients who weigh more than 198 lb (90 kg) should be aware that patches may be less effective in preventing pregnancy.

The contraceptive vaginal ring is inserted, releases estrogen and progesterone very slowly for 3 weeks, and is removed during the menstrual cycle.

New mothers who are nursing full time can use the lactational amenorrhea method of birth control. This option is best for mothers within a 6-month postpartum period and not experiencing menstruation.

Emergency Contraception

Emergency contraception may be used when no contraceptive method was used during sexual intercourse. A copper T IUD can be inserted within 5 days after unprotected intercourse. A second option is the "morning after" pill. The pill can be taken within 3 days after unprotected sex. The pill should be taken as a single dose within 72 hours after unprotected sexual intercourse.

Male Reproductive Diseases

The most common diseases of the male reproductive system are those affecting the prostate gland. The gland can become inflamed or enlarged as a result of bacteria and can cause urinary problems. Common symptoms are:

- any urinary symptoms, such as frequency, urgency, incontinence, and dysuria
- pain, swelling, or enlargement of any of the reproductive organs
- any sexual dysfunction, such as ED/impotence

Epididymitis

Description

Epididymitis is inflammation of the epididymis, the excretory duct of the testicles.

ICD-10-CM Code	N45.1 (Epididymitis)
	N45.2 (Orchitis)
	N45.3 (Epididymo-orchitis)

The above code may be valid as a principal diagnosis. Use an additional code to identify the causative organism. Refer to the physician's diagnosis and then to the current edition of the ICD-10-CM coding manual to ensure the greatest specificity of pathology.

Symptoms and Signs

Symptoms of inflammation of the epididymis can include scrotal pain and discomfort that radiates into the groin and pain with ejaculation. It is the most common cause of scrotal pain in men seen in the outpatient setting. The epididymis may become enlarged, tender, and firm to palpation. The patient may have groin and scrotal tenderness with severe pain in the testes. Walking may be difficult for the patient as he tries to protect a painful scrotum.

Patient Screening

The patient often experiences great discomfort during the acute phase, requiring a same-day appointment, if possible.

Etiology

The most common cause of epididymitis is an infection; however, it can also be a result of noninfectious etiologies, including trauma or autoimmune disease. STIs by *N. gonorrhoeae* and *C. trachomatis* are the most common bacterial causes of epididymitis. *Escherichia coli* and *Pseudomonas* are other bacterial causes of this condition in older men. Urinary tract infections, tuberculosis, mumps, removal of the prostate gland (prostatectomy), trauma, and the prolonged use of an indwelling catheter also may predispose the patient to epididymitis. A viral infection associated with HIV infection can also cause epididymitis.

Diagnosis

Physical examination, urinalysis, urine culture, and urethral swabs for chlamydia and gonorrhea are used to make the diagnosis of epididymitis. The patient also may have an elevated white blood cell (WBC) count.

Treatment

Antibiotic treatment for infectious causes, combined with the administration of antiinflammatory drugs and rest, is beneficial. Use of scrotal support or elevation also may help. Epididymitis usually responds well to treatment. Scarring may occur, which can lead to sterility if treatment is delayed. This is especially true if the disease is bilateral.

Prognosis

The prognosis is usually good with early treatment. Possible complications include sterility.

Prevention

The best prevention for epididymitis is the early treatment of urinary and STIs. Condom use during sexual intercourse also is recommended.

Patient Teaching

Advise using comfort measures, including ice packs, scrotal support, lightweight clothing, and elevation of the scrotum while at rest. List the warning signs of complications: increased pain, swelling, or discharge.

Orchitis

Description

Orchitis is infection of the testis.

ICD-10-CM Code	N45.1 (Epididymitis)
	N45.2 (Orchitis)
	N45.3 (Epididymo-orchitis)

The above code may be valid as a principal diagnosis. Use an additional code to identify the causative organism. Refer to the physician's diagnosis and then to the current edition of the ICD-10-CM coding manual to ensure the greatest specificity of pathology.

Symptoms and Signs

Inflammation of the testes is caused by viral or bacterial infection and injury. It may affect one or both testes, causing swelling, tenderness, and acute pain. The patient also may experience chills, fever, nausea, vomiting, and general malaise.

Patient Screening

Prompt treatment to alleviate pain and appropriate antibiotic therapy are indicated.

Etiology

Isolated orchitis may be a consequence of infection by the mumps virus and most often affects boys younger than 10 years of age. Other viruses and bacteria also can cause this condition, and it may follow epididymitis in sexually active men older than 15 years of age. About one-half of severe cases result in atrophy of the affected testicle. Sterility results when both testicles are affected.

Diagnosis

The clinical history to determine the patient's exposure to mumps or other related diseases and a physical examination usually indicate the diagnosis. Further testing in sexually active men should include urethral swabs for chlamydia and gonorrhea. Urinalysis, serologic study, throat culture, or serum antibody testing may be used to isolate or identify causative agents, such as the mumps virus, but is rarely necessary. Immediate differentiation of orchitis from testicular torsion can be accomplished with Doppler ultrasonography.

Treatment

If the cause of orchitis is bacterial, appropriate antibiotic treatment with cephalexin or ciprofloxacin should be started immediately. Orchitis caused by the mumps virus has no specific treatment other than supportive care. Bed rest usually is prescribed, along with certain antiinflammatory drugs to reduce fever and swelling in severe cases. The use of scrotal support also may help.

Prognosis

Healing follows successful treatment with antibiotics, but scarring may compromise fertility.

Prevention

Risk factors for STDs should be avoided. To prevent orchitis related to the mumps virus, all adult men who have not had mumps should be vaccinated.

Patient Teaching

Emphasize the importance of finishing the entire course of antibiotics as prescribed. Suggest comfort measures, such as scrotal support and the use of ice packs. Explain the importance of follow-up appointments for urologic care.

Torsion of the Testicle

Description

Torsion of the testicle is a condition in which one testicle is twisted out of its normal position (Fig. 12.10A).

| ICD-10-CM Code | N44.00 (Torsion of testis, unspecified) |
| | (N44.00-N44.04 = 5 codes of specificity) |

Symptoms and Signs

The primary symptom is a sudden, severe pain in one testicle. The pain can be so severe that it causes nausea and vomiting, and it is usually constant. When the torsion occurs, the scrotum becomes swollen, red, and tender. Torsion can cause the blood vessels supplying the testicle to become kinked, which, in turn, prevents the blood flow to and from the affected testicle.

Patient Screening

Emergency treatment is required.

Etiology

This condition occurs when the testis rotates on the spermatic cord, causing a sudden, extreme twist or torsion. It can happen spontaneously or as a result of trauma. The arteries and veins are compressed, ischemia develops, and the scrotum swells.

Diagnosis

Diagnosis is based on the patient history and a gentle physical examination by the physician. The testicle usually has an abnormal horizontal lie in the scrotum. Because the symptoms of testicular torsion and epididymitis are similar, Doppler ultrasonography may be performed to determine whether testicular torsion is the cause of the pain and swelling. In torsion of the testicle, ultrasonography shows little or no blood flow to the testicle.

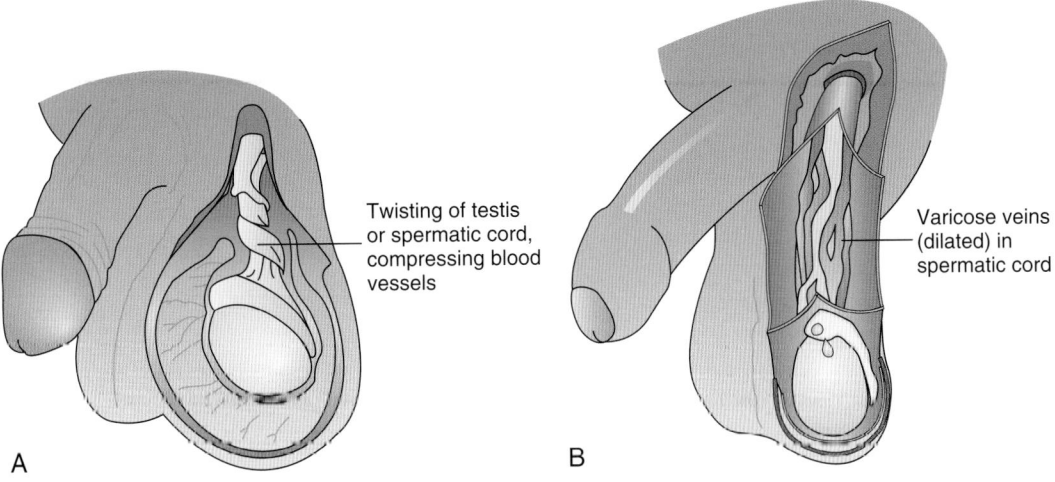

Twisting of testis
or spermatic cord,
compressing blood
vessels

Varicose veins
(dilated) in
spermatic cord

A   B

• **Fig. 12.10** (A) Torsion of testis. (B) Varicocele. (From Gould BE, Dyer RM: *Pathophysiology for the health professions,* ed 4, St Louis, 2012, Saunders.)

Treatment

Immediate consultation with urology is required, followed by surgical intervention for both testes. Surgery should never be delayed, because the delay may result in permanent damage to the testicle. Even if detorsion is accomplished, the patient still requires bilateral orchiopexy (untwisting and stitching the testes into proper position) for fixation to reduce the risk of torsion in the future.

Prognosis

The prognosis is good if treatment is given promptly when the torsion does not correct itself. Even if the condition corrects itself and pain is relieved, the torsion may recur; orchiopexy helps limit the possibility of recurrence.

Prevention

No prevention is known.

Patient Teaching

Surgical intervention, if necessary, is performed on an emergency basis. Give as much preoperative information as possible by answering questions and giving directions to the patient or the family. The patient also will need information about postoperative care.

Varicocele

Description

In varicocele, the veins of one of the testicles become abnormally distended, causing swelling around the testicle that expands within the scrotal sac (see Fig. 12.10B).

ICD-10-CM Code	I86.1 *(Scrotal varices)*

Symptoms and Signs

This is a rather mild disorder that is more uncomfortable than painful. A varicocele may be especially uncomfortable in hot weather or after exercise and may be relieved temporarily by lying down. Because the increased presence of venous blood raises the temperature within the scrotum, varicocele may contribute to a lower sperm count. It is more common on the left side because of the anatomy of the vascular supply.

Patient Screening

The condition often is asymptomatic. If a vein ruptures as a result of local injury, pain and swelling in the scrotum cause the patient to seek prompt medical intervention.

Etiology

Incompetent venous valves can cause dilation of the large scrotal veins and venous stasis. The condition may be congenital and usually becomes symptomatic in the 15- to 25-year age group.

Diagnosis

Patient history, physical symptoms, and examination by the physician confirm the diagnosis.

Treatment

Treatment consists of measures to relieve the symptoms. These can include the wearing of tight-fitting underwear or the use of an athletic supporter. If the varicocele affects fertility, surgery can remove the distended veins, but the results may not justify the risks of the surgery. Results vary, depending on the severity of the distention.

Prognosis

In some cases, surgical repair has been reported to improve fertility and decrease pain.

Prevention

No prevention is known.

Patient Teaching

Encourage the patient to use comfort measures to relieve the symptoms. If the patient undergoes surgical repair, review the postoperative care.

Prostatitis

Description

Prostatitis is acute or chronic inflammation of the prostate gland.

ICD-10-CM Code	N41.0 *(Acute prostatitis)*
	N41.1 *(Chronic prostatitis)*

Refer to the physician's diagnosis and then to the current edition of the ICD-10-CM coding manual to ensure the greatest specificity of pathology.

Symptoms and Signs

Inflammation of the prostate gland is more common in men older than 50 years of age but can occur in men of any age. The prostate may be enlarged and tender, and in some instances, pus may be seen at the tip of the penis. The patient may be asymptomatic or may experience acute symptoms in mild or sporadic forms and has pain and a burning sensation during urination. Other common symptoms include low back pain, perineal pain, fever, muscular pain or tenderness, and urinary frequency with urgency. There may be blood in urine.

Patient Screening

When a patient has acute symptoms of pain and other urinary symptoms, prompt medical evaluation is indicated.

Etiology

The cause of inflammation of the prostate is usually infection but is not always known. Infection may be either bacterial or nonbacterial. Bacterial causes may include, most commonly, *E. coli* that has caused a urinary tract infection, gonococci from a patient with gonorrhea, *Staphylococcus*, *Streptococcus*, or *Pseudomonas*.

Diagnosis

The prostate gland is gently palpated on physical examination. Urinalysis, blood culture, and a WBC count are ordered. Ultrasonography to measure post-void residual urine may be ordered.

Treatment

The usual treatment of acute prostatitis is fluoroquinolone or trimethoprim-sulfamethoxazole therapy. The physician also may order sitz baths, rest, an increase in fluid intake, and the administration of analgesics and antiinflammatory drugs. Patients acutely ill on presentation are hospitalized for IV fluids and antibiotics.

Chronic prostatitis can potentially develop from recurrent urinary tract infections, urethral obstruction, and acute urinary retention.

Prognosis

The prognosis for acute prostatitis is good because it responds well to treatment. The outlook for the less common chronic prostatitis is not as favorable. Complications, such as epididymitis, bacteremia, or prostatic abscesses, can occur.

Prevention

The best prevention for prostatitis is the early treatment of urinary tract infections with the prescribed antibiotics.

Patient Teaching

Emphasize the need for strict adherence to the prescribed medications. Encourage the practice of comfort measures ordered by the physician (see the Treatment section).

Benign Prostatic Hyperplasia

Description

Benign prostatic hyperplasia (BPH) is nonmalignant, noninflammatory hypertrophy of the prostate gland.

ICD-10-CM Code	N40.0 *(Enlarged prostate without lower urinary tract symptoms [LUTS])*
	N40.1 *(Enlarged prostate with lower urinary tract symptoms [LUTS])*

Symptoms and Signs

Enlargement of the prostate gland is a common condition in men older than 50 years of age, and the frequency increases with age. BPH usually progresses to the point of causing compression of the urethra with urinary obstruction and resulting urinary retention (Fig. 12.11). Common signs and symptoms may include difficulty starting urination, a weak stream of urine, or inability to empty the bladder completely. Urinary frequency, including nocturia, and in severe cases, inflammation and symptoms of renal disease have been observed.

Patient Screening

A routine physical examination is appropriate to evaluate BPH.

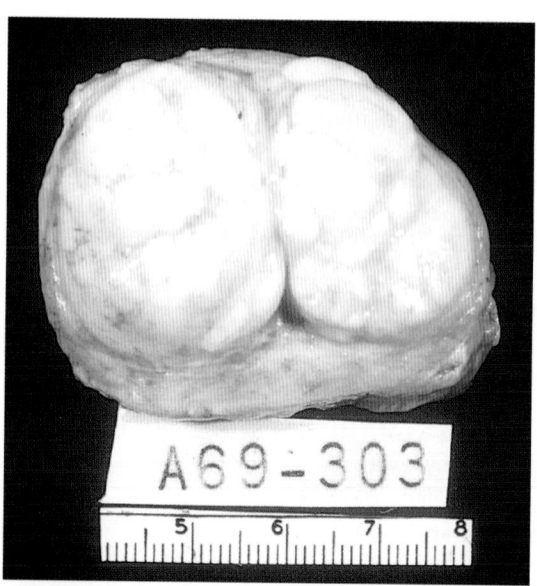

• **Fig. 12.11** Benign prostatic hyperplasia (BPH). (From Kumar V, Cotran RS, et al: *Robbins basic pathology,* ed 7, Philadelphia, 2003, Saunders.)

Etiology

The cause of BPH is not completely understood, but the condition seems to be associated with the aging process and hormonal and metabolic changes. As the prostate gland enlarges, it compresses either the neck of the bladder or the urethra, causing obstruction of the urinary flow.

Diagnosis

The usual diagnosis is based on patient history and a rectal examination for prostatic abnormalities. Routine tests include urinalysis, urine culture, renal function studies, and prostate-specific antigen (PSA) serum level to screen for prostatic cancer. These tests help differentiate BPH from other possible causes of lower urinary tract symptoms, including urinary tract infection, stones in the urinary tract, or possible malignancy, such as prostate cancer.

In many cases, the international prostate symptom score (IPSS) is used to determine the subjective degree of symptoms and the impact of the symptoms on the patient's quality of life. This score can be used to determine the best therapeutic approach.

Treatment

Treatment of BPH may be watchful waiting when symptoms are not bothersome. Lifestyle changes that are recommended include control of fluid intake before bedtime and avoiding medication that may cause urinary retention, such as decongestants. Drug therapy with alpha-adrenergic blockers, including tamsulosin hydrochloride (Flomax), doxazosin mesylate (Cardura), and terazosin hydrochloride (Hytrin), may be prescribed to relax the tightened muscles inside the prostate and relieve symptoms. Another class of drugs is the 5-alpha-reductase inhibitors, which are dutasteride (Avodart) or finasteride (Proscar) that work by reducing the size of the prostate by about 30%. When symptoms are moderate to severe, a highly effective surgical treatment, transurethral resection of the prostate (TURP), may be performed to remove the obstructive part of the prostate.

Prognosis

The prognosis for BPH is good with intervention. Severe symptoms, if left untreated, can progress to urinary retention and infection, which may reach the kidneys. Complications of this condition may include cystitis, dilation of the ureters, pyelonephritis, hydronephrosis, and uremia.

Prevention

Prevention of BPH is unknown. Physicians strongly recommend that older men have regular prostate examinations to detect any enlargement.

Patient Teaching

Inform the patient that ingestion of decongestants, antidepressants, tranquilizers, alcohol, and anticholinergics tends to increase urinary obstruction.

If a prostatectomy is scheduled, review with the patient the physician's explanation of the procedure, and give appropriate information about presurgical and postsurgical care, including possible complications that should be reported to the physician.

Prostate Cancer

Description

Prostate cancer is a malignancy of the small gland located below the bladder and anterior to the rectum in men, known as the *prostate gland*. Although this is a very common cancer, it grows so slowly that only 1 of 41 men diagnosed with prostate cancer will die as a result of it. Nonetheless, after lung cancer, prostate cancer is the second leading cause of cancer-related death in men (Fig. 12.12).

ICD-10-CM Code	C61 *(Malignant neoplasm of prostate)*

Symptoms and Signs

Prostate cancer is often asymptomatic at diagnosis because it is usually detected clinically by abnormalities on routine digital rectal examination (DRE) or by detecting a high concentration of PSA in serum. Asymmetric areas of induration and nodules felt on DRE suggest prostate cancer, and malignant prostate tissue generates more PSA than normal or hyperplastic tissue does (refer to Table 12.1 for PSA values). The usual symptoms, when present, are those associated with urinary obstruction. These include weak or interrupted urine flow, urinary frequency, urinary retention, dysuria, and hematuria. However, these symptoms also often are common to BPH or an infection or inflammation of the prostate gland. New onset of ED also should raise suspicion for prostate cancer.

Patient Screening

Schedule a physical examination with screening for prostate cancer annually for patients 50 years of age or older or when a patient reports urinary symptoms or new-onset ED.

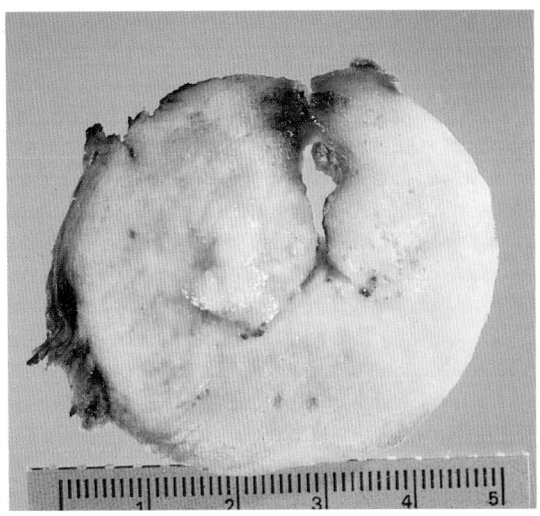

• **Fig. 12.12** Cancer of the prostate. (From Kumar V, Cotran RS, et al: *Robbins basic pathology,* ed 7, Philadelphia, 2003, Saunders.)

TABLE 12.1	Age-Specific Reference Ranges for Serum Prostate-Specific Antigen		
	Reference Range (ng/mL)[a]		
Age Range (years)	Blacks	Caucasians	Japanese
40–49	0.0–2.0	0.0–2.5	0.0–2.0
50–59	0.0–4.0	0.0–3.5	0.0–3.0
60–69	0.0–4.5	0.0–4.5	0.0–4.0
70–79	0.0–5.5	0.0–6.5	0.0–5.0

[a]Prostate-specific antigen (PSA) blood tests are reported as ng/mL.

Etiology

Risk factors for prostate cancer include race, ethnicity, age, gene changes or heredity, geographic location, and lifestyle. Prostate cancer is more common in older men and rarely occurs before age 40 years. Ethnicity is also important, because prostate tumors are much more common in African American men than in white or Hispanic men. Risk is also higher in men who have particular mutations in the *BRCA1* or *BRCA2* genes (breast cancer susceptibility genes). Although many dietary risk factors have been studied, a diet high in animal fat is the most consistent link. Many studies are being done to evaluate other genetic factors, exposures, and infections as possible risk factors.

Diagnosis

Although abnormally high PSA level and abnormal DRE are highly suggestive findings, prostate biopsy is necessary to diagnose cancer. Biopsy is advised if the PSA level is greater than 4 ng/mL and should be performed at lower values if clinical suspicion is high. A transrectal ultrasound-guided biopsy is usually performed. If the biopsy result is negative but the PSA level remains high, a repeat biopsy is often performed several weeks to months later, because prostate cancer can be missed on the initial biopsy. If a biopsy specimen is found to contain carcinoma, further evaluation and clinical staging is needed to select the appropriate treatment strategy. The TNM (tumor–node–metastasis) staging system proposed by the American Joint Committee on Cancer (AJCC) is the most popular method used for staging. Clinical staging uses DRE, PSA measurement, and imaging studies. Analysis of the tumor histology (the Gleason score) leads to a scoring system based on the degree of glandular differentiation and structural architecture. The Gleason score and the PSA level are incorporated into the TNM stage determination as well.

See Chapter 1 for information about the staging and grading systems used to assess malignant neoplasms.

Treatment

Treatment of prostate cancer depends on the stage of the disease, the Gleason score, the PSA level, the age and physical condition of the patient, and the risks and benefits of each treatment option. Options for early-stage prostate cancer include radical prostatectomy, radiation therapy, brachytherapy (the direct implantation of a radiation source into the prostate), or active surveillance. Radical prostatectomy and radiation have potential complications of ED/impotence and urinary symptoms. Active surveillance with initiation of treatment at any sign of disease progression may be preferred for those with low-risk disease or significant comorbidities.

For patients with metastatic prostate cancer, first-line treatment involves androgen deprivation therapy (ADT) by either surgical orchiectomy (removal of a testicle) or medical orchiectomy (use of hormones to suppress the release of testosterone). The purpose of ADT is to reduce the amount of androgen hormones in the body or prevent the body from responding to them as a method to inhibit growth of cancer cells. If the cancer becomes resistant to ADT, there are a number of other recently approved medicines that can be tried, with or without chemotherapy, including the Sipuleucel-T cancer vaccine. Regardless of the therapy selected and the disease stage, patients should be followed up with PSA measurements every 3 to 12 months to monitor the efficacy of treatment and to detect recurrences.

Prognosis

The most important predictors of disease progression are TNM stage, Gleason score of the biopsy specimen, and serum PSA level. For early-stage tumors, radiation therapy and prostatectomy offer similar 10-year survival rates. The overall 5-year survival rate is nearly 100%, because many prostate cancers are diagnosed in early stages as a result of the current screening procedures. The survival rate declines, however, with longer follow-up.

Prevention

It is unclear whether routine screening for prostate cancer decreases morbidity and mortality from the disease. All men should be involved in the decision-making process to determine whether screening is right for them. Clinicians should explain the benefits of early detection of prostate cancer, the risk of false-positive and false-negative results, and the significant risks associated with aggressive treatment should prostate cancer be detected before offering testing. Screening consists of serum PSA measurement with or without a DRE, followed by a transrectal ultrasound-guided prostate biopsy if either test is positive. Screening can be offered beginning at age 50 years to men who have a life expectancy of at least 10 years. Men considered at high risk for prostate cancer (African American men and men with two or more first-degree relatives with prostate cancer) can begin screening at age 40 to 45 years. Screening is generally not beneficial if the patient's life expectancy is less than 10 years.

Eating a healthy diet is recommended, although no dietary supplement has a known definite link to prostate cancer prevention at this time.

Patient Teaching

Emphasize the risks and benefits of annual screening for prostate cancer after age 50 years. Describe and explain diagnostic procedures. Review the information given by the physician about the mode of treatment and the likely side effects. Explain the warning signs of complications that should be reported to the physician. Encourage the patient to ask questions and voice concerns about sexual function and prognosis.

Testicular Cancer

Description

The testicles are the male gonads that produce sperm and are the primary source of male hormones. Cancer of the testicle is one of the most curable solid neoplasms, but it still has a significant effect on the physical and emotional status of the young population it usually affects. Nearly all testicular tumors are germ cell tumors (GCTs), equally distributed between two main types: seminomas and all others, termed *nonseminomatous germ cell tumors (NSGCTs).*

ICD-10-CM Code	C62.10 *(Malignant neoplasm of unspecified descended testis)* (C62.10-C62.12 = 3 codes of specificity) C62.90 *(Malignant neoplasm of unspecified testis, unspecified whether descended or undescended)* (C62.90 C62.92 – 3 codes of specificity)

Symptoms and Signs

The most common presentation is a nodule or painless swelling of one testicle. Some patients complain of a dull ache or a heavy sensation in the abdomen, perianal area, or scrotum. Fewer patients have acute pain or gynecomastia. Symptoms of advanced disease include enlarged lymph nodes in the neck, dyspnea or cough, anorexia, bone pain, and lower extremity swelling.

Patient Screening

When a patient reports any nodule or swelling of a testicle, the next available appointment should be scheduled for a medical evaluation.

Etiology

Testicular neoplasms are most common in men between ages 15 and 45 years (Fig. 12.13). Risk factors include cryptorchidism (undescended testicle), personal and family histories of testicular cancer, previous GCT(s), infertility, and HIV infection. Down syndrome and Klinefelter syndrome may predispose affected men to the development of testicular cancer. Children with cryptorchidism are at a higher risk for the disease, even if the testicle is brought to its anatomic position in the scrotum.

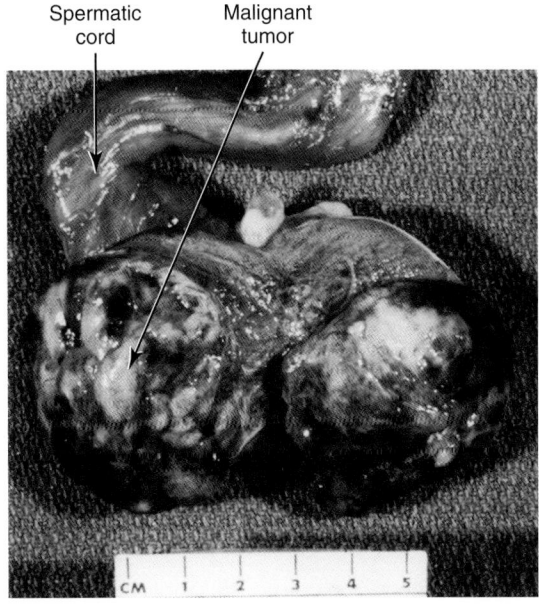

Spermatic cord   Malignant tumor

• **Fig. 12.13** Cancer of the testes. (From Gould BE, Dyer RM: *Pathophysiology for the health professions,* ed 4, St Louis, 2012, Saunders.)

Diagnosis

Diagnosis begins with physical examination of the testes and palpation for nodal involvement. Any firm, hard area in the affected testis is cause for concern. The diagnostic evaluation of suspected testicular cancer continues with scrotal ultrasonography, computed tomography (CT) of the abdomen and pelvis, chest radiography, and measurement of serum tumor markers. Radical orchiectomy also is performed to provide histologic evaluation of the tumor, and retroperitoneal lymph node dissection identifies nodal metastasis. Biopsy is not attempted because of the risk of causing tumor spread. In young men for whom future fertility is important, efforts should be made to perform a baseline sperm count and sperm banking before radiographic procedures so that radiation does not damage sperm. Serum tumor markers that are elevated in many testicular cancers are alpha-fetoprotein (AFP), the beta-subunit of human chorionic gonadotropin (beta-hCG), and lactate dehydrogenase (LDH). These markers help in initial diagnosis, but they are more useful for subsequent disease follow-up. (Tumor markers are explained in Chapter 1 in the Cancer section.)

The TNM staging system for testicular cancer developed by the AJCC considers the primary tumor, nodal involvement, distant metastases, and the serum tumor marker values for AFP, beta-hCG, and LDH. These parameters define stages I to III, which define good, intermediate, and poor prognoses, respectively. Metastatic tumors are staged under a separate system.

Treatment

Testicular NSGCTs are highly chemosensitive. Cisplatin-based combination chemotherapy can cure up to 80% of patients, even those with distant metastases. For those with advanced disease, residual masses may remain after chemotherapy. Surgical resection may be performed to excise the masses, remove any histologically malignant elements, and prevent compression of adjacent structures. Seminomas are radiosensitive, so the patient may be treated with radiation, with or without chemotherapy. For men with elevated levels of a serum tumor marker, monitoring the level throughout treatment often produces the best indication of treatment effectiveness.

As a result of the high cure rate for testicular cancer, post-treatment follow-up is an important part of the care for these patients. Periodic follow-up includes history and physical examination, serum tumor marker measurement, and radiographic studies for a minimum of 5 years after orchiectomy. The optimal surveillance schedule is determined by tumor type and pretreatment disease stage.

Prognosis

Patients with good (60% of GCTs), intermediate (26% of GCTs), and poor (14% of GCTs) prognoses are defined on the basis of the stage. Overall, however, the 5-year survival rate is greater than 95%. Factors that affect the prognosis include initial serum concentration of tumor markers, time between diagnosis and treatment, age of the patient, extent of visceral organ involvement, and number of distant metastases.

Prevention

There is no known prevention for testicular cancers. Routine screening with testicular self-examination or measurement of tumor markers is not recommended because the risks of screening do not outweigh potential benefit of early detection, given the good prognosis even with advanced disease.

Patient Teaching

Explain all diagnostic and treatment procedures. Review the physician's explanations, and encourage questions. Give the patient information about fertility and sexual potency. Emphasize the importance of the long-term surveillance schedule.

Female Reproductive Diseases

The female reproductive organs are affected by disease in several ways: (1) Microorganisms can invade the pelvis or vagina, causing infection. (2) Tumors, either benign or malignant, may occur anywhere in the reproductive tract. Symptoms that may require further evaluation are:
- symptomatic vaginal discharge, with or without odor
- lower pelvic or abdominal pain
- pelvic symptoms, such as menstrual pain (dysmenorrhea), absence of menstruation (amenorrhea), scanty menstruation (oligomenorrhea), bleeding between menses (metrorrhagia), and heavy or prolonged menstrual flow (menorrhagia)
- Fever

- Pain during sexual intercourse (dyspareunia) or other sexual dysfunction

Premenstrual Syndrome

Description

Premenstrual syndrome (PMS) is a constellation of physical and emotional symptoms that may appear shortly after ovulation and subside with the onset of menstruation or shortly thereafter.

ICD-10-CM Code	N94.3 *(Premenstrual tension syndrome)*

Symptoms and Signs

During the menstrual cycle, fluctuating hormone levels alter mood, sexual desire, and energy levels and may affect physical functioning. Troublesome symptoms related to these hormone shifts include anxiety, anger, sadness, bloating, food cravings, breast pain, irritability, and fatigue. Some women experience edema (swelling related to fluid retention), bloating, and abdominal pain as well. When these cyclic symptoms become severe and fit certain psychological criteria, the diagnosis shifts from PMS to premenstrual dysphoric disorder (PMDD).

Patient Screening

Consultation with a physician and a pelvic examination are scheduled.

Etiology

PMS is related to fluctuations in the levels of estrogen and progesterone and their subsequent impact on levels of neurotransmitters, such as dopamine, serotonin, and norepinephrine in the brain and other parts of the body. There are also alterations in other compounds in the body leading to sodium and fluid retention. PMS occurs only in ovulating women.

Diagnosis

One of the best ways to make the diagnosis is to have the patient keep a record of her symptoms as they relate to her menstrual cycle. There are no specific medical tests to diagnose PMS, but blood tests, careful history, and physical examination may help rule out other medical conditions. Symptoms usually subside shortly after the onset of menses.

Treatment

The treatment of PMS is directed toward the relief of symptoms. Reduced dietary intake of sodium, increased calcium consumption, moderate exercise, use of mild analgesics and diuretics, and emotional support all help. In addition, some women notice less breast tenderness when they eliminate caffeine from their diet. In some cases, treatment with antidepressants, such as fluoxetine or sertraline, may be indicated, especially if the patient meets the criteria for PMDD. Medical treatment may include a prescription for birth control pills. Other therapies include using extended-cycle birth control pills. These contraceptives are packaged so that the woman will have only four periods per year compared with the normal 12 per year.

Prognosis

Most PMS can be managed with dietary modification. In some women, PMS worsens with age, and for others, it does not appear until they are older. PMS resolves when a woman reaches menopause.

Prevention

There is no prevention available.

Patient Teaching

Some women benefit from a stress-reduction program or counseling to better cope with symptoms. Assure the patient that an estimated 50% of menstruating women experience PMS in some form.

Amenorrhea

Description

The absence of menstrual periods, whether temporary or permanent, is known as *amenorrhea.*

ICD-10-CM Code	N91.2 *(Amenorrhea, unspecified)*
	(N91.0-N91.2 = 3 codes of specificity)

Symptoms and Signs

Primary amenorrhea is no menses by age 16 years. Secondary amenorrhea is no menses after a woman has been having menstrual cycles. Short periods of amenorrhea may be normal between menarche (the onset of menstruation) and regular menstrual cycling, which is established usually by age 18 years or later. Amenorrhea has no symptoms, and the only sign is lack of cyclic bleeding.

The term *post-pill amenorrhea* refers to failure to resume menses within 3 months of discontinuation of oral contraception.

Patient Screening

A medical consultation and physical examination are indicated for a female having amenorrhea.

Etiology

In primary amenorrhea, the cause is generally late onset of puberty. It also can be caused by an abnormality in the reproductive system or hormonal imbalances. These conditions usually are not suspected unless the girl has reached age 16 years and is still not having her periods. Obstruction of the uterus or vagina or chromosomal/developmental/endocrine abnormalities are ruled out as a cause of primary amenorrhea. Cases of secondary amenorrhea are mainly hormone related. After pregnancy is ruled out, other conditions (e.g., thyroid disease, excess weight loss, poor nutrition, excessive athletic training, psychological stress, or pituitary tumors) should be ruled out.

Diagnosis

Pregnancy should be ruled out in all sexually active women in their reproductive years. Premature ovarian failure should be ruled out in women younger than 40 years of age. The diagnosis of amenorrhea is based on the patient history, whereas the etiology requires blood tests, physical examination, and occasionally radiographic evaluation.

Treatment

The treatment of primary or secondary amenorrhea is to correct the underlying condition that caused it, if possible. When this is not possible, then contraceptive hormones or cyclic progesterone may be used to induce menstruation.

Prognosis

The prognosis of amenorrhea is excellent when the underlying cause is corrected or if cyclic hormones are used to induce menses.

Prevention

Management of weight, proper nutrition, and reducing stress can help prevent amenorrhea.

Patient Teaching

Reinforce any medical regimen as prescribed, and review any adverse effects of hormonal therapy that should be reported to the physician.

Dysmenorrhea

Description

Dysmenorrhea, a common gynecologic disorder, is pain and cramping associated with menstruation and affects about 50% of postpubertal women.

ICD-10-CM Code	N94.6 *(Dysmenorrhea, unspecified)*
	(N94.4-N94.6 = 3 codes of specificity)

Symptoms and Signs

Dysmenorrhea is pain or cramping that begins either shortly before or shortly after the onset of the menstrual flow. Primary dysmenorrhea describes the onset with the initiation of menses, and secondary dysmenorrhea occurs later, after years of normal nonpainful menses. The discomfort can be located just in the uterine area or diffusely throughout the lower pelvis and back, and with occasional radiation to the thighs or buttocks. Painful bowel or bladder function may be experienced. The symptoms normally lessen and abate by the end of menstruation.

Patient Screening

Severe pain associated with menstruation can result in loss of time at work or inability to perform usual daily activities. An appointment should be scheduled for an initial evaluation to diagnose the cause and select the proper management.

Etiology

In primary dysmenorrhea, the cause is thought to be the underlying muscular structure of the uterus and how it reacts to the various chemicals produced during the cycle. Secondary dysmenorrhea is more likely to be caused by an underlying disorder or disease condition, including pelvic infections, fibroids, cervical stenosis, but most commonly by endometriosis.

Diagnosis

The diagnosis is made from patient history. Medical causes of dysmenorrhea should be eliminated first. The etiology may be determined from careful history and physical examination, pelvic ultrasonography, and even diagnostic laparoscopy. In some cases, psychiatric evaluation may be indicated.

Treatment

Nonsteroidal antiinflammatory drugs (NSAIDs), whether prescription or over-the-counter, and hormonal birth control are generally beneficial for pain relief. Using a heating pad on the abdomen also may help. If an underlying organic reason that is causing the pain is found, then that disease process is treated. For endometriosis, birth control pills, progestins, gonadotropin-releasing hormone (GnRH) analogues, and surgery may all be used to alleviate pain. Fibroids may be removed surgically or reduced in size with high-frequency ultrasound ablation or embolization. Newer techniques, such as laparoscope-guided fibroid diathermy,

are just becoming available for the right patient. Progesterone receptor antagonists have also shown promise in clinical studies and may soon be available to manage fibroids.

Prognosis

The prognosis for dysmenorrhea is good when the underlying causes are corrected. Even when a cause is not found, the response to NSAIDs and birth control pills is excellent. Primary dysmenorrhea often improves after childbirth.

Prevention

The initial occurrence of dysmenorrhea cannot be prevented; however, if menses are eliminated, then recurring dysmenorrhea can be eliminated.

Patient Teaching

Comfort measures are individualized in mild cases. Help the patient understand the use of analgesics or hormonal contraceptives. When surgery is required, provide preoperative and postoperative counseling.

Ovarian Cysts

Description

Ovarian cysts are fluid-filled, semisolid, or solid masses that originate on or within the ovary. Follicles that occur during a normal menstrual cycle are often called *cysts* during radiologic evaluation, but it is best to think of them as follicles unless they are outside the physiologic norm in size or appearance (Fig. 12.14).

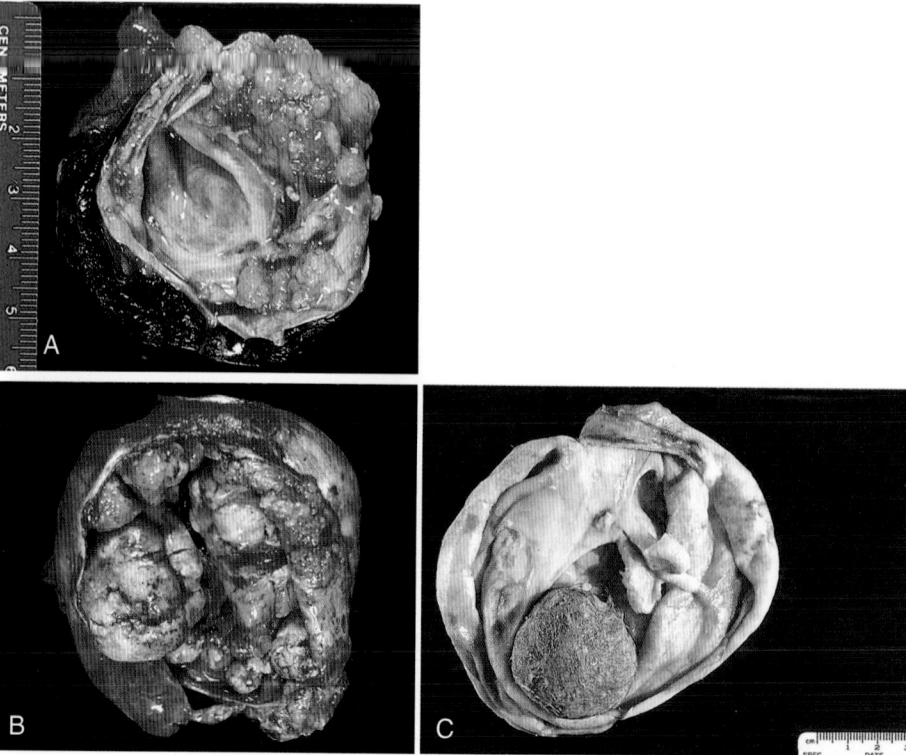

• **Fig. 12.14** (A, B) Ovarian serous tumors. (C) Dermoid cyst of the ovary. (Courtesy Dr. Christopher Crum, Brigham and Women's Hospital, Boston, Massachusetts.)

ICD-10-CM Code   N83.20 *(Unspecified ovarian cysts)*
         N83.29 *(Other ovarian cysts)*

Refer to the physician's diagnosis and then to the current edition of the ICD-10-CM coding manual to ensure the greatest specificity of pathology.

Symptoms and Signs

Most small cysts will go unnoticed by the patient. The size at which a cyst becomes symptomatic depends on many factors, including how quickly it develops, the underlying cause, and association with adjacent structures or other intrapelvic pathology. Rarely, urinary retention can result when a large cyst presses on the area near the bladder. If the cyst produces hormones, then it can affect the body functions associated with those hormones. Larger cysts can undergo a process known as *torsion* or *twisting*, which can cause pain, nausea, and vomiting. Torsion is resolved with surgery and occasionally removal of the ovary. Torsion of the ovary can be as serious as torsion of the testicle.

Patient Screening

The pain and other symptoms associated with an ovarian cyst, or possible complications, prompt the call for medical intervention.

Etiology

There are two basic types of ovarian cysts: physiologic cysts (those caused by normal functioning of the ovary) and neoplastic cysts. Neoplastic cysts are either benign or malignant. Occasionally cancer from other parts of the body metastasizes to the ovary. Most ovarian cysts are physiologic, resulting from ovarian follicle growth or a corpus luteum that persists too long. Cysts that occur in a postmenopausal woman and those greater than 10 cm in size are more concerning with regard to possible malignancy. The cause of malignant or benign ovarian tumors is not certain.

Diagnosis

A pelvic mass may be noted during a pelvic or rectal examination. Ultrasonography is the best way to assess the presence and nature of ovarian cysts. Magnetic resonance imaging (MRI) or CT can also help detect cysts. Laparoscopy with direct vision of the ovaries may be appropriate if a cyst must be removed.

Treatment

Benign physiologic cysts are common, and small cysts seldom require any treatment. Large cysts sometimes can be drained during laparoscopy or even removed. This often can be performed without affecting the ovary. Cysts that are drained are more likely to recur than those that are removed. Small physiologic cysts usually disappear spontaneously. Birth control pills were once believed to help cysts resolve; however, their effectiveness has recently been called into question. Cysts that are cancerous require surgery, often with removal of the uterus, omentum, appendix, and lymph nodes.

Prognosis

For nonmalignant cysts, the outcomes are generally excellent. For cysts related to endometriosis, the outcome depends on the success of treating the endometriosis, and these cysts have a high percentage of recurrence. In the case of cancerous cysts, the prognosis depends on the stage of the disease and origin of the tumor's cell line and degree of cellular abnormality.

Prevention

No prevention is known, although taking birth control pills may reduce the occurrence of physiologic cysts.

Patient Teaching

Explain the nature of the cyst. Encourage the patient to use the analgesic medication, as prescribed, for comfort. Offer appropriate assurance about the prognosis. Give preoperative and postoperative instructions when surgery is scheduled.

ENRICHMENT

Mittelschmerz

Mittelschmerz is the term used to refer to unilateral pain occurring in the region of an ovary during ovulation, usually midway through the menstrual cycle. This dull pain has a duration of a few minutes to a few hours and can indicate the time of ovulation for couples attempting to conceive.

Although the etiology is unknown, leakage of follicular fluid into the abdomen during ovulation or stretching and rupturing of the ovarian cortex may be the cause. The pain occasionally is severe enough for the woman to seek medical care. A history of occurrence at the midpoint of the menstrual cycle and the elimination of other pelvic or abdominal causes lead to the diagnosis of mittelschmerz. Mild analgesics provide pain relief.

Endometriosis

Description

Endometriosis is a chronic condition characterized by extrauterine endometrial tissue. The implants of endometrium are found most commonly in the pelvis but may occur in distant sites (Fig. 12.15).

ICD-10-CM Code   N80.9 *(Endometriosis, unspecified)*
         (N80.0-N80.9 = 9 codes of specified)

Endometriosis may be coded by site and the pathology. Refer to the physician's diagnosis and then to the current edition of the ICD-10-CM coding manual to ensure the greatest specificity of pathology.

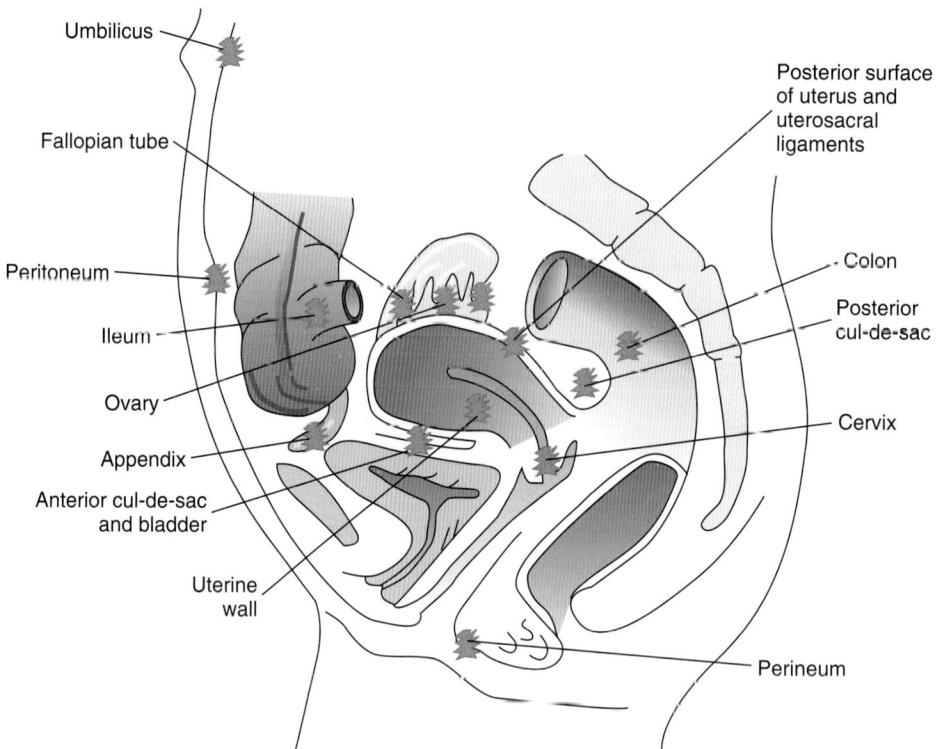

- **Fig. 12.15** Endometriosis (ectopic sites). (From Gould BE, Dyer RM: *Pathophysiology for the health professions,* ed 4, St Louis, 2012, Saunders.)

Symptoms and Signs

Although endometriosis is considered a benign condition, it can be acute or chronic. Secondary dysmenorrhea is a classic symptom. Painful intercourse, painful defecation, and even infertility can be related to this disease. The cyclical inflammation and scarring eventually can lead to symptoms even when a woman is not menstruating. Complications include infertility, ectopic pregnancy, pelvic scarring, and adhesion formation.

Patient Screening

When a patient has progressively painful menstruation, a pelvic examination should be scheduled. Infertility may be the only complaint in some patients.

Etiology

There are differing theories regarding the cause of endometriosis. Retrograde menstruation is believed to be the most likely cause for most cases of this condition. When functioning endometrial tissue grows outside the uterine cavity, it responds to the ovarian hormones as the endometrium (lining of the uterus) does during the normal menstrual cycle. The cyclic swelling, inflammation, bleeding, and subsequent scarring are the reasons for the pain. Risk factors include a family history of the disease, menstrual cycles being shorter than 28 days or lasting longer than 7 days, and uterine structural abnormalities that interfere with the normal flow of menstrual blood out of the uterus. Fibroids and diseases of the immune system, such as systemic lupus erythematosus (SLE), have also been associated with an increased incidence of endometriosis.

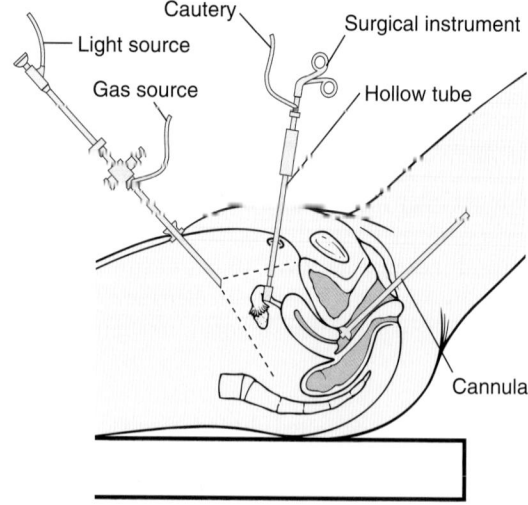

- **Fig. 12.16** Laparoscopy.

Diagnosis

During the pelvic examination, the physician may be able to detect tender areas, nodules, or even thickened scar tissue. Enlarged ovaries may represent endometriomas, and a retroflexed uterus may be scarred and immobile. Good history and physical examination, combined with ultrasonography, can help accurately diagnose advanced endometriosis in the majority of patients. Laparoscopy may be used to confirm the diagnosis and help stage the extent of disease (Fig. 12.16). Treatment can then be tailored to the woman's needs depending on her age, general health, and severity of symptoms.

Treatment

Conservative treatment with various hormones is indicated for younger patients who wish to have children. Hormonal contraception, GnRH analogues, and progestin-releasing intrauterine devices (IUDs; Fig. 12.17) or subdermal progestin-releasing implants can all be used to manage the symptoms associated with this disease. Danazol (a testosterone derivative) is rarely used because of the high frequency of unacceptable side effects. Another alternative is the use of aromatase inhibitors. Although these agents are normally used for the treatment of breast cancer, they can decrease the conversion of other hormones to estrogen. Blocking estrogen may prevent the endometriosis from growing. Surgery can remove endometrial implants, deep nodules, and adhesions. Although there is no cure, pregnancy, breastfeeding, or menopause may bring remission of symptoms because the aberrant tissue tends to shrink under these conditions. Surgery can be used to remove or destroy endometrial growths. In severe cases, a total hysterectomy with bilateral salpingo-oophorectomy may be indicated.

Prognosis

Although no cure for endometriosis is known, a variety of treatment options are available. Generally the prognosis is good.

Prevention

The mechanisms that cause the disease are not clear, so no effective prevention is known. Eliminating menstruation may help reduce disease recurrence.

Patient Teaching

Review with the patient the issues surrounding the disease and inform her that it can progress or even regress over time. Discuss treatment options and the importance of adherence to prescribed treatments.

Pelvic Inflammatory Disease

Description

PID is infection of a woman's pelvis. The tubes, ovaries, and surrounding tissue are involved in the infection, which can be self-limiting or, in cases of abscess formation, life threatening (Fig. 12.18).

ICD-10-CM Code	N73.9 *(Female pelvic inflammatory disease, unspecified)* (N73.8-N74 = 3 codes of specificity)

Symptoms and Signs

The infection is most common in young sexually active women, especially those with more than one sexual partner. Initially, the patient may experience low abdominal pain. Other symptoms are those of an active infection: fever, chills, malaise, a foul-smelling vaginal discharge, backache, and a painful, tender abdomen. Often even walking is painful, and the patient may walk with a shuffling gait. If an abscess has developed, a soft, tender pelvic mass may be palpated. The WBC count and the erythrocyte sediment rate (ESR) are usually elevated.

Patient Screening

The patient with PID reports constitutional symptoms and pain. When symptoms are severe, arrange for immediate medical intervention.

Etiology

The initial infection usually is an STI (e.g., gonorrhea, chlamydia), but then the etiology becomes multibacterial, with involvement of both aerobic and anaerobic organisms.

Diagnosis

The pelvic examination demonstrates tenderness, usually bilaterally. Most commonly, the cervix is tender to manipulation or movement. Cervical cultures may or may not be positive for an STI. Ultrasonography can help rule out abscess formation. Fever, elevated WBC count, and physical examination usually are sufficient to make the diagnosis and begin treatment. Sometimes the symptoms or signs are not clear; in that case, laparoscopy can be helpful in confirming the diagnosis.

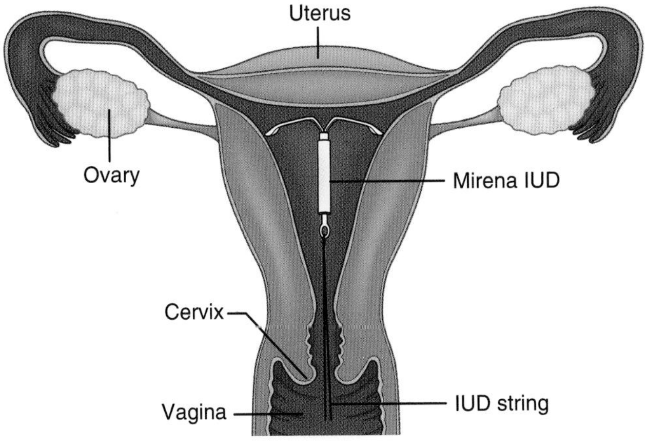

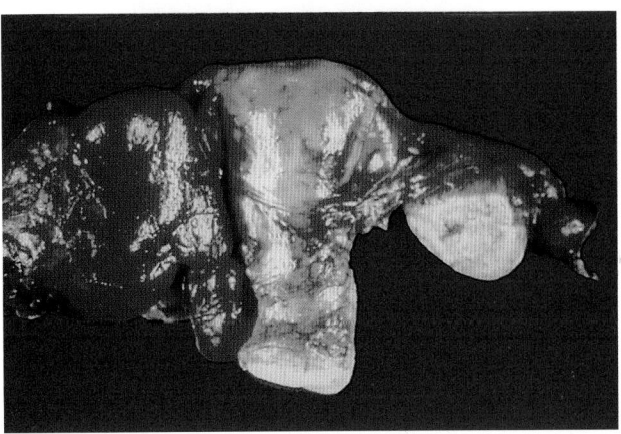

• **Fig. 12.17** Mirena IUD. (From Proctor D, et al: *Kinn's the medical assistant,* ed 13, St. Louis, 2017, Elsevier.)

• **Fig. 12.18** Pelvic inflammatory disease. (From Kumar V, et al: *Robbins basic pathology,* ed 10, St. Louis, 2018, Elsevier.)

Treatment

Early diagnosis and prompt treatment lessen the damage to the reproductive system. Treatment consists of antibiotics given either intravenously or orally, depending on the severity of the infection. The inflammation of the female reproductive organs can cause scar tissue (adhesions) to form. If adhesions form in or around the fallopian tubes, they can cause infertility or increase the risk of ectopic pregnancy.

Prognosis

Without effective treatment, serious complications may develop. Peritonitis can spread the infection throughout the abdominal cavity, or if the infection becomes bloodborne, septicemia and even death may result. Recurrent or severe PID can cause scarring of the fallopian tubes, obstruction, and infertility. Early and aggressive therapy can improve the prognosis.

Prevention

The best prevention of PID is to not acquire an STI. Condom use and reducing the number of sexual partners both help. Douching has also been associated with an increase in PID.

Patient Teaching

Inform the patient that infection typically begins intravaginally and ascends through the entire genital tract. Review all risk factors. Sexually active women with multiple partners should be told that PID is frequently associated with STIs. Insertion of an IUD is also a risk factor.

Uterine Leiomyomas (Fibroids)

Description

Leiomyomas (fibroids) are noncancerous (benign) tumors of the smooth muscle within the uterus. They may vary in number, size, and location within the uterus. They are the most common tumors of the female reproductive tract and can occur in up to 40% of women before menopause (Fig. 12.19).

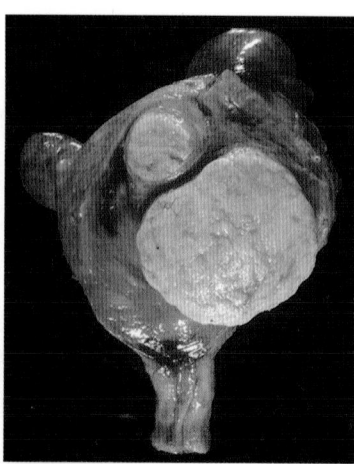

• **Fig. 12.19** Leiomyomas. (From Cotran RS, Kumar V, Collins T: *Robbins pathologic basis of disease,* ed 6, Philadelphia, 1999, Saunders.)

ICD-10-CM Code	D25.9 *(Leiomyoma of uterus, unspecified)*
	(D25.0-D25.9 = 4 codes of specificity)

Leiomyomas are coded according to site. Refer to the physician's diagnosis and then to the current edition of the ICD-10-CM coding manual to ensure the greatest specificity of pathology.

Symptoms and Signs

Most fibroids are asymptomatic. If symptoms do occur, they may include pelvic pain, pressure, constipation, urinary frequency, abnormal bleeding, and heavy or prolonged periods. The latter symptom is the most common. The severity of symptoms is related to the number, size, and location of the tumors.

Patient Screening

Schedule a gynecologic examination and medical consultation for a woman experiencing the symptoms mentioned previously. Ask the woman if she is pregnant or could be pregnant.

Etiology

The cause of leiomyomas and fibroids is unknown. Their development is stimulated by estrogen, and they typically regress after menopause. Birth control pills and hormone replacement therapy do not appear to have much of an impact on the growth or size of fibroids.

Diagnosis

The diagnosis is based on pelvic examination and patient history. Definitive diagnosis is based on ultrasonography and tissue biopsy.

Treatment

Treatment generally depends on the severity of the symptoms, the patient's age, and her desire to have children. In women of childbearing age, surgery can be performed to remove the tumors. In the woman who does not want to have children, MRI-guided high-frequency ultrasound ablation may be useful. Uterine artery embolization, once considered useful only in women who are through with childbearing, may be finding a niche in women who want to have children. Hysterectomy is the only definitive treatment because fibroids can recur after other procedures. The route of hysterectomy depends on many factors; however, modern techniques allow for many women to undergo the surgery as an outpatient.

Prognosis

In general, fibroids do not need to be removed. The rate of malignancy within a fibroid is about 0.27%. In cases where they are removed, there is a 10% to 50% recurrence rate. The risk of recurrence is greater when multiple fibroids are present. With removal of the uterus, there is essentially no risk of recurrence.

Prevention

No method for the prevention of leiomyomas is known.

Patient Teaching

Teach the patient about the signs of complications, such as hemorrhage or sudden onset of pain and fever.

Vaginitis

Description

Vaginitis is inflammation and/or infection of the vaginal tissues.

ICD-10-CM Code	N76.0 *(Acute vaginitis)*
	N76.1 *(Subacute and chronic vaginitis)*
	N76.2 *(Acute vulvitis)*
	N76.3 *(Subacute and chronic vulvitis)*

Refer to the physician's diagnosis and then to the current edition of the ICD-10-CM coding manual for an additional code to identify the causative organism.

Symptoms and Signs

Inflammation of the vagina is common, and all age groups are at risk. It is generally not perilous, but it can be irritating and painful. Vaginal discharge, with local itching, burning, and odor is the principal symptom. Depending on the causative agent, the discharge may be white, gray, or green, almost absent to copious, and odorless or malodorous. The discharge may cause irritation and soreness of the vulva. Fever may be present.

Patient Screening

The discomfort and irritation secondary to vaginal infection prompt the earliest possible appointment for a pelvic examination, diagnosis, and treatment.

Etiology

Fungal infections are the most common cause of vaginitis. Other causes may include bacterial overgrowth when the balance of "good" and "bad" bacteria normally found in the vagina is affected. Another infection is caused by a protozoan called *Trichomonas*. Cervical infections in chlamydia or gonorrhea can produce a discharge that is irritating and may be mistaken for vaginitis. In postmenopausal women, the absence of estrogen can cause thinning of the vaginal lining and alterations in the normal flora, leading to increased susceptibility to infections. This condition is referred to as *atrophic vaginitis*.

Diagnosis

After taking the medical history, the physician performs a pelvic examination and swabs the vagina. Specimens from the vagina and cervix are analyzed for the presence of bacteria and fungus, and the pH of the discharge is assessed. The discharge can also be assessed for odor. Specifically, *Gardnerella* infection causes a strong "fishy" odor. If the diagnosis is in doubt, a specimen can be sent to the laboratory for culture.

Treatment

Depending on the results of culture and wet preparation examination, treatment may consist of an antifungal, antibacterial, or hormone therapy (in the case of atrophic vaginitis). More specifically, appropriate treatment for bacterial vaginosis would be metronidazole or clindamycin (oral or vaginal). Yeast infections may be treated with miconazole, clotrimazole (vaginally), or fluconazole (orally). Trichomoniasis may be treated with metronidazole or tinidazole. Patients taking metronidazole or tinidazole are cautioned not to consume any alcohol-based products in any form.

Prognosis

With proper treatment, the inflammation usually clears up in about a week. However, vaginitis may be a recurring problem in some women.

Prevention

Preventive measures are directed toward known causes, avoidance of STDs, maintenance of good hygiene, avoidance of known chemical irritants, and recognition of risk factors for postmenopausal women. Douching interrupts the normal pH of the vagina and may contribute to *Gardnerella* infection.

Patient Teaching

Give information to the patient according to the determined etiology. Emphasize the importance of complying with the prescribed antibiotic therapy exactly as directed after the infection has been identified. Review the risk factors for STDs, if appropriate. Advise the patient to avoid mechanical or chemical irritants, which may be found in douches, deodorant sprays, spermicides, latex condoms, detergents, or bubble bath products. Tight, nonporous underclothing and poor personal hygiene can promote bacterial growth. The use of a nonirritating vaginal lubricant during intercourse may help the postmenopausal woman.

Toxic Shock Syndrome

Description

Toxic shock syndrome (TSS) is an acute, systemic infection with *Staphylococcus aureus* or streptococcal toxic-like syndrome. The condition occurs in young, healthy persons age 20 to 50 years.

ICD-10-CM Code	A48.3 *(Toxic shock syndrome)*

Refer to the physician's diagnosis and then to the current edition of the ICD-10-CM coding manual for an additional code to identify the bacterial agent.

Symptoms and Signs

The sudden onset is characterized by high fever, headache, sore throat, and a rash. The syndrome progresses rapidly to hypotension and shock. Other symptoms and signs that the patient might experience are gastrointestinal (GI) symptoms, diarrhea, neuromuscular disturbances, abnormal kidney function, and an elevation of the liver enzyme levels. Without treatment, the disease may become life threatening.

Patient Screening

Immediate medical treatment is indicated.

Etiology

The cause of TSS is thought to be an increase in *S. aureus* colonization on superabsorbent tampons. The toxins produced by the bacteria create the illness. The initial infections were primarily associated with a single brand of tampons, which have since been removed from the market. TSS can also occur in women using contraceptive sponges or even diaphragms.

Diagnosis

A diagnosis of TSS is based on clinical evaluation and laboratory tests. The CDC has listed specific diagnostic criteria for TSS.

Treatment

Therapy for TSS is supportive and includes replacement of fluids to counteract shock and the use of antibiotics to treat the infection. Currently, physicians are treating staphylococcal toxic shock with IV vancomycin to cover methicillin-resistant *Staphylococcus aureus* (MRSA). If treatment is delayed, death can result from overwhelming shock.

> **NOTE**
>
> Use of universal precautions against all body secretions is necessary.

Prognosis

Prompt diagnosis followed by antibiotic treatment offers the best prognosis. However, TSS can result in neurologic, renal, and respiratory complications and death.

Prevention

Although the synthetic fiber composition of tampons has changed, physicians advise women to use tampons that are just absorbent enough to handle their menstrual flow and to avoid the superabsorbent type. Tampons are best used during the daytime and should be changed frequently. Storing tampons in a cool, dry area also helps avoid creating an environment prone for bacterial growth.

Patient Teaching

Review the preventive measures mentioned previously and other advice given by the health care provider. Explain the importance of taking the entire course of antibiotics as prescribed.

Menopause

Description

Menopause (change of life, or *climacteric*) is the cessation of menstrual periods for 1 year, with evidence of ovarian failure. The average age of menopause is between ages 50 and 51 years, and it is not considered premature unless it occurs before age 40 years.

ICD-10-CM Code   N95.1 *(Menopausal and female climacteric states)*
(N95.0-N95.9 = 5 codes of specificity)

Symptoms and Signs

Many women experience the onset of menopause between ages 45 and 55 years. Fluctuation in the menstrual cycle and flow is noted, with periods often becoming lighter and less frequent. Hot flashes and night sweats often are reported as a mild to intolerable nuisance in about 30% of women going into menopause; vaginal dryness and skin changes may appear. Many women experience transient to troublesome psychological symptoms, including depression, poor memory, anxiety, sleep disorders, and loss of interest in sex. By definition, women who are still menstruating but having symptoms of menopause are not menopausal. They are more properly classified as perimenopausal. Once they have stopped menstruating, then they are considered menopausal.

Patient Screening

Schedule a medical examination and consultation with the physician. Inform the patient that a pelvic examination may be required.

Etiology

Starting as early as age 30 years, changes occur in the ovarian production of certain hormones. This creates alterations in the pituitary levels of follicle-stimulating hormone (FSH), driving the failing ovary to produce more follicles. This altered balance between ovarian estrogen, follicle generation, and pituitary level of FSH leads to fluctuations in the menstrual cycle hormones. These changes create the symptoms that women experience as they approach menopause. Once the ovarian reserve has been exhausted and the ovary can no longer produce viable eggs, then ovulation halts and menstruation ceases. Chemotherapy or radiation treatment for certain cancers can also bring on menopause. Surgical menopause (i.e., a total hysterectomy) is a sudden event and may be associated with an increase in hot flashes and nuisance symptoms compared with natural menopause, if not treated with hormones.

Diagnosis

Patient history suggests menopause. The blood serum levels of FSH are elevated, and the estrogen levels are low.

Treatment

The treatment of menopause is really the management of the symptoms related to the condition. Hot flashes and other symptoms related to estrogen withdrawal may be managed with estrogen products or a low-dose selective serotonin reuptake inhibitor (SSRI) (paroxetine mesylate [Brisdelle]). Because there is ongoing debate regarding the potential for cancer with hormone treatment, the patient should be involved in the final decision regarding whether or not to use hormones. Estrogen may not be recommended for long-term use in all patients. Vaginal changes can be managed with local estrogen products and lubricants or the newer selective estrogen receptor modulator (SERM) ospemifene (Osphena). Bone loss can be effectively treated with bisphosphonates alendronate (Fosamax), risedronate (Actonel), ibandronate (Boniva), SERMs (raloxifene [Evista]), or salmon calcitonin. With very low bone density, other agents, such as denosumab (Prolia, a rank ligand inhibitor) or teriparatide (Forteo, a synthetic parathyroid hormone), may be required. Weight-bearing exercise and dietary calcium or calcium supplementation with adequate vitamin D_3 can also help reduce the rate of bone loss in sedentary patients or those with poor calcium intake and low vitamin D levels.

Prognosis

Menopause is a normal condition with a variable course. Cigarette smokers experience menopause about 2 years earlier compared with nonsmokers.

Prevention

Menopause cannot be prevented. Patients who have a total hysterectomy experience menopause after surgery as a result of removal of the ovaries.

Patient Teaching

Give the patient informative brochures about menopause, the pros and cons of hormone replacement therapy, and alternatives to hormone replacement therapy. Encourage questions about symptoms being experienced. Recommend a healthy lifestyle as the first line of defense against changes related to aging.

Uterine Prolapse

Description

Prolapse of the uterus is the downward displacement of the uterus from its normal location in the pelvis.

ICD-10-CM Code	N81.2 (Incomplete uterovaginal prolapse) (N81.2-N81.4 = 3 codes of specificity)

Symptoms and Signs

Most patients with mild degrees of prolapse have no symptoms. On occasion, the patient may feel increased vaginal or pelvic pressure as the uterus descends into the vagina. When the prolapse is at the point where the cervix is exiting the vagina, the woman may feel it while wiping herself after urination. Sometimes the prolapsed uterus can cause pain during intercourse or generalized pelvic discomfort.

Patient Screening

Schedule a routine appointment and a pelvic examination for the patient.

Etiology

Uterine prolapse occurs when the normal support of the uterus weakens as a result of trauma (childbirth), aging, or genetic factors. The weakening of these supports allows the uterus to move down the vaginal canal, pulling the vagina with it (the cervix is attached along with it). When the uterus is completely outside the vagina, it is termed *complete procidentia* (Fig. 12.20). If it is less than complete, then it is graded on the basis of the distance that it has traveled down the vagina in comparison with the normal anatomic position in relation to the introitus (opening of the vagina).

Diagnosis

The prolapse is visible on pelvic examination. It helps to have the patient stand or, more commonly, perform the Valsalva maneuver or cough to elicit the prolapse.

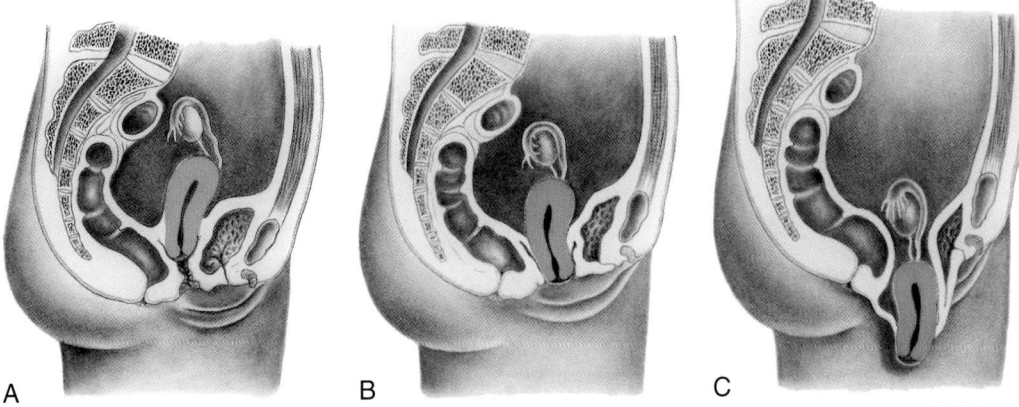

• **Fig. 12.20** Uterine Prolapse. (A) First degree. (B) Second degree. (C) Complete prolapse. (From Seidel HM, et al: *Mosby's guide to physical examination,* ed 8, St Louis, 2014, Mosby.)

Treatment

There is no way to have the prolapse reverse itself once it has occurred. Losing weight, reduction of coughing, correction of constipation by using the Valsalva maneuver, or targeted physical therapy can help slow down the progression of the process. The use of a pessary may help alleviate some of the symptoms of prolapse, but it does not correct the problem. This device is inserted into the vagina to support the uterus and prevents it from prolapsing. Surgery is the only way to correct prolapse. In women who no longer need the uterus, a hysterectomy is commonly performed, with or without reattaching the vaginal apex to the sacrum or to the sacrospinous ligaments.

Prognosis

The prognosis is good even if surgery is required.

Prevention

Exercises that strengthen the muscles of the pelvic floor after childbirth are recommended. Smoking cessation to reduce coughing and high-fiber diets with adequate fluid intake to reduce constipation can help.

Patient Teaching

Review the anatomy and nature of the condition, and make sure the patient understands how to perform Kegel exercises. If applicable, answer questions about surgical correction of the condition.

Cystocele

Description

Cystocele is the downward displacement and protrusion of the urinary bladder into the anterior wall of the vagina (Fig. 12.21).

ICD-10-CM Code	N81.9 *(Female genital prolapse, unspecified)* (N81.10-N81.12 = 3 codes of specificity)

Symptoms and Signs

This disorder causes the female patient to experience pelvic pressure. It may cause bladder symptoms, such as urinary leakage, urgency, or discomfort during intercourse. In severe cases with urethral or bladder neck kinking, the bladder cannot be emptied completely. This can cause overdistension of the bladder with resultant nerve and/or muscle damage or increased incidence of bladder infections.

Patient Screening

Schedule a routine appointment and a pelvic examination for the patient. Symptoms of cystitis, such as painful and frequent urination, may require an earlier appointment.

Etiology

This condition results from trauma to the fascia, muscle, and pelvic support structures during pregnancy and delivery or from atrophy of these structures as a result of aging and genetic predisposition.

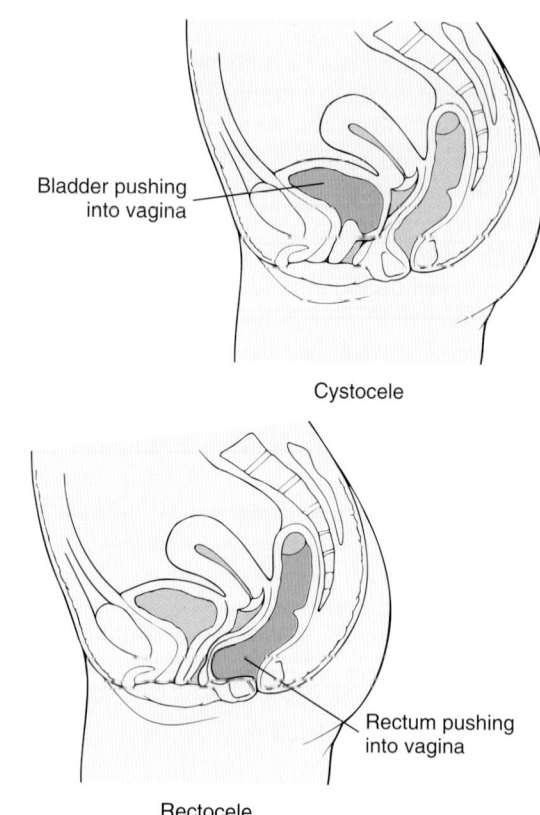

Cystocele

Rectocele

• **Fig. 12.21** Cystocele and rectocele.

Diagnosis

Diagnosis is based on the clinical picture and findings of the physical examination.

Treatment

The treatment options for cystocele are the same as those for uterine prolapse. Symptoms of incontinence may be improved by performing Kegel exercises; however, surgery or pessary insertion are the current methods of treatment. Surgery to return the bladder to its normal position may be done with or without applying surgical mesh. Each type of mesh carries its own benefits and risks. A candid discussion of these risks and benefits is necessary before surgical intervention.

Prognosis

The prognosis is good.

Prevention

Exercises that strengthen the pelvic floor muscles after childbirth may help. The tissue changes associated with aging cannot be prevented. Avoiding traumatic vaginal delivery may also help reduce the incidence of this condition.

Patient Teaching

Review the prescribed exercises. Give preoperative and postoperative instructions to candidates for colporrhaphy, a surgical procedure that involves suturing of the vagina to narrow it.

Rectocele

Description
A rectocele is the protrusion of the rectum into the posterior wall of the vagina.

| ICD-10-CM Code | N81.6 (Rectocele) |

Symptoms and Signs
The rectocele causes the female patient to experience a bearing-down feeling, fullness in the vagina, back pain, pelvic pressure, and difficulty evacuating the rectum (see Fig. 12.21).

Patient Screening
Schedule a routine appointment and a pelvic examination as soon as possible.

Etiology
Similar to a cystocele, a rectocele occurs when the posterior wall of the vagina is weakened, allowing protrusion of the rectum into the vagina. This most commonly occurs as a result of childbirth, aging, or genetic predisposition.

Diagnosis
Diagnosis is based on the clinical picture and the findings of the physical examination.

Treatment
Treatment consists of surgical repair of the posterior wall of the vagina (posterior colporrhaphy). A pessary can also be used if surgery is not desired.

Prognosis
The prognosis is good with surgical repair.

Prevention
No prevention is known. Reduction in coughing and in constipation may help decrease the severity or delay onset in predisposed patients.

Patient Teaching
Give the patient appropriate preoperative and postoperative instructions. Anticipate questions, and reassure the patient concerned about how the procedure may affect sexual intercourse.

Cervical Cancer

Description
The cervix is the lower part of the uterus, extending from the uterine isthmus into the vagina. It functions to allow sperm into the uterine cavity and the infant to pass into the birth canal. Most cervical cancers are either squamous cell carcinomas that arise in the transitional zone between the different epithelial types of the uterus corpus and the vagina or adenocarcinoma (Fig. 12.22).

| ICD-10-CM Code | C53.9 (Malignant neoplasm of cervix uteri, unspecified) |
| | (C53.0-C53.9 = 4 codes of specificity) |

Symptoms and Signs
The two main symptoms of cervical cancer are (1) a watery, bloody, or purulent vaginal discharge that may be heavy and foul smelling and (2) bleeding between menstrual periods, after intercourse, or after menopause. The most common sign is the abnormal Pap smear test result. The appearance of the cervical lesion varies, but it is often a mass or an ulcer on the surface of the cervix. Signs and symptoms of advanced disease include pelvic or lower back pain, hematuria, dysuria, or rectal bleeding.

Patient Screening
Encourage women to have regular screening with cervical Pap smear tests. Schedule a gynecologic examination for the female experiencing abnormal vaginal bleeding, prolonged or intermittent periods, or bleeding after intercourse.

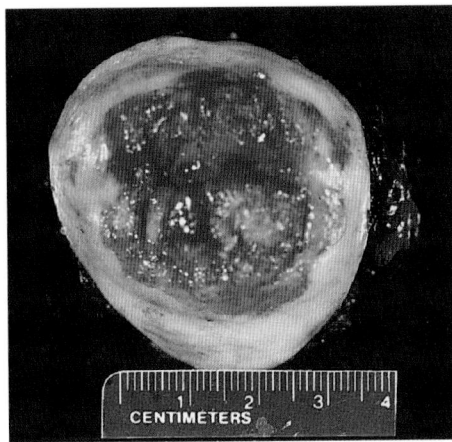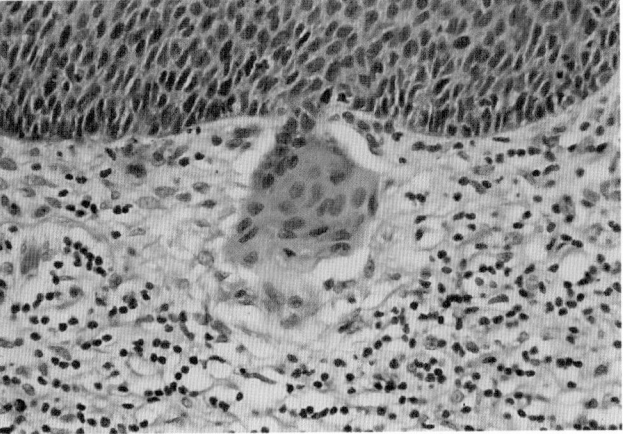

• **Fig. 12.22** Cancer of the cervix. (From Cotran RS, Kumar V, Collins T: *Robbins pathologic basis of disease,* ed 6, Philadelphia, 1999, Saunders.)

Etiology

Invasive cervical cancer is often considered a preventable disease because it has a long premalignant stage (often 10 years or longer) and an effective screening program and effective therapies. Therefore the biggest risk factor for invasive cervical carcinoma is lack of regular screening with cervical Pap smear tests. The other major risk factor is exposure to oncogenic types of HPV, such as HPV-16, -18, -31, and -45. Infections by these HPV types are more common in individuals who have had early and frequent unprotected sexual activity with multiple partners. HPV DNA is detected in nearly all invasive cervical cancers. HPV infection is often found with other risk factors, such as smoking, immunosuppression, low socioeconomic status, early and multiple parity, prolonged use of oral contraceptives, and/or other STDs. The most common age at diagnosis is 45 to 55 years, but it is also a significant problem in women older than 65 years of age, who are less likely to undergo Pap smear tests. The premalignant lesion for cervical cancer is called *cervical intraepithelial neoplasia* (CIN), and it involves dysplasia or atypical changes in the cervical epithelium.

Diagnosis

The Pap smear test was developed specifically to detect cervical cancer. By obtaining scrapings from the cervix and cervical os and examining them microscopically, cellular abnormalities can be detected. HPV testing is often done to detect the oncogenic types of HPV. The diagnosis of cancer is then confirmed through colposcopy and directed biopsy of the cervical lesion. The stage is determined clinically through physical examination of the patient, chest x-ray, intravenous pyelography (IVP), cystoscopy, and proctoscopy. Lymph node sampling also may be performed. The International Federation of Gynecologists and Obstetricians developed the staging system that is currently used. It differs from the commonly used TNM system in that it relies on clinical evaluation rather than the pathologic features of the tumor. This is because cervical cancer is most common in developing countries where more modern techniques are not available for staging of the tumor. See the Cancer section in Chapter 1 for more information on staging systems used to evaluate malignancy.

Treatment

Treatment is determined by stage. Low-grade CIN is followed with repeat cytology at 6 and 12 months. For high-grade CIN, loop electrosurgical excision procedure (LEEP) is preferred, and other treatments include laser therapy and cryoablation. Radical hysterectomy (removal of the uterus, cervix, and upper vagina) is usually performed to treat CIN in the early invasive stages. For carcinomas that have invaded the pelvic wall or have distant metastases, radiation therapy is included in the treatment. Cisplatin-based chemotherapy often is used in conjunction with radiotherapy. Patients should be followed up with periodic physical examination and Pap smear tests to detect recurrences.

Prognosis

Stage is the most important determinant of prognosis, followed by lymph node status, tumor volume, and depth of tumor invasion. HPV subtype also may affect the prognosis, with HPV-18 having a poorer prognosis compared with the other subtypes. The 5-year survival rate ranges from 98% for women at stage IA1 to 9% for those at stage IVB. Recurrence is usually local (e.g., cervix, uterus, and/or vagina) and carries a very poor prognosis.

Prevention

Primary prevention of cervical cancer can be achieved through vaccination with one of the two FDA-approved vaccines against HPV (see the Enrichment box about Human Papillomavirus Vaccine and Cervical Cancer). Regardless of vaccination history, however, all sexually active women should undergo an annual Pap smear test and pelvic examination starting 3 years after the first sexual intercourse or at age 21 years, whichever comes first. After three or more consecutive normal Pap smear test results or after age 30 years, screening can be performed less often, at the discretion of the physician, but should be done at least every 3 years. HPV testing can be performed at the same time as the Pap smear test to detect infection by high-risk subtypes of HPV. Women with a Pap smear test result suggesting CIN should be evaluated with colposcopy and biopsy of any lesion detected. For women with no risk factors and at least three normal smear test results, screening can cease around age 65 or 70 years. Unfortunately often screening programs are lacking in developing countries. Other risk-reducing methods include use of barrier contraception, limiting the number of sexual partners, and smoking cessation.

Patient Teaching

Emphasize that with early diagnosis, the survival rate for cervical cancer is excellent. Review the recommendations listed under Prevention section. Women diagnosed with invasive stages of cervical cancer require information about treatment and possible complications. Explain preoperative and postoperative instructions for hysterectomy, radiation therapy, and/or chemotherapy. Encourage the patient to express feelings associated with loss of body image, changes in sexual functioning, and changes in fertility. Provide referral to a support group.

Vaginal Cancer

Description

Primary cancer of the vagina is rare, and malignancy usually results from metastasis from neoplasms of adjacent structures. Most primary tumors are squamous cell carcinomas, but other types, such as melanoma or adenocarcinoma, may be seen.

| ICD-10-CM Code | C52 *(Malignant neoplasm of vagina)* |

Symptoms and Signs

Most patients have vaginal bleeding, usually postcoital or postmenopausal bleeding. Other symptoms include a malodorous or watery vaginal discharge; urinary symptoms, such as dysuria or frequency; constipation; melena; or a vaginal mass. The tumor itself presents as a mass, plaque, or ulcer on the vaginal wall. The posterior wall of the upper one-third of the vagina is the most common site.

Patient Screening

Unusual vaginal bleeding, pelvic pain, or the symptoms mentioned earlier require diagnostic evaluation. Advise the patient that she should be prepared for a gynecologic examination.

Etiology

Risk factors for primary vaginal cancer include HPV infection (particularly subtypes 16 and 18), prior history of gynecologic malignancy, advanced age, multiple lifetime sexual partners, early age at first intercourse, and cigarette smoking. Vaginal intraepithelial neoplasia (VAIN), which comprises atypical squamous cells without invasion, may be a premalignant lesion for vaginal cancer. It is usually asymptomatic but can be associated with postcoital spotting or vaginal discharge.

For squamous cell carcinoma, the average age at diagnosis is 60 years. Adenocarcinomas usually occur in women younger than 20 years of age and have been linked to the synthetic hormone diethylstilbestrol (DES). DES has been used in the past to prevent spontaneous abortions and manage pregnancies in patients with diabetes. The cancer tends to develop in the daughters of mothers who received DES during pregnancy.

Diagnosis

Diagnosis is difficult because the malignant lesion may be small and missed on gynecologic examination. Pap smear tests may reveal malignant cells of the vagina incidentally when screening for cervical cancer. Definitive diagnosis is accomplished through colposcopic examination and direct biopsy of the lesion. Cervical biopsy also must be performed to rule out primary cervical cancer. Carcinomas are staged by means of physical and pelvic examinations, cystoscopy, proctoscopy, chest radiography, and bone scanning. The TNM staging system is used, where T reflects the extent of tumor penetration through the vaginal wall. See Chapter 1 for information about the staging and grading systems used to assess malignant neoplasms.

Treatment

Treatment is based on the location, size, and clinical stage of the tumor. Surgery usually includes hysterectomy, upper vaginectomy, and bilateral pelvic lymphadenectomy and may be performed with adjuvant radiation therapy. Radiotherapy alone may be sufficient to treat early-stage vaginal cancers.

Prognosis

The major indicator of prognosis is stage at the time of diagnosis, although lymph node status, age, and lesion location also are important. Because many vaginal cancers are diagnosed at an advanced stage and because a high percentage of locally advanced cancers recur within 6 months of initial treatment, the overall 5-year survival rate for squamous cell vaginal cancer is around 50%.

Prevention

Undergoing regular screening with Pap smear tests, using barrier contraceptives, and limiting the number of sexual partners may reduce the risk of vaginal cancer. Diagnosis and treatment of VAIN with surgical excision, laser ablation, or topical 5-fluorouracil may prevent progression to invasive disease. Periodic follow-up should be performed to look for recurrent VAIN or invasive disease.

Patient Teaching

Emphasize the importance of early diagnosis and treatment. Enforce the physician's recommendation for a screening schedule based on the patient's history of risk factors. If treatment is required, review with the patient the physician's explanation of procedures and possible complications of therapy. Help the patient with referrals to care and support groups.

Labial or Vulvar Cancer

Description

The vulva is the area of the female external genitalia. Any condition that can affect the skin on other parts of the body can affect the vulva. Greater than 90% of vulvar malignancies are squamous cell carcinomas.

ICD-10-CM Code	C51.0 *(Malignant neoplasm of labium majus)*
	C51.1 *(Malignant neoplasm of labium minus)*
	C51.9 *(Malignant neoplasm of vulva, unspecified)*

Symptoms and Signs

Most patients have a nodule or ulcer, usually on the labia majora. The lesion may be associated with pruritus. Less common symptoms and signs include vulvar bleeding, discharge, dysuria, and enlarged lymph nodes in the groin.

Patient Screening

The patient may complain of a sore or nodule on the labia causing discomfort; schedule a gynecologic examination.

Etiology

Vulvar neoplasms are encountered most often in postmenopausal women. The average age at diagnosis is 65 years. Risk factors include cigarette smoking; HPV (usually subtypes 16 and 33) or HIV infection; multiple sexual partners;

prior history of cervical cancer; and northern European ancestry. Vulvar intraepithelial neoplasia (VIN), which is noninvasive epithelial dysplasia of the vulva, is thought to be a premalignant lesion for invasive carcinoma.

Diagnosis

Diagnosis requires biopsy of the lesion. Colposcopy may be used to define areas for biopsy. After the diagnosis of cancer is confirmed, physical examination for involvement of regional lymph nodes is mandatory. Evaluation also includes colposcopy to assess for multifocal lesions and MRI or positron emission tomography (PET) with CT. A Pap smear test is performed to check for cervical cancer. The tumor is staged surgically, because lymph node involvement is the most important prognostic indicator.

Treatment

The usual treatment of vulvar carcinoma is either surgical removal of the growth and surrounding skin or removal of all or part of the vulva itself. The latter procedure is known as *vulvectomy*. Inguinofemoral lymphadenectomy is usually performed. Depending on the stage of disease, radiation therapy, with or without chemotherapy, is added. Patients with distant metastases or recurrences typically have a poor rate of response. Because of the risk of recurrence, patients should be followed up with periodic gynecologic examinations.

Prognosis

Inguinofemoral lymph node status is the most important indicator of prognosis, regardless of stage. Tumor size and depth of invasion are also important. The overall 5-year survival rate ranges from 25% to greater than 90%, depending on the stage.

Prevention

The risk for vulvar carcinoma is reduced by the use of barrier contraceptives, regular gynecologic examinations, and treatment of VIN with excision, laser therapy, or topical 5-fluorouracil. Close follow-up is necessary after a diagnosis of VIN because of the high risk of recurrence.

Patient Teaching

Inform the patient of the purpose of biopsy and when to expect the results. Explain the medical treatment, when indicated; this may include preoperative and postoperative instructions, the use of analgesics, and the side effects to expect from radiation therapy or chemotherapy. Explain sitz baths, as directed, and the application of sanitary napkins, as needed. Support the patient in the presence of any anxiety or concerns about sexuality and body image. Emphasize the importance of follow-up care.

Ovarian Cancer

Description

Ovarian cancer accounts for more deaths than any other gynecologic malignancy. Because of the location of the ovaries deep within the pelvis, the cancer is often asymptomatic until the more advanced stages.

ICD-10-CM Code	C56.9 *(Malignant neoplasm of unspecified ovary)* (C56.1-C56.9 = 3 codes of specificity)

Symptoms and Signs

Ovarian neoplasms may cause nonspecific symptoms, such as lower abdominal discomfort, bloating, constipation, lower back pain, irregular menstrual cycles, urinary frequency, or dyspareunia. The most common sign is enlargement of the abdomen caused by accumulation of fluid (ascites), but this usually indicates advanced disease. Persistent, vague digestive disturbances (e.g., discomfort, gas, or distention that cannot be explained by any other cause) should be evaluated for ovarian cancer.

Patient Screening

For a woman experiencing the nonspecific symptoms listed previously, schedule a physical examination, including a pelvic examination. Women who are at high risk need regular gynecologic examinations.

Etiology

Most ovarian cancers occur in women older than 40 years of age. The etiology is largely unknown, but multiple risk factors have been identified. Women who have had breast cancer or who have a family history of breast or ovarian cancer have an increased risk. They may have mutations in BRCA1 or BRCA2, the breast cancer susceptibility genes. People with hereditary nonpolyposis colon cancer (HNPCC) also have an increased risk for ovarian cancer. Pregnancy, breastfeeding, prolonged use of oral contraceptives, and tubal ligation may reduce the risk of development of ovarian cancer.

Diagnosis

Early-stage ovarian cancer is sometimes diagnosed on palpation of an abnormal adnexal mass during a routine pelvic examination. Because of the deep anatomic location of the ovary, however, early-stage tumors often are not discovered. The finding of a pelvic mass usually leads to pelvic ultrasonography and the use of serum tumor markers to help distinguish malignant masses from benign masses. If not clinically suggestive of malignancy, the mass should be monitored for 2 months to see whether it resolves. Serum CA-125, a glycoprotein tumor marker that is elevated (> 65 units/mL) in greater than 80% of ovarian cancers, should be measured. Tumors are staged by using the TNM system. The stage is based on surgical evaluation during a surgical diagnostic procedure (usually laparotomy). Therapeutic cytoreduction (surgical reduction of tumor volume) also is performed at this time. Abdominal or pelvic CT may be used to identify distant metastases.

Treatment

Optimal therapy for ovarian cancer is determined by the extent of disease at the time of diagnosis and by the size and location of any residual tumor after the surgical staging procedure. Early stage disease (stages I and II) is treated with surgical removal of the ovaries and fallopian tubes (bilateral salpingo-oophorectomy) and the uterus (hysterectomy), although only one ovary may be removed if the cancer is diagnosed in a very early stage and the woman still wishes to have children. The risk of relapse is reduced by adjuvant chemotherapy with platinum-based compounds. Treatment for advanced disease may also include intraperitoneal chemotherapy. The efficacy of treatment is evaluated through radiography and is indicated by a decline in the serum CA-125 level. Patients should be followed up regularly with physical examinations and CA-125 level measurements to detect recurrent disease.

Prognosis

The overall 5-year survival rate for epithelial ovarian cancer is about 50%, because greater than 75% of cancers have spread beyond the ovary at the time of diagnosis. The stage at diagnosis guides the prognosis, with women diagnosed at stage I having a 5-year survival rate of 89%, and those with metastatic disease having a 5-year survival rate of 18%. Other important factors for a better prognosis include young age, absence of ascites, and low volume of residual disease after surgery. Women with ovarian cancer and *BRCA1* or *BRCA2* mutations often have a more favorable prognosis because of better response to chemotherapy.

Prevention

Periodic pelvic examinations are very important so that ovarian cancer could be detected at an early stage. Screening is recommended only for women with known *BRCA1* or *BRCA2* gene mutations after discussions with their physicians about the benefits and risks of screening. Screening is done with transvaginal ultrasonography and serum CA-125 measurements every 6 to 12 months, beginning at age 30 to 35 years, or 5 to 10 years before the earliest age at the first ovarian cancer diagnosis in the family. Alternatively, women at high risk for ovarian cancer may choose to have prophylactic oophorectomy by age 35 years, although it does not completely eliminate the risk of cancer.

Patient Teaching

Emphasize the importance of regular gynecologic examinations. If a pelvic mass is found, provide a complete explanation of the diagnostic procedures. Explain the presurgical and postsurgical instructions, and explain the terminology particular to the staging and grading of cancer, when appropriate. Refer all questions about the prognosis to the physician. Make referral, as needed, for psychological support.

Endometrial Cancer

Description

Endometrial cancer (also known as *uterine cancer*) involves the lining of the uterus, which undergoes cyclic changes as

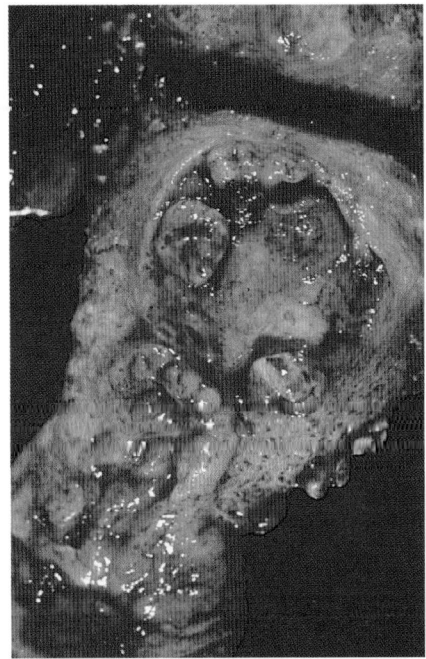

• **Fig. 12.23** Endometrial cancer. (From Cotran RS, Kumar V, Collins T: *Robbins pathologic basis of disease*, ed 6, Philadelphia, 1999, Saunders.)

a result of hormonal stimulation. It is the most common gynecologic malignancy (Fig. 12.23).

ICD-10-CM Code	C54.1 (Malignant neoplasm of endometrium)
	C54.2 (Malignant neoplasm of myometrium)
	C54.3 (Malignant neoplasm of fundus uteri)
	C54.9 (Malignant neoplasm of corpus uteri, unspecified)

Symptoms and Signs

Endometrial cancer causes ulcerations in the uterus. As blood vessels erode, vaginal spotting or bleeding occurs. The most common presenting symptom is abnormal perimenopausal or postmenopausal uterine bleeding. This occurs even in the early stages of the disease. Late manifestations of this cancer include pain and systemic symptoms. The disease may be revealed by the presence of atypical endometrial cells observed on routine Pap smear testing.

Patient Screening

Schedule a gynecologic examination and a Pap smear test for the woman having abnormal uterine bleeding. Any uterine bleeding in postmenopausal women should prompt evaluation for malignancy.

Etiology

There are two types of endometrial cancer. The most common type is related to high cumulative exposure to estrogen and usually presents as a low-grade adenocarcinoma. Excess estrogen may come from such sources as estrogen replacement therapy in postmenopausal women, tamoxifen therapy for breast cancer, obesity, early onset of menarche, late menopause, never having children, and chronic anovulation. Endometrial hyperplasia with cellular atypia caused by endometrial exposure to continuous estrogen unopposed by progesterone is a precursor lesion for this type of carcinoma. The second type is unrelated to estrogen exposure or hyperplasia and often presents as a high-grade papillary serous or clear cell carcinoma and has a poorer prognosis.

Endometrial cancer is primarily a disease of postmenopausal women. The median age at diagnosis is 61 years. Women with HNPCC syndrome are at high risk for endometrial cancer. Type 2 diabetes, obesity, and hypertension also lead to an increased risk. Pregnancy and the use of oral contraceptives for at least 12 months appear to offer a protective effect.

Diagnosis

After a pelvic examination to assess for pelvic masses or other causes of uterine bleeding, endometrial biopsy is usually performed on all women with abnormal uterine bleeding or abnormal endometrial cells observed on the Pap smear test. Transvaginal ultrasonography may be helpful as an initial study in postmenopausal women. Dilation and curettage (D&C) remains the gold standard and is usually performed when endometrial biopsy is nondiagnostic. The staging system developed for endometrial cancer is based on the TNM system. Staging requires total hysterectomy with bilateral salpingo-oophorectomy, along with lymph node dissection to fully evaluate the extent of disease. The serum tumor marker CA-125 also may be measured to predict the spread of disease beyond the uterus.

Treatment

Very-early-stage endometrial cancer is treated with surgery alone, whereas adjuvant radiation therapy with or without chemotherapy is recommended for those with more advanced disease. A radioactive implant can be inserted into the vagina and left in place for the duration of treatment while the patient is in the hospital (vaginal brachytherapy). The risk of recurrent disease is greatest within the first 3 years of diagnosis. Follow-up physical examination, including pelvic examination, should be performed initially every 3 to 6 months to detect recurrence.

Prognosis

The prognosis is determined by the stage of the disease and the tumor grade. The 5-year survival rate ranges from 20% to 90%, depending on the stage at diagnosis.

Prevention

Routine screening is not recommended for most women, because no good noninvasive test is available. For those with HNPCC, however, annual endometrial biopsy is recommended, starting at age 35 years. These women also should be counseled about prophylactic hysterectomy with salpingo-oophorectomy after completion of childbearing.

Patient Teaching

Counsel patients about the symptoms of endometrial cancer, and instruct them to report any abnormal bleeding or spotting to the health care provider. After endometrial cancer is diagnosed, give preoperative and postoperative instructions. Provide additional information about procedures to patients who have more advanced disease and are receiving adjunctive radiation therapy. Explain the purpose, duration, and possible side effects of any therapeutic regimen. Offer referrals for every possible avenue of support, especially in more advanced cases.

Conditions and Complications of Pregnancy

Most pregnancies progress to term uneventfully (Fig. 12.24). Complications ranging from worrisome or annoying conditions to life-threatening conditions affecting the mother or the fetus occasionally occur. Complications can develop at any point during pregnancy, which underscores the importance of early and continual prenatal care and patient education.

Prenatal diagnostic tests can help identify fetal genetic or chromosomal abnormalities and detect complications:

- Amniocentesis: A small amount of amniotic fluid is extracted for laboratory analysis (Fig. 12.25)
- Chorionic villus sampling (CVS): A biopsy procedure to excise placental tissue for laboratory analysis
- Maternal serum fetal free DNA analysis
- Doppler ultrasonography: Noninvasive real-time, three-dimensional (3D) fetal imaging (see Fig. 12.25)

The first two procedures carry a low risk for miscarriage and infection; the maternal serum test has no risk of fetal loss. Recent recommendations regarding ultrasonography are that it should be performed only for medical reasons, with time and power output kept to a minimum.

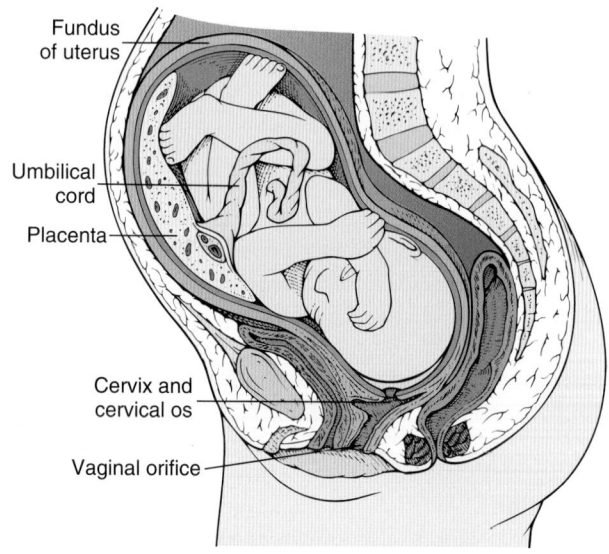

Fundus of uterus

Umbilical cord

Placenta

Cervix and cervical os

Vaginal orifice

• **Fig. 12.24** Normal uterine pregnancy.

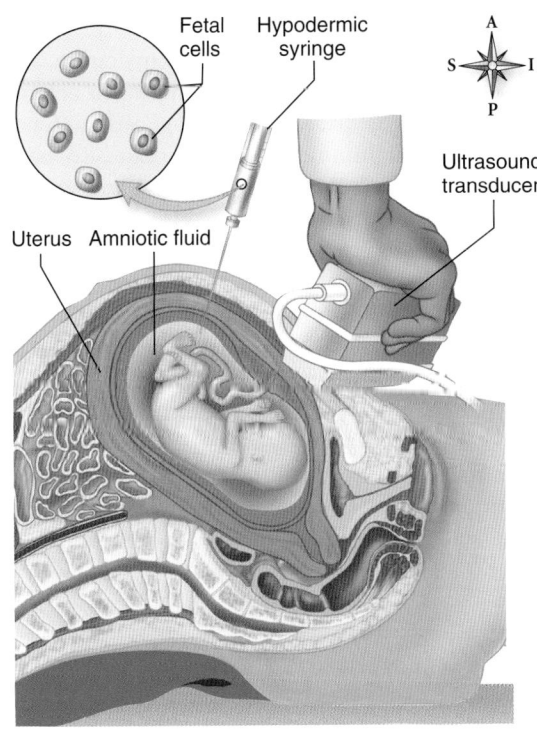

• **Fig. 12.25** Amniocentesis. In amniocentesis, a syringe is used to collect amniotic fluid. Ultrasound imaging is used to guide the tip of the syringe needle to prevent damage to the placenta and fetus. Fetal cells in the collected amniotic fluid can then be chemically tested or used to produce a karyotype of the developing baby. (From Patton KT, Thibodeau GA: *The human body in health and disease,* ed 6, Maryland Heights, MO, 2014, Elsevier.)

◆ ENRICHMENT

Ultrasonography

Ultrasonography is a technique in which high-frequency intermittent sound waves are reflected off tissues and are read by scanners. The various densities of the tissue then are displayed on a screen, and still pictures can be taken to record the real-time image.

Pelvic ultrasonography is specific for the lower abdominal tissues, including the uterus, adnexa, and fetus. This noninvasive, nonradiating, painless technique helps diagnose fetal anomalies; determine fetal age, size, and position; evaluate the condition and placement of the placenta; and identify many other conditions of the female reproductive system (Fig. 12.26A).

A more recent advance is 3D prenatal ultrasonography, which produces 3D, crystal-clear images of the fetus as photographs (see Fig. 12.26B). Four-dimensional (4D) ultrasonography adds the dimension of time to the process. Parents can now see live-action images of their unborn child or of any internal anatomy. Ultrasonography is considered harmless for both mother and baby and is of particular value in high-risk obstetrics.

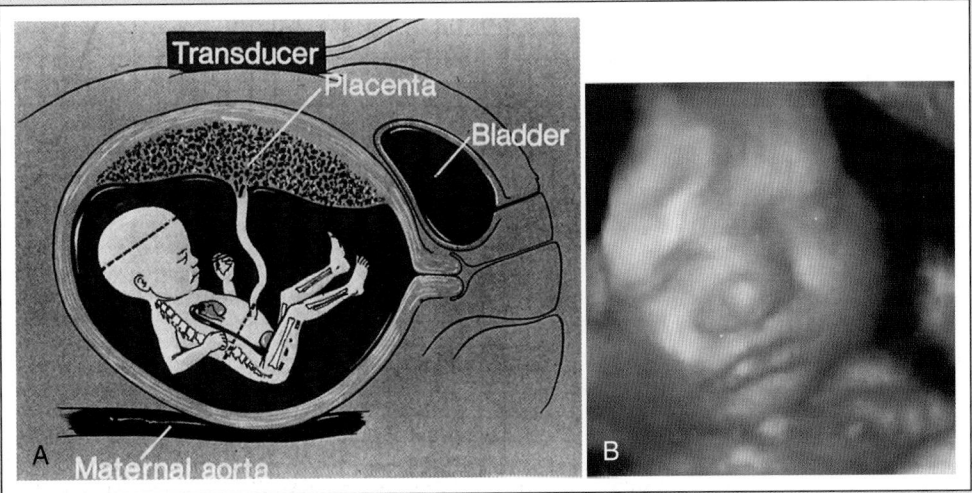

• **Fig. 12.26** (A) Ultrasonography. (B) 28-week three-dimensional (3D) ultrasonography. Note distortion of the right forehead, which is caused by the uterine wall. (A, From Hadlock FP: The role of fetal biometry in obstetric sonography. In Putman CE, Ravin CE, editors: *Diagnostic imaging,* Philadelphia, 1988, Saunders. B, Courtesy Carli Reed.)

Morning Sickness

Description

Morning sickness is the nausea and vomiting associated with pregnancy. It is quite common, affecting up to 80% of pregnant women. The symptoms may begin before the first missed menses but normally resolve by 12 to 16 weeks of pregnancy. Only 1% of pregnant women will have persistent morning sickness beyond the 20th week of pregnancy. If the nausea and vomiting are severe enough to cause excessive weight loss or metabolic imbalance, then it is called *hyperemesis gravidarum (HG)*. This condition affects only 0.5% to 3% of pregnant women.

ICD-10-CM Code	O21.0 *(Mild hyperemesis gravidarum)*
	(O21.0-O21.9 = 5 codes of specificity)

Symptoms and Signs

The symptoms of nausea and vomiting occur during the day, with only 2% of women experiencing true "morning" symptoms. Sometimes the nausea is short-lived and occurs in waves; at other times, the patient may feel nauseated for hours at a time. If she is dehydrated, urine can look dark; ketones may be present on urine testing; and if the vomiting is severe enough, blood tests may show evidence of metabolic and electrolyte abnormalities. Thyroid testing is usually not performed, because these laboratory tests can be abnormal as a result of this condition and not because of underlying thyroid disease. Signs to watch for are rapid pulse, poor skin turgor, decreased urine output, and constipation. These are all signs of dehydration.

Patient Screening

Follow office policy for scheduling an examination for possible pregnancy. If the patient is experiencing excessive nausea and vomiting, make a prompt appointment for a regular pregnancy checkup. The patient's weight is important and helps measure the degree of her condition. If a woman experiences weight loss greater than 10% of her prepregnancy weight, she may need to have a more complete evaluation and management in a hospital setting.

Etiology

The etiology of morning sickness has yet to be clearly defined; however, it is believed that human chorionic gonadotropin (hCG) or one if its forms and estrogen (estradiol) are the main culprits responsible for this condition. Psychological problems can also cause nausea and vomiting in pregnancy or make it worse. Patients with underlying GI conditions may also experience more nausea and GI symptoms.

Diagnosis

The diagnosis is based on symptoms and a positive pregnancy test result.

Treatment

In most cases of simple morning sickness, hydration, rest, and eating small amounts of food are sufficient to help the woman cope with the process. Avoiding certain foods, smells, and other environmental triggers can also be of benefit. Use of ginger, hypnosis, wristbands, and vitamin B_6 and B_{12} all can help reduce the severity of this condition. If the patient needs assistance beyond these measures, there are various drugs that can be used to help alleviate symptoms. Most of these drugs are considered safe in pregnancy, although none has undergone specific testing for this indication.

Prognosis

The condition usually is self-limiting and resolves gradually. If the condition becomes severe, it can lead to esophageal tears, peripheral neuropathies, encephalopathy, and even death.

Prevention

No prevention is known.

Patient Teaching

Instruct the pregnant woman to keep her scheduled appointments and to notify the nurse or physician of any worsening of nausea and vomiting.

Hyperemesis Gravidarum

Description

HG is the more severe stage of morning sickness; it usually does not respond to over-the-counter remedies and requires prescription medications and even hospitalization. It is associated with weight loss of greater than 10% and associated metabolic disturbances and dehydration.

ICD-10-CM Code	P05.2 *(Newborn affected by fetal [intrauterine] malnutrition not light or small for gestational age)*
	(P05.00-P05.9 = 20 codes of specificity)
	O21.1 *(Hyperemesis gravidarum with metabolic disturbance)*

Symptoms and Signs

HG, excessive vomiting in pregnancy occurs when the pregnant patient experiences frequent, severe episodes of nausea and vomiting, weight loss, and dehydration and is unable to keep either food or liquid in the stomach. If left untreated, fluid and electrolyte imbalances can cause acid–base disturbances in the fetus and the mother. Abnormal urine osmolality, the excretion of moderate or high levels of ketones into urine, is usually noted during the evaluation of these patients. Laboratory tests may indicate an increase in the number of red blood cells (hemoconcentration), mild elevations in the WBC count and abnormalities in other blood chemistries as a result of excessive vomiting and dehydration. Abnormal liver enzymes and thyroid laboratory values may also be present.

Patient Screening

Severe nausea and vomiting during pregnancy require prompt medical evaluation.

Etiology

The etiology is unknown. As with morning sickness, elevated estrogen and hCG levels are believed to be responsible for this condition. Emotions may play a part in the onset and severity of vomiting. The patient is unable to ingest any food or liquid without resultant vomiting. Patients with underlying emotional disturbances or those in abusive relationships have a higher incidence of this condition.

Diagnosis

Diagnosis is based on symptoms, weight loss, and signs of dehydration, which disturb the serum electrolyte balance. Any pregnant patient with severe nausea and vomiting not responding to standard measures and who continues to lose weight can be classified as having HG.

Treatment

In severe cases, the patient is hospitalized for reversal of dehydration with IV fluids. Any electrolyte imbalance can also be corrected with proper infusion of necessary salts. Other metabolic disturbances, such as hyperthyroidism, can be ruled out at this time. Antiemetics can be given intravenously until the woman feels able to take oral liquids. Once the patient is able to tolerate oral agents without vomiting and when her weight stabilizes, she may be sent home. Home nursing then can be used to continue any IV treatments. Most patients are managed outside of the hospital for this condition.

Prognosis

The prognosis is excellent because the condition resolves spontaneously as the pregnancy progresses. As long as the patient is treated in an expedient fashion, complications from dehydration and excessive electrolyte disturbances should be avoidable. If treated nonaggressively or unsuccessfully, profound maternal and fetal complications can result.

Prevention

Timely medical intervention can prevent complications from affecting the mother and her fetus. Treating nausea and vomiting in pregnancy aggressively early on in the course of the disease may help prevent progression to HG.

Patient Teaching

After the patient's condition becomes stable, instruct the patient to eat small, frequent meals of bland food. Suggest that portions be increased as tolerated. Warn the mother to report signs of dehydration or recurrence of symptoms.

Spontaneous Abortion (Miscarriage)

Description

Spontaneous abortion is a naturally occurring loss of a fetus before the 20th week of pregnancy. Spontaneous abortions are classified as missed (no tissue has passed), incomplete (some tissue has passed), or complete (all tissue has passed).

ICD-10-CM Code	O03.9 (Complete or unspecified spontaneous abortion without complication)
	(O00.0 O03.0 – 28 codes of specificity)

Coding spontaneous abortion requires modifiers to identify stage. Refer to the physician's diagnosis and then to the current edition of the ICD-10-CM coding manual to ensure the greatest specificity of pathology.

Symptoms and Signs

In cases of incomplete or complete abortion, the patient has vaginal bleeding and pelvic cramping (Fig. 12.27).

Excessive bleeding may lead to hypovolemia, which causes a rapid pulse and low blood pressure. In the hospital, a complete blood count (CBC) will verify the extent of blood loss. In severe cases with extensive hemorrhage, shock can ensue. A positive pregnancy result on urine or blood tests is important to verify that the patient is/was pregnant. Examination of the cervix may reveal blood in the vagina, with or without any visible products of conception. It is always important to realize that a patient with an ectopic pregnancy may have very similar symptoms.

Patient Screening

Vaginal bleeding and cramping during pregnancy should be reported to the attending physician immediately, and the patient should be directed to prompt medical care.

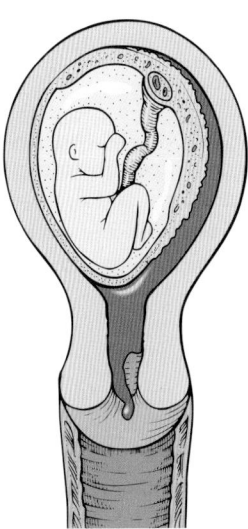

• **Fig. 12.27** Miscarriage.

Etiology

The etiology is usually unknown, with about 10% to 20% of all pregnancies ending in spontaneous abortion. The majority of spontaneous miscarriages result from abnormal chromosomes. Infection, metabolic disturbances, and maternal antibody production (e.g., in SLE or clotting disorders) have been associated with an increased risk of abortion. Drugs and most prescribed medications do not normally cause abortions. Travel, exercise, and intercourse are also not associated with miscarriage. Women who work as anesthesiologists have been noted to have a higher rate of spontaneous abortion.

Diagnosis

The diagnosis is based on the clinical picture and pelvic ultrasonography. Ultrasonography can help determine fetal viability or amount of remaining tissue within the uterus. Depending on the level of serum hCG, it may also be helpful in ruling out ectopic pregnancy.

Treatment

If bleeding is not severe, the mother is treated conservatively by allowing the products of conception to pass on their own. The woman may also be given medications to help expedite the passage of fetal and placental tissues. In cases of complete abortion, there usually is no need for medications. If bleeding is severe or the expulsion of the contents of the uterus is incomplete, surgical intervention (D&C) may be indicated. In many instances of missed abortion, the woman may elect to have surgical removal of the products of conception to avoid the uncertainty and discomfort associated with spontaneous passage of the pregnancy. It is important to know the woman's blood type, because Rho(D) immune globulin (RhoGAM) may be indicated if she is Rh negative.

Prognosis

The prognosis in all three types of spontaneous abortion is excellent. Even when a D&C is required or requested, the impact on future pregnancies is minimal.

Prevention

The cause often is not certain, but good prenatal care is recommended. All restricted substances, including alcohol, tobacco, abuse of inhalants, and drugs, are contraindicated during pregnancy. Herbs are not necessarily safe as pregnancy remedies. Herbs and prescription drugs should be taken with caution.

Patient Teaching

Instruct the patient to report any increased vaginal discharge, bleeding, or progressive cramping to the nurse or the physician. In mild cases, advise bed rest and abstinence from sexual intercourse. After spontaneous abortion, alert the patient to the signs of infection, which should be reported immediately. Provide referral for grief counseling, which may be helpful.

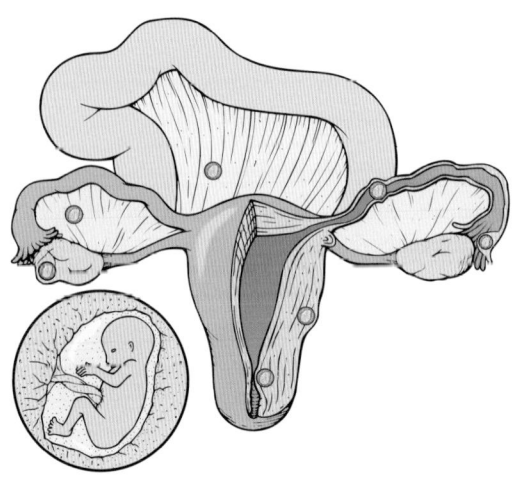

• **Fig. 12.28** Sites of ectopic (tubal) pregnancy.

Ectopic Pregnancy

Description

An ectopic pregnancy occurs when the fertilized ovum implants and grows outside the endometrial canal, most often the fallopian tube (Fig. 12.28).

ICD-10-CM Code	P01.4 *(Newborn [suspected to be] affected by ectopic pregnancy)*
	O00.9 *(Ectopic pregnancy, unspecified)*
	(O00.0-O00.9 = 5 codes of specificity)

Symptoms and Signs

The woman with a positive pregnancy test result and pelvic pain is the most common presentation for an ectopic pregnancy. However, there may be no pain, and the urine test may yield a negative result for pregnancy. When pain is present, it is usually on one side. Cramping of the uterus, with or without bleeding, can also occur. If there is bleeding into the abdomen, then the patient may experience diffuse pelvic pain. If there is a large amount of internal bleeding, the patient may become hypotensive and go into shock. If not treated promptly, an actively bleeding ectopic pregnancy can cause death. A level of the serum beta-hCG greater than 1500 to 2500 units, with an empty uterus seen on transvaginal ultrasonography, is suspicious for ectopic pregnancy. An abnormal rise in the level of beta-hCG over 48 hours can also be an early sign of an ectopic pregnancy.

Patient Screening

The sudden onset of severe lower abdominal pain accompanied by vaginal bleeding signals the need for prompt medical evaluation. Defer to the physician or nurse for instructions.

Etiology

Any fertilized egg that cannot make it into the uterus but is able to implant itself and grow will become ectopic. The cause of most ectopic pregnancies is generally unknown.

Pelvic adhesions, the presence of damaged fallopian tubes, progesterone contraception, previous tubal ligation, previous pelvic infection, prior pelvic surgery, and IUDs are all associated with an increased incidence of ectopic pregnancy.

Diagnosis

The diagnosis of ectopic pregnancy can be very difficult. If it is not ruptured and not causing pain, then serial ultrasound examinations with serial blood pregnancy tests may help make the diagnosis. In cases of ruptured ectopic pregnancies or those associated with pain, the diagnosis may be less difficult. Transvaginal ultrasonography is the mainstay in diagnostic imaging. In areas where the diagnosis remains unclear or ultrasonography is not available, then a frozen D&C may be performed to look for evidence of intrauterine gestational tissue. Culdocentesis (placing a needle into the space behind the uterus) can likewise be used in some unusual cases where the diagnosis is uncertain. If the diagnosis still remains in question, then laparoscopy may be performed to directly visualize the pelvis and the fallopian tubes.

Treatment

The treatment of ectopic pregnancy depends on many factors. In early unruptured ectopic pregnancies, a medication (methotrexate) may be administered. This drug causes the placenta to die and the products to be reabsorbed by the body. Laparoscopic surgery is one of the most common ways of treating ectopic pregnancy. If the tube is unruptured, then tubal conservation may be possible. In many cases, the tube is sacrificed, but rarely is it necessary to remove the ovary. Even when there has been internal bleeding, surgery can still be accomplished through the laparoscope. Blood transfusion is rarely needed unless the blood loss has been excessive. If the fallopian tube is preserved, then the woman is at increased risk for another ectopic pregnancy in that tube. In some instances of known ectopic pregnancy with falling beta-hCG levels, close observation may be warranted without the use of methotrexate or surgery. This is, however, clearly reserved for special circumstances.

Prognosis

The prognosis is good with prompt medical intervention. The chances of conception and a normal intrauterine pregnancy are generally excellent. If there is underlying tubal disease or extensive pelvic adhesions, then the chances of pregnancy are reduced. A prior ectopic pregnancy increases the risk of subsequent ectopic pregnancies. Clearly, massive internal bleeding from ruptured ectopic pregnancy can be life threatening.

Prevention

One of the major risk factors for ectopic pregnancy is a history of PID. Preventing this infection can reduce the risk of ectopic pregnancy. Most causes of ectopic pregnancy cannot be altered.

Patient Teaching

During emergency medical care, provide reassurance to the patient in pain and distress through frequent updates and explanations of the procedures being performed and the reasons. Give analgesics as prescribed. Anticipate the normal emotional response to a terminated problem pregnancy.

Premature Labor

Description

Premature labor is contractions leading to cervical change occurring before 37 completed weeks of pregnancy.

ICD-10-CM Code	O60.00 *(Preterm labor without delivery, unspecified trimester)* (O60.00-O60.23 = 10 codes of specificity)

Symptoms and Signs

Premature labor occurs when the pregnant woman begins experiencing contractions that are generally regular and painful and that lead to changes in the size of the cervical opening or length of the cervix. Sometimes the woman has contractions that she cannot feel and are only evident on a fetal monitor. She may have an increase in vaginal discharge or spotting. Vaginal examination may reveal cervical changes, as mentioned previously. Ultrasonography can also be used to assess cervical length and can reveal dynamic changes in this length with abdominal pressure or contractions.

Patient Screening

A patient with premature contractions must be brought to the attention of the physician or the nurse for immediate instructions for medical intervention.

Etiology

Most cases of premature labor are of unknown etiology. Predisposing conditions include maternal infection, uterine abnormalities, uterine fibroids, uterine bleeding, prior history of preterm birth, multifetal pregnancy, advanced maternal age, gum disease, vaginal colonization with certain bacteria, lack of prenatal care, and preterm cervical dilation or effacement. Other possible contributing factors include smoking, stress, and domestic violence.

Diagnosis

The diagnosis is made by demonstrating cervical change in the presence of uterine contractions. Many physicians treat painful regular contractions even when there is no cervical change if risk factors are present. Newer tests for a substance produced by the fetal membranes called *fetal fibronectin* can help predict the risk of preterm delivery and may be used to manage the patient who is experiencing contractions without cervical change, depending on the risk profile. A cervical length change on ultrasonography is as useful as a pelvic examination to make the diagnosis.

Treatment

There is no effective treatment for preterm labor. Most studies show that true preterm labor can, at best, be delayed by 48 to 72 hours. Preterm contractions may be managed with terbutaline (while the patient is in the hospital), indomethacin (Indocin), or calcium channel blockers; and magnesium sulfate. Current data have called into question the use of magnesium sulfate, although it may be neuroprotective in premature infants. Intramuscular injections of steroids are given to the mother to reduce the complications of prematurity to the fetus if labor cannot be stopped and the patient is about to deliver a very premature fetus ($\leq$ 34 weeks). The only clear treatment for women with a prior history of preterm birth is the use of weekly intramuscular progesterone injections. These injections can reduce the incidence of premature birth by around 30% in selected patients. These injections do not appear to work in multifetal pregnancies.

Prognosis

The outcome for the fetus depends on the age at delivery, underlying presence of infection, birth defects, and cause of the labor. The earlier the gestational age, the more guarded is the prognosis. The addition of steroids before birth can improve neonatal outcomes.

Prevention

The causes of premature labor are not clearly understood. Treatment of underlying infections; bed rest; judicial use of tocolytics (to inhibit uterine contractions); use of steroids, when appropriate; and enhanced fetal surveillance may all help prevent some cases of preterm labor and preterm birth. Intramuscular progesterone is the only proven agent for the prevention of preterm birth, but its success is limited.

Patient Teaching

Present all elements of good prenatal care, with attention to individual needs and the medical history, clearly with as many teaching aids as possible. Help the patient set goals for a healthy outcome for mother and infant. Give written instructions about signs of possible complications or early onset of labor to report.

ENRICHMENT

Fetal Movement

Studies have shown fetal movement is an indicator of the oxygenation and well-being of the fetus. Some physicians have the expectant mother chart fetal kicks beginning at 28 weeks of gestation and continuing until the day of delivery (see Fig. 12.28). Kick counting methods vary; the attending physician or the nurse midwife provides the guidelines. For example, the mother should lie comfortably, relax, and concentrate on her baby. She can rest her hands on her abdomen to help feel the fetal movements. The mother then jots down the date and time of the baby's first kick and the time the number of kicks reaches 10. According to the Perinatal Guidelines of the American Academy of Pediatrics and the American College of Obstetricians and Gynecologists, an expectant mother should be able to feel 10 kicks in 2 hours or less at 28 weeks' gestation. The number of perceptible fetal movements varies from patient to patient, but the mother becomes familiar with her baby's pattern of kicks and can notice any reduction in movement. The mother is instructed to contact her physician if she notices fewer kicks or absence of fetal movements. Any concerns or questions about performing the kick chart are to be referred to the physician, who can investigate and further evaluate the fetal status (Fig. 12.29).

• **Fig. 12.29** Sample kick count chart. (Courtesy Pamela Hood, RN, MSN CNE.)

Preeclampsia and Eclampsia

Description

The term *preeclampsia* refers to a serious disease of pregnancy characterized by hypertension and proteinuria. This condition occurs most commonly in the third trimester but can occur any time after 20 completed weeks of pregnancy.

Eclampsia is the occurrence of a seizure in a patient with preeclampsia.

ICD-10-CM Code	O14.00 *(Mild to moderate preeclampsia, unspecified trimester)*
	O14.90 *(Unspecified preeclampsia, unspecified trimester)*
	(O14.00-O14.93 = 12 codes of specificity)
	O15.9 *(Eclampsia, unspecified as to time period)*
	(O15.00-O15.9 = 6 codes of specificity)

Symptoms and Signs

Preeclampsia can be preceded by increased weight gain, usually noted as peripheral swelling or edema. Not all patients with preeclampsia will have edema. Elevation of blood pressure to a level greater than 140/90 mm Hg is a sign that also indicates this condition. When there is greater than 300 mg of protein in urine over a 24 hour period, then the conditions for the diagnosis of preeclampsia are present. The presence of other symptoms, such as persistent headache, visual disturbances, or epigastric pain, can also be present. When blood pressure and urinary protein levels become markedly elevated, the disease may have a more severe course and a potentially worse prognosis. The deep tendon reflexes may also be more exaggerated; and in patients who are severely affected, clonus may be present. If the patient has a seizure, it is usually of the grand mal type and can demonstrate the usual postictal manifestation of confusion and disorientation. These patients are also at increased risk for stroke, and thus any symptom of a central neurologic nature needs to be evaluated for the presence of stroke.

Patient Screening

The woman who is pregnant or suspects pregnancy and reports the onset of edema, sudden weight gain, headaches, or sudden elevation of blood pressure should be evaluated by the physician promptly. The onset of seizures requires emergency intervention.

Etiology

The etiology of preeclampsia remains unknown. It occurs in about 7% of pregnant women in the United States and is more common in first pregnancies, young women, women with multiple fetuses, women older than 35 years of age, and women with underlying hypertension or vascular disease, such as diabetes and SLE. The actual causative agent or agents is unknown; however, the presence of a placenta is necessary for this condition to occur. Once the placenta is delivered, the condition typically begins to resolve after 24 to 48 hours, although there are cases of persistent preeclampsia that last for 7 days or even up to 6 weeks after delivery.

Diagnosis

The diagnosis is based on the clinical picture, history, elevated urinary protein level, elevated blood pressure, neurologic symptoms, and/or abnormal laboratory results.

Treatment

The treatment for preeclampsia is delivery of the infant and the placenta. If the disease is mild and the woman is far from her due date, then bed rest, frequent monitoring of the fetus and the mother, monitoring of blood tests, and delay of delivery until fetal lung maturity may be necessary. In cases of more severe disease, immediate delivery may be warranted. In fetuses younger than 34 weeks of age, steroids may be given to the mother to help accelerate fetal lung maturity before delivery. Laboring women with preeclampsia may require medications, such as magnesium sulfate, which dramatically reduce the risk of a seizure. There is currently some debate as to whether or not to give magnesium sulfate to women who have mild preeclampsia and are in labor. After delivery, the disease usually remits; however, it may worsen over the immediate 24 to 48 hours before improving. There can even be new-onset disease up to 6 weeks after delivery.

Prognosis

Early diagnosis and treatment of preeclampsia offer the best prognosis for mother and baby. The prognosis is poorer with severe disease, which may result in maternal and/or fetal death.

Prevention

Possible preventive steps currently being explored are calcium supplementation and low-dose aspirin therapy, although, to date, there are no preventative measures. Good nutrition may also be of some value.

Patient Teaching

Emphasize the advantages of early and regular prenatal care to monitor weight, blood pressure, and urinary protein levels. If a pregnant woman is considered to be at risk for eclampsia, educate the woman about the warning signs to report: sudden weight gain, edema, headache, and increased blood pressure. Early signs can be managed to prevent hospitalization and the onset of complications.

Abruptio Placentae

Description

Abruptio placentae is premature detachment of a normally positioned placenta during pregnancy.

ICD-10-CM Code   P02.1 *(Newborn [suspected to be] affected by other forms of placental separation and hemorrhage)*
O45.8X9 *(Other premature separation of placenta, unspecified trimester)*
(O45.001-O45.93 = 24 codes of specificity)

Symptoms and Signs

When the placenta separates prematurely from the uterine wall, it can cause hemorrhage, abdominal pain, fetal distress, and even fetal death. The degree of bleeding can vary quite considerably, with most cases being mild to moderate. The uterus usually contracts when there is an abruption, and these painful contractions are often very closely spaced and come on rather suddenly. Monitoring of the fetal heart rate may show some abnormalities; however, early on, there may be a normal heart rate and pattern. If the abruption is extensive, then fetal death may ensue, and the large clot that forms under the placenta may lead to excessive blood loss in the mother and consumption of clotting factors, leading to a coagulopathy. In more severe cases, the mother's blood is unable to clot. Some abruptions do not have any associated external bleeding, and the only signs are fetal heart rate abnormalities or even fetal death. Occasionally, a large abruption may be detected with ultrasonography.

Patient Screening

The signs of abruptio placentae represent a medical emergency for mother and fetus. The physician is contacted immediately, and the patient is directed to the emergency room.

Etiology

Abruptio placentae is a complete or partial separation of the placenta from the uterine wall (Fig. 12.30). In many cases, the cause is unknown; however, hypertension, preeclampsia, trauma, maternal vascular disease, infection, drug use (cocaine), and multiple gestation all predispose a woman to placental abruption.

Diagnosis

The diagnosis is usually made by the constellation of risk factors, fetal heart rate pattern, the mother's symptoms, contraction pattern, and presence of bleeding. In many instances, the diagnosis is only suspected and is confirmed or refuted at the time of delivery. Ultrasonography rarely helps in the diagnosis of small or moderate abruptions, but it can identify large subplacental bleeds.

Treatment

The care of the patient with suspected abruption depends on the degree of placental separation, proximity to the due date of delivery, and maternal and fetal stability. In mild cases, labor may continue with anticipated vaginal delivery. An operating room must be readily available in these cases, because the clinical picture may deteriorate rapidly in these patients. In significantly preterm patients not in labor, hospitalization with careful monitoring may be appropriate. Most cases are treated by immediate surgical delivery. Massive blood loss and coagulopathy are treated with replacement of blood and clotting factor.

Prognosis

Prognosis depends on the degree of abruption and the gestational age of the fetus. As long as the abruption is small and the fetus is beyond 34 weeks' gestation, then the outlook is excellent. In very premature infants and those in whom the abruption compromises oxygenation, the prognosis may be more guarded.

Prevention

Good prenatal care with individualized attention to risk factors may help prevent abruptions in some cases.

Patient Teaching

Reinforce the principles of prenatal care, and instruct the patient to report unexpected symptoms, such as sudden bleeding or abdominal pain, immediately.

Placenta Previa

Description

Placenta previa is the placenta covering the opening to the cervix. In a partial previa, the majority of the placenta is away from the opening (os), and in a complete or central previa, the more central portion of the placenta covers the os.

ICD-10-CM Code   O44.00 *(Placenta previa specified as without hemorrhage, unspecified trimester)*
(O44.00-O44.13 = 8 codes of specificity)

Symptoms and Signs

The patient experiences painless, bright vaginal bleeding, usually in the first or second trimester of pregnancy.

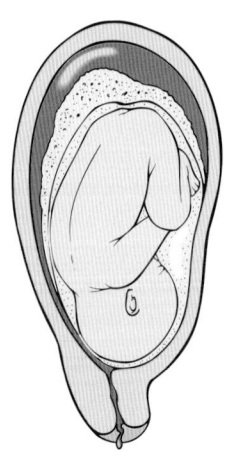

• **Fig. 12.30** Abruptio placentae.

Occasionally the patient experiences painless vaginal bleeding in the third trimester as the first sign. The abdomen is soft and nontender. In cases of excessive bleeding, vital signs may indicate shock, with a rapid and thready pulse and falling blood pressure. The fetal heart rate may indicate that the blood supply to the fetus is compromised.

Patient Screening
The onset of bright-red vaginal bleeding during pregnancy requires immediate attention, close observation, and diagnostic evaluation. The attending physician is notified.

Etiology
This condition is caused by low implantation of the blastocyst in the uterine cavity. A prior cesarean delivery increases the risk of previa, as does previous childbirth or multiple gestation.

Diagnosis
The diagnosis is based on a pelvic ultrasonogram showing the placenta being implanted over the cervical os. In a complete placenta previa, the placenta totally overlies the os

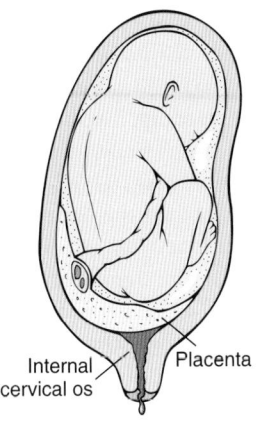

Internal cervical os   Placenta

• **Fig. 12.31** Placenta previa.

(Fig. 12.31). In a partial placenta previa, the placenta is implanted low in the uterus but does not entirely overlie the os. As the cervix begins to dilate, the vessels tear loose, and the placenta bleeds. It is critical that a cervical examination not be performed until the location of the placenta has been verified on ultrasonography.

❖ ENRICHMENT

Usual and Unusual Presentations

Most fetuses present in the cephalic, or vertex (head first), position, but some present in other positions, such as footling breech (feet first), frank breech (buttocks), or transverse lie (across the uterus). Even some of the cephalic presentations

(brow or chin) cause complications that may preclude normal vaginal delivery (Fig. 12.32). In cases of abnormal presentations, delivery is accomplished with cesarean section.

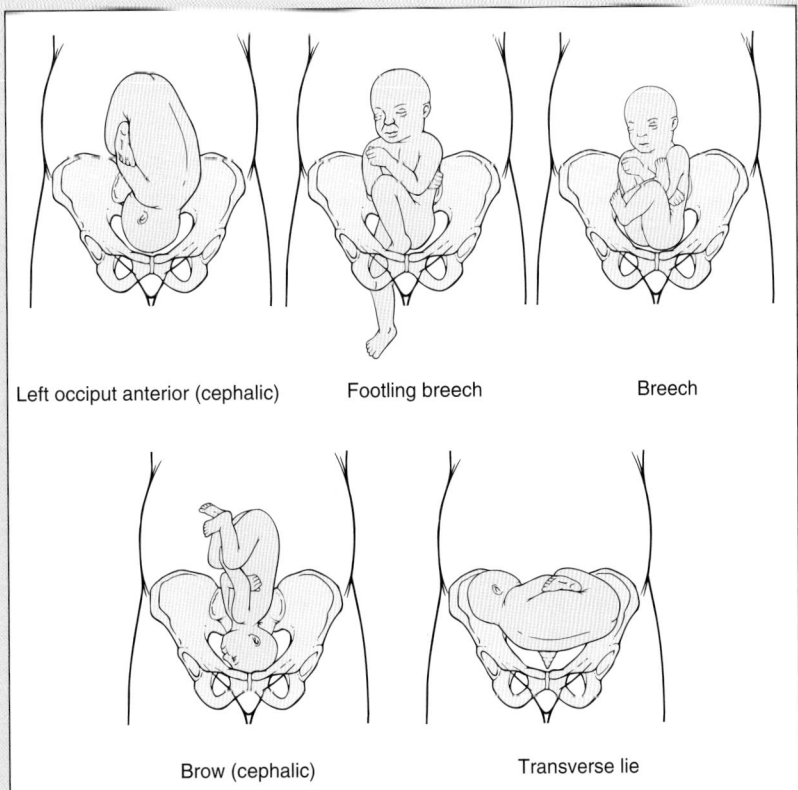

Left occiput anterior (cephalic)   Footling breech   Breech

Brow (cephalic)   Transverse lie

• **Fig. 12.32** Fetal presentations.

Treatment

In many pregnancies with a known history of placenta previa, the woman may go about her daily activities as long as she is not bleeding. Exercise and intercourse are avoided; and if bleeding occurs, then prompt evaluation in the hospital is usually warranted. If the bleeding stops and the fetus is stable, then the patient may be monitored as an outpatient, with activity restriction and regular visits. If the bleeding is more significant, then hospitalization may be required until the fetus is deemed mature. Often, in stable previa, delivery is accomplished around the 36th week to avoid the potential for catastrophic bleeding that may occur if labor ensues. For any massive hemorrhage with fetal or maternal compromise, immediate delivery by cesarean section is warranted. At no time is vaginal delivery of a viable fetus allowed when there is placenta previa present.

Prognosis

In most cases of previa, the outcomes are excellent. Clearly the prognosis becomes more guarded if there is excessive blood loss and fetal compromise requiring immediate delivery, especially if the infant is premature.

Prevention

No prevention is known.

Patient Teaching

Conditions requiring surgical intervention to save the life of the mother and/or the infant give rise to strong emotional responses that require recognition and care by the medical team. Explain all procedures, and offer reassurance throughout. Conservative treatment may require bed rest and lifestyle modification for an extended period during pregnancy; reinforce the purpose of the treatment, and address the need for home care referrals. Vaginal intercourse may be contraindicated.

◆◆ ENRICHMENT

Problems Associated with Multiple Pregnancies

The incidence rate of multiple (gestation) pregnancies is increasing. Infertility treatment contributes to this increase because fertility drugs, such as follicle-stimulating hormone (FSH; Follistim), are given to stimulate ovulation. These drugs often cause several ova to be released at ovulation, thus giving sperm multiple opportunities for fertilization. During the process of in vitro fertilization (IVF), several fertilized ova are implanted in the hope that at least one successful pregnancy will result. The ovaries sometimes release more than one ovum in the natural course of events. Finally, a fertilized zygote sometimes divides to produce identical twins (Fig. 12.33).

Many problems are associated with multiple (gestation) pregnancies. The mother is at greater risk for toxemia (preeclampsia) and for complications such as dyspnea, urinary frequency, constipation, edema of the feet and legs, and heartburn earlier in the pregnancy compared with the mother with a single fetus. The expectant mother of triplets, quadruplets, quintuplets, or sextuplets often is hospitalized by the beginning of the third trimester and restricted to bed rest. The fetuses are monitored frequently and usually must be delivered by cesarean section. The size of the multiple pregnancy generally prevents the pregnancy from continuing to term. This may result in very small, immature infants who need intensive nursing care and monitoring. See Chapter 2 for a discussion on conjoined twins.

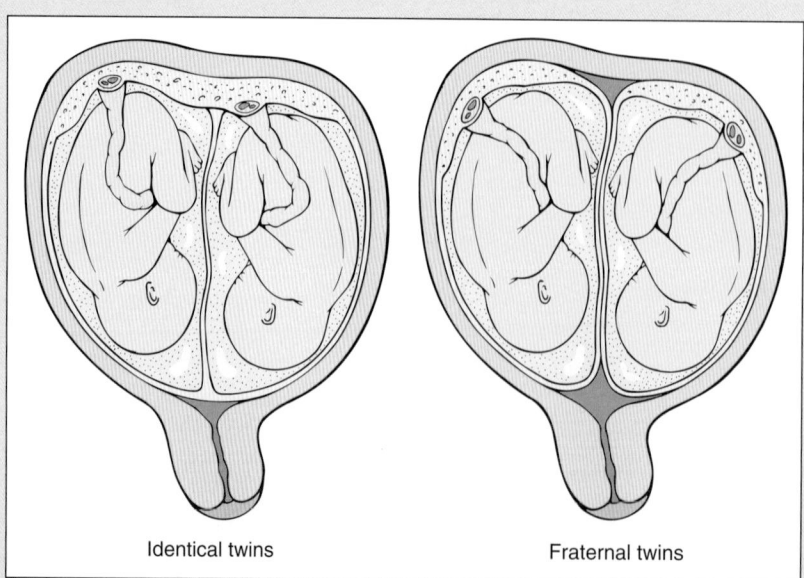

Identical twins   Fraternal twins

• **Fig. 12.33** Twin pregnancies.

Hydatidiform Mole

Description

A hydatidiform mole is an abnormal proliferation of the placental tissue that can take on the characteristics of a malignancy. The placenta has a "cluster of grapes" type of appearance on ultrasonography, or the diagnosis may be based on pathologic evaluation after a miscarriage or pregnancy termination.

ICD-10-CM Code	O01.9 *(Hydatidiform mole, unspecified)*
	(O01.0-O01.9 = 3 codes of specificity)
	D39.2 *(Neoplasm of uncertain behavior of placenta)*

Symptoms and Signs

The patient with a hydatidiform mole experiences symptoms just like any other pregnant woman. Occasionally there may be more nausea and vomiting and more vaginal bleeding than usually seen. On physical examination, the uterus may feel larger than expected, based on the last menstrual period. In cases of complete molar pregnancy, no fetus develops, and ultrasonography shows an empty or absent sac and an abnormal-appearing placenta. An incomplete mole is one that occurs with a living fetus, so it may be more difficult to detect. If the blood hCG level is measured, it may be greatly elevated, out of proportion to what would be expected on the basis of the stage of pregnancy.

Patient Screening

If a pregnant woman reports vaginal bleeding, an appointment for ultrasonography is scheduled to evaluate the uterus.

Etiology

The cause of a molar pregnancy is a genetic anomaly in fertilization. The placenta develops abnormally as a mass of clear grapelike vesicles (Fig. 12.34). Usually no fetus is present.

Diagnosis

The diagnosis is based on the clinical picture; the absence of fetal heart tones (FHTs) in a complete mole; abnormally elevated hCG levels; and, most importantly, the appearance of the placenta on the ultrasonogram. On occasion, the diagnosis is made during microscopic examination of the placenta by the pathologist after delivery or pregnancy termination or miscarriage.

Treatment

The mole normally is not expelled spontaneously, so surgical intervention is indicated, the usual treatment being evacuation of the uterus by D&C. Observation for hemorrhage is important. If the molar tissue persists after evacuation, then chemotherapy may be indicated to prevent further growth and spread of the tissue. On occasion, persistent trophoblastic tissue that does not respond to chemotherapy may necessitate hysterectomy. In cases of uterine evacuation, then serial beta-hCG assessments are required until the values fall below detectable amounts. Pregnancy should be avoided for at least 6 months after removal of a hydatidiform mole.

Prognosis

Most hydatidiform moles do not persist, and the prognosis is good with early treatment. Complications, such as infection and bleeding, can occur. When a fetus is present, preeclampsia may occur before 20 weeks' gestation, raising concerns about an incomplete mole. This condition can be a precursor to choriocarcinoma, and the patient must be instructed to have frequent follow-up examinations.

Prevention

No prevention is known. Hydatidiform moles occur in about 1 in 1500 pregnancies in the United States.

Patient Teaching

Explain the surgical procedure. Anticipate emotional responses to the diagnosis of a "false pregnancy." Emphasize the importance of follow-up care. The condition usually

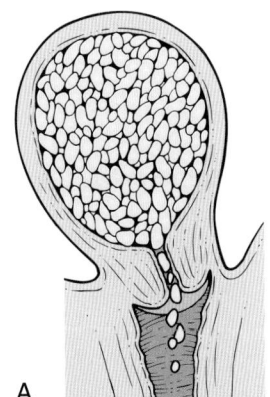
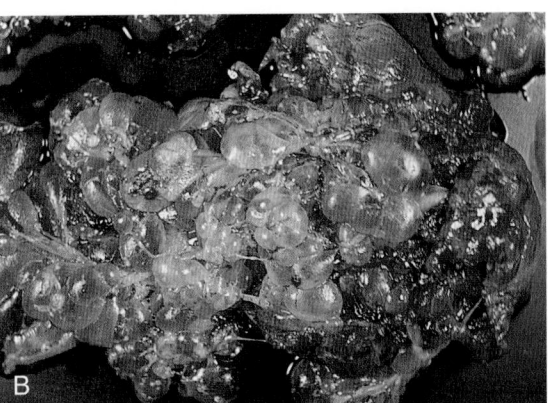

• **Fig. 12.34** **Hydatidiform Mole.** (A) Abnormal proliferation of placental tissue in a hydatidiform mole. (B) "Cluster of grapes" type appearance of hydatidiform mole. (B, From Damjanov I, Linder J: *Pathology: a color atlas,* St Louis, 1999, Mosby.)

does not affect fertility, but advise the patient not to become pregnant for 1 year.

Diseases of the Breast

Ranging from mild to fatal, diseases of the breast necessitate age-appropriate screening, with routine mammography, as prescribed by the physician. Although diseases of the breast are most common in women, diseases of the breast occur also in men. Any changes in the breast tissue, such as lumps, indentations, nipple crusting, or leaking, should be cause for concern and investigation.

Fibrocystic Breast Condition

Description
Fibrocystic breast condition is a common, benign breast disorder.

ICD-10-CM Code	N60.19 *(Diffuse cystic mastopathy of unspecified breast)* (N60.11-N60.19 = 3 codes of specificity)

Symptoms and Signs
The female patient with mammary fibroplasia experiences an uncomfortable feeling in the breasts. Lumps and cysts, single or multiple, smooth and rounded, can be palpated in one or both breasts. The breasts are tender on palpation, and the patient may experience shooting pains in the breast tissue. Tenderness is usually more intense during the premenstrual period. After menopause, the condition becomes less of a problem.

Patient Screening
A female who discovers one or more breast lumps is scheduled for a breast examination.

Etiology
The etiology of this condition is unknown. An increase in the formation of fibrous tissue and hyperplasia of the epithelial

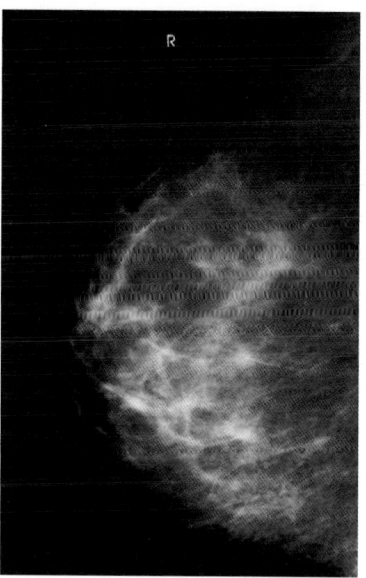

• **Fig. 12.35** Mammogram. (From *Mosby's medical, nursing, and allied health dictionary,* ed 8, St Louis, 2010, Mosby.)

cells of the ducts and glands result in dilation of the ducts. Cystic disease is the most common disease of the female breast, usually occurring between ages 30 and 50 years, and is related to normal hormonal variations.

Diagnosis
Prompt diagnosis is based on palpation and mammography (Fig. 12.35 and Table 12.2) to differentiate cystic disease from a malignant neoplasm. Ultrasonography may be performed to determine whether the lump is solid or hollow. This can help distinguish between cysts and tumors of the breasts.

Treatment
No specific treatment for this condition is known. The goal of treatment is to relieve breast pain and correct menstrual irregularity. Antiinflammatory medication or oral contraceptives may be ordered. In some cases, physicians aspirate the cysts with a needle. The patient is advised to wear a firm, supporting bra and restrict caffeine intake.

TABLE 12.2 Breast Cancer Screening

Test	American Cancer Society	U.S. Preventive Services Task Force
Mammography		
40–49 years	Annual	Insufficient evidence to support
> 49 years	Annual, if healthy	Every 2 years; 50–75 years
Clinical breast examination	Every 3 years; 20–39 years Annually, ≥ 40 years	Insufficient evidence to support
Breast self-examination	Optional	Not recommended

(From Goldman L, Schafer AI: *Goldman's Cecil medicine,* ed 24, Philadelphia, 2012, Elsevier/Saunders.)

Prognosis

The condition is benign, and most fibrocystic breast conditions never result in malignancy; however, microscopic findings that show atypical cells or hyperplasia are associated with an increased risk for breast cancer.

Prevention

No universal means of prevention is known. Some women notice an improvement with caffeine restriction.

Patient Teaching

Teach the patient about the importance of breast self-examination and of annual mammography. Emphasize the need for careful surveillance, because the lumps and cysts of the disease can mask malignancy.

Mastitis

Description

Mastitis is inflammation of one or more mammary glands of the breast.

ICD-10-CM Code	N61 (Inflammatory
	disorders of breast)

Symptoms and Signs

Acute puerperal (postdelivery) mastitis is inflammation of breast tissue during postpartum lactation. The nursing mother experiences sudden pain, redness, and heat in the breasts at either the beginning or the end of lactation. The breasts are hot and feel doughy and rough, and the axillary lymph nodes may be enlarged. There is a discharge from the nipple. Other symptoms are fever and malaise.

Patient Screening

Schedule a same-day appointment for a woman experiencing symptoms of mastitis.

Etiology

Mastitis often is caused by a streptococcal or staphylococcal infection. Bacteria invade the milk ducts and cause inflammation and occlusion. Milk stagnates in the lobules, producing a dull pain. The baby, the nursing staff, or even the mother's own body may be the source of the infection.

Diagnosis

The diagnosis is based on the clinical picture.

Treatment

A firm, supportive bra should be worn, heat may be applied to the area, progesterone may be prescribed, and drug therapy in the form of antibiotics is implemented. Palliative care includes rest, analgesia, and warm soaks. Breast-feeding need not be discontinued if there is improvement.

Prognosis

The prognosis for this benign condition is good with treatment. Abscesses may form with inadequate treatment.

Prevention

Anyone in contact with a nursing mother should practice infection prevention techniques.

Patient Teaching

Instruct the mother in good personal hygiene, especially in hand-washing technique. Emphasize the importance of taking the complete course of antibiotics as prescribed. Patients may benefit from referral to a lactation expert or to a support group, such as the La Leche League.

Fibroadenoma of the Breast

Description

Fibroadenoma is a nontender benign tumor of the breast (Fig. 12.36).

ICD-10-CM Code	D24.9 (Benign neoplasm of
	unspecified breast))
	(D24.1-D24.9 = 3 codes of
	specificity)

Symptoms and Signs

Fibroadenoma of the breast is the most frequent breast tumor in adolescents and young women, with the peak incidence at age 30 to 35 years. The female patient in her late teens or early 20s feels a firm, round, encapsulated, movable mass in the breast. She experiences no pain or only slight tenderness.

Patient Screening

Schedule an appointment for a breast examination to evaluate the breast mass.

Etiology

The etiology is unknown, but fibroadenomas are hormonally responsive, growing in size during the late phases of the menstrual cycle or during pregnancy.

Diagnosis

The diagnosis is based on palpation, the clinical picture, and mammography. Core biopsy is highly specific to

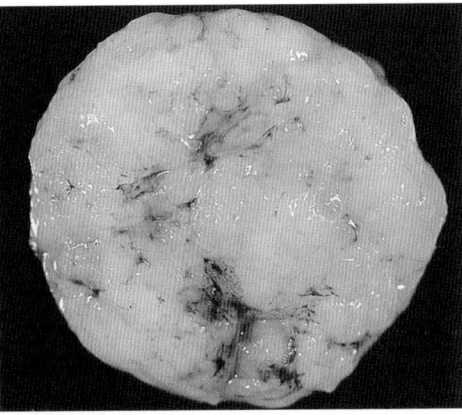

• **Fig. 12.36** Fibroadenoma of the breast. (From Damjanov I, Linder J: *Pathology: a color atlas*, ed 6, St Louis, 2006, Mosby.)

distinguish breast masses, such as fibroadenoma, from malignancy.

Treatment

Treatment of this benign tumor of the breast is surgical removal of the tumor with the patient under local anesthesia. The pathology report confirms the diagnosis.

Prognosis

The prognosis is usually good, and there are no complications.

Prevention

No prevention is known.

Patient Teaching

Discuss the surgical course of action with the patient. Assure the patient that the physician or the nurse will tell her the results of the pathology report as soon as possible.

Cancer of the Breast

Description

Breast cancer usually arises from the terminal ductal lobular unit (TDLU) of the breast, the functional unit of the breast tissue, which is very hormonally responsive.

ICD-10-CM Code	C50.919 *(Malignant neoplasm of unspecified site of unspecified female breast)* (C50.011-C50.919 = 27 codes of specificity) C50.929 *(Malignant neoplasm of unspecified site of unspecified male breast)* (C50.021-C50.929 = 27 codes of specificity)

Symptoms and Signs

Physical symptoms and signs of breast cancer include a lump, swelling, or tenderness of the breast; irritation or dimpling of the breast skin *(peau d'orange);* and pain,

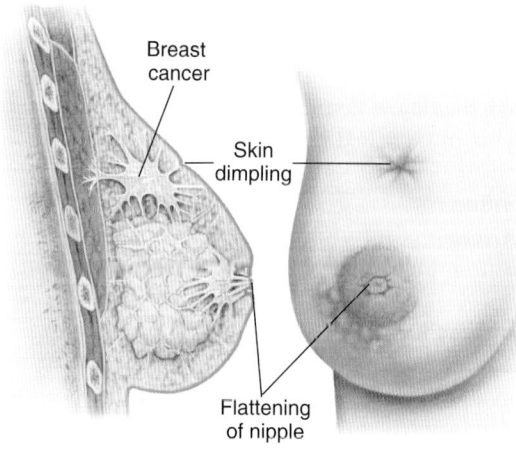

• **Fig. 12.37** Clinical signs of breast cancer. (From Seidel HM, et al: *Mosby's guide to physical examination,* ed 8, St Louis, 2014, Mosby.)

ulceration, or retraction of the nipple (Fig. 12.37). Visual examination may reveal that the breasts are asymmetric. The earliest sign, however, is an abnormality seen on a mammogram, which usually appears before the woman or her physician can feel a lump. In advanced stages of untreated lesions, the nodule becomes fixed to the chest wall, and axillary masses and ulceration develop (Fig. 12.38). Breast pain is not a common factor in early breast cancer.

Patient Screening

A woman (or man) presenting with any lump, nodule, dimpling, abnormal nipple discharge, or change in breast shape, with or without pain, should be given the first available appointment for diagnostic evaluation. The same applies for a patient with abnormal findings on screening mammography.

Etiology

Breast cancer is the most common cancer and the second leading cause of cancer-related death among women in the United States. Mortality rates are highest among those younger than 35 years of age (because of more aggressive tumors) and those older than 75 years of age (because their

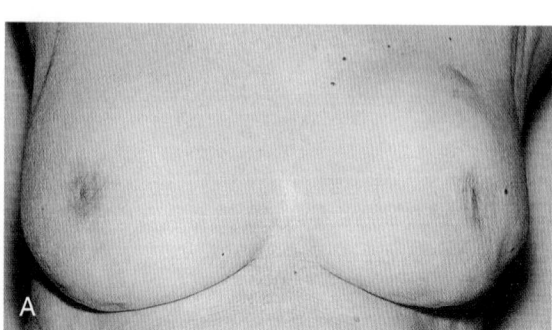
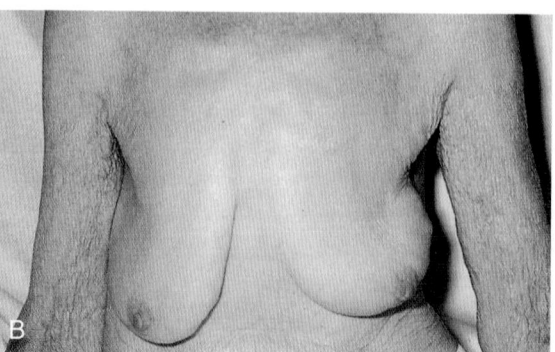

• **Fig. 12.38** (A) Patient with lump and nipple retraction in left breast. (B) Patient with altered nipple height resulting from breast cancer in left breast. (From Seidel HM, et al: *Mosby's guide to physical examination,* ed 7, St Louis, 2011, Mosby.)

bodies are less able to fight the cancer and handle the side effects of treatment). The two greatest risk factors for breast cancer are increased age and female gender. Breast cancer is 100 times more common in women than in men.

Other risk factors have to do with hormonal, reproductive, and genetic factors. Prolonged exposure to and higher concentrations of endogenous estrogen increase the risk of breast cancer. Therefore, younger age at menarche, older age at first full-term pregnancy, and older age at menopause are risk factors. Long-term (> 5-year) use of combined estrogen/progesterone hormone replacement therapy causes a modest increase in the risk of breast cancer. Those with a history of breast cancer have an increased risk of breast cancer in the other breast. The use of alcohol increases the risk. Family history is important in determining risk, although only 15% to 20% of women diagnosed with breast cancer have a positive family history. About 5% of breast cancers are associated with mutation of *BRCA1* or *BRCA2*, the inherited breast cancer susceptibility genes.

Ductal carcinoma in situ (DCIS), defined as a malignant population of cells that lack the capacity to invade through the basement membrane, is a precursor lesion for breast cancer. These cells can spread through the duct system to involve an entire sector of the breast, or they can even migrate up to involve the nipple skin, possibly leading to Paget disease of the breast. The presence of DCIS multiplies the risk of invasive carcinoma by 8 to 10 times.

The risk of breast cancer is lower in men because the male breast is much less sensitive to hormonal influences. In addition, the normal male breast does not have lobules; thus it has no TDLU. Risk factors for male breast cancer are Klinefelter syndrome, gynecomastia, testicular dysfunction, and *BRCA2* gene mutation.

Diagnosis
Greater than 90% of breast cancers are diagnosed on the basis of abnormal findings on mammography, with the remainder being detected on physical examination. Because not all mammographic findings indicate cancer, further evaluation (e.g., diagnostic mammography and ultrasonography) are used to determine the need for biopsy. Ultrasonography is used to differentiate solid masses from cystic masses and to determine whether malignant features are present, although contrast-enhanced MRI may need to be performed in women with dense breasts. Biopsy of all suspicious lumps should be performed for a definitive diagnosis. Breast cancer is staged according to the TNM system. Staging mammography for both breasts is important in patients considering breast-conserving therapy (BCT). See Chapter 1 for information about the staging and grading systems used to assess malignant neoplasms.

If the disease is suspected to be at an advanced stage, CT of the chest and/or the abdomen and the pelvis and bone scanning should be performed, depending on the patient's symptoms. Estrogen receptor and progesterone receptor status of the tumor and expression of the oncogene *c-erbB-2* and its protein product HER2/neu should be measured because they have both predictive value and prognostic value.

Treatment
DCIS should be treated with either mastectomy or BCT (wide excision followed by radiation therapy) and, in many cases, tamoxifen to prevent progression to invasive cancer. Treatment of invasive breast cancer takes into account stage and patient preferences. Surgical resection of the tumor via mastectomy or BCT with removal of any affected axillary lymph nodes is almost always part of the treatment plan. Surgery is usually combined with radiation therapy, hormone therapy (depending on the estrogen/progesterone receptor status of the tumor), and/or chemotherapy. Trastuzumab (Herceptin) is a humanized monoclonal antibody directed against *c-erbB-2* and may be effective against tumors that overexpress this oncogene. Patients with hormone receptor-positive tumors may benefit from treatment with an aromatase inhibitor. Close follow-up after completion of treatment is necessary to assess for disease recurrence.

Prognosis
Axillary lymph node positivity is the most important prognostic indicator. The presence of estrogen and progesterone receptors is associated with a better prognosis and tumor responsiveness to hormone therapy, although this difference is becoming smaller as a result of advances in chemotherapy. Expression of *c-erbB-2* is usually associated with a poorer prognosis. Other factors associated with prognosis are tumor size and grade. Many new prognostic factors are in use or being studied. One such test, the 21-gene recurrence score assay, is performed on breast tissue in patients with newly diagnosed, lymph node negative, estrogen receptor-positive breast cancer to predict recurrence risk. It can also be used to predict response to chemotherapy and identify those who may benefit from prolonged endocrine therapy.

Localized breast cancer has a 5-year survival rate of nearly 100%. Regional spread reduces the rate to 50% to 70%, and distant metastasis results in a 5-year survival rate of around 20%. Some women may report a condition called *post-breast therapy pain syndrome* (PBTPS) after surgery for breast cancer. The pain can develop weeks or years after surgery, and nerve damage is suspected to be the cause.

Prevention
Some lifestyle changes may reduce the risk of breast cancer, such as having a child before age 25 years, breastfeeding for at least 6 months, avoiding weight gain, and limiting alcohol consumption. Women at very high risk can reduce their risk by 50% by taking tamoxifen or raloxifene for 5 years. Both drugs are approved by the FDA for the prevention of breast cancer. General screening of the population for *BRCA1* or *BRCA2* mutations is not recommended.

Regular screening with mammography can reduce the risk of death from breast cancer. Mammography can identify breast cancer at an early stage, before physical symptoms develop. Tomosynthesis, also referred to as *3D mammography*, is a new technology providing a clearer, more accurate, and detailed view of the breast. The screening recommendation from the American Cancer Society is for women age 40 years and older to undergo mammography every 1 to 2 years and an annual clinical breast examination by a health professional (preferably before the scheduled mammography). The recommendation for women age 20 to 39 years is to have a clinical breast examination every 3 years. Performance of monthly breast self-examinations is no longer recommended, but women should report any changes in their breasts to their health care provider whether they do regular self-examinations or not. In addition to breast mammography, annual MRI should be offered to patients at high risk of breast cancer. For patients with *BRCA1* or *BRCA2* mutations, prophylactic double mastectomy can reduce breast cancer risk by 90%. The risks and benefits of this procedure need to be discussed in detail with an experienced health care provider.

Patient Teaching

Review and reinforce the preventive measures mentioned earlier. Provide information to women diagnosed with localized tumors about the local resection procedure and the importance of follow-up care, including regular mammography and/or ultrasonography, and clinical breast examination by a health care professional.

More aggressive therapy for invasive or metastatic disease requires a great deal of teaching. Explain the purpose of the procedures and any discomfort that normally may be experienced as a result of surgery, radiation, chemotherapy, or hormone therapy. Psychological concerns about loss of the breast and the entire recovery process are best placed in the hands of volunteers from cancer survival support groups. Most patients express great concern about their prognosis; this issue is always referred to the attending physician, as are questions about breast reconstruction.

Paget Disease of the Breast

Description

Paget disease of the breast is a characteristic breast lesion that signifies the presence of malignant adenocarcinoma cells. Underlying carcinoma of the breast is present in up to 90% of cases. It accounts for up to 3% of new breast cancers.

ICD-10-CM Code	C50.019 *(Malignant neoplasm of nipple and areola, unspecified female breast)*

Symptoms and Signs

The skin of the nipple develops an erythematous, eczematous, scaly, or ulcerated lesion (Fig. 12.39). The lesion, often unilateral, may heal spontaneously, or topical treatments may mask the inflammation, but this does not mean that Paget disease is not present. Signs of more advanced disease include bloody discharge from the nipple and nipple retraction. Some patients may have only persistent pain or

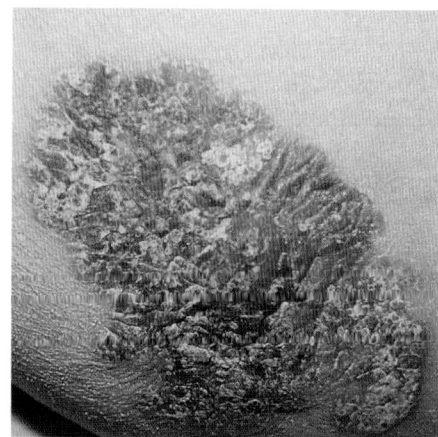

• **Fig. 12.39** Paget disease of the breast. (From Habif T: *Clinical dermatology,* ed 4, Philadelphia, 2004, Mosby.)

pruritus of the nipple. The patient also may have a palpable breast mass or abnormality on mammography.

Patient Screening

Schedule a breast examination for any patient reporting redness, scaling, or lesions of the nipple, discharge from the nipple, or changes in the shape of the nipple; this is important even when the patient reports an eventual improvement in the condition.

Etiology

It is not known whether Paget cells arise from underlying mammary adenocarcinoma (the most widely accepted theory) or whether they represent a carcinoma in situ that is independent of any underlying carcinoma. The peak age of disease onset is 50 to 60 years.

Diagnosis

The diagnosis can be established by means of biopsy or nipple scrape cytology. Mammography or MRI can be used to detect an associated breast mass. Paget cells are often tested for estrogen and progesterone receptor positivity and for overexpression of HER2.

Treatment

Historically, treatment has consisted of simple mastectomy, but breast-conserving surgery used to treat breast cancer is now being used to treat Paget disease as well. Axillary lymph node dissection should also be performed if carcinoma is suspected. Whole-breast irradiation may be performed in addition to surgery. The underlying breast carcinoma must also be treated.

Prognosis

The prognosis is affected by the presence of invasive ductal carcinoma and by metastasis to the axillary nodes. Women with a palpable mass have a 5-year survival rate ranging from 20% to 60%, and those without a mass have a survival rate of 90% to 100%.

Prevention

Women should be educated to report nipple changes to aid in the detection of lesions in the early stages of the disease.

Patient Teaching

Review the value of reporting nipple and breast changes, especially for women between ages 50 and 60 years. Clarify the purpose and the procedure of biopsy of the nipple lesion. Additional teaching should be provided to explain the treatment decision; this could include patient preparation for breast surgery and radiation therapy. The value of woman-to-woman support is again emphasized.

Review Challenge

Answer the following questions:

1. What are the risk factors for sexually transmitted diseases (STDs)?
2. Why is chlamydia called the *silent STD*?
3. What are the possible complications of untreated gonorrhea?
4. What is meant by the term *ping-pong vaginitis*?
5. What is the pathologic course of genital herpes? How is it treated? Can it be cured?
6. How is genital herpes contracted?
7. Why is early diagnosis and treatment of syphilis important?
8. List the causes of dyspareunia in men and women.
9. Which drugs may contribute to male impotence?
10. What are the possible causes of male and female infertility? Are any preventable?
11. How is benign prostatic hyperplasia (BPH) treated? What are the possible complications?
12. What are the possible causes of epididymitis? Of orchitis?
13. What are the symptoms and signs of torsion of the testicle?
14. What is a varicocele? How may it be a factor in male infertility?
15. Why is prostate specific antigen (PSA) screening valuable? Why is early detection of prostatic cancer vital? Name the diagnostic criteria.
16. What is often the first sign of testicular cancer?
17. List the common symptoms of female reproductive diseases.
18. Explain the difference between primary and secondary dysmenorrhea.
19. How is mittelschmerz related to ovulation?
20. What is the pathology associated with endometriosis?
21. Why is pelvic inflammatory disease (PID) a serious condition? What is the etiology?
22. What are the most common tumors of the female reproductive system?
23. What organism is commonly the cause of vaginitis?
24. What is toxic shock syndrome (TSS)?
25. How has medical opinion changed recently regarding the use of hormone replacement therapy during menopause?
26. Which etiologic factor do uterine prolapse, cystocele, and rectocele have in common?
27. What are the risk factors for cervical cancer? How is cervical cancer detected by the Papanicolaou (Pap) smear?
28. What is the leading cause of death attributed to female reproductive system disorders? Why is it called a *silent cancer*?
29. What are the possible causes of ectopic pregnancy?
30. What are the clinical indications of toxemia?
31. What is the life threatening complication that may occur in abruptio placentae? In placenta previa?
32. What are the factors that place women at a higher risk for cancer of the breast?

Real-Life Challenge: Benign Prostatic Hyperplasia

A 60-year-old man reports urinary frequency and nocturia three to four times a night. On questioning, he reveals having difficulty starting urination and a weak stream of urine. He also reports that he thinks he is not completely emptying his bladder. The symptoms have had an insidious onset.

The examination reveals a well-nourished, 60-year-old man with vital signs as follows: temperature, 98.6°F; pulse, 72 beats per minute; respirations, 14 breaths per minute; and blood pressure, 116/78 mm Hg. His skin is warm, dry, and pink. The prostate-specific antigen (PSA) test is ordered, and results return at 5 ng/mL. The subsequent digital rectal examination (DRE) reveals an enlarged prostate gland with no nodules or depressions. The urinalysis results are normal, and the urine culture results are negative.

Drug therapy with tamsulosin hydrochloride (Flomax) is ordered. The patient is instructed to have a repeat PSA test in 6 weeks and to return for follow-up DRE. The diagnosis is possible benign prostatic hyperplasia (BPH).

Questions

1. What is the underlying reason for the urinary symptoms?
2. What are normal results for PSA?
3. What causes the prostate to enlarge?
4. Why is the PSA drawn before the DRE?
5. What are treatment options other than drug therapy?
6. What are possible side effects of drug therapy?
7. What might be the side effects of surgical treatment of BPH?
8. What symptoms of BPH are similar to symptoms of prostate cancer?

Real-Life Challenge: Endometriosis

A 35-year-old woman has dysmenorrhea, often having onset of pain the day before onset of menses. The pain occasionally continues a few days after the end of menses. She describes the pain as a constant cramping type of pain in the lower abdomen, vagina, and back. The patient describes her menstrual flow to be unusually heavy and also states that she has pain during defecation.

The patient is a gravida III, para II, with a history of a miscarriage 5 years ago. Her living children are 7 and 11 years of age. The patient also states that she has been unable to conceive after 3 years of unprotected intercourse. She also reveals a history of tampon use during the past 10 years.

The pelvic examination reveals generalized tenderness throughout the pelvis. Vital signs are temperature, 98.8°F; pulse, 88 beats per minute; respirations, 16 breaths per minute; and blood pressure, 106/74 mm Hg. Endometriosis is suspected, and the patient is given the choice of conservative treatment with hormones or laparoscopy to visualize the condition of the reproductive organs. The Pap smear result is negative.

Questions

1. What is the cause of endometriosis?
2. What is the significance of the obstetric history?
3. Why would the patient experience pain before menses?
4. What other pelvic organs might be involved?
5. Why would hormone therapy be prescribed?
6. What other types of treatment may be used?
7. What is the significance of the patient being unable to conceive?

Internet Assignments

1. Explore a medical website, such as Medicinenet.com, to research the latest findings on hormone replacement therapy for women experiencing menopause or perimenopause.
2. Visit the Women's National Health Resource Center website, select a health topic of interest to you, and research it. Report a summary of your findings to the class.
3. Visit the National Centers for Disease Control and Prevention (CDC) website, and research the latest campaign to stop the spread of genital herpes through a sexually transmitted disease (STD) awareness outreach.
4. Visit the American Society for Reproductive Medicine website, and go to *Headlines in Reproductive Medicine* to research a topic of current interest, such as the risks of midlife motherhood.

Critical Thinking

1. Breast cancer is the most common cancer, except for skin cancer, and the second leading cause of cancer-related death among women in the United States. Explain the facts you know about what factors, such as age, affect the mortality rate. Discuss the risk factors for breast cancer. What percentage of breast cancers are diagnosed through abnormal mammography findings?
2. Name some specific symptoms and signs that may signal the onset of certain complications of pregnancy.
3. There are many causes of infertility. Are the causes more easily identified in men or in women? Which causes are preventable? In many cases, can a couple seeking help to achieve pregnancy be offered reasonable hope?
4. In a patient teaching session with a woman with a trichomoniasis infection, why is it necessary to explain how to avoid "ping-pong" vaginitis?
5. For patients with metastatic prostate cancer, how would you explain how first-line treatment with androgen deprivation therapy (ADT) works against the cancer?

Prepare to discuss Critical Thinking case study exercises for this chapter that are posted on Evolve.

13

Neurologic Diseases and Conditions

CHAPTER OUTLINE

Orderly Function of the Nervous System, 534

Disorderly Function of the Nervous System, 537

    Vascular Disorders, 537

    Head Trauma, 544

    Spinal Cord Injuries, 548

Intervertebral Disk Disorders, 549

Functional Disorders, 556

Peripheral Nerve Disorders, 563

Infectious Disorders, 566

Intracranial Tumors (Brain Tumors), 570

LEARNING OBJECTIVES

After studying Chapter 13, you should be able to:

1. Name the main components of the nervous system.
2. Describe how data are collected during a neurologic assessment.
3. Name the common symptoms and signs of a cerebrovascular accident (CVA).
4. Name the three vascular disorders that may cause a CVA.
5. Define a transient ischemic attack (TIA).
6. List some of the problems to which the nervous system is susceptible.
7. Distinguish between (1) epidural and subdural hematomas and (2) cerebral concussion and cerebral contusion.
8. Describe three mechanisms of spinal injuries.
9. Name the goals of treatment of spinal cord injuries.
10. Explain the neurologic consequences of the deterioration or rupture of an intervertebral disk.
11. Explain why cephalalgia sometimes is considered a symptom of underlying disease.
12. Describe the symptoms of a migraine.
13. Describe first aid for seizures.
14. Explain how the symptoms of Parkinson disease are controlled.
15. Describe the progression of amyotrophic lateral sclerosis (ALS).
16. Discuss restless legs syndrome (RLS).
17. Discuss transient global amnesia.
18. Distinguish between trigeminal neuralgia and Bell palsy.
19. List the diagnostic tests used for meningitis and explain how the causative organism is identified.
20. Name the common causes of encephalitis.
21. Explain the pathologic course of Guillain-Barré syndrome.
22. Explain what is meant by post-polio syndrome.

KEY TERMS

aphasia (ah-**FAY**-zee-ah)
aura (**AW**-rah)
autonomic (aw-toe-**NOM**-ic)
cephalalgia (sef-ah-**LAL**-jee-ah)
chorea (ko-**REE**-ah)
concussion (kon-**KUSH**-un)
contusion (kon-**TOO**-zhun)
contrecoup (**KON**-trah-koo)
craniotomy (**kray**-nee-**OTT**-toe-me)
demyelination (dee-**my**-eh-lih-**NAY**-shun)
diplopia (dip-**LOW**-pee-ah)

epidural (ep-ih-**DUR**-al)
fasciculation (fa-**sik**-you-**LAY**-shun)
hematoma (hem-ah-**TOE**-mah)
hemiparesis (**hem**-ee-**PAR**-ee-sis)
hemiplegia (**hem**-ee-**PLEE**-jee-ah)
neurotransmitter (**new**-roh-**TRANS**-mit-er)
paraplegia (par-ah-**PLEE**-jee-ah)
parasympathetic (**par**-ah-**sim**-pa-**THET**-ik)
paresis (pah-**REE**-sis)
quadriplegia (**kwod**-rih-**PLEE**-jee-ah)
tetraplegia (tet-ra-PLEE-jee-ah)

Orderly Function of the Nervous System

The nervous system is a complex, sophisticated, and elaborate network of many interlaced nerve cells (neurons) that make up the brain (Fig. 13.1A), the spinal cord (see Fig. 13.1B), and the nerves. Electrical impulses are carried throughout the body by the neurons (see Fig. 13.1C; Fig. 13.2). This entire system regulates and coordinates the body's activities and produces responses to stimuli, which help the body adjust to changes in its environment, both internal and external.

The nervous system is composed of two divisions: the central nervous system (CNS) and the peripheral nervous system (PNS). The CNS includes the brain and spinal cord. Its function is to process and store sensory and motor

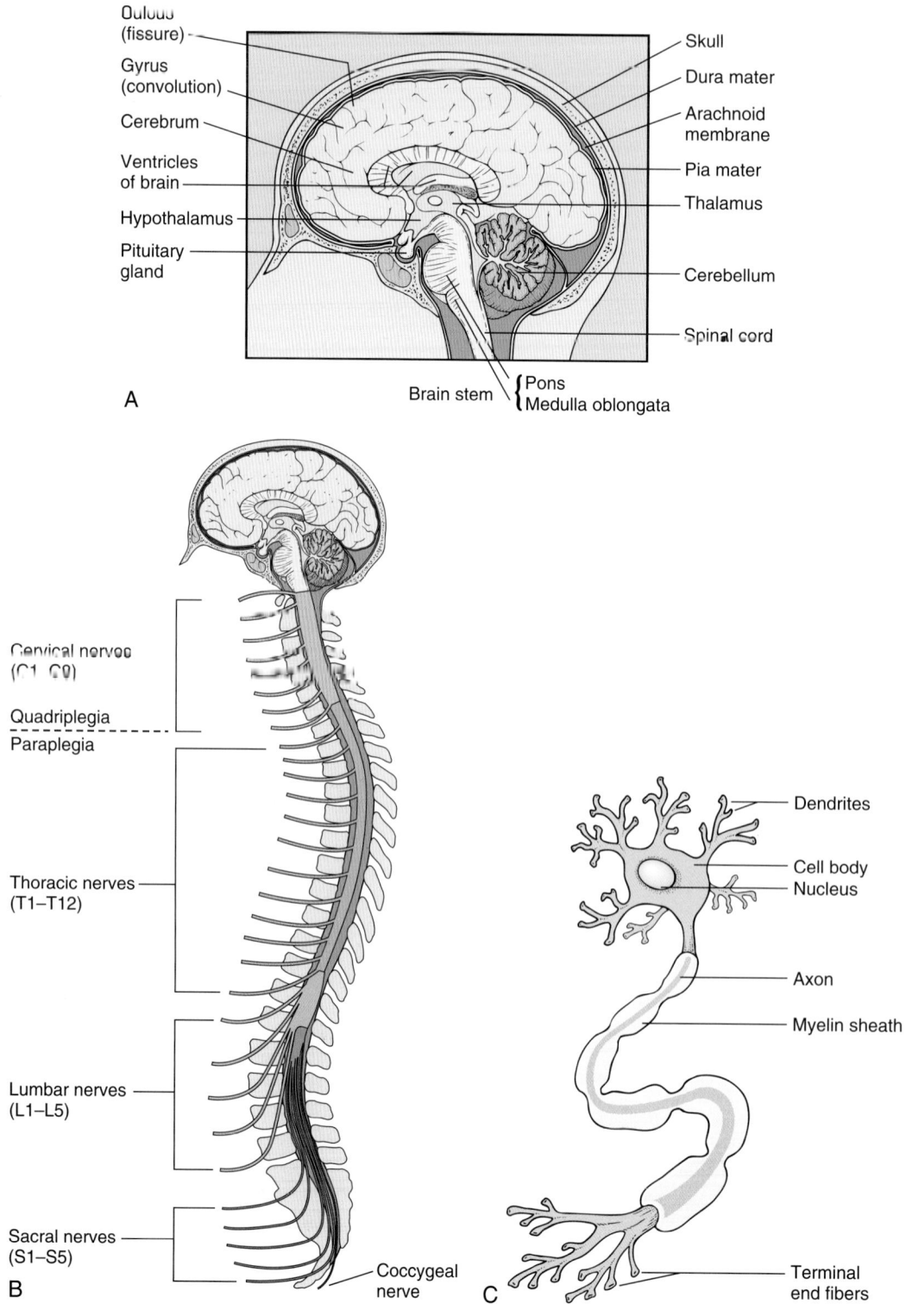

• **Fig. 13.1** (A) Normal brain. (B) Spinal cord. (C) Neuron.

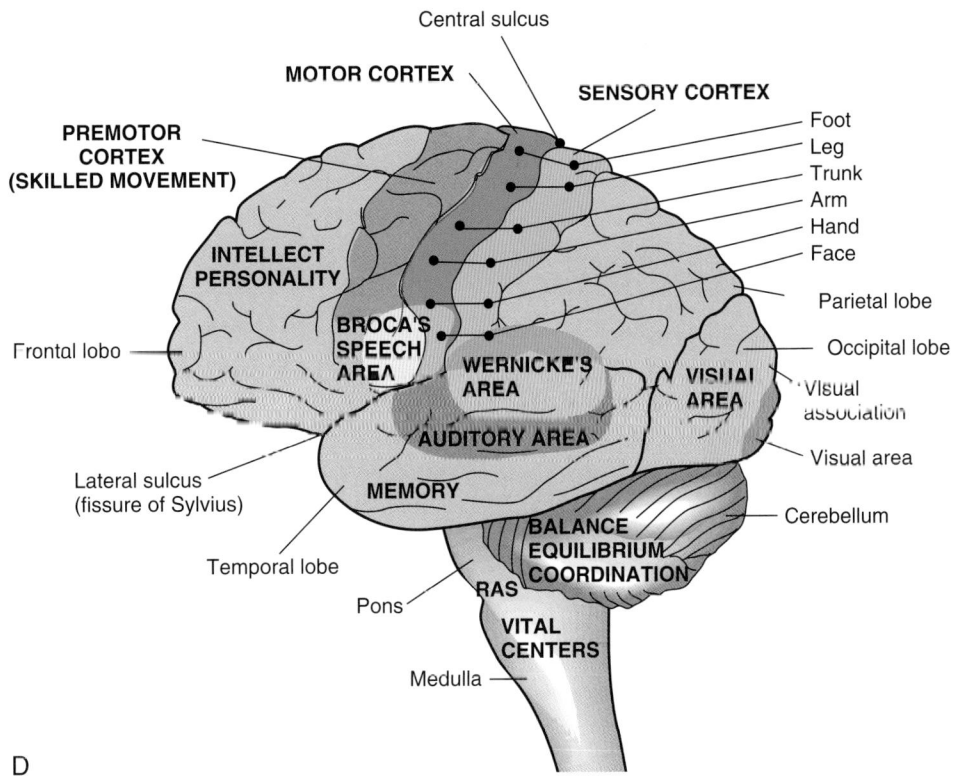

D

• **Fig. 13.1, cont'd** (D) Functional areas of the brain. *RAS,* Reticular activating system. (D, From Gould BE, Dyor RM: *Pathophysiology for the health professions,* ed 4, St Louis, 2012, Saunders.)

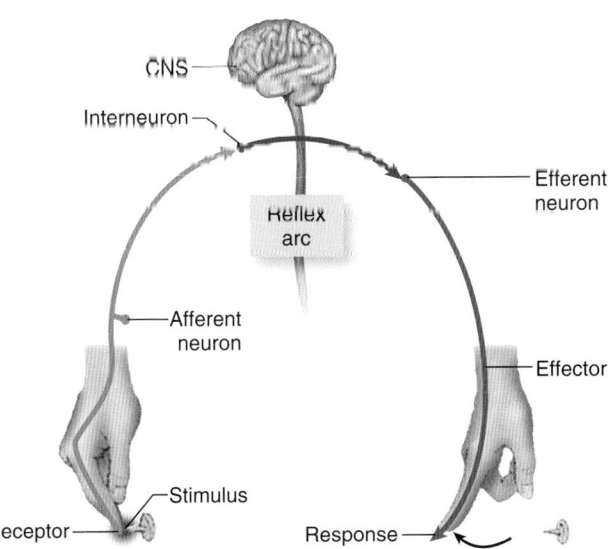

• **Fig. 13.2** Functional classification of neurons. Neurons can be classified according to the direction in which they conduct impulses. The most basic route of signal conduction follows a pattern, called *reflex arc. CNS,* Central nervous system. (From Patton K, Thibodeau G: *Anatomy & physiology,* ed 9, St Louis, 2016, Mosby.)

information and to govern the state of consciousness. The frontal lobe of the cerebrum controls intellectual functions, such as thinking, willing, remembering, and deciding, and those that control personality. Coordination, equilibrium, and posture are coordinated in the cerebellum area of the brain. The hypothalamus regulates the secretion of hormones from the pituitary gland and regulates many visceral activities.

The medulla oblongata contains vital centers that help regulate heart rate, blood pressure, and respiration. Five pairs of the 12 cranial nerves originate in the medulla oblongata. It is considered an extension of the spinal cord. All the sensory and motor nerve fibers pass through the medulla oblongata, connecting the brain and the spinal cord. The spinal cord, a continuation of the medulla oblongata, extends to the first lumbar vertebra. It is divided into 31 segments, each giving rise to a pair of spinal nerves that act like a telephone switchboard, or reflex center, carrying impulses to and from the brain (see Fig. 13.1D).

The vast network of nerves throughout the rest of the body is part of the PNS (Fig. 13.3A). Peripheral nerves connect with the spinal cord at many levels, and the information (impulses) they carry travels to and from the brain and spinal cord. Sensory (afferent) nerves transmit impulses from parts of the body (e.g., skin, eye, ear, and nose) to the spinal cord and brain. Motor (efferent) nerves transmit impulses away from the CNS and produce responses in muscles and glands. The PNS contains 12 pairs of cranial nerves (see Fig. 13.3B), and 31 pairs of spinal nerves (see Fig. 13.3C). Refer to Fig. 6.14 to compare innervations of spinal nerves and the sympathetic and parasympathetic nerves.

The sympathetic and parasympathetic nerves make up the autonomic nervous system (ANS), which regulates the involuntary muscle movements and glandular actions of the body. The PNS also controls all conscious activities, which greatly affect unconscious processes, such as heart rate, breathing, and bowel functions (see Fig. 13.3D).

Four major blood vessels on each side of the head supply the brain with essential oxygen and nutrients. The carotid arteries (two internal and two external) originate from the two common carotid arteries and are located in the anterior portion of the neck; the two vertebral arteries, located within the vertebral column (Fig. 13.4), join with the two anterior and posterior cerebral arteries and the two anterior and posterior communicating arteries to form the brain's vascular system in a roughly circular configuration of arteries known as the *circle of Willis*. Branches from the circle of Willis supply blood to all portions of the brain (Fig. 13.5). Areas of the brain that depend on a single branch for survival are especially susceptible to any disruption in the blood flow (e.g., thrombus or embolus) (see the Vascular Disorders section).

Like the rest of the body, the nervous system is susceptible to a variety of problems. Defects in the circulatory system of the brain can lead to vascular disorders and damaged brain cells. The brain also can be damaged by injuries, infections, metabolic derangement, inherited defects, congenital defects, degeneration, and tumors. Because of the complex nature of the CNS and the PNS, damage to either of the systems can cause extremely diverse symptoms.

Common problems within the nervous system that necessitate attention from health care providers include the following:

- headaches
- dizziness
- muscle weakness
- tremors
- motor disturbances, other disturbances of movement, or paralysis
- radiating pain
- memory impairment
- altered levels of consciousness
- drowsiness
- sensory disturbances or numbness
- speech disturbances
- visual disturbances

◆ ENRICHMENT

Neurologic Assessment

Neurologic assessment relies on a step-by-step collection of data to evaluate the neurologic status and cognitive function of a person. The examination is appropriate after head trauma occurs, cranial surgery is performed, or when a neurologic disorder, such as a brain tumor or stroke, is suspected. Observations and findings are graded on a scale and documented. The assessment is done within the constraints of circumstances (e.g., the location [the scene of an accident or a physician's office] and the patient's state of consciousness).

Neurologic assessment begins with a thorough medical history, noting past and current problems and recording of medications, vitamins, and supplements being taken. The patient's comprehension and judgment are noted during the examination.

The patient's mental status may be graded with the Glasgow coma scale, which is a standardized system for assessing responses to stimuli.

Next the more sophisticated mental functions, including speech, language, and writing skills, are tested. Is the patient having difficulty putting words together, or is speech slurred? Do the patient's ideas and thoughts make sense? Behavior, emotional state, long-term and recent memory, and attention span are observed.

The cranial nerves are assessed by testing the patient's sense of smell, visual acuity, eye movements, muscles of mastication, taste perception, facial muscles, hearing, and tongue movements and swallowing.

Motor function is evaluated by testing muscle tone and strength. Asymmetry in size, shape, or strength of corresponding muscles may be significant. Changes in the extension and flexion of muscles and the spasticity or flaccidity of muscles are noted.

Coordination and balance are assessed by watching for unsteadiness or a shuffling gait or the dragging of a foot. The patient is asked to perform rapid alternating movements and tasks to demonstrate fine motor coordination. A reflex hammer is used to test deep tendon reflexes in the arms and legs; any depression or hyperactivity is recorded.

Sensory examination determines diminished or abnormal sensation. A cotton ball is brushed against the skin at different points. A slight pin stick tests for superficial pain. Temperature and vibration tests also are done.

Findings lead the clinician to begin focusing on any problem area. The need for further testing also is indicated as abnormal assessment findings emerge.

GLASGOW COMA SCALE

Score	1	2	3	4	5
Eye opening	No response	To pain	To voice	Spontaneously	
Best motor response (movement of arms and legs)	No response	Extension to pain	Flexion to pain	Localizes to pain	Follows commands
Best verbal response	No response	Incomprehensible sounds	Inappropriate words	Disoriented and converses	Oriented and converses

Scoring: 13 to 15, mild head injury; 9 to 12, moderate head injury; 3 to 8, severe head injury.

From Proctor D, et al: *Kinn's the medical assistant*, ed 13, St Louis, 2017, Elsevier.

◆ **ENRICHMENT—cont'd**

Major Components of Cranial Nerves

NUMBER	NAME	TYPE OF FIBERS	FUNCTION
I	Olfactory	Sensory	Special sensory—smell
II	Optic	Sensory	Special sensory—vision
III	Oculomotor	Motor	Eye movements
			Four extrinsic eye muscles
			Upper eyelid—levator palpebrae muscle
		PNS	Iris—pupillary constrictor muscle
			Ciliary muscle—accommodation
IV	Trochlear	Motor	Eye movements—superior oblique eye muscle
V	Trigeminal	Sensory	General sensory—eye, nose, face and oral cavity, teeth
		Motor	Muscles of mastication with sensory proprioceptive fibers; speech
VI	Abducens	Motor	Eye movements—lateral rectus eye muscle
VII	Facial	Sensory	Special sensory—taste, anterior two-thirds of tongue
		Motor	Muscles of facial expression
			Scalp muscles
		PNS	Lacrimal gland, nasal mucosa, salivary glands (sublingual and submandibular)
VIII	Vestibulocochlear	Sensory	Special sensory—hearing and balance (inner ear)
IX	Glossopharyngeal	Sensory	Special sensory—taste, posterior one-third of tongue
			General sensory—pharynx and soft palate (gag reflex)
			Sensory—carotid sinus for baroreceptors and chemoreceptors
		Motor	Pharyngeal muscles—swallowing
		PNS	Salivary gland (parotid)
X	Vagus	Sensory	Special sensory—taste, pharynx, posterior tongue
			General sensory—external ear and diaphragm
			Visceral sensory—viscera in thoracic and abdominal cavities
		Motor	Pharynx and soft palate—swallowing and speech
		PNS	Heart and lungs, smooth muscle, and glands of digestive system
XI	Spinal accessory	Motor	Voluntary muscles of palate, pharynx, and larynx
			Head movements—sternocleidomastoid and trapezius muscles
XII	Hypoglossal	Motor	Muscles of tongue

PNS, parasympathetic nervous system.
From Gould: *Pathophysiology for the Health Professions*, ed 4, St. Louis, 2011, Saunders.

Disorderly Function of the Nervous System

Vascular Disorders

Cerebrovascular Accident (Stroke)

Description

A cerebrovascular accident (CVA), or stroke, is a neurologic emergency, which occurs when the brain is damaged by a sudden disruption in the flow of blood to a part of the brain (embolic) or by bleeding inside the head (hemorrhagic). Sometimes a stroke may be referred to as a *brain attack*.

ICD-10-CM Code   I63.50 *(Cerebral infarction due to unspecified occlusion or stenosis of unspecified cerebral artery)*
(I63.00-I63.9 = 72 codes of specificity)

Symptoms and Signs

CVAs are the number one cause of adult disability. Because of the inadequate blood supply, the physical and mental functions controlled by the affected area of the brain fail to operate properly (Fig. 13.6A).

The symptoms and signs of a stroke reflect the portion of the brain affected (see Fig. 13.6B). Common stroke symptoms include the following:
- sudden severe headache
- sudden aphasia, *dysphasia,* or difficulty understanding language
- sudden weakness, numbness, or paralysis of the face, including one-sided drooping mouth and eyelid (hemiparesis)
- sudden confusion or impaired consciousness
- sudden loss of vision, blurred vision, unequal pupils, or diplopia
- sudden onset of dizziness, loss of balance, or loss of coordination

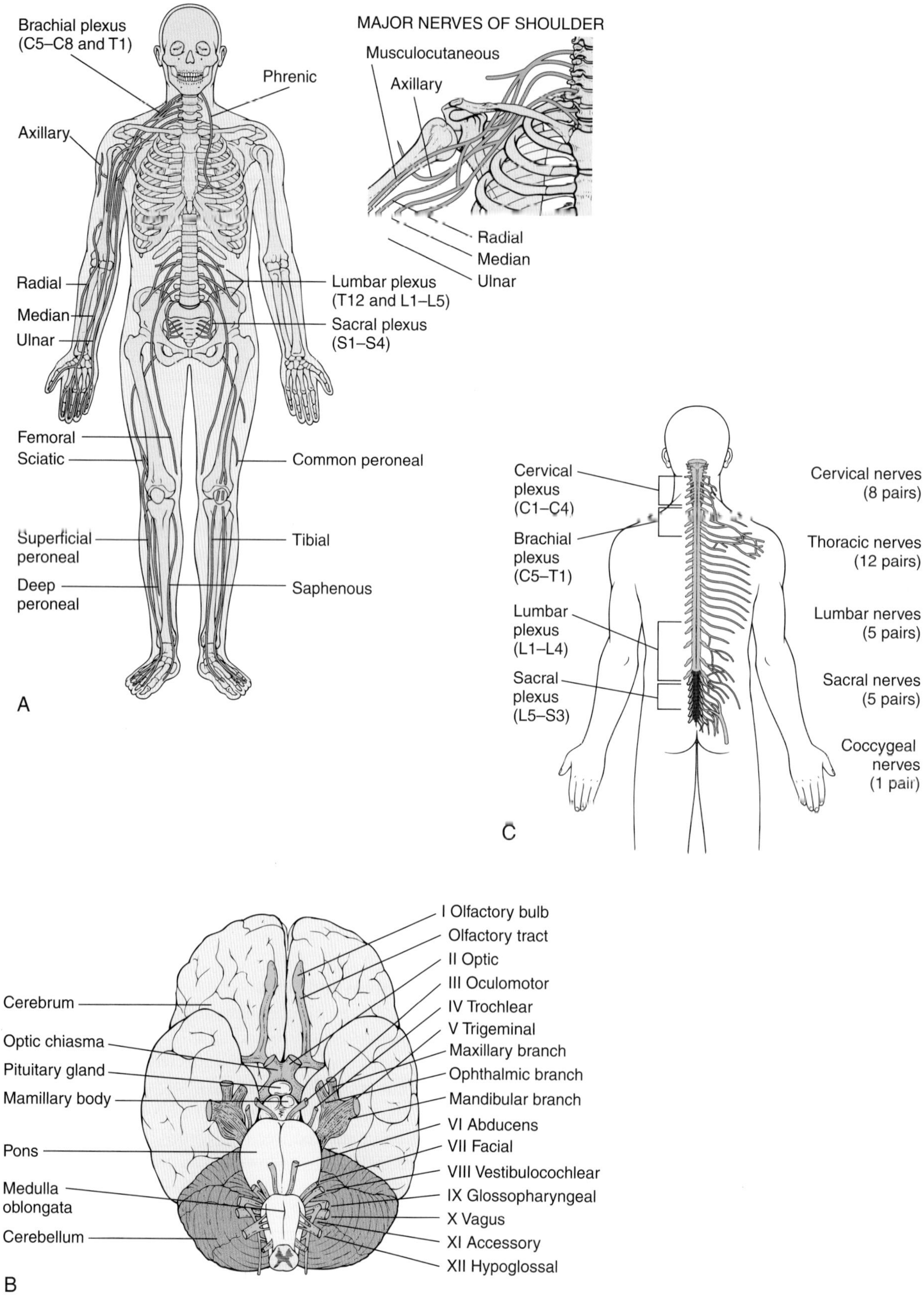

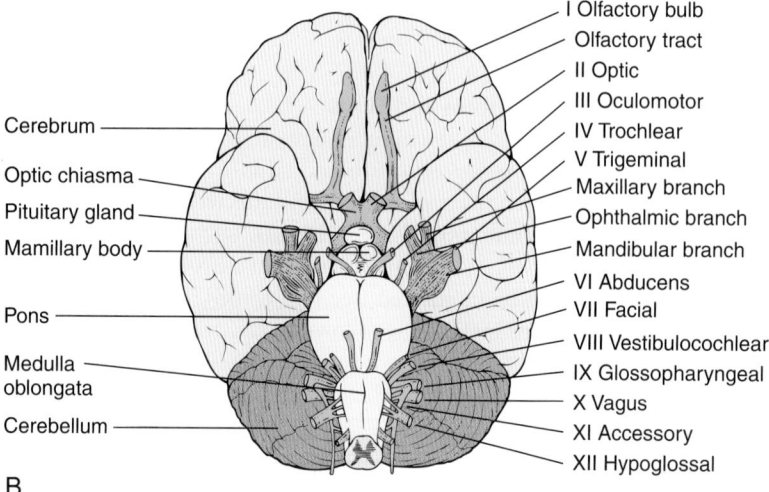

Brachial plexus
(C5–C8 and T1)

Phrenic

Axillary

Radial

Median

Ulnar

Lumbar plexus
(T12 and L1–L5)

Sacral plexus
(S1–S4)

Femoral

Sciatic

Common peroneal

Superficial
peroneal

Tibial

Deep
peroneal

Saphenous

A

MAJOR NERVES OF SHOULDER

Musculocutaneous

Axillary

Radial
Median
Ulnar

Cervical
plexus
(C1–C4)

Brachial
plexus
(C5–T1)

Lumbar
plexus
(L1–L4)

Sacral
plexus
(L5–S3)

Cervical nerves
(8 pairs)

Thoracic nerves
(12 pairs)

Lumbar nerves
(5 pairs)

Sacral nerves
(5 pairs)

Coccygeal
nerves
(1 pair)

C

Cerebrum

Optic chiasma

Pituitary gland

Mamillary body

Pons

Medulla
oblongata

Cerebellum

B

I Olfactory bulb
Olfactory tract
II Optic
III Oculomotor
IV Trochlear
V Trigeminal
Maxillary branch
Ophthalmic branch
Mandibular branch
VI Abducens
VII Facial
VIII Vestibulocochlear
IX Glossopharyngeal
X Vagus
XI Accessory
XII Hypoglossal

• **Fig. 13.3** (A) Peripheral nervous system (PNS). (B) Cranial nerves. (C) Spinal nerves.

Sympathetic division

Parasympathetic division

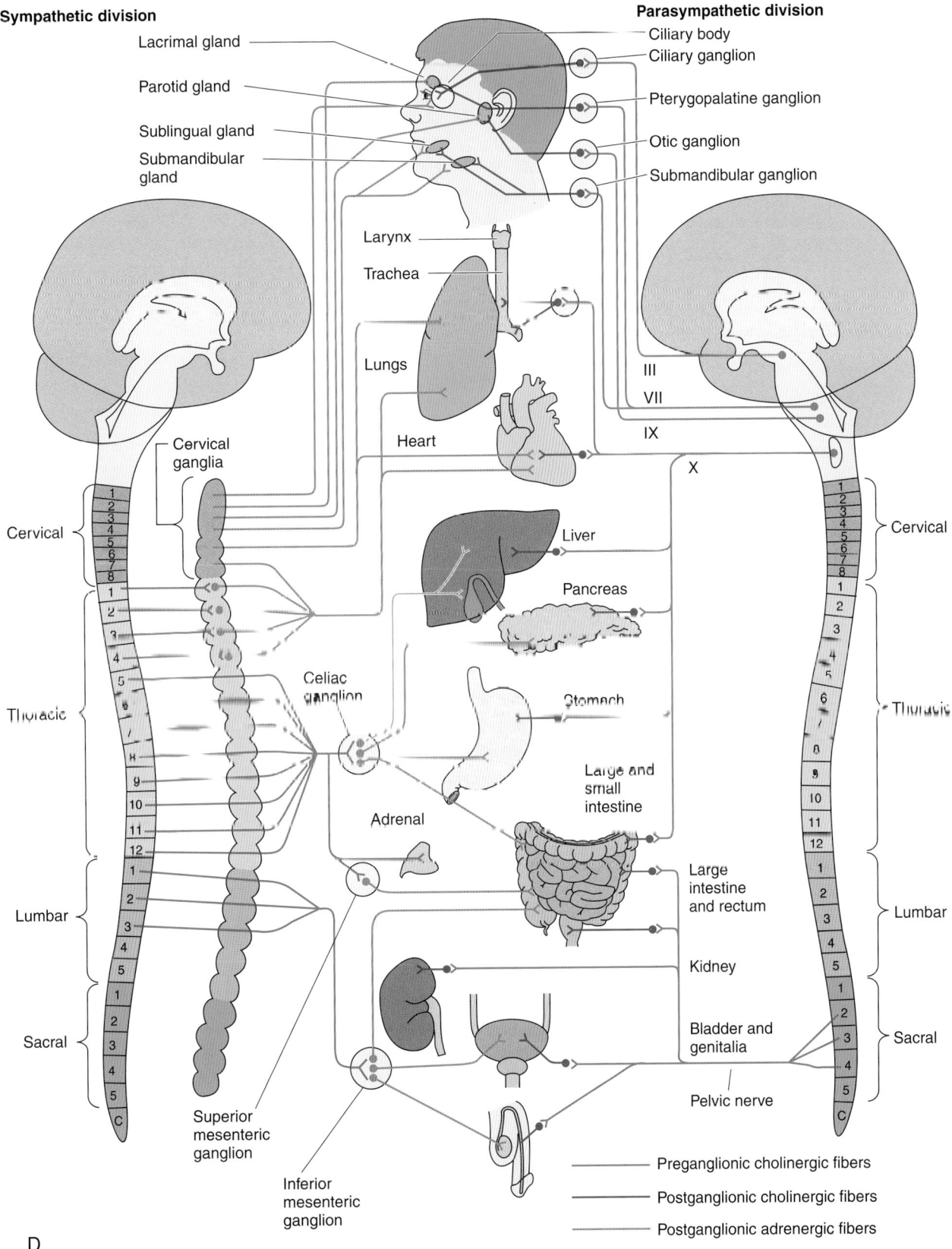

Lacrimal gland

Parotid gland

Sublingual gland

Submandibular gland

Ciliary body
Ciliary ganglion

Pterygopalatine ganglion

Otic ganglion

Submandibular ganglion

Larynx

Trachea

Lungs

Heart

III

VII

IX

X

Cervical ganglia

Cervical

Liver

Pancreas

Thoracic

Celiac ganglion

Stomach

Large and small intestine

Adrenal

Lumbar

Large intestine and rectum

Kidney

Sacral

Bladder and genitalia

Pelvic nerve

Superior mesenteric ganglion

Inferior mesenteric ganglion

Cervical

Thoracic

Lumbar

Sacral

Preganglionic cholinergic fibers

Postganglionic cholinergic fibers

Postganglionic adrenergic fibers

D

• **Fig. 13.3, cont'd** (D) Autonomic nervous system (ANS).

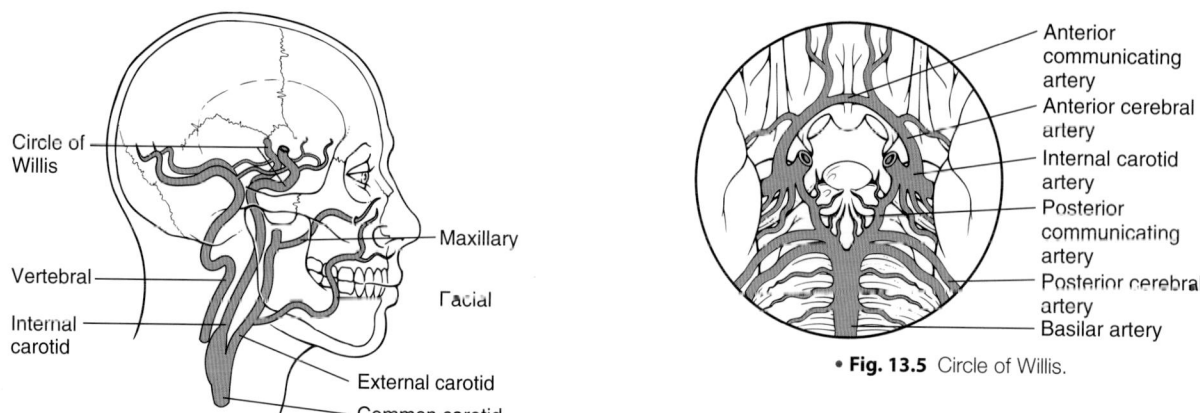

Circle of Willis

Vertebral

Internal carotid

Maxillary

Facial

External carotid

Common carotid

• **Fig. 13.4** Cerebral circulation. Major arteries of the head and neck.

Anterior communicating artery

Anterior cerebral artery

Internal carotid artery

Posterior communicating artery

Posterior cerebral artery

Basilar artery

• **Fig. 13.5** Circle of Willis.

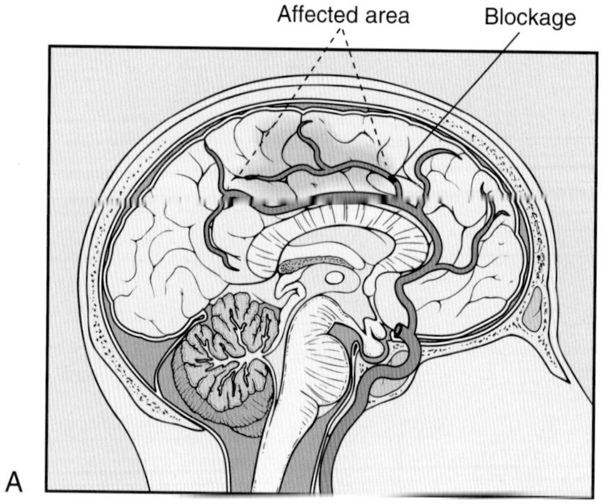

Affected area   Blockage

A

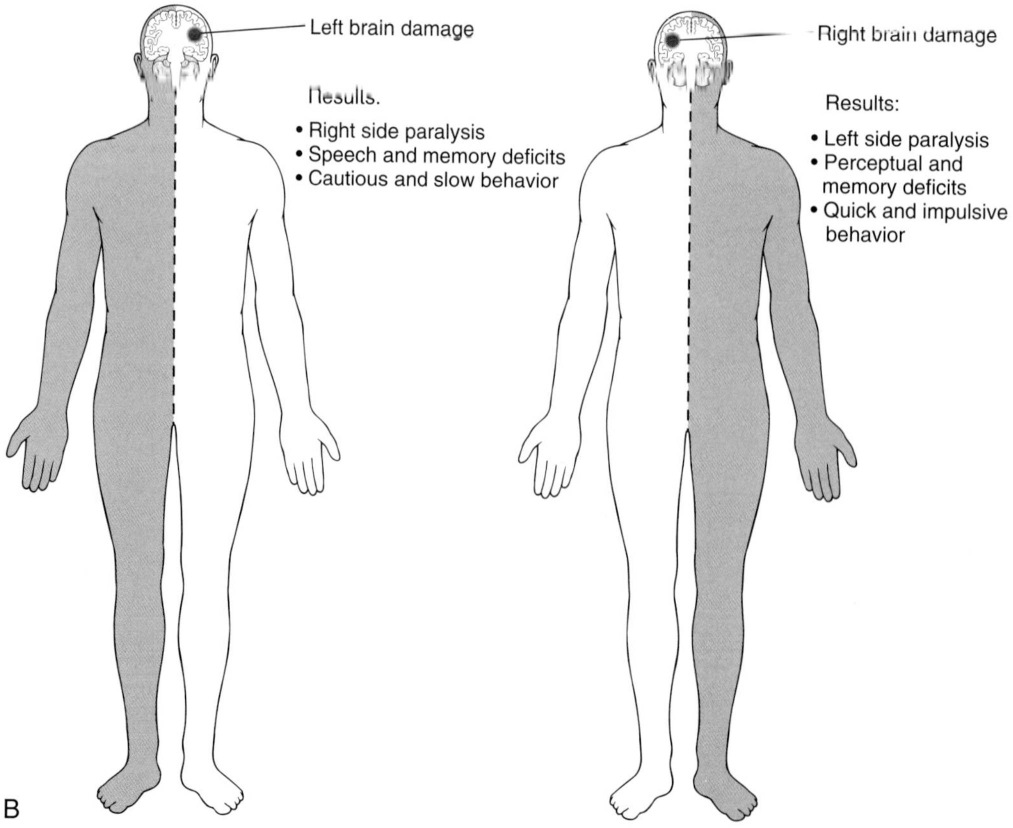

Left brain damage

Results:
• Right side paralysis
• Speech and memory deficits
• Cautious and slow behavior

Right brain damage

Results:
• Left side paralysis
• Perceptual and memory deficits
• Quick and impulsive behavior

B

• **Fig. 13.6** (A) Cerebrovascular accident (CVA). (B) Areas of the body affected by CVA.

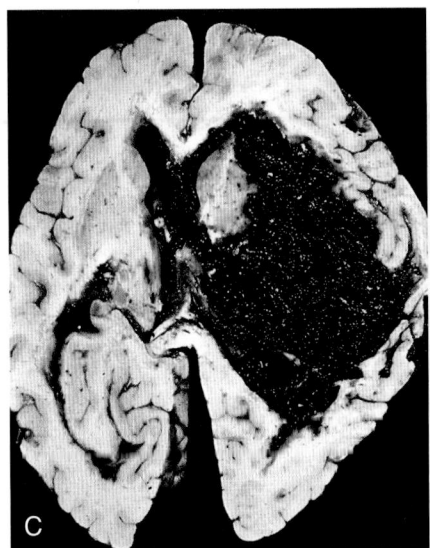
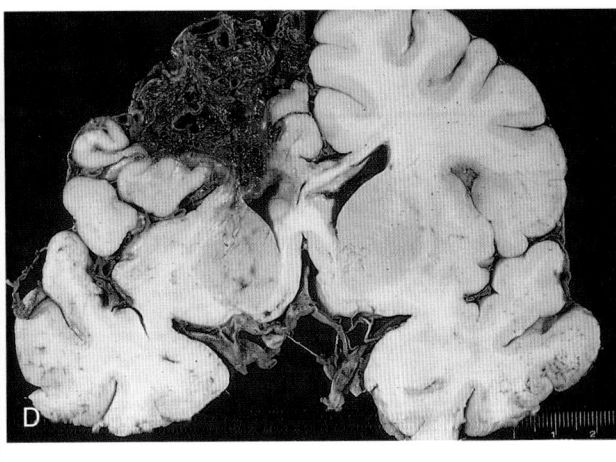

• **Fig. 13.6, cont'd** (C) Cerebral hemorrhage. Massive hypertensive hemorrhage rupturing into a lateral ventricle. (D) Arteriovenous malformation. (C and D, From Kumar V, et al: *Robbins basic pathology,* ed 8, Philadelphia, 2009, Saunders.)

A severe stroke can result in coma and death. Early recognition of symptoms and prompt medical intervention can help reduce the risks of disability and death.

Patient Screening

Any individual experiencing sudden onset of weakness, numbness or paralysis, difficulty speaking or understanding language, confusion or loss of consciousness, loss of vision or double vision, loss of balance or coordination, or dizziness requires immediate assessment and aggressive intervention. These individuals should be immediately entered into the emergency medical system (EMS) by the medical office or a family member. Occasionally the onset of symptoms may be insidious over a period of a few hours or even a day.

ⓘ *ALERT!*

FAST Method for Recognizing and Responding to Stroke Symptoms

F (Face): Ask the person to smile. Is the person's smile uneven or lopsided?

A (Arms): Ask the person to raise both arms. Does one arm drift downward?

S (Speech): Is the person unable to speak or hard to understand? Ask the person to repeat a simple sentence.

T (Time): If the person shows any of these symptoms, even if the symptoms go away, call 911, and get them to the hospital immediately.

Stroke symptoms, act FAST. National Stroke Association website: https://www.stroke.org/en/about-stroke/stroke-symptoms. Accessed August 25, 2019.

Etiology

A CVA is usually the result of one of three types of vascular disorders: (1) occlusion of an artery caused by an atheroma; (2) sudden obstruction by an embolus, including a cerebral thrombosis (clot), embolism (moving clot), or other moving emboli; or (3) cerebral bleeding. These vascular disorders most often are caused by atherosclerosis (see the Atherosclerosis section in Chapter 10) and hypertension (high blood pressure). Strokes also can result from blood disorders, arrhythmias, systemic diseases (e.g., diabetes mellitus and syphilis), hyperlipidemia, rheumatic heart disease, or head trauma. A high-fat diet, lack of exercise, cigarette smoking, obesity, and a family history of atherosclerotic disease are contributing factors.

CVAs caused by an embolus or hemorrhage often have a sudden onset, whereas strokes caused by a thrombus may appear more gradually. Cerebral thrombosis occurs if one of the cerebral arteries becomes narrowed because of plaque buildup from atherosclerotic disease. This thrombus, or clot, can enlarge until it partially or completely blocks blood flow to the artery, thereby starving the tissue it feeds of oxygen.

Cerebral embolism is also a blockage, but it is caused by a foreign object, or embolus. This embolus can be a piece of arterial wall, a small blood clot from a diseased heart, or a bacterial clot; usually platelet fibrin from an ulcerated arterial wall of the heart or valve of the heart is the causative factor. Atrial fibrillation may be a cause of the release of the embolus from the inner chambers of the left side of the heart. It is carried in the bloodstream until it becomes wedged in a blood vessel and obstructs the flow of blood to an area of the brain.

With cerebral hemorrhage, the cerebral artery is not blocked but instead ruptures, flooding the surrounding brain tissue with blood (see Fig. 13.6D). Initial effects of a hemorrhage may be more severe than those of a thrombosis or embolism, and the long-term effects are much more serious (see Fig. 13.6E) (refer to the Enrichment box about Arteriovenous Malformations).

Diagnosis

Physical examination of the patient leads the physician to suspect a CVA and to gauge the impairments on a functional scale. It can be confirmed with magnetic resonance imaging (MRI), computed tomography (CT), cerebral angiography, or electroencephalography (EEG). Blood tests for bleeding and clotting disorders may be performed. Cardiac monitoring may show atrial fibrillation or other arrhythmias.

Treatment

Immediate appropriate medical intervention (within 3 hours) from onset of stroke symptoms may limit brain damage and thereby improve the prognosis. Anticoagulants (heparin, enoxaparin), thrombolytic agents, and antiplatelet medications (aspirin, dipyridamole in a loading dose) may be given orally, or the thrombolytic agent heparin may be administered intravenously. A recently introduced protocol includes having the individual immediately chew an aspirin tablet, if possible. Surgery to improve circulation within the cerebral arteries or to remove clots is considered.

Other therapeutic measures include surgery to repair broken or bleeding blood vessels and drugs to prevent or reverse brain swelling. Antiarrhythmic drugs are administered for arrhythmias. Long-term treatment for CVA depends on the size and location of the stroke and the presence and severity of impairments. The goal of medical treatment is to restore lost functions and treat underlying disorders. A team approach to rehabilitation includes help from family members and a medical team of speech, physical, and occupational therapists; nurses; and physicians.

Prognosis

Recovery varies in rate of improvement and degree of rehabilitation. Some permanent disability may remain even after rehabilitation efforts. Brain cells that are destroyed do not recover and are not replaced; patients can learn new ways of functioning by using other undamaged brain cells.

Prevention

Prevention of stroke includes positive lifestyle changes to reduce controllable risk factors, such as smoking, excesses in diet and alcohol consumption, untreated high blood pressure, and uncontrolled diabetes. Other risk factors over which the individual has no control include age and family history of stroke. Approximately 80% of CVAs are preventable with patient education and control or modification of risk factors. Control of atrial fibrillation is important.

Patient Teaching

Review the warning signs of a stroke with the patient and the family, and instruct them about the importance of quickly seeking medical intervention for any signs of impending stroke.

Assist the family in finding appropriate medical equipment for home use that will facilitate the home care and safety of the patient. Talk with the family about achievable goals. Assist the family by providing referrals to support groups and encouraging them to seek available help in the community. Generate print-on-demand electronic materials, when possible, as teaching tools.

Transient Ischemic Attack

Description

Transient ischemic attacks (TIAs) are temporary episodes with duration of less than 24 hours of impaired neurologic functioning caused by inadequate flow of blood to a portion of the brain.

ICD-10-CM Code	G45.0 *(Vertebro-basilar artery syndrome)*
	(G45.0-G45.9 = 7 codes of specificity)

Symptoms and Signs

Transient cerebral ischemia can occur in various sites, and therefore various diagnostic codes are used. After the physician has diagnosed the site of the ischemia, refer to the current edition of the *International Classification of Diseases, 10th revision, Clinical Modification* (ICD-10-CM) coding manual to confirm the appropriate code for transient cerebral

---

 ENRICHMENT

Arteriovenous Malformations

Formed during fetal development, arteriovenous malformations (AVMs) are abnormal structures of the blood vessels (see Fig. 13.6E). The etiology of this congenital condition, which is rarely discovered before age 20 years, is unknown. Although usually found in the brain, AVMs may be located in any vascular structure. Blood normally flows from the artery through the capillaries to the veins. In AVMs, there is an abnormal connection in which the capillaries are lacking. As a result, arterial blood moves directly into the veins, giving the blood vessels the appearance of a tangled mass of arteries and veins. These fragile vascular structures have a tendency to bleed, and this often results in hemorrhage. When AVMs are located in the brain, the symptoms of bleeding are similar to those of a stroke. The patient complains of generalized or region-specific headache or the worst headache of their life. Nausea and/or

vomiting, stiff neck, confusion, lethargy, generalized weakness, visual problems, and irritability may be noted. As the bleeding progresses, speech may become impaired, muscle weakness and paralysis may be noted in the face, ringing in the ears may be reported, and dizziness and syncope may follow. Some patients may lose consciousness.

Diagnosis is made through assessment of the clinical signs and imaging studies, including CT and MRI of the brain. Prompt treatment is required and includes surgical intervention, radiation therapy, or embolization of the involved vessel. Cerebral AVMs have a mortality rate of approximately 10%. Additionally residual conditions caused by the insult of oxygen and nutrition deprivation of the brain tissue are possible. Seizure activity and other neurologic problems may follow. No method of prevention is known for this condition.

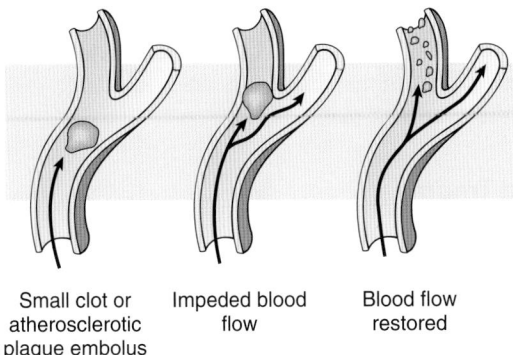

• **Fig. 13.7** Embolus causing transient ischemic attack.

(Labels: Small clot or atherosclerotic plaque embolus · Impeded blood flow · Blood flow restored)

ischemia. TIAs often are referred to as *little strokes* or *mini-strokes* because they resemble a stroke caused by an embolism. The individual may report sudden weakness and numbness down one side of the body, dizziness, dysphagia, confusion, difficulty seeing with one eye, and/or loss of balance. The individual may complain of a sudden onset headache. Usually TIAs do not cause unconsciousness. These "little strokes" often manifest as recurring episodes, lasting from just seconds to possibly hours, with symptoms gradually subsiding. The symptoms of a true stroke (or CVA) last longer than 24 hours, but TIAs should not be dismissed as a minor condition because often they are important signals of an impending stroke (CVA). The symptoms, like those of a stroke, depend on which part of the brain is affected. Differentiation between a stroke and a TIA is the duration of symptoms and the absence of permanent brain damage.

Patient Screening

As with individuals complaining of CVA type of symptoms, individuals experiencing TIAs require immediate assessment and intervention to reduce residual effects. Instruct them or their families to contact the EMS or to be transported immediately to an emergency facility.

Etiology

The most common cause of a TIA is a piece of plaque, formed by atherosclerosis, which breaks away from the wall of an artery or heart valve and travels to the brain (Fig. 13.7). This is known as an *embolus,* or a moving clot. Platelet fibrin emboli from an arterial ulcer are often the causative factor. Arterial vascular spasms and minute blood clots also may be etiologic factors. Unlike strokes, TIAs do not normally cause permanent damage to the brain tissue.

Diagnosis

Physical examination and history are the first steps in diagnosing the problem. Next is determining the source of a possible embolus. The carotid arteries are a likely source of emboli. Cranial MRI, CT, carotid ultrasonography, and EEG are all helpful in confirming the diagnosis; however, all results can appear normal.

Treatment

Treatment depends on the location of the TIA and the underlying cause. Anticoagulants commonly are used during an episode to lessen the frequency or risk of recurrences. Anticoagulant therapy may include heparin, enoxaparin, warfarin, aspirin, ticlopidine, dipyridamole, apixaban, and clopidogrel. Current protocol is to have the patient chew an aspirin tablet as soon as symptoms appear. In certain cases, surgery may be attempted to increase the blood flow to the affected area.

Prognosis

The prognosis varies, depending on the extent and duration of the ischemia. Most attacks resolve with minimal residual effects. TIAs should be considered warning signals for future CVAs. Stress reduction and lifestyle changes to reduce risk factors should be implemented.

Prevention

As with CVAs, prevention includes positive lifestyle changes to reduce controllable risk factors, such as smoking, excesses in diet and alcohol consumption, untreated high blood pressure, and uncontrolled diabetes. Other risk factors over which the individual has no control include age and family history of stroke. Oral contraceptives may increase the risk of strokes. Women taking oral contraceptives must be made aware of the symptoms and signs of a stroke and instructed to seek immediate medical attention if experiencing any symptoms.

Patient Teaching

As with patients who have suffered a stroke, instructions should be given concerning possible symptoms of an impending stroke. Family members should be instructed to seek immediate medical intervention for the patient at the first sign of a stroke. Give instructions for monitoring blood pressure, and emphasize the importance of complying with the prescribed drug therapy. Use customized electronically generated educational materials, when available, to reinforce the treatment plan.

Head Trauma

Head trauma may result in brain injury, also known as a traumatic brain injury (TBI). Ranging from mild to life-threatening or fatal, TBIs may be the result of several types of insults to the head. Included in the forms of TBI are concussions, contusions, closed head injuries, open head injuries, linear fractures, comminuted fractures, compound fractures, and contrecoup injuries. Concussions, contusions, and injuries in which the cranial vault is not violated are types of closed head injuries; fractures to the cranial vault are open head injuries and include linear, depressed, comminuted, compound, and basilar skull fractures (see Fig. 13.11).

Professional sports organizations are now actively exploring the results of TBIs and concussions that have occurred and are occurring in various sport activities. Recommendations are forthcoming on how long an individual should be kept inactive after a TBI. Research is also being done into the residual and/or cumulative effects of TBI.

Epidural and Subdural Hematomas

Description

An epidural hematoma is a collection or mass of blood that forms between the skull and the dura mater, the outermost of the three meningeal layers covering the brain. With a subdural hematoma, the blood collects or pools between the dura mater and the arachnoid membrane, the second meningeal membrane (Fig. 13.8).

ICD-10-CM Code	S06.6X0A *(Traumatic subarachnoid hemorrhage without loss of consciousness, initial encounter)* (S06.6X0[7th digit]-S06.6X9[7th digit] = 10 codes of specificity) S06.4X0A *(Epidural hemorrhage without loss of consciousness, initial encounter)* (S06.4X0[7th digit]-S06.4X9[7th digit] = 10 codes of specificity) S06.5X0A *(Traumatic subdural hemorrhage without loss of consciousness, initial encounter)* (S06.5X0[7th digit]-S06.5X9[7th digit] = 10 codes of specificity)

Intracranial injuries are coded according to site, type of wound, state of consciousness, or length of unconsciousness. Refer to the current edition of the ICD-10-CM coding manual for verification of the appropriate code once the diagnosis has been confirmed.

Symptoms and Signs

Pressure on the brain resulting from either of these hematomas can result in impaired functioning of the brain or possibly death.

Symptoms of an epidural hematoma typically appear within a few hours of head trauma. They include sudden headache, dilated pupils, nausea and often vomiting, increased drowsiness, and perhaps hemiparesis. If the hematoma is not treated promptly, unconsciousness, coma, and death occur. Deterioration of the patient's condition can be rapid. This is a neurologic emergency.

Subdural hematomas often exhibit symptoms similar to those of an epidural hematoma, except the onset is delayed because of slower accumulation of blood. This delayed onset may mimic the symptoms of a TIA, stroke, or dementia. Diplopia is a common occurrence in patients with a subdural hematoma.

Patient Screening

Most trauma victims with closed and open head injuries are transported to an emergency facility for treatment. When a head injury is not obvious, the onset of symptoms may be insidious. When a family member, or possibly the injured individual himself or herself, calls in complaining of pain in the head and onset of other neurologic symptoms after head trauma, instruct the family member to have the trauma victim transported to an emergency facility for immediate assessment. Emphasize that the victim should not drive. The victim of any acceleration-deceleration type injury, such as motor vehicle accidents (MVAs) or falls, requires prompt assessment and intervention.

Etiology

Both types of hematomas can result when blood from ruptured vessels seeps into and around the meningeal layers. Head trauma is the usual cause; a blow to the head can cause an epidural hematoma, or the head striking an immovable object (sudden acceleration or deceleration injury) can cause a subdural hematoma. Sudden acceleration or deceleration injury results in the brain striking the skull or tearing of the vessels within the brain or meninges. Subdural hematomas often occur among older adults or alcoholics as a result of falls. Cerebral hematoma often follows a skull fracture.

Diagnosis

The clinical findings noted on examination of the patient, along with a history of recent head trauma, suggest to the physician the possibility of either an epidural hematoma or a subdural hematoma. Cranial radiography, CT, and cerebral arteriography help locate the hematoma and rule out other causes of the symptoms. Prompt investigation of the condition is vital. Obtaining the history of the mechanism of injury and time of the initial insult is an additional aid in determining the diagnosis.

Treatment

If the person loses consciousness because of head trauma, rapid medical attention is needed. A craniotomy and/or

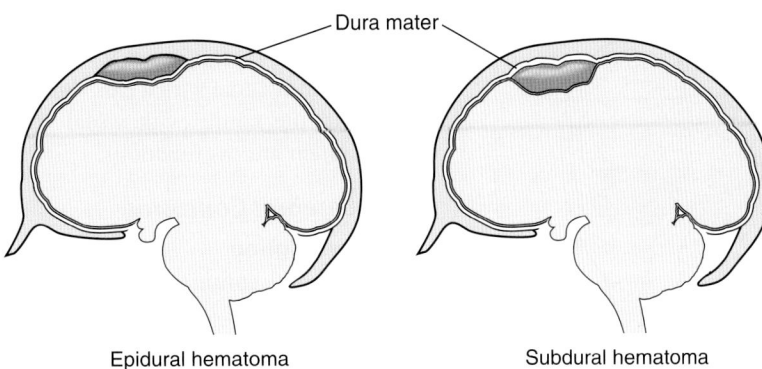

Dura mater

Epidural hematoma   Subdural hematoma

• **Fig. 13.8** Hematomas (two types).

cranial *trephination* (i.e., making a burr hole in the skull with a drill to relieve pressure by draining off the blood that has accumulated), may be necessary. This procedure is performed to remove the accumulated blood and to cauterize the bleeding vessels if increasing intracranial pressure indicates a life-threatening situation. When this procedure is performed promptly, complete recovery is possible. A patient not losing consciousness but displaying symptoms, either immediate or delayed, should be seen by a physician as soon as possible for evaluation.

Prognosis
Unchecked bleeding enlarges the hematoma and increases pressure on the blood vessels supplying the brain tissue, depriving it of oxygen. Additionally, when pressure is allowed to build within the skull, herniation of the brain tissue downward through the foramen magnum compresses the brainstem and vital centers, resulting in death. Prompt assessment and intervention are the keys to a good prognosis.

Patient Teaching
Provide postsurgical instructions for care of the incision. Instruct caregivers to assess for indications of neurologic changes and other signs of increased intracranial pressure. Encourage the use of seat belts, child restraint seats, and helmets in contact sports and cycling, skiing, boarding, or any such activity. Generate print-on-demand electronic materials, when possible, as teaching tools.

Cerebral concussion
Description
Cerebral concussion is bruising of the cerebral tissue caused by back-and-forth movements of the head, as in an acceleration-deceleration insult. Blunt force trauma also may result in cerebral concussion.

ICD-10-CM Code   S06.0X9A *(Concussion with loss of consciousness of unspecified duration, initial encounter)*
(S06.0X0[7th digit]-S06.0X9[7th digit] = 10 codes of specificity)

Cerebral concussions have various codes according to the level of consciousness and duration of any periods of unconsciousness and are designated by the addition of the fourth digit. Refer to the current edition of the ICD-10-CM coding manual to determine the appropriate code.

Symptoms and Signs
With cerebral concussion, patients may experience loss of consciousness. It often is referred to as *being knocked out.* This state may last from a few seconds to several minutes and may be followed by periods of amnesia, lasting from 12 to 24 hours or longer. Respirations become shallow, the pulse rate drops, and muscle tone is flaccid. Symptoms appearing after the person has regained consciousness may include headache, nausea, vomiting, diplopia or blurred vision, and photophobia (sensitivity to light). Persons with this injury may exhibit irritability, decreased levels of concentration, and amnesia.

Patient Screening
Individuals who have suffered a head injury and experienced loss of consciousness need immediate assessment and intervention. In most cases, treatment at an emergency care facility is the optimal choice. The unconscious individual should be transferred to the EMS for immediate assessment and transport to an emergency facility.

Etiology
Cerebral concussion is an injury resulting from impact with a blunt object, either by receiving a blow to the head or by falling. This results in disruption of the normal electrical activity in the brain, but the brain itself usually is not permanently injured (Fig. 13.9). *Mild traumatic brain injury (MTBI)* is a term that can be applied to this injury.

Diagnosis
A complete neurologic examination, along with history of the injury, is required. CT indicates no evidence of damage to the brain tissue. History from others (e.g., relatives, friends, observers, and ambulance staff) is vital.

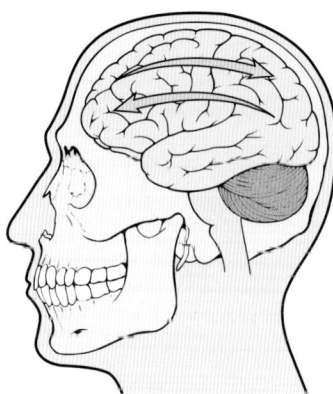

Concussion

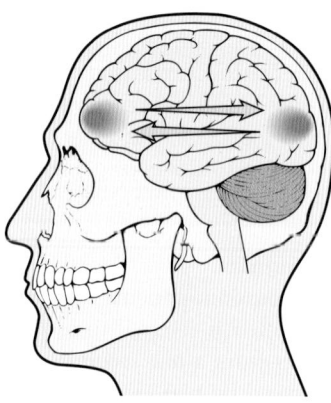

Contusion

• **Fig. 13.9** Head injuries.

Treatment

The usual treatment for concussion is quiet bed rest, with observation of the patient for signs of behavioral changes. Current recommendations suggest that it is acceptable to allow the patient to sleep, but it is important to make sure that the patient awakens fully when roused. Any changes noted, including changes in the level of consciousness, could indicate a progressive brain injury.

Prognosis

Prognosis is unpredictable and depends on the extent of the insult and any additional trauma. Cumulative effects may occur with successive MTBIs, resulting in more severe symptoms. Although most symptoms disappear after a few days or weeks, some individuals may experience postconcussion syndrome for weeks or months. Many people recover with no residual damage.

Prevention

Cerebral concussions are difficult to prevent. Consistent use of seat belts, child restraint seats, and helmets may help reduce the severity of the injury. Individuals who have experienced concussion are encouraged to avoid situations where another blow to the head could occur.

Patient Teaching

Encourage all patients to consistently use seat belts, secure children in child restraint seats, and wear helmets while playing contact sports or cycling. Provide family members or other caregivers with written information about care of the individual with a closed head injury. Provide the patient and the family with visual aids depicting the neurologic system and its functions.

Cerebral Contusion

Description

Cerebral contusion is more serious than concussion. This injury to the brain involves bruising of tissue along or just beneath the surface of the brain. It may also be termed a *contrecoup insult.*

ICD-10-CM Code	S06.330A *(Contusion and laceration of cerebrum, unspecified, without loss of consciousness, initial encounter)*
	(S06.300[7th digit]- S06.389[7th digit] = 90 codes of specificity)

Cerebral lacerations and contusions are coded according to site, type of wound, state of consciousness, or length of unconsciousness. Once the diagnosis has been confirmed, refer to the current edition of the ICD-10-CM coding manual for assistance in verifying the appropriate code.

Symptoms and Signs

The symptoms and signs of contusion vary, depending on the site and extent of the injury, and persist for longer than 24 hours. They may range from temporary loss of consciousness to coma. When conscious, the person may report a severe headache and hemiparesis. The symptoms may be progressive in nature. The person may appear drowsy and lethargic or hostile and combative.

Permanent damage to the brain may result from cerebral contusions caused by subdural and epidural hematomas (see the Epidural and Subdural Hematomas section), causing impaired intellect, dysphasia, paralysis, epilepsy, impaired gait, and continuing stupor.

Patient Screening

Individuals who have suffered a head injury and complain of severe headache experience one-sided paralysis and a period of unconsciousness and are in need of immediate assessment and intervention. In most cases, treatment at an emergency care facility is the optimal choice. The unconscious individual should be transferred to the EMS for immediate assessment and transport to an emergency facility.

Etiology

Contusion of the brain is caused by a blow to the head or by impact against a hard surface, as occurs in an automobile accident. The twisting or shearing force against the two hemispheres of the brain that occurs when it collides with the cranial bones may damage the structures deep within the brain (see Fig. 13.9). Cerebral contusion often is associated with a skull fracture. This TBI may be observed in child, spouse, partner, or elder abuse.

Diagnosis

A thorough neurologic examination is necessary, along with obtaining the history of the mechanism of the injury. CT reveals the location and extent of brain damage (Fig. 13.10). Cranial radiography helps rule out a possible skull fracture.

Treatment

Patients with cerebral contusion need to be hospitalized so that their vital signs can be monitored and rapid medical intervention can be provided, if required. Specific treatment depends on the site and severity of the contusion.

Prognosis

The prognosis is unpredictable and depends on additional trauma and the health of the individual. Underlying pathology may compromise the possibility of a favorable outcome. Increased intracranial pressure and possible herniations are complications that may follow the injury.

Prevention

As with cerebral concussions, cerebral contusions are difficult to prevent. The consistent use of seat belts, child restraint seats, and helmets may help reduce the severity of the injury.

Patient Teaching

As with cerebral concussions, all individuals should be encouraged to consistently use seat belts, secure children in child restraint seats when traveling by car, and wear helmets when engaging in contact sports or cycle riding. Provide family members or caregivers with written information about the care of a victim with a closed head injury. Instruct family members or caregivers to seek immediate medical attention for the victim if the symptoms worsen. Provide the patient and the family with visual aids depicting the neurologic system and its functions.

Depressed skull fracture

Description

A fractured skull occurs with a break or fracture in one of the bones of the cranium (Fig. 13.11). When the skull bones are depressed or torn loose, they are pushed below the normal surface of the skull.

ICD-10-CM Code	S02.91XA *(Unspecified fracture of skull, initial encounter for closed fracture)*
	(S02.0[7th digit]–S02.92[7th digit] = 32 codes of specificity)

Once a diagnosis has been made specifying site and type of skull fracture, refer to the current edition of the ICD-10-CM coding manual to determine the highest specificity.

Symptoms and Signs

When a portion of the skull is broken and is pushed in on the brain, causing injury, it is said to be a *depressed skull fracture* (see Fig. 13.11). The symptoms depend on the site of the fracture. For example, a bone fragment pressing on the motor area of the brain may cause hemiplegia (Fig. 13.12). Characteristically, symptoms from a depressed fracture are not progressive. They tend to remain static until the depressed bone is elevated and the pressure is relieved. Seizures are a common complication of depressed skull fractures (see Fig. 13.11 for additional types of skull fractures).

Signs include bleeding from the wound, ears, nose, or around the eyes; changes in pupils (either nonreactive or unequal); bruising behind the ears *(Battle sign)* or around and under the eyes *(raccoon eyes* [see Fig. 2.53, a photo of "raccoon eyes"]); and clear or bloody drainage from the ears

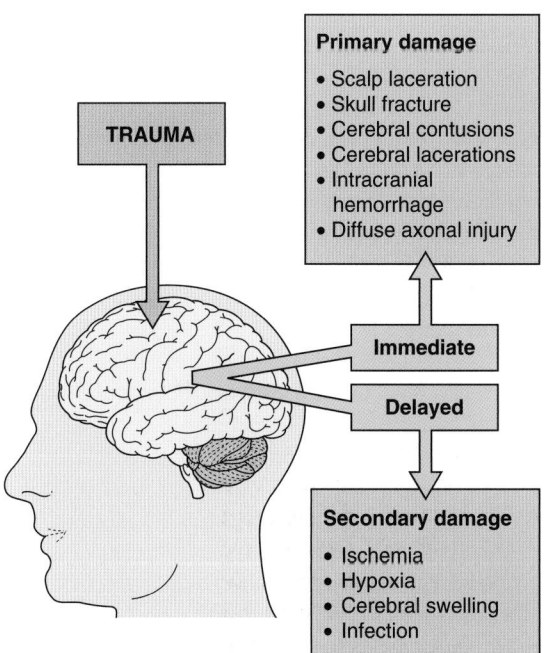

• **Fig. 13.10** Closed head injury. (From Stevens A, et al: *Core pathology,* ed 3, London, 2010, Mosby/Elsevier.)

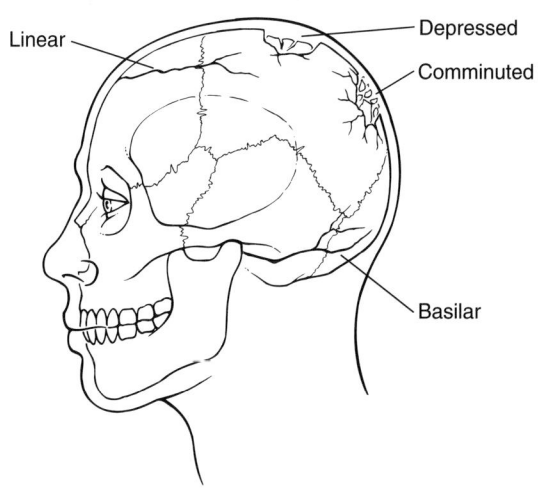

• **Fig. 13.11** Skull fractures.

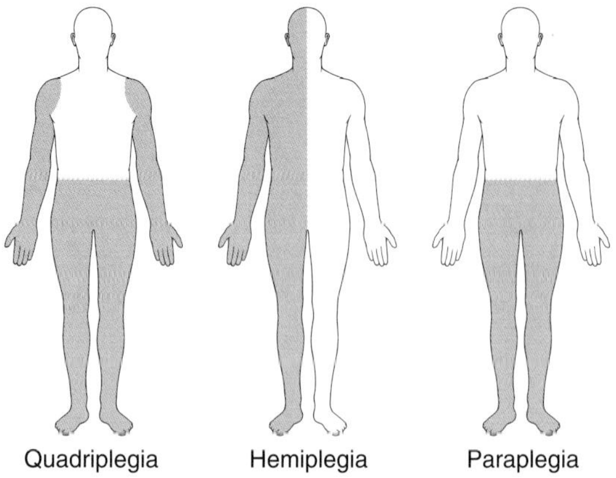

Quadriplegia   Hemiplegia   Paraplegia

• **Fig. 13.12** Types of paralysis.

or the nose. Other signs include headache, stiff neck, nuchal rigidity, nausea, vomiting, visual disturbances, slurred speech, confusion, restlessness, irritability, difficulty balancing, drowsiness, seizures, and/or loss of consciousness.

Patient Screening

Patients with head injuries are in need of prompt intervention. Immediate transfer to the EMS for transportation to an emergency facility is recommended. Head injuries should always be considered life threatening until ruled otherwise.

Etiology

Direct impact on the skull by a blunt object is the most common cause of depressed fractures. Industrial and automobile accidents are two of the many possible causes. Child, domestic, intimate partner, or elder abuse may also be a causative factor. The fractured bone may cut an artery or vein, causing hemorrhage in the brain.

Diagnosis

Physical examination of the patient most likely reveals a defect in the skull. Cranial radiography indicates whether and where the brain is being crushed. CT shows the presence of life-threatening cerebral edema.

Treatment

Treatment is aimed at relieving intracranial pressure. Craniotomy is performed, and the depressed bone is elevated back into place. Head protection is worn until the fracture has healed at least partially.

Prognosis

The prognosis is unpredictable; it depends on the extent of the insult, timely intervention, possible complications, additional trauma, and any underlying medical conditions. Successful surgical intervention to relieve intracranial pressure and arrest bleeding usually has a positive outcome.

Prevention

Prevention is difficult because of the accidental nature of the fracture. Consistent use of seat belts and child restraint seats when in motor vehicles; wearing helmets during cycling, skiing, skateboarding, or similar activities; and wearing full protective gear when playing contact sports will all help reduce the extent of damage in a head injury.

Patient Teaching

Reinforce to parents the potential dangers of head injuries in children, and remind them of the importance of children wearing helmets while cycling, skiing, skateboarding, or similar activities and while playing contact sports. Advise parents and others to seek professional emergency intervention in the event of a head injury in their children. Provide the patient and the family with visual aids depicting the neurologic system and its functions.

❖ ENRICHMENT

Basilar Skull Fracture

A basilar skull fracture is a fracture of the bones of the floor of the cranial vault (see Fig. 13.11). This injury usually results from a massive insult to the cranium during a motor vehicle accident (MVA) or other violent trauma in which the head is struck anteriorly or laterally in the midportion. As with other head injuries, symptoms, signs, and treatment depend on the area involved and the extent of the fracture. "Raccoon eyes" and "battle sign" are manifestations of basilar skull fracture and alert the physician to order imaging of the cranial vault for further investigation. Cerebrospinal fluid (CSF) flowing from the ears or nares may be associated with a skull fracture. The level of consciousness is assessed, as are other neurologic signs. Treatment is like that of head injuries, including surgical intervention to relieve intracranial pressure. Occasionally the severity of the fracture causes severing of the pituitary stalk, resulting in panhypopituitarism.

Spinal Cord Injuries

Paraplegia and quadriplegia (tetraplegia)

Description

Injuries to the spinal cord affect the innervation of any spinal nerves distal to the point of insult. The extent of the injury and consequential edema often result in the failure of spinal nerve functioning, with resulting loss of motor and sensory function. Paraplegia is loss of nerve function in areas below the waist and paralysis of the lower trunk and legs. Quadriplegia/Tetraplegia is loss of nerve function at the cervical region resulting in paralysis of the arms, hands, trunk, and legs.

ICD-10-CM Code	G82.20 (Paraplegia, unspecified) (G82.20-G82.22 = 3 codes of specificity) G82.50 (Quadriplegia, unspecified) (G82.50-G82.54 = 5 codes of specificity)

Quadriplegia/Tetraplegia is coded by site and type. Once diagnosis confirms site and type, refer to the current edition of the ICD-10-CM coding manual for the appropriate code.

Symptoms and Signs

When the spinal cord is injured, one or more parts of the body inferior to the point of injury may be affected. The damage to the cord may be only temporary, but it usually leads to some degree of permanent disability, because nerve pathways control many body functions and actions. Paraplegia results in the loss of motor and sensory control of the trunk of the body and lower extremities. Loss of bowel, bladder, and sexual function is also common. Quadriplegia/tetraplegia results in paralysis of the lower extremities and usually the trunk, with either partial or total paralysis of the upper limbs. Hypotension, hypothermia, bradycardia, and respiratory problems also may be present. In some patients, respiration is maintained or assisted by mechanical ventilation.

Patient Screening

Individuals who sustain the acceleration-deceleration type of injury require stabilization for transport to an emergency care facility. Once families are advised of their loved one's condition, they contact the office for an appointment to request information from the physician concerning the condition of their loved one. The family will be experiencing extensive anxiety, and the next available appointment should be scheduled for them to see the physician. Appointments for recovering patients will be scheduled for follow-up as necessary.

Etiology

Generally spinal cord injuries that cause paraplegia and quadriplegia/tetraplegia are the result of vertebral fractures or vertebral dislocation. The site of the injury, the type of trauma to the cord, and the severity of the trauma determine whether paraplegia or quadriplegia/tetraplegia will occur (see Fig. 13.12).

Trauma to the thoracic and lumbar regions of the spine (T1 and below) usually results in paraplegia (see Fig. 13.1B). Vertical compression and hyperflexion of the spine usually produce this injury. Trauma to the cervical vertebrae (C5 or above) may result in quadriplegia/tetraplegia. Injuries between C5 and C7 in the cervical vertebrae may produce varying degrees of paresis to the shoulders and arms. Damage occurring above C3 is usually fatal. The usual cause of this fatal injury is hyperextension or flexion of that portion of the spine. Mechanisms of spinal cord injury are presented in Fig. 13.13.

Diagnosis

A complete assessment of neurologic functioning is needed. Spinal radiography, MRI, and CT are ordered to determine the type and extent of injury. Figs. 13.14A and B show the effects of spinal cord damage.

Treatment

The goals of treatment for all spinal cord injuries include restoration of the normal alignment and stability of the spine; decompression of the spinal cord, nerves, and vertebrae; and early rehabilitation of the patient. These goals may involve surgery or using specialized medications and procedures.

Immediate spinal cord trauma intervention includes stabilization of the neck and spine before any movement to prevent secondary damage. After the patient is stabilized, corticosteroid medications (e.g., methylprednisone) may be administered to prevent or slow edema. Another intervention may include inducing a hypothermic state to the injured area in hopes of preventing edema of the spinal cord area. The location of the injury will also bear an impact on treatment.

Prognosis

The prognosis for a person with a spinal cord injury always is guarded. However, the earlier treatment is begun, the better is the prognosis. Research focused on improving outcomes for spinal cord injuries is ongoing. Partial or total severing of the spinal cord results in permanent, irreversible damage and paralysis of areas below the insult.

Prevention

Absolute prevention of spinal cord injury is not possible. Preventing injury beyond the initial insult is helped by immediate stabilization of the injured person before any form of movement is attempted.

Patient Teaching

Assist patients and families in locating and contacting available community resources. Encourage patients to continue with recommended therapy. Generate print-on-demand electronic materials, when possible, as teaching tools.

ENRICHMENT

Wounded Warrior Project

The Wounded Warrior Project provides opportunities to veterans with quadriplegia or other physical or emotional injury to stay in an underwater cage and interact with some species of sharks and to swim with whale sharks, manta rays, and other species of fish, in conjunction with rehabilitative therapy after injury. In cases of paralysis, water therapy allows these individuals, who are no longer able to move on land, to move in the water. There are some programs that involve dives while in underwater cage, and other programs, such as the one at the Georgia Aquarium, in which allow swimming in the water with marine life species, but without the use of cages.

Intervertebral Disk Disorders

Degenerative Disk Disease

Description

The degeneration or deterioration of an intervertebral disk may result in pain in the areas served by the spinal nerves exiting at or below that disk space. Degenerative disk disease is a natural part of aging, occurring in almost everyone over time.

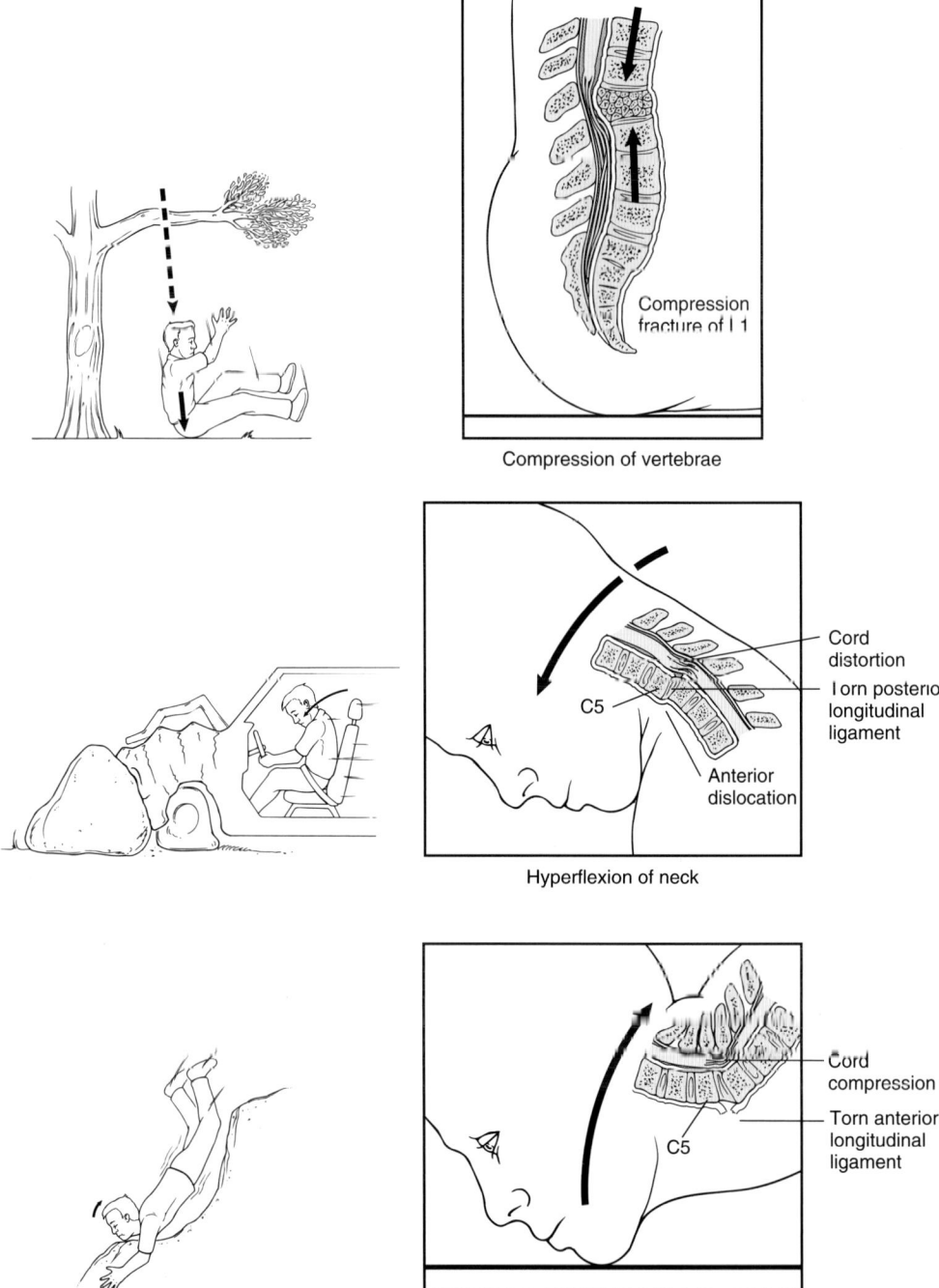

Compression of vertebrae

Hyperflexion of neck

Hyperextension of spine

• **Fig. 13.13** Spinal injuries.

ICD-10-CM
Code

M51.34 *(Other intervertebral disk
 degeneration, thoracic region)*
M51.35 *(Other intervertebral disk
 degeneration, thoracolumbar region)*
M51.36 *(Other intervertebral disk
 degeneration, lumbar region)*
M51.37 *(Other intervertebral disk
 degeneration, lumbosacral region)*

*Degenerative disk disease is coded by site. Once the
site is confirmed by diagnosis, refer to the current
edition of the ICD-10-CM coding manual for the
appropriate code.*

Symptoms and Signs

When pain occurs, it radiates down the nerve path (dermatome); may be described as burning; and can become
intractable (refer to Fig. 6.14 for an illustration of dermatomes). The constant back pain and the severe pain that
radiates down one or both legs may be accompanied by loss
of some motor functions in the legs. Additionally, the individual may also experience some numbness and tingling
associated with weakness. There can also be bowel or bladder issues. Ask about any incontinence (urinary or fecal) or
constipation.

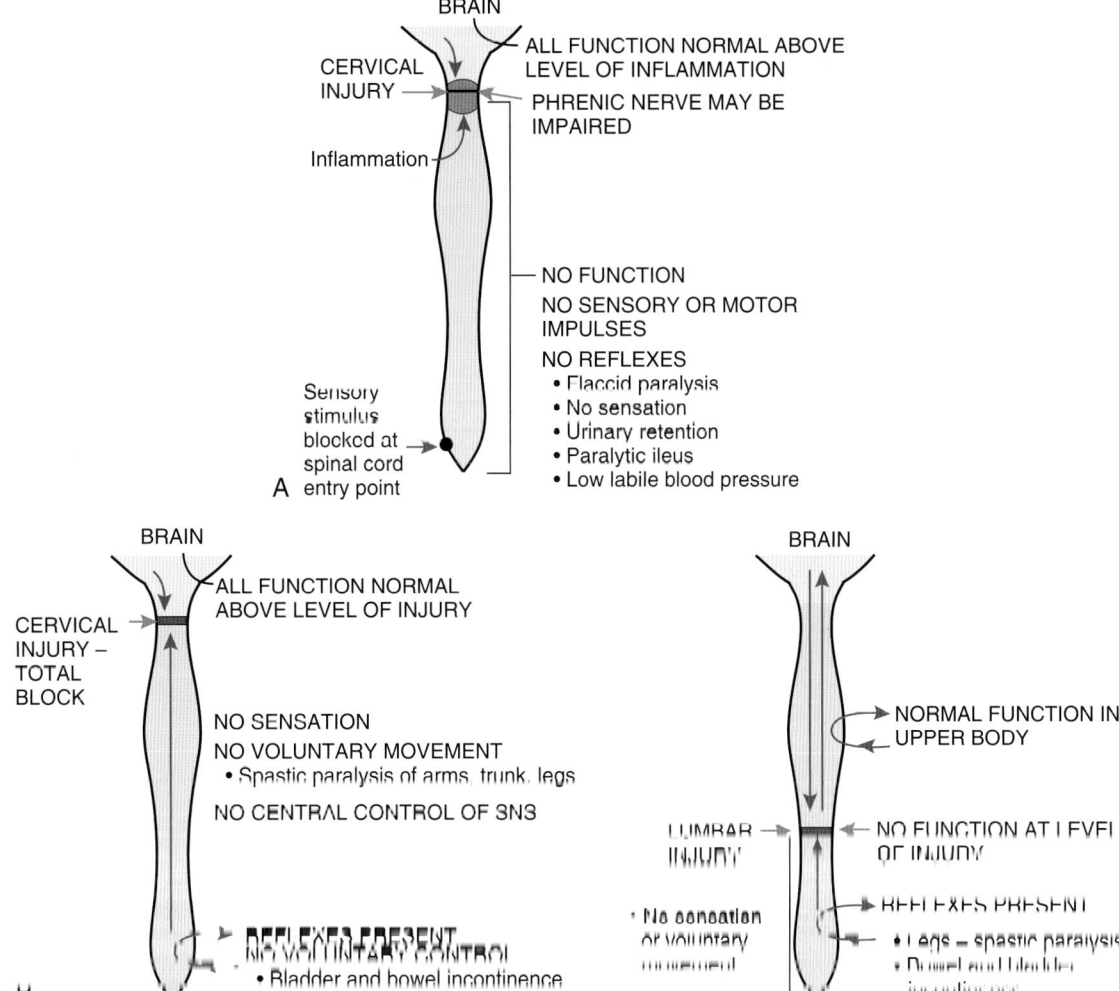

BRAIN

CERVICAL INJURY —

— ALL FUNCTION NORMAL ABOVE LEVEL OF INFLAMMATION

— PHRENIC NERVE MAY BE IMPAIRED

Inflammation —

— NO FUNCTION

NO SENSORY OR MOTOR IMPULSES

NO REFLEXES
• Flaccid paralysis
• No sensation
• Urinary retention
• Paralytic ileus
• Low labile blood pressure

Sensory stimulus blocked at spinal cord entry point

A

BRAIN

CERVICAL INJURY – TOTAL BLOCK

— ALL FUNCTION NORMAL ABOVE LEVEL OF INJURY

NO SENSATION
NO VOLUNTARY MOVEMENT
• Spastic paralysis of arms, trunk, legs

NO CENTRAL CONTROL OF SNS

REFLEXES PRESENT
NO VOLUNTARY CONTROL
• Bladder and bowel incontinence

B

BRAIN

— NORMAL FUNCTION IN UPPER BODY

LUMBAR INJURY

— NO FUNCTION AT LEVEL OF INJURY

• No sensation or voluntary movement

REFLEXES PRESENT
• Legs – spastic paralysis
• Bowel and bladder incontinence

• **Fig. 13.14** Effects of spinal cord damage. (A) During spinal shock (partial immediately after injury). (B) Overview of permanent effects (after spinal shock). *SNS,* Sympathetic nervous system. (From Gould BE, Dyer RM: *Pathophysiology for the health professions,* ed 4, St Louis, 2012, Saunders/Elsevier.)

Patient Screening

Patients complaining of severe back pain require prompt assessment. An appointment should be scheduled for them as soon as possible or according to office policy. A report of loss of motor function in the legs requires prompt assessment. That patient should be referred to an emergency treatment facility.

Etiology

As a person ages, the fluid in the disk decreases, causing degenerative disk disease. The degeneration may be mechanical and the result of constant wearing on the disk. Misalignment of vertebrae causes continual rubbing on the disk involved, resulting in inflammation and gradual destruction of the disk. The resulting inflammation eventually involves the spinal nerve roots and may cause scarring. A sequela is spinal stenosis, in which there is narrowing of the vertebral canal, the nerve root canals (foramen), or intravertebral foramina, causing the nerve roots to become trapped in the foramen as they leave the spinal canal.

Diagnosis

The clinical findings and a history of previous back injury leads to investigation with various types of imaging. This may include radiography, most often MRI, myelography with contrast to show the disk status, and rarely, CT. The narrowing of the intervertebral spaces is consistent with the condition. Electromyography (EMG) and neurologic examinations demonstrate the involvement of the dependent nerves and also measure nerve conduction. The observation of neurologic deficits, including footdrop and the dragging of a leg when walking, adds to suspicion of nerve damage.

Treatment

Current treatment includes advising patients to be as active as possible. Narcotic analgesics and nonsteroidal antiinflammatory drugs (NSAIDs) are prescribed for pain relief. Oral steroids also may be prescribed. Epidurals or selective nerve root blocks for disk pain or spinal stenosis may be recommended. Physical therapy is also very helpful. Transcutaneous electrical nerve stimulation (TENS) is used with positive results. (Refer to Enrichment box about Transcutaneous Electrical Nerve Stimulation; and see the Enrichment box about Physical Therapy later in the text.) Bracing of the back may be helpful. Surgical intervention includes spinal fusion and freeing of the spinal nerve roots from entrapment. When surgical intervention is not an option, lidocaine topical (Lidoderm) patches may be prescribed for placement over the affected area of the back for some relief. Although still considered experimental, internal TENS units are offering a measure of relief to some individuals. Ablation is done for the medial branch to treat facet pain, not nerve impingement. Pain pumps are the last resort. A continuous infusion of morphine, via a pump, into the epidural space may be employed as the last resort to treat intractable pain. (Refer to Chapter 14 for a discussion on intractable pain.) Implantation of a spinal cord stimulator (SCS), a device that masks pain, is used to control chronic pain that cannot be relieved surgically or medically.

Prognosis

The prognosis varies, depending on the extent of the degenerative process and the response of the patient to treatment.

Prevention

Prevention is difficult because this is a degenerative process and common in aging. Encouraging proper body mechanics may be helpful.

Patient Teaching

Encourage patients to be compliant with physical therapy prescribed and to take medications as prescribed. Provide them with information about pain control measures. When a surgical procedure is involved, discuss wound care

Herniated and Bulging Disk

Description

A herniated disk, also known as a *ruptured* or *slipped disk,* is the rupture of the nucleus pulposus through the annular wall of the disk and into the spinal canal (Fig. 13.15A and C).

ICD-10-CM Code	M51.9 *(Unspecified thoracic, thoracolumbar, and lumbosacral intervertebral disk disorder)* (M51.84-M51.9 = 5 codes of specificity)

Herniated intervertebral disk disorders are coded according to sites and involvement of myelopathy. Once diagnosis has been confirmed, refer to the current edition of the ICD-10-CM coding manual for the appropriate code.

Symptoms and Signs

Intervertebral disks are soft pads of cartilage and gelatinous material located between each of the vertebrae that make up

ENRICHMENT

Transcutaneous Electrical Nerve Stimulation

Transcutaneous electrical nerve stimulation (TENS) is prescribed as a nondrug alternative pain relief intervention. This involves use of small electronic units that operate with 9-volt power to produce high frequency electrical impulses, which are transmitted to the surface of the skin through electrodes placed on the skin into underlying nerve fibers. This concept of electrotherapy allows for placement of a unit where the pain occurs.

Two concepts are thought to be involved in pain relief. First the impulse or stimulation that is transmitted to the nerve fibers blocks the pain signal from being sent to the brain. When the signal is blocked, pain is not perceived. Second, the body has its own method to suppress pain by releasing endorphins, natural chemicals that have analgesic activity. The impulses transmitted by the TENS unit stimulate the release of the endorphins.

Use of TENS, a nondrug therapy option, permits many with chronic pain to return to a fairly normal life and activities. The unit is small, measuring 2 to 2½ inches wide, 4 to 4½ inches long, and less than 1 inch thick. The units are programmable for strength and frequency of impulse to be delivered. Dual-chamber units have two lead wires that can be attached to the unit, and each has the capacity to be attached to two electrode leads. The electrodes are attached into the lead wires by small connecting wires. The unit can be hung from the waistband or from a belt. The electrodes are patches of various sizes, with adhesive on the back for attachment to the skin.

TENS units may be ordered for relief of chronic back pain, spinal stenosis, sciatica, arthritis, and postherpetic neuralgia. TENS units should *not* be used on patients with pacemakers or implantable cardiovertor defibrillators. Caution is recommended regarding their use in a pregnant woman, especially around the developing fetus. The physician or physical therapist will provide instructions regarding use, settings, and safety measures.

the spine. Each disk acts as a shock-absorbing cushion for the vertebrae and gives the back its flexibility for movement. Within each of these disks is a gelatinous center called the *nucleus pulposus,* which is surrounded by an annulus, a circular wall-like structure. The nucleus pulposus is contained within the annular wall in a bulging disk (see Fig. 13.15B); thus the protrusion into the spinal canal is not as severe. The rupture can cause severe back pain and even disability if it presses against or pinches the spinal nerves. Sudden, sharp pain that worsens with movement or in certain positions may radiate from the back to the buttocks, thighs, and legs following the course of the impinged nerve, causing pain, paresthesia, and muscle weakness in the leg, in a dermatomal pattern. When this pain results from pinching of the nerve roots that form the sciatic nerve, it is known as *sciatica* (Fig. 13.16). In most cases, herniation of disks occurs in the lower back, between the fourth and fifth lumbar vertebrae or between the fifth lumbar and first sacral vertebrae (lumbosacral area). Ruptured disks in the cervical region of the spine often produce pain and

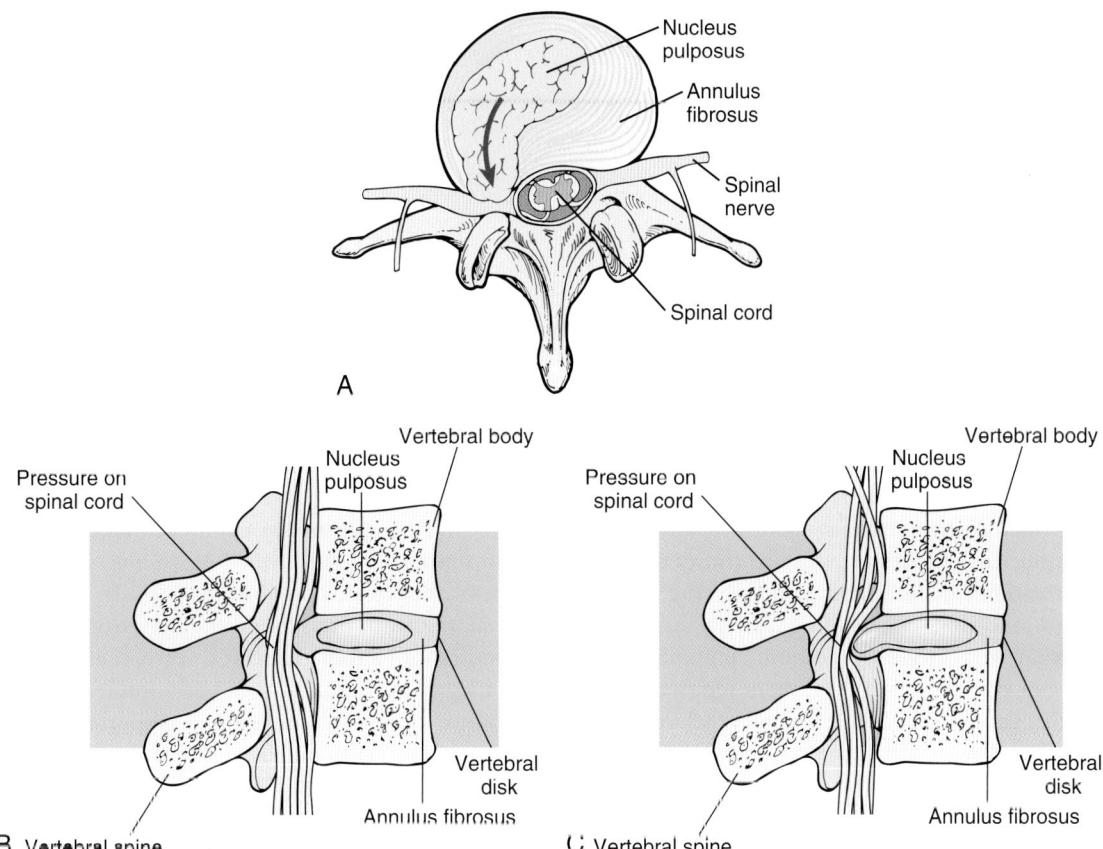

• **Fig. 13.15** (A) Herniated disk. Nucleus pulposus protrudes through the annulus fibrosus, putting pressure on the spinal cord and the spinal nerve. (B) Bulging disk (lateral view). Nucleus pulposus contained in the annulus fibrosus. (C) Herniated disk (lateral view). Nucleus pulposus through the annular wall (annulus fibrosus) and pressure on the spinal cord.

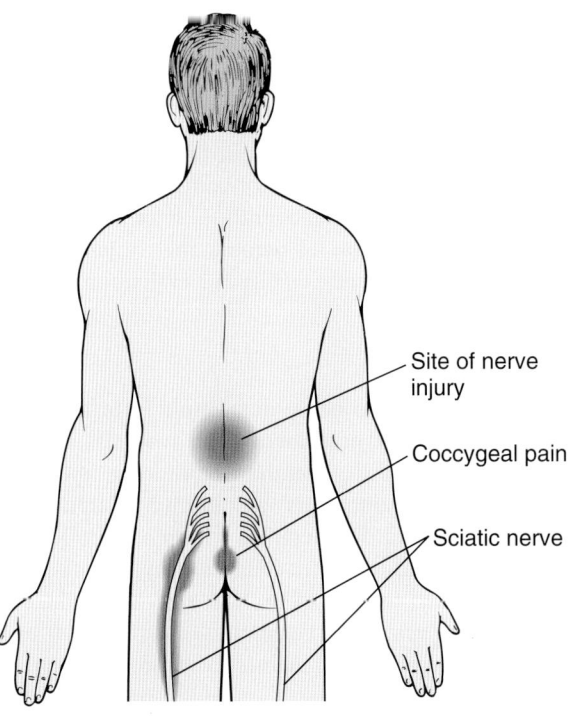

• **Fig. 13.16** Radiation of sciatic nerve pain.

weakness in the arms and the neck. Pain from injury to a disk can be either unilateral or bilateral.

Patient Screening

Herniated disk is a painful and serious condition and necessitates immediate medical attention. It occurs more often in men than in women.

Etiology

Herniated and bulging intervertebral disks usually result from accumulated trauma (e.g., improper body mechanics when lifting) or sudden impact. Poor posture and the aging process can cause the disks to degenerate. The rupture may occur at the time of the trauma or shortly thereafter.

Diagnosis

A thorough history of the back pain is important. Physical examination of the back is performed to rule out other possible causes of the patient's symptoms. A diagnosis of lumbar disk herniation can be considered if the patient has sciatic pain when the physician performs the straight leg raise test. The physician may order MRI, CT, or myelography to help confirm the diagnosis.

In a bulging disk, the disk material is herniated through the inner annulus but not the outer annulus, so the contained material can still distort the path of the nerve with resulting pain. In more severe herniation, which is considered noncontained, the nucleus pulposus penetrates both the inner and outer layers of the annulus.

Treatment

Conservative treatment consists of the use of hot or cold packs and the administration of muscle relaxants and analgesics, such as aspirin, ibuprofen, or oral prednisone. Additional conservative treatment includes epidural injections and physical therapy.

When conservative treatment is not successful, surgical excision of the herniated disk may be needed. Procedures include percutaneous diskectomy, in which a needle is introduced into the intravertebral space and the encroaching portion of the nucleus pulposus is aspirated (for uncomplicated disk herniation); microdiskectomy, involving a small surgical incision, allowing the offending material to be aspirated; diskectomy as a surgical procedure combined with laser ablation and evaporation of the disk; or removal of the disk along with a laminectomy, with fusion of the vertebrae.

Often the pain from bulging disks resolves with rest and drug therapy.

Prognosis

The prognosis varies, depending on the extent and duration of herniation. In many cases, the herniation resolves with conservative care. When surgical intervention is necessary, the outcome usually is favorable.

Prevention

Use of good and proper body mechanics is helpful in prevention; however, accidental slips and falls cannot always be avoided.

Patient Teaching

Provide these patients with information about good and proper body mechanics. Encourage those for whom rest and physical therapy are prescribed to be compliant. Generate print-on-demand electronic materials, when possible, as teaching tools.

Sciatic Nerve Injury—Spinal Stenosis

Description

Sciatic nerve injury is a pathologic condition. It is caused by trauma, degeneration, or rupture of the nucleus pulposus within the intervertebral disks. Spinal stenosis, a narrowing of the spinal canal or the nerve root foramen, is often termed *sciatica* because of the compression on the spinal cord and spinal nerve roots.

ICD-10-CM Code	S74.00XA (Injury of sciatic nerve at hip and thigh level, unspecified leg, initial encounter)

(S74.00[7th digit]–S74.92[7th digit] = 15 codes of specificity)

Spinal stenosis is coded by region. Once the diagnosis has confirmed the affected region, refer to the current edition of the ICD-10-CM coding manual for the appropriate code.

Symptoms and Signs

Degeneration or rupture of the nucleus pulposus causes pressure to be exerted directly on the sciatic nerve or on other closely positioned spinal nerves, sending impulses down the nerves. Rupture of one or more disks or their nuclei produces severe, sharp pain radiating from the sciatic nerve down the leg and to the foot (see Fig. 13.16). The pain may be continuous or intermittent, and areas of the skin supplied by the affected nerves may feel numb. A rupture of the nucleus pulposus posteriorly, toward the neural canal, results in pressure on the nerve root, causing sciatica symptoms or affects the sciatic nerve, causing low back pain and leg pain. Anterior or lateral ruptures may or may not produce symptoms. Resulting symptoms depend on the extent of the rupture and the proximity of the nerves to the site. Nerve injury can produce severe disability, which may be temporary or permanent. Persons with sciatic nerve involvement may be so uncomfortable that they are unable to sit or stand.

Patients with spinal stenosis also report pain in the back, radiating down the legs, and pain in the buttocks, thighs, or calves; the pain increases with standing, walking, or exercise. Additionally, they may experience numbness in these areas that becomes worse when standing, walking, or exercising. A weakness in the legs may be noted. Reflexes in the lower extremities often are asymmetric, and sensation may be decreased.

Patient Screening

Patients reporting lower back pain that radiates down the leg require prompt assessment for pain relief and to prevent further exacerbation of the condition. If an appointment is not available on the day of request, the patient should be referred to an emergency facility for evaluation and treatment.

Etiology

Trauma to the sciatic nerve may result from a fall, poor body mechanics, or gunshot or stab wounds. The aging process can lead to degeneration of disks or the nucleus pulposus. An inflammatory autoimmune response may prompt more rapid degeneration within a disk. The aging process, along with arthritic changes, may cause a narrowing of the spinal canal and the foramen where the spinal nerves exit the vertebrae. Formation of osteophytes on the foramen where the spinal nerves exit also can cause pain that radiates down the leg. Congenital narrowing of the spinal canal may be involved as well.

Diagnosis

After obtaining the medical history and performing a physical examination, the physician may order several diagnostic tests. These tests may include spinal radiography, MRI, CT, myelography, and blood serum studies. Vascular integrity is assessed, and insufficiency is ruled out. Often radiography of the spine shows degenerative changes along with a narrowed spinal canal. EMG studies may show neurologic changes.

Treatment

Conservative treatment may include oral corticosteroids (prednisone, methylprednisolone) and physical therapy, including ultrasound diathermy with massage or acupuncture. After the acute pain and inflammation have subsided, an exercise program to strengthen the back and abdominal muscles may be ordered. Drug therapy consists of analgesics (e.g., acetylsalicylic acid [aspirin] and acetaminophen [Tylenol]), muscle relaxants (e.g., diazepam, cyclobenzaprine, and methocarbamol), and antiinflammatory medications (e.g., ibuprofen, naproxen, indomethacin, celecoxib, or meloxicam). For severe pain not controlled by the aforementioned medications, tramadol (Ultram), hydrocodone-acetaminophen (Norco), or oxycodone-acetaminophen (Percocet) are used.

Physical therapy, including applications of heat and cold or gentle massage (myofascial release), may help relieve acute pain. Corticosteroid epidural injections may relieve pain and reduce inflammation of the spinal nerve. This option, many times, does not cure the spinal stenosis or sciatica. Leaning forward or sitting often helps relieve the back pain.

Disabling pain or increasing weakness may necessitate surgical intervention. If a disk is causing the pain, then removal of part or all of the disk or nucleus pulposus (diskectomy or microdiskectomy); spinal fusion; or chemical dissolving with an enzyme of the nucleus pulposus (chemonucleolysis) may be helpful. Decompression of the spinal nerve foramen can be used to free the trapped spinal nerves. Surgery may not relieve low back pain caused by underlying conditions, such as osteoarthritis.

See the Enrichment box about Physical Therapy.

Prognosis

The prognosis varies, depending on the extent of the degeneration and traumatic insult. Surgical intervention may provide relief from pain.

Prevention

Preventing injury associated with traumatic insults is difficult. Degeneration of disks in aging is unavoidable.

Patient Teaching

Provide instructions for good and proper body mechanics. Encourage compliance with prescribed physical and drug therapy. Generate print on demand electronic materials when possible, as teaching tools.

❖ ENRICHMENT

Physical Therapy

Normal physical activity and function can be compromised by the aging process and by disease or injury. Physical therapy is a branch of rehabilitative health used to help patients maintain or restore their physical abilities. Physical therapists are trained and certified to help plan programs and set goals for improvement in the individual's body strength and ability to function in daily activities. This process of rehabilitation can be challenging, but many experience positive physical and psychological rewards with good compliance.

Physical therapy is prescribed to help with recovery from insult to the musculoskeletal and/or the nervous system. Trauma to the musculoskeletal system often involves injury to the nerves in proximity. These insults may be traumatic in nature, resulting from a motor vehicle accident (MVA), a fall, a strain or sprain, or any other type of trauma. After surgical procedures with joint replacement or stabilization of fractures, physical mobility and healing often are improved with regular therapy. Sports injuries and work-related injuries are common reasons for use of the intervention techniques of physical therapy. The aging process brings about mechanical changes to the body and causes interference in the individual's normal daily activities. The condition of individuals who are in the poststroke phase or who have other neurologic conditions often improves with physical therapy.

After assessment of the individual's gait, posture, range of motion, reflexes, strength, and the physical insult to the tissue, the therapist develops a plan of action discussing this with the individual. Realistic goals are identified, along with time that can be committed to the therapy. The goal of the therapy is to improve the use of bones, joints, muscles, and nerves and to reduce the level of pain experienced by the individual. Restoration of function, improving the ability to move, and prevention of disability are also part of the goal. The therapist incorporates treatment modalities, including specially designed exercise; heat, light, massage, or ultrasound therapy; electrical stimulation; and/or aquatic therapy. Instruction and advice on proper body mechanics, posture, and motion may be included in the therapy. Individuals are provided with instructions for home exercise and exercise techniques for continuing therapy at home.

Physical therapists also provide assistive devices for ambulation and instruction in the use of the devices. Individuals requiring ambulation devices are measured for the device, and the device is then assembled to fit the patient. Crutch use, walker use, and cane walking will be taught for safe ambulation by the individual.

Functional Disorders

Headache

Description

Headache (**cephalalgia**) is pain in the head that is not confined to any one specific nerve distribution area.

ICD-10-CM Code	G44.1 *(Vascular headache,*
	not elsewhere classified)
	(G44.1 G44.09 – 20 codes
	of specificity)
	R51 (Headache)

Symptoms and Signs

Headaches may be acute or chronic and located in the frontal, temporal, or occipital regions of the head or a combination of these. Cephalalgia also may be confined to only one side of the head or may be located above one or both eyes. The type of pain may vary from dull and aching to almost unbearable. It can be an intense intermittent pain, throbbing pain, pressure pain, or penetrating pain driving through the head. Brain tissues themselves never ache because they do not contain sensory nerves; however, the meninges do have pain receptors. Sensitivity in this area exists in only the meninges, the skin and muscles covering the skull, and the numerous nerves that travel from the brain to the head and the face.

Headaches are commonly experienced and usually are self-limiting. Cephalalgia, or secondary headache, is sometimes a symptom of an underlying disorder or disease (e.g., sinus infection or congestion, temporomandibular joint [TMJ] syndrome, hypertension, stroke, brain tumor, and encephalitis). In most cases, however, headaches are caused by nothing more serious than fatigue or tension.

Some types of headaches are not symptoms of underlying disorders but are considered a specific disease. One of these is cluster headache. In a cluster headache, the pain is generally severe, developing around or behind one eye, and having abrupt onset and cessation. The affected eye may tear. Cluster headaches usually occur at night, continue occurring for several weeks or months, and then disappear for some time, even years. Cluster headaches are more common in men and are associated with nasal congestion and partial Horner syndrome. Another example of a severe type of headache is migraine (see the Migraine section).

Patient Screening

Patients complaining of intractable head pain require prompt assessment. An appointment should be scheduled as soon as possible. If a same-day appointment is not possible, the patient should be referred to an emergency treatment facility. An appointment should be scheduled as soon as possible for other types of headaches.

Etiology

Many factors, either alone or in combination, can irritate the pain-sensitive tissues or structures in the head and produce headaches. Examples are stress; too little or too much sleep; overeating or overdrinking; a stuffy or noisy environment; and heavy physical labor, either indoors or outdoors. Some affected individuals may also be suffering from caffeine withdrawal or sensitivity to scents. From a physiologic standpoint, however, there are only two causes of headaches. The first cause is strain on the facial, neck, and scalp muscles resulting from tension. The headache that results is called a *tension headache*. The second cause is edema within the blood vessels of the head, which results in a change in arterial size. The headache that results is called a *vascular headache*.

Diagnosis

The medical history is vitally important in identifying a pattern to the headaches and is helpful in detecting any underlying causes. Physical examination and neurologic testing are necessary if a recurring pattern of headaches is revealed. Cranial and spinal radiography, EEG, and cranial CT may be ordered to rule out organic causes.

Treatment

The cause of the headache determines the type of treatment chosen. If the physician does not find an underlying cause of the headache, the use of analgesics (e.g., aspirin, acetaminophen, and NSAIDs), muscle relaxants, minor tranquilizers, muscle massages, and relaxation with a warm bath are effective in providing temporary relief from headache.

Prognosis

The prognosis for the typical headache is good. The prognosis for intractable head pain varies, depending on the cause. Drug therapy often helps relieve the pain. Stress reduction and relaxation techniques may lead to a positive outcome.

Prevention

Prevention involves avoiding known or suspected trigger factors.

Patient Teaching

Provide patients with information on relaxation techniques and stress reduction. Use customized electronically generated educational materials, when available, to reinforce the treatment plan.

Migraine

Description

Periodic severe headaches that may be completely incapacitating and almost always are accompanied by other symptoms, such as nausea and vomiting, sensitivity to light and sound, anorexia, intense hemicranial or bilateral throbbing pain, and visual signs and symptoms (or auras), are known as *migraine headaches*.

ICD-10-CM Code	G43.909 *(Migraine, unspecified,*
	not intractable, without status
	migrainous)
	(G43.001-G43.919 = 40 codes
	of specificity)

Refer to the current edition of the ICD-10-CM coding manual for the most specific code.

Symptoms and Signs

Before the onset of headache, many persons who experience migraine headaches have visual auras: flashing lights, zigzagging lines, or areas of total darkness. Photophobia is another warning sign. The nature of each attack varies from person to person, but usually there is a warning period during which the person feels abnormally fatigued and irritable. Other less common symptoms that occur occasionally are numbness or tingling in one arm or on one side of the body, dizziness, and temporary mental confusion.

These headaches may begin in adolescence or early adulthood, becoming less frequent and less intense with age. They affect women nearly three times as often as men.

Patient Screening

Patients known to experience migraine headaches and those reporting typical migraine headache symptoms require prompt treatment. If an office appointment is not immediately available, the patient should be referred to an emergency treatment facility.

Etiology

Despite much medical research, it is not known why some people are prone to migraines or what triggers these headaches. Certain factors do appear to be involved in many cases. Susceptibility to migraines, for instance, tends to appear in families, leading to a strong suspicion of inherited or genetic aspects of the disorder. In some cases, certain foods (e.g., aged cheese, chocolate, and red wine) have been found to induce an attack.

The biologic cause of migraines may be changes in the cerebral blood flow. This is presumably attributable to vasoconstriction followed by vasodilation of the cerebral and cranial arteries.

Diagnosis

A medical history of recurring, severe headaches, preceded by any combination of the aforementioned symptoms or signs, suggests the diagnosis. EEG, CT, and possibly MRI may be ordered to rule out any organic conditions.

Treatment

In some cases, the treatment is simply bed rest in a quiet, darkened room and the use of analgesics at the first sign of attack. For other patients, drug therapy in the form of vasoconstrictors to constrict dilated blood vessels is effective in relieving pain. Antiemetics to control vomiting may be needed. The use of *ergot* preparations has been effective in some patients to prevent an impending attack or lessen the symptoms of an ongoing attack. Migraine treatment is multifaceted and may include many different drug classes. Initial treatment is usually with triptans (sumatriptan, zolmitriptan, eletriptan, naratriptan, and frovatriptan). Other medications include ergotamine, dihydroergotamine, acetaminophen, ibuprofen, propranolol, verapamil, amitriptyline, nortriptyline, topiramate, gabapentin, and diphenhydramine. Antiemetics may include ondansetron, prochlorperazine, or promethazine. Relaxation therapy or biofeedback has been used successfully to lessen the frequency of migraines in some patients. A new class of migraine medications was approved by the U.S. Food and Drug Administration (FDA) in 2018. They are called calcitonin gene-related peptide (CGRP) inhibitors, which interfere with CGRP, which is produced in nerve cells in the brain and spinal cord. This peptide makes nerve cells more sensitive to painful stimuli. The medications used inhibit some of that activity to reduce migraine frequency and are indicated for patients who experience four or more migraine days per month. Currently three of these drugs are available: erenumab (Aimovig), galcanezumab (Emgality), and fremanezumab (Ajovy).

Prevention

Patients should be advised to avoid the "trigger" factors, if possible. The value of implementing drug therapy and relaxation techniques at the first sign of a headache should be stressed. If additional drug therapy is required for pain relief, it should be employed as soon as possible. The prognosis is usually favorable when the patient complies with drug therapy and the instruction to rest.

Patient Teaching

Provide patients with information on stress reduction. Advise them on the importance of taking preventive medications on a regular basis. Use customized electronically generated educational materials, when available, to reinforce the treatment plan.

Epilepsy

Description

Epilepsy, a seizure disorder, is a chronic brain disorder, characterized by sudden episodes of abnormal intense electrical activity in the brain, which results in seizure activity.

ICD-10-CM Code	G40.901 *(Epilepsy, unspecified, not intractable, with status epilepticus)*
	G40.909 *(Epilepsy, unspecified, not intractable, without status epilepticus)*
	(G40.301-G40.919 = 21 codes of specificity)

Epilepsy is coded according to type. Both fourth and fifth digits are required. Once the diagnosis has been confirmed, refer to the current edition of the ICD-10-CM coding manual for the appropriate code.

Symptoms and Signs

Epilepsy has many forms and a variety of manifestations; greater than 30 types of seizures are known, and it is possible for a person to have more than one type. The recurring seizures may entail involuntary contractions of muscles (convulsions) with disturbances in consciousness and sensory phenomena. Epileptic seizures are classified as partial or generalized. Status epilepticus is a complication involving prolonged seizure activity.

Partial seizures do not involve the entire brain but arise from a localized area in the brain. The effects may involve the hand or face, with motor signs, such as a rhythmic twitching of a group of muscles or compulsive lip smacking or picking at clothing. Behavioral, psychic, and sensory manifestations (auras) can occur. The patient usually experiences amnesia of the attack. However, no loss of consciousness occurs.

Generalized seizures cause a diffuse electrical abnormality within the brain and include absence (petit mal) and tonic-clonic (grand mal) attacks. Absence seizures, also called *petit mal epilepsy* or *petit mal seizures,* consist of a brief change in the level of consciousness indicated by staring, blinking, or blankly staring with loss of awareness of surroundings. The episodes last only a few seconds and can occur many times a day, if not treated. Absence seizures occur most often in children and young adults.

Tonic-clonic seizures (grand mal epilepsy) may begin with a loud cry, followed by falling to the ground and loss of consciousness. During the tonic phase, the body stiffens, and the tongue may be bitten. Prolonged contraction of the respiratory muscles causes the patient to become cyanotic. Then in the clonic phase, generalized rhythmic muscle spasms occur, followed by relaxation. The patient may be incontinent of urine and/or feces. The seizure subsides in 1 to 2 minutes, but consciousness may be regained slowly. The person may be drowsy, confused, and weak; report a headache; and have no memory of the event afterward. This time is referred to as the *postictal period,* in which the patient experiences a level of awareness.

Status epilepticus occurs when one seizure follows another with no recovery of consciousness between attacks. This is considered a medical emergency that requires immediate anticonvulsant therapy to prevent cerebral anoxia, hyperpyrexia, vascular collapse, and even death.

Patient Screening

Patients experiencing any form of seizure activity need immediate assessment and intervention.

Etiology

In idiopathic epilepsy, no apparent cause for the abnormal electrical discharge is found, although a greater incidence may be found in some families.

In symptomatic epilepsy, a known abnormality in the brain resulting from a pathologic process, genetic or acquired, seems to trigger seizures. Pathologic conditions associated with seizure disorder include scar tissue on the cerebral cortex from infection or trauma, cortical neoplasms, cerebral edema, TIAs, and CVAs (strokes). Other possible causes are birth trauma (cerebral palsy), drug toxicity (e.g., alcohol), diabetes, hypoglycemia, and other conditions that deprive the brain of oxygen.

Diagnosis

Not all seizures imply epilepsy; thus a medical history is essential for determining the diagnosis. EEG shows semispecific brain activity, suggesting epilepsy; MRI also may be helpful. Classification of epilepsy is based on the location of the abnormal activity and its duration. CT shows structural changes in the brain, such as tumors, scars, and malformations. Cerebral angiography may identify vascular changes in the brain. Skull radiography may reveal evidence of fracture, separation of cranial sutures, or movement of the pineal gland. Blood serum chemistry changes may indicate metabolic disease, drug toxicity, or hypoglycemia.

Treatment

Anticonvulsant medications are the treatment of choice for epilepsy; the more commonly used drugs include phenytoin, carbamazepine, valproic acid, divalproex, levetiracetam, gabapentin, phenobarbital, topiramate, and oxcarbazepine. Close monitoring and adjustments of dosage to attain good therapeutic control are essential. Patients are instructed to adhere to their medication schedules and take their medications as directed.

Side effects from anticonvulsants can vary, and patients should be instructed to review concerns with their prescribers. In rare cases, surgical intervention may be necessary to excise an identified lesion in the brain. Certain restrictions may be necessary. For instance, depending on state regulations, a license to drive a motor vehicle may not be issued unless the person has been seizure free, with treatment, for a specific period. Emotional support for the patient and the family is made available.

Another treatment option is an implanted vagus nerve stimulator (VNS), which sends impulses of electrical energy through the vagus nerve to the brain to prevent seizures. Different models that can be implanted are available.

Prognosis

The prognosis varies. Drug therapy often can control seizure activity. Status epilepticus is a life-threatening event. Immediate intervention may afford a positive outcome.

Prevention

Prevention of the initial onset of seizure activity is impossible. Compliance with drug therapy has a positive effect on the ultimate outcome.

Patient Teaching

Because this disease often is feared and misunderstood, education is necessary to dispel myths. Talk about first aid instructions that are available and can teach family members how to care for the patient in the event of grand mal seizures (Fig. 13.17). Emphasize abiding by local restrictions regarding driving a motor vehicle. Additionally, stress the importance of drug therapy compliance. Assist the patient and the family in locating and contacting support groups in the community. Generate print-on-demand electronic materials, when possible, as teaching tools.

Parkinson Disease

Description

Parkinson disease is a common, slowly progressive neurologic disorder characterized by the onset of recognizable

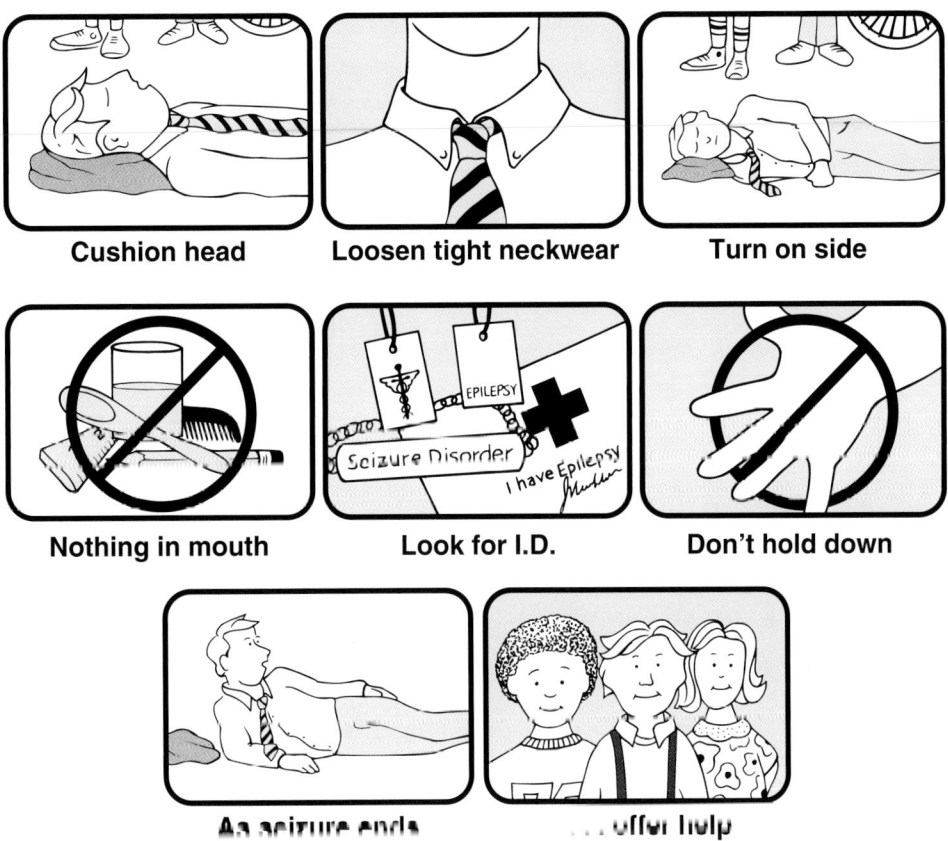

Cushion head   **Loosen tight neckwear**   **Turn on side**

Nothing in mouth   **Look for I.D.**   **Don't hold down**

As seizure ends   **. . . offer help**

Most seizures in people with epilepsy are not medical emergencies. They end after a minute or two without harm and usually do not require a trip to the emergency room.

But sometimes there are good reasons to call for emergency help. A seizure in someone who does not have epilepsy could be a sign of serious illness.

Other reasons to call an ambulance include:

• A seizure that lasts more than 5 minutes
• No "epilepsy" or "seizure disorder" I.D.
• Slow recovery, a second seizure, or difficulty breathing afterward
• Pregnancy or other medical I.D.
• Any signs of injury or sickness

• **Fig. 13.17** First aid for seizures. *ID,* Identification. (Courtesy Epilepsy Foundation, www.epilepsy.com.)

disturbances: "pill rolling" tremor of the thumb and forefinger, muscular rigidity, slowness of movement, and postural instability.

ICD-10-CM Code   G20 (*Parkinson's disease*)

Symptoms and Signs

Usually insidious in onset, Parkinson disease symptoms, which vary from person to person, may be associated with aging until the recognizable paradigm of Parkinson disease emerges. A primary symptom is tremor or trembling in hands, arms, jaws, face, and legs. Additionally there is rigidity or stiffness of limbs and trunk, causing a stooped posture. The patient moves slowly, with a peculiar shuffling gait: the head is bowed, the body is flexed forward, the knees are slightly bent, and the patient tends to fall as a result of impaired balance and coordination

(Fig. 13.18). The face takes on a masklike or expressionless appearance, speech is muffled, and swallowing is difficult. Gradual changes in behavior and mental activity are noted in some patients as the disease progresses. The mean age at onset is 60 years, but many cases appear in younger persons. Parkinson disease afflicts men more than it affects women, and the usual lifespan after diagnosis is 10 years.

Patient Screening

Because of the insidious onset of Parkinson disease, patients and family members may contact the office for an appointment because of the vague neurologic symptoms. The next available appointment should be scheduled for these individuals. Those already identified as having the disease will have appointments scheduled for routine follow-up care.

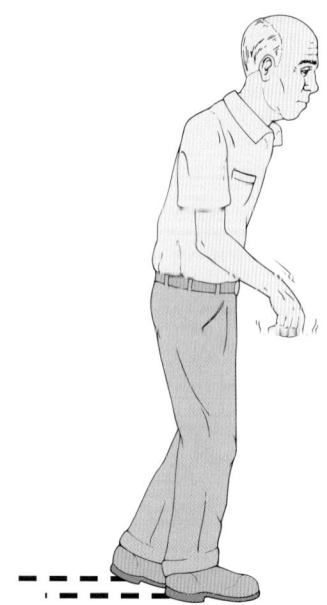

• **Fig. 13.18** Typical shuffling gait and posture of patients with Parkinson disease.

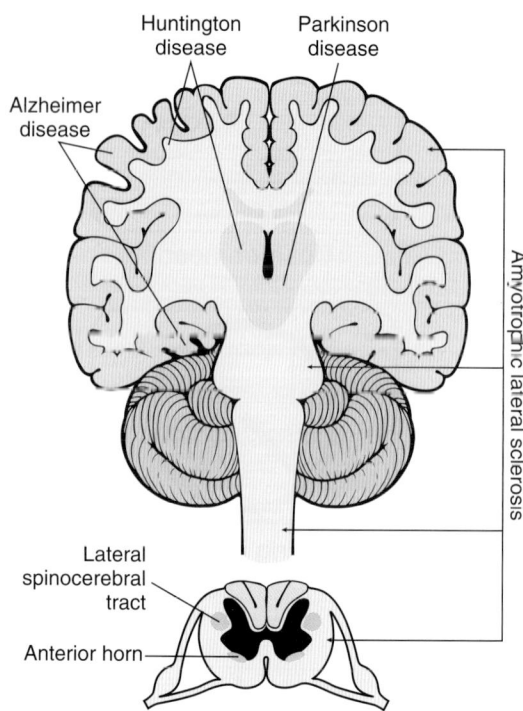

• **Fig. 13.19** Degenerative diseases of the brain involve preferentially various parts of the brain. Alzheimer disease causes atrophy of the frontal and occipital cortical gyri. Huntington disease affects the frontal cortex and basil ganglia. Parkinson disease is marked by changes in the substantia nigra. Amyotrophic lateral sclerosis (ALS) affects the motor neurons in the anterior horn of the spinal cord, brainstem, and the frontal cortex of the brain. (From Damjanov I: *Pathology for the health-related professions,* ed 4, St Louis, 2011, Saunders/Elsevier.)

Etiology

What causes the degeneration of nerves in the motor system of the brainstem is not known. A deficiency of dopamine, a **neurotransmitter** manufactured in the midbrain, has been clinically demonstrated in patients with Parkinson disease. Parkinsonism (as a syndrome) also can occur after ingestion of poison, after encephalitis, and after taking certain major tranquilizers and certain antihypertensive drugs (Fig. 13.19). Degenerative diseases of the brain involve preferentially various parts of the brain. Although Parkinson disease is a neurodegenerative brain disorder that progresses slowly in most people, the term *parkinsonism* refers to a group of neurologic disorders that cause movement problems, such as tremors, slow movement, and stiffness, similar to those seen in Parkinson disease.

Diagnosis

The diagnosis is based on the characteristic history and a careful neurologic examination. Decreased dopamine levels in urine may be noted.

Treatment

Because Parkinson disease has such a wide variety of symptoms, treatment is individualized for each patient. Parkinson disease cannot be cured; therefore medical management consists of supportive measures and control of symptoms with the use of drugs, such as levodopa, carbidopa, bromocriptine, pramipexole, ropinirole, selegiline, or rasagiline. Physical therapy helps the patient maximize mobility within the limitations of the disease. The patient is given every possible supportive measure to encourage independence and self-care.

A new treatment called *deep brain stimulation (DBS)* was recently approved by the FDA. Electrodes are implanted into the brain and connected to a small pulse generator, which can reduce the need for levodopa and result in a decrease in involuntary movements (dyskinesias). The pulse generator is carefully programmed externally to lessen the symptoms.

Prognosis and Prevention

At the present time, no cure for Parkinson disease is known. There is ongoing research to find a cure. No method of preventing Parkinson disease is known.

Patient Teaching

Assist the patient and family in locating and contacting available community resources. Encourage family members to be supportive of therapy prescribed to help the patient remain independent as long as possible. Generate print-on-demand electronic materials, when possible, as teaching tools.

Huntington Chorea

Description

Huntington **chorea** (Huntington disease) is a hereditary degenerative disease of the cerebral cortex and basal ganglia, resulting in progressive atrophy of the brain.

ICD-10-CM Code   G10 *(Huntington's disease)*

Symptoms and Signs

The chronic, progressive chorea (ceaseless, uncontrolled, involuntary movements) has an insidious onset, with loss of musculoskeletal control exhibited by subtle, semipurposeful movements. Typically the arms and the face are the first areas to be involved, with movements ranging from mild fidgeting to tongue smacking. Difficulty swallowing may occur. Speech difficulties are experienced, and the emotional state deteriorates, and dementia occurs eventually. Disruption of personality is displayed by the untidy and careless appearance of the individual. Personality changes noted are described as apathetic, moody behavior; loss of memory; and onset of paranoia. The onset of symptoms typically begins in early middle age.

Patient Screening

The insidious onset of Huntington chorea results in vague symptoms; therefore, the condition may be found by chance during a routine visit. Because it is a familial-type disease, patients with a family history of the disease may be aware of the progression of symptoms and request an appointment. Although not considered an emergency, the occurrence of symptoms can create high levels of anxiety in patients, so the next available appointment should be scheduled for them.

Etiology

Although the exact etiology of this condition is uncertain, it is transmitted by an autosomal dominant trait that can be inherited by either gender.

Diagnosis

No definitive method of diagnosis is known, except by careful neurologic appraisal and by detection of the defective gene through deoxyribonucleic acid (DNA) analysis. A history of progressive chorea and dementia, along with a familial trait for the disease, leads to further investigation. Cerebral CT shows brain atrophy.

Treatment

No cure for this progressively deteriorating condition is known; therefore treatment is supportive, symptomatic, and protective. Haloperidol (Haldol) and fluphenazine (Prolixin) are prescribed in an attempt to control choreic movements and to reduce agitation. An orphan drug (tetrabenazine) has been available since 2008 in the United States. It is also used to treat the symptoms of chorea. Selective serotonin reuptake inhibitor (SSRI) antidepressants, benzodiazepines, and atypical antipsychotic medications are used to treat the psychiatric symptoms of the disease. Some authors have advocated using physical therapy, occupational therapy, speech therapy, and psychosocial support.

Prognosis

At the present time, no cure for Huntington chorea is known. Drug therapy may help control agitated behavior. Eventually, institutionalization may be necessary to provide the care required to manage the deteriorating condition of the patient.

Prevention

Because this is an inherited familial type disorder, no method of prevention is known.

Patient Teaching

Provide the patient and the family with information about the disease. Assist them in locating and contacting community resources.

Amyotrophic Lateral Sclerosis

Description

Amyotrophic lateral sclerosis (ALS), also known as *Lou Gehrig disease,* is a progressive, destructive motor neuron disease that results in muscular atrophy.

ICD-10-CM Code	G12.21 *(Amyotrophic lateral sclerosis)*
	(G12.20-G12.29 = 4 codes of specificity)

Symptoms and Signs

Fasciculations (small local involuntary muscular contractions) and accompanying atrophy and weakness are noted in the forearms and hands. This condition progresses to cause difficulties in speech, chewing, swallowing, and breathing; eventually, a ventilator is required. No sensory neuron involvement is noted, and functioning of the mind is not affected. ALS characteristically affects men slightly more often than women, with onset occurring after the age of 50 to 60 years.

Patient Screening

Patients complaining of weakness and involuntary muscular contractions of the hands and arms should be assessed promptly. Anyone complaining of difficulty breathing and swallowing requires immediate assessment and should be transferred into the EMS for immediate treatment and transport to an emergency facility.

Etiology

Although the etiology of ALS is uncertain, in some cases, it may be caused by autosomal inherited traits.

Diagnosis

Clinical findings, including upper and lower motor neuron involvement without any sensory neuron involvement, will lead to further investigation. EMG and muscle biopsy are employed to confirm nerve, not muscle, involvement. Over a period of several months, the diagnosis is confirmed by the typical progression of the disease.

Treatment

Because no cure for the condition is known, treatment involving a team of caregivers consists of supportive measures and therapy directed at controlling symptoms. Riluzole (Rilutek) is a new entity that has shown promise in slowing progression of the disease and extending life. Other drug therapy includes tizanidine and baclofen, which are muscle relaxants that help relieve muscle spasticity. Other medications are used to reduce fatigue, spasticity, pain, sleep difficulties, and excess salivation. Pulmonary management is vital.

Prognosis

No cure for ALS is known, and death usually occurs within 6 to 10 years after diagnosis.

Prevention

No method of prevention is known; the disease is thought to be caused by autosomal inherited traits.

Patient Teaching

Provide the patient and the family with information about the disease. Assist them in locating and contacting community resources. Generate print-on-demand electronic materials, when possible, as teaching tools.

Restless Legs Syndrome

Description

Restless legs syndrome (RLS) is a neurologic condition characterized by an overwhelming urge to move the legs. This irresistible urge to move the legs or body part is to stop an uncomfortable or odd sensation.

ICD-10-CM Code	G25.81 (Restless legs syndrome)

Symptoms and Signs

RLS is characterized by a group of symptoms that cause the individual to move the legs. There are feelings that often are described as itching, burning, jittery, creepy-crawly, pulling, tugging, and/or painful sensations in the legs. Occasionally the sensations may be felt in the arms, hips, or face. The awareness of the sensations may be intermittent, or it may occur on a daily basis. The inability to sit for extended periods often interferes with normal activities of life. These symptoms usually occur at night; during the day, they usually occur after long periods of sitting. Walking or moving the legs often relieves the symptoms. Many patients with RLS also experience periodic limb movement disorder (PLMD) during sleep.

Patient Screening

Patients requesting an appointment for difficulty and pain in the legs while sitting still may be experiencing RLS. They may also complain of unusual feelings in the legs that are relieved by standing and moving. Schedule an appointment as soon as convenient for both patient and physician. Request that the patient keep a daily record of symptoms, noting when they occur and what helps provide relief.

Etiology

The exact cause of RLS is unknown. The incidence of RLS appears to increase after age of 40 or 50 years. Anemia may play a part in the disorder. Stressful events may precipitate the onset of symptoms.

Diagnosis

Medical history and physical examination are useful in making the diagnosis. Symptoms occur most frequently in the evening or at night while the individual is relaxed or sleeping. Movement of the legs provides only temporary relief. A daily diary of symptoms noting when they occur and what helps provide relief is helpful in diagnosis.

Blood tests may show low blood iron levels. Secondary causes, including iron deficiency, varicose veins, folate and magnesium deficiencies, sleep apnea, uremia, diabetes, peripheral neuropathy, Parkinson disease, thyroid disease, and certain autoimmune disorders, need to be identified. Some drugs also may cause the symptoms.

Treatment

There is no cure for this condition. Treatment involves identifying the underlying cause of the disorder and treating that disorder. Drug therapy, including levodopa, dopamine agonists, and ropinirole, does not help achieve a cure but may help alleviate or lessen some symptoms. Opioids and benzodiazepines may also be prescribed. Often the side effects of the drugs outweigh the benefits, and the drugs must be stopped. Regular exercise, including leg stretching and massage along with application of heat, may provide relief. Cold application may be an alternative for some individuals.

Prognosis

Although there is no cure for this lifelong disorder, it is possible that symptoms may worsen as the individual ages. Therapies currently available may provide control and minimize symptoms. Some patients may experience periodic remissions of symptoms. There is no known prevention for this disorder.

Patient Teaching

Encourage patients to be compliant with recommended medications and exercises. Provide information concerning possible side effects of medications, and instruct patients to report any side effects as soon as possible. Provide them with contact information for support groups.

Transient Global Amnesia

Description

Transient global amnesia, although frightening and anxiety provoking, usually is a benign event. As the name implies, the event is transient or temporary, with a duration of 1 to 6 (maybe even up to 12) hours. It is global in nature because it encompasses the entire memory of current events. The amnesia manifests as a total loss of recent memory; the learning process is completely blocked. Memory disturbances are involved.

ICD-10-CM Code   G45.4 *(Transient global amnesia)*

Symptoms and Signs
The individual experiencing the onset of transient global amnesia has a sudden onset of memory loss, primarily of both current and recent events. Repetitive asking of such questions as "Where are we going?" "Why are we going there?" "Where am I?" and "Why did we do that?" is typical. Confusion is apparent; nevertheless the individual has recall of personal identity and orientation to place if the place is a normal environment. Memory loss may encompass the preceding 3 to 5 years and specific events. Usual tasks, including those requiring mechanical abilities, often are performed without difficulty. Neurologic signs are normal; no numbness, tingling, or weakness (unilateral or total) is noted; PERLA (*p*upils are *e*qual and *r*eact to *l*ight and *a*ccommodation) and vocalization are normal. Communication skills concerning current events and status are affected by the amnesic event, which begins and ends abruptly. Memory usually returns within 6 to 12 hours; however, the period of amnesic experience will remain unavailable to any recall. This also may be true of events that occurred a few hours to a few days before the amnesic event. Some patients complain of headache.

Patient Screening
The patient should be seen as soon as possible if the office schedule will allow. This permits observation of the symptoms and helps reduce anxiety in both patient and family. Neurologic signs need to be observed, evaluated, and recorded. If an immediate appointment is not possible, the patient should be referred to an emergency facility for prompt observation and to rule out TIA and CVA.

Etiology
The etiology is unknown; however, evidence points to the precursors such as, experiencing stress or emotional events, swimming or immersion in cold water, driving a motor vehicle, or having sexual intercourse. The individual may have experienced migraine headaches on previous occasions, usually without nausea, vomiting, or photosensitivity.

Diagnosis
Diagnosis is made by observing the symptoms and signs and obtaining a negative result on neurologic examination. TIA, CVA, and seizure activity are to be ruled out first.

Prognosis
The prognosis is good; recurrence is very unlikely. The individual probably will never regain memory of the events that occurred during the episode or during the hours or days immediately preceding the episode.

Treatment
Treatment is supportive; the patient is given reassurance during and after the episode.

Prevention
No method of prevention is known. All patients are encouraged to reduce stress factors in their lives.

Patient Teaching
Provide patient and family with reassurance that this event is transient in nature and likely will not occur again. Additionally, instructions should be provided to the family to return if symptoms do recur.

◆ ENRICHMENT

Chiari Malformation

Chiari malformation is diagnosed when the brain tissue is pressed down into the spinal cord. This is caused by an abnormally shaped or smaller-than-normal skull. The skull puts pressure on the brain and displaces it into the spinal cord. Chiari malformation is classified as type I, II, or III, depending on the severity of displacement of the brain. Type I involves the smallest amount of brain tissue in the spinal cord. Type II involves more brain tissue displacement than in type I. Type III is congenital and is the rarest of the three types. A portion of the brainstem or cerebellum extends out from the skull through an abnormal opening. Type III has the worst outcome, with a high rate of death. It should also be noted that type II is also seen in the myelomeningocele form of spina bifida. Typically severe headache, which occurs after a person sneezes, coughs, or strains, is one main symptom. Lack of fine skill coordination, difficulty balancing, neck pain, tingling of feet and hands, numbness, dizziness, difficulty swallowing, and other neurologic symptoms may be experienced.

Peripheral Nerve Disorders

Peripheral Neuritis/Neuropathy

Description
Peripheral neuritis/neuropathy is degeneration of the peripheral nerves.

ICD-10-CM Code   G60.9 *(Hereditary and idiopathic neuropathy, unspecified)*
(G60.0-G60.9 = 6 codes of specificity)

Symptoms and Signs
Peripheral neuritis, the degeneration of peripheral nerves, affects the distal muscles of the extremities. Unless the precipitating factors are severe infection or chronic alcohol intoxication, the onset is insidious. Clumsiness and loss of sensation in the hands and feet are followed by a flaccid paralysis and a wasting of muscles in these areas. Deep tendon reflexes become diminished, and tenderness is noted in the atrophied muscles. The skin may take on a glossy, red

appearance, and sweating is decreased. With leg and foot involvement, foot drop may be experienced. Some patients have pain in the affected regions.

Patient Screening

Patients reporting loss of sensation in the hands and feet should be promptly assessed. Schedule an immediate appointment, according to office policy.

Etiology

Chronic alcohol intoxication; toxicity from arsenic, lead, carbon disulfide, benzene, or phosphorus; infectious diseases, including mumps, pneumonia, and diphtheria; metabolic or inflammatory disorders, including diabetes, rheumatoid arthritis, gout, and systemic lupus erythematosus; and certain nutritional deficiency diseases are all causative factors. The nerve degeneration leads to muscle weakness and sensory loss.

Diagnosis

The history, combined with the clinical findings characteristic of motor and sensory involvement, leads to additional investigation. Motor and sensory nerve impairment usually is detected by EMG and a nerve conduction study (NCS).

Treatment

The first step in effective treatment is to ascertain the cause and, if possible, to correct or eliminate the condition. Toxic substances need to be removed, if possible, and vitamin and nutritional deficits corrected. Underlying disease processes, especially diabetes, are treated or controlled. When chronic alcoholism is the cause, the patient must avoid all alcohol in any form. Supportive measures, such as administration of anticonvulsants and tricyclic antidepressants and getting rest and physical therapy, are employed to relieve pain.

Prognosis

Control of underlying causes may provide relief of symptoms. Proper nutrition is helpful.

Prevention

Prevention is difficult when the etiology is a preceding disease process or exposure to toxic substances. Avoidance of alcohol may help prevent recurrence of neuritis.

Patient Teaching

Encourage patients to be compliant with drug and physical therapy as prescribed.

Trigeminal Neuralgia (Tic Douloureux)

Description

Trigeminal neuralgia, or tic douloureux, is pain of the area innervated by the cranial nerve V (CN V), the trigeminal nerve.

ICD-10-CM Code	G50.0 *(Trigeminal neuralgia)*
	(G50.0-G50.9 = 4 codes of specificity)

Symptoms and Signs

The transient, excruciating pain of trigeminal neuralgia radiates along the distribution of the CN V and can affect any of the three CN V branches, although it usually affects the second and third branches (Fig. 13.20). When the ophthalmic branch is affected, pain is experienced in the eye and the forehead. The maxillary branch involves the nose, upper lip, and cheek. The mandibular branch involves the lower lip, the outer portion of the tongue, and the area of the cheek close to the ear. Additionally, more than one branch may be involved. The pain is always unilateral and does not cross the midline because only one side of the face is involved. The sudden onset of pain is triggered by mechanical or thermal stimulation. An affected person sleeps poorly and may be undernourished and dehydrated because chewing, swallowing, or any touching of the area may set off the pain.

Patient Screening

The pain of trigeminal neuralgia is so severe that affected individuals require immediate pain relief. When an immediate appointment is not available, the patient should be referred to an emergency facility for assessment and treatment with medications for pain relief.

Etiology

The cause is uncertain, although in some cases, trigeminal neuralgia has been found to be related to compression of a nerve root by a tumor or vascular lesion. Occasionally trigeminal neuralgia is a sequela of multiple sclerosis or herpes zoster. Most cases have no identified cause.

Diagnosis

The reports of an excruciating pain that has an abrupt onset and duration of seconds to minutes on one side of the face suggest trigeminal neuralgia. Observation of the patient,

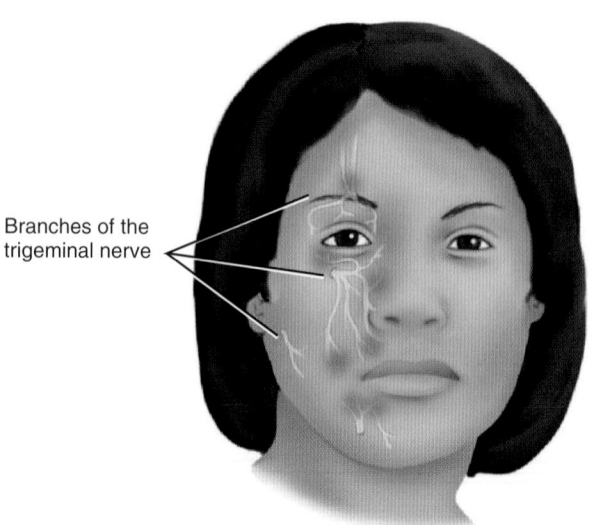

Branches of the trigeminal nerve

• **Fig. 13.20** Trigeminal nerve (cranial nerve V) and branches. (From Shiland B: *Mastering healthcare terminology*, ed 5, St Louis, 2015, Elsevier.)

both during an attack and at normal times, demonstrates the presence of pain. The patient avoids touching the face to prevent triggering an attack.

Because even a draft or gentle breeze may set off the pain, the face should be protected and temperature extremes avoided. No impairment of sensory or motor function is noted. The episodes may last from months to years and then subside. Infection of a sinus or a tooth and tumors must be ruled out.

Treatment

Analgesics are prescribed for pain. Some authors have reported that many patients respond well to carbamazepine. Current drug therapy includes the use of anticonvulsant drugs to control the pain. However, after some time, the effectiveness may decrease. Side effects may include dizziness, nausea, double vision, and sleepiness. The addition of muscle relaxants may be more effective; however, side effects include depression, confusion, and severe drowsiness.

When relief cannot be obtained, surgical intervention to dissect the nerve roots is performed. Patients who smoke are advised to cease smoking.

Prognosis

The prognosis varies, depending on the underlying causative factors. Some cases resolve spontaneously, and some others may respond to drug therapy. Surgical intervention, as a last resort, affords pain relief; however, the function of the affected nerve may be compromised as a result.

Prevention

No method of prevention is known. Smokers are encouraged to stop smoking.

Patient Teaching

Provide information about the condition to the patient and the family. Assist them in locating and contacting community support groups.

Bell Palsy

Description

Bell palsy is a disorder of the facial nerve (CN VII) that causes a sudden onset of weakness or paralysis of facial muscles.

ICD-10-CM Code	G51.0 (Bell's palsy)

Symptoms and Signs

The severity of paralysis in Bell palsy varies widely. The patient may be aware of pain or a drawing sensation behind the ear, followed by an inability to open or close the eye and drooping of the mouth and drooling of saliva. Often the disorder is first noticed in the morning, having developed overnight. Initially the patient is unable to smile, whistle, or grimace, and the facial expression is distorted (Fig. 13.21).

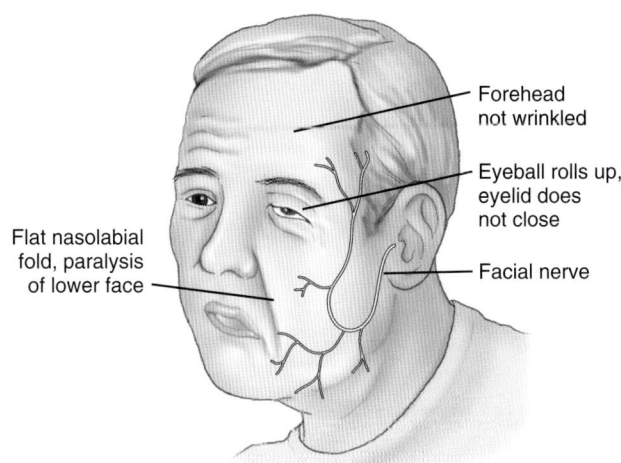

• **Fig. 13.21** Bell palsy. (From Shiland B: *Mastering healthcare terminology,* ed 5, St Louis, 2015, Elsevier.)

Taste perception may be diminished, contributing to loss of appetite. The condition is usually unilateral. It may be transient or permanent and usually occurs between ages 20 and 60 years, in men and women alike.

Patient Screening

The individual reporting sudden onset of one-sided facial paralysis requires prompt assessment to rule out a CVA. Referral is usually to an emergency facility for diagnosis. Anxiety will be high in the individuals and their families, so the next available appointment should be scheduled to discuss the condition after diagnosis.

Etiology

The cause of Bell palsy is not always certain. The symptoms result from blockage of impulses from the facial nerve (CN VII) caused by compression of the nerve in the bony canal. Bilateral facial paralysis has been noted in a small percentage of people with Lyme disease.

Diagnosis

Bell palsy is diagnosed from symptoms and signs and the characteristic history. The differential diagnosis includes CVA (stroke) and autoimmune disease.

Treatment

Early treatment is critical. The application of warm moist heat, gentle massage, and facial exercises to stimulate muscle tone is recommended. Prednisone may be prescribed to reduce inflammation of the facial nerve. Analgesics also may be required. Inability to close the eye may result in dry, sore eyes; artificial tears and an eye patch for protection from outside elements may be needed unless symptoms are mild. Electrotherapy stimulates the nerve and prevents atrophy of muscles.

Prognosis

Complete recovery is possible if the disease is treated early, and recovery often occurs spontaneously, especially in younger individuals. Nevertheless, residual effects may remain for an undetermined period. Patients who smoke are advised to cease smoking.

Prevention
No method of prevention is known.

Patient Teaching
Provide information about the condition to the patient and the family. Assist them in locating and contacting community support groups.

Infectious Disorders

Meningitis

Description
Meningitis is inflammation of the meninges, the membranous coverings of the brain, and spinal cord.

ICD-10-CM Code	G03.9 *(Meningitis, unspecified)*
	(G03.0-G03.9 = 5 codes
	of specificity)

Meningitis is coded according to cause or type. Once the diagnosis has confirmed the cause and type, refer to the current edition of the ICD-10-CM coding manual for the appropriate code.

Symptoms and Signs
Early symptoms of meningitis include vomiting and a headache that increases in intensity with movement or shaking of the head. Attempts of the examiner to move the head reveal nuchal rigidity, which is stiffness of the neck with resistance to any sideways or flexion-extension movements of the head; this is a classic sign. Positive *Kernig sign* (resistance to leg extension after flexing the thigh on the body) and *Brudzinski sign* (neck flexion causing flexion of the hips from the supine position) indicate meningeal irritation. Deep tendon reflexes increase, and the patient exhibits irritability, photophobia, and hypersensitivity of the skin. Seizures caused by cortical irritation can be late manifestations of the process. Drowsiness may progress to stupor and coma.

Patient Screening
Early symptoms of meningitis are easily overlooked and may not appear severe enough to demand immediate assessment at first. As the symptoms and signs increase in nature, prompt assessment and intervention are necessary. The patient should be referred to an emergency facility without delay.

Etiology
Meningitis can be either bacterial or viral. The infection can originate directly from the brain, spinal cord, or sinuses. Open head injuries are additional portals of entry for the offending bacteria. *Haemophilus influenzae, Neisseria meningitidis,* and *Streptococcus pneumoniae* are the bacteria

responsible for most meningeal infections; however, the causative microorganism can be either bacterial or viral (Fig. 13.22).

Diagnosis
The clinical findings alert the physician to the possibility of meningitis. Diagnostic lumbar puncture reveals increased CSF pressure and the presence of white blood cells (WBCs), protein, and glucose in CSF. Culture of CSF showing growth of microbes confirms the diagnosis. CSF may appear cloudy because of the presence of WBCs.

Treatment
Bacterial meningitis is treated aggressively with intravenous (IV) antibiotic therapy. Anticonvulsive drugs are administered to control seizure activity. Glucocorticoids (dexamethasone, prednisone, and methylprednisolone) may be administered to reduce cerebral inflammation and edema. Aspirin, an NSAID, or acetaminophen is given for the headache. External stimuli are kept to a minimum and the room dark and quiet.

Prognosis
The prognosis is unpredictable and depends on the source of the infection and patient response to drug therapy. Bacterial forms respond well to aggressive antibiotic therapy. Most viral forms run their course. The degree of residual damage, if any is noted, also depends on patient response to drug intervention.

Prevention
Prevention is difficult. Those who have had contact with known cases are often prescribed prophylactic antibiotics. Good hand washing techniques are always helpful in preventing the spread of any bacterial or viral infection. Vaccines are now available as a preventive measure against some types of meningococcal meningitis. Many health departments are

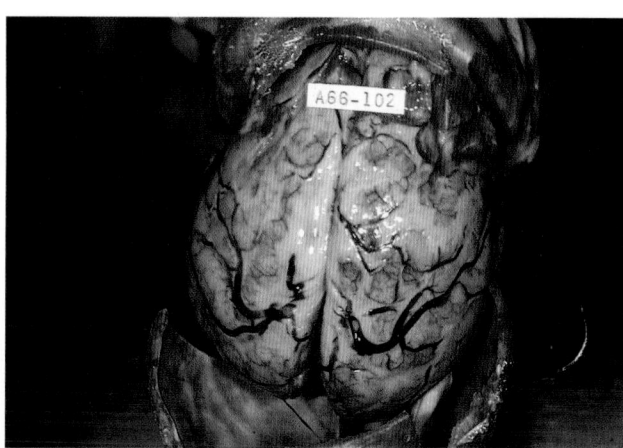

• **Fig. 13.22** Bacterial meningitis. The surface of the brain is covered with pus. (From Kumar V, Cotran RS, Robbins SL: *Robbins basic pathology*, ed 7, Philadelphia, 2003, Saunders.)

now suggesting administration of the vaccines when an outbreak of meningitis occurs.

Patient Teaching

Stress the importance of completing a prescribed regimen of antibiotics. Provide the patient and the family with visual aids depicting the meningeal system and its functions.

Encephalitis

Description

Encephalitis is inflammation of the brain tissue.

> ICD-10-CM Code   G04.90 (Encephalitis and
>   encephalomyelitis, unspecified)
>   G04.91 (Myelitis, unspecified)
>   (G04.00-G04.01; G04.81-
>   G04.91 = 6 codes of
>   specificity)
> Once the diagnosis has confirmed the cause and type, refer to the current edition of the ICD-10-CM coding manual for the appropriate code.

Symptoms and Signs

Encephalitis, an inflammation of the brain tissue, may have an insidious or sudden onset. Primary symptoms include headache and an elevated temperature. The patient experiences stiffness of the neck and back, muscular weakness, restlessness, visual disturbances, and lethargy. Mental confusion progresses to disorientation and even coma.

Patient Screening

Individuals reporting stiffness in the neck and back, muscle weakness, accompanied by headache, fever, restlessness, visual disturbances, and lethargy should be referred to an emergency facility without delay.

Etiology

Inflammation leads to cerebral edema and subsequent cell destruction. It is caused by viruses or the toxins from chickenpox, measles, or mumps. Most cases are the result of a bite from an infected mosquito. Eastern equine, Western equine, and Venezuelan equine encephalomyelitis and St. Louis encephalitis are forms of encephalitis encountered in the United States. Recently, West Nile viral encephalitis, a form of encephalitis that is not *endemic* to the United States, has evolved and is spreading across the country.

Diagnosis

The clinical findings lead the physician to further investigation, including a lumbar puncture; CSF pressure is elevated. Blood and CSF studies reveal the presence of the virus. EEG is abnormal. MRI is ordered to look for herpes simplex virus (HSV) encephalitis and rule out other pathology.

Treatment

Antiviral agents are effective against only HSV encephalitis. Otherwise, treatment is symptomatic, with mild analgesics for pain, antipyretic drugs for elevated temperature, anticonvulsants for seizure activity, and antibiotics for any intercurrent infection.

Prognosis

The prognosis is unpredictable and depends on the type of infection and response to drug therapy. Most viral forms run their course. Residual damage to the brain tissue may result.

Prevention

Prevention is difficult. Avoiding environments heavily populated by mosquitoes may prevent the bites. Use of mosquito spray and wearing long-sleeved shirts and long pants may prevent bites. Preventing mosquito breeding sites by eliminating standing water helps control the mosquito population. Community boards of health monitor the mosquito population and those of other vectors, such as birds that carry the West Nile virus.

Patient Teaching

Prevention is important. Stress the use of mosquito repellant when in an outdoor environment. Encourage patients and their families to be aware of encephalitis outbreaks in the community. Generate print-on-demand electronic materials, when possible, as teaching tools.

Guillain-Barré Syndrome

Description

Guillain-Barré syndrome is an acute, rapidly progressive disease of the PNS.

> ICD-10-CM Code   G61.0 (Guillain-Barré syndrome)

Symptoms and Signs

The individual with Guillain-Barré syndrome experiences numbness and tingling of the feet and hands at the onset of the disease, followed by increasing muscle pain and tenderness. Progressive muscle weakness and paralysis usually start in the lower extremities and move up the body in 24 to 72 hours. Although most patients experience ascending paralysis, occasionally some patients experience descending weakness and paralysis. Respiratory insufficiency is possible, as is difficulty swallowing.

Patient Screening

Individuals reporting numbness and tingling of the feet and hands, followed by increasing muscle pain and tenderness and subsequent progressive muscle weakness and paralysis, need immediate assessment and intervention. The patient should be referred to an emergency facility for prompt care.

Etiology

Knowledge of the etiology is limited, but the syndrome is thought to have an autoimmune basis. The condition has been known to follow a respiratory infection or gastroenteritis in 10 to 21 days. Demyelination of nerves occurs with the syndrome.

Diagnosis

Confirmation is made by the finding of an elevated protein level in CSF, with the level peaking in 4 to 6 weeks after onset. The leukocyte count is normal, as is CSF pressure.

Treatment

Hospitalization usually is required for observation. Treatment is supportive. Plasmapheresis washes plasma to remove antibodies, thereby shortening the time required for recovery. IV human immune globulin (IVIG) may be beneficial.

Prognosis

The prognosis varies, but recovery is usually complete.

Prevention

No method of prevention is known.

Patient Teaching

Encourage patients to keep follow-up appointments as scheduled. Generate print-on-demand electronic materials, when possible, as teaching tools.

Brain Abscess

Description

A brain abscess, a collection of pus, can occur anywhere in the brain tissue (Fig. 13.23).

ICD-10-CM Code	G06.0 *(Intracranial abscess and granuloma)*

Symptoms and Signs

The primary symptom of a brain abscess is headache. Other symptoms and signs depend on the location and extent of the abscess. Generally the patient exhibits symptoms and signs of increased intracranial pressure, including nausea and vomiting, visual disturbances, unequal pupil size, and seizures. Many times, the eyes look toward the area of insult, that is, toward the side of the head where the abscess is located. *Nuchal rigidity* (stiffness of neck with resistance to moving head side to side or up and down) may be noted.

Patient Screening

Individuals who complain of an unusual headache should be given an appointment as soon as possible. When reports of nausea, vomiting, visual disturbances, stiff neck, unequal pupil size, and possible seizures are relayed, the disease has progressed to a stage that requires prompt assessment and intervention. The patient should be referred to an emergency facility or advise the individual or the family to call 911 and enter the individual into the EMS system.

Etiology

CNS abscesses may be the result of a local infection or may be secondary to infections elsewhere in the body. The common causative organisms are staphylococci, streptococci, and pneumococci. Any occurrence that breaches the integrity of the CNS, including head trauma and a craniotomy wound, may be the portal of entry for the microorganisms. The abscess may be secondary to another infectious process, such as sinusitis, otitis, dental abscess, subdural empyema, and bacterial endocarditis (Fig. 13.24).

Diagnosis

A history of infection, especially of the sinuses or the ear, or an insult to the CNS, coupled with the characteristic clinical features of increased intracranial pressure, suggests an abscess. EEG and CT are used to verify the diagnosis. Lumbar puncture is contraindicated because the resulting increase in intracranial pressure may cause the brainstem to herniate, resulting in death. Blood cultures may also be ordered.

Treatment

IV antibiotics are administered to resolve the infection. Mannitol or steroids are prescribed to reduce cerebral edema. Surgical drainage of the abscess may be necessary to

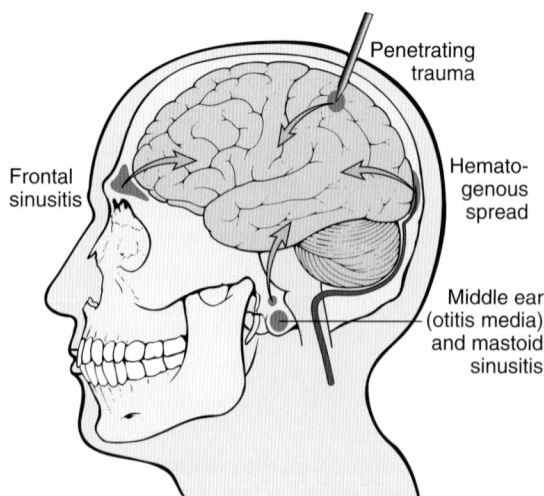

• **Fig. 13.24** Bacterial infections of the central nervous system (CNS). Infectious organisms may reach the brain through several routes: hematogenously; by direct entry because of penetrating trauma; or by direct spread from adjacent structures, such as the inner ear or the nasal sinuses. (From Damjanov I: *Pathology for the health-related professions,* ed 4, St Louis, 2011, Saunders/Elsevier.)

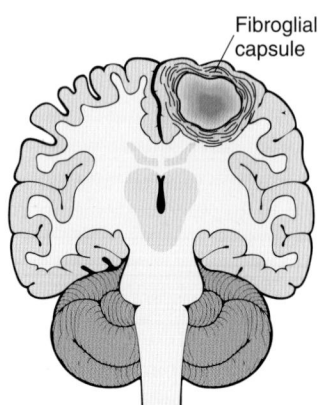

• **Fig. 13.23** Brain abscess.

relieve intracranial pressure and to culture the offending organism. Additional treatment is supportive.

Prognosis

The prognosis varies, depending on the location, size, and causative agent of the abscess. Underlying pathology and the health status of the patient also affect the recovery process. When intracranial pressure cannot be controlled, death may result.

Prevention

Prevention is difficult because of the numerous possible sources of infection. Prompt treatment of potential secondary sources or another infectious process, including sinusitis, otitis, dental abscess, subdural empyema, and bacterial endocarditis, helps in prevention.

Patient Teaching

Encourage prompt reporting of infectious processes involving the head so that treatment can resolve these potential sources of the abscess in a timely manner. Generate print-on-demand electronic materials, when possible, as teaching tools.

Poliomyelitis and Post-Polio Syndrome

Description

Poliomyelitis, a viral infection of the anterior horn cells of the gray matter of the spinal cord, causes selective destruction of the motor neurons.

ICD-10-CM Code	A80.9 (Acute poliomyelitis, unspecified)
	(A80.0-A80.9 = 7 codes of specificity)
	B91 (Sequelae of poliomyelitis)
	G14 (Postpolio syndrome)

Poliomyelitis is coded according to type and paralytic involvement. Once the diagnosis has been confirmed, refer to the current edition of the ICD-10-CM coding manual for the appropriate code and fourth and fifth digits.

Symptoms and Signs

This highly contagious disease is no longer the threat to humankind that it was before the 1960s. The Salk and Sabin vaccines have virtually eliminated poliomyelitis in the Western world, making its occurrence rare.

The patient with poliomyelitis has a low-grade fever, a profuse discharge from the nose, and malaise. These symptoms are followed by progressive muscle weakness, stiff neck, nausea and vomiting, and flaccid paralysis of the muscles involved. Atrophy of the muscles follows, with decreased tendon reflexes, followed by muscle and joint deterioration.

Poliomyelitis that involves the muscles supplied by the spinal nerves is termed *spinal poliomyelitis,* whereas involvement of the muscles supplied by cranial nerves (gray matter of the medulla) is termed *bulbar poliomyelitis.*

Patient Screening

Any individual complaining of progressive muscle weakness, stiff neck, nausea and vomiting, and flaccid paralysis of the muscles involved requires prompt assessment. The patient should be referred to an emergency facility. For individuals who are known to have previously contracted polio (usually 30 years earlier) and report onset of progressive weakness in the already affected muscles, the next available appointment should be scheduled.

Etiology

Poliovirus enters the body through the nose and throat, crosses into the gastrointestinal tract, and reproduces in the lymphoid tissue. Traveling by way of the bloodstream, the virus moves to the CNS and assaults the motor neurons of the spinal cord. The incubation period is 7 to 21 days. Poliovirus is transmitted from person to person through infected oropharyngeal secretions or feces that contain the virus.

Diagnosis

The clinical symptoms and a history of possible exposure to an infected person are the primary tools of diagnosis. Isolation of poliovirus from throat washings or feces confirms the diagnosis. When the CNS is involved, the results of CSF culture are positive for poliovirus.

Treatment

Treatment is supportive. Analgesics are administered for pain relief, along with moist heat applications. Bed rest is indicated until the acute stage is resolved. Physical therapy, including the use of braces, may be necessary. When respiratory difficulty is present, respiratory support with mechanical ventilation may be necessary. Prevention by means of Sabin and Salk vaccines has rendered poliomyelitis almost nonexistent in the world.

Three distinct serotypes of poliovirus exist: types 1, 2, and 3. All three types can be found worldwide, and immunization with the Sabin trivalent oral vaccine affords immunity to all three forms. A monovalent Sabin vaccine grants immunity to only one form, as does the Salk vaccine. Persons with immunosuppressive conditions should not be given the trivalent vaccine because they are at risk for contracting poliomyelitis. Additionally, any immunosuppressed person should not come in contact with the feces or nasal secretions of a recently vaccinated person. Two poliovirus vaccines currently are licensed in the United States: inactivated poliovirus vaccine (IPV) and oral poliovirus vaccine (OPV).

Post-polio syndrome occurs later in life in persons who have previously experienced the disease. Functional deterioration of muscles is accompanied by loss of strength. Progressive weakness begins 30 years or more after the initial attack and involves the already affected muscles. Fasciculations and muscular atrophy may accompany the weakness. Treatment is supportive.

Prognosis

The prognosis is fair, depending on which muscles are involved. Muscles involved in respiration may require intervention to maintain ventilation. Muscles in the arms and legs require intensive rehabilitation with physical therapy. The prognosis for those with post-polio syndrome is good.

Prevention

Administration of the polio vaccines has helped to significantly reduce the incidence of polio. The World Health Organization's goal is to eradicate polio throughout the world with immunization.

Patient Teaching

Encourage all parents to have their children vaccinated according to the recommended inoculation schedule.

Intracranial Tumors (Brain Tumors)

Description

Brain tumors can be primary tumors, neoplasms that originate in the brain itself, or secondary tumors, cancers that have metastasized from another area of the body, such as the lung, liver, kidney, or skin. Primary tumors can arise from any cell within the CNS (Fig. 13.25). They are named according to the tissues from which they originate.

ICD-10-CM Code   D49.6 (Neoplasm of
                                       unspecified behavior of
                                       brain)

Symptoms and Signs

Regardless of the tumor cell type, symptoms and signs result from displacement and compression of normal brain tissue by the tumor, causing progressive neurologic deficits, expansion of the brain (cerebral edema), and increased intracranial pressure, leading to possible herniation (Fig. 13.26). Common symptoms include headache (usually dull, constant, and worse at night); focal or generalized seizures (common in gliomas and secondary tumors); nausea and vomiting; syncope; cognitive dysfunction (including memory problems

and personality changes); muscle weakness; sensory loss; aphasia; and visual dysfunction. The classic symptoms of cerebellar tumors (e.g., medulloblastoma) often are gait disturbance, nystagmus, lethargy, dysarthric speech pattern, and balance difficulty. Glioblastoma causes such symptoms as seizures, nausea, vomiting, and headache. This type of tumor is very aggressive and difficult to treat.

Patient Screening

Symptoms of early brain tumors are somewhat vague. Individuals complaining of constant headaches with increasing severity and worsening at night require prompt assessment. Reports of seizures, loss of consciousness, and reduced cognitive functioning also require prompt assessment, and the patient should be referred to an emergency facility.

Etiology

Primary brain tumors are classified histologically according to the predominant cell type: Gliomas, tumors derived from glial cells; meningiomas, tumors arising from the arachnoid membrane; and embryonal tumors, neoplasms that arise in children. Together they account for 75% of all cancerous primary brain tumors in the population. The incidence of gliomas and meningiomas increases after age 45 years. Among children under age 15 years, brain tumors are the most common solid malignancy.

The incidence of brain tumors is greater in developed, industrialized countries, such as the United States, Western Europe, and Australia. Caucasians are affected more often than any other race. Many risk factors for brain tumors have been proposed and are under investigation, but so far only

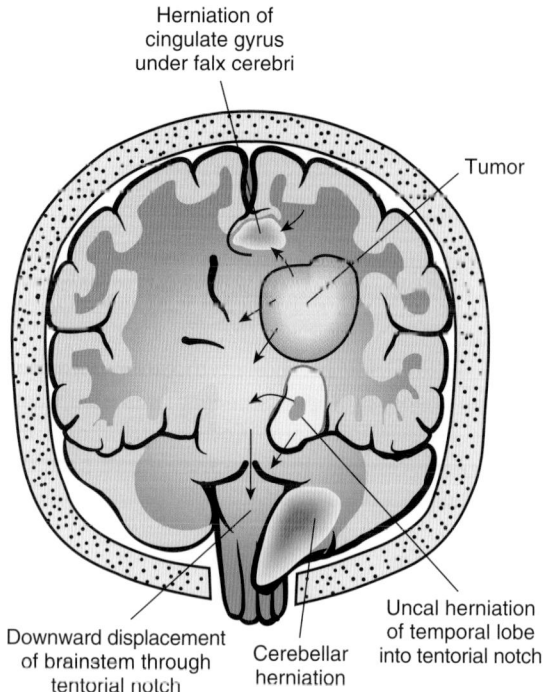

Herniation of cingulate gyrus under falx cerebri

Tumor

Downward displacement of brainstem through tentorial notch

Cerebellar herniation

Uncal herniation of temporal lobe into tentorial notch

• **Fig. 13.26** Increased intracranial pressure and possible herniations. (From Gould BE, Dyer RM: *Pathophysiology for the health professions,* ed 4, St Louis, 2012, Saunders/Elsevier.)

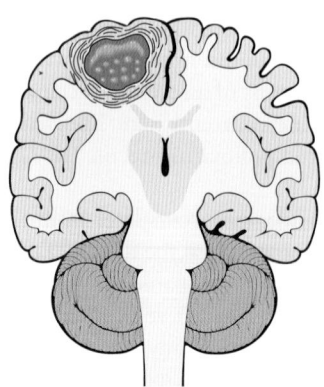

• **Fig. 13.25** Brain tumor.

therapeutic ionizing radiation and genetic predisposition through inherited cancer syndromes, such as neurofibromatosis and von Hippel-Lindau syndrome, have been established as risk factors. However, these risk factors account for only a fraction of cases.

Diagnosis

The evaluation of a patient with a suspected brain tumor includes a detailed history, a neurologic examination, and diagnostic neuroimaging studies. Neurologic examination findings are associated with particular regions affected by destruction of neural tissue. Cranial MRI is the diagnostic imaging modality of choice. Functional MRI, which measures blood flow through regions of the brain during various activities, or positron emission tomography (PET) can be helpful in preoperative planning. Tissue obtained during surgery or through stereotactic biopsy is necessary for correct histologic diagnosis of the tumor type. Only tumor grade and histologic classification are considered definitive factors to determine the malignant potential of the tumor. (Refer to Chapter 1 for staging and grading of cancer.)

Although brain tumors can be malignant or benign, the distinction is blurred. Unlike benign neoplasms in other locations of the body, benign brain tumors may cause the same symptoms as malignant tumors, such that distinguishing between the benign and malignant types on clinical grounds can be very difficult. Even a benign tumor with little to no metastatic potential can be lethal if it occurs in a region of the brain that precludes full surgical resection.

Treatment

Benign and malignant neoplasms are often treated similarly. Patients with primary brain tumors must be treated for their symptoms and for the neoplasm. Symptomatic treatment includes use of anticonvulsants to treat seizures and corticosteroids to decrease intracranial pressure. Surgery is the initial treatment for most tumors. It provides tissue samples for definitive diagnosis and relieves symptoms by reducing tumor bulk. The extent of surgery is limited by the goal of not inflicting incapacitating neurologic damage on the patient. Surgery is usually followed by radiotherapy and/or chemotherapy, depending on the tumor type and stage. Staging of most brain tumors uses the modified TNM (tumor-node-metastasis) system. The N component of the staging system is not very informative because the

CNS does not contain lymphatic structures. Although still experimental, immunotherapy is showing promise as an additional modality to treat brain tumors.

Treatment of secondary brain tumors focuses on relief of neurologic symptoms and long-term tumor control. Treatment choice is based on the location, size, and number of metastases; patient age; the patient's neurologic status; and the extent of systemic cancer. In general, patients with solitary brain lesions and no metastases at other sites are candidates for treatment with surgery and whole brain radiation therapy (WBRT). Although the patient may still be affected by extracranial disease, this treatment improves quality of life and reduces the likelihood of death resulting from neurologic causes. Patients with multiple or recurrent metastases are often treated with surgery or radiation with palliative intent.

It is important to remember that patients, especially children, may be affected by the long-term complications of surgery, radiation, and chemotherapy in the years after treatment. Problems include neurocognitive defects, growth hormone deficiency, learning disability, loss of vision, and secondary malignancies.

Prognosis

The overall 5-year survival rate for all types of brain tumors combined varies, depending on the type of tumor and the age and gender of the patient. Poor prognostic indicators include a high tumor grade, presence of mental changes at the time of diagnosis, large tumor size, and inability to fully resect the tumor during surgery. Despite continued research to successfully treat gliomas, the 5-year survival rate is only 5.5%.

Prevention

No methods are known to prevent intracranial neoplasms, and no screening programs are available for early detection.

Patient Teaching

Assist the patient and the family members in locating and contacting available community resources. Discuss the neurocognitive functional deficits resulting from insults to the brain and the delayed growth and learning disabilities that may occur in children. Encourage compliance with any prescribed drug or physical therapy. Use customized electronically generated educational materials, when available, to reinforce the treatment plan.

Review Challenge

Answer the following questions:

1. What is the central nervous system (CNS) composed of? The peripheral nervous system (PNS)?
2. What are some possible causes of diseases of the nervous system?
3. How is the nervous system evaluated during a diagnostic examination?
4. What are the three vascular disorders that may result in a cerebrovascular accident (CVA)?
5. How does a transient ischemic attack (TIA) differ from a CVA?
6. What are some of the likely causes of epidural and subdural hematomas? Which condition is more likely to have a delayed onset of symptoms?
7. Which condition is more serious, cerebral concussion or cerebral contusion? Why?
8. What is the relationship between the location of a spinal cord injury and the signs and symptoms?

9. Which diagnostic findings may indicate degeneration or rupture of an intervertebral disk?
10. How does spinal stenosis contribute to sciatic pain?
11. Are headaches always a symptom of an underlying disease? What are some causative factors of cephalalgia?
12. What are the classic signs and symptoms of migraine?
13. What are the different types of epileptic seizures? What are the first aid guidelines?
14. What are the characteristic signs and symptoms of (1) Parkinson disease, (2) Huntington chorea, and (3) amyotrophic lateral sclerosis (ALS)?
15. What are suggested causes of and treatment interventions for transient global amnesia?
16. What are some causative factors of peripheral neuritis?
17. How does a patient with trigeminal neuralgia typically describe the pain?
18. What is the clinical appearance of a person with Bell palsy?
19. What is the diagnostic significance of nuchal rigidity in the presence of headache and photophobia?
20. What are the possible etiologic agents of encephalitis?
21. What is the pathologic progression of Guillain-Barré syndrome?
22. How do infectious organisms reach the brain? How is a brain abscess treated?
23. What is post-polio syndrome?
24. How are intracranial tumors classified, and what determines the symptomatology?
25. What is the 5-year survival rate for brain tumors identified as gliomas?

Real-Life Challenge: Epilepsy

A 26-year-old man had been (2 weeks earlier) in a motor vehicle accident (MVA) and had suffered a closed head injury. Recovery was uneventful, and the patient was discharged from the hospital. The patient returned to work 2 days ago. The patient's wife called the office to state that she had awakened this morning to find her husband having a seizure. The patient was responsive but appeared confused.

The patient was transported to a hospital. Vital signs were temperature, 98.4°F; pulse, 72 beats per minute;

respirations, 18 breaths per minute; and blood pressure, 116/78 mm Hg. The patient was responsive but not oriented to time, place, or person and appeared postictal. EEG was ordered, as was cerebral CT. The patient was diagnosed with seizure activity (epilepsy) secondary to the cerebral trauma suffered in the MVA. The patient was placed on antiseizure medication and admitted for observation.

Questions

1. What patient or family teaching regarding patient activity is indicated?
2. What is the significance of the cerebral trauma to the onset of seizure activity?
3. As what type of epilepsy is this seizure activity classified?
4. Compare the three types of epilepsy with regard to seizure activity, treatment, and predisposing factors.
5. Which other diagnostic tests might be ordered?
6. Describe appropriate first aid intervention for a patient with grand mal seizure.
7. Explain status epilepticus.

Real-Life Challenge: Transient Ischemic Attack

The wife of a 67-year-old man called the office and reported that her husband awoke this morning with weakness and numbness of the right side. He had difficulty getting out of bed and complained of intermittent episodes of dizziness. He also was experiencing difficulty speaking. The patient had a history of hypertension and was taking enalapril (Vasotec) and propranolol (Inderal). The wife was advised that her husband should be seen in an emergency care facility, and an ambulance was called for transport.

On examination in the emergency facility, the patient was found to have diminished strength in the right hand and foot, diminished movement in the right arm and leg, and slurred speech. Vital signs were temperature, 98.6°F;

pulse, 106 beats per minute and irregular; respirations, 22 breaths per minute; and blood pressure, 172/96 mm Hg. Oxygen therapy was started. Reflexes were diminished, as was pain response on the right side, including the extremities.

Cerebral MRI, CT, EEG, skull radiography, and ECG were ordered. ECG showed atrial fibrillation. Approximately 6 hours after onset, the symptoms began to resolve, with improvement seen in feeling and movement of the right extremities. Speech slowly became less slurred. The patient was diagnosed as having a transient ischemic attack (TIA), and an appointment was scheduled for follow-up evaluation. He was started on anticoagulant therapy.

Questions

1. What is the importance of the right-side involvement and slurring of speech?
2. Why would ambulance transportation to an emergency facility be recommended?
3. What is the significance of the elevated blood pressure?
4. Explain the differences between a TIA and a CVA.
5. In what area of the brain would the diminished circulation and subsequent reduced oxygenation be anticipated?
6. Why would anticoagulant therapy be prescribed?
7. Research the importance of the ECG results indicating atrial fibrillation.

Internet Assignments

1. Go to the National Spinal Cord Injury Association to research advances in the treatment of spinal cord injuries.
2. Go to the National Parkinson Foundation to research the latest developments in treatment interventions for Parkinson disease.
3. Research the diagnostic tests used by neurosurgeons at the American Association of Neurological Surgeons. What other procedures are used to treat head trauma and CVAs?
4. Research the American Neurological Association, and write a report on a discussion of a disease entity or condition you find there. (Some topic suggestions are pain management, headache treatment, cancers of the neurologic system, encephalitis, and West Nile virus encephalitis.)

Critical Thinking

1. According to the Glasgow coma scale in Fig. 13.1, what would you consider severe coma?
2. According to the figure shown in the Neurologic Assessment Enrichment box at the beginning of the chapter, what test is used to evaluate ocular movement?
3. Unilateral cerebral bleeding and refusal of treatment often have what kind of outcome?
4. Identify some of the incidents where individuals may have a sudden onset of life-threatening emergencies.
5. A 74-year-old man has been diagnosed with a cerebrovascular accident (CVA). Although his speech is not affected, he has trouble with the use of nouns in sentences. Most of the time, he is able to groom himself and to feed himself. He has difficulty making decisions and following complex commands. What would you recommend that his wife, the caretaker, do about obtaining help in his care? Would there be financial assistance for the couple? What kind of home health care might be available?
6. A 17-year-old man recently was involved in a motorcycle crash. He was not wearing a helmet and sustained a head injury and fractured lumbar vertebrae. As a result, he is a paraplegic and is unable to move his legs and to control elimination. What type of care will this young man require? How will this affect his education? How will his family find assistance for care and for financial needs?
7. A 78-year-old woman has been diagnosed with Parkinson disease. She does not exhibit the usual symptoms of hand tremors with "pill rolling" activity. Her mental status has been compromised, and she requires constant watching for her instability and her inability to perform activities of daily living. Her husband is her caretaker. What type of teaching will you provide to assist the family in the care of the patient? What can they expect in the future?
8. A 50-year-old woman has been diagnosed with peripheral neuropathy. What kind of teaching would you provide to encourage her to get her diabetes under control? How would you assist her with dietary management? What resources would you encourage her to seek to get assistance?
9. What type of patient teaching would you provide to parents about the importance of childhood immunizations? Polio still may occur, so it is important for all children to receive the polio vaccine.

Prepare to discuss Critical Thinking case study exercises for this chapter that are posted on Evolve.

14

Mental Disorders

CHAPTER OUTLINE

Mental Wellness and Mental Illness, 575

Intellectual Developmental Disorder, 577

Learning Disorders, 578

Communication Disorders, 578

Pervasive Development Disorders, 579

Attention-Deficit/Hyperactivity Disorder, 581

Oppositional Defiant Disorder, 582

Tic Disorders, 583

Dementia, 584

Substance-Related Disorders, 589

Schizophrenia, 592

Mood Disorders, 598

Anxiety Disorders, 603

Pediatric Autoimmune Neuropsychiatric Disorders
Associated With Streptococcal Infections (PANDAS), 606

Somatoform Disorders, 608

Gender Dysphonia, 611

Sleep Disorders, 612

Personality Disorders, 615

LEARNING OBJECTIVES

After studying Chapter 14, you should be able to:

1. Name some contributing factors to mental disorders.
2. List some of the many causes of intellectual developmental disorder.
3. Describe the characteristic manifestations of pervasive development disorders (PDDs), including autism.
4. List criteria for diagnosis of attention-deficit/hyperactivity disorder (ADHD).
5. List some examples of tic disorders.
6. Describe the progressive degenerative changes in an individual with Alzheimer disease.
7. Explain important factors in the treatment of Alzheimer disease.
8. Explain the cause of vascular dementia.
9. Relate treatment options for alcohol abuse.
10. Name the classic signs and symptoms of schizophrenia. Explain what is included in the multidimensional treatment plan.

11. Explain why bipolar disorder is considered a major affective disorder. Describe the treatment approach.
12. Discuss normal grieving process phases.
13. Discuss how each type of anxiety disorder prevents a person from leading a normal life.
14. Explain how posttraumatic stress disorder (PTSD) differs from other anxiety disorders.
15. Explain how a somatization disorder is diagnosed.
16. Discuss the relationship between anxiety and conversion disorder.
17. Describe factitious syndrome.
18. Contrast insomnia to narcolepsy.
19. List and discuss personality disorders, including the distinguishing characteristics.
20. Discuss the predisposing factor(s) of PANDAS syndrome.
21. Discuss options of animal therapy.

KEY TERMS

affect (**AF**-feckt)

amyloid (**AM**-ih-loyd)

anhedonia (an-hee-**DOH**-nee-ah)

autism (**AW**-tism)

catatonic (kat-ah-**TOH**-nic)

circadian (sir-**KAY**-dee-an)

cognitive (**KOG**-nih-tive)

deficit (**DEAF**-ih-sit)

delusion (dee-**LOO**-zhun)

endarterectomy (**end**-ar-ter-**EK**-toh-me)

hallucination (ha-loo-sih-**NAY**-shun)

hypoxia (**hi-POX**-ee-ah)

ischemia (is-**KEY**-me-ah)

mutism (**MYOO**-tizm)

narcissistic (nar-sis-**SIST**-ik)

paranoid (**PAR**-ah-noid)

psychotic (sigh-**KOT**-ik)

schizoid (**SKIZ**-oyd)

Mental Wellness and Mental Illness

At some time in life, almost everyone is affected by mental disorders, either personally or by the involvement of a family member or friend. Stress is considered a contributing factor that causes exacerbation of mental disorders. Other factors are hereditary or congenital, accidental, traumatic, psychosocial, socioeconomic, or related to drug toxicity. Chemical imbalances in the brain and its neurotransmitters also are postulated to be causative factors. The specific causes of mental illness remain unclear in many cases. Power and control along with bullying contribute to many forms of mental illnesses.

Mental illness has been linked to the patient's inability to cope with stress imposed by modern society. Pressures imposed by life circumstances can be a source of personal pain and distress. The definition of mental wellness, or being in a good state of mental health, varies and is a relative state of mind. When healthy people have the capacity to cope and adjust in a reasonable manner to the ongoing stresses of everyday life, they are considered to be in a state of equilibrium, known as *mental wellness.*

Psychological pain is real, is intense, and can affect physical health. Subsequently, impaired or pathologic coping skills emerge in people's behavior. Some coping behaviors are conscious, and some are not easily controlled because they are unconscious. Certain disorders in thinking, perceiving, and behaving can be organized into clusters of signs and symptoms. These clusters become diagnostic criteria and a part of a total physical and psychological evaluation.

The American Psychiatric Association's *Diagnostic and Statistical Manual of Mental Disorders,* fifth edition (DSM-V) is the accepted reference that offers guidelines for criteria to be used in the clinical setting when diagnosing a mental disorder (Fig. 14.1). The DSM-V replaces the previous edition, and some diagnoses have been removed or changed. In addition to diagnostic criteria, the DSM-V gives the practitioner a standardized diagnostic code, similar to the *International Classification of Diseases,* ninth and tenth revisions, Clinical Modification (ICD-10-CM) coding systems.

Mental disorders include those of congenital and hereditary origins. Other categories, such as maladaptive disorders, phobias, anxiety, depression, addiction, and psychotic disorders, have uncertain or unknown causes and possibly more than one contributing factor. Psychosis, a symptom of a mental disorder, may be indicative of a severe mental disorder where the individual loses touch with reality. The individual may experience verbal or visual hallucinations, irrational thoughts, delusions, regressive behavior, and degeneration of personality.

Mental disorders cause mild to severe disruption in a person's ability to function in interpersonal relationships, self-care, and occupational settings. In some disorders, the person may experience incapacitating psychotic symptoms. The DSM-V also includes substance-related, eating, and sleep disorders. In some mental disorders, oxygen and nutrient deprivation with necrosis result in the death of brain cells; these are known as *organic disorders* and are permanent and cannot be reversed. Supportive therapy and custodial care often are the only available interventions.

Modern therapeutic approaches include control of symptoms with psychotropic drugs, including antipsychotic drugs, antidepressants, anxiolytics (antianxiety agents), central nervous system (CNS) stimulants, and mood stabilizing medications. Additionally, hospitalization during acute episodes, psychotherapy, electroconvulsive therapy, and group therapy are used to stabilize and treat patients. Outpatient treatment is available and preferred in many cases (Fig. 14.2). Play therapy is included in counseling sessions for some children. See the Enrichment box about The Child, the Therapist, and Play Therapy. Patients with mental illnesses and conditions need established routines and consistency in treatment and daily living activities.

Pet therapy and service animals are also used as options in treatment of various disorders. As defined by the U.S. Department of Justice, Civil Rights Division *Disability*

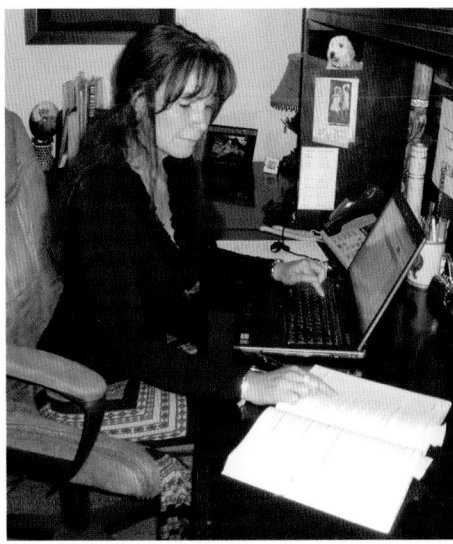

• **Fig. 14.1** Counselor reviewing criteria for diagnosis. (Courtesy Mark Boswell, 2015.)

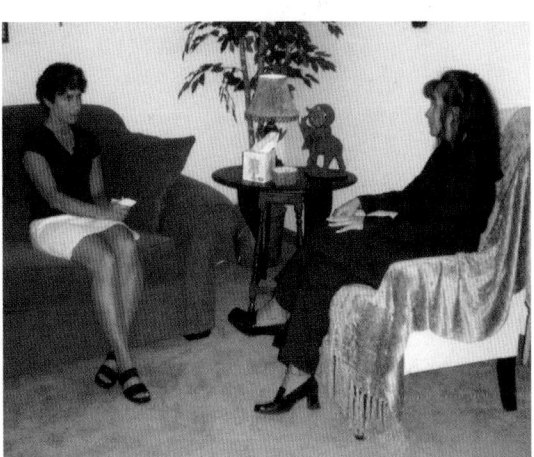

• **Fig. 14.2** Counseling session in progress. (Courtesy Mark Boswell, 2003.)

Rights Section, "Service animals are defined as dogs that are individually trained to do work or perform tasks for people with disabilities. Examples of such work or tasks include guiding people who are blind, alerting people who are deaf, pulling a wheelchair, alerting and protecting a person who is having a seizure, reminding a person with mental illness to take prescribed medications, calming a person with post-traumatic stress disorder (PTSD) during an anxiety attack, or performing other duties. Service animals are working animals, not pets. The work or task a dog has been trained to provide must be directly related to the person's disability. Dogs whose sole function is to provide comfort or emotional support do not qualify as service animals under the Americans with Disability Act (ADA). Service, emotional support, and therapy animals are often used to assist in treatments of individuals. Service animals require intensive training in behavior and response to provide their handler with assistance for the disability. Many veterans with PTSD and others have service, emotional support, or therapy animals to help them deal with their disorder. Comfort and support of the emotional support animal furnishes the individual with nonjudgmental relief. Therapy animals (usually dogs) supply comfort and affection to people in various facilities or situations. All types require training with their handler.

Traumatic events, including mass shootings, can cause anxiety and fear in many members of society. Children are being taught in schools how to protect themselves with books and backpacks in the event of an active shooter in the room. Students and school personnel are trained in school lockdowns. Parents recognize school lockdowns as safety measures for their children. Numerous individuals have expressed apprehension about being in crowded places or at overcrowded events to the point of avoiding occasions where they might feel they are in danger. In many cases, worry has turned into fear that is based on recent events in the United States, such as mass shootings at schools, public events, churches, and even rural areas. Schools for

---

❖ ENRICHMENT

The Child, the Therapist, and Play Therapy

Play is a natural means of expression for a child and a way for children to learn and develop a variety of skills. Therapists working with children use play therapy in assessment and treatment interventions, assisting the child to cope with emotional stress and trauma. Children often cannot verbalize their thoughts and feelings, and play therapy becomes a nonverbal avenue for them to communicate with the therapist. This type of therapy creates a nonthreatening atmosphere for the children. Play therapy may be employed on a one-to-one basis or in a group setting. Children are allowed, and occasionally encouraged, to act out or express feelings and experiences. During play therapy sessions, the therapist establishes rapport with the child and encourages the child to act out any feelings of anxiety and tension he or she may be experiencing. The therapist's goals are to give the child an opportunity to reveal feelings that he or she cannot verbalize, to understand the child's interactions and relationships with the important people in his or her life, and to teach the child appropriate coping mechanisms and adaptive socialization skills.

Children who have been exposed to abuse often respond to the therapist in the nonthreatening environment of play therapy. The use of dolls and various toys gives the child a means of acting out the abuse and offers an avenue for positive interaction.

Therapists may use objects and toys during play therapy. All kinds of dolls, doll houses, stuffed animals, puppets, soft balls and foam bats, toy vehicles, punching toys, a sand tray, and paper and markers or crayons may be used during play therapy. During these play sessions, family interactions and dynamics may become apparent. Sand therapy may include small plastic animals or people and allows the child to act out feelings (Fig. 14.3).

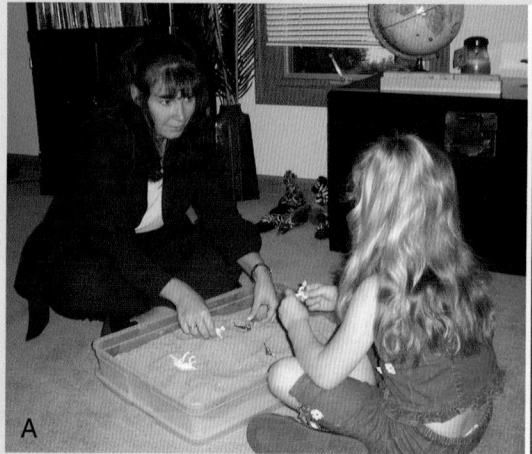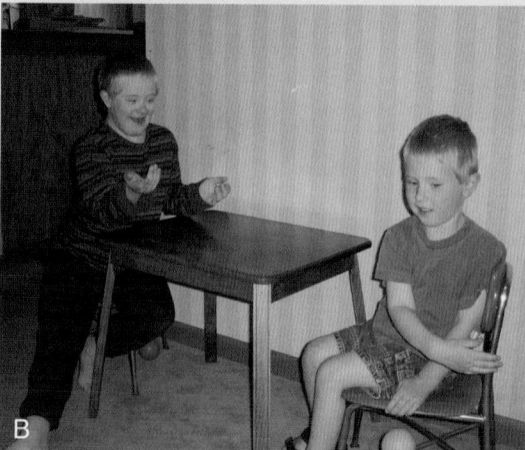

• **Fig. 14.3** Play therapy sessions with children. (Courtesy David L. Frazier, 2003.)

pre-kindergarten to 12th grade are hiring resource officers to provide security in case of such events. Bomb threats are another concern facing schools because each one must be taken seriously, even though at times they are hoaxes. The children, however, are still affected by this type of threat.

Intellectual Developmental Disorder

Description

Intellectual developmental disorder, or developmental disability, is not a disease but a wide range of conditions with many causes. A causative factor interferes with the developmental processes, resulting in changes in the acquisition of intellectual skills and adaptive functioning in a variety of areas, including social and interpersonal skills, self-care, communication, self-direction, health, and safety. In addition, the level of behavioral performance is reduced. General intellectual functioning is subaverage, and the individual has noticeable deficits in adaptive behavior. This condition is manifested during the developmental period and before age 18 years.

ICD-10-CM Code	F70 (Mild intellectual disabilities)
	F71 (Moderate intellectual disabilities)
	F72 (Severe intellectual disabilities)
	F73 (Profound intellectual disabilities)
	F79 (Unspecified intellectual disabilities)

Symptoms and Signs

Intellectual disability disorder is identified by impairments that have an impact on a person's adaptation or function in three domains of their life. These domains include practical, social, and conceptual. Conceptual domain includes skills in reading, writing, language, math and reasoning as well as memory and knowledge. Social domain includes interpersonal communication skills with others, being able to make friends, and an ability to show empathy to others and use good social judgment. The practical domain includes being able to take care of oneself and use good hygiene, manage money, participate in life activities or recreation, and being able to organize tasks associated with school or work.

Patient Screening

Signs of intellectual developmental disorder may appear on well-baby examinations or during preschool routine checkups. The first significant indications of intellectual developmental disorder sometimes appear when the child begins school or preschool. When these parents contact the office, an appointment should be made for the earliest possible date when schedules will allow sufficient time for the physician to conduct a thorough assessment. The parents possibly will be feeling great anxiety, and the child should be assessed as soon as possible.

Etiology

Intellectual developmental disorder has a variety of causes, many of which are unidentifiable. The predisposing factors include heredity (inborn errors of metabolism, genetic disorders, or chromosomal abnormalities); early alterations of embryonic development (Down syndrome or damage from toxins); prenatal, perinatal, or postnatal conditions (prematurity, hypoxia, viral infections, or trauma); general medical conditions (infections, trauma, or poisoning); and environmental influences. Any condition that compromises the blood supply to the developing brain, depriving it of oxygen and nutrients, can result in neurologic damage and intellectual developmental disorder. Some examples are placental insufficiency, cord or head compression during the perinatal period, failure to breathe at birth, premature birth, and viral infections in the mother in the prenatal period or in the infant or child after birth. Trauma of any type that causes hypoxia or anoxia also may contribute to the deficit. Fetal alcohol syndrome also may result in intellectual developmental disorder. Pregnant women should be told that any alcohol ingestion during pregnancy is to be avoided.

Diagnosis

Diagnosis requires observation and confirmation of the intellectual capabilities and adaptive behavior of the child. The individual must have symptoms which begin during the developmental period, but there is not a specific age requirement for making a diagnosis.

Standardized testing of intelligence in the conceptual, social, and practical domains will help ensure the healthcare provider makes a decision on diagnosis determined by functioning needed for everyday life.

Treatment

When the deficit occurs, the brain cells die and cannot be restored. The child can be taught to perform tasks at various levels. Underlying causes should be treated and intervention may prevent or delay progression. The full treatment plan is based on the areas of deficit, once identified.

Prognosis

The prognosis varies, depending on identifiable etiology and adaptive skills.

Prevention

Preventing all intellectual developmental disorder might not be possible, but early and good prenatal care and nutrition are encouraged for all pregnant women to reduce the occurrence. Fetal monitoring during labor may alert the labor and delivery staff when the fetus is deprived of adequate oxygen. In such a case, immediate intervention is necessary. Prompt attention to head injuries in children may prevent the onset of intellectual developmental disorder during childhood. Genetic counseling may be desirable before pregnancy for parents with a family history of intellectual developmental disorder.

Patient Teaching

Parents require encouragement to recognize that there is no cure. Some individuals with intellectual developmental disorder may be educable or trainable. Routines and consistency are important in enabling the individual to function at the highest possible level. Provide parents and family with electronically obtained data explaining various tests used to evaluate IQ.

Learning Disorders

Description

Learning disorders, sometimes referred to as *learning differences* or *learning disabilities,* are conditions that cause children to learn in a manner that is not normal. Performance on standardized tests is lower than expected for age, schooling, and intelligence level. The brain's ability to receive and process information is affected.

ICD-10-CM Code	F81.81 *(Disorder of written expression)*
	F81.89 *(Other developmental disorders of scholastic skills)*

Symptoms and Signs

The person with a learning disorder exhibits difficulty in acquiring a skill in a specific area of learning, such as reading, writing, or mathematics. This lower level of achievement occurs despite the child's normal (sometimes above-normal) intelligence and adequate schooling. Many of these individuals become school dropouts, have low self-esteem, and feel demoralized. They also may exhibit deficits in social skills. Individuals with learning disabilities may have problems listening or paying attention, reading or writing, speaking, and/or performing arithmetic problems. Individuals with learning disabilities experience difficulties performing specific types of skills or completing tasks. The disability is no indication of intelligence level.

Patient Screening

Most learning disorders are noted as the child begins the formal education process. Typically a teacher will notice that the child is not learning at the standard pace, or family members may be concerned about a child's progress and grades at school. At this time, the child is tested by the school system to evaluate for any discrepancy between ability and performance. The school system develops an individualized education plan (IEP) for teachers to adhere to when providing instruction to the student. The parents or guardians are involved in the process, too; and if a learning disability is identified, the child receives reasonable accommoda-

tions to enable him or her to achieve the highest potential. When parents demand an appointment, schedule it as soon as possible, because their anxiety level will be high.

Etiology

The etiology of this condition is uncertain, but there may be underlying abnormalities in cognitive processing. Deficits in visual perception, language processes, attention, or memory may contribute to the problem.

Diagnosis

When the school, after intensive testing, notifies parents of their findings, the physician will establish that the child has met all the diagnostic criteria listed in the DSM-V, and further evaluation may be performed. In addition to ruling out normal variations in academic attainment, the physician eliminates inadequate schooling, language barriers, lack of opportunity, and poor teaching as causes. Hearing and vision must be tested. Other mental disorders are ruled out.

Treatment

Some children who have learning disabilities also may be diagnosed with hyperactivity and therefore may respond to drug therapy, usually with stimulants. Other children may respond favorably to special instructional techniques (Fig. 14.4). Continuing research is attempting to help develop additional treatments for children with learning disabilities.

Prognosis

The prognosis varies, depending on the etiology and support of the community, school system, and family.

Prevention

Other than good prenatal care and close monitoring during labor, no specific prevention for learning disorders is known.

Patient Teaching

Parents are encouraged to seek out community and educational resources and support groups in the community. Help parents to learn about special services provided by the state through the school systems. Generate print-on-demand electronic materials, when possible, as teaching tools.

Communication Disorders

Children often exhibit difficulties in communication. These disorders may be psychologically based and are listed in the DSM-V. There are a variety of expressive language disorders, including mixed receptive or expressive language disorders.

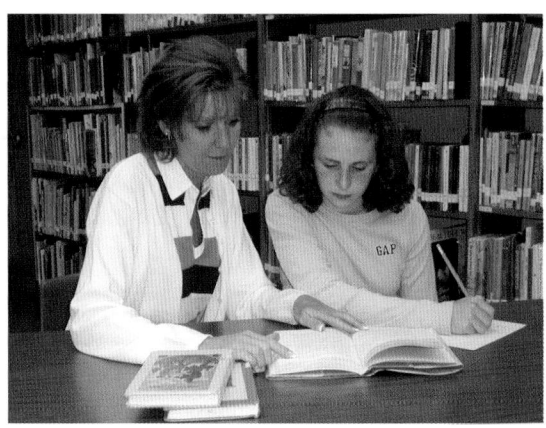

• **Fig. 14.4** Tutoring session in progress. (Courtesy Mark Boswell, 2003.)

Stuttering

Description

Stuttering, a phonological or communication disorder, is defined as frequent repetitions or prolongations of sounds or syllables. Stuttering is considered a speech disorder.

ICD-10-CM Code	F98.5 (Adult onset fluency disorder)

Symptoms and Signs

The frequent repetition or prolongation of sounds or syllables constitutes a disturbance of the pattern and fluency of speech, a disturbance that is inappropriate for the child's age. There also may be broken words filled or unfilled pauses in speech, word substitutions, or word repetitions. The onset usually occurs between ages 2 and 7 years. When stuttering occurs suddenly in a teenager or an adult, a thorough physical examination should be performed to rule out neurologic causes.

Patient Screening

Although this is not an emergency, when a parent calls for an appointment for a child who is stuttering, the next available regular appointment should be given. The family's anxiety level will be high, and they should be seen as soon as is convenient.

Etiology

Although the etiology is uncertain, recent research has confirmed that genetic factors are involved, and specific genes have been identified. Stuttering appears to have a familial tendency, with the condition occurring more often in men. Parents also may unwittingly cause anxiety in their child by overreacting to a mild speech limitation. Anxiety appears to be a major factor that creates and maintains stuttering.

Diagnosis

Observation of the speech pattern usually is all that is needed for the diagnosis. Hearing should be assessed, however, and any hearing difficulty should be ruled out.

Treatment

Speech therapy helps in the treatment. The condition may resolve spontaneously.

Prognosis

Although there is no cure for stuttering, the prognosis is good with intervention.

Prevention

No prevention is known.

Patient Teaching

Parents should be supportive and noncritical of the child. In addition, they should be encouraged to seek out support groups in their community. Generate print-on-demand electronic materials, when possible, as teaching tools.

Pervasive Development Disorders

Children diagnosed with pervasive development disorders (PDDs) differ widely in abilities, intelligence, and behaviors. The principal characteristics of PDDs are severe impairments in several areas of development, including communication and social interaction skills. The disorders can include particular behaviors that cause the failure to develop peer relationships and interactions with others, including lack of nonverbal communication and lack of reciprocation of emotions. This impairment is related directly to the person's developmental level or mental age. A category of disorders is referred to as *autism* spectrum, encompassing the broad group of developmental delays and disorders having an effect on social communication skills and possibly, to a larger or smaller degree, motor and language skills. The disorders listed as pervasive development type disorders are as follows: autism; pervasive development disorder, not otherwise specified (PDD-NOS); Rett syndrome; childhood disintegrative disorder (CDD); and Asperger syndrome.

Autism spectrum disorder (autism)

Description

Autism spectrum disorder (autism) is a syndrome in which individuals are likely to have communication deficits, including responding inappropriately in conversations. They also may misread nonverbal interactions. Additionally, they may experience difficulty in establishing age-appropriate relationships. These individuals exhibit some symptoms in early childhood, although they may not be noticed until later in life. Symptoms may vary in intensity and be different in individuals. Many are very sensitive to changes in environment and are found to depend on routines. Autism is considered to be highly heritable.

> ICD-10-CM Code   F84.0 (Autistic disorder)
> Autism is coded by active or residual status. When the activity status of the autism has been determined by diagnosis, refer to the physician's diagnosis and then to the current edition of the ICD-10-CM coding manual to ensure the greatest specificity of pathology

Symptoms and Signs

The child with autism exhibits noticeable impairment in socialization, communication, activities, and other interests. Impairment in nonverbal behaviors, such as eye-to-eye gaze, facial expressions, and other forms of nonverbal communication, is also noted. In addition, the child fails to establish normal peer relationships and to seek shared enjoyment. Communication impairments include delayed or absent verbal communication, inability to initiate a conversation, and repetitive use of inappropriate language. The child does not initiate age-appropriate play activities. Repetitive motions, often self-destructive, may be noted along with inflexibility toward change and a compulsion for sameness. These youngsters display a persistent preoccupation with objects and may have a memory for certain lists or facts.

Four symptoms that are nearly always present are social isolation, cognitive (based on knowledge) impairment, language deficits (shortages or missing), and repetitive naturalistic motions. Aversion to physical contact or cuddling also can be a sign. The autistic child resists any change or transition or has difficulty transitioning. The signs and symptoms can be in varying degrees.

Patient Screening

The parent of the child with autistic behavior often is aware of problems that are developing. Studies show that parents often know there is a problem before the child's first birthday. Often this issue is discussed on regular well-child (toddler) visits. When the parents first become aware of a problem, an appointment should be scheduled as soon as possible for an extensive examination and history.

Etiology

The etiology is uncertain, but evidence indicates a possible organic factor or possible predisposing factors that may include maternal rubella, encephalitis, and phenylketonuria. In fact, research on autism suggests that autism is not a single disorder and that there is not a singular cause. The occurrence is four times more common in men than in women. Much scientific research has been done to determine whether or not ingredients in vaccines are the cause of autism because parents and other individuals have posed this question. Studies show that there is no link between childhood immunizations and autism. Most children are diagnosed after age 4 years; however, it can be diagnosed as early as age 2 years.

Diagnosis

Observation of the behavior usually is all that is needed for the diagnosis. The child exhibits impairment in social interaction and communication; restricted, repetitive patterns of behavior; and delayed or abnormal patterns of symbolic or imaginative play. The physician may order blood and imaging studies to rule out any underlying physical cause.

Treatment

Behavioral therapy and self-instructed training have helped some children with autism. This therapy is most beneficial when parents also are trained in behavioral techniques and have the goal of helping these children to learn some adaptive responses, thus enabling the children to function outside of custodial care. Risperidone is the first drug approved for use in autism. Risperidone decreases irritability, tantrums, aggression, and mood swings. Although risperidone is still being prescribed, it has a severe side effect, that is, breast development and lactation. Other drugs that may be used for autism (but are not approved) include selective serotonin reuptake inhibitor (SSRI) antidepressants, antiepileptics (especially valproic acid for impulse control), and stimulants. SSRI antidepressants (fluvoxamine) are believed to decrease repetitive thoughts and behaviors. Antiepileptics may help treat impulsivity and decrease aggression. Stimulants are useful for the treatment of attention-deficit/hyperactivity disorder (ADHD), which is often a comorbid condition to autism spectrum disorders.

Prognosis

The prognosis depends on the severity of the disorder. Research is ongoing, but currently there is no specific drug therapy or known cure for this disorder. Greater public awareness is being generated to support additional research to cure the disorder. The prognosis is actually good for children on the autism spectrum. It appears that many children can learn adaptive behaviors and eventually "grow out" of some of the behaviors. Usually, by the early 20s, the patient is showing improvement and functioning with support quite well. Early intervention is essential to prognosis. Many children are being diagnosed earlier than they were years ago. Another key to prognosis is the severity of the diagnosis on the spectrum. There are also positive statistics in that almost half of children diagnosed with autism spectrum disorder have average to above-average intelligence.

Prevention

No prevention for this disorder currently is known. Children born to older parents are at a higher risk for this condition.

Patient Teaching

Encourage parents to investigate community and educational resources and to seek out support groups. Use customized electronically generated educational materials when available to reinforce the treatment plan.

Asperger Syndrome, Childhood Disintegrative Disorder, Rett Syndrome, and Pervasive Development Disorder, Not Otherwise Specified

Asperger Syndrome

Similar to children with autism, children with Asperger syndrome experience problems with social interaction and communication. Additionally, they usually have a narrow range of interests. Usually children experiencing Asperger syndrome tend to have average or above-average intelligence. They also appear to develop normally in the spheres of language and cognition. Many times, those with Asperger syndrome may have difficulty concentrating and may experience poor coordination. Children with Asperger syndrome seem to adjust better as they get older.

Childhood Disintegrative Disorder

A rare condition, childhood disintegrative disorder (CDD) allows children to start developing normally in all areas, both physical and mental. Typically between ages 2 and 10 years, the child may lose many of the skills he or she has acquired. Additionally, the child tends to lose language and social skills and may lose control of body functions, including bowel and bladder control. The long period of normal development before regression helps differentiate CDD from Rett syndrome.

Rett Syndrome

A very rare disorder, Rett syndrome, causes the child to experience symptoms associated with a pervasive development disorder (PDD). Additionally, the child also experiences problems with physical development. The child who commonly suffers the loss of many motor or movement skills, including ambulation and use of hands, along with development of poor coordination, is placed in this category. The condition, usually affecting only girls, appears to be associated with a defect on the X chromosome.

Pervasive Development Disorder, Not Otherwise Specified

The child who does not meet all of the criteria for autism or Asperger but demonstrates several of the traits or symptoms is considered to have pervasive development disorder, not otherwise specified (PDD-NOS).

As previously mentioned, similar to autistic disorder, there is no known cure for PDD. Drug therapy may be used as a symptomatic treatment for irritability, aggression, serious behavioral problems, obsessive-compulsive behavior, anxiety, depression, seizure activity, inattention, and hyperactivity. Behavioral therapy is beneficial but should be specialized to the child's needs. Specialized classrooms with a small class size and one-on-one instruction are sometimes helpful to certain children, whereas regular classroom education serves others.

Attention-Deficit/Hyperactivity Disorder

Description

ADHD, previously referred to as attention-deficit disorder (ADD), is a condition of persistent inattention leading to hyperactivity and impulsivity. ADHD is traditionally considered a hyperactivity issue, but many children and adults simply have difficulty maintaining attention and have no hyperactivity problems. Therefore ADHD has been classified into subtypes: ADHD, predominately inattentive type; ADHD, predominately hyperactive-impulsive type; and ADHD, combined type.

ICD-10-CM Code	F90.0 (Attention-deficit hyperactivity disorder, predominantly inattentive type)
	F90.1 (Attention-deficit hyperactivity disorder, predominantly hyperactive type)
	F90.2 (Attention-deficit hyperactivity disorder, combined type)
	F90.8 (Attention-deficit hyperactivity disorder, other type)
	F90.9 (Attention-deficit hyperactivity disorder, unspecified type)

Symptoms and Signs

Typical ADHD behavior can be observed at any age, but symptoms are usually present before age 7 years. Failure to pay close attention to details, careless mistakes, messy work, performed carelessly, and difficulty sustaining attention and completing tasks are manifestations of the condition. The child avoids activities that require sustained attention, effort, concentration, and organization. Inability to sit quietly without fidgeting or squirming, or even to remain seated, denotes hyperactivity. Inappropriate running and climbing, difficulty in playing, and excessive talking are other signs of the condition. The American Psychological Association (APA) has established criteria for each of these disorders.

Display of impatience, difficulty waiting for one's turn, frequent interruptions, and failure to listen to directions are manifestations of impulsivity. The inability to organize activities and define goals creates difficulty in performing simple tasks, such as picking up toys. Sexual and relationship problems may occur as the child grows older.

Any aspect of this behavior may be displayed at home, school, work, or social occasions. The behavior seems to be exaggerated in group situations.

The three subtypes are listed as follows:

- ADHD, predominantly inattentive type: This subtype is used if six (or more) symptoms of inattention (but fewer than six symptoms of hyperactivity-impulsivity) have persisted for at least 6 months.
- ADHD, predominantly hyperactive-impulsive type: This subtype should be used if six (or more) symptoms of hyperactivity-impulsivity (but fewer than six of inattention) have persisted for at least 6 months.

- ADHD, combined type: This subtype should be used if six (or more) symptoms of inattention and six (or more) symptoms of hyperactivity-impulsivity have persisted for at least 6 months.

Patient Screening

Similar to learning disorders, most ADHDs are first noted as the child begins the formal education process. At that time, the parent usually contacts the physician's office for an evaluation and a treatment plan. The appointment should be scheduled as soon as there is enough time for the physician to conduct a thorough assessment. The parents may be feeling a great deal of anxiety, so the child should be assessed as soon as possible.

Etiology

The cause is uncertain, but there appears to be a familial pattern. Observers now postulate that this condition is genetic, with definite brain malfunction.

Diagnosis

The diagnosis is based on observation of behavior and an evaluation concluding that the inattention is not age appropriate. The inattention must last for longer than 6 months and appear in at least two of the following settings: home, school, work, and social activities. Persistent hyperactivity and impulsivity also must meet the aforementioned criteria. Some of the symptoms are present before age 7 years. The behavior severely impairs functioning.

According to the DSM-V criteria, "children must have at least six symptoms from either (or both) the inattention group of criteria and the hyperactivity and impulsivity criteria, while older adolescents and adults (over age 17 years) must present with five." Although the criteria have not changed from DSM-IV, examples have been included to illustrate the types of behaviors that children, older adolescents, and adults with ADHD might exhibit. The descriptions will help clinicians better identify typical ADHD symptoms at each stage of the patients' lives.

According to DSM-V, several of the individual's ADHD symptoms must be present before age 12 years, compared with 7 years as the age at onset in DSM-IV.

Treatment

An effective treatment for some children is the use of stimulants, such as dextroamphetamine (Dexedrine), methylphenidate (Ritalin), and mixed salts of a single-entity amphetamine and dextroamphetamine product (Adderall). The most commonly used stimulants now are extended-release methylphenidate (Concerta), extended-release amphetamine and dextroamphetamine salts (Adderall XR), and lisdexamfetamine (Vyvanse). A methylphenidate transdermal patch (Daytrana) is gaining popularity. An alternative to stimulant therapy is the noncontrolled agent atomoxetine (Strattera). Atomoxetine provides similar results to stimulant therapy without many of the unwanted side effects (weight loss and so on). Other successful treatments,

such as guanfacine (Intuniv), are gaining popularity. Guanfacine (Intuniv) is typically used as supplemental therapy in conjunction with stimulant medications. It is not used often as stand-alone therapy.

Because some believe that ADHD may be worsened by poor nutrition and specifically lack of melatonin or zinc, vitamin supplementation is being promoted for ADHD treatment. At this time, there are no large-scale studies that substantiate this line of thought. If supplementation is requested, a multivitamin that includes zinc and melatonin is suggested.

Prognosis

Prompt diagnosis with appropriate management via medication leads to an excellent prognosis. Compliance with the medication dosage and frequency, however, is imperative. Effective parenting skills improve the prognosis.

Prevention

ADHD is genetic and therefore has no prevention.

Patient Teaching

Parents who use effective discipline and consistent routines are most successful in managing the condition. In addition, when medical treatment calls for drug therapy to treat the disorder, compliance is imperative. Proper nutrition with low amounts of sugar and red dye is helpful. Customized electronically generated educational materials should be used, when available, to reinforce the treatment plan. For children, regular weight monitoring is essential, because many psychostimulants decrease appetite which can slow growth. Children usually "catch up" on growth by age 18 years.

Oppositional Defiant Disorder

Description

Oppositional defiant disorder (ODD) is a behavior disorder in which children demonstrate behaviors that are oppositional toward adults. This is the most common referral complaint to counselors and a major source of family stress, as ODD behaviors occur hundreds of times per week. Comorbid conditions include ADHD (incidence increases with age), conduct disorder, PTSD, learning disabilities, school underperformance, poor social skills, dysthymia, and major depression. ODD is a strong predictor of poor outcomes (i.e., school underachievement, poor peer relations, delinquency, major depression, early substance initiation and abuse, and school expulsion and dropout).

ICD-10-CM Code	F91.3 (Oppositional defiant disorder)
	(F91.0-F91.9 = 6 codes of specificity)

Symptoms and Signs

Children with ODD often demonstrate behaviors, such as losing their tempers, arguing with adults, defying or refusing to comply with the adult's requests or rules, deliberately annoying others, and blaming others for mistakes and behaviors. In addition, they are irritable and easily annoyed, are angry and resentful, and are spiteful and vindictive. Additionally, these children may be involved in theft, vandalism, and bullying. They are negative and defiant.

Patient Screening

The appointment should be made as soon as schedules allow time for a thorough assessment by the physician. The parents may be experiencing great anxiety, and the child should be assessed as soon as possible.

Etiology

ODD has four main causes. These are negative child temperament and ADHD, negative parent temperament, ineffective child management, and parent and family stress events.

Diagnosis

Many parents report that their child never came out of the "terrible twos." Thus some symptoms may appear as early as age 3 years. Patients generally present at about ages 8 to 10 years. Patients must often (at least three times per week) demonstrate at least one of the eight symptoms listed above for at least 6 months.

Treatment

Mood stabilizers, such as risperidone (Risperdal) and olanzapine (Zyprexa), are often prescribed and are helpful for these patients. The most effective form of treatment is family therapy incorporating parent training and psychotherapy for the child.

Prognosis

Treatment is effective for children who demonstrate behaviors of ODD. If the child begins to demonstrate conduct disorder (a more severe disorder), the outcome is poor.

Prevention

Reducing family chaos and improving parenting skills helps control the onset of ODD.

Patient Teaching

Encourage parent training courses and education. The child's lack of acceptance of responsibility for behaviors is somewhat indicative of this disorder. Use customized electronically generated educational materials, when available, to reinforce the treatment plan.

Tic Disorders

Tic disorders appear as sudden, rapid, recurrent motor movement or vocalization that is nonrhythmic. Resistance against tics is not possible, but they may be suppressed for varying lengths of time and diminish during sleep. Eye blinking, facial grimacing, coughing, and neck jerking are examples of simple motor tics. Making facial gestures, jumping, touching, and stamping are examples of complex motor tics. Simple vocal tics include throat clearing, sniffing, snorting, and grunting. The repetition of words out of context, the use of socially unacceptable words, and the repetition of one's own words or of the last sound heard are examples of complex vocal tics. Tic disorders may be motor or vocal and may be chronic.

Tourette Disorder

Description

Tourette disorder, also known as *Gilles de la Tourette syndrome*, is a syndrome of multiple motor tics coupled with one or more vocal tics, which may appear simultaneously or at different times.

ICD-10-CM Code	F95.2 *(Tourette's disorder)*
	(F95.0-F95.9 = 5 codes of specificity)

Symptoms and Signs

The location, nature, and number of tics tend to change over time. The head typically is involved. Other body parts, such as the torso or the upper and lower limbs, may be involved. Clicks, grunts, yelps, barks, and snorts are examples of vocal tics. The vocal tics also may include the uttering of obscenities.

Patient Screening

The appointment should be made for the earliest date when schedules will allow sufficient time for a thorough assessment by the physician. The parents possibly will be feeling great anxiety, and the child should be assessed as soon as possible.

Etiology

Although the etiology is uncertain, some observers postulate that Tourette disorder is inherited. Some research has associated the onset of Tourette syndrome with streptococcal infections caused by a reaction of antibodies to group A beta-hemolytic *Streptococcus* and nerve tissue. The incidence is higher in men.

Diagnosis

The observation of symptoms is usually enough for diagnosis. The onset may be as early as age 2 years and occurs before age 18 years. Remissions may occur, but the syndrome is of lifelong duration. The severity of the symptoms usually diminishes, and the symptoms may even disappear by early adulthood.

To meet the diagnostic criteria, both motor and vocal tics must occur, although not necessarily at the same time. They occur several times a day over a period of a year without a tic-free period of longer than 3 months. The patient has significant impairment in functioning at work and in socialization, and the condition is not the result of substance use or a general medical condition.

Treatment

Pharmacologic treatment is the only proven effective treatment for tics. Some patients with Tourette disorder have improved with the administration of haloperidol (Haldol). Other treatment options include clonidine and clonazepam for their calming effects. Additionally, fluoxetine (Prozac) may be helpful in treating repetitive and obsessive behaviors that occur with Tourette syndrome.

Prognosis

Although there is no cure for Tourette disorder, some patients experience lessening of symptoms as they reach maturity. However, this usually is a lifelong, chronic condition.

Prevention

No prevention is known for this disorder.

Patient Teaching

Encourage the patient and the family to seek out support groups and to access information from community health organizations. All those involved should work with the educational system to help the young person exhibiting Tourette syndrome to obtain all possible educational assistance. Use customized electronically generated educational materials, when available, to reinforce the treatment plan.

Dementia

Description

Dementia causes progressive, general deterioration of mental faculties, including decline in perceiving, thinking, remembering, and cognitive functioning. Dementia, which is *not* a part of normal aging, represents a pathologic development. The irreversible brain damage may be the result of compromised blood flow to the brain resulting from atherosclerosis, thrombi, or trauma. In addition, toxins, metabolic conditions, organic disorders, infections, tumors, Parkinson disease, or Alzheimer disease may be responsible for the deterioration (see Fig. 13.19). The onset may be slow and insidious or may be sudden, depending on the cause.

Parkinson Disease

Refer to Chapter 13 for a discussion of Parkinson disease.

Alzheimer Disease

Description

Alzheimer disease, a progressive degenerative disease of the brain, produces a typical profile of lost mental and physical functioning. It is the most common cause of deterioration in intellectual capacity, or dementia. It is most common in people older than 65 years of age, and its incidence increases in people older than 80 years of age.

ICD-10-CM Code	G30.9 *(Alzheimer's disease, unspecified)* (G30.0-G30.9 = 4 codes of specificity)

Symptoms and Signs

The onset of Alzheimer disease is gradual and insidious, with early signs including loss of short-term memory, inability to concentrate, incapacity to learn new information, impairment of reasoning, and subtle changes in personality. Progression of symptoms corresponds with stages ranging from very mild decline (patients note memory lapses) to severe decline (patients frequently lose their capacity for recognizable speech and/or lose the ability to walk without assistance or sit without support). Staging provides useful frames of reference for making future plans of care. As the disease course continues, communication skills decline, and the patient struggles to find the right words, uses meaningless words, or interjects nonsensical phrases. Over a span of 5 to 10 years, there is profound deterioration of intellectual and physical ability. The patient becomes increasingly dependent on a caregiver. Response to stimuli from the outside world diminishes, and the patient seems emotionally detached. The patient may exhibit restlessness, sleep disturbances, disorientation, hostility, or combativeness. The patient eventually becomes bedridden and ultimately dies as a result of undercurrent infection or other complications.

Patient Screening

The onset is insidious, and symptoms may be uncovered during routine office visits. When a family member notices obvious signs and calls for an appointment, the appointment should be scheduled as soon as schedules will allow for a thorough assessment. Anxiety levels will be high, so the next available appointment should be provided.

Etiology

The cause of Alzheimer disease is not known, but the disease is age related and may have a genetic basis in some families. Research has focused on an abnormality found on chromosome 21 as a genetic link. Patients with Down syndrome (a syndrome also linked to an abnormality on chromosome 21) show the same brain changes as do patients with Alzheimer disease. In later life, people with Down syndrome have the clinical symptoms of Alzheimer disease. Other theories for the cause of Alzheimer disease include biochemical changes in brain growth, an autoimmune reaction, infection by a slow virus, toxic chemical excess, chemical deficiency, blood vessel defects, and a deficiency of neurochemical factors in the brain. Research has shown a higher rate of occurrence in people with a history of head trauma.

Diagnosis

Obtaining direct evidence of Alzheimer disease is difficult. When other causes of organic brain disease have been ruled out, the diagnostic criteria for Alzheimer disease include evidence of memory and cognitive disturbances. As the disease progresses, neurologic examination reveals sensory and motor deficits. In later stages, diagnostic studies include brain scans, which may detect brain atrophy, widened sulci, and enlarged cerebral ventricles. Positive diagnosis is possible after death, when evidence of brain atrophy and characteristic lesions in the cerebral cortex can be found on pathologic examination of the brain (Fig. 14.5).

The brain shows loss of neurons and the presence of senile plaques, which include microscopic deposits of amyloid material. Neurofibrillary tangles also are evident (Fig. 14.6). Some of the same postmortem anomalies may be found, however, in people who never were diagnosed with or exhibited symptoms of Alzheimer disease. Alzheimer disease is one of the most overdiagnosed or misdiagnosed disorders of mental functioning of older adults because it is not easily distinguished from other dementias that result from excessive use of medication, depression, brain tumors, subdural hematomas, and certain other metabolic diseases.

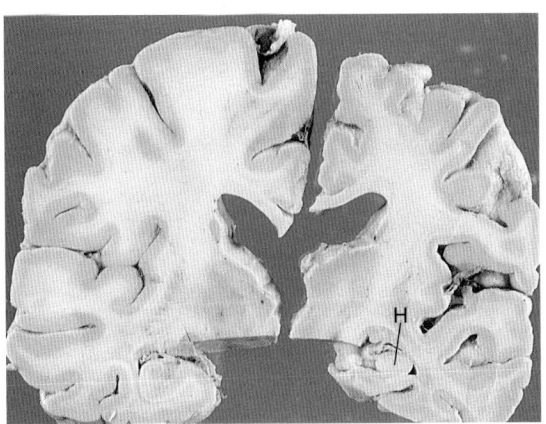

• **Fig. 14.5** Alzheimer disease. The diseased brain tissue (H) shows loss of cortex and white matter (From Stevens A, et al: Core pathology ed 3, St Louis, 2010, Mosby/Elsevier.)

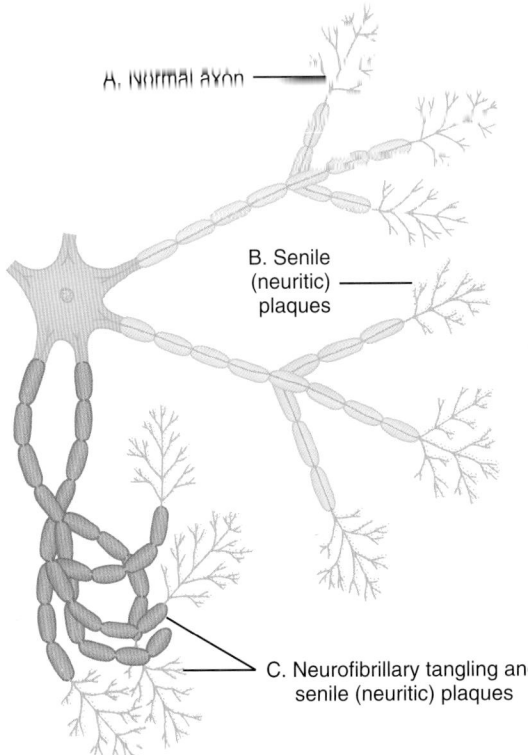

A. Normal axon

B. Senile (neuritic) plaques

C. Neurofibrillary tangling and senile (neuritic) plaques

• **Fig. 14.6** Neurofibrillary tangles and senile plaques found in patient with Alzheimer disease. (From Black JM, Matassarin-Jacobs E: *Medical-surgical nursing,* ed 7, Philadelphia, 2004, Saunders.)

Treatment

No cure is known for Alzheimer disease, so treatment is supportive and is geared toward helping alleviate symptoms.

Drug therapy to alleviate cognitive symptoms includes the use of cholinesterase inhibitors, with the primary drug being donepezil (Aricept). Rivastigmine (Exelon) is a newer medication thought to prevent the breakdown of acetylcholine in the brain, although its exact mechanism is unknown. Memantine (Namenda) is an N-methyl-D-aspartate (NMDA) inhibitor; that is, because the persistent activation of CNS NMDA receptors by the excitatory amino acid glutamate has been hypothesized to contribute to symptoms, inhibition of this reaction is thought to alleviate symptoms. Antipsychotic or neuroleptic agents, including haloperidol; antianxiety agents, including buspirone (BuSpar); and SSRI antidepressants, including paroxetine (Paxil), are used to manage behavioral symptoms. Research has suggested that benzodiazepams may be linked to an increased risk for Alzheimer disease.

Other drugs used to treat the agitation associated with Alzheimer disease are risperidone and olanzapine in those who start to have delusional symptoms caused by Alzheimer progression. Divalproex sodium (Depakote) and gabapentin (Neurontin) are used as mood stabilizers and to help. Trazodone sometimes is used for "sundowning," a condition associated with Alzheimer disease in which patients become confused and disoriented after dark.

In addition to reducing symptoms and suffering, treatment aims to increase the patient's ability to cope and to reduce the patient's frustration level. As the patient's ability for self-care declines, general management of fluid intake, adequate nutrition, and personal hygiene is necessary. Treatment gives the patient opportunities to be mobile and to maintain his or her remaining mental abilities for as long as possible. Provisions are employed to protect the patient from injury. Finally, emotional support for the patient and the family or the caregiver is vital, because caring for the person with the disease forces them to make enormous adjustments.

Research continues to delve into the etiology of Alzheimer disease. Researchers hope that identifying the cause may lead to prevention, because currently there is no way to reverse the neurologic damage caused by the disease. Early diagnosis and drug therapy may help slow the course of the disease. It is necessary to avoid giving certain drugs to patients with dementia (Box 14.1).

Prognosis

No cure is known for Alzheimer disease. Drug therapy may help delay the progression of the disorder. Cholinesterase inhibitors should be discontinued when patients can no longer care for themselves. Advanced status of the disease usually indicates the need for custodial care.

• BOX 14.1 Drugs To Avoid In Patients With Dementia

The following abbreviated list includes some of the medications that should be avoided in patients with Alzheimer disease and patients with other types of dementia. When selecting medications for this patient group, the following medications should be avoided or at least be used in a limited manner. Generally, these medications may worsen cognitive function in patients with dementia.

Narcotic Analgesics

Meperidine, pentazocine, propoxyphene

Antiarrhythmics

Disopyramide

Tricyclic Antidepressants

Amitriptyline, clomipramine, doxepin, imipramine, protriptyline

Antiemetics

Cyclizine, dimenhydrinate, meclizine, promethazine, trimethobenzamide

Antipsychotics

Chlorpromazine, clozapine, pimozide, promazine, thioridazine, triflupromazine

Antihistamines

Azatadine, brompheniramine, chlorpheniramine, clemastine, cyproheptadine, diphenhydramine, hydroxyzine, promethazine

Benzodiazepines

Alprazolam, chlordiazepoxide, diazepam, lorazepam, triazolam

Gastrointestinal/Urinary Antispasmodics

Belladonna alkaloids, atropine, hyoscyamine, scopolamine, dicyclomine, flavoxate, oxybutynin, tolterodine

Muscle Relaxants

Carisoprodol, chlorzoxazone, cyclobenzaprine, metaxalone, methocarbamol, orphenadrine

---

Prevention

No prevention for Alzheimer disease is currently known. Research is showing that exercise, socialization, and brain exercises actually do reduce the risk of Alzheimer disease. It is possible that even stress level management and nutrition play a part in prevention.

Patient Teaching

Advise the caregiver to be consistent in planning daily activities for the patient and to keep the activities simple. Emphasize the importance of complying with the prescribed drug therapy regimen. Encourage the family to use community resources and local support groups. Generate print-on-demand electronic materials, when possible, as teaching tools. Encourage caregivers to provide themselves with respite time. The continuous care demanded of a caregiver can be draining both physically and emotionally.

Vascular Dementia

Description

A reduction in blood flow to the brain can result from narrowed and stenosed arteries. The functional areas of the cerebrum are shown in Fig 14.7. The resulting hypoxia and

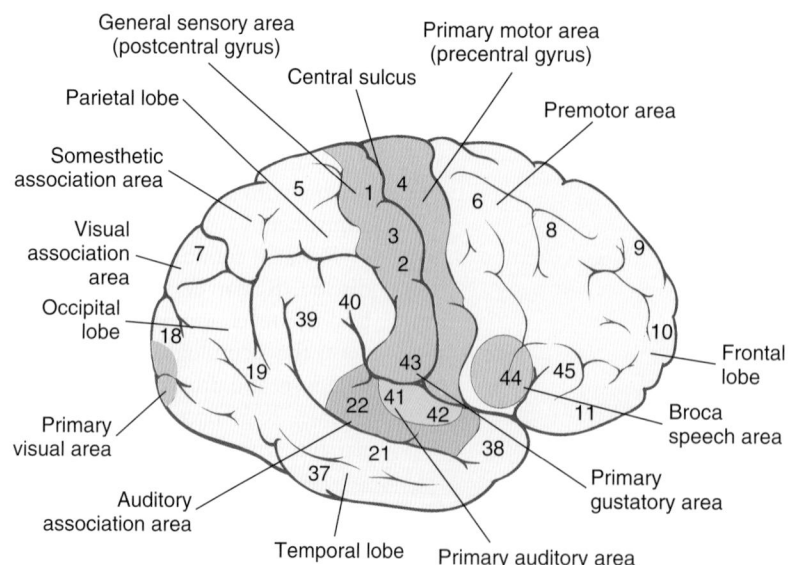

• **Fig. 14.7** Map of the lateral surface of the cerebral cortex showing some of the functional areas. Areas 4, 6, and 8 are motor areas; areas 1, 2, 3, 41, 42, and 43 are primary sensory areas; and areas 9, 10, 11, 18, 19, 22, 38, 39, and 40 are association areas. (From Solomon EP: *Introduction to human anatomy and physiology,* ed 3, St Louis, 2009, Saunders/Elsevier.)

reduced nourishment to the brain cells cause a general loss in intellectual abilities.

ICD-10-CM Code F01.50 *(Vascular dementia without behavioral disturbance)*
(F01.50-F03 = 6 codes of specificity)
I67.2 *(Cerebral atherosclerosis)*
F03 *(Unspecified dementia)*
Refer to the physician's diagnosis and then to the current edition of the ICD-10-CM coding manual to ensure the greatest specificity of pathology.

Symptoms and Signs

Along with the general loss of intellectual abilities in the patient, changes in memory, judgment, abstract thinking, and personality can be noted. A disregard for personal hygiene is observed, along with apathy, disorientation, and inappropriate responses. Depression, anxiety, and irritability often are noted. Restlessness, sleeplessness, hallucinations, and psychotic tendencies appear as the condition advances. Stupor and coma are the final stages (Fig. 14.8).

Patient Screening

Similar to the onset of Alzheimer disease, the onset of vascular dementia is insidious, and symptoms may be uncovered during routine office visits. When a family member notices obvious signs and calls for an appointment, enough time should be allowed for a thorough assessment. Anxiety levels will be high, so the next available appointment should be provided.

Etiology

As atherosclerotic plaque grows in the carotid and cerebral arteries, blood flow to brain tissue is reduced. Prolonged hypoxia with resulting ischemia leads to irreversible

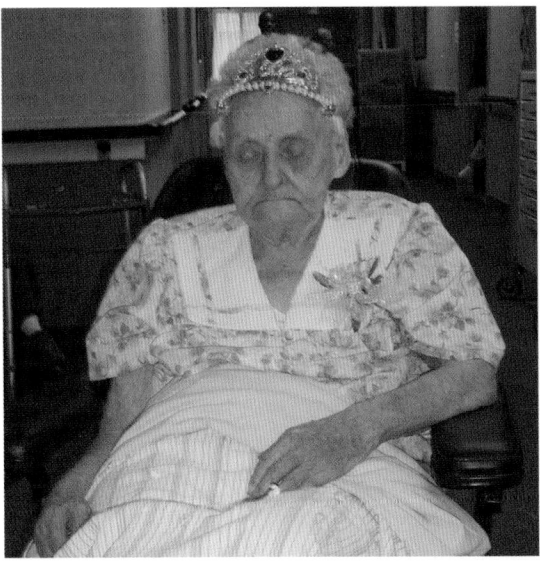

• **Fig. 14.8** A 103-year-old woman after several "mini strokes." (Courtesy David L. Frazier, 2003.)

necrosis and death of the brain cells. When an embolism causes the blockage, the hypoxia is sudden and complete. Small aneurysms may be responsible for minute cerebral bleeds. When the cerebral cortex is involved, cognitive capabilities are compromised. See the Cerebrovascular Accident [Stroke] section in Chapter 13.

Diagnosis

Because symptoms of atherosclerotic involvement have an insidious onset, the family often does not notice the subtle changes taking place. When the patient's personal hygiene deteriorates, along with memory and judgment, family members may notice a problem. A thorough history, with physical and neurologic examinations, is necessary to rule out other causes of altered behavior. Vascular assessment of the carotid and cerebral arteries may yield information about compromised blood flow. Cerebral arteriography or magnetic resonance imaging (MRI) arteriography confirms the presence of the condition. When the patient has a pacemaker, pacemaker readings may provide indications of periods of reduced blood flow to the brain with resulting ischemia.

Treatment

Treatment aims to increase the blood supply to the brain. Low dose aspirin, clopidogrel (Plavix), prasugrel (Effient), and cilostazol (Pletal) all are used for their antiplatelet effect in preventing stroke or its recurrence, especially in patients who have hypertension or have had a myocardial infarction. Drug therapy may help increase blood flow. When the carotid arteries are compromised, surgical intervention in the form of carotid endarterectomy may limit the progress of the condition. Brain cell death is irreversible. As the condition progresses, the patient may need to be institutionalized to ensure safety and care.

Prognosis

Improvement is guarded and depends on the extent of the cerebral insult. Many of these patients are trainable with rehabilitation and can function in the community.

Prevention

Very little is known about preventing this condition. Early diagnosis and treatment may slow the progress of the dementia.

Patient Teaching

As previously mentioned in the discussion about patient teaching for the patient with Alzheimer disease, consistency in patient activities and therapy is necessary. Caregivers should encourage patients to do what they can do for themselves. Advise the family that improvement is not likely and that they should prepare themselves and the patient for that possibility. Generate print-on-demand electronic materials, when possible, as teaching tools. As with Alzheimer disease and any other long-term condition, encourage caregivers to provide themselves with respite time. The continuous care demanded of caregivers can be draining both physically and emotionally.

Dementia Caused by Head Trauma

Description

A traumatic insult causing reduced blood flow to the cerebrum may result in dementia. Deprivation of oxygen and nutrition (ischemia) results in the death of brain cells. Both closed and open head injuries, hematomas, and skull fractures are examples of insults that cause reduced blood flow to the cells (Figs. 14.9 and 14.10).

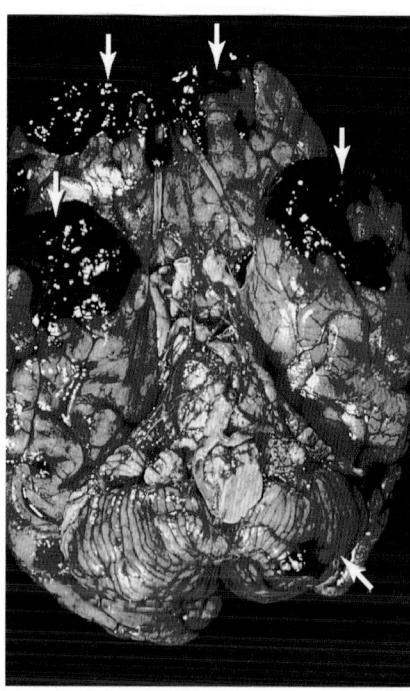

• **Fig. 14.9** Contusion. Contrecoup lesions in the frontal and temporal poles *(arrows)* are located opposite to a small coup lesion over the cerebellum *(bottom right arrow).* (From Damjanov I, Linder J: *Pathology: a color atlas,* St Louis, 1999, Mosby.)

ICD-10-CM Code	S09.8XXA *(Other specified injuries of head, initial encounter)*
	S09.90XA *(Unspecified injury of head, initial encounter)*
	F02.80 *(Dementia in other diseases classified elsewhere, without behavioral disturbance)*
	(F02.80-F03 — 3 codes of specificity)

Symptoms and Signs

Reductions in intellectual capabilities and cognitive functioning may result from trauma to the head. After a head injury, the patient exhibits reduced mental status and is unable to perform many of the cognitive tasks that were possible before the injury. Intelligence testing shows reduced capabilities.

Patient Screening

The patient probably is in an inpatient facility because of the head trauma. After discharge, when the patient needs outpatient medical assessment and treatment, an appointment should be arranged as soon as the schedules allow time for a complete assessment.

Etiology

Trauma to the head causes an insult to the brain as a result of edema, increased intracranial pressure, or damage to the vessel walls. The insult results in compromise of the cerebral blood supply. The hypoxia is followed by ischemia and eventually irreversible necrosis of brain cells. See the Head Trauma section in Chapter 13.

Diagnosis

Obtaining a history of head trauma with a reduced level of mental functioning is complemented by a thorough physical and neurologic examination. Imaging studies may

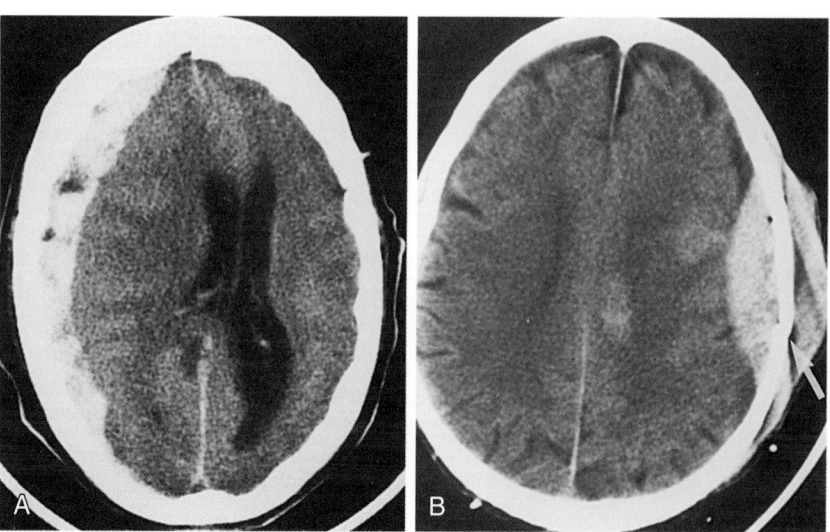

• **Fig. 14.10** (A) Subdural hematoma. (B) Epidural hematoma. (From Vincent JL, et al: *Textbook of critical care,* ed 7, St Louis, 2017, Elsevier.)

include skull radiography, computed tomography (CT) of the brain, and MRI of the brain and cerebral vessels. Subdural or epidural hematomas and any type of skull fracture may be noted.

Ventricular shift indicates increasing intracranial pressure. Any neurologic deficit, such as unequal pupils, unequal grips, hemiparesis, and posturing, indicates insult to the brain tissue. As the condition progresses, reduced intellectual functioning is noted.

Treatment

Treatment includes correcting the insult to the brain to prevent further damage. After the necrosis has evolved, the damaged tissues cannot be repaired. Therapy and training to maintain the remaining functions are attempted.

Prognosis

Similar to the prognosis for vascular dementia, improvement is guarded and depends on the extent of the cerebral insult. Many of these patients are trainable with rehabilitation and can function in the community. When the damage is severe, the patient may need to be institutionalized for care and safety.

Prevention

Prevention depends on the causative factors and the extent and type of the injury. Consistent use of seat belts in motor vehicles is known to reduce the severity of head injuries. Use of helmets when cycling and playing contact sports has a similar benefit. Professional football associations are attempting to provide information about head trauma and cumulative brain injury. Guidelines are being developed and/or in place to protect the athlete from receiving head injury and periods of rest before returning to the contact sport.

Patient Teaching

As previously mentioned in the discussion of patient teaching for other dementias, consistency in patient activities and therapy is necessary. Urge caregivers to encourage patients to do what they can for themselves. Rehabilitation and therapy may lead to improvement in the condition. Families may need encouragement to recognize the fact that there is no cure. Some patients who have experienced dementia caused by head trauma may be educable or trainable. Routines and consistency are important in enabling the patient to function at the highest possible level. Advise the family that improvement is not likely and that they should prepare themselves and the patient for that possibility. Generate print-on-demand electronic materials, when possible, as teaching tools.

Substance-Related Disorders

> ICD-10-CM Code   F10.10 (Alcohol abuse,
> uncomplicated)
> (F10.1-F10.99 = 47 codes of
> specificity)

> F19.20 (Other psychoactive
> substance dependence,
> uncomplicated)
> (F19.20-F19.99 = 41 codes of
> specificity)

Alcohol Abuse

Description

Alcohol abuse or alcoholism is a disorder of physical and psychological dependence on daily or regular excessive intake of alcoholic beverages. The onset of this chemical dependency can be insidious or can be accelerated by an acute traumatic event.

> ICD-10-CM Code   F10.20 (Alcohol dependence,
> uncomplicated)
> (F10.1-F10.99 = 47 codes of
> specificity)

Symptoms and Signs

Alcohol acts on the CNS as a depressant. Individuals under the influence of alcohol may experience a decrease in activity, tension, and normal inhibitions. Ingestion of a few drinks of alcohol may change behavior, decrease the ability to think clearly, slow motor skills, and impair judgment and concentration. Excessive use of alcohol often is associated with anxiety, depression, insomnia, impotence, and behavioral disorders both before and during intoxication. Amnesia often occurs after intoxication. Repeated heavy drinking of alcohol produces symptoms and signs in nearly every organ system (Fig. 14.11). Chronic alcoholism causes

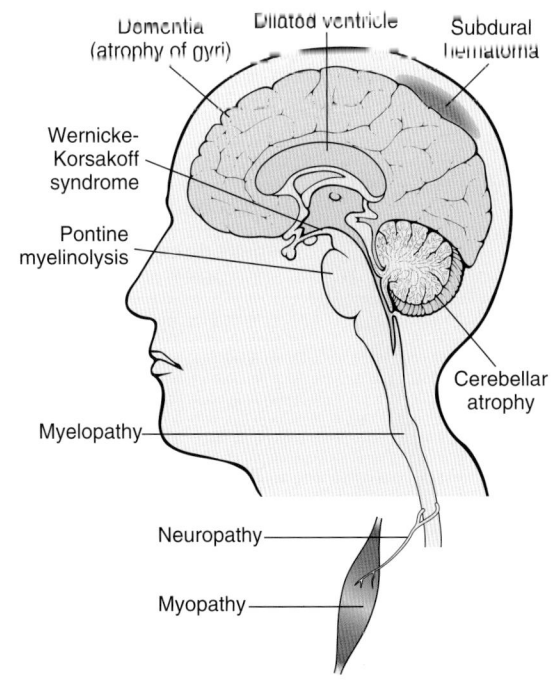

• **Fig. 14.11** Pathologic changes in the nervous system caused by chronic alcoholism. (From Damjanov I: *Pathology for the health related professions*, ed 4, St Louis, 2011, Saunders.)

pathologic changes in the nervous system. Common physical findings include frequent infections, hypertension, and gastrointestinal (GI) problems. Some individuals experience confusion, abdominal pain, and nausea and vomiting. The patient may report unexplained seizure activity or symptoms of alcohol withdrawal. Prolonged heavy use of alcohol may cause cirrhosis of the liver, pancreatitis, and peripheral neuropathy, resulting in muscle weakness and paresthesia. The risk of cancer of the esophagus, stomach, and other parts of the GI system also is increased. The consequences of chronic alcohol abuse include dysfunction within family and social relationships and disruption in occupational responsibilities. Some people are prone to aggressive or violent behavior, accidents, and threatened or attempted suicide. The patient often denies his or her inability to control or discontinue alcohol abuse.

Patient Screening

When the patients themselves call for the appointment, they require prompt assessment and intervention. When they state that they are in a crisis and are unable to be seen in the office right away, they should be referred to an emergency facility.

Etiology

Alcohol abuse has no single cause but a cluster of possible causative factors. The origin may include genetic or biologic factors, depression, emotional conflict, social factors, and cultural attitudes. Because the patient history frequently includes a familial pattern of alcohol abuse, genetic factors pose a recognized statistical risk.

Diagnosis

Screening tests for alcohol abuse include questionnaires that attempt to identify pathologic behavior. Test results may be altered by the patient's attempts to deny or hide the addiction. Diagnostic information gathered during physical examination and a medical history may fit the profile of alcohol abuse. Laboratory findings may help confirm the diagnosis. One sensitive indicator of heavy alcohol intake is the level of high gamma-glutamyltransferase (GGT) in blood. The amount of alcohol consumed may be calculated through the use of a chart, such as those used by law-enforcement agencies. Table 14.1 lists the effects of various levels of blood alcohol on the brain. Table 14.2 shows how an individual's weight and the amount of alcohol consumed determine blood alcohol content. Fig. 14.12 compares the alcohol contents of various forms of alcohol. Other abnormal laboratory findings emerge with organ system complications resulting from chronic alcohol abuse (i.e., liver profile).

Treatment

Rehabilitation consists of a specialized treatment plan that meets the patient's physical and psychological needs and supports abstinence from alcohol. After detoxification, most patients benefit from psychotherapy or group therapy and participation in the 12-step program of Alcoholics

TABLE 14.1	Effects Of Rising Blood Alcohol Level[a]
Blood Alcohol Level	**Effects**
0.02	Mild euphoria, reduced inhibitions, slight body warmth, talkativeness
0.05	Noticeable relaxation, reduced alertness, increased self-confidence
0.08	**Legally drunk in 45 states;** impairment in coordination, judgment, memory, and comprehension
0.10	**Legally drunk in remaining states;** behavior becomes loud or embarrassing; mood swings are noticeable, and reaction time is reduced
0.15	Impaired balance and coordination; appears intoxicated
0.20	Disorientation, mental confusion, dizziness, lethargy, exaggerated emotional states
0.30	Staggering gait, slurred speech, visual disturbances, possible loss of consciousness
0.40	Inability to walk or stand, reduced response to stimuli, vomiting, incontinence, loss of consciousness, possible death ("dead drunk")
0.50	Respiratory effort depressed to point of ceasing, lack of reflexes, body temperature drops, impairment of circulation, possible death; immediate intervention and intense life-support measures required to sustain life
0.60	Death usually occurs or has occurred

[a]Blood alcohol level (BAL) is measured in milligrams of alcohol per 100 mL of blood and reported as a percentage. An individual with a BAL of 0.10 has one-tenth of 1% (1/1000) of total blood volume as alcohol. BAL depends on the blood volume (blood volume increases with weight) and the amount of alcohol consumed over a given time.

TABLE 14.2 Blood Alcohol Content[a]

Body Weight (lb)	Number of Drinks (1 oz 86-Proof Liquor, 3 oz Wine, or 12 oz Beer)								
	1	2	3	4	5	6	7	8	9
100	0.032[a]	0.065[b]	0.097[c]	0.129[c]	0.162[c]	0.194[c]	0.226[c]	0.258[c]	0.291[c]
120	0.027[a]	0.054[b]	0.081[c]	0.108[c]	0.135[c]	0.161[c]	0.188[c]	0.215[c]	0.242[c]
140	0.023[a]	0.046[a]	0.069[b]	0.092[c]	0.115[c]	0.138[c]	0.161[c]	0.184[c]	0.207[c]
160	0.020[a]	0.040[a]	0.060[b]	0.080[c]	0.101[c]	0.121[c]	0.141[c]	0.161[c]	0.181[c]
180	0.018[a]	0.036[a]	0.054[b]	0.072[b]	0.090[c]	0.108[c]	0.126[c]	0.144[c]	0.162[c]
200	0.016[a]	0.032[a]	0.048[a]	0.064[b]	0.080[c]	0.097[c]	0.113[c]	0.129[c]	0.145[c]
220	0.015[a]	0.029[a]	0.044[a]	0.058[b]	0.073[b]	0.088[c]	0.102[c]	0.117[c]	0.131[c]
240	0.014[a]	0.027[a]	0.040[a]	0.053[b]	0.067[b]	0.081[c]	0.095[c]	0.108[c]	0.121[c]

[a]Blood alcohol content to 0.05%: Caution.
[b]Blood alcohol content 0.05% to 0.079%: Driving impaired.
[c]Blood alcohol content 0.08% and up: Presumed under the influence in most states.

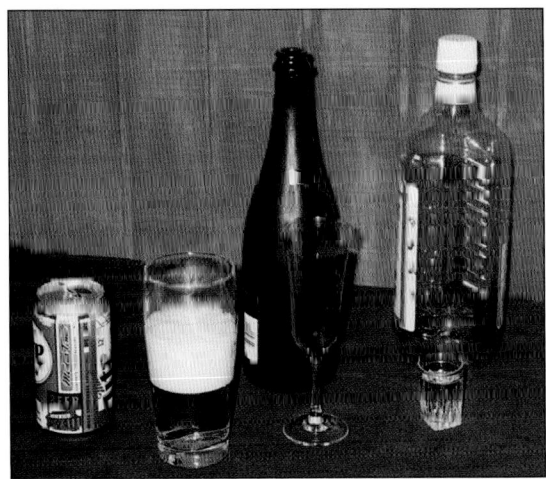

• **Fig. 14.12** Comparison of the amounts of beer (12 oz), wine (6 oz), or 86-proof liquor (1 oz) that contain 10 to 15 mL of pure alcohol. (Courtesy David L. Frazier, 1999.)

available as an injectable medication, which must be given monthly by a health care professional. It works by binding to opioid receptors in the brain resulting in an inability of the alcohol user to achieve a "high."

Prognosis

The prognosis varies depending on the duration of the alcoholism and motivation of the person to work a program of recovery.

Prevention

No prevention is known for alcoholism.

Patient Teaching

Encourage patients and family members to be aware of the dangers related to excessive ingestion of alcohol. Generate print-on-demand electronic materials, when possible, as teaching tools.

Anonymous (AA). Ongoing therapy usually can continue on an outpatient basis. Willing participation in a recovery program on a sustained, as-needed basis usually offers a promising prognosis. Relapses are common and need not represent failure of treatment as long as the patient returns to a program of recovery and abstinence from alcohol. Only a small percentage of patients can ever become "social" or moderate drinkers again, but that is not the goal of treatment. (Some alcoholics volunteer to take the drug disulfiram [Antabuse], which causes nausea and vomiting when alcohol is consumed. Other alcoholics are ordered by a court to use this drug.) Total abstinence is the goal of treatment. As of June 2006, naltrexone (Vivitrol) has become

♦ ENRICHMENT

Blood Alcohol Levels

After alcohol is ingested, it is absorbed from the gastrointestinal (GI) tract and distributed to all tissues. The rich blood supply to the brain results in a concentration of alcohol in the central nervous system (CNS) proportional to blood alcohol concentration. The rate at which alcohol is metabolized in the liver is constant, and only 10 to 15 mL of pure alcohol can be metabolized in 1 hour. Fig. 14.12 compares the amount of beer (12 oz), wine (6 oz), and 86-proof liquor (1 oz) that contains 10 to 15 mL of pure alcohol.

Substance Abuse

Substance abuse is a significant social and medical concern. Altered behavior and medical complications of substance abuse are found in all social, economic, ethnic, racial, educational, and professional groups. Some substances that are abused on a regular but episodic basis are alcohol, sedatives, stimulants, opioids, cannabis (marijuana), synthetic cannabis (spice), hallucinogens (including bath salts), inhalants, caffeine, nicotine, illicit synthetic (designer) drugs, and other chemical substances (Table 14.3). These substances, prescribed or illegal, give the user a stimulant or depressant effect. The overindulgence in or dependence on chemical substances often produces a detrimental effect on the user's physical and psychological well-being and on the welfare of others.

During substance abuse, tolerance to the chemical or drug often develops, necessitating increased amounts of the substance to achieve the desired effect. In addition to tolerance, both physical and psychological dependence can develop. Rapid withdrawal from certain drugs can cause life-threatening and even fatal reactions.

The individual under the influence of drugs often exhibits inappropriate behavior. Judgment often is impaired, and users are at risk for injury to themselves or others when driving or operating machinery while under the influence. They experience multiple social and interpersonal problems. While under the influence of mood-altering drugs, some may appear intoxicated, but others may exhibit a fairly normal pattern of behavior. Over an extended period, performance and relationships deteriorate. Dependability decreases, legal problems develop, and desperation for more of the desired substance may lead to criminal behavior.

Many employers require applicants and employees to undergo drug screening. This type of drug screening usually is performed in one of two noninvasive methods. In the first method, a urine sample can be analyzed for drug content. Urine drug screening typically reveals drug use only during the preceding 3 to 4 days. An individual may be able to abstain from the drug for 4 days and produce negative test results.

The second method is analysis of a hair sample (Fig. 14.13). Evidence of drug use stays in the hair shaft for about 90 days and is the only drug test that gives this length of drug use history. Hair shaft testing is different from follicle testing, which requires "pulling" the hair from the follicle instead of cutting a lock of hair. Drugs are absorbed into the bloodstream and circulated in blood, which nourishes the hair follicle, leaving trace amounts of residue entrapped in the core of the hair shaft. Washing, bleaching, or dying the hair does not remove the drug residue. Thus abstinence for a few days does not affect the results of the test. Finally, these tests do not reveal a pattern of use or the presence of dependence, so results should be interpreted and integrated into other clinical data. Some facilities have adopted cheek swabbing for rapid results.

Law enforcement officers use a breath analyzer to measure blood alcohol levels quickly. Qualitative or quantitative drug assay tests (blood tests to detect the presence or level of specific drugs) also are performed. General toxicology drug screening determines only the presence or absence of a drug. Any identified drugs should be confirmed and their levels determined through a test specific for that drug. Blood screening for nonspecific drugs usually is accompanied by urine drug screening.

Drugs of Abuse

The misuse of various drugs that modify mood or behavior is called *drug abuse*. Many types of drugs, including depressants, stimulants, opiates, opiate-like drugs, hallucinogens, volatile substances, cannabinoids, steroids, tobacco, and prescription drugs may be suspected in abuse and dependence (see Table 14.3). Some of these drugs have been used for centuries and often are called *recreational drugs*.

Peer pressure, a chaotic home environment, and poor coping skills can lead to drug abuse by individuals. The use of a prescription drug to treat illness and mental disorder often introduces the individual to the drug of abuse.

Table 14.3 presents popular drugs of abuse, their common names, and their many potential adverse effects. A new drug combination has been approved for opioid addiction. Suboxone is the combination of buprenorphine (a narcotic used for pain relief) and naloxone (an opioid antagonist). This combination decreases the symptoms of opioid withdrawal and reduces the cravings for the opioid high.

According to recent statistics, an opioid crisis exists. Steps are being taken to reduce the amount of opioids that are being prescribed. Suggested criteria include a prescription for only 1 week of the medication and no refills. Patients with chronic or severe pain are often referred to a pain specialist for long-term relief from pain with use of an opioid-containing medication.

Schizophrenia

Description

Schizophrenia, a major psychiatric disturbance, is a group of disorders that may result in chronic mental dysfunction, producing varying degrees of impairment.

ICD-10-CM Code   F20.9 *(Schizophrenia, unspecified)*

Symptoms and Signs

Schizophrenia is a mental disorder characterized by the presence of either positive manifestations (an excess or distortion of normal functions) or negative manifestations (a loss of normal functions). Positive symptoms include delusions (fixed, false beliefs), hallucinations, disorganized speech, and grossly disorganized or catatonic behavior. Negative symptoms are affective flattening, alogia, and avolition.

Schizophrenia is very disabling for the affected individual. In most cases, a person with schizophrenia will have difficulty finishing their education, maintaining employment,

TABLE 14.3 Drugs of Abuse

Drug Name	Classification	Other Names	How Consumed	Effects
Alcohol	Depressant	Beer, wine, liquor, cooler, malt liquor, booze	Orally	Addiction (alcoholism), dizziness, slurred speech, disturbed sleep, nausea, vomiting, hangovers, impaired motor skills, violent behavior, impaired learning, fetal alcohol syndrome, respiratory depression and death (high doses)
Amphetamines	Stimulant	Speed, uppers, ups, hearts, black beauties, pep pills, copilots, bumble bees, Benzedrine, Dexedrine, footballs, biphetamine	Orally, injected, snorted, smoked	Addiction, anxiety, agitation, confusion, increased blood pressure, aggression, insomnia, dizziness, dilated pupils and blurred vision, loss of appetite, malnutrition, hyperthermia, rages, violent behavior, psychotic features, withdrawal syndrome, progressive deterioration with heavy use
Methamphetamines	Stimulant	Speed, meth, crank, crystal, ice (street name for smokable type), fire, croak, cryptol, white cross, glass	Orally, injected, snorted, smoked	Addiction, irritability, anxiety, increased blood pressure, paranoia, psychosis, aggression, nervousness, hyperthermia, compulsive behavior, stroke, depression, convulsions, heart and blood vessel toxicity, insomnia, anorexia, hallucinations, formication (crawling sensation)
Ecstasy	Stimulant	XTC, Adam, MDMA known as a club drug	Orally	Psychiatric disturbances (including panic, anxiety, depression, and paranoia), muscle tension, nausea, blurred vision, sweating, tachycardia, hypertension, tremors, hallucinations, anorexia, sleep problems, marked hyperthermia, drug craving, fainting, chills, dehydration
Methylphenidate (Ritalin)	Stimulant	Speed, west coast (Note: Used legally to treat attention-deficit/hyperactivity disorder [ADHD])	Tablet is crushed and is snorted or injected	Loss of appetite, fevers, convulsions, severe headaches, irregular heartbeat and respiration, paranoia, hallucinations, delusions, excessive repetition of movements and meaningless tasks, tremors, muscle twitching
Herbal ecstasy/ephedrine	Stimulant	Cloud 9, Rave, Energy, Ultimate Xphoria, X	Orally	Increased heart rate, increased blood pressure, seizures, heart attacks, stroke, death (Note: Active ingredients are caffeine and ephedrine)
Designer drugs (fentanyl-based)	Stimulant	Synthetic heroin, goodfella	Injected, sniffed, or smoked	Instant respiratory paralysis; potency creates strong possibility of overdose; many of same effects as heroin
Gamma-hydroxybutyric acid (GHB)	Stimulant	Liquid ecstasy, somatomax, scoop, Grievous Bodily Harm, liquid x, Georgia Home Boy, goop	Snored orally in liquid form, smoked, or mixed drinks	Liver failure, vomiting, tremors, seizures, coma, fatal respiratory problems
Cocaine	Stimulant	Coke, snow, nose candy, flake, blow, big C, lady, white, snowbirds; crack with heroin is "speedball"	Snorted or dissolved in water and injected; freebase form (crack) is smokable	Addiction, pupil dilation, elevated vital signs, paranoia, seizures, heart attack, respiratory failure, constricted peripheral blood vessels, restlessness, irritability, anxiety, loss of appetite, hallucinations, insomnia, hyperthermia, altered judgment, erratic behavior, death from overdose

Continued

TABLE 14.3 Drugs of Abuse—cont'd

Drug Name	Classification	Other Names	How Consumed	Effects
Heroin (processed from morphine)	Opiate	Smack, horse, mud, brown sugar, junk, black tar, big H, dope	Injected, smoked, or snorted	Addiction, intense euphoria, slowed and slurred speech, slow gait, constricted pupils, droopy eyelids, impaired night vision, vomiting after first use and at very high doses, reduced sexual pleasure, reduced appetite, constipation, respiratory depression or failure, dry and itching skin, skin infections
Rohypnol (flunitrazepam)	Opiate-like	Roach, roofie, the forget pill, rope, rophie, ruffies, R2, roofinol, la roche, rib; known as the "date rape" drug	Orally in pill form, dissolved in a drink, or snorted	Blackouts with a complete loss of memory, sense of fearlessness and aggression, dizziness and disorientation, nausea, difficulty with motor movements and speaking, creates a drunk feeling
Ketamine hydrochloride	Opiate-like	Special K, Vitamin K, new ecstasy, psychedelic heroin, Ketalar, Ketaject, Super-C, breakfast cereal, used as a rave drug	Snorted or smoked	Delirium, amnesia, impaired motor function, potentially fatal respiratory problems
Lysergic acid diethylamide (LSD)	Hallucinogen	Acid, microdot, tabs, doses, trips, hits, sugar cubes	Tablets taken orally or gelatin/liquid put in eyes	Unpredictable effects, emotional swings (fear to euphoria), elevated body temperature and blood pressure, suppressed appetite, sleeplessness, tremors, flashbacks, drug-induced psychosis, chronic recurring hallucinations. (Note: LSD is the most common hallucinogen. LSD tablets are often decorated with colorful designs or cartoon characters.)
Phencyclidine (PCP)	Dissociative drug	Angel dust, ozone, rocket fuel, peace pill, elephant tranquilizer, dust, boat, dummy dust, zombie	Snorted, smoked, taken orally, or injected	Out-of-body experience, impaired motor coordination, inability to feel pain, anxiety, disorientation, fear, panic, paranoia, altered perception of body image, mental turmoil, delusions, delirium, agitation, unpredictable violent outbursts, and death. (Note: Marijuana joints may be dipped into PCP.)
Mushrooms (psilocybin)	Hallucinogen	Shrooms, caps, magic mushrooms	Eaten or brewed and drunk in tea	Increased blood pressure, sweating, nausea, hallucinations
Inhalants Vapors Aerosols	Volatile substances	Nitrous oxide, laughing gas, whispers, aerosol sprays, cleaning fluids, solvents, many household products	Sniffed, direct spray, bagging, huffing (from soaked rag), inhaling	Intoxication similar to alcohol, headache, muscle weakness, abdominal pain, severe mood swings, violent behavior, numbness and tingling of hands and feet, nausea, nosebleeds, liver, lung, and kidney damage, dangerous chemical imbalances in the body, anorexia, fatigue, decreases in heart and respiratory rates, hepatitis or peripheral neuropathy
Marijuana/hash	Cannabinoid	Weed, pot, reefer, grass, dope, ganja, Mary Jane, sinsemilla, herb, Aunt Mary, skunk, boom, kif, gangster, chronic, 420	Smoked or eaten	Bloodshot eyes, dry mouth and throat, impaired comprehension, altered sense of time, reduced ability to perform tasks requiring concentration and coordination (e.g., driving a car), paranoia, intense anxiety or panic attacks, altered cognition, impaired learning, memory, thinking, perception, speaking, listening, problem solving, and forming of concepts

Drug Name	Classification	Other Names	How Consumed	Effects
Steroids	Steroidal	Rhoids, juice	Oral, or injected into muscle, gels or creams rubbed into the skin; may be "stacked" by mixing oral and inject-able types	Mood swings ranging from euphoria to depression, acne, cardiovascular disease, liver tumors, liver cancer, irritability and aggression, sterility, increased energy, masculine traits in women and feminine traits in men
Tobacco and nicotine	Other	Smoke, bone, butt, coffin nail, cancer stick	Cigarettes, cigars, pipes, smokeless tobacco (chew, dip, snuff)	Addiction; heart and cardiovascular disease; cancer of the lung, larynx, esophagus, bladder, pancreas, kidney, and mouth; em-physema and chronic bronchitis; spontaneous abortion; preterm delivery, low birth weight
Prescription drugs	Others	Opioids (narcotics), central ner-vous system (CNS) depres-sants, stimulants	Orally, without supervision of a physician	General types of effects from commonly abused prescription drugs may include: physical stimulants dependence, addiction, with-drawal symptoms, mood alteration, sleep disorders, seizures, psychological changes, cardiovascular failure, neurologic disorders
Oxycodone (OxyContin)	Painkiller, highly addictive		Crushed and swallowed or mixed combined with methamphetamine to create a speedball	Similar to morphine, heroin; euphoria
Caffeine	Other		Coffee tea, chocolate, soft drinks, energy drinks medications	Stimulant, blood vessel effects
K2 (Incense) Spice	Synthetic cannabis	K2 Citron K2 Blonde K2 Pink	Usually smoked	Similar to cannabis
Dextromethorphan		Dex, Orange Crush	Oral syrup	Euphoria and impaired judgment when taken in large amounts

General principles of treatment for addiction to various drugs:
- A treatment plan must meet the individual's needs and be tailored to the drug of abuse.
- The program or facility appropriate for the individual should be identified so that it can be accessed when needed.
- Effective treatment begins with a medical, psychological, and social assessment.
- Medical detoxification may be required.
- Treatment requires adequate time, individual and/or group counseling, support, and medication in some cases.
- Behavior therapy and a support program, such as the 12-step program, are crucial to recovery.
- Relapses can occur, so monitoring for drug use is important.
- Note: If the drugs of abuse have been injected, the patient has increased risk of exposure to human immunodeficiency virus (HIV), hepatitis B and C, tuberculosis, and other infectious diseases.
- Education about drug abuse, the nature of addiction, and the importance of recovery as a long-term process is beneficial to family and friends but essential to the recovering addict.

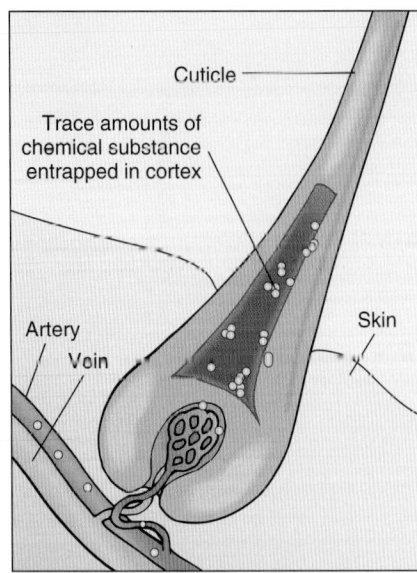

• **Fig. 14.13** The scientific principle behind hair analysis is that as drugs are ingested, they enter the bloodstream, which nourishes the hair follicles. In this way, trace amounts of drugs are deposited in the hair shaft, and, when analyzed, they can reveal a person's drug history. (With permission from Psychemedics Corporation, www.phychemedics.com.)

and participating in relationships. Many experience trouble with activities of daily living. Schizophrenia is rarely seen in children. Most symptoms begin to manifest in the mid- to late 20s. Careful consideration must go into the diagnosis of schizophrenia, because some cultures and religions may regard some symptoms as normal. The onset of schizophrenia is usually insidious during adolescence or young adulthood.

Prodromal signs, such as withdrawal, odd behavior, disheveled appearance, and loss of interest in school or work may be noted. The patient may report feeling confused, isolated, anxious, and afraid. In the active phase of schizophrenia, a vast range of severe behavioral and perceptual manifestations is present, with notable social and occupational dysfunction.

One important feature is disorganized thinking, usually reflected by the patient's speech and by disturbances in language and communication. For example, the patient may switch from one topic to another, speak incoherently, give an unrelated answer to a question, or experience difficulty speaking at all.

Distortions in perception called *hallucinations* are a common characteristic of schizophrenia. Hallucinations may be auditory, visual, olfactory, or sensory. The patient with auditory hallucinations acknowledges hearing voices that may be threatening, instructive, or conversational. Delusions, which are erroneous beliefs, represent exaggerations or distortions of perceptions or experiences. In persecutory delusion, for instance, people may believe that they are being mistreated, deceived, or stalked. More bizarre delusions may include belief that one's thoughts are controlled by an "alien."

Inappropriate **affect** (feeling) is another identifying characteristic of schizophrenia. Lack of emotional expression (flat affect) or unreasonable outbursts of emotions may be noted. Eye contact is minimal.

Behavior may be bizarre or grossly disorganized, unpredictable, agitated, or violent. The patient may assume rigid posturing (catatonic posturing), dress in an odd manner, and neglect self-care. Any of these behaviors can stem from the patient's delusional thinking. As the symptoms and signs persist, the patient's ability to function in interpersonal, social, or occupational relationships deteriorates.

Schizophrenia has subtypes, which are determined by a clustering of characteristics, as shown in the table below.

ICD-10-CM Code   F20.0 (*Paranoid schizophrenia*)
Paranoid schizophrenia features anger, hostility, violence, grandiose or persecutory delusions, or hallucinations. The patient may be intelligent and well informed.
ICD-10-CM Code   F20.1 (*Disorganized schizophrenia*)
The patient is blatantly incoherent, with delusions that are not systematized into a theme. The patient's feelings are dull, inappropriate, or greatly exaggerated. Behavior may be odd or regressive. The patient has a history of extreme social impairment, poor functioning, and poor adaptation. The condition has a chronic course.
ICD-10-CM Code   F20.2 (*Catatonic schizophrenia*)
Catatonic schizophrenia features either excitement or stupor with mutism, negativism, rigidity, and posturing.
ICD-10-CM Code   F20.9 (*Schizophrenia, unspecified*)
The behavior is grossly disorganized, and the patient is obviously incoherent, grossly delusional, and hallucinatory. Prominent symptoms of psychosis may fit more than one subtype.
ICD-10-CM Code   F20.5 (*Residual schizophrenia*)
(F20.0-F20.9 = 8 codes of specificity)
The patient has experienced at least one episode of schizophrenia but is currently without prominent symptoms. Continuing evidence of illness, such as illogical thinking and odd behavior, may prevent the patient from functioning in the workplace.

Patient Screening

Scheduling of the appointment for the patient with schizophrenia varies, depending on the situation. When the patient or family member reports a crisis, they should be asked to report to an emergency facility.

Etiology

The cause of schizophrenia is unknown, but evidence suggests that genetic factors play a substantial role. Close biologic relatives of patients with schizophrenia have a 10-fold greater risk of schizophrenia. The incidence of schizophrenia is two to three times higher among men than among women. Vulnerability to stress and environmental factors are considered contributing catalysts.

Diagnosis

The diagnosis of schizophrenia requires recognizing a group of psychotic signs and symptoms, including delusions, hallucinations, disorganized speech, grossly disorganized behavior, affective flattening, alogia, and avolition. Previously, no laboratory findings had been identified as diagnostic of schizophrenia. Recent advances in medical imaging of the brain now provide images of brain activity. These include positron emission tomography (PET), functional magnetic resonance (FMR), and magnetic encephalography (MEG). These tests, applied to patients with schizophrenia by researchers, have produced an insight into brain activity in these patients and in those without the disease.

Psychological tests that may help in diagnosis include the Rorschach (inkblot) test, the Thematic Apperception Test (TAT), and the Minnesota Multiphasic Personality Inventory (MMPI). Organic causes, such as toxic psychosis associated with substance abuse, cerebral arteriosclerosis, and hyperthyroidism, should be ruled out.

Treatment

During the acute phase of schizophrenia, antipsychotic drugs are used to control symptoms and to allow early release from the hospital. The minimal dose that produces remission of symptoms without troublesome side effects associated with antipsychotic medications is desirable. Subsequent long term multidimensional treatment combines supportive psychotherapy, drugs, and family involvement. After the patient is stabilized, the goal of treatment is helping the patient to establish a better sense of self through personal, social, and vocational achievements.

Atypical antipsychotics are first-line therapy and include risperidone, olanzapine, asenapine (Saphris), clozapine (Clozaril), iloperidone (Fanapt), paliperidone (Invega), ziprasidone (Geodon), quetiapine (Seroquel), and lurasidone (Latuda). Some of these medications are supplied as injectable long-acting preparations. Atypical antipsychotics have less chance of causing extrapyramidal side effects compared with older drug entities, although most atypical antipsychotics carry a black box warning regarding mortality risk in dementia-related psychosis and suicidal tendencies. Atypical antipsychotics also have varying degrees of metabolic side effects, QT prolongation, and risk of interaction with cytochrome P450 3A4 (CYP3A4) inhibitors. Older antipsychotic drugs are used for those who do not respond well to atypical drugs and in cases where the patient has been on the older drugs for a long time and reports no unmanageable side effects. These drugs include chlorpromazine (Thorazine), haloperidol (Haldol), fluphenazine (Prolixin), and many more that are used less often. Intramuscular injections increase compliance because the medication can last for a month. Rexulti (brexpiprazole) is another medication which may be used to treat symptoms. Potential side effects of the neuroleptic agents used to treat schizophrenia are known as *extrapyramidal side effects (EPSs)*, which are manifested as involuntary motor movements. Tardive dyskinesia is a type of EPS characterized by repetitive, involuntary, purposeless movements. Features may include grimacing, tongue protrusion, lip smacking, puckering and pursing of the lips, and rapid eye blinking. Weekly laboratory tests should be ordered and performed.

Patients, families, and caretakers should be alert for side effects caused by risperidone. The physician should be notified if any of the following are noted in the individual taking risperidone: fever, confusion, rapid or irregular pulse, seizures, fainting, difficulty swallowing or breathing, or unusual, uncontrollable movements of the mouth or body. Refer to the Enrichment box about Neuroleptic Malignant Syndrome.

◆ ENRICHMENT

Neuroleptic Malignant Syndrome

Neuroleptic malignant syndrome (NMS), a unique life-threatening reaction to antipsychotic drugs, is suspected when patients suddenly develop a fever, muscle rigidity, altered mental status, and autonomic dysfunction. This is a danger that may accompany all neuroleptics, such as newer atypical antipsychotics and a range of other medications that have an effect on central dopaminergic neurotransmission. NMS is an important factor in the diagnosis of patients who suddenly experience fever, muscle rigidity and mental status changes. NMS needs prompt identification to prevent significant morbidity and death. Recommended treatment is to immediately stop the offending drug and to begin supportive treatment. Additionally, drug intervention may be required in more severe cases.

Prognosis

The prognosis is moderate if the patient takes prescription drugs regularly and if the family is supportive and willing to participate in treatment. Treatment in a community support program also is beneficial. Responses to treatment vary, and relapses may occur.

Prevention

Schizophrenia is genetic, so no prevention is known. Compliance in taking medications reduces psychotic breaks, helping to prevent the illness from worsening. Each time a patient has a psychotic break, baseline functioning is reduced.

Patient Teaching

Instruct patients to comply with the medication regimen despite the frequent unpleasant side effects. Because noncompliance can be an issue, involving the family is helpful. Advise family members and support persons that patients with schizophrenia are not bad people but are simply people with a bad illness. In addition, encourage family members to help the patient with activities of daily living.

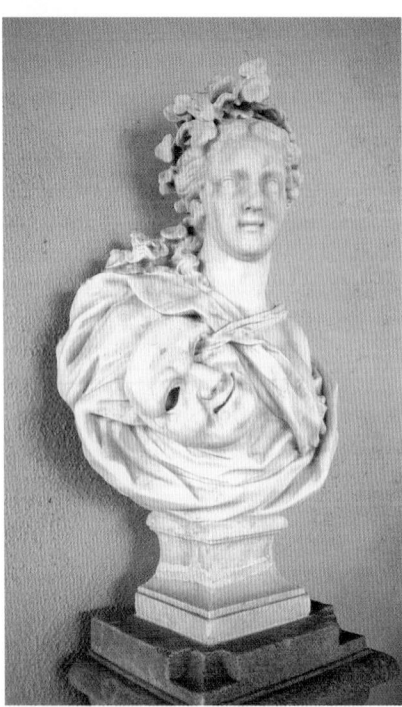

• **Fig. 14.14** Representation of bipolar disorder. (Courtesy David L. Frazier, 2003.)

Mood Disorders

In a mood disorder, a person experiences a pathologic disturbance in mood that affects all aspects of his or her life. The terms *affect* and *mood* are used interchangeably to refer to the outward manifestation of a person's feeling or tone.

Bipolar Disorder

Description
Bipolar disorder is a major affective disorder with abnormally intense mood swings from a hyperactive, or manic, state to a depressive syndrome (Fig. 14.14). In some cases, symptoms of hyperactivity and depression may coexist. This is known as a "mixed" episode. The patient may remain manic for days, weeks, or months before experiencing depression. Assessment findings vary with the type of episode (manic, depressive, or mixed) that the patient is experiencing at the time of medical evaluation.

ICD-10-CM Code	F31.9 *(Bipolar disorder, unspecified)*
	(F31.0-F31.9 = 28 codes of specificity)

Symptoms and Signs
During a manic episode, the patient is excited, euphoric, and expansive. The person speaks rapidly with great certitude and conviction. Evidence of thought disorders, such as frequent changes of topic or flight of ideas, may be noted. Patients sleep little and seem to have excessive energy, which leads to overinvolvement in activities. Judgment is impaired, and they may spend money extravagantly. Behavior may appear bizarre, grandiose, or promiscuous. The patient may be delusional or experience auditory hallucinations.

During an episode of depression, the patient's mood becomes lowered, sad, or notably indifferent (flat affect). Thoughts and speech are slow, and the patient may avoid communication. The patient becomes withdrawn and demonstrates loss of interest in life. Reports of sleep disturbance, loss of appetite, and feelings of guilt are common. The patient experiences a substantial decrease in physical activity. Suicide may be threatened or attempted.

Patient Screening
Most often, help will be sought during the depressive portion of the illness. Depressed individuals require immediate assessment.

Etiology
Bipolar disorder has no clear cause. Biochemical factors, such as alterations of neurotransmitter levels in the brain, endocrine disorders, and electrolyte imbalances, may play a role. The risk of mood disorders is higher among close relatives of the patient. Emotional or physical trauma may precipitate the onset of bipolar disorder in a predisposed person.

Diagnosis
A thorough family history and patient history of symptoms is obtained. The patient may appear to be experiencing only depression.

Bipolar disorder is identified when certain prescribed diagnostic criteria can be documented during physical and psychological evaluations. The mood disturbance must be pervasive and persistent and cause substantial impairment over a distinct period. Other medical causes, such as organic diseases, thyroid disorders, and psychiatric conditions, must be ruled out.

Treatment
After diagnosis, therapeutic treatment is dictated by the specific form of behavior the patient exhibits. Lithium carbonate is the drug of choice during an acute manic phase of bipolar disease. It may even abate a swing into the depressive phase. Valproate sodium and carbamazepine (Tegretol) are good drugs for add-on therapy in stabilizing manic episodes. During an episode of depression, antidepressants are used with caution, because they may trigger a manic episode. Antidepressants are best used in conjunction with anticonvulsants for optimal mood stabilization. Many of the drugs that fall into the category of anticonvulsant also function well to provide mood stabilization. Examples include lamotrigine (Lamictal) and gabapentin, and the aforementioned valproate sodium and carbamazepine. Atypical antipsychotics are often used for mood stabilization (especially lurasidone [Latuda], which is approved by the U.S. Food and Drug Administration [FDA]

for treatment of bipolar type II disorder). Treatment includes a therapeutic milieu, or environment, that meets the patient's physical needs, encourages personal responsibility, and sets reasonable limits and goals for behavior. During this time, the patient may need to be protected from self-injury.

Prognosis

The prognosis is good with treatment and drug therapy. Compliance is the key to successful treatment.

Prevention

No prevention is known.

Patient Teaching

Encourage patients to take medications and to keep the appointments with their therapist. Blood studies may be necessary, depending on the medications prescribed and taken. Use customized electronically generated educational materials, when available, to reinforce the treatment plan.

Major Depressive Disorder

Description

Major depressive disorder is a mood disorder characterized by one or more major depressive episodes. Persons with major depressive disorders have no history of a manic or hypomanic episode.

ICD-10-CM Code	F32.9 (Major depressive disorder, single episode, unspecified)
	(F32.0 F33.9 17 codes of specificity)

Symptoms and Signs

Major depressive disorder is a serious alteration in mood that may be described as deep and persistent sadness, despair, and hopelessness (Fig. 14.15). Symptoms develop gradually over several days, during which an anxious or brooding appearance may be noted. The person may experience an empty or heavy feeling inside accompanied by a vague sense of loss. The person also may have an attitude of self-blame, remorse, guilt, or loss of self-esteem. Other symptoms include sleep disturbance (insomnia or hypersomnia), physical sluggishness or fatigue, loss of concentration, and inability to experience pleasure. In addition, a depressed person may have a variety of physical symptoms. Appetite disturbance results in a change in weight. The patient withdraws socially and may admit to having suicidal thoughts; suicidal behavior is common in major depression (Table 14.4).

Patient Screening

People experiencing symptoms of depression, often reported by family members, require immediate assessment. A risk of suicide requires immediate assessment and intervention.

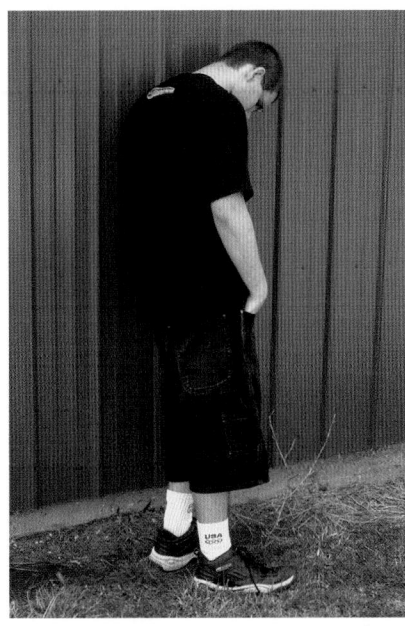

• **Fig. 14.15** Depression. (Courtesy David L. Frazier, 2003.)

Etiology

Major depressive disorder is thought to have a biologic basis and a familial pattern, but the precise cause is not understood. Psychosocial pressures, chronic physical illness, and alcohol dependence are considered predisposing factors. Although many patients blame their environment, it is not considered a cause of the disease.

Diagnosis

Major depressive disorder must be differentiated from a reactive type of depression that results from a difficult or stressful life circumstance, such as a grief syndrome. Diagnostic criteria used in psychiatric evaluation include a prominent and persistent depressed mood lasting at least 2 weeks, with at least four of any of the aforementioned symptoms documented. A family history of depression is included in the assessment.

Treatment

The most effective treatment is a combination of medication and psychotherapy. Most patients have relief of symptoms and a good prognosis if they respond favorably to antidepressant therapy. SSRIs, including fluoxetine, are the first-line agents, but many patients with major depression also might be prescribed the tricyclics amitriptyline/nortriptyline along with the SSRI. Atypical antipsychotics may be used in severe cases of major depressive disorder. Depression may occur as a single episode or may be recurrent. Electroconvulsive therapy helps when a patient is severely incapacitated, has psychotic features, or does not respond to other therapeutic measures. Family support and education are considered important in the recovery process.

TABLE 14.4	Depression on a Continuum

Mild to Moderate	Severe
Communication	
• Slow speech • Long pauses before answering • Monotone	• Slow in extreme • May be mute and not talk at all
Affect	
• Crying and weeping, slumping in chair, drooping shoulders, look of gloom and pessimism • Anxiety may or may not be manifested • Anhedonia (inability to experience pleasure)	• May appear without affect • May be experiencing "nothingness" • Can sit for hours staring into space • Anhedonia
Thinking	

• No impairment in reality testing
• Thinking is slow; concentration and memory are poor; interest narrows; perspective in situations is lost:
  • "Everyone always lets me down."
  • "No one cares."
  • Thoughts reflect doubts and indecisions; thinking is often repetitive in negative cycle:
  • "Why was I born?
  • "What's life all about?"
• Mild feelings of guilt and worthlessness
 	
• *May have suicidal ideation*
	• Grasp of reality may be tenuous
	• Thoughts may indicate delusional thinking, reflecting feelings of:
	  • Low self-esteem
	  • Worthlessness
	  • Helplessness
	  • "I'm no good."
	  • "God is punishing me for my terrible sins."
	  • "My insides are rotting."
	  • "My heart has stopped beating."
	  • Concentration is extremely poor
	  • Preoccupation with bodily symptoms
	
	• *May have suicidal ideation*

Physical Behavior	
• Fatigue and lethargy are hallmark symptoms; they do not prevent the person from working, but the person often works below potential; initiative and creativity are impaired • Grooming and hygiene usually are neglected	• Severe and extreme chronic fatigue and lethargy greatly interfere with occupational functioning, social activities, or relationships with others • Client may show extreme neglect of personal grooming and hygiene
Vegetative Signs	
• Sleep: Middle or late insomnia, hypersomnia; EEG studies show shortened REM latency • Energy is often highest in the morning, lowest in the evening • Eating: May have anorexia or overeat • Sexual appetite is diminished • Bowels: Constipation if psychomotor impairment is present; may have diarrhea if psychomotor agitation is present • Psychomotor impairment (slow motor movements): Everything is an effort *Or* • Psychomotor agitation (agitated depression); pacing up and down halls, wringing hands	• Sleep: Usually insomnia; early morning waking at 3 or 4 AM • Energy is often lowest in the morning, highest in the evening • Eating: Usually has anorexia; weight loss of more than 5% in 1 month • Loss of libido • Bowels: Usually constipation • Psychomotor impairment (most common) *Or* • Psychomotor agitation

EEG, Electroencephalogram; *REM,* rapid eye movement.
(From Varcarolis EM: *Foundations of psychiatric mental health nursing,* ed 3, Philadelphia, 1998, WB Saunders. Used with permission.)

Patients who commit suicide have a high incidence of the hopelessness of acute depression. The suicidal patient often wishes to discuss suicidal fears and does not want to die but sees suicide as the only escape from an intolerable situation. A reluctance to discuss suicidal thoughts makes it important for the examiner to explore the patient's preoccupation with death or such comments as, "People would be better off without me" or "I am better off dead."

Suicide intervention is an attempt by medical, mental health, and community organizations to help the depressed individual through the crisis situation. Most telephone directories list crisis intervention centers. Hospital emergency departments and law enforcement agencies have professionals immediately available to offer support and personal contact to this individual. Mental health agencies routinely offer their clients a 24-hour "hotline" number for contacting a counselor. Structures that are often used as jumping points, such as bridges, have

strategically placed signs that offer crisis intervention telephone numbers (Fig. 14.16).

The increase in suicide rates continues to rise. It was the fourth leading cause of death for ages 35–54 in the United States in 2018. Occurrences of suicides among veterans and law enforcement officers have been increasing recently.

• **Fig. 14.16** The Golden Gate Bridge, where many suicide jumps have been made. (Courtesy David L Frazier, 1999.)

❖ ENRICHMENT

Grief Response

The grief response is initiated primarily by the death of a loved one, but grieving also is a normal sequela to any loss, including loss of a function, body part, employment, or other important entity. The patient with a terminal illness faces the prospect of total separation and also must work through the various stages of grief.

The normal grieving process passes through several phases. The most recognized stages are those identified by Elisabeth Kübler-Ross. The first is denial: "No, I don't believe it." Second is anger: "Why did he or she do this to me?" or "Why is God letting this happen?" The third stage is bargaining: "If only this task can be accomplished or I can achieve this goal (live long enough), I will do this." Fourth is depression, in which people retreat within themselves and have little or no involvement with their environment. Finally, in the fifth stage, acceptance comes. Not everyone is able to move through these steps, and not everyone moves through them at the same pace or in the same order. Some people cannot express anger at the dead person or at God and do not move on. Many of these people never complete the grieving process, so they remain in a depressed state and have reduced coping mechanisms. Medical intervention may help during depression, but most people recover with minimal treatment.

Different cultures grieve in different ways. Many groups grieve quietly and privately, whereas others cry, moan, rant, and even throw themselves on the funeral pyre. The important goal of funerals and the viewing of the remains is to allow closure of the relationship and to allow loved ones to say good-bye (Table 14.5 and Fig. 14.17).

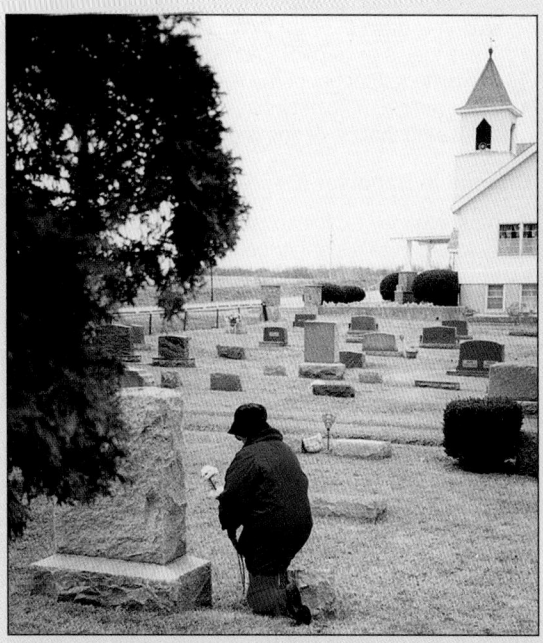

• **Fig. 14.17** Grief response. (Courtesy David L. Frazier, 1999.)

TABLE 14.5 Phenomena Experienced During Mourning

Symptoms	Examples
Sensation of Somatic Distress	
• Tightness in throat, shortness of breath, sighing, "mental pain," exhaustion. • Food tastes like sand; things feel unreal. • Pain or discomfort may be identical to the symptoms experienced by the dead person. • Symptoms normally are brief.	A woman whose husband died of a stroke complains of weakness and numbness on her left side.
Preoccupation with the Image of the Deceased	
• The bereaved brings up, thinks, and talks about many memories of the deceased. • The memories are positive. • This process goes on with great sadness. • The idealization of the deceased lets the bereaved relive the gratifications associated with the deceased and helps resolve any guilt the bereaved has toward the deceased. • The bereaved also may take on many of the mannerisms of the deceased through identification. • Identification serves the purpose of holding onto the deceased. • Preoccupation with the dead person takes many months before it lessens.	A man whose wife just died states, "I just can't stop thinking about my wife. Everything I see reminds me of her. We picked up this seashell on our honeymoon. I remember every wonderful moment we had together. The pain is so great, but the memories just keep coming." His friends notice that when he talks, his hand gestures and expressions are very like those of his recently deceased wife.
Guilt	
The bereaved reproaches himself or herself for real or fancied acts of negligence or omissions in the relationship with the deceased.	"I should have made him go to the doctor sooner." "I should have paid more attention to her, been more thoughtful."
Anger	
• The anger the bereaved experiences may not be toward the object that gives rise to it. • The anger often is displaced onto the medical or nursing staff. It is often directed toward the deceased. • The anger is at its height during the first month but is often intermittent throughout the first year. • The overflow of hostility disturbs the bereaved, resulting in the feeling that he or she is going "insane."	"The doctor didn't operate in time. If he had, Mary would be alive today." "How could he leave me like this...? How could he?"
Change in Behavior (Depression, Disorganization, Restlessness)	
• A person may exhibit substantial restlessness and an inability to organize his or her behavior. • Routine activities take a long time to perform. • Depressive mood is common as the year passes and as the intensity of the grief declines. • Absence of depression is more abnormal than its presence. • Loneliness and aimlessness are most pronounced 6 to 9 months after the death.	Six months after her husband died, Mrs. Faye stated, "I just can't seem to function. I have a hard time doing the simplest tasks. I can't be bothered with socializing." "I feel so down... so, so empty."
Reorganization of Behavior Directed Toward a New Object or Activity	
• The person gradually renews his or her interest in people and activities. • The grieving thus releases the bereaved from one interpersonal relationship, and new ones are free to take its place.	Twenty months after her husband's death, Mrs. Faye tells a friend, "I'll be away this weekend. I am going fishing with my brother and his friend. This is the first time I've felt like doing anything since Harry died."

(From Varcarolis EM: *Foundations of psychiatric mental health nursing*, ed 6, St Louis, 2010, Saunders.)

Seasonal Affective Disorder

Seasonal affective disorder (SAD), also known as *seasonal pattern specifier,* is a depressive condition that is manifested on a cycle at regular times of the year. The depression usually begins in the fall of the year, extends through the winter months, and then improves or goes into remission during the spring before returning in the fall. The individual may have an occasional summer episode. The episode pattern occurs over successive years. Symptoms include lack of energy, excessive sleeping, overeating, a craving for carbohydrates, and weight gain. The incidence of SAD is greater in women than in men, and younger people appear to be at higher risk than older adults. The geographic latitude appears to be involved, with the occurrence increasing with higher latitudes and shorter daylight hours. In addition, a lack of sunshine and presence of snow and cloudy days tend to foster the condition (Fig. 14.18).

The cause of SAD has been proposed to be an increase in the amount of the hormone melatonin secreted by the pineal gland. Melatonin is produced during dark hours, so observers speculate that an excessive amount affects certain people. The secretion of this hormone is suppressed by light. Increased amounts of melatonin are associated with lethargy and drowsiness. Drugs have been used to suppress melatonin secretion with some success. Another theory suggests that the body's circadian rhythm is delayed in people with SAD, causing the "vegetative" symptoms. This theory supports the use of light therapy, exposing the patient to artificially reproduced light for periods of time in the morning during the winter months. This treatment also has produced good results and improved the depressed state of people with SAD.

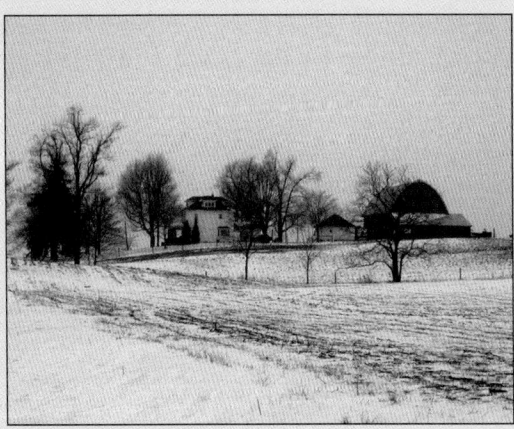

• **Fig. 14.18** Desolate farm house during a snowstorm. (Courtesy David L. Frazier, 2003.)

Postpartum Depression

Postpartum depression (PPD), often labeled "baby blues," ranges from mild depression, to moderate depressive mood, to severe postpartum psychosis. Depressive symptoms after the birth of a baby have been recorded for centuries. Although no specific cause has been identified, abrupt changes in the levels of hormones, including estrogen and progesterone, have been proposed as the cause of this condition. In addition, changes in thyroid status may play a role in some cases. The responsibility of caring for a helpless newborn along with other demands of motherhood can be overwhelming. The frustration felt during feeding attempts along with the sleep disruption caused by the neonate add to the mother's despair. A previous history of depression or other mental health conditions may increase the risk of PPD.

Symptoms usually begin within 24 to 48 hours after birth or during the first 6 weeks after giving birth. The symptoms may subside in a few days or a few weeks or may last for several months. The new mother experiences fatigue, changes in normal appetite and sleep patterns, feelings of worthlessness and despair, crying episodes, poor personal hygiene, despair about her ability as a mother, feelings of anger, and recurrent thoughts of suicide. She also feels sad, has a flat affect, appears excessively angry, lacks interest in normal daily events, and experiences difficulty in concentrating and making decisions. One may express the desire to run away from everything, fears of being alone, and concern about potentially harming the baby. In the more severe cases of PPD, the mother may have thoughts of homicide, especially of killing the infant.

Maternal-child health care providers must be alert for any symptoms of PPD. Prenatal teaching of both parents should include the typical symptoms of PPD and instructions to seek prompt medical intervention if and when they occur. Early intervention with medication and therapy helps to reduce symptoms and to prevent harm to the mother or child. The teaching also should urge parents not to feel any stigma for experiencing the condition, because it is a very common occurrence in many postpartum periods. Postpartum psychosis is considered a rare outcome, and when it does occur, it may bring about serious events.

Anxiety Disorders

Description

Anxiety is a common form of psychological disorder. For most people, anxiety is just a temporary response to stress. For some people, however, anxiety becomes a chronic problem, and they regularly experience excessive levels of anxiety. They often exhibit anxiety that is inappropriate to the circumstance. Only when anxiety persists and prevents the person from leading a normal life does it become an illness. As a group, anxiety disorders represent the single largest mental health problem in the United States. They can lead to more severe disorders, such as depression and alcoholism.

Anxiety disorders, previously known as *neuroses,* include four specific disorders or syndromes that are different in behavioral manifestations but share the fact that the person's behavior is dominated by anxiety. The four disorders are generalized anxiety disorder, panic disorder, phobic disorder, and obsessive-compulsive disorder (OCD).

Symptoms and Signs

Symptoms can range from worry and stress to extreme panic, depending on which anxiety disorder the patient is experiencing. Mild to moderate levels of anxiety can easily be mistaken for depression because of the similarity in symptoms, such as irritability, difficulty concentrating, and disturbance in sleep patterns.

Some symptoms of anxiety disorders are observed behaviors (e.g., nail biting), compulsive rituals (e.g., hand washing and checking), and other nervous movements.

Generalized anxiety disorder and panic disorder

ICD-10-CM Code   F41.0 *(Panic disorder [episodic paroxysmal anxiety] without agoraphobia)*
F41.1 *(Generalized anxiety disorder)*
(F41.0-F41.9 = 5 codes of specificity)

Patients with generalized anxiety disorder have a condition known as *free-floating anxiety* and live in a constant state of apparently causeless anxiety. They constantly worry about previous mistakes and future problems. These individuals dislike making decisions and worry about the decisions they have made. Their constant worrying often is accompanied by physiologic symptoms, such as diarrhea, elevated blood pressure, and sustained muscular tension. Inability to sleep and nightmares are common. Some patients are even prone to panic attacks.

In panic disorder, the anxiety also is unfocused. With a panic attack, the anxiety begins suddenly and unexpectedly, reaching a peak within 10 minutes. The attack often is accompanied by a sense of impending doom and a feeling that the person is "going crazy," losing control, or dying. The world may seem unreal (derealization), or patients may seem unreal to themselves (depersonalization). In addition, these patients may experience palpitations, rapid pulse, pounding heart, sweating, trembling, shortness of breath, chest pain, nausea, paresthesia, dizziness, and chills or hot flashes.

The anxiety characteristic of a panic disorder can be differentiated from generalized anxiety by its sudden, intermittent nature and greater severity. A person is said to have panic disorder if he or she has four panic attacks within a month's time or if one or more attacks have been followed by a persistent fear of having another attack.

Phobic disorder

Description

A phobic disorder is marked by excessive, persistent, and irrational fear and the avoidance of the phobic stimulus. In

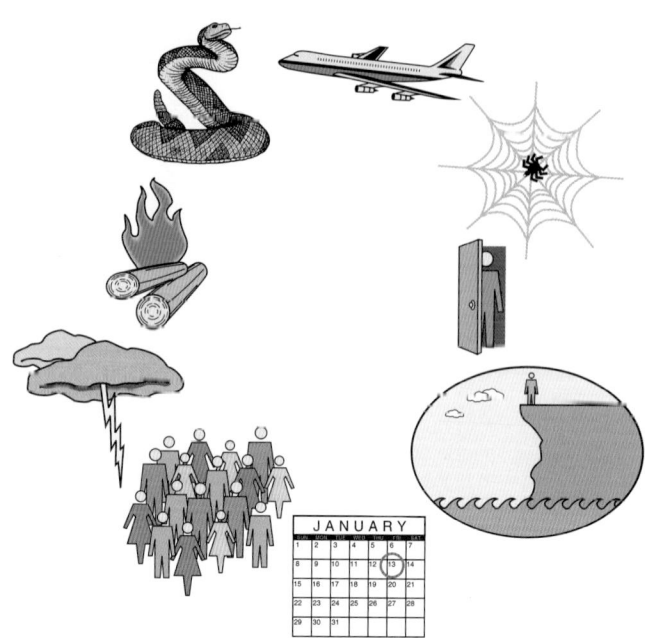

• **Fig. 14.19** Phobias.

phobic disorders, the person's excessive anxiety has a specific focus (Fig. 14.19), some object or a situation that presents no real danger. Many people with phobias realize that their fears are irrational but feel powerless to control or prevent them. Individuals with phobias must design their lives to avoid the things that they fear. When they confront an object or situation that causes them anxiety, they often have a severe attack of anxiety. Phobias can develop from or against almost anything (Table 14.6).

ICD-10-CM Code   F40.9 *(Phobic anxiety disorder, unspecified)*
(F40.00-F40.9 = 23 codes of specificity)

Obsessive-compulsive disorder

Description

OCD is marked by the presence of obsessions (persistent unwanted thoughts) and compulsions (persistent urges to carry out specific actions).

ICD-10-CM Code   F42 *(Obsessive-compulsive disorder)*

Symptoms and Signs

Obsessions are persistent intrusions of unwanted thoughts, and compulsions are uncontrollable urges to carry out certain actions. The two features of this disorder usually, but not always, occur together. People with obsessions often have thoughts of harming others, committing suicide, or performing sexual acts considered immoral. These people feel as though they have lost control of their minds, which causes them great anxiety. People with compulsions develop senseless actions or rituals that relieve their anxiety temporarily (e.g., excessive hand washing). Examples include an

TABLE 14.6 Phobias

Name	Description	Name	Description
Acrophobia	Fear of high places	Olfactophobia	Fear of odor
Agoraphobia	Fear of open spaces	Ombrophobia	Fear of rain
Algophobia	Fear of pain	Ophidiophobia	Fear of snakes
Androphobia	Fear of men	Pathophobia	Fear of disease
Arachnophobia	Fear of spiders	Pharmacophobia	Fear of drugs
Astrophobia	Fear of storms, thunder, and lightning	Phasmophobia	Fear of ghosts
Aviophobia	Fear of flying	Phobophobia	Fear of fear
Claustrophobia	Fear of closed or narrow spaces	Ponophobia	Fear of work
Hematophobia	Fear of blood	Pyrophobia	Fear of fire
Hodophobia	Fear of travel	Sitophobia	Fear of food
Hydrophobia	Fear of water	Thanatophobia	Fear of death
Iatrophobia	Fear of physicians	Toxiphobia	Fear of being poisoned
Kainophobia	Fear of change	Traumatophobia	Fear of injury
Kakorrhaphiophobia	Fear of failure	Triskaidekaphobia	Fear of the number 13
Lalophobia	Fear of speaking in public	Xenophobia	Fear of strangers
Monophobia	Fear of being alone	Zoophobia	Fear of animals
Ochlophobia	Fear of crowds		

obsession with germs that results in a compulsion to clean or wash one's hands and an obsession with fire or theft that results in a compulsion to check doors, appliances, and outlets.

Patient Screening

Patients with complaints of persistent intrusion of unwanted thoughts and compulsions and uncontrollable urges to carry out certain actions require prompt assessment.

Etiology

Many theories attempt to explain the causes of anxiety disorders. Some anxiety disorders are caused by severe stress. In people who are anxiety prone, only slight stress, or none at all, can be a cause. A physical condition, such as hyperthyroidism (overactive thyroid gland) or a cerebrovascular disorder, also can produce the symptoms of anxiety. The role of neurotransmitters and genetic factors has been studied. OCD also may be related to dysfunction in the frontal lobe of the brain.

Diagnosis

Anxiety disorders are diagnosed after much investigation into the patient's symptoms and history, family history, and level of stress. In some cases, metabolic testing indicates abnormalities. PET to detect chemical activity or metabolism of the brain and biochemical studies also have been used. Using the DSM-V criteria during assessment is important in arriving at a diagnosis, one must ask whether the individual meets the requirements for the diagnosis.

Treatment

If the anxiety prevents the person from living a normal life, a psychiatrist or a practitioner trained in treating psychological problems (e.g., psychologist or psychoanalyst) should be consulted. These therapists use many forms of treatment, depending on their perspective. Hypnosis sometimes is used to help the patient and the therapist to gain access to the subconscious mind. If the anxiety is caused by a specific stress (e.g., job related), steps should be taken to minimize or eliminate the problem.

Various methods of relaxation (e.g., systematic desensitization, progressive relaxation, breathing exercises, and guided imagery) can lessen the symptoms. Relaxation exercises (e.g., biofeedback) to relax tense muscles or a physical activity (e.g., brisk walking, jogging, or swimming) may be beneficial. In addition, or as an alternative, the physician may prescribe an anxiolytic drug. SSRIs are first-line therapy (fluvoxamine [Luvox] is FDA approved for the treatment of OCD), but many patients with major depression also may have been prescribed a tricyclic amitriptyline/nortriptyline along with the SSRI and recommended psychotherapy. Benzodiazepines are also frequently prescribed. Examples are lorazepam (Ativan), clonazepam (Klonopin), and alprazolam (Xanax). These medications should be prescribed on an "as needed," short-term basis for severe anxiety, because dependence can occur. In severe cases of anxiety, a period of hospitalization also may be necessary. If severe anxiety is not treated, psychotic depression may develop.

Prognosis
The prognosis is proportional to the patient's compliance with recommended medications and therapy interventions.

Prevention
No prevention is known.

Patient Teaching
Encourage patients to attempt relaxation techniques. When drug therapy is prescribed, encourage compliance and follow-up with therapy as recommended. Use customized electronically generated educational materials, when available, to reinforce the treatment plan.

Pediatric Autoimmune Neuropsychiatric Disorders Associated With Streptococcal Infections (PANDAS)

Description
PANDAS, a form of obsessive compulsive disorder with abrupt onset, follows the occurrence of a group A beta-hemolytic streptococcal infection (GABHS).

ICD-10-CM Code	D89.89 (Other specified disorders involving the immune mechanism, not elsewhere classified)

Symptoms and Signs
An abrupt emotional personality change appears in 3-year-olds to prepubertal children, . They may experience severe mood swings, separation anxiety, and abrupt, obsessive, and unusual behavior. Some may show signs of detachment to parents or caregivers, hyperactivity, or uncontrollable ADHD symptoms. They may encounter sleep disturbances, motor or vocal tics, and nighttime fears.

Patient Screening
The patient experiencing PANDAS suffers acute emotional pain and anxiety and requires prompt medical attention.

Etiology
The condition usually occurs after a bacterial streptococcal infection.

Diagnosis
Diagnosis is confirmed through patient history of a previous streptococcal infection and physical examination.

Treatment
Treatment with antibiotics to eliminate the streptococcal infection is primary. Short-term cognitive behavioral therapy may help deal with current behavioral changes. Medical intervention may involve managing OCD symptoms by prescribing the use of SSRIs. Additional options may include steroids.

Prognosis
The prognosis is good with therapy and medications; however, the reoccurrence of a streptococcal infection may trigger another episode.

Prevention
Prevention is to complete the course of prescribed antibiotics.

Patient Teaching
Parents should be instructed to make sure the child takes all of the antibiotics prescribed as treatment for any streptococcal infection.

Posttraumatic stress disorder

Description
PTSD is a delayed response to an external traumatic event that produces signs and symptoms of extreme distress.

ICD-10-CM Code	F43.0 (Acute stress reaction)
	F43.10 (Post-traumatic stress disorder, unspecified)
	F43.12 (Post-traumatic stress disorder, chronic)
	(F43.10-F43.12 = 3 codes of specificity)

Symptoms and Signs
PTSDs are different from other anxiety disorders because the cause of the stress is an external event of an overwhelmingly painful nature (Fig. 14.20) The person may experience this disorder for weeks, months, or even years (transitory episode) after the event through painful recollections or nightmares. People with PTSD go out of their way to avoid being reminded of the painful event. They may be unable to respond to affection and have insomnia and irritability. These individuals also may exhibit strong physiologic responses to any reminder of the event. PTSDs can also be experienced by adults who were victims of child abuse and repress those memories until something triggers them during adulthood.

Symptoms of PTSD usually appear within a short time of the event. In some cases, however, the person has a delayed response (onset). The person may be symptom-free for days or months after the event before signs of response to the painful event begin to appear. The symptoms disappear spontaneously, however, in about 6 months. Not all people exposed to severely traumatic events have such symptoms. The likelihood of developing PTSD appears to depend, to some degree, on the person's psychological strength before the event. The likelihood of this disorder also depends on the nature of the event.

Patient Screening
The patient experiencing PTSD suffers acute emotional pain and anxiety and requires prompt medical attention.

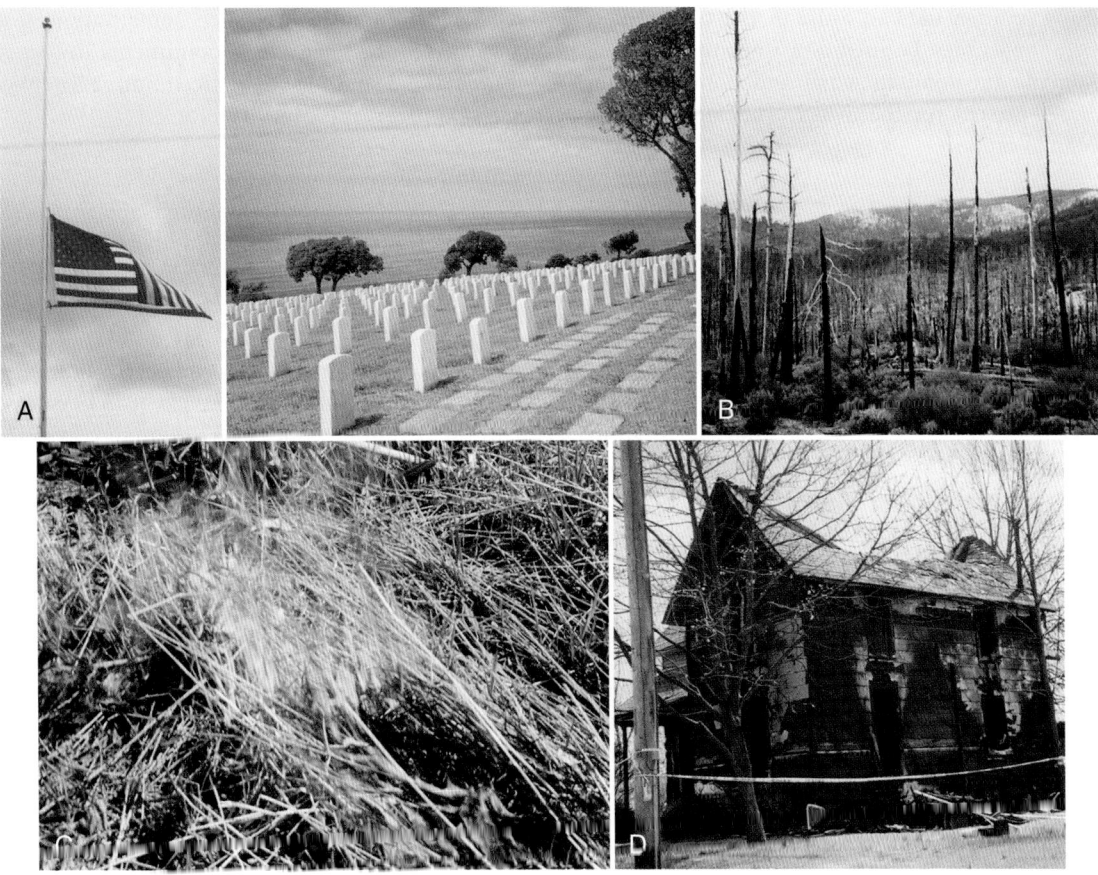

• **Fig. 14.20** Posttraumatic stress disorder (PTSD) sources. (A) Overwhelming numbers of violent deaths, as in wars. (B) Destruction of one's environment by fire, as by forest fires encroaching on communities. (C) Brush fires suddenly erupting on community property. (D) Fire deaths with children and property. (Courtesy David L. Frazier, 1998.)

Etiology

PTSD caused by human actions (e.g., rape, acts of war, and continued abuse) tends to precipitate more severe reactions compared with PTSD caused by natural disasters (e.g., hurricanes, earthquakes, and floods). In the case of natural disasters, the greater the threat of death and the greater the number of people affected, the greater the likelihood of severe PTSD. The overwhelming experience of a threat to the individual's life is a causative factor.

Children also may be affected by experiencing or observing horrific events in their lives. Traumatic events include acts of war, in which they have observed family members being killed or being separated from the family unit. In addition, catastrophic events of nature, in which the children have witnessed violent destruction of homes and surroundings, may make them fearful and withdrawn. Abuse also is known to cause PTSD, especially sexual abuse. Recognizing traumatic events in children's lives is essential, as is involving them in therapy decisions.

Diagnosis

The diagnosis is confirmed when the patient experiences intrusive symptoms and both recurrent and distressing recollections of the event, including recurrent dreams and flashbacks of the event. An additional factor in the diagnosis is the individual's persistent avoidance of stimuli associated with the traumatic experience. The patient usually experiences hyperarousal in the form of rapid heartbeat, dyspnea, and panic.

Children often will reenact the event, have recurrent dreams or nightmares of the event, or have repetitive patterns of the event in their play.

Treatment

The goal of treatment of PTSD is to restore the individual's sense of control. Counseling and drug therapy are used in the treatment. The counseling therapy helps those with PTSD to accept the overwhelming memories without rearranging their lives to avoid the memories. They work to develop a sense of safety and control. Feelings of guilt and self-blame need to be addressed. Cognitive behavior training to increase self-esteem and self-control is employed.

Sleep disturbances must be recognized and treated. Benzodiazepines may be prescribed to help the patient regain normal sleep patterns. In addition, antianxiety agents or SSRIs may be used as drug therapy. Recovery may be complete in some individuals in a short time, whereas others may never recover completely.

Pet therapy is often used to assist in the treatment of PTSD. The animals may be used as a substitute for drug therapy. Animals are nonjudgmental and nonthreatening and are always present for the owner. They are unconditional emotional support.

Prognosis

The prognosis is good with therapy and medications.

Prevention

No prevention is known.

Patient Teaching

Encourage compliance with therapy and medication. Generate print-on-demand electronic materials, when possible, as teaching tools.

Somatoform Disorders

Somatoform disorders are a group of mental disorders in which the person experiences physical symptoms without the underlying organic cause. These symptoms are not under voluntary control and are real to the affected person. The opposite is true of factitious disorders (Munchausen syndrome) or malingering, in which the patient presents with feigned symptoms for personal or emotional gain. There is no confirmed, diagnosable, general medical condition that accounts for the symptoms of somatoform disorders.

Somatization disorder

Description

Somatization disorder is also known as *Briquet syndrome.* This disorder is multisymptomatic, occurring before age 30 years. Extending over a number of years, it is typified by complaints of pain and GI, sexual, and neurotic symptoms without a clinical basis.

> ICD-10-CM Code   F45.0 (Somatization disorder)
> (F45.0-F45.1 = 2 codes of specificity)

Symptoms and Signs

In somatization disorder, the patient experiences multiple, recurring somatic symptoms that have no underlying clinical pathologic basis. These symptoms appear before age 30 years and continue for several years. Symptoms include pain related to four or more areas or functions of the body. In addition, the patient reports GI symptoms (nausea, vomiting, and blood in the stool) other than pain, a symptom related to the reproductive system (e.g., for women, irregular or heavy menses; and for men, erectile or ejaculatory problems), and a neurologic symptom that is without a clinical basis.

Patient Screening

Patients with initial complaints of severe pain and symptoms, as mentioned earlier, should be given the next available appointment. After somatization disorder has been diagnosed, routine appointments can be scheduled. Patients demanding to be seen immediately should be referred to an emergency facility.

Etiology

The etiology is uncertain, but there appears to be a familial pattern. This nonspecific condition tends to have symptoms that intensify after a loss and during periods of severe stress.

Diagnosis

The diagnosis is made after medical conditions are ruled out. Criteria include the presence of four pain symptoms, two GI symptoms, one sexual symptom, and one pseudoneurologic symptom. The onset occurs early in life, before age 30 years, and the condition is chronic, without a symptom-free period of longer than 1 year. Clinically, there is no pathologic change, and no laboratory findings support the symptoms.

Treatment

Treatment includes investigation of symptoms and ruling out of any underlying general medical condition. Psychotherapy including behavior modification is a helpful treatment option.

Prognosis

The prognosis for cure is very poor. This chronic condition rarely has complete remission.

Prevention

Because the etiology is unknown and a familial tendency for the disorder exists, no prevention is known. Encourage the patient to develop skills for dealing with stress.

Patient Teaching

Encourage patients to keep the regularly scheduled appointments. Support the patient through the condition. Explain any diagnostic test results. Generate print-on-demand electronic materials, when possible, as teaching tools.

Conversion disorder

Description

Conversion disorders formerly were termed *hysteria.* Anxiety is changed (converted) to a physical or somatic symptom. The anxiety is too difficult to face, and as a defense mechanism, the physical symptoms allow the person to escape or avoid a stressful situation.

> ICD-10-CM Code   F44.4 (Conversion disorder with
> motor symptom or deficit)
> F44.6 (Conversion disorder with
> sensory symptom or deficit)

Symptoms and Signs

Symptoms include deficits in voluntary motor or sensory functions (paralysis) that are unintentional and preceded by conflicts or other stressors. Clinically significant social and occupational functioning is present.

Sensory symptoms may include anesthesia, hyperesthesia, analgesia, and paresthesia. Motor symptoms may include paralysis, tremors, tics, contractures, and ambulation disturbances. Speech disturbances may include aphonia and mutism, and visceral symptoms may include headaches, difficulty in swallowing and breathing, choking, coughing, nausea, vomiting, belching, cold and clammy extremities, weight loss, and pseudocyesis. Blindness and seizures also may be noted.

Patient Screening

Patients with initial symptomology, as previously described, require prompt attention. Many of the complaints warrant referral to an emergency facility. Careful neurologic and psychological screening will reveal the diagnosis of conversion disorder.

Etiology

The cause of this psychiatric syndrome is usually a highly stressful situation.

Diagnosis

The diagnosis is based on a history of the preceding event and the classic pattern of acute onset of symptoms. A complete physical examination rules out underlying pathologic conditions.

Treatment

Treatment is supportive and symptomatic. The course of this disorder is usually short, with many cases resolving in a few weeks, especially when the stressful situation is eliminated. Recurrence is common. Psychotherapy and hypnosis are treatment options.

Prognosis

The prognosis varies, depending on the intensity of the stress. Most cases do resolve within a few weeks, but recurrence is common.

Prevention

Avoiding extremely stressful situations may prevent the condition.

Patient Teaching

Encourage patients and families to find ways to reduce stressful situations. Help them find support groups, and encourage them to become involved in the groups.

Pain disorder

Description

Pain disorder manifests as pain that causes significant distress and physical and social impairment. This pain is very real to the patient and takes control of the patient's activities.

ICD-10-CM Code	F45.41 *(Pain disorder exclusively related to psychological factors)* (F45.41-F45.42 = 2 codes of specificity)

Symptoms and Signs

Pain disorders include the subtypes that are associated with psychological factors, those associated with both psychological factors and general medical conditions, and those associated with only general medical conditions. The pain is severe and lasting and may have a clinical basis. The response to pain depends on the patient's interpretation, but this type of pain interferes with life activities (e.g., occupational, social, and other areas of functioning). The pain may be associated with musculoskeletal disorders (herniated disk, osteoporosis, and arthritis), neuropathies, and malignancies. Chronic pain often causes depression.

Patient Screening

Pain is very real in these patients. Underlying clinical factors should be assessed. These patients require prompt attention.

Etiology

The pain may be related to underlying clinical pathologic conditions. Psychological factors may play a role in the onset and severity of the pain. Occasionally, both clinical pathologic and psychological factors contribute to the manifestation of the condition. This condition is not intentionally produced, as is malingering.

Diagnosis

Diagnostic studies may reveal pathologic change. Because pain is subjective and pain disorder may or may not have a clinical basis, determining the extent of the pain and psychological involvement is difficult. Longstanding pain may cause depression and even lead to suicide.

Treatment

Any underlying identifiable pathologic change is treated. Patients with terminal disease may be given narcotics to relieve intractable pain. Psychotherapy may be of some help.

Prognosis

The prognosis varies, depending on underlying pathology. Pain of terminal disease may be treated, but the only relief is death.

Prevention

Because this condition is not intentionally produced, prevention depends on the underlying pathology.

Patient Teaching

Patient teaching includes information about accepted methods of pain relief. Suggest to those with intractable pain that they take prescribed pain medication as scheduled, especially before the pain becomes severe. Relaxation techniques along with methods of psychological distraction may help. Pain management clinics have been established to help patients with chronic pain to follow various forms of treatment. These include lifestyle adjustment, relaxation rooms, physical therapy, and group psychotherapy. Generate print-on-demand electronic materials, when possible, as teaching tools.

Hypochondriasis

Description

The patient with hypochondriasis is preoccupied with fear of having a serious disease. The patient has this excessive fear despite negative medical tests and reassurance that there is no clinical basis for the symptoms. Patients mistake body system symptoms or aches and pains without clinical basis for serious illnesses.

> ICD-10-CM Code   F45.21 (Hypochondriasis)
> F45.22 (Body dysmorphic disorder)
> (F45.20-F45.29 = 4 codes of
> specificity)

Symptoms and Signs

Hypochondriasis is characterized by patients' reports and symptoms of possible physical illness without any identifiable evidence of the illness. These patients have a preoccupation with illness and an abnormal fear of disease. The patients provide a generalized history, their symptoms are vague, and they have difficulty with specifics. They do not consciously fake symptoms; these patients really do feel the conditions that they complain about.

Patient Screening

Until underlying clinical causes are eliminated, these patients require prompt attention.

Etiology

The etiology of hypochondriasis is uncertain.

Diagnosis

The diagnosis is difficult because these people change physicians when a health care provider does not affirm their illness. Laboratory and diagnostic studies often reveal no underlying condition. When a condition does exist, it may be overlooked. Social and occupational relationships suffer from the constant abnormal preoccupation with health. The complaints of the disorders will last more than 6 months.

Treatment

Treatment of any underlying conditions is necessary, but these conditions easily can be missed because of the vagueness of the symptoms reported and the changing of health care providers. Some patients may benefit from psychotherapy.

Prognosis

The prognosis varies according to the amenability of the patient to psychotherapy.

Prevention

Because the etiology is uncertain, no specific prevention is known.

Patient Teaching

Encourage the patient to learn to live with the symptoms. A supportive attitude of the health care provider builds confidence. Regular appointments should be scheduled, and the patient should be persuaded to keep these appointments.

Factitious disorder

Description

Factitious disorder, formerly called *Munchausen syndrome*, is a mental illness in which the patient simulates symptoms of illness and presents for no apparent reason other than to get special attention and empathy given to those who are truly ill.

> ICD-10-CM Code   F68.12 (Factitious disorder with
> predominantly physical signs
> and symptoms)
> (F68.10-F69 = 6 codes of
> specificity)

Symptoms and Signs

Patients with factitious disorder know that they are not ill but seek medical attention so that they can draw attention to themselves. They believe they have no other way to get this type of attention. They exaggerate and feign symptoms and actually can make themselves ill by injecting foreign material to cause a fever or doing other things to cause illness. They make up medical histories and may also tamper with instruments or results. These patients generally have extensive knowledge of medical terminology and hospital routines.

Factitious disorder imposed on another occurs when someone, usually a parent, projects the symptoms to the child, usually a preschooler. This parent often stimulates or causes the illness in the child and then presents the child for treatment. The parent denies any knowledge of actual cause and relates the symptoms to be GI, genitourinary, or CNS in nature. As in factitious disorder, the degree of the complaint is limited only by the caregiver or parent's medical knowledge.

Patient Screening

Until underlying clinical causes are eliminated, these patients require prompt attention.

Etiology

The cause of this behavior is uncertain. The patient has no external motive other than to assume the sick role and draw attention to himself or herself.

Diagnosis

These patients present at a hospital or physician's office with reports of fever, anemia, dermatitis, or seizure activity expecting to receive medical attention. The symptoms have an atypical clinical course with laboratory findings that are inconsistent with the symptoms. They have a dramatic flair but give vague answers when questioned closely. When the initial workup indicates no particular disease entity, symptoms change. The patient eagerly undergoes multiple invasive procedures. The patient has a history of repeated hospitalizations with no firm evidence of an underlying disease process. In addition, the patient has no motive of financial gain, only that of attention.

Treatment

Eventually the behavior is revealed, and when these patients are confronted with this fact, they seek attention at another facility. Some physicians believe this condition is untreatable.

Prognosis

The prognosis varies, depending on the duration of the condition. Those who have experienced the condition on a long-term basis are the least amenable to treatment. Intervention is necessary in factitious disorder imposed on another, and in many situations, the child is removed from the care of the adult who is inflicting the source of the illness. This is a form of child abuse.

Prevention

If one could detect the need for attention and then fulfill that need, the disorder might be prevented or at least reduced.

Patient Teaching

A nonjudgmental attitude by the health care provider may help reduce the severity of the condition. Discuss the condition with the family, and advise them that this disorder often requires therapeutic intervention. Generate print-on-demand electronic materials, when possible, as teaching tools.

◆ ENRICHMENT

Malingering

Malingering is the feigning of symptoms for financial or personal gain. The action is deliberate and fraudulent, and the symptoms usually are exaggerated. The patient may report these symptoms to avoid or delay various undesirable events. The diagnosis is difficult because the symptoms often are subjective and cannot be disproved.

Gender Dysphonia

Description

Gender dysphonia or gender identity disorders are conditions in which an individual feels a powerful connection with the opposite sex and wants to be the other sex.

ICD-10-CM Code   F64.2 *(Gender identity disorder of childhood)*
                   F64.1 *(Gender identity disorder in adolescence and adulthood)*
                   (F64.1-F64.9 = 4 codes of specificity)

Symptoms and Signs

Gender identity is a person's inner sense of maleness or femaleness. In this disorder, the person feels as if she or he really should be the opposite sex. Evidence of strong cross-gender identification is present, and the person has a discomfort about the assigned sex. These people also experience a sense of inappropriateness in their gender role.

Boys have a substantial preoccupation with feminine activities, including dressing in feminine clothing and playing with traditionally girl toys. Competitive sports and typical boy activities and play are avoided. Some boys state that they do not want their penis and would prefer to have a vagina.

Girls display a dislike for feminine attire and prefer boy type of clothing and short hair. They prefer boys as playmates and engage in typical boy sports and games. Many claim that they will grow a penis and do not want breast growth or menses.

During adulthood, these persons have a strong desire to adopt the role of the opposite sex and to seek out physical change through hormonal or surgical intervention. They are not comfortable in the gender role defined by society and prefer to act out as the opposite sex. They take on the characteristics of the other sex and dress accordingly.

Regardless of age, many of these patients experience social isolation and ostracism. They frequently have low self-esteem.

Patient Screening

Although not an emergency, gender identity disorder becomes a very important issue in the individual's and his or her parents' lives. When a parent recognizes that the child has a medical issue needing to be addressed and calls for an appointment, one should offer understanding and validation of the issue by scheduling an appointment at the earliest available time.

Etiology

The etiology of the syndrome is uncertain.

Diagnosis

Observation of the behavioral patterns leads to suspicion of gender identity disorder, but there is no known diagnostic test for this syndrome. Psychological evaluation may reveal the tendency. Strong cross-gender identification persists, along with a discomfort with one's sex or a sense of inappropriate gender identification.

Treatment

Psychological counseling to recognize and acknowledge the feelings may be of value. Sex reassignment through hormone treatment and surgical intervention often helps these patients. Unisex bathrooms make such individuals feel more at ease in the office setting.

Prognosis

The prognosis varies, depending on the extent of the feeling and the extent of the action taken. Many sex change surgical procedures are successful when accompanied by intense psychotherapy. Family and employment relationships may affect the success of treatment.

Prevention

No prevention is known.

Patient Teaching

Help the patient to find support groups. Encourage family members to accept the condition as an illness and thereby accept the patient's choice, which will help the patient. Generate print-on-demand electronic materials, when possible, as teaching tools.

Sleep Disorders

Sleep disorders include insomnia, parasomnias, sleep apnea, and narcolepsy. Sleep disorders are assessed through polysomnography, which measures rapid eye movement (REM) and the four non-rapid eye movement (NREM) sleep stages: stages 1, 2, 3, and 4. Stage 1 NREM sleep is considered transitional and occupies 5% of normal sleep time. Stage 2 occupies about 50% of normal sleep time and is a deeper sleep. Stages 3 and 4 (slow-wave sleep) are the deepest states and occupy 10% to 20% of sleep time. Stages 3 and 4 lessen in duration with aging and even disappear in some people older than age 55 years. The average adult requires 6 to 8 hours of continuous sleep, with younger people requiring more and older adults needing less.

The disorders can be caused by functional or organic disorders, so underlying pathologic conditions must be ruled out or treated.

Insomnia

Description

The individual experiencing insomnia has difficulty in falling asleep and/or staying asleep.

ICD-10-CM Code	G47.00 *(Insomnia, unspecified)*
	(G47.00-G47.09 = 3 codes of specificity)

Symptoms and Signs

Insomnia, difficulty in falling asleep or staying asleep, tends to cause the individual to feel physically and mentally tired, groggy, tense, irritable, and anxious on awakening. In addition, some people experience extremely early morning awakening and report that their sleep was not restorative.

Patient Screening

Although not an emergency, chronic insomnia becomes a very important issue in the individual's life. When the patient recognizes that he or she has a medical issue needing to be addressed and calls for an appointment, the health care provider understands and validates the issue by scheduling an appointment at the earliest available time.

Etiology

The cause may be related to a situation, a medical problem, or time zone changes (e.g., jet lag), or the cause may be a change to high altitudes. Additional causes are pain, cardiovascular problems, thyroid conditions, and fever. Stimulants, including caffeine, amphetamines, steroids, alcohol, nicotine, and bronchodilators, tend to cause drug-related insomnia. Psychological causes include anxiety, stress, and even the fear of sleeplessness itself.

The older generation, shift workers, travelers experiencing jet lag, and those with chronic pain often experience periods of difficulty sleeping. Other causative factors may be environmentally related and include room temperature that is too hot or too cold, noise, brightness or light, an uncomfortable bed, or a sleep partner who snores, is restless, or has restless legs syndrome.

Diagnosis

To be diagnosed as insomnia, the sleeplessness must have been present for longer than 1 month and must interfere with normal functioning in social, occupational, or other areas. A study is conducted of the 24-hour sleep and wakefulness periods, along with an examination of any underlying factors. Polysomnography, a recording of several physiologic variables related to sleep made while the patient is sleeping, indicates poor sleep patterns, including increased stage 1 and reduced stage 3 and 4 periods, along with increased muscle tremors. The patient appears fatigued and exhibits no other abnormalities. The incidence of insomnia increases with age and is higher in women.

Treatment

The first step in treatment is to identify and remove the cause; this is followed by an attempt to improve sleep hygiene. Patients are counseled to change their lifestyle to relieve tension and reduce stress. They are encouraged to keep a regular sleep schedule, to consider the bedroom only for sleep, and not to worry about stressful situations. Noise and disruptions during the normal sleep time should be eliminated, and daily activities should be increased. Caffeine, nicotine, and stimulants should be avoided in late afternoon and evening. Strenuous physical exercise also should be avoided in the few hours before retiring. A darkened and quiet environment would help. The patient should keep a regular bedtime and a regular time for arising. Psychotherapy may be indicated to help relieve anxiety and stress. As a last resort, hypnotics of the benzodiazepine class may be prescribed. Although benzodiazepines are still used for this purpose, a newer class of hypnotics is used more often for sleep disorders. Zolpidem (Ambien), zaleplon (Sonata), eszopiclone (Lunesta), and ramelteon (Rozerem) are medications used to induce restful sleep. Other therapies include use of melatonin, trazodone, and benzodiazepines. When these do not work, patients usually are referred to sleep disorder clinics.

Prognosis

The prognosis varies, depending on the cause. Adjusting late afternoon and early evening activities and eliminating any drugs that interfere with sleep may relieve insomnia.

A favorable outcome depends on the patient's ability to modify the sleep environment and to reduce stressors.

Prevention

Eliminating the ingestion of caffeine, nicotine, and other stimulants during late afternoon and evening hours helps prevent insomnia. Developing good sleep habits, such as keeping regular hours to retire, also helps in prevention. Avoiding watching television or reading in bed also may prevent insomnia.

Patient Teaching

Instruct patients about normal sleep patterns and about avoiding caffeine, nicotine, and other stimulants in the late afternoon and evening hours. As previously mentioned, patients should be encouraged to avoid the habit of watching television or reading in bed. Help them to identify environmental changes they could make to improve the sleep environment. Generate print on demand electronic materials, when possible, as teaching tools.

Parasomnias

Description

Parasomnias are a group of sleep disorders that include sleepwalking, night terrors, and nightmares. Parasomnias may also be termed *sleep arousal disorders* and often include dreams.

ICD-10-CM Code	G47.9 *(Sleep disorder, unspecified)* (G47.50-G47.9 = 12 codes of specificity)

Symptoms and Signs

Parasomnias usually occur in children early in the night. When they affect older adults and have a late onset, a CNS pathologic process is responsible. People who sleepwalk generally have no memory of the event. They awake confused, with blank expressions on their faces, and are unaware of the environment. Those experiencing nightmares often have vivid recall and remember dreams of fear of attack, falling, and death. These dreams occur late at night.

Patient Screening

Although usually not an emergency, parasomnia becomes a very important issue in the individual's life. When the patient recognizes that he or she has a medical issue that

needs to be addressed and calls for an appointment, the health care provider should understand and validate the issue by scheduling an appointment at the earliest available time. When safety is an issue, prompt attention is essential.

Etiology

Several elements, including possible genetic, developmental, psychological, and organic factors, may precipitate the incidents. Febrile episodes or brain tumors may be causes. Lithium and certain drugs precipitate the condition. There is evidence that certain medications cause increased REM sleep periods and rebound REM sleep.

Diagnosis

Reports of the episodes lead to further investigation. A thorough history should include any drug consumption. Any underlying cause in older adults and mature adults should be investigated and diagnosed.

Treatment

Protection from injury is primary for the sleepwalking person. The sleepwalking person should not be interrupted or awakened. Minimizing the exposure to terror, especially from movies, videos, and television programs, reduces the occurrence of night terrors. Children usually outgrow these conditions. Adults often are treated initially with zolpidem or zaleplon, because these drugs do not leave patients feeling drugged when they wake up in the morning. When drugs are suspected as a contributing factor, alternative drug therapy is considered.

Prognosis

The prognosis varies, depending on the cause. Many children will outgrow parasomnia. When the etiology is drug related, eliminating the causative drug helps.

Prevention

Minimizing stimulating factors, such as exposure to frightening movies, helps prevent this condition. Additionally, having a regular bedtime and a comfortable environment conducive to sleep and avoiding caffeine and other stimulants is helpful in prevention.

Patient Teaching

Family members should be advised not to interrupt or attempt to awaken the sleepwalking person. Parents are advised to use caution when discussing terrorist activities or catastrophic events and to prevent children from hearing about such events.

Narcolepsy

Description

Narcolepsy, irresistible daytime sleep episodes, can have duration of a few seconds to a half hour.

ICD-10-CM Code	G47.419 *(Narcolepsy without cataplexy)* (G47.411-G47.429 = 4 codes of specificity)

Symptoms and Signs

Narcolepsy, a chronic neurologic condition, is an overwhelming recurring compulsion to fall asleep. Usually precipitated by sedentary, monotonous activity, narcolepsy attacks occur while driving, sitting in a lecture, or even eating. The onset normally is before age 25 years. A period of sleep paralysis lasts about 1 minute; the person is unable to move, but breathing continues.

Patient Screening

The patient experiencing episodes of narcolepsy requires prompt attention.

Etiology

The condition appears to have a familial incidence, and those with narcolepsy may have a genetic aberration in REM sleep time.

Diagnosis

The history of repeated episodes suggests narcolepsy. Seizure activity and sleep apnea should be ruled out. The onset usually is during adolescence, producing disturbed night sleep. Sleep studies help in confirming the diagnosis.

Treatment

The patient should take therapeutic naps and establish a normal night sleep pattern. Drug therapy helps. Stimulants including methylphenidate and dextroamphetamine are prescribed. Modafinil (Provigil) and armodafinil (Nuvigil) are nonamphetamine stimulants and wakefulness-promoting drugs and may be prescribed for excessive daytime sleepiness. These patients must be warned of the dangers of falling asleep while driving or operating machinery. This chronic disorder is not under voluntary control.

Prognosis

The prognosis varies, depending on the adaptation techniques the patient develops. The patient's response and tolerance to drug therapy also may dictate the outcome of this condition.

Prevention

No prevention is known.

Patient Teaching

Patients and families should be told that this is a disease that may be treatable. They also need to understand the dangers that could arise, however, if the narcolepsy occurs while driving or operating machinery. Students are encouraged to discuss this condition with counselors and request special assistance in the classroom setting. Patients may be helped by scheduling classes for times when they are not sleepy. They should enlist the help of another student in note taking.

Those who are in the workplace should look for jobs that will keep them active and allow for interaction with others. Patients should avoid jobs that require them to make long drives or operate dangerous equipment. Encourage and help both patients and families to become involved in support groups.

Sleep apnea

Description

Sleep apnea is intermittent short periods of breathing cessation during sleep.

ICD-10-CM Code	G47.30 *(Sleep apnea, unspecified)*
	(G47.30 G47.39 = 9 codes of specificity)

Symptoms and Signs

Sleep apnea is considered a potentially life-threatening condition. During normal nocturnal sleep, the patient has periods in which breathing ceases, followed by snorting and gasping. This condition occurs more often in men than in women and may be associated with obesity, hypertension, or an airway obstructive condition. The patient does not feel rested even after several hours of sleep.

Sleep apnea may be categorized as either obstructive or central. The more common type is obstructive, in which air is unable to flow in or out of the upper airway. Attempts to breathe continue. During central episodes, the brain does not send appropriate messages to the intercostal muscles and the diaphragm to initiate the breathing process. The patient can experience 20 or more periods of apnea in 1 hour. The individual with sleep apnea occasionally will complain of choking episodes.

Patient Screening

The patient experiencing episodes of sleep apnea requires prompt attention.

Etiology

Patients appear to have an inherent predisposition to this condition. Nasal obstruction often is the cause. Alcohol ingestion, smoking-related bronchitis, and sleep deprivation are other causes. Obesity can cause extra tissue to develop in the throat, creating a mechanical obstruction. As levels of oxygen (O_2) drop and levels of carbon dioxide (CO_2) increase, the brain is alerted to stimulate the breathing process, and the individual usually gasps for air.

Diagnosis

The diagnosis begins with a sleep history. The onset usually occurs in middle age. Daytime sleepiness, sleep attacks, and snoring and snorting episodes also suggest sleep apnea. Sleep laboratory studies and polysomnography confirm the diagnosis by observing periods of breathing cessation while the patient is sleeping (Fig. 14.21).

Treatment

Weight loss is encouraged. Protriptyline is prescribed. Continuous positive air pressure (CPAP) or dental appliances may be tried (Fig. 14.22). Any underlying pathologic condition should be diagnosed and corrected. The patient is

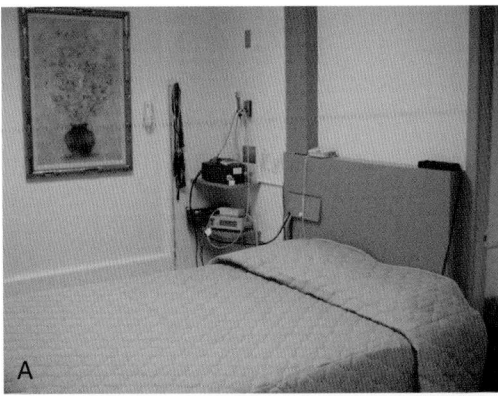

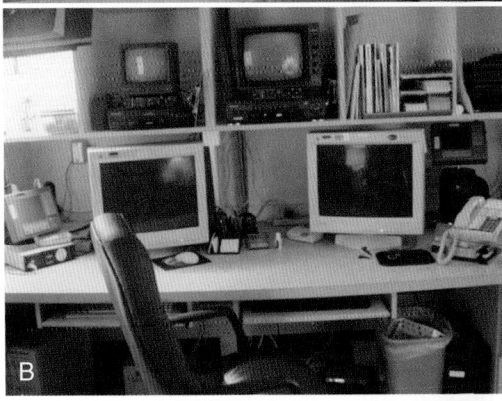

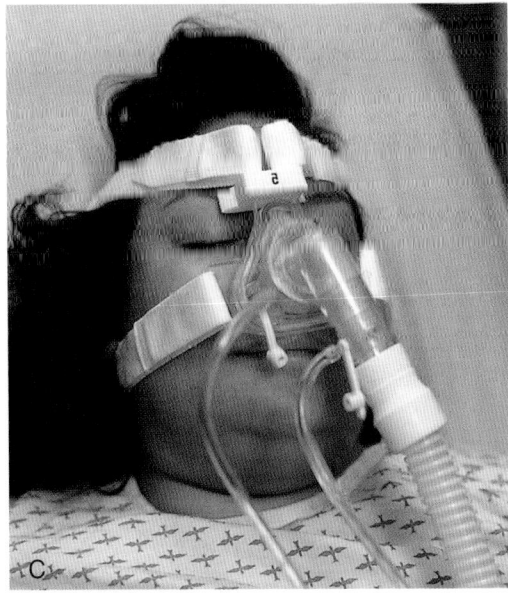

• **Fig. 14.21** (A and B) Sleep laboratory. (C) Nasal CPAP mask. (A and B, Courtesy Saint Joseph's Hospital, Fort Wayne, IN, 2003. C, From Cobbett SL, et al: *Canadian clinical nursing skills & techniques,* St Louis, 2020, Elsevier.)

advised to avoid the use of any drugs that depress the CNS. Uvulopalatopharyngoplasty (UPPP), a surgical procedure to remove portions of the uvula, soft palate, and posterior pharyngeal mucosa, is attempted as a last resort. Alcohol, tobacco, and sedatives tend to cause collapse of the upper airway passages during sleep and therefore should be avoided.

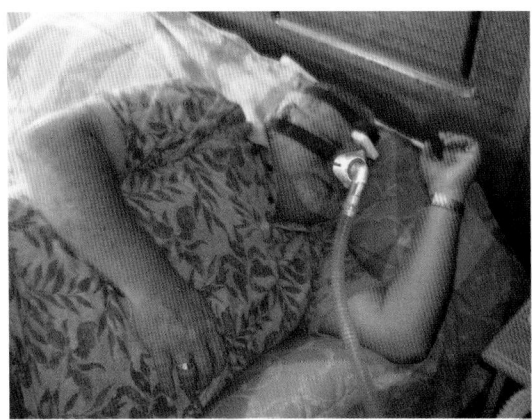

• **Fig. 14.22** Patient using continuous positive airway pressure (CPAP). (Courtesy David L. Frazier, 2003.)

Prognosis
The prognosis varies, depending on the cause. When overweight patients lose weight, they often experience significant improvement. Use of CPAP usually relieves symptoms and reduces the danger of respiratory arrest.

Prevention
No prevention is known.

Patient Teaching
Patients using CPAP will need instructions on the use of the equipment. If overweight, they should be encouraged to lose weight. Offer weight-reduction diets, or help the patient find support groups. Use customized electronically generated educational materials, when available, to reinforce the treatment plan.

Personality Disorders

Description
A personality disorder is a pattern of behavior that deviates from society's norms. In addition, a person with a personality disorder typically has thoughts about the self and the world that cause inappropriate behavior. Signs of a personality disorder become evident in adolescence. There are 10 named personality disorders, categorized into three clusters. These clusters are cluster A, patients who appear odd or eccentric; cluster B, patients who appear dramatic, emotional, or erratic; and cluster C, patients who appear anxious and fearful.

ICD-10-CM Code   **Cluster A**
F60.0 *(Paranoid personality disorder)*
F60.1 *(Schizoid personality disorder)*
F21 *(Schizotypal disorder)*
Cluster B
F60.2 *(Antisocial personality disorder)*
F60.3 *(Borderline personality disorder)*
F60.4 *(Histrionic personality disorder)*
F60.81 *(Narcissistic personality disorder)*

Cluster C

F60.6 *(Avoidant personality disorder)*

F60.7 *(Dependent personality disorder)*

F60.5 *(Obsessive-compulsive personality disorder)*

F60.9 *(Personality disorder, unspecified)*

Symptoms and Signs

Personality disorders influence the mental affect of a person and produce chronic, ingrained, maladaptive behavior. Disordered patterns of relating, thinking, and perceiving impair social and occupational performance. Personality disorders typically begin to appear in adolescence. Personality disorders should not be diagnosed until adulthood. A history of longstanding problems in interpersonal relationships and occupational difficulties is likely. Personality traits may give the person a reputation of arrogance or painful shyness and of rejecting responsibility for his or her behavior. The person tends to project negative feelings and blame others. Many types of personality disorders are recognized, each with unique distinguishing characteristics. Examples of personality disorders include **paranoid**, **schizoid**, antisocial, histrionic, and **narcissistic** disorders.

Antisocial disorder

Behavior patterns of the antisocial personality cause frequent conflicts with societal values. Troublesome conduct usually emerges by age 15 years, with truancy, fighting, stealing, a history of running away, or cruel behavior. Antisocial persons do not express guilt or learn from their mistakes. Other traits include a propensity for irresponsible and impulsive actions.

Cluster A

Cluster A personality disorders should be assessed and distinguished from delusional disorders and psychotic disorders.

Paranoid Personality Disorder

Those with paranoid personality disorder do not trust others and are suspicious of others. They assume others will exploit, harm, or deceive them. Individuals with paranoid personality disorder often misinterpret the meaning behind others' behaviors by thinking others are deliberately trying to exploit them.

Schizoid Personality Disorder

Individuals with schizoid personality disorder (SPD) appear to lack, or show emotions of, pleasure or pain. They tend to be loners and do not enjoy relationships with others. They appear to be indifferent, flattened, or detached.

Schizotypal Personality Disorder

Persons with schizotypal personality disorder are similar to those with SPD in that they have difficulty with social relationships. Individuals with schizotypal personality disorder, however, typically have ideas of reference; they may be superstitious or preoccupied with paranoid phenomena. In addition, they may believe they have magical control over others. More often, they seek treatment for associated symptoms of anxiety or depression.

Cluster B

Antisocial Personality Disorder

Individuals with antisocial personality disorder (APD) have a disregard for, and tend to violate, the rights of others. They fail to conform to societal norms and often engage in behavior that could be grounds for arrest. These individuals are aggressive, manipulative, and reckless. They generally do not show remorse or make amends for their behavior.

Borderline Personality Disorder

A person with borderline personality disorder (BPD) has a pattern of unstable interpersonal relationships, self-image, and affects (feelings). Impending separation or rejection are central concerns for individuals with BPD. When those with BPD believe they are being rejected or abandoned, they often react with extreme emotions, such as anger, panic, or despair. They may display extreme sarcasm and verbal outbursts. They are impulsive and manipulative in their behavior.

Histrionic Disorder

Individuals with histrionic disorder display overly dramatic and theatrical mannerisms. They have a conscious or unconscious pervasive need to be the center of attention. People with this disorder are immature and dependent, constantly seeking approval and reassurance. Behavior or appearance may be inappropriately seductive.

Narcissistic Disorder

The narcissistic personality demonstrates pathologic self-love or grandiose self-admiration. When criticized, the person reacts with rage or humiliation, based on an exaggerated sense of self-importance. These individuals lack empathy and tend to exploit others. They exhibit preoccupation with fantasies of unlimited success.

Cluster C

Avoidant Personality Disorder

The person with avoidant personality disorder avoids any social situation because of fears of criticism, disapproval, or rejection. Individuals with avoidant personality disorder view themselves as socially inept, personally unappealing, and inferior to others. They are preoccupied with being judged or criticized by their peers.

Dependent Personality Disorder

Individuals with dependent personality disorder (DPD) have a pattern of excessively relying on others to make decisions for them. They are passive and have trouble disagreeing with others because they fear losing support or approval.

Obsessive-Compulsive Personality Disorder

Individuals with obsessive-compulsive personality disorder have an extreme pattern of preoccupation with orderliness, perfection, and mental and interpersonal control. They are preoccupied with details or lists to the point that they never finish a task.

Patient Screening

Individuals displaying these behaviors or family members reporting the behavior and requesting an appointment should be given an appointment as soon as convenient.

Etiology

The cause of personality disorders has not been identified. Various theories include possible biologic, social, or psychodynamic origins.

Diagnosis

The diagnosis of personality disorders is based on the documentation of diagnostic criteria defined in DSM-V.

Treatment

The treatment of personality disorders depends on the symptoms and includes psychotherapy and, in some cases, drug therapy. Pharmacologic treatments are often prescribed to address specific symptoms demonstrated by the individual. For example, antidepressants may be helpful for those with a depressed or labile mood. Improved coping mechanisms and control of symptoms are the goals of therapy. A trusting relationship between patient and therapist is advantageous, because some people with these disorders tend to be noncompliant and resist therapy. Specialized psychotherapy incorporating specific limits and boundaries (dialectical behavioral training [DBT]) has been shown to be effective in helping these clients feel more secure and in control. Hospitalization may be required during acute episodes that incapacitate the person. Family involvement in group therapy has proved beneficial for some patients. Treatment of comorbid conditions, such as anxiety and depression, with medications is essential. Personality disorders themselves do not respond to drug therapy.

Prognosis

The prognosis for cure is very poor. Treatment of comorbid conditions improves outcome. Long-term treatment is necessary.

Prevention

Treatment in adolescence when symptoms first appear and ongoing treatment into adulthood seem to lessen the frequency of behaviors. No prevention is known.

Patient Teaching

Compliance with continued treatment and drug therapy is an issue. Encourage the patient to continue with treatment and drug therapy. Use customized electronically generated educational materials, when available, to reinforce the treatment plan.

Review Challenge

Answer the following questions:
1. What are the contributing factors to mental disorders?
2. What observations may indicate intellectual developmental disorder??
3. What variants are considered in the diagnosis of a learning disorder?
4. What are the characteristics of a child with autism?
5. What are the diagnostic criteria for attention-deficit/hyperactivity disorder (ADHD)?
6. What are the diagnostic criteria for a tic disorder?
7. Under what conditions may dementia occur?
8. Why is Alzheimer disease so difficult to diagnose?
9. How may vascular dementia be related to atherosclerosis?
10. How might head trauma cause dementia?
11. How does repeated heavy alcohol abuse harm the body?
12. What are some effects of a rising blood alcohol level on the brain?
13. Why is schizophrenia considered a major psychiatric disturbance?
14. How do bipolar disorders affect an individual?
15. What is thought to cause a major depressive disorder?
16. What are the phases of the grief process?
17. What are some of the longstanding problems typical of personality disorders?
18. How are the major anxiety disorders classified? How do they differ from each other?
19. What condition may result as a delayed response to an external painful event?
20. What is a somatization disorder?
21. How is anxiety related to a conversion disorder?
22. What condition results from preoccupation with illness and abnormal fear of disease?
23. Can severe pain cause illness?
24. How is factitious disorder diagnosed?
25. What is the typical pattern of sleep disorder in (1) insomnia, (2) narcolepsy, and (3) sleep apnea?
26. What are the three clusters of the 10 personality disorders?

Real-Life Challenge: Alzheimer Disease

A 75-year-old man is diagnosed with Alzheimer disease. The retired businessman noticed many memory lapses, primarily in the area of short-term memory and the inability to concentrate. His family states that his verbalization appears somewhat diminished in that he has difficulty expressing his thoughts in an appropriate manner and interjects nonsensical phrases. He becomes agitated quite easily and has very little interest in grooming and self-appearance. The family has been advised that they may need help in the future to care for the patient and that he probably will have to be institutionalized.

Because the patient has exhibited both cognitive and behavioral symptoms of Alzheimer disease, he is treated with donepezil (Aricept) and alprazolam (Xanax).

Questions

1. Who is most likely to exhibit symptoms of Alzheimer disease?
2. List the typical symptoms.
3. What interventions may be taken?
4. What are some of the theories that have been advanced regarding the cause of Alzheimer disease?

5. How is Alzheimer disease diagnosed?
6. What is the anticipated prognosis for this patient?
7. What differentiates Alzheimer disease from senile dementia?
8. To what class of drugs does Xanax belong and what is the expected outcome of its administration?

Real-Life Challenge: Sleep Apnea

The wife of a 48-year-old man complains that she cannot sleep because of her husband's loud snoring. Questioning reveals she has noticed that he appears to stop breathing for periods of about 30 seconds when sleeping. The patient has a history of mild alcohol consumption and also of smoking. He is approximately 30 pounds overweight.

Sleep studies are ordered because sleep apnea is suspected. He also says he does not feel rested after sleeping 8 to 9 hours a night.

Questions

1. What is the significance of the loud snoring?
2. Why is a history of social habits (smoking and alcohol consumption) important?
3. What are sleep studies?

4. What may happen if the sleep apnea is not diagnosed?
5. Which treatment may be prescribed?
6. What is the anticipated outcome of the treatment?

Internet Assignments

Ascertain what services are available at the Alzheimer Association for families of individuals diagnosed with Alzheimer disease. Write a report listing and explaining these services and how the family may obtain the services.

Locate meeting sites for Alcoholics Anonymous (AA) in your community and the regular meeting times and days.

Critical Thinking

1. List some of the methods of play that a therapist might use with children who have been abused.
2. List some of the causes of intellectual developmental disorder.
3. What are acceptable terms to describe intelligence based on the intelligence quotient (IQ) determined by the Stanford-Binet test?
4. What are some of the suggested ways to prevent intellectual developmental disorder?
5. Learning disorders, conditions that cause children to learn in a manner that is not normal, affect performance on standardized tests causing lower than expected scores for age, schooling, and intelligence level as a result of the brain's ability to receive and process information. List and define some of the learning disorders.
6. What might be some of the psychological effects on the individual with learning disorders even after childhood? How may the diagnosis of learning disorders affect the family? How does this diagnosis affect the educational system?

7. Children often exhibit difficulties in communication. These disorders may be psychologically based and are a variety of expressive language disorders, including mixed receptive or expressive language disorders. List some of the disorders along with how they may affect the child, the parents, the rest of the family, and the educational system
8. The individual who experiences stuttering may be made fun of in school. What might the school do about this form of "bullying"?
9. What is the prognosis for the autistic individual in society?
10. List some of the symptoms of attention-deficit/hyperactivity disorder (ADHD). How may this disorder affect individuals in adult life?
11. Oppositional defiant disorder (ODD) is a strong predictor of poor outcomes in children. List some of the possible poor outcomes.
12. List and describe some of the tic disorders.

13. An older individual has been diagnosed with early onset dementia. The person's judgment and reaction times are slightly reduced. How would you approach the topic of cessation of driving?
14. List possible causes of dementia.
15. Alcoholism contributes to many crises in life. List some of the problems. How does alcoholism affect your community?
16. The misuse of various drugs that modify mood or behavior is called *drug abuse.* List various drugs that are commonly abused. How are these drugs obtained? What is the effect of drug abuse on your community?
17. What are some of the effects of drug abuse on the individual and the family?
18. How does schizophrenia affect the individual? What is a prognosis for the individual who has been diagnosed with schizophrenia?
19. In a mood disorder, a person experiences a pathologic disturbance in mood that affects all aspects of his or her life. List the mood disorders.
20. What is meant by a manic episode? List some of the activities an individual experiencing a manic episode may do.
21. What is the opposite of a manic episode? How does this affect the individual's life?
22. What is a major concern for the individual experiencing major depressive disorder?
23. How does depression affect the individual's family? How does it affect his or her employment?
24. What are causes of major depression disorder?
25. List types of depression, their causes, and possible outcomes of the disorders.
26. What may be the cause of panic disorder?
27. List phobias, and describe how they are treated.
28. Posttraumatic stress disorders (PTSDs) are different from other anxiety disorders because the cause of the stress is an external event of an overwhelmingly painful nature. List some of the reactions of individuals experiencing PTSD.
29. How is PTSD treated? How does this disorder affect your community?
30. What are somatoform disorders? List the types and describe their symptoms.
31. How does factitious disorder affect the family?
32. How are individuals experiencing gender identity difficulties accepted in the families and their community?
33. List the types of parasomnias.
34. What are treatment options for sleep apnea?
35. Personality disorders are patterns of behavior that deviate from society's norms. There are three clusters of these disorders. List the three clusters and each disorder within the cluster.
36. Research gender dysphoria, and create an informational handout for patients to share with their family members and friends.

Prepare to discuss Critical Thinking case study exercises for this chapter that are posted on Evolve.

15

Disorders and Conditions Resulting from Trauma

CHAPTER OUTLINE

Trauma, 621
    Open Trauma, 621
    Foreign Bodies, 626
    Thermal Insults, 630

Bites, 640
Cumulative Trauma (Repetitive Motion Trauma, Overuse Syndrome), 646
Physical and Psychological Assault Trauma, 651

LEARNING OBJECTIVES

After studying Chapter 15, you should be able to:

1. List the major types of trauma.
2. List the environmental factors that may result in trauma or other conditions.
3. Distinguish between an abrasion and an avulsion injury.
4. Describe conditions that require prophylaxis with tetanus toxoid.
5. Name three factors that generally need to be addressed in open trauma.
6. Explain the risk of puncture wounds to health care workers.
7. Describe management of foreign bodies in the ear, eye, and nose.
8. Name the conditions classified as thermal insults.
9. Explain the "rule of nines" in adults with burns and how it is used.
10. Describe the possible injuries caused by (1) electrical shock and (2) lightning.
11. Define *hypothermia* and list those most at risk.
12. Describe the guidelines for treating (1) frostbite, (2) insect bites, and (3) snakebites.
13. Discuss various conditions resulting from cumulative trauma.
14. Explain the pathology that results in the pain and numbness of carpal tunnel syndrome.
15. Explain the importance of immediate intervention in shaken infant (baby) syndrome.
16. Name the best management strategies for child abuse and neglect and elder abuse and neglect.
17. Discuss special concerns in the diagnosis of (1) intimate partner violence (IPV), (2) sexual abuse, and (3) rape/sexual assault.
18. Discuss the signs of impending suicide and possible interventions.

KEY TERMS

abrasion (ah-**BRAY**-shun)
analgesic (**an**-ahl-**GEE**-sik)
antipyretic (an-tee-pye-**RET**-tic)
antiseptic (**an**-tih-**SEP**-tic)
avulsion (ah-**VUL**-shun)
cautery (**KAW**-ter-ee)
débride (day-**BREED**)
ergonomic (**er**-go-**NOM**-ic)

hyperabduction (**high**-per-ab-**DUCK**-shun)
hyperthermia (**high**-per-**THERM**-ee-ah)
hypothermia (**high**-poh-**THERM**-ee-ah)
laceration (**lass**-er-**AY**-shun)
prophylaxis (proh-fih-**LACK**-sis)
tendinitis (**ten**-deh-**NYE**-tis)
vector (**VECK**-tor)

Trauma

Although they are not specific disease entities, traumatic occurrences do include physical and psychological injuries that are derived from external force or violence; trauma may be self-inflicted, accidental, or the result of an act of violence. Regardless of the cause, trauma can interfere with body functions or the homeostatic status of the body, it can inflict a permanent disability, or it may be life threatening. Major types are open trauma, assault trauma, thermal trauma, and psychological trauma. Whether physical or emotional, trauma (including abuse and sexual attack) is prevalent in every society. Physical trauma is a leading cause of death in the United States among people ages 1 to approximately 44 years.

Environmental factors sometimes result in traumatic circumstances. Weather-related conditions are often contributing factors in the occurrence of thermal insults and motor vehicle accidents (MVAs), along with accidents involving other types of machinery or accidents caused by natural elements (e.g., lightning strikes or tornadoes). Severe wind and changes in barometric pressure are responsible for trauma to the tissues and to the respiratory system in those exposed to these elements. Poisons may come from contaminated ground water, toxins in the air, ingestion of seafood gathered from contaminated locations, or chemical spills. Bites from animals, insects, reptiles, or humans may occur under particular environmental circumstances. High altitudes also can affect body functions. Precaution and prevention are of primary concern whenever people are subjected to potentially traumatic circumstances.

Triage means "to sort or pick" and is a process used to determine the severity of injury or illness in each patient who enters any medical facility. The goal of an effective triage system is rapid identification of patients' needs and the ability to identify urgent and life-threatening conditions.) Placing a patient in the right place at the right time to use the proper resources and appropriate level of health care to meet the patient's medical needs is mandatory. A system should be in place in every medical facility to provide a communication system and support team to facilitate the needs of the patient. Trauma centers can provide specialized critical care on a 24-hour basis for those seriously injured. Services include a specially trained medical team, medical devices to provide intensive care measures, and a facility equipped for surgical intervention, if needed.

Open Trauma

Open trauma may involve only the skin surface, or it may extend to the soft tissue and structures far below the skin surface. It may be in the form of an abrasion, in which the skin surface is scraped away, or it may be an avulsion, in which the tissue or an appendage is torn away. The injury can involve only a small area of the skin, as with a puncture wound, a slightly larger area as in an injury caused by a missile, or encompass substantially larger areas, as with crushing injuries. All incidents of open trauma have a commonality:, the risk of infection if the wound is not appropriately cleansed and dressed. Pain also is usually involved in most open trauma.

Open wounds can be the source of tetanus infection; therefore tetanus prophylaxis must be provided. Those who have completed the initial inoculation series for tetanus require a booster dose every 10 years. Those with no previous inoculation history are given tetanus immune globulin (human) and referred to a physician for the complete series of tetanus toxoid inoculations. When the patient has not had a booster injection within the past 10-year period, the booster injection of tetanus, diphtheria, and pertussis (Tdap) is recommended and/or administered.

Bleeding can be a factor in open trauma and must be addressed at once. Some injuries need only basic first aid, whereas others require medical intervention and surgical repair. Regardless of the severity of the injury, appropriate treatment aids healing and lessens scarring. Orthopedic and neurologic traumas are addressed in Chapters 7 and 13, respectively.

Abrasions

Description

Abrasions have occurred when the outer layers of the skin have been scraped away or roughed up and deeper layers are exposed.

| ICD-9-CM Code | 919.0 (Abrasion or friction burn without mention of infection) |
| ICD-10-CM Code | T07 (Unspecified multiple injuries) |

(Injuries/wounds are coded by site and type. Since the diagnosis has been confirmed, refer to the current editions of the ICD-9-CM and ICD-10-CM coding manuals for the appropriate code.)

Symptoms and Signs

The injured area appears raw and reddened, is painful, and has a small amount of bleeding (Fig. 15.1).

The exposure of sensitive nerve endings causes a burning type of pain in the injured area; small foreign particles may be embedded in it.

Patient Screening

Abrasions require prompt cleansing. Current tetanus prophylaxis should be confirmed.

Etiology

Abrasions are caused by friction created when a rough, hard surface comes in contact with skin as a consequence of a scraping or sliding type of motion, often the result of a fall or scrape. An example is when a child falls off a bicycle and "skins" the knee. Such injuries are often referred to as *friction burns*, *floor burns*, *rug burns*, or *road rash*.

Diagnosis

Diagnosis is made on the basis of subjective information (what the patient says), history, and visual inspection.

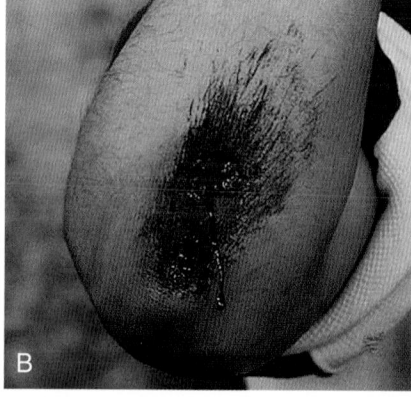

• **Fig. 15.1** Abrasion. (A) Outer layers of the skin are scraped away. (B) Abrasion wounds of the elbow. (From Browner BD, Fuller RP: *Musculoskeletal emergencies,* Philadelphia, 2012, Saunders.)

Treatment

Treatment consists of gentle washing and irrigation of the area with a germicidal soap and water to remove any bacteria and contamination. Any foreign particles, such as gravel and dirt, which have not been removed by cleansing should be removed carefully with forceps. Failure to remove foreign particles left in the skin can stain the epidermis and cause scars or a tattoo. Next a germicidal ointment or cream may be applied. A dressing may be applied as well, depending on the size and location of the abrasion. Prophylaxis with Tdap injection is confirmed or administered, if necessary. Benzocaine spray, a topical anesthetic can be purchased over the counter and used to lessen the pain when an abrasion or similar wound needs cleaning.

Prognosis

The prognosis for healing is good once cleansing to remove any foreign bodies or bacteria is accomplished. The extent of scarring depends on the depth and extent of the insult.

Prevention

Prevention is difficult, especially in active individuals. Protective gear or leather clothing worn sometimes by cyclists helps prevent extensive "road rash" abrasions.

Patient Teaching

Instruct the patient regarding appropriate wound care and the importance of keeping the wound clean and dry. Reinforce the value of maintaining up-to-date tetanus prophylaxis. Instruct the patient to avoid direct sunlight and to protect the new fragile skin with sunscreen or clothing for 6 months to prevent pigment changes in the skin. Provide written instructions to the patient regarding signs and symptoms of infection and when to report concerns. Generate print-on-demand electronic materials as teaching tools, when possible, to explain or depict proper applications of dressings.

Avulsion

Description

With avulsion injuries, a portion of the skin and possibly underlying tissue is torn away, either completely or partially (Fig. 15.2). At times, the injury may include separation of the bone area, which is a more serious injury.

ICD-10-CM Code	S31.000A *(Unspecified open wound of lower back and pelvis without penetration into retroperitoneum, initial encounter)*

Open wounds are coded by site and type. Once the diagnosis has been confirmed, refer to the current edition of the ICD-10-CM coding manual for the appropriate code.

Symptoms and Signs

An avulsion injury can involve a limb, an appendage, or any soft tissue area anywhere on the surface of the body. The patient usually has severe pain in the area. Bleeding from the wound is common. When the avulsion is partial, the avulsed tissue is still partially attached to the injured area. Larger avulsed areas are considered a serious injury and may require split-thickness grafting. One type of severe avulsion is a "degloving" injury, in which the full thickness of skin is peeled away from the body, such as the skin on the hand or foot.

Patient Screening

Avulsion injuries require prompt cleansing and closure of the open wound. When the avulsed tissue is available (i.e., still partially attached to the body or retrieved from the accident site, as in the case of a severed fingertip) and reattachment is possible, the surgical procedure is performed as quickly as possible. Current tetanus prophylaxis should be confirmed.

Etiology

The mechanism of this kind of injury is usually one in which the affected body part becomes entangled in machinery, clothing, or some other means of entrapment, causing the skin, tissue, and possibly bone to be torn and pulled away from the body. If the limb or appendage is severed completely from the body, it is termed an *amputation*.

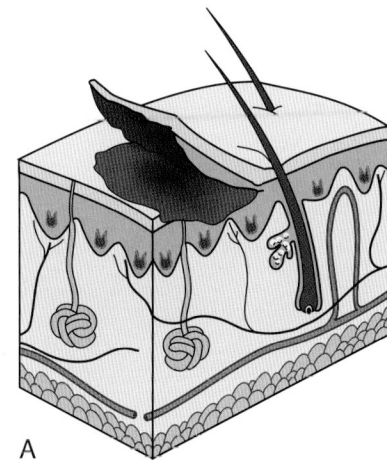

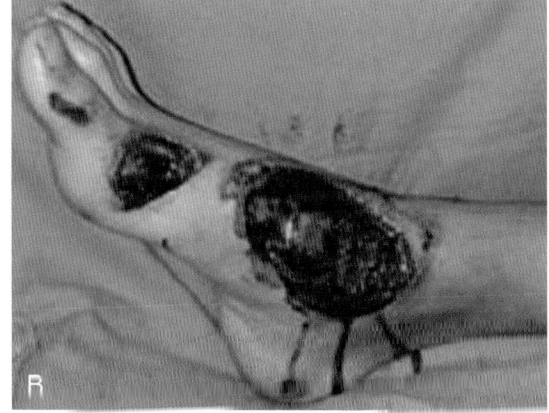

• Fig 15.2 Avulsion. (A) A flap of skin has been torn away. (B) Avulsions over the foot and ankle. (From Browner BD, Fuller RP: Musculoskeletal emergencies, Philadelphia, 2012, Saunders.)

Diagnosis

Diagnosis is made by performing a visual inspection of the affected part and on the basis of the history of the injury mechanism.

Treatment

Treatment consists of controlling the bleeding, cleansing the area, and surgically repairing the tissue. If an amputation has occurred, the stump or remaining area must be cleansed and surgically repaired. The patient probably will be treated prophylactically with antibiotics to prevent infection. Obtain information on the patient's history of medicine allergies. A sterile dressing is applied to the repaired wound. Tetanus prophylaxis is confirmed, or Tdap injection is administered, if necessary. Pain medication is prescribed and administered, when necessary. Revascularization is needed for increased blood supply in some instances when repairing with a skin graft. Application of basic fibroblast growth factor (bFGF) is also used to promote epithelialization in severe cases.

Prognosis

Prognosis depends on the extent of the insult. Prompt intervention helps promote the healing process.

Prevention

Prevention is difficult, and the likelihood of injury is unpredictable. Following safety guidelines when operating machinery, especially wearing clothes that are fitted and not loose, is important, as is confining long hair that could be pulled into equipment and cause a scalp or facial avulsion.

Patient Teaching

Reinforce the importance of following safety guidelines. Instruct the patient on wound care and the importance of keeping the wound clean and dry. Reinforce the value of being up to date with tetanus prophylaxis. Provide the patient written instructions regarding the signs and symptoms of infection. Encourage patients to keep any follow-up appointments as scheduled. Generate print-on-demand electronic materials, when possible, as teaching tools regarding treatment of wound.

Crushing injuries

Description

Crushing injuries occur when a part of the body is compressed with extreme force between two surfaces.

ICD-10-CM Code	S77.20XA
	(Crushing injury of unspecified hip with thigh, initial encounter)
	(S77.00-S77.22 = 9 codes of specificity)

Symptoms and Signs

A crushing injury may involve any body part, but most often, a finger, hand, toe, or foot is the involved part. The patient experiences pain and may not be able to move the injured part. Soft tissue is compressed or crushed, and depending on the amount of pressure involved in the mechanism of injury, bone, nerves, and vessels may also be crushed.

Patient Screening

Crushing injuries require prompt assessment and intervention. Many individuals that sustain such an injury are transported to an emergency facility. If not, they should be seen as soon as possible on the day of the injury or referred to an emergency facility.

Etiology

The crushing injury occurs when the affected body part becomes pressed between two hard surfaces. Examples of such injuries are fingers shut in doors, hands or fingers caught in presses, heavy objects being dropped on feet or toes, and compression of any body part as a result of an MVA. Falling debris, such as building parts broken loose in a storm or earthquake, can also cause crushing injuries.

Diagnosis

Diagnosis is made on the basis of history, visual inspection of the body area, and physical examination. Radiographic studies of the injured part also aid in the diagnosis.

Treatment

Treatment depends on the severity and location of the injury. When an open wound is present, the area is cleansed, irrigated, and débrided, if necessary. Immobilization of the affected limb or appendage follows any surgical repair that is indicated. Sterile dressings will probably be applied to any open wound or surgical area. If the crushing injury involves the head or trunk of the body, appropriate triage of the patient, monitoring of vital signs, and surgical intervention is undertaken. Tetanus prophylaxis is confirmed, or Tdap injection is administered, if necessary, and antibiotics may be prescribed as an additional prophylactic measure.

When a crushing injury occurs at the workplace, workers' compensation forms and any mandatory drug and alcohol screening must be completed. Witnesses may be interviewed if the patient is unable to give details.

Prognosis

Prognosis depends on the extent of the insult. Prompt intervention helps hasten the healing process.

Prevention

Prevention is difficult, and the likelihood of injury is unpredictable. Following safety guidelines, especially that of not wearing loose clothing while operating machinery, is a prudent practice. Other such Occupational Safety and Health Administration (OSHA) guidelines should be followed whenever engaging in high-risk activities.

Patient Teaching

Reinforce safety guidelines. Instruct the patient on wound care and the importance of keeping the wound clean and dry. Reinforce the value of being up to date with tetanus prophylaxis. Encourage patients to keep any follow-up appointments as scheduled.

◆ ENRICHMENT

Needlesticks

Health care providers are at risk for puncture wounds from contaminated needlesticks. U.S. Occupational Safety and Health Administration (OSHA) guidelines and the facility guidelines must be followed to lessen the risk of occurrence. This also reduces the likelihood of transmitting acquired immunodeficiency syndrome (AIDS), hepatitis B, hepatitis C, and any other bloodborne diseases.

Puncture wounds

Description

Puncture wounds result when a pointed or sharp foreign object penetrates the soft tissue (Fig. 15.3). Animal bites, discussed later in this chapter, also may be considered puncture wounds.

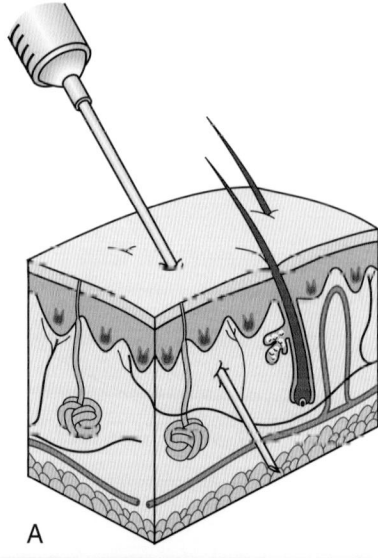

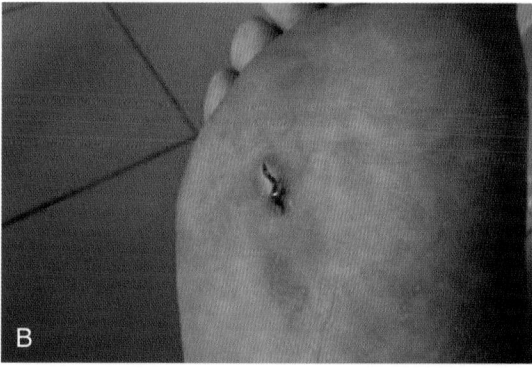

• **Fig. 15.3** Puncture wound. (A) A pointed object has punctured the skin. (B) Puncture wound of the foot. (From Browner BD, Fuller RP: *Musculoskeletal emergencies*, Philadelphia, 2012, Saunders.)

ICD-10-CM Code	S31.000A (Unspecified open wound of lower back and pelvis without penetration into retroperitoneum, initial encounter)

Open wounds are coded by site and type. Once the diagnosis has been confirmed, refer to the current edition of the ICD-10-CM coding manual for the appropriate code and modifier.

Symptoms and Signs

Puncture wounds cause pain and usually very little bleeding. Redness at the site may be noted, or there may be no indication of the wound other than the pain. A puncture wound may not have a dramatic appearance; therefore meticulous inspection of the area and underlying structures should be carefully performed. If the foreign body that caused the injury is protruding out of the wound, it is described as an *impaled object* (Fig. 15.4).

Patient Screening

Puncture wounds require prompt assessment and cleansing. Tetanus prophylaxis needs to be confirmed. Impaled objects

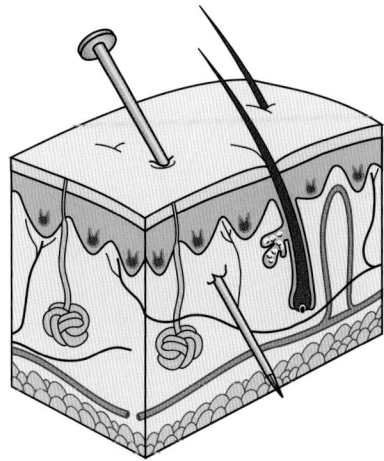

• **Fig. 15.4** Impaled object. A nail is impaled in the skin.

require stabilization to keep the object in the same position until assessment and treatment are accomplished. Removing an impaled object may cause more damage to tissues, nerves, and vessels.

Etiology

A puncture wound occurs when a sharp, pointed object penetrates the skin and underlying soft tissue. The offending object may be a needle, a nail, a splinter of glass, wood or metal, a knife, or even a bullet. The object first penetrates the skin, and then the skin closes around the object or point of entry. As a result, bleeding is minimal. In some situations, bleeding will occur as the penetrating object is removed. Puncture wounds near joints are at risk for bacterial infection, and wounds on the bottom of the foot are at risk for cellulitis.

Diagnosis

Diagnosis is made by visual examination, history, and sometimes radiographic studies (if the object can be visualized by imaging). An embedded organic object, such as a small twig, can be visualized only by using magnetic resonance imaging (MRI). An impaled object is easily observed because it protrudes from the injured site.

Treatment

Treatment involves removal of the foreign body, along with copious irrigation of the wound with sterile fluid. A sterile dressing is applied. Tetanus prophylaxis is confirmed or Tdap injection is recommended and/or administered, if necessary, and antibiotics may be prescribed as an additional prophylactic measure. Impaled objects are stabilized until they can be removed by the physician. As with other work-related injuries, workers' compensation forms and any required drug or alcohol screening testing must be completed. Some puncture wounds are allowed to heal from the inside out to prevent infection. If bacteria are present in the wound, the wound may become infected after it is closed with sutures.

Prognosis

The prognosis varies, depending on the extent and depth of the puncture wound.

Prevention

Prevention is difficult. Health care providers should follow OSHA guidelines when handling sharps and needles. Construction workers are encouraged to use air tools with great caution and wear recommended safety devices, such as steel-toed safety shoes, hard hats, and safety goggles.

Patient Teaching

Instruct the patient on wound care and on keeping the wound clean and dry. Provide the patient with instructions on signs and symptoms of infection. Reinforce the importance of tetanus prophylaxis. Encourage enforcement of OSHA guidelines, when appropriate.

◆ ENRICHMENT

Penetrating Injuries

Violence in today's society results in various forms of penetrating injuries. These injuries may be the result of knife wounds (stabbings), gunshot wounds, and accidental or intentional impaling of a pointed or sharp object or instrument. Although the victims are not usually seen in an office setting, families often seek appointments to speak with the physician about the injury and prognosis. Some patients may be seen in the office after release from emergency care and/or during rehabilitation for treatment.

Lacerations

Description

Lacerations result when a sharp object cuts the skin and possibly underlying soft tissue.

> ICD-10-CM Code   S31.000A *(Unspecified open wound of lower back and pelvis without penetration into retroperitoneum, initial encounter)*
> *Open wounds are coded by site and type. Once the diagnosis has been confirmed, refer to the current edition of the ICD-10-CM coding manual for the appropriate code.*

Symptoms and Signs

Lacerations result when a sharp object cuts the skin and possibly the underlying soft tissue as well. Lacerations cause pain and moderate to severe bleeding. The edges of the cut may be smooth or jagged, depending on what object did the cutting. The bleeding is generally proportionate to the depth and length of the laceration.

Patient Screening

Lacerations require prompt cleansing and repair.

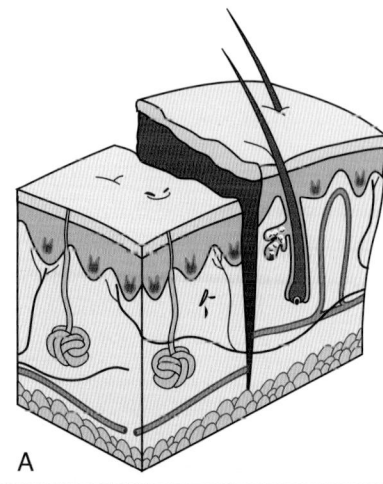

A

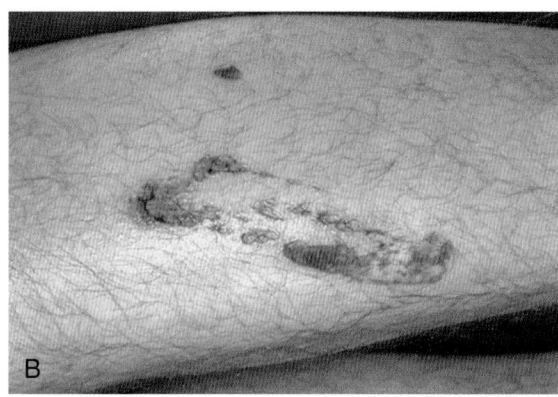

B

• **Fig. 15.5** Laceration. (A) Skin is cut by a sharp object. (B) Laceration. (B, From Klatt EC: *Robbins and Cotran atlas of pathology,* ed 3, Philadelphia, 2015, Saunders.)

Etiology

Lacerations occur when a sharp instrument, such as a knife or sharp piece of glass or metal, cuts the skin and underlying soft tissue (Fig. 15.5).

Diagnosis

Diagnosis is made on the basis of visual examination. History may reveal the type of sharp object that caused the injury. A laceration with smooth edges that can be approximated cleanly is termed an *incision* (Fig. 15.6).

Treatment

Lacerations should be cleansed gently with germicidal soap and water. If the laceration is not too deep and bleeding is controlled, approximating and securing the edges with tape, a butterfly dressing, or sterile adhesive strips (Steri-Strips) may be the only intervention necessary other than a sterile dressing application. In some cases, a new type of "glue" is used to hold the edges together, thereby eliminating the need for sutures. Lacerations that are deep, have jagged edges, or continue to bleed need to be débrided and have the edges trimmed to facilitate good approximation. Bleeding should be controlled by either coagulation or suture. Suturing of the wound will probably be necessary. If the laceration is over a movable joint, immobilization of the

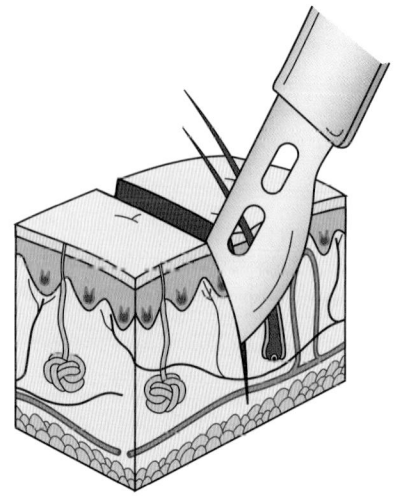

• **Fig. 15.6** Incision. A laceration with smooth edges.

area is indicated. A sterile dressing should be applied. Tetanus prophylaxis is confirmed, and Tdap injection is recommended and/or administered, if necessary, and antibiotics may be prescribed as an additional prophylactic measure.

As with other work-related injuries, workers' compensation forms and any required drug or alcohol screening testing must be completed.

Prognosis

The prognosis varies, depending on the location, length, depth, and condition of the laceration. The degree of approximation of the edges of the wound may determine the extent of the scarring.

Prevention

Prevention is difficult. Care when using knives should be stressed. Following OSHA guidelines when using power tools is a prudent practice.

Patient Teaching

Instruct the patient on wound care and the importance of tetanus prophylaxis. When sutures have been used for closure, instruct the patient regarding when to return for suture removal and that signs and symptoms of infection should be reported promptly.

Foreign Bodies

Anything that enters a portion of the body where it does not belong is considered a foreign body. Common sites for entrapped foreign bodies include the ears, the eyes, and the nose, but any surface area of the body can be involved.

Foreign bodies in the ear

Description

Foreign bodies in the ear typically range from bugs, pebbles, and bits of cotton to anything small enough to fit in the ear canal.

ICD-10-CM Code   T16.1XXA *(Foreign body in right ear,*
                             initial encounter)
                     T16.2XXA *(Foreign body in left ear,*
                             initial encounter)
                     T16.9XXA *(Foreign body in ear,*
                             unspecified ear, initial encounter)

Symptoms and Signs

The patient complains of feeling stuffiness and something in the ear. If the foreign object is a bug, the patient also may complain of a buzzing sound in the ear. Complaints of pain in the ear canal and decreased hearing capability may be expressed. Anything small enough to fit in the ear could be the offending foreign body. Visualization of the ear canal usually shows an apparent object.

Patient Screening

Although not a life-threatening condition, individuals with foreign bodies in the ear require prompt assessment and intervention.

Etiology

Flying insects may enter the ear canal accidentally in the course of flight, and instances of a bug crawling into the ear when an individual is lying down have been reported. Children have a tendency to place small objects in their ear canals and typically do not report the event in a timely manner. Small toys, cereal, grapes, peas, beans, and pebbles are examples of some of the objects commonly found in the ear canals of children. Vegetative foreign bodies, such as wood or thorns, may lead to infection and computed tomography (CT) may be required for diagnosis. Foreign bodies in the ear should be removed as quickly as possible. Cotton from cotton-tipped applicators also may be the offending object; the cotton inadvertently comes off of the applicator stick during a cleaning process. Anything small enough to be placed into the ear canal could be the problem, especially in the case of children.

Diagnosis

Diagnosis is made on the basis of history and visual and/or otoscopic inspection of the ear canal (Fig. 15.7).

Treatment

The goal of treatment is removal of the offending object without damaging the ear canal or the tympanic membrane. Many times, the object simply may be grasped by forceps and removed. Food and cereal can absorb moisture from the ear canal and swell to the point of being compressed against the walls of the ear canal. Such objects may require removal by a physician with the use of gentle, controlled suctioning. The individual with a live bug in the ear should be placed in a dark room and have a flashlight shined in the ear. Bugs that are alive will crawl out of the ear toward the light. Bugs that are not responsive to the light technique may have to be washed out of the ear. In that case, the ear canal is gently irrigated with a warm solution of 50% water and 50% hydrogen peroxide or mineral oil; the bug usually flows out with the solution. If this is not successful, then gentle suction may be necessary to remove the foreign body. Caution is taken not to scratch or damage the ear canal or the tympanic membrane.

Prognosis

The prognosis is good with prompt removal of the foreign body with no consequential damage to the ear canal or the tympanic membrane.

Prevention

Prevention includes educating children about not putting anything in their ears. A good rule to teach them is "Never place anything in your ears that is smaller than your elbow." Cotton-tipped applicators should be kept out of the reach of children and extreme caution used when attempting to cleanse the ears with them.

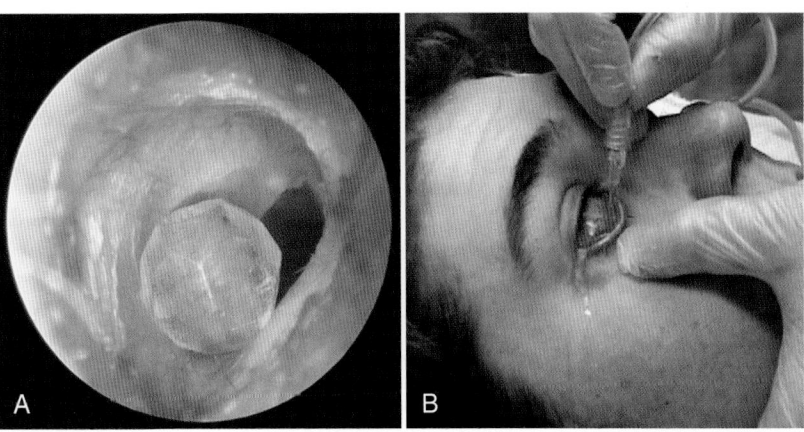

• **Fig. 15.7** (A) Foreign body in the ear. (B) Eye irrigation. (A, From Swartz MH: *Textbook of physical diagnosis,* ed 5, Philadelphia, 2006, Saunders. B, From Eagling and Roper-Hall: *Eye injuries: an illustrated guide,* 1986, Butterworth-Heinemann.)

Patient Teaching

Stress the dangers of putting small objects in the ears. Encourage parents to seek medical intervention when a child has a foreign body in the ear canal.

Foreign bodies in the eye

Description

Foreign bodies in the eye are objects that would not normally be found in the eye. Common offenders are bugs, rust, dust, sand, hair, small pieces of metal, or small pieces of brush or tree branches. Chemicals may be accidentally splashed in the eye.

ICD-10-CM Code   T15.90XA *(Foreign body on external eye, part unspecified, unspecified eye, initial encounter)*
T15.91XA *(Foreign body on external eye, part unspecified, right eye, initial encounter)*
T15.92XA *(Foreign body on external eye, part unspecified, left eye, initial encounter)*
(T15.00[7th digit]-T15.92[7th digit] = 12 codes of specificity)

Foreign bodies in the eye are coded by site. Once the diagnosis has been confirmed, refer to the current edition of the ICD-10-CM coding manual for the appropriate code.

Symptoms and Signs

The individual complains of scratching or irritation of the eye. The patient may experience pain in the eye and report blurred or compromised vision. Tearing is usually present.

Patient Screening

Foreign objects in the eye require prompt evaluation and intervention. If the injury involves splashed chemicals, immediate irrigation of the eye is advised. If an immediate appointment is not available, the individual should be referred to an emergency facility. Patients should be encouraged to have someone else provide their transportation; they should not attempt to drive. If the object is impaled and sticking out of the eye, the emergency medical service (EMS) is the recommended mode of transport to the hospital after stabilization of the impaled object has been accomplished.

Etiology

Foreign bodies in the eyes can result from a number of sources and routes of entry. A common source of rust and metal particles in the eye is the undercarriage of a car; the person working under a car may inadvertently knock loose rust particles or minute scraps of metal that then fall into the eye. Industrial accidents involving objects that have been propelled through the air, possibly as the result of an explosion, also can result in a foreign body entering the unprotected eye. Foreign objects also may be propelled into the eye as a result of an MVA or sports injury. Dust and other debris in the environment may be blown into open unprotected eyes. A bug flying into the eye is a common occurrence. Occasionally just rubbing the eyes with dirty hands can be the source of entry for dirt or a chemical. Working with caustic liquids without wearing eye protection, resulting in splashing, and dust trapped under a contact lens are other sources of foreign substances in the eye.

Diagnosis

Diagnosis is made by visual and ophthalmoscopic examinations of the eye. A history of feeling something in the eye combined with the circumstance of possible exposure to foreign bodies is helpful. Staining the eye with fluorescein to visualize a corneal abrasion confirms the presence or previous presence of a foreign body. Refer to Chapter 5 for discussion on corneal abrasion.

Treatment

Treatment involves removal of the offending material. Many times, gentle irrigation of the eye with normal saline will flush dust, bugs, or debris out of the eye (see Fig. 15.7B).

When the foreign body is embedded in the eye, the physician may attempt removal with surgical instruments or an eye spud. If these procedures are unsuccessful, immediate referral to an ophthalmologist or emergency department is made. Ophthalmic antibacterial drops or ointments may be placed in the eye, and the eye is usually covered with a patch. Because eyes have sympathetic movement, it is usual procedure to bandage both eyes. Metal pieces or rust fragments falling from the undercarriage of a motor vehicle may result in eventual rust rings forming in the eye. These may have to be removed by an ophthalmologist.

Prognosis

The prognosis varies, depending on the offending material and the depth and involvement of the eye structures. Many injuries caused by bugs and dust will resolve after cleansing irrigation. Extensive corneal abrasions may result in residual scarring and compromised vision. Chemical burns may result in blindness.

Prevention

The best prevention for occupational and other possible insults by foreign objects to the eye is wearing approved eye protection. Many accidental incidents can be prevented in this way.

Patient Teaching

Encourage the use of eye protection whenever any possible hazard to the eye is anticipated. When a foreign object other than minute dust particles enters the eye and is not removed successfully by gentle irrigation, encourage the individual to seek professional treatment. When one eye is patched or covered with a bandage, make the patient aware that depth perception will be absent, and encourage care in navigating steps.

Patients who have experienced metal in their eyes will need to be advised that in the future, should they require an MRI, the information about the metal having been in eye as a foreign body must be shared with the radiology technician.

◆ ENRICHMENT

Emergency Medical Service

The emergency medical service (EMS) provides prehospital care in emergency situations. Those responding may be paramedics, emergency medical technicians (EMTs), or first responders. This system is designed to provide early or lifesaving medical intervention for those who have a need for urgent and immediate medical care. This emergency care is followed by rapid transport to an emergency facility for further evaluation or advanced medical care.

Initially, the person experiencing a medical problem, or someone at the scene, can quickly survey the situation and determine whether entry into the EMS system is warranted. Access to the EMS system is achieved by telephone and dialing 911. This number is a free call on cell phones and on pay phones.

It is important to realize that once an individual is entered into the system, emergency care will be provided until a physician orders it to cease. When a valid *Do Not Resuscitate* order exists for an individual, medical care is managed accordingly.

Illnesses for which the system may be called include chest pain, shortness of breath, unconsciousness; possible stroke; accidental injuries, including possible poisoning; possible suicide, severe falls with neck, back, or leg injuries; serious motor vehicle crashes with serious injuries; burns; lightning injuries; electrocutions; possible or near-drownings; impaled objects; and gunshot wounds. Impending precipitous childbirth, severe bleeding, near-choking, and asthma attacks may require immediate emergency care provided by the EMS.

The caller will be asked to supply the phone number from which the call is being made, the location of the individual requiring the emergency treatment, and the nature of the emergency. Additionally, the caller will be instructed to remain on the line until help arrives. This is to maintain contact for updates of the individual's status, to provide instructions for treatment that can be rendered until help arrives, and for additional location information. In cases of cardiac arrest or cessation of breathing, the caller will be provided with instructions on beginning and performing cardiopulmonary resuscitation (CPR).

◆ ENRICHMENT

Mock Disaster Drills

Emergency medical management, emergency departments, police departments, fire departments, and emergency medical transport services conduct mock disaster drills. During these drills, mock disasters or accidents are orchestrated to provide as realistically as possible incidents for simulated events and health care professionals' training. Mock patients are transported to emergency facilities, and extra staff is called in to help provide service. Triage is practiced, and patients are assigned on the basis of their injuries or trauma to a health care provider.

Foreign bodies in the nose

Description

Any object or foreign material that is causing an obstruction in the nares should be considered a foreign body in the nose, and medical intervention for removal should be sought. Foreign bodies often found wedged in the nares of children are cereals, dried peas or beans, grapes, Styrofoam particles, pebbles, and cotton.

| ICD-10-CM Code | T17.0XXA *(Foreign body in nasal sinus, initial encounter)* |
| | T17.1XXA *(Foreign body in nostril, initial encounter)* |

Symptoms and Signs

Children have the most occurrences of foreign bodies wedged or stuck in the nares. Parents usually note mucus running from one of the nares, swelling near the bridge of the nose, and congested breathing. On investigation, they are able to confirm that one of the nares is constricted and that air is not moving through the affected side.

Patient Screening

Foreign bodies in the nose require prompt assessment and treatment.

Etiology

Children have a tendency to insert foreign objects into their noses. These foreign bodies include but are not limited to cereals, dried peas or beans, grapes, Styrofoam particles, pebbles, toys or small doll shoes, and anything else small enough to fit in the nares. Dry materials, such as dried peas, beans, and cereal, have a tendency to absorb moisture from the mucous membrane and then swell, creating an obstruction.

Diagnosis

Diagnosis is made on the basis of history and visualization of the foreign body in the nares. Often mucus is dripping from the unobstructed nares and may be foul smelling.

Treatment

The child is encouraged to blow the nose in the hopes that the object will be expelled. If the offending foreign substance is a bit of cereal, squeezing the nose usually will crush the cereal bit and permit it to be expelled by blowing the nose. The child should be old enough to understand not to inhale, or the child may inhale the crushed cereal. A physician may need to grasp the object with forceps for removal or use a suction device if the forceps will not reach far enough.

Prognosis

The prognosis is good when removal of the offending object is uncomplicated and complete.

Prevention

Prevention is difficult because children often have a tendency to insert small objects into their noses.

Patient Teaching

Counsel children not to place any objects in their noses. Emphasize that dried objects will swell and that medical intervention may be needed to correct the situation.

Thermal Insults

Thermal insults can be caused by either heat or cold, which includes burns or frostbite. Extremes in temperatures cause conditions such as hypothermia, hyperthermia, heat stroke, and heat exhaustion. Regardless of the variance in temperature (hot or cold), most conditions resulting in a severely altered state can be life threatening if left untreated. However, hypothermia may be a protective factor in the case of a near-drowning in cold water.

Burns

Description

Burns are the result of thermal insults to tissue. The insults may be caused by heat, chemical sources, electrical sources, or radiation. Heat sources that cause injury may be in the form of dry heat, steam, or hot substances; sun rays are also capable of causing a burn.

ICD-10-CM Code	T30.0 *(Burn of unspecified body region, unspecified degree)*
	T30.4 *(Corrosion of unspecified body region, unspecified degree)*

Burns are coded by site, degree, and body surface involved. Once the diagnosis has been confirmed, refer to the current edition of the ICD-10-CM coding manual for the appropriate code.

Symptoms and Signs

The patient who has experienced a burn usually has pain. The extent of the burn, along with the percent of body surface involved, usually is related proportionately to the degree of pain. Depending on the depth and nature of the burn, the skin surface may be reddened, blistered, or charred (Fig. 15.8).

Patient Screening

Burns require prompt assessment and intervention. After evaluation and stabilization, patients with major burns are referred to burn centers for treatment. Knowing the mechanics of the injury is important in determining the type of treatment intervention required; this includes assessment of respiratory status, wound contamination, eye involvement, and fluid management.

Etiology

Burns can be caused by flame, dry heat, liquid scalds, radiation, chemicals, or electricity. Exposure of the skin to any of these sources can cause destruction of the skin. Injury to the underlying soft tissue is proportionate to the duration of the exposure and the intensity of the thermal source.

Diagnosis

Diagnosis is made on the basis of visual examination and history. In the type of burn caused by flames, it is necessary to determine whether the burn occurred inside an enclosed space or out in the open. The respiratory state of any patient with this type of burn must be assessed. The status of the eyebrows, eyelashes, and nasal hair must be determined. Any singeing of these hairs indicates that the patient inhaled the flame or superheated air and that the respiratory status may be in grave danger.

Determination of the depth (Fig. 15.9) and extent (Fig. 15.10) of burns is important. Pain intensity depends on the amount of nerve tissue that is involved or destroyed.

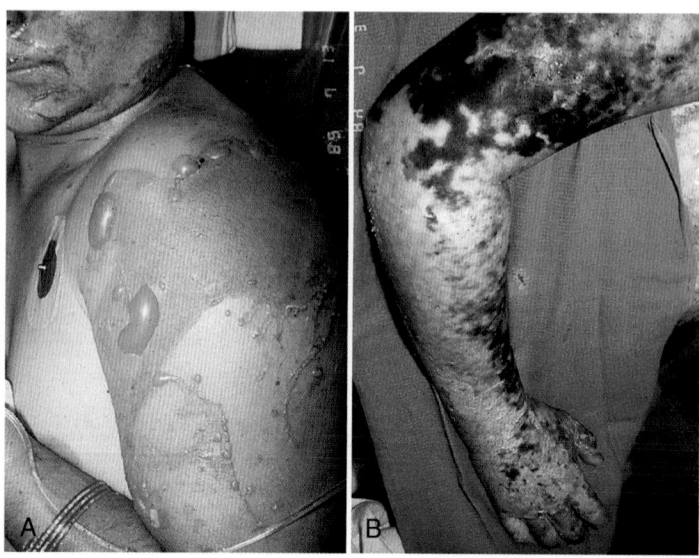

• **Fig. 15.8** (A) Examples of burns. Partial-thickness burn; note the blisters. (B) Full-thickness burn; note the dark color. (Courtesy Judy Knightton, Ross Tilley Burn Center, Sunnybrook and Women's College Health Center, Toronto, Ontario, Canada.)

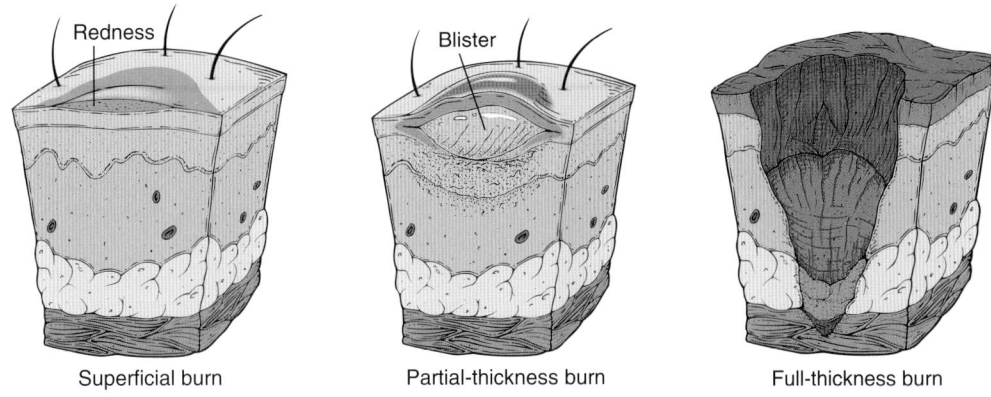

• **Fig. 15.9** Depths of burns. The extent of involvement of layers of the skin.

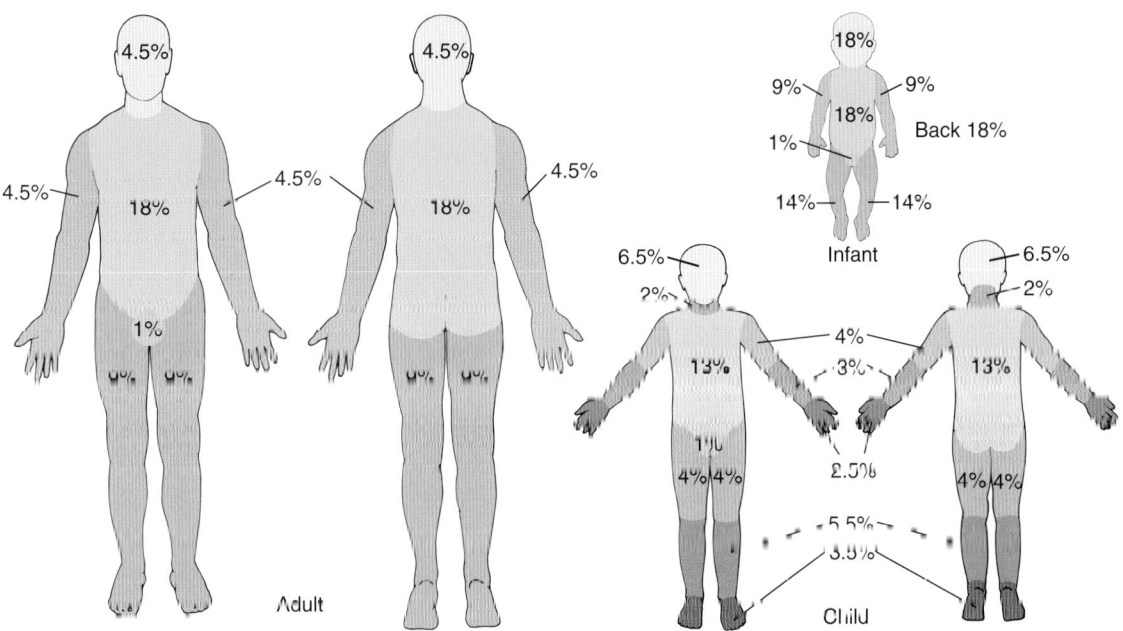

• **Fig. 15.10** Rule of nines.

Superficial burns involve only the outer layers of the skin, which usually appear only reddened, and yet these burns are painful. Partial-thickness burns involve all layers of the skin; they produce blisters and are quite painful. Full-thickness burns involve both the skin and the underlying subcutaneous tissue. Resultant destruction of nerve endings often results in minimal pain in that particular area; however, pain may be reported in areas around the periphery of the burn site. Prompt assessment of the percent of skin surface area involved in the burn injury is achieved by applying the "rule of nines." The "rule of nines" provides a fast and fairly accurate calculation of the body surface involved. Percentages used to ascertain the burned tissue area in the adult are as follows: head, 9%; anterior trunk, 18%; posterior trunk, 18%; entire right arm, 9%; entire left arm, 9%; anterior surface right leg, 9%; posterior surface right leg, 9%; anterior surface left leg, 9%; posterior surface left leg, 9%; and perineum, 1%. Percentages in children and infants are slightly different. Another method of designating a percentage

of body surface involvement is used by the *International Classification of Diseases,* 10th revision, Clinical Modification (ICD-10-CM) code books. Refer to the current edition of the ICD-10-CM code books for these percentages.

Treatment

Treatment depends on the source of burns. Heat burns (from flames, liquid scalds, or superheated air) should be cooled with cool water and covered with dry sterile dressings until the patient can be seen by a physician. Sunburns should be treated with the application of cool water, and the damaged skin may be sprayed with **antiseptic** and **analgesic** sprays (Fig. 15.11). Over-the-counter (OTC) medications, including aspirin, ibuprofen, and naproxen, may be used for relief of sunburn pain. Cool compresses applied to the areas of sunburned skin may also provide pain relief.

Skin burned with chemicals other than lime must first be brushed away, should be flushed with cool water for at least 15 minutes, covered with a sterile dressing, and treated by a

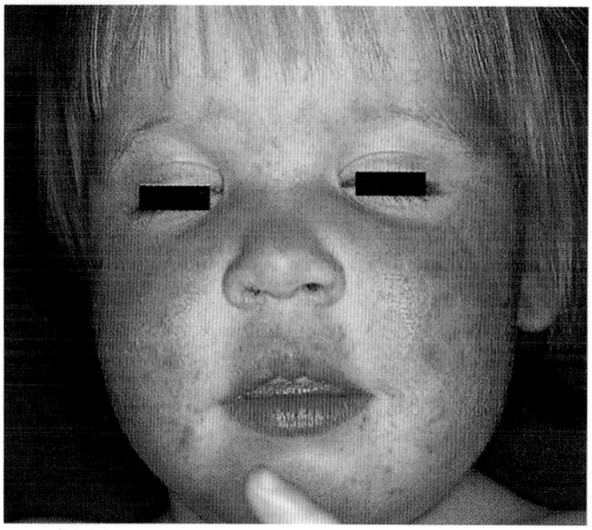

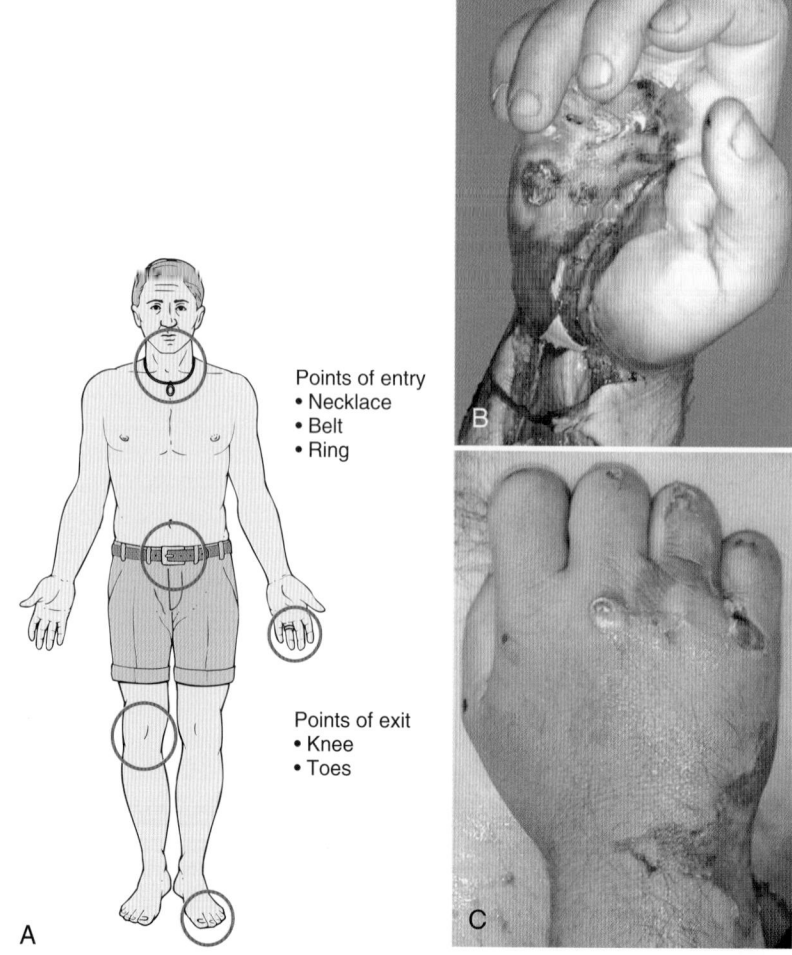

• **Fig. 15.11** Sunburn. (From Weston WL, et al: *Color textbook of pediatric dermatology,* ed 4, St Louis, 2008, Mosby.)

physician. Electrical burns should be examined for points of entry (rings, belts, necklaces) and exit (knees, fingers, and toes) (Fig. 15.12). These areas should be covered with dry sterile dressings and treated by a physician.

Analgesics are given to treat the pain. Minor burns usually are treated with an antibacterial cream or ointment. Severe burns require specialized treatment with surgical débridement of the burned tissue and skin grafts, if necessary.

Patients with severe large-area burns, older adults, the very young with burns, and those with severe burns to the face, hands, feet, or perineal area usually are admitted to a burn center, where they receive specialized burn care. Respiratory status (if the respiratory tract is involved), fluid and electrolyte balance, and vital signs are monitored. Pain control is accomplished with the use of narcotic analgesics. Tetanus prophylaxis is confirmed or administered, if necessary, and antibiotics may be prescribed as an additional prophylactic measure. A list of the patient's medicine allergies should be obtained. Skin grafting, including the use of cloned skin and

Points of entry
• Necklace
• Belt
• Ring

Points of exit
• Knee
• Toes

A

B

C

• **Fig. 15.12** (A) Points of entry and exit for electrical burns. (B) Entry wound from electrocution on the palm of the hand. (C) Exit wound of the same injury on the dorsum of the hand. (B and C, From Klatt EC: *Robbins and Cotran atlas of pathology,* ed 2, Philadelphia, 2010, Saunders.)

the use of autografts and adjacent tissue grafts, is used for treatment of extensive destruction of tissue.

The American Burn Association's National Burn Repository requests that forms be completed and submitted. These forms collect information for statistics about burns as well for research. The information submitted includes the name of the facility; admission year; patient age, gender, and race; admission type; discharge date; external causes; and total body surface area percentage.

Some communities request or require completion and submission of a burn incident report, often to the fire department.

Work-related burns must be reported to state workers' compensation. As with other work-related injuries, drug and alcohol testing may be required.

Prognosis

The prognosis varies, depending on the cause and extent of the burned tissue and other organ or system involvement.

Prompt intervention helps promote a positive outcome. Scarring is typical (refer to the Enrichment box about Radiation Exposure).

Prevention

Prevention is difficult. Prudent use of fire or combustible materials is helpful. Being proactive to avoid situations where burns may occur is wise. Application of sunscreens is strongly recommended when prolonged exposure to the sun is anticipated.

Patient Teaching

Stress the importance of keeping follow-up appointments and compliance with prescribed therapy. Provide instruction on wound care and the signs and symptoms of infection. Emphasize the importance of being current with tetanus prophylaxis.

◆ ENRICHMENT

Sunburn

Exposure to the ultraviolet alpha- and beta-rays from the sun can cause sunburn, ranging from mild to severe. The person who has experienced at least three severe sunburns with blistering is at risk for the development of skin cancer. Prevention of sunburn includes avoiding exposure from 10 a.m. to 2 p.m., which is when the sun's rays are the strongest, applying a sunscreen to exposed skin areas, and wearing a hat to protect the scalp and eyes. Those at greatest risk have light or fair skin and freckles and blond or red hair. Fig. 15.13 illustrates the short-term and long-term effects of prolonged sun bathing. Acute injury results

in hyperemia of the dermis and blister formation. Long-term exposure may stimulate pigmentation but may also promote carcinogenesis and aging of the epidermis and the dermis.

Sun protection factor (SPF) is the technical name for measurement of ultraviolet B (UVB; shortwave) protection provided by sunscreen. The numbers assigned to a product designate the length of time it takes to redden the skin compared with no protection. An SPF of at least 15 is recommended by the Skin Cancer Foundation as protection against the sun's harmful rays, or UVB.

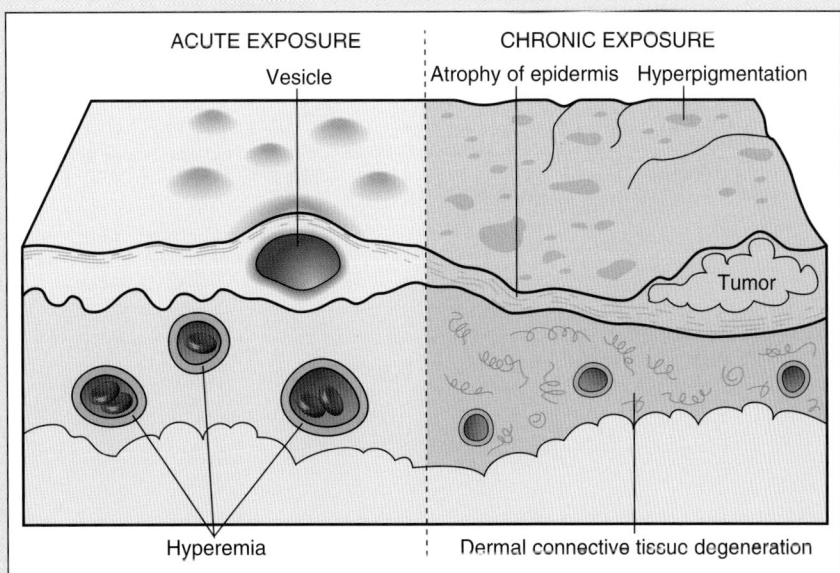

• **Fig. 15.13** Short-term and long-term effects of sunbathing. (From Damjanov I: *Pathology for the health related professions,* ed 4, St Louis, 2011, Saunders.)

Radiation Exposure

Exposure to radioactive material is another threat to society. "Dirty bombs" may contain radioactive particles that can be released into the environment on explosion of the bomb. The three main types of exposure to ionizing radiation are slow, cumulative whole-body exposure; sudden whole-body exposure; and high-dose localized exposure. Sudden whole-body exposure is the most likely form of ionizing radiation exposure for the general public in a terrorist type of event. The body's exposure to radiation may be external irradiation of all or part of the body from an external source, including radiation therapy for cancer treatment, contamination by radioactive material in gases, liquids, or solids that have been released into the environment causing external, internal, or both types of contamination, or by incorporation of the radioactive material as a sequela to other contamination. Symptoms of radiation exposure include nausea, vomiting, and diarrhea; redness and blistering of skin burns; dehydration; weakness, fatigue, exhaustion, and fainting; hair loss, ulceration of oral mucosa, esophagus, and gastrointestinal (GI) tract; vomiting blood and experiencing bloody stools; bruising; sloughing of the skin; and bleeding from nose, mouth, and gums. The extent of the toxicity of ionizing radiation depends on the dose, the distance from the source of radiation, and the length of time of the exposure. Body responses and long-term effects as an overview of major morphologic consequences are presented in Figs. 15.14 and 15.15.

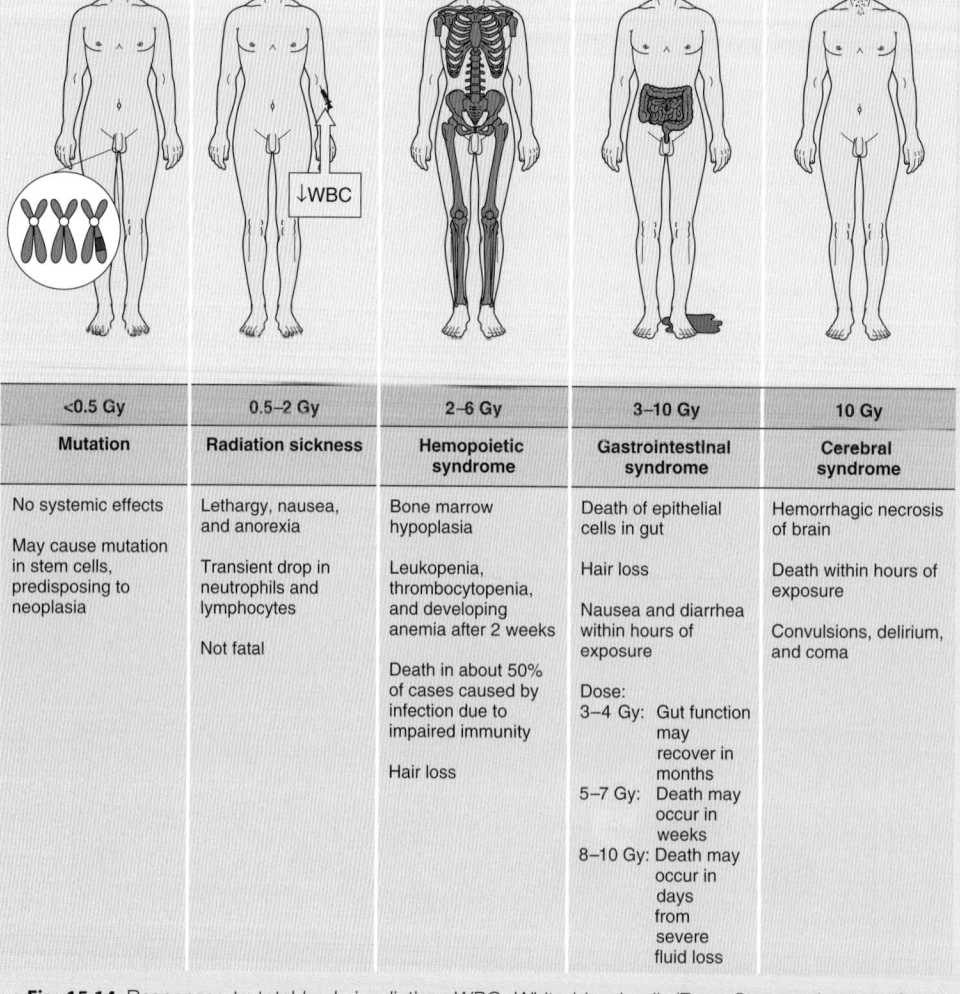

<0.5 Gy	0.5–2 Gy	2–6 Gy	3–10 Gy	10 Gy
Mutation	**Radiation sickness**	**Hemopoietic syndrome**	**Gastrointestinal syndrome**	**Cerebral syndrome**
No systemic effects May cause mutation in stem cells, predisposing to neoplasia	Lethargy, nausea, and anorexia Transient drop in neutrophils and lymphocytes Not fatal	Bone marrow hypoplasia Leukopenia, thrombocytopenia, and developing anemia after 2 weeks Death in about 50% of cases caused by infection due to impaired immunity Hair loss	Death of epithelial cells in gut Hair loss Nausea and diarrhea within hours of exposure Dose: 3–4 Gy: Gut function may recover in months 5–7 Gy: Death may occur in weeks 8–10 Gy: Death may occur in days from severe fluid loss	Hemorrhagic necrosis of brain Death within hours of exposure Convulsions, delirium, and coma

• **Fig. 15.14** Responses to total-body irradiation. *WBC,* White blood cell. (From Stevens A, et al: *Core pathology,* ed 3, London, 2010, Mosby.)

◆ ENRICHMENT—cont'd

Radiation Exposure

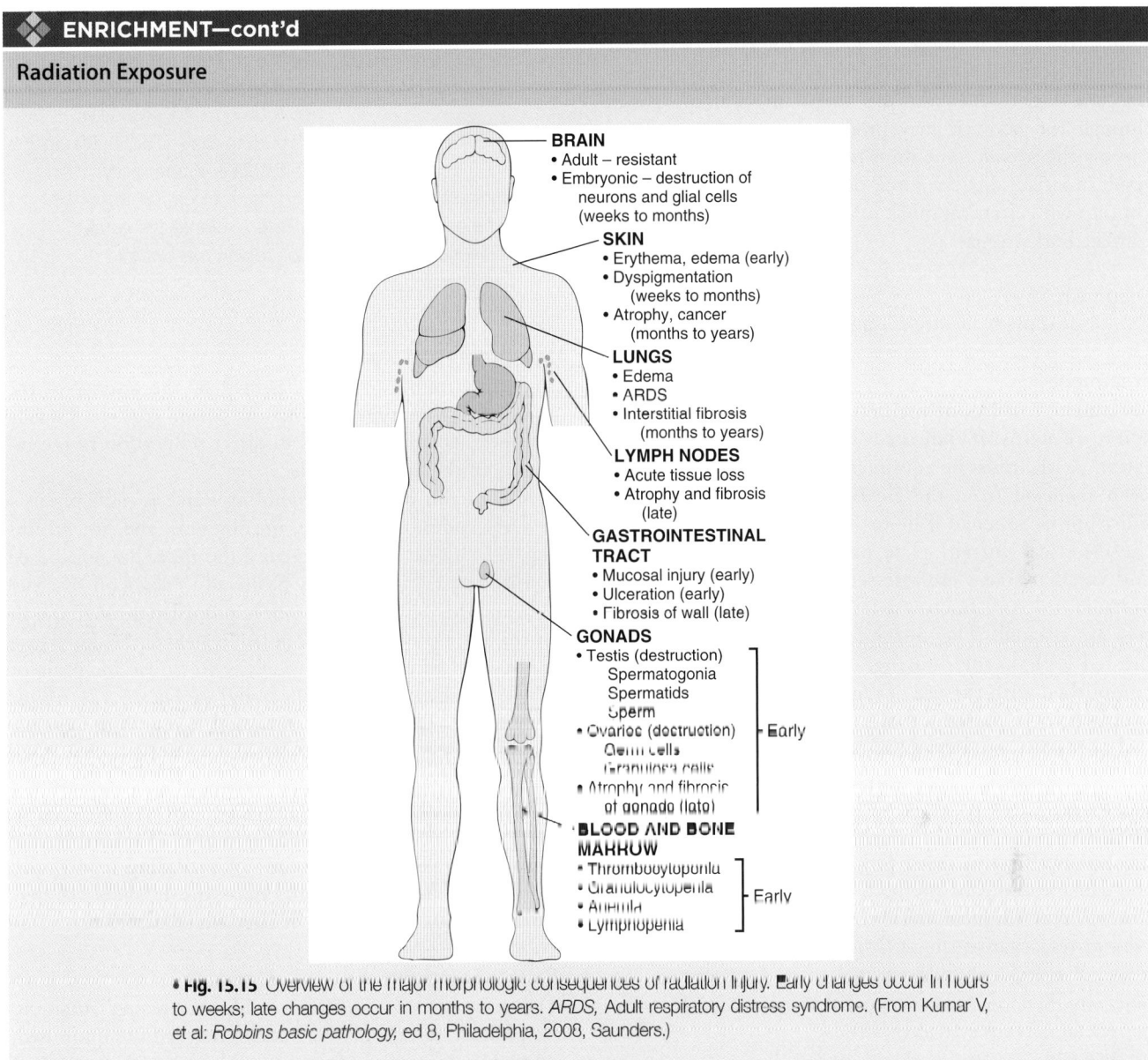

BRAIN
- Adult – resistant
- Embryonic – destruction of neurons and glial cells (weeks to months)

SKIN
- Erythema, edema (early)
- Dyspigmentation (weeks to months)
- Atrophy, cancer (months to years)

LUNGS
- Edema
- ARDS
- Interstitial fibrosis (months to years)

LYMPH NODES
- Acute tissue loss
- Atrophy and fibrosis (late)

GASTROINTESTINAL TRACT
- Mucosal injury (early)
- Ulceration (early)
- Fibrosis of wall (late)

GONADS
- Testis (destruction)
  Spermatogonia
  Spermatids
  Sperm
- Ovaries (destruction)
  Germ cells
  Granulosa cells
- Atrophy and fibrosis of gonads (late)   } Early

BLOOD AND BONE MARROW
- Thrombocytopenia
- Granulocytopenia
- Anemia
- Lymphopenia   } Early

• **Fig. 15.15** Overview of the major morphologic consequences of radiation injury. Early changes occur in hours to weeks; late changes occur in months to years. *ARDS,* Adult respiratory distress syndrome. (From Kumar V, et al: *Robbins basic pathology,* ed 8, Philadelphia, 2008, Saunders.)

Electrical shock

Description

Electrical shock is an injury that occurs as the result of exposure to or contact with electricity.

ICD-10-CM Code	T75.4XXA *(Electrocution, initial encounter)*

Burns are coded by site, degree, and body surface involved. Once the diagnosis of a burn has been confirmed, refer to the current edition of the ICD-10-CM coding manual for the appropriate code.

Symptoms and Signs

Patients who have experienced electrical shock may be in cardiac or respiratory failure. They have a visible burn at the entrance wound and at the exit wound. If conscious, they experience pain at these sites. Charred tissue may be noted.

Patient Screening

Individuals who have suffered electrical shock constitute a life-threatening emergency. They need to be entered into the EMS for transport to an emergency care facility. Resuscitation and life support may be required during transport.

Etiology

The person who has sustained electrical shock experiences tissue damage from the point of entry of the electricity to the point of exit. The electrical current follows the path of least resistance through the body, usually along nerve routes. The current enters the body at the point of contact with the electrical source and exits at the point of grounding (see Fig. 15.12). As the alternating current passes through the body, it may produce muscle contractions, causing the person to be thrown from the source. This can result in lacerations, fractures, or head trauma. One major concern with electrical shock injuries is the development of cardiac dysrhythmias.

Diagnosis

Diagnosis is made by visual examination and history.

Treatment

Treatment consists of maintaining the cardiac and respiratory status. If indicated, cardiopulmonary resuscitation (CPR) must be administered after the patient has been removed from the electrical source. The patient must not be touched if he or she is still in contact with the electrical current. The patient's neurologic status and vascular status are assessed for the extent of tissue destruction. Any fractures, lacerations, and head injuries are treated. The burned areas are débrided and dressed with sterile dressings. Pain management is accomplished with the use of narcotic analgesics. Tetanus prophylaxis is confirmed or administered, if necessary, and antibiotics may be prescribed as an additional prophylactic measure.

Prognosis

The prognosis varies, depending on the extent of the insult and damage to organs and body systems. When cardiac arrest has occurred, prognosis may not be favorable, even with prompt resuscitative efforts. It is important to realize that electrical energy will follow nerves on its path through the body and therefore has the potential to cause damage to the peripheral nervous system (PNS).

Prevention

Extreme care should be taken in situations that involve repair of or close proximity to electrical power, and people should be alert for possible electrical accidents at all times. Electrical outlet covers should be used when the outlets are not in use. It is prudent to avoid standing in water when there is a risk of nearby electrical wires coming in contact with the water.

Patient Teaching

Advise patients to follow the OSHA guidelines when working with electricity. Encourage them to be aware of potential sources of electrocution in the workplace and in the home environment.

Lightning injuries

Description

Lightning injuries occur when an individual is struck directly or indirectly (splash effect) by lightning.

ICD-10-CM Code	T75.00XA (Unspecified effects of lightning, initial encounter)
	T75.01XA (Shock due to being struck by lightning, initial encounter)
	(T75.00-[7th digit]-T75.09-[7th digit] = 3 codes of specificity)

Burns are coded by type and site. Once the diagnosis of a burn has been confirmed, refer to the current edition of the ICD-10-CM coding manual for additional burn codes.

Symptoms and Signs

Lightning injuries can be classified by the severity of the injury or by the type of strike the person receives. Usually the severity of the injury is in direct proportion to the intensity of the lightning strike.

The victim of a direct lightning strike is probably in a severely compromised state, unconscious, and not breathing. A heartbeat may be present if the apnea has not caused cardiac arrest. Clothing may be literally "blown off" the victim, and the victim may have been propelled through the air by the jolt. Burns usually are noted in areas of the skin where moisture is normally found, such as the axillae and groin or where metal was touching the body (see Fig. 15.12). Motor and sensory disturbances are noted, along with possible ruptured tympanic membranes. The patient who has experienced moderate contact will have less severe symptoms but with an altered level of consciousness and skin burns. The person with minor injuries exhibits fairly normal vital signs, some confusion, amnesia of preceding events, and some minor muscle or sensory nerve disturbances. All may experience some hearing or visual difficulties.

Patient Screening

Lightning strikes constitute a life-threatening situation. Respiratory efforts of the patient may be compromised; providing immediate rescue breathing is imperative. If apnea has caused cardiac arrest, CPR must be instituted immediately. It is important to call 911 promptly to enter the victim into the EMS.

Etiology

Lightning can strike a person in five different ways: (1) When the person is struck directly by a lightning discharge, it is termed a *direct strike.* (2) When lightning strikes an object that the person is touching, resulting in transference of the energy, it is termed a *contact strike.* (3) If lightning strikes an object, travels a certain distance, then "jumps" through the air and strikes the person, it is termed a *side flash.* (4) If the current enters the leg of the person, travels through the lower part of the body, and exits out the other leg, it is termed *stride potential.* (5) When the lightning bolt hits the ground and travels to the person by way of the ground, it is termed *ground current.*

Lightning tends to flow over the surface of the body, often sparing the deeper tissues.

Diagnosis

Diagnosis is made on the basis of visual examination and a history of the person having been outdoors when lightning occurred or inside a structure that was hit by lightning and in contact with a conductive or grounding source. A detailed neurologic assessment and a thorough examination of the surface of the body for burns should be completed. A classic fernlike pattern of burn may be noted on the skin. An eye examination should be conducted for retinal, optic nerve, or occipital lobe damage. Baseline visual acuity should be measured, because cataracts, corneal ulcers, or hemorrhage may occur. The ears should be examined for ruptured tympanic membranes. Vital signs should be assessed, including screening for hypertension. The cervical spine and the entire musculoskeletal system should be evaluated for injury.

Treatment

The patient should be entered into the EMS without delay. Treatment consists of restoring or maintaining the patient's respiratory effort. If the person is apneic, cardiac function ceases in a few minutes. If the person is in cardiac arrest, CPR must be initiated and continued for an extended period. Cardiac monitoring is indicated, along with observation for cerebral edema and respiratory insult. Fractures and lacerations, burns, and other injuries need to be treated according to the facility protocol. Tetanus prophylaxis must be confirmed or administered if necessary. Follow-up eye examinations should be conducted, because cataracts may develop in the year after the lightning strike. Treatment of ruptured tympanic membranes should be instituted.

Prognosis

The prognosis varies, depending on the extent of the insult. When respiratory efforts are maintained, survival may be possible. Cardiac dysrhythmias are a potential lethal complication of lightning injuries. Prompt institution of CPR when respiratory efforts are found to be absent also may result in survival of the victim. Those who do not have respiratory or cardiac activity cessation usually survive, but they require follow-up examinations of the eyes and the ears for late-onset problems. Burn treatment of points of entry and exit and treatment of any other skin burns are required.

Prevention

Seeking shelter during a thunder storm and lightning is wise. It is best to avoid seeking shelter under a tree. When no shelter is available, positioning oneself as low as possible on the ground is a prudent action.

Patient Teaching

Provide patients and family members with safety information regarding lightning and thunderstorms. Emphasize the importance of having CPR training and of providing immediate intervention to a lightning strike victim when doing so is safe and possible.

Extreme heat (hyperthermia)

Description

Hyperthermia occurs when an individual's core body temperature is much higher than the normal body temperature of 98.6°F. Accidentally occurring hyperthermia is the consequence of prolonged exposure to extreme environmental heat.

ICD-10-CM Code   T67.9XXA *(Effect of heat and light, unspecified, initial encounter)* (T67.0[7th digit]-T67.9[7th digit] = 10 codes of specificity)

Effects of heat are coded by type. Once the diagnosis has been confirmed, refer to the current edition of the ICD-10-CM coding manual for the appropriate code.

Symptoms and Signs

The person with hyperthermia may be experiencing heat stroke or heat exhaustion as a result of prolonged exposure to extremely hot temperatures. Heat stroke occurs when the person has a body temperature of 105°F or greater. The skin is hot, red, and usually dry. The patient may have a dry mouth, headache, nausea or vomiting, dizziness and weakness, and shortness of breath. The pulse is rapid and strong at the onset, gradually becoming weak, and blood pressure decreases. The pupils are constricted. Patients exhibit anxiety, mental confusion, irritability, aggression, and even hysterical behavior. In extreme cases, the person collapses and experiences altered levels of consciousness and may have seizure activity.

Heat exhaustion produces profuse sweating, fatigue, headache, weakness, nausea, dizziness, and possible heat or muscle cramps. The pulse is weak and rapid; the skin is pale, cool, and moist; and the body temperature is normal or subnormal. The pupils are dilated.

Patient Screening

Hyperthermia is a life-threatening emergency. The individual should be entered into the EMS without delay. Until emergency care arrives to transport the person to an emergency facility, family, friends, or coworkers should move the individual from the extremely hot environment to a colder environment, loosen the victim's clothing, and place cool, moist cloths on the individual's face, neck, arms, and hands.

Etiology

Heat stroke results when the body's heat-regulating systems are unable to cope with the exposure to severe external heat sources. As the body overheats, its temperature rises to 105°F to 110°F. Approximately one-half of patients in these circumstances fail to perspire. Because no effective cooling mechanism is functioning, the body stores the heat, eventually resulting in damage to the brain cells and subsequently permanent brain damage or death. Older adults, infants, children, and malnourished and debilitated people are the most susceptible to heat stroke. Others who experience heat stroke are those who work near furnaces and intense sources of heat and athletes who are exposed to the combination of high temperatures and high humidity.

Heat exhaustion is the result of salt or water depletion. Generally the person is involved in strenuous activity in a hot, humid environment. As a result, the person experiences prolonged and profuse sweating, causing the loss of excessive amounts of salt and water. This mimics a mild state of shock.

Diagnosis

The diagnosis of heat stroke is made by the presence of symptoms, especially the elevated body temperature. The history of exposure to high temperatures and humidity, along with the altered level of consciousness, aids in the diagnosis.

Diagnosis of heat exhaustion is made from the history and clinical findings, specifically the moist, pale skin and normal or below-normal body temperature of the patient.

Treatment

Treatment of heat stroke, possibly a life-threatening condition, must be aggressive and instituted promptly. It consists of cooling the body down. The first step is to move the person to a cooler environment, to remove what clothing is possible, and to cool the body by pouring cool water over it or soaking it with a cool wet cloth. If the person begins to shiver, the cooling process should be slowed. It is imperative to bring the core temperature of the body below 100°F. The person should be transported to an emergency facility where vital signs can be monitored.

Treatment heat exhaustion consists of moving the victim to a cool place and applying cool compresses. The individual should be made to lie down with the feet elevated. If the person is fully conscious, 4 ounces of cool water should be given every 10 to 15 minutes.

Many emergency departments are equipped with "Bair Huggers" used to heat or cool patients.

Prognosis

The prognosis varies, depending on the duration of the exposure and any underlying pathology. Prompt intervention with effective cooling may afford a positive outcome.

Prevention

All persons should be encouraged to avoid lengthy exposure to hot environments and advised of the importance of staying hydrated during hot weather or when working in hot environments. Drinking fluids before going outside to work will help with hydration status. Older individuals and parents of young children should be provided education on the dangers of heat exposure.

Patient Teaching

Provide printed material to the patient or family on precautions to take to prevent hyperthermia.

Extreme cold (hypothermia)

Description

Hypothermia is generalized cooling of the body in which the core temperature of the body drops below 95°F (35°C).

ICD-10-CM Code	T68.XXXA (Hypothermia, initial encounter)

Symptoms and Signs

Hypothermia, which is generalized severe cooling of the body, causes the person to shiver and have a feeling of extreme cold or numbness. Fatigue is followed by loss of coordination, thick speech, and disorientation. The skin appears blue (in light-skinned people) or ash-colored (in dark-skinned people) and puffy, with the pulse being slow and weak. Core body temperature drops below 95°F. Breathing is slow and shallow, and the pupils are dilated. As the body temperature drops, the person experiences confusion, stupor, and unconsciousness.

Etiology

Hypothermia can occur when a person is exposed to cold wind, a cold environment, or cold water for prolonged periods. Older, very young, exhausted, and physically debilitated persons have the greatest risk of hypothermia. Lack of adequate clothing or becoming wet, as in a rainstorm, can add to the risk. Sudden immersion in cold water can cause hypothermia.

Diagnosis

Diagnosis is made on the basis of history, the clinical picture, and the finding of below-normal body temperature.

Treatment

Treatment of hypothermia, a life-threatening condition, must be aggressive and immediate. Any wet clothing must be removed, and gradual rewarming of the body is begun by wrapping the person in warm blankets and keeping the body dry. If auxiliary sources of heat, such as hot packs or warm stones, are not available, the warmth from another person's body as he or she embraces the patient can also help warm the patient. If the person is conscious, warm liquids should be given orally in small quantities. The patient should be transported to an emergency facility where vital signs can be monitored.

Prognosis

The prognosis varies, depending on the duration of the exposure to cold and any underlying pathology.

Prevention

Prevention involves avoiding extremely cold temperatures.

Patient Teaching

Encourage patients to avoid situations in which they may be exposed to extreme cold for long periods. Advise them to wear adequate layers of clothing when they must be in an extremely cold environment.

Frostbite

Description
Frozen or extremely cold tissue, usually on the face, ears, fingers, and toes, is termed *frostbite*.

ICD-10-CM Code   T33.90XA *(Superficial frostbite of unspecified sites, initial encounter)*
T33.99XA *(Superficial frostbite of other sites, initial encounter)*
T34.90XA *(Frostbite with tissue necrosis of unspecified sites, initial encounter)*
T34.99XA *(Frostbite with tissue necrosis of other sites, initial encounter)*
(T33.011[7th digit]-T34.99[7th digit] = 74 codes of specificity)
Frostbite is coded by site. Once the diagnosis has been confirmed, refer to the current edition of the ICD-10-CM coding manual for the appropriate code.

Symptoms and Signs
Frostbite, usually occurring on the face, fingers, toes, and ears causes the skin in the affected area to become white in light skinned people or when in dark skinned people (Fig. 15.16).

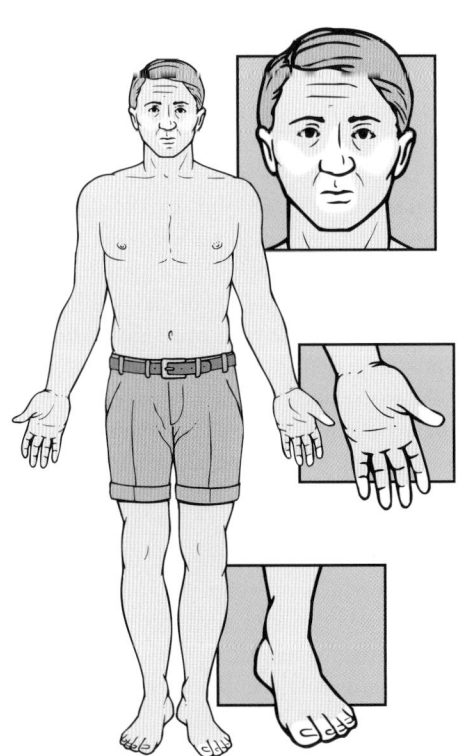

• **Fig. 15.16** Usual sites of frostbite.

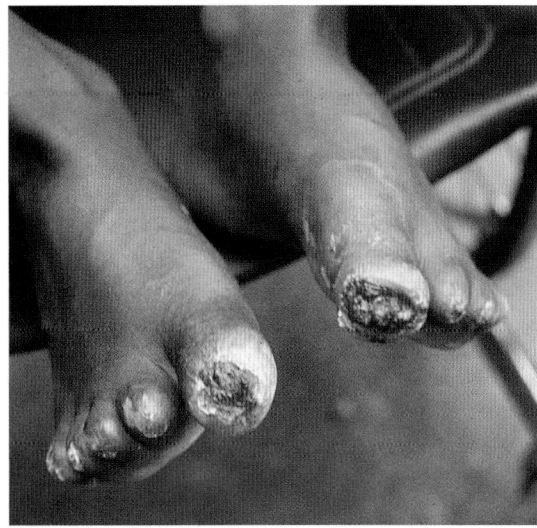

• **Fig. 15.17** Frostbite of the toes. Similar changes also may occur in the fingers. (From Stevens A, et al: *Core pathology*, ed 3, London, 2010, Mosby.)

The person does not realize that the condition is occurring because little or no pain is felt as the tissue freezes. As the freezing deepens, the underlying tissue becomes firm, and the skin takes on a waxy appearance (Fig. 15.17).

Patient Screening
Frostbite requires prompt assessment and intervention. Most individuals will be seen in an emergency facility and assessed for additional hypothermal insults.

Etiology
Frostbite occurs when tissue is exposed to cold air, water, or objects. Ice crystals form between the cells of the skin. As the freezing continues, fluid that is drawn from the cells subsequently freezes. People who have undergone trauma, older adults, newborns, and those wearing wet clothing or tightly laced footwear are at greatest risk when exposed to cold temperatures.

Diagnosis
Diagnosis is made on the basis of visual examination and a history of exposure to cold. The depth or degree of the frostbite is determined by the color and appearance of the skin.

Treatment
Treatment consists of removing the patient from the cold environment. People suffering from superficial frostbite should be warmed with an external source of even heat. The temperature of the heat source should not be above 105°F. The affected skin area should *never* be rubbed. Patients suffering from frostbite should be treated by a physician, if possible. Rewarming of deep frostbite (frozen tissue) should not begin

until professional medical care can be provided. The person should be kept warm, vital signs should be monitored, and alcohol should *never* be given. Pain medication may be administered. Additionally, dehydration may occur and require treatment with intravenous (IV) fluids.

Prognosis

The prognosis varies, depending on the length of exposure and the depth of the insult. Additional variables are the patient's age, general health status, and underlying pathology.

Prevention

Encourage patients to wear gloves, hats, scarves, and heavy socks when prolonged exposure to cold is anticipated. Advise them to replace any wet clothing with dry clothing to prevent additional trauma resulting from the cold temperature.

Patient Teaching

Provide patients with written information concerning prevention of frostbite. Advise parents to dress children in adequate gloves, hats, and scarves when they are engaged in outside winter activities.

◆ ENRICHMENT

Rehabilitation

As recovery begins, many patients begin rehabilitation. The goal of rehabilitation is to help the patient regain some of the functions, both physical and mental, lost or diminished by the injury. The state of recovery depends on many things and often takes months or even years to regain most of the diminished functions. Factors involved include the mechanics of the injury, emotional challenges, family and social support, and complications from the injury. Before rehabilitation can begin, a thorough assessment of the physical state of the patient along with identification of lost or diminished functions must be made. The assessment is followed by the setting of obtainable and realistic goals. The sooner patients are entered into the rehabilitative stage, the more likely they are to succeed in returning to a near-preinjury state.

Bites

Bites can occur at any time and to any part of the body. They range from the annoying insect bite to those by domestic animals, reptiles, or even other humans. Insect bites may be insignificant or life threatening. It has been reported that insect bites are the most common cause of anaphylaxis in the United States. Mosquito bites can cause only itching, or they can cause encephalitis resulting from

infection. An example is the West Nile virus, which is contracted through a bite from an infected mosquito. Additionally tick bites can cause Rocky Mountain spotted fever, malaria, or Lyme disease. Animal bites range in severity from mere nips that do not break the skin and cause no serious disease to life-threatening bites that carry the risk of rabies and infection.

Some states have reportable incident forms to be completed. It is important for medical professionals to recognize the reportable communicable diseases and conditions, as listed in the state board of health guidelines. Some of the reportable diseases and conditions are animal bites, anthrax, cholera, diphtheria, encephalitis, Lyme disease, measles, mumps, pertussis, poliomyelitis, rabies, rubella, smallpox, tetanus, and varicella.

Insect bites

Description

An insect bite, the puncture of the skin by the bite or sting of any insect or arthropod, may involve the injection of venom into the tissue of the individual. Examples of insects that commonly bite humans include fleas, mosquitoes, lice, horseflies, fire ants, and mites. Bees, wasps, and hornets can sting an individual and inject venom, thereby causing localized pain and swelling. Spiders also bite or sting humans and inject venom.

| ICD-10-CM Code | T07 *(Unspecified multiple injuries)* |

Insect bites are coded by mention of infection. Once the diagnosis has been confirmed, refer to the current edition of the ICD-10-CM coding manual for the appropriate code.

Symptoms and Signs

The symptoms and signs of an insect bite or sting vary, depending on the type of insect that has bitten or stung the individual (Figs. 15.18 and 15.19). Usually a sharp, stinging pain is felt and may be followed by itching, redness, or swelling at the site. If the patient experiences a systemic reaction to the bite, he or she will have itching on the palms of the hands or soles of the feet, the neck, or the groin or may experience generalized itching, along with a rash over the entire body. As the allergic reaction progresses, the patient experiences generalized edema, dyspnea, weakness, nausea, shock, and unconsciousness.

Patient Screening

Individuals reporting insect stings or bites require prompt assessment. Some bites or stings may precipitate an allergic reaction, often a very rapid and life-threatening reaction. Those with a known severe allergic response to certain types of bites or stings usually require emergency intervention as a life-saving measure. Many such individuals and their families are aware of the potential danger and carry a "bee-sting" kit containing an epinephrine injection (EpiPen)

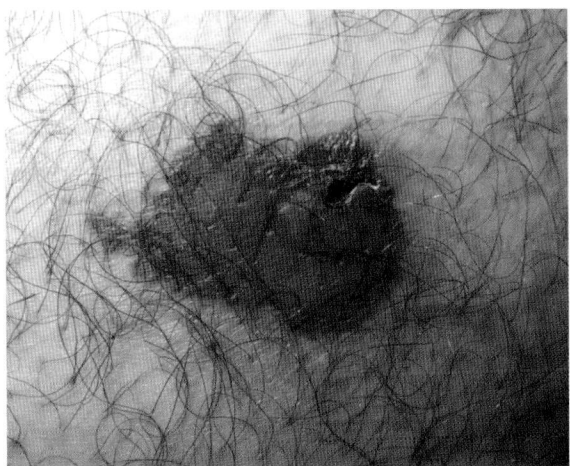

• **Fig. 15.18** Brown recluse spider bite after 48 hours of treatment. (From Miller JJ, Marks JG: *Lookingbill and Marks' principles of dermatology,* ed 6, Philadelphia, 2019, Elsevier.)

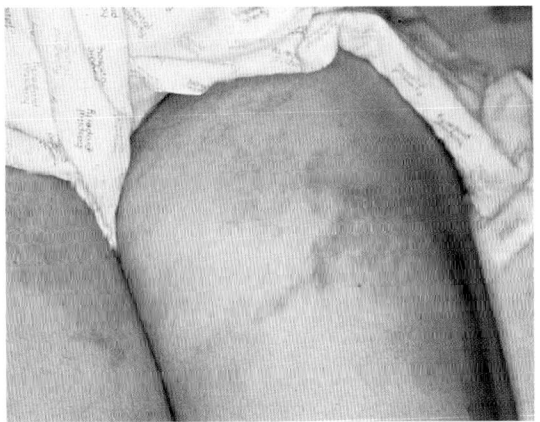

• **Fig. 15.19** Multiple bites of imported fire ants. (From [illegible] *disorders—Mosby's clinical nursing series,* St Louis, 1994, Mosby. Courtesy Dermatology Department, University of Texas Southwestern Medical School, Dallas, TX.)

with them at all times for emergency injection to reverse the allergic response. Follow-up appointments should be scheduled to educate the patient and the family about the dangers of insect stings and about taking preventive measures.

Etiology

The injury occurs when the insect either bites or stings the individual. Venom is injected into the tissue, resulting in the body's response to a foreign protein. Some of the more common types of bites or stings are those of mosquitoes, bees, wasps, hornets, spiders, fire ants, ticks, and fleas. Bites by black widow spiders, brown recluse spiders, and scorpions occur less often. Ocean animal bites cause pain and swelling and may be mild; however, sometimes they cause swelling of lymph nodes and difficulty breathing, depending on the type of bite.

Diagnosis

The diagnosis is made on the basis of visual examination and patient history. It is hoped that the patient can identify or give a description of the offending insect. Some insect bites or stings leave characteristic signs.

Treatment

The first step in treating an insect sting is to determine whether the stinger is still present in the bite wound. If it is present, it must be removed to prevent further damage. The best method of removal is scraping across the site of the sting with a plastic card or a fingernail. (The use of forceps or tweezers squeezes more venom into the site.) The area is then cleansed with soap and water. Application of dry dressing, cold packs, or anesthetic sprays affords some comfort. The person should be observed for any signs of allergic reaction to the sting or bite. Lyme disease, the result of a tick bite, and encephalitis, the result of a mosquito bite, are discussed in Chapters 7 and 13, respectively.

People with black widow spider or brown recluse spider bites or scorpion stings should be transported to an emergency facility. Aggressive treatment includes cleansing of the wound, administration of medication for pain relief, cold applications, and antivenin, and monitoring of vital signs.

Prognosis

The prognosis varies, depending on the degree to which the person is sensitized to the offending foreign protein injected during the bite or sting. Many bites or stings resolve without treatment and no sensitization occurs. In those with much can in severe reaction, recovery may be speedy or slow, depending on any underlying pathology. Refer to Chapters 7 and 13 for additional information about Lyme disease and encephalitis.

Prevention

Prevention includes avoiding situations where exposure to the offending insect may occur. Use of insect repellant may be helpful. Education of family members and coworkers regarding possible severe reactions and the measures that are necessary to counteract a potentially life-threatening allergic response is beneficial.

Patient Teaching

Provide the patient with information pertaining to prevention of insect bites and stings. Instruct the family about procedures to follow in case of an emergency situation involving a severe reaction.

Rocky Mountain Spotted Fever/Tick Bite

Description. Rocky Mountain spotted fever, a tick-borne disease, is a severe systemic infection. It is the most commonly reported rickettsial disease in the United States.

ICD-10-CM Code	A77.0 *(Spotted fever due to Rickettsia rickettsii)* (A77.0-A77.3 = 4 codes of specificity)

Symptoms and Signs. The patient may recall being bitten by a tick, typically during outdoor activity, such as camping and hiking. Patients are frequently unaware of the presence of the insects on their bodies because they are flat and small and may be hidden in an area covered by hair. Several days to 2 weeks later, a sudden onset of fever, severe headache, vomiting, malaise, and myalgia occur. Four days after the onset of fever, a characteristic maculopapular rash is noted, and the rash spreads over the body. Small hemorrhages appear under the skin, the characteristic sign that gives the disease its name. Inflammation of blood vessels (vasculitis) affects the skin and other organs, leading to systemic manifestations in the heart, lungs, kidneys, and nervous system. After 2 to 3 weeks, the skin begins to peel (Fig. 15.20).

Patient Screening. Individuals reporting symptoms of fever, severe headache, vomiting, malaise, and myalgia require prompt assessment.

Etiology. The causative agent, *Rickettsia rickettsii,* is transmitted by the wood tick and is carried in the feces of infected ticks. It is introduced into the bloodstream of a person during a prolonged tick bite (duration of 4 to 6 hours). Once it is in the bloodstream, the organism, an intracellular parasite, reproduces in certain cells and destroys them. The disease cannot be transmitted from person to person.

Diagnosis. Although Rocky Mountain spotted fever is difficult to diagnose, a history of a tick bite or recent outdoor activity in tick-infested areas and the onset of severe systemic symptoms, with the appearance of the characteristic rash, suggest the diagnosis (Fig. 15.21). Laboratory findings include a positive complement fixation reaction, which measures the antigen-antibody reaction occurring in the body, and thereby the severity of infection. Changes in the clotting components in blood may be noted. Isolation of the organism in a blood culture confirms the diagnosis.

Treatment. The treatment of choice for Rocky Mountain spotted fever is antibiotic therapy with tetracycline or

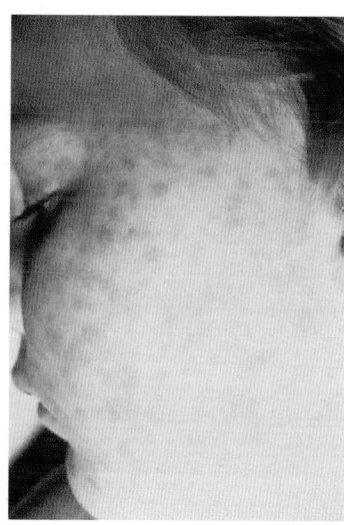

• **Fig. 15.21** Rocky Mountain spotted fever rash on side of face 9 days after onset. (From Grimes D: *Infectious diseases—Mosby's clinical nursing series,* St Louis, 1994, Mosby.)

doxycycline and symptomatic relief with the administration of analgesics. Infection confers lifetime immunity.

Prognosis. The prognosis is good with rapid diagnosis and treatment with antibiotic regimen. Underlying pathology or concurrent health problems may complicate the outcome.

Prevention. Preventive measures include wearing protective clothing and applying insect repellent to clothing and exposed skin. Visual inspection of the skin for the presence of ticks should be made every few hours during and after outdoor activity in infested areas. If a tick is found, it should be removed carefully with tweezers, avoiding handling of the tick.

Patient Teaching. Encourage individuals to wear proper protective clothing when in environments where ticks may reside. Also instruct them to make a visual inspection of the skin for ticks or apparent tick bites every few hours.

Malaria/Mosquito Bite

Description. Malaria is a severe generalized infection caused by the bite of an *Anopheles* mosquito that is infected by a *Plasmodium* type of protozoa.

ICD-10-CM Code	B54 *(Unspecified malaria)*
	(B50.0-B54 = 13 codes of specificity)

Symptoms and Signs. Malaria is an acute, sometimes chronic, serious infectious illness. It is characterized by a classic cycle of chills, fever, and sweats, occurring in that order. The patient also may have headache, nausea, fatigue, and myalgia. Although the course and severity of the disease can vary, bouts of malaria usually last from 1 to 4 weeks. Signs include an enlarged spleen, an enlarged liver, and

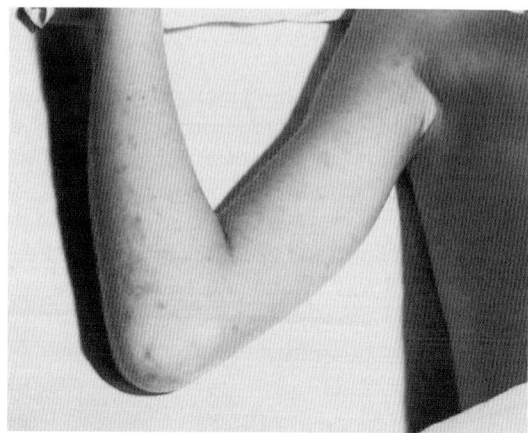

• **Fig. 15.20** Rocky Mountain spotted fever rash on arm. (From Grimes D: *Infectious diseases—Mosby's clinical nursing series,* St Louis, 1994, Mosby.)

anemia. The symptoms have a tendency to recur and may persist for years.

Patient Screening. An individual reporting symptoms of chills, fever, and sweats, possibly combined with headache, nausea, fatigue, and myalgia, requires prompt assessment.

Etiology. Malaria is caused by four species of the protozoan *Plasmodium*, which is transmitted from infected human to human by the bite of mosquito vectors or, less commonly, by blood transfusion or IV drug use. After they are introduced into the body, the protozoan parasites feed on hemoglobin and reproduce within red blood cells (RBCs). Malaria is endemic in tropical and subtropical areas, such as South and Central America, Asia, and Africa, and usually is brought to the United States by travelers returning from these areas.

Diagnosis. Laboratory testing of infected individuals reveals decreased hemoglobin level, decreased platelet count, prolonged prothrombin time (PT), and a positive serum antibody test result. Diagnosis is confirmed by identifying the *Plasmodium* organism in a blood smear.

Treatment. Malaria is treated with chloroquine, an antimalarial drug, given orally. Other drugs may include mefloquine, atovaquone-proguanil (Malarone), artemether-lumefantrine (Coartem) and quinine. Tetracycline, doxycycline, and clindamycin may be used in conjunction with quinine. Artesunate is another drug that is available but not licensed for use in the United States. This drug is available through the Centers for Disease Control and Prevention (CDC). Antipyretics are given for fever. Infusion of packed RBCs may be required to treat anemia. Each new case of malaria must be reported to the local board of health.

Prognosis. The prognosis varies, depending on the response to treatment and any underlying pathology.

Prevention. A prophylactic course of chloroquine may be given before travel to known endemic areas.

A number of medications may be used for chemoprophylaxis, although some of these medications may cause serious or fatal side effects. Current CDC guidelines recommend the combination drug atovaquone/proguanil (Malarone), which seems to work well without causing serious side effects. Current CDC guidelines should be checked for dosage and duration of therapy instructions.

Patient Teaching. Provide patients who may be traveling to endemic areas with information on prophylactic medications. Also instruct them regarding possible symptoms of malaria, and encourage them to seek medical treatment at the onset of any such symptoms.

Animal bites/Human bites

Description

An animal bite is any bite inflicted on an individual by another animal. The source may be another human, a domestic pet, or any wild animal.

 ENRICHMENT

Altitude Sickness

Altitude sickness, or acute mountain sickness, is a disorder associated with the low oxygen content of the atmosphere at high altitudes. It occurs when individuals make a rapid ascent into high altitudes, usually greater than 8000 feet. Symptoms include loss of appetite, nausea and vomiting, headache, dizziness, rapid pulse, fatigue, difficulty sleeping, shortness of breath on exertion, and air hunger. Mild symptoms that mimic jet lag or the flu can subside as the body adjusts to the higher altitude. More severe symptoms include cough, chest tightness or congestion, confusion, cyanosis, decreased level of consciousness, pale or grayish skin, difficulty walking, and shortness of breath at rest. Life-threatening altitude sickness can cause prostration, cardiac disturbances, and cerebral edema, with possible seizures and death. Pulmonary edema is another severe state in altitude sickness. It is possible for those with heart problems to experience angina and subsequent myocardial infarction triggered by the high-altitude conditions (Fig. 15.22). In addition, dehydration is a contributing factor. Those who experience symptoms should descend to a lower altitude and drink plenty of water. Rest and curtailing stressful activities help relieve symptoms and are necessary interventions for shortness of breath and increased heart rate.

Prevention includes acclimating oneself to the higher altitudes slowly over a period of a few days, drinking extra fluids, and avoiding alcohol and smoking. When at elevations greater than 8000 feet, it is best not to climb greater than 0000 feet a day.

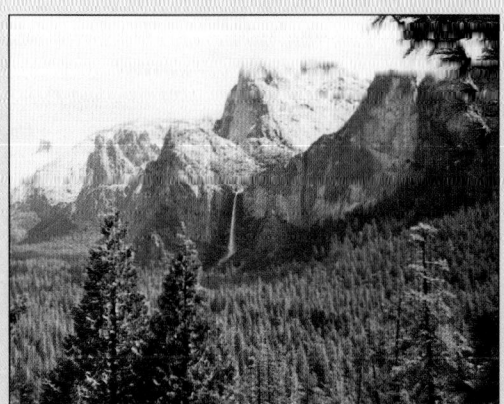

• **Fig. 15.22** Typical site for onset of altitude sickness. (Courtesy David L Frazier, 1999.)

ICD-10-CM Code   S codes by site
Refer to the current edition of the ICD-10-CM coding manual for additional information and appropriate codes according to site.

Symptoms and Signs

Broken skin with evidence of teeth marks is the usual clinical finding related to an animal bite. Puncture wounds are present, with possible tearing of the skin. Bleeding is usually evident, and the flesh actually may be bitten away. Discoloration of the surrounding skin indicates bruising to the area. The patient usually reports pain at the site.

Patient Screening

Individuals reporting animal bites require prompt assessment. The extent of the bite requires evaluation so that prompt treatment can begin. It is also important that information about the animal be obtained for animal control to confine the animal until possible rabies infection is ruled out. The patient should be given the next available same-day appointment. If this is not possible, the patient should be sent to an outpatient clinic or to an emergency department.

Etiology

Typically the bite occurs when the offending animal is agitated, frightened, threatened, or angry. Bites can be from domestic animals, such as cats and dogs; farm animals; or wild animals, such as skunks, bats, raccoons, and foxes (Fig. 15.23). Human bites have been recorded. Shark bites are also a potential source of injury in some areas with an increase in shark presence.

Diagnosis

The diagnosis is made on the basis of history and physical examination. The pattern of the teeth marks is helpful in determining the type of bite, whether human or animal, and the type of animal that did the biting, if not immediately known.

Treatment

Treatment begins with cleansing of the wound to remove bacteria and contamination. If bleeding cannot be controlled, hemostasis is achieved with cautery or suturing. Depending on the site and severity of the wound, plastic surgery may be indicated for optimal repair.

Rabies is transmitted through the saliva of infected animals. If the offending animal is a domestic pet, it usually is not too difficult to confirm the most recent date of rabies inoculation or to quarantine the animal for the

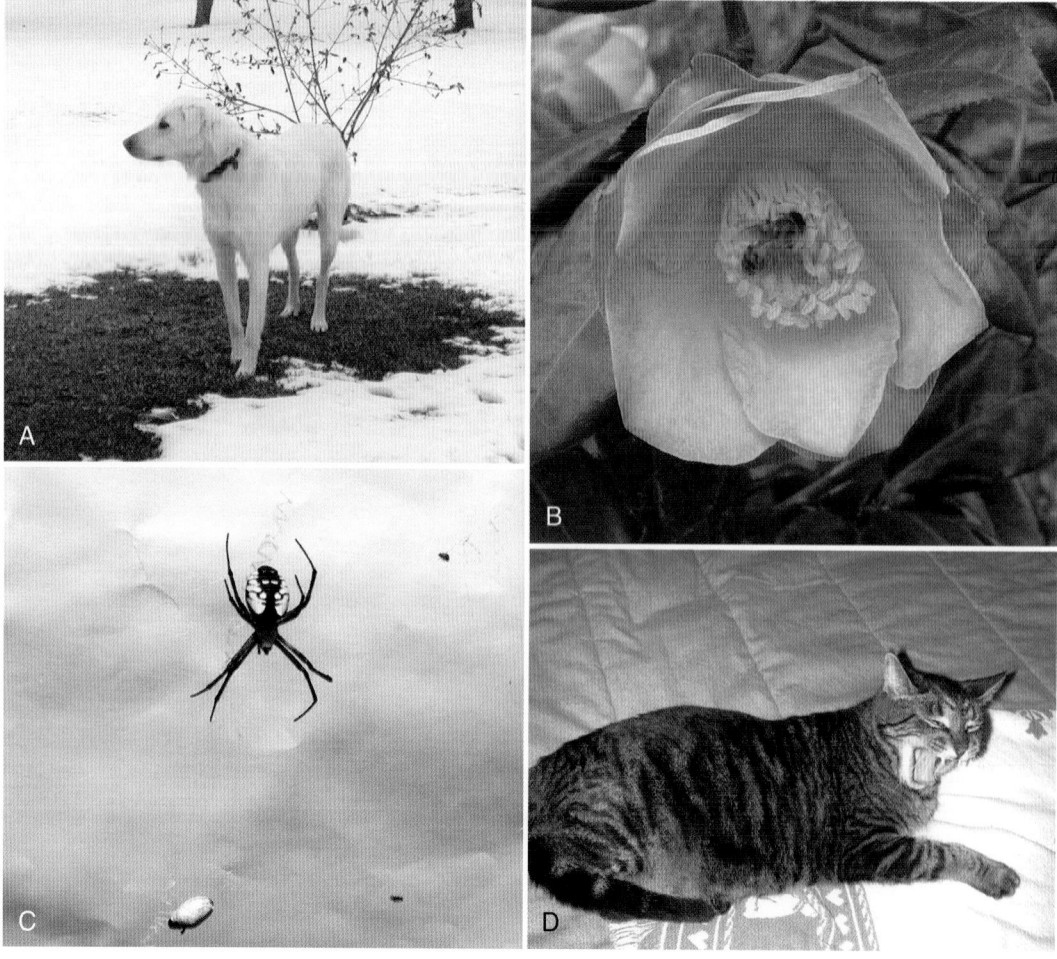

• **Fig. 15.23** Insects and animals possibly capable of inflicting bites. (A to C, Courtesy David L. Frazier, 2003. D, Courtesy Mark Boswell, 2003.)

time necessary to rule out rabies infection. Most communities require reporting animal bites to the local animal control agency or a local law enforcement agency that will follow through on determining the rabies inoculation status of the animal. If it is not possible to determine if the animal is rabid, the injured person probably will have to undergo a series of injections to confer immunity against rabies. Human bites are dangerous because of the organism that may contaminate the wound.

As with most invasive trauma, a sterile dressing should be applied. Tetanus prophylaxis is confirmed or administered, if necessary, and antibiotics may be prescribed as an additional prophylactic measure.

Prognosis

The prognosis varies, depending on the extent of the damage to the tissue and on any underlying pathology. If the animal is rabid, the prognosis is guarded.

Prevention

Prevention often is difficult, especially when the bite is not knowingly provoked by the actions of the victim.

Patient Teaching

Encourage children not to approach or touch animals, even those that are in a restrained environment. Advise individuals with pets to keep the animal's inoculations, especially for rabies, current. Instruct the patient or his or her family members on wound care and also on the importance of completing any antibiotic therapy that has been prescribed.

Snakebites

Description

A snakebite is a penetrating tissue wound made by the fangs or teeth of a snake.

ICD-10-CM Code	(T63.001A-T63.94XA =
	152 codes of
	specificity)

Refer to the current edition of the ICD-10-CM coding manual for additional information and appropriate codes according to site.

Symptoms and Signs

The patient may have actually seen the snake that gave the bite or may not have been aware of the snake at the time the bite happened. In either event, the patient will have a noticeable bite to the skin or possibly only a slight skin discoloration at the site of injury. Burning pain is present, and swelling begins around the bite; however, this reaction may be delayed, developing slowly over time. Pulse rate becomes rapid, and the patient begins to experience weakness, visual difficulties, and nausea and vomiting. Signs and symptoms of the poisoning may take 30 minutes to several hours to develop. Coral snakes are extremely poisonous and leave small chew type of teeth marks rather than the two distinct fang marks made by other poisonous snakes (Fig. 15.24).

Patient Screening

Complaints reporting a possible snakebite require prompt assessment and intervention. The EMS should be activated for transportation of the victim to the nearest emergency care facility.

Etiology

The poisoning from the snakebite usually takes 1 to 2 days to develop unless the person is allergic to the foreign protein of the venom, which will speed up the reaction time. Four kinds of poisonous snakes are known to inhabit the United States: rattlesnakes, copperheads, water moccasins, and coral snakes. Rattlesnakes account for the greatest number of poisonous snakebites. Some bites are the work of nonpoisonous snakes, but all snakebites should be treated as poisonous by the first aid provider.

Diagnosis

Diagnosis is made by history and visual examination of the affected area. Typically, two fang marks in the skin are indicative of poisonous snakebites; the exception is the bite of a coral snake, which appears as a chew type of bite that leaves teeth marks (see Fig. 15.24).

Some physicians request, if possible, that the snake head be brought in for assisting in treatment. Any rescuer must always remember that their own safety is a priority, and they *must never* jeopardize their own safety in a rescue. Attempting to obtain a snake head could be dangerous and should only be done if the snake is dead.

Treatment

First aid and intervention at the scene consists of removing the person from the injury site to prevent further risk and keeping her or him calm and quiet. The EMS system should be activated. The bitten area is cleansed with soap and water. Any jewelry, including rings or other constricting objects, should be removed from the affected limb. The extremity should be immobilized and, if possible, kept below the level of the heart. Transport to the nearest emergency facility should be initiated as soon as possible so that aggressive treatment can begin immediately. If it is not possible to reach emergency care within 30 minutes, consideration should be given to suctioning the bite with equipment from a snakebite kit. Antivenin may be given to the patient and vital functions supported, as needed. The protocol for snakebite treatment indicates that cold should *not* be applied, the wound should *not* be cut, tourniquets should *not* be applied, and electrical shock should *not* be applied.

Prognosis

The prognosis varies, depending on how poisonous the snake is. Bites from nonpoisonous snakes usually resolve and heal

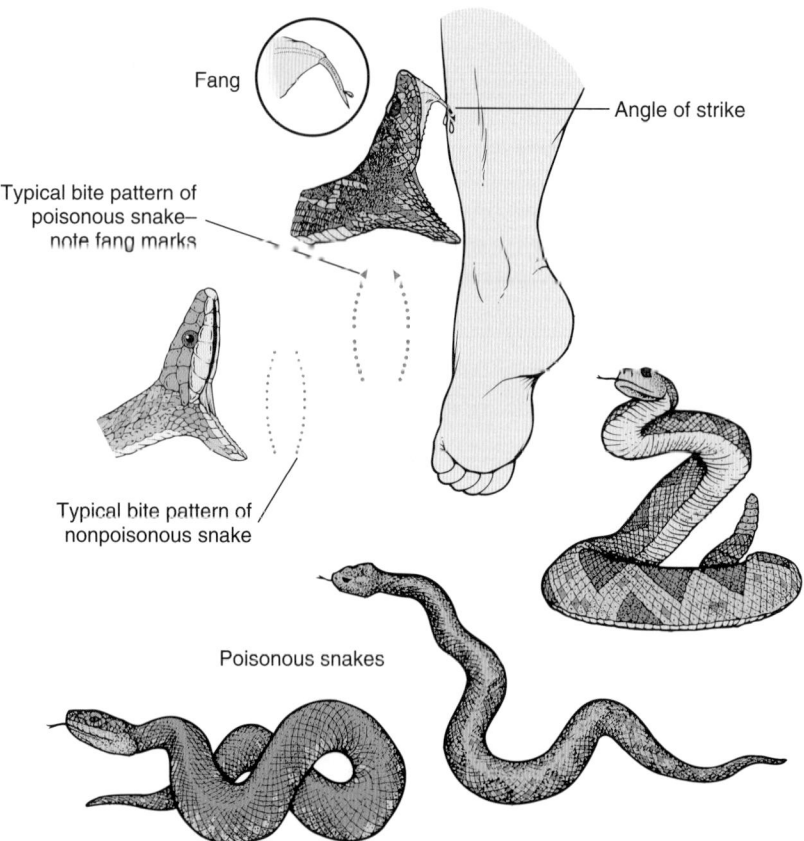

Fang

Angle of strike

Typical bite pattern of poisonous snake— note fang marks

Typical bite pattern of nonpoisonous snake

Poisonous snakes

• **Fig. 15.24** Snakebite. (Redrawn with permission of *Patient Care Magazine,* Montvale, NJ, 1976, Patient Care Publications.)

with few complications. Recovery from bites of poisonous snakes depends on the availability of antivenin, the promptness of the treatment, and the location of the bite on the body. Preexisting pathology of the patient may dictate the outcome.

Prevention

Using caution in areas known to be inhabited by snakes is prudent (Fig. 15.25). When in an area where snakes are likely to be present, heavy "snake" boots should be worn to prevent possible bites from penetrating tissue. Grassy, wet areas should be avoided, if possible.

Patient Teaching

Encourage individuals to regard all snakes as being potentially poisonous. Provide information about areas in the community that snakes are likely to inhabit, and recommend avoidance of these areas. If travel within or occupation of these areas is necessary, encourage wearing of heavy boots to prevent bites around feet and lower legs.

Cumulative Trauma (Repetitive Motion Trauma, Overuse Syndrome)

Cumulative trauma disorders, or repetitive motion injuries, are common to numerous occupations. They account for

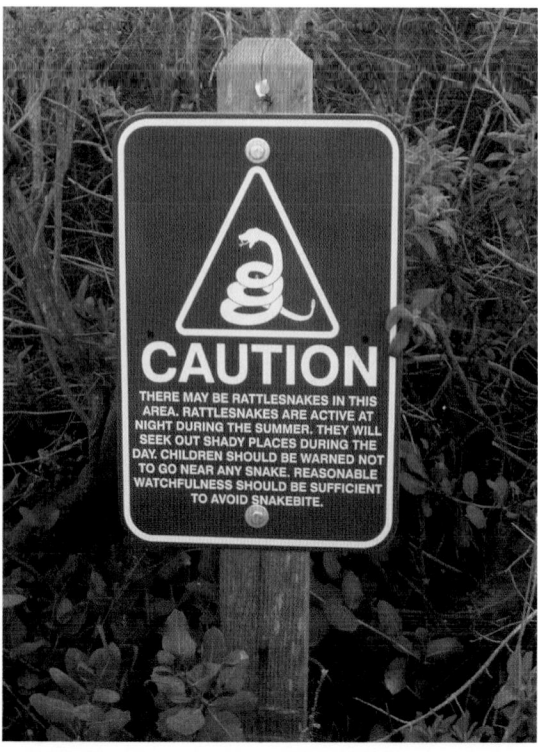

• **Fig. 15.25** Warning sign concerning presence of rattlesnakes. (Courtesy David L. Frazier, 2003.)

Poisoning

Poisons are any substances that, when introduced into the body, cause illness or injury; many cause death. Poisoning can be accidental or intentional. Poisons can be introduced into the body by absorption through the skin, ingestion through the GI tract, inhalation through the respiratory system, and injection through a sting, bite, or hypodermic needle. The signs and symptoms vary according to the poison and the method of introduction into the body. Many poisons are found in the domestic setting and often are the cause of exposure. Refer to Table 15.1 for a list of common chemicals found in the domestic setting.

Ingested or swallowed poisons can include food, alcohol, chemicals, medications, and plants.

Refer to Table 15.2 for a list of poisonous plants. Inhaled poisons include gases, such as carbon monoxide, carbon dioxide, nitrous oxide, chlorine, and fumes from chemicals or drugs. Absorbed poisons include chemicals or oils from certain plants. Injected poisons include venom injected by bites from insects, spiders, ticks, snakes, or drugs given via a hypodermic needle.

Because of the vast number of poisons and methods of introduction into the body, it is impossible to identify symptoms, etiology, diagnosis, and treatment for each toxic substance. General guidelines include (1) identification of the toxic substance and (2) contacting a poison control center or emergency facility for assistance. Of utmost importance is that the rescuer or care provider not compromise his or her own safety, especially when inhalation of toxic fumes could be involved.

Poison control centers are available on the phone and the Internet. Poison control center hotlines are available 24 hours a day, 7 days a week. Many families contact poison control centers for recommended tests and managements.

TABLE 15.1 Common Chemical Toxins Present In Domestic Settings

Agent	Effects
Methyl alcohol	• Metabolic acidosis • Neurologic damage
Ethylene glycol	• Metabolic acidosis • Oxalate deposition in kidneys • Acute tubular necrosis
Carbon tetrachloride	• Centrilobular necrosis in liver • Tubular necrosis in kidneys
Carbon monoxide	• Tissue hypoxia by forming carboxyhemoglobin • Headache, dizziness, and confusion (early features) • Delayed damage to basal ganglia and white matter • Coma and death with high saturation
Strong alkalis	• Ulceration of oropharynx and esophagus

(From Stevens A, et al: *Core pathology,* ed 3, London, 2010, Mosby.)

TABLE 15.2 Poisonous Plants

Plant	Toxic Parts
Apple	Leaves, seeds
Apricot	Leaves, stem, seed pits
Azalea	All parts
Buttercup	All parts
Cherry (wild or cultivated)	Twigs, seeds, foliage
Daffodil	Bulbs
Dumb cane (dieffenbachia)	All parts
Elephant ear	All parts
English ivy	All parts
Foxglove	Leaves, seeds, flowers
Holly	Berries, leaves
Hyacinth	Bulbs
Ivy	Leaves
Mistletoe[a]	Berries, leaves
Oak tree	Acorn, foliage
Philodendron	All parts
Plum	Pit
Poinsettia[b]	Leaves
Poison ivy, poison oak	Leaves, fruit, stems, smoke from burning plants
Pothos	All parts
Rhubarb	Leaves
Tulip	Bulbs
Water hemlock	All parts
Wisteria	Seeds, pods
Yew	All parts

[a]Eating one or two berries or leaves is probably nontoxic.
[b]Toxic if ingested in massive quantities.
(From Hockenberry MJ, Wilson D: *Wong's nursing care of infants and children,* ed 9, St Louis, 2011, Mosby.)

more time lost from work than any other single factor. At risk are those working in industries where repetitive tasks have to be performed, including those who work on computers on a regular and continuous basis, cashiers who scan products on conveyor belts, and those who engage in target practice and in certain other sports.

Cumulative trauma disorders are muscular conditions that result from repeated motions performed in the course of daily activities. These conditions are caused by repetitive movement that is unnatural or awkward, such as overexertion, twisting, or muscle fatigue. Soft tissue injuries that develop over time as a result of repetitive activities cause continuing stress on specific muscles or nerves. These injuries can result from improper posture of the wrist, arm, back, shoulder, or legs. Many occur because of pressure centered on the hand or the wrist, with frequent repetitive motions for an extended period. In the industrial setting, improper use of handheld tools, especially with excessive or improper grip, can cause cumulative trauma disorders. Additionally, continuous vibration contributes to increased occurrence of trauma. The characteristics of cumulative trauma disorders are pain, tingling, numbness, swelling, redness, loss of flexibility and strength. These disorders include but are not limited to white finger (Raynaud phenomenon), trigger finger, carpal tunnel syndrome, tennis elbow, thoracic outlet syndrome, de Quervain disease, synovitis, tenosynovitis, and nonspecific tendinitis. Cumulative trauma develops over an extended period, so the onset of symptoms is insidious. Much investigation may be necessary to pinpoint the repetitive task that has caused the trauma. Ergonomics is an assessment of how a person performs tasks. During the assessment, the individual is observed in a work situation or other action where a repetitive task is performed. An attempt is made to determine whether a subtle or other change in the way the task is done may help relieve symptoms or prevent an injury from occurring.

As with other work-related injuries, workers' compensation forms must be completed.

Carpal tunnel syndrome

Description
Entrapment and compression of the median nerve in the carpal tunnel causes pain and numbness in the wrist, hands, and fingers.

ICD-10-CM Code	G56.00 (Carpal tunnel syndrome, unspecified upper limb) (G56.00-G56.02 = 3 codes of specificity)

Symptoms and Signs
The patient experiences numbness of hands and fingers, with pain more pronounced at night. Swelling of the wrist or hand and "fluttering" of the fingers are additional symptoms. The patient often is observed cradling the arm or rubbing the hand or arm. Temporary relief is sometimes obtained by shaking or moving the wrist.

Patient Screening
Although not an emergency, assessment of this painful condition should be accomplished at the earliest available and convenient time.

Etiology
Tendons, blood vessels, and the median nerve pass through a narrow fibrous tunnel that extends from the wrist to the hand (Fig. 15.26). Carpal tunnel syndrome results when the tendons within the tunnel become inflamed from repetitive overuse of the hand, wrist, or fingers, thereby causing entrapment of the median nerve as it passes through the wrist, which results in the pinching of the median nerve (Fig. 15.27). Any condition that exerts pressure on the median nerve can cause carpal tunnel syndrome.

Diagnosis
The clinical findings, along with the history of the repetitive motion activities, suggests carpal tunnel syndrome. Patients with carpal tunnel syndrome typically feel symptoms of numbness and tingling of the hand in the area of the thumb, index finger, middle finger, and part of the fourth finger. Two specific minor tests aid in the confirmation of the diagnosis. One is the median nerve percussion test (Fig. 15.28), in which the examiner taps his or her fingers along the inside of the affected wrist, eliciting a pins-and-needles sensation in the hand and the fingers. The other is the Phalen wrist flexor test, in which the patient presses the backs of the hands together to bend the wrists as far downward as possible, without applying force, and holds them together for 60 seconds. The fingers should be kept pointing toward the floor. In a patient with a positive test result, numbness and tingling of the hand or fingers is present.

Treatment
Treatment consists of physical therapy and identification and cessation of the repetitive motion to rest the wrist and the hand. Antiinflammatory drugs are prescribed; ice packs and a splint may be applied to maintain the wrist in a neutral position. Oral corticosteroids or a local injection into the affected area by an experienced clinician may quickly relieve symptoms. As a final resort, surgery to divide the carpal ligament is performed in an attempt to relieve pressure on the nerve.

Prognosis
The prognosis is usually favorable. If the conservative measures are not successful, surgical intervention may be indicated. Compliance with the suggested or prescribed therapy is helpful to achieve a positive outcome.

Prevention
Prevention is important, so ergonomic studies and correction of improper repetitive activities should be implemented.

Prevention involves using ergonomically correct devices and positions when engaging in activities that tend to cause the repetitive motion injury.

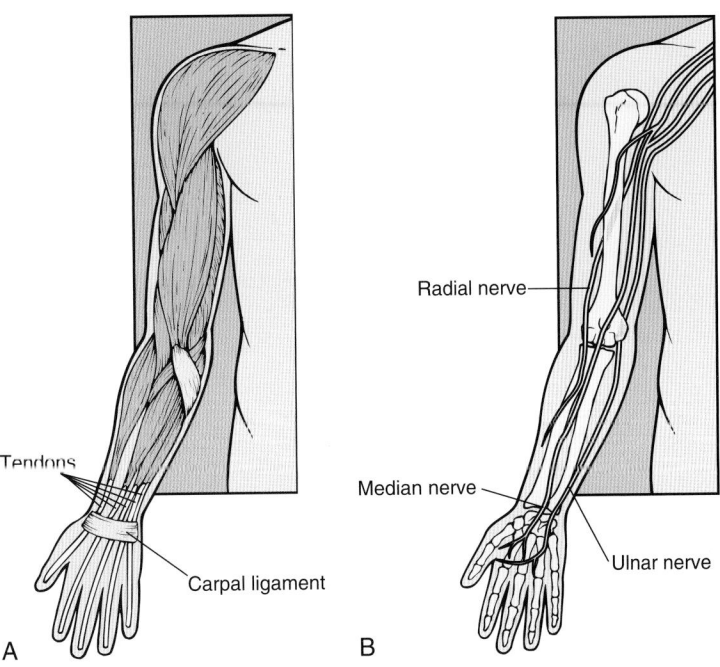

• **Fig. 15.26** Anatomy of arm, wrist, and hand. (A) Muscles, tendons, and carpal ligament. (B) Nerves.

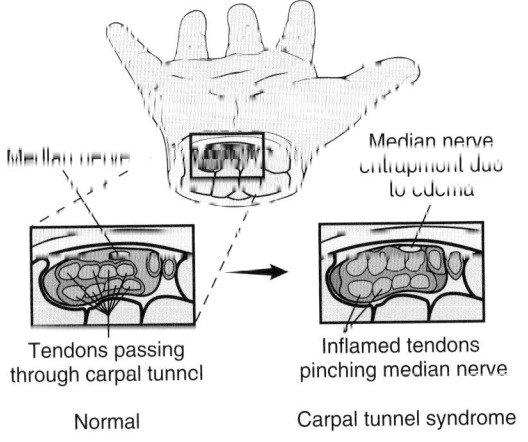

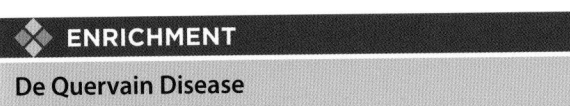

• **Fig. 15.27** Entrapment of the median nerve in the carpal tunnel space.

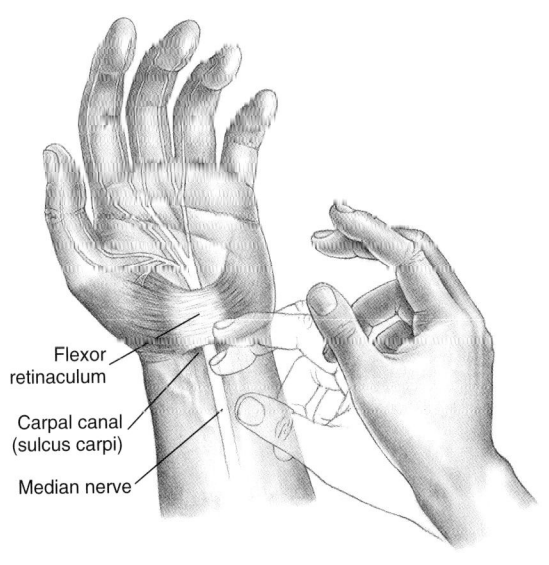

• **Fig. 15.28** Elicitation of Tinel sign. (From Seidel HM, et al: *Mosby's guide to physical examination,* ed 8, St Louis, 2014, Mosby.)

Patient Teaching

Encourage patients to avoid repetitive motion that places the arm, hand, and wrist in compromised positions. Work with employers to eliminate or modify tasks requiring repetitive motion that places the median nerve at risk. Provide the patient visual aids depicting the anatomy and physiology of the wrist, hand, and lower arm.

◆ ENRICHMENT

De Quervain Disease

De Quervain disease is an inflammation of the tendons of the thumb. It is caused by irritation of the long abductor and short extensor tendons. Repetitive motion causes edema and tenderness in the thumb and its base.

Tennis elbow

Description

Tennis elbow, technically known as *lateral humeral epicondylitis,* is the result of repetitive movement involving flexion of the wrist against resistance. The result of this repetitive action is an inflammatory condition of the tissue at the distal portion of the humerus.

ICD-10-CM Code   M77.10 *(Lateral epicondylitis, unspecified elbow)*
                      (M77.00-M77.12 = 6 codes of specificity)

Symptoms and Signs

The patient has pain in the outer (lateral) aspect of the elbow and lower arm. Weakness is exhibited in the affected extremity.

Patient Screening

Tennis elbow is not an emergency but can be quite painful. Schedule the patient to be seen at the next available appointment.

Etiology

The extensor attachment to the lateral humeral condyle becomes inflamed. Repetitive motion in the elbow, usually with accompanying stress to the joint, causes this inflammatory condition.

Diagnosis

Diagnosis is made by evaluating the clinical findings and by physical examination.

Treatment

Treatment consists of stopping the repetitive task and resting the affected arm. An elastic brace can be placed distal to the elbow to alter the fulcrum of the activity. Nonsteroidal antiinflammatory drugs (NSAIDs) and ice packs to the area are also helpful in decreasing the inflammation. Steroid injections into the joint space may quickly afford relief.

Prognosis

Prognosis is good when the repetitive motion is alleviated. Resting the affected limb usually affords pain relief, and the condition may resolve by itself. When steroid injections are provided, the condition usually improves.

Prevention

Use of proper body mechanics when engaging in activities involving the shoulder and arm is helpful as a preventive measure. Recognition of stressful activities and modification of the activity also may be helpful in prevention. If the condition is the result of an occupational task, explore ergonomically correct methods for performing the task.

Patient Teaching

Provide the patient with information and suggestions regarding ergonomically correct methods of performing activities that place stress on the elbow joint. When physical therapy is prescribed, encourage compliance with the recommended exercises. Provide the patient visual aids depicting the anatomy and physiology of the elbow and the upper and lower arm.

Trigger finger

Description

The technical term for trigger finger is *stenosing tenosynovitis*. The index finger has a lump or knot that appears on the flexor tendon. Flexion or extension of the finger may be interrupted and then begin again in a jerking or snapping type of motion when the hand is opened and closed.

| ICD-10-CM Code | M65.30 *(Trigger finger, unspecified finger)* |
| | (M65.30-M65.35 = 16 codes of specificity) |

Symptoms and Signs

A lump or knot appears on the flexor tendon of the affected index finger. Movement of the finger may be temporarily interrupted and then continues on with a jerking type of motion. Trigger finger can also affect the thumb. Closing the hand often causes pain at the base of the finger on the palm of the hand.

Patient Screening

The next available appointment should be given to the patient.

Etiology

The cause of trigger finger is excessive use of the index finger resulting from difficult repetitive finger movement or trauma to the tendon sheath. Trigger finger is caused by local swelling from inflammation or scarring around the tendons that provide the flexion motion of the finger.

Diagnosis

The diagnosis is made by evaluating the clinical findings, history, and physical examination results.

Treatment

As with other cumulative trauma, cessation of the repetitive activity and rest of the affected part is the prescribed course of treatment. Placing ice packs on the inflamed area, stretching exercises, using NSAIDs, and injecting cortisone into the inflamed tendon are effective treatments. Surgical intervention may be considered if all other conservative treatments fail.

Prognosis

The prognosis is good when the repetitive motion is halted.

Prevention

No method of prevention, other than avoiding the repetitive activity, is known.

Patient Teaching

Encourage the patient to allow the finger to rest. Generate print-on-demand electronic materials, when possible, as teaching tools.

Thoracic outlet syndrome (brachial plexus injury)

Description

Thoracic outlet syndrome is the compression of the brachial plexus nerves.

| ICD-10-CM Code | G54.0 *(Brachial plexus disorders)* |

Symptoms and Signs

Thoracic outlet syndrome causes the patient to experience pain in the arm of the affected side. Paresthesia of the fingers also is experienced, along with weakness and diminished grasp capability in the fingers and the thumb. The small muscles of the hand may even begin to waste away.

Patient Screening

Although not an emergency, the condition will cause the patient pain and possibly apprehension because of the numbness in the fingers and the continual dropping of items. Schedule the next available appointment for the patient.

Etiology

The performance of repetitive tasks that cause continual hyperabduction of the arm is one of the causative factors of this condition. Other causes include a continual dropping of the shoulder girdle, a cervical rib, or a fibrous band that develops around the nerve plexus.

Diagnosis

The diagnosis is made by evaluating the clinical findings, history, and physical examination results. Electromyography (EMG) aids in the confirmation of the diagnosis.

Treatment

The cessation of any continued hyperabduction of the arm helps relieve symptoms. Specific types of exercises or physical therapy may improve the condition. When a cervical rib is the cause, it may be surgically removed. Entrapment of the brachial plexus in cases by the anterior scalene muscle usually necessitates a surgical release of any fibrous band or entrapping tissue.

Prognosis

When the condition is the result of hyperabduction of the arm, cessation of the movement is helpful in resolution of the pain. When the condition is caused by a cervical rib or entrapped nerve, the prognosis is good with surgical intervention to release the entrapped nerve or to remove the cervical rib.

Prevention

Cessation of the offending movement of the arm may prevent the continuation of the condition. For a structural cause, there is no prevention.

Patient Teaching

Discuss causative factors with the patient. Provide instructions for care of the incision if surgery is the chosen treatment. Use customized electronically generated educational materials, when available, to reinforce the treatment plan.

Tendinitis

Description

Tendinitis (tendonitis) is inflammation of a tendon that is usually caused by insult or injury to the tendon.

ICD-10-CM Code   M77.9 *(Enthesopathy, unspecified)*
(M77.5-M77.9 = 5 codes of
specificity)

Symptoms and Signs

The patient experiences nonspecific pain anywhere along the route of the tendon or its attachments. The most common symptom is acute pain.

Patient Screening

The patient experiencing severe pain requires prompt assessment. Schedule an appointment as soon as possible.

Etiology

Tendinitis is inflammation of a tendon. It is caused by an insult to the tendon resulting from prolonged or improper activity of the affected part. Calcium deposits often are associated with tendinitis, and the bursa around the tendon also may be involved.

Diagnosis

Nonspecific tendinitis is difficult to diagnose. A careful history indicates the event or events that caused the stress to the involved area. If the shoulder is involved, a 50- to 130-degree abduction of the affected arm causes pain.

Treatment

Treatment is aimed at reducing pain, decreasing inflammation, and preserving the integrity of the joint involved. Resting the involved area is important, as is administering oral antiinflammatory drugs and applying ice. Steroids may be injected into the joint space. If the joint (e.g., the shoulder) becomes fixed (frozen shoulder), the adhesions that have formed may need to be released surgically to allow full range of motion (ROM) of the joint.

Prognosis

The prognosis is unpredictable because of the tendon being involved and the uncertain response to treatment and rest.

Prevention

Prevention involves avoiding the strenuous activity that initiates and subsequently aggravates the condition. With calcium deposit involvement, prevention is unlikely.

Patient Teaching

Encourage patients to be compliant with the prescribed drug therapy, physical therapy, and resting of the affected part. Use customized electronically generated educational materials, when available, to reinforce the treatment plan.

Physical and Psychological Assault Trauma

Violence inflicted on a victim by others takes many forms, including child abuse, intimate partner violence (IPV), elder abuse, psychological abuse, sexual abuse, and rape.

Victimization of individuals has become so prevalent that health care providers are now trained to identify people who have been victimized, to treat their physical and emotional trauma, and to report incidents or suspicion of abuse, as required by law.

Violence occurs in all areas of society, affecting both sexes, occurring at all socioeconomic levels, and including the entire age spectrum. The number of occurrences continues to increase, even though societal and cultural values typically expressed in the United States do not condone such behavior. Health care providers are encouraged to provide unconditional support to victims and to direct them to support groups or counseling for appropriate therapy.

Violence has taken on a new dimension in the past few years in the form of terrorist attacks and bioterrorism. (Refer to the Alert box about Bioterrorism for additional information.)

ⓘ ALERT!

Bioterrorism

Bioterrorism is a source of great public concern. Anthrax, smallpox, plague, botulism, and radiation exposure are possible sources of danger. Government agencies and health care providers are researching these conditions and exploring treatment options. Silent and deliberate attacks can seriously threaten life and cause social disruption. Awareness of the likelihood of the threats and knowledge of these conditions and possible intervention measures may prevent a potentially catastrophic final outcome. Updates about these conditions will be provided by the health care communities and government agencies.

The following are thumbnail sketches of bioterrorism agents that a terrorist group would be likely to choose:

Anthrax

Anthrax is a bacterial infection caused by *Bacillus anthracis;* it can affect the skin, intestinal tract, or respiratory system. Anthrax traditionally has affected mainly agricultural animals and their handlers. However, pulmonary anthrax has recently been reported in the United States and has been suspected to be the result of terrorist activity.

Pulmonary anthrax begins when a sufficient amount of spores suspended in the air is inhaled into the lungs. Once infected, victims complain of fever, fatigue, muscle aches, chest pain, cough, and severe respiratory distress; without very early medical intervention, most will die. As soon as exposure to the disease is confirmed, administration of vaccine and antibiotic therapy is begun. Diagnosis is confirmed by examination of blood, skin lesions, or respiratory secretions. Presence of the anthrax bacterium or elevated antibodies causes increased amounts of the protein to be produced directly as a response to the infection. Every effort is made to find the source of the infection. This form of anthrax is not considered contagious.

Skin anthrax starts as a raised, itching lesion; within a day or two, the lesion resembles a blister that ulcerates and develops a coal-black center.

Caregivers must wear gloves because the skin lesions may be infectious with direct skin contact. This disease is usually not fatal if treated promptly with antibiotics.

Plague

A bioterrorism outbreak of plague would most likely be brought about by the inhalation of the causative bacteria, causing a severe life-threatening lung disease within a few days of exposure. The onset is sudden and includes very severe respiratory symptoms. Prompt antibiotic treatment is required to save the infected person. Precautions are necessary to prevent the spread of the disease via face-to-face contact.

Smallpox

Smallpox is a highly contagious viral infection caused by the variola virus (a member of the poxvirus family) that can be spread in aerosol form as a biologic weapon. It was once eradicated worldwide through vaccination, but now there is growing concern because people younger than 30 years of age have never been vaccinated, and some adults vaccinated as children may no longer be immune.

Early symptoms resemble a mild viral infection. After a variable incubation (7 to 17 days), symptoms worsen and include high fever, malaise, headache, delirium, and a rash that begins over the face and spreads to the extremities. The rash turns into pustules that leave pitted scars. No cure has been developed, and the only treatment is supportive. Immediate isolation of the infected individual is required, and every case must be reported to health authorities. Vaccine is once again available and is being given or has been given to the military, certain public safety providers, and some health care providers. Provisions are in progress to accomplish mass citizen vaccination should there be an endemic occurrence.

Botulism

Botulism toxin, a powerful poison, is easy to make and store and can be easily aerosolized. Although other forms of botulism exist, it is the inhalation form that could possibly be used in a bioterrorist attack.

Within a day or two after exposure to the toxin, the infected person experiences a cluster of flulike symptoms. Shortly thereafter, rapid progression of neurologic symptoms begins and can result in complete respiratory failure. Early intervention with an antitoxin may be helpful in cases in which the toxin is attached to nerve endings. Additionally, treatment with human botulism immune globulin may be used. No other drugs are available to treat botulism toxin or poisoning at this time.

Child abuse/neglect

Description

Physical, psychological, or sexual injury to a child is considered child abuse. The most commonly observed form is physical abuse because the resulting injuries are usually apparent. Signs of psychological abuse may be evidenced in the actions of the child. Sexual abuse may be discovered incidentally and investigated when the child complains of discomfort in the genital region or if the child reports the abuse. Neglect also may be considered a form of child abuse.

ICD-10-CM Code   T74.92XA *(Unspecified child maltreatment, confirmed, initial encounter)*

                                T76.92XA *(Unspecified child maltreatment, suspected, initial encounter)*

Additional codes may be required to identify any injury, the nature of the abuser or perpetrator, or the type of abuse. Once the diagnosis has been confirmed, refer to the current edition of the ICD-10-CM coding manual for additional appropriate codes.

Symptoms and Signs

Often children who are victims of child abuse are identified as such by teachers, day care providers, or health care providers. The injuries to the child encompass many forms, including bruises, fractures, burns, bites, and welts. The injuries can even be fatal (Fig. 15.29).

Bruising can have many telltale appearances, such as finger marks, which wrap around the child's limb and may show evidence of rings worn by the perpetrator; imprints of electrical cords or hangers; and horizontal wraparound marks left by belts or straps, and possibly buckle marks. These bruises appear on soft tissue and not over bony prominences where normal falls would have caused them to be. The bruising often is in areas normally covered by clothing and the bruises are in various stages of healing.

Burns from cigarettes appear as small circles (the diameter of a cigarette) often on hands, feet, buttocks, or genitals. These are at various stages of healing. Another form of burn is the scald burn with the pattern of "dipping," straight lines

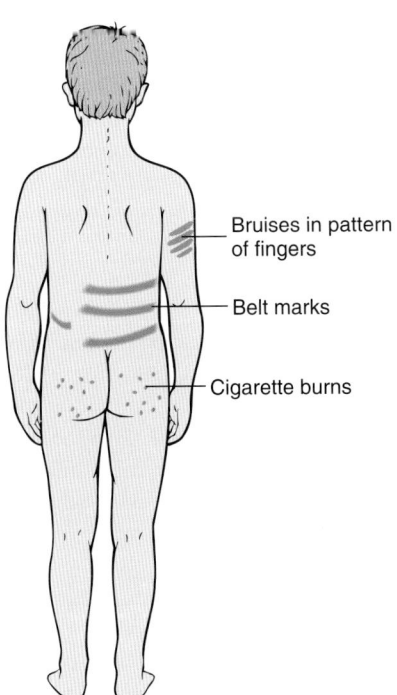

• **Fig. 15.29** Typical marks of child abuse.

Bruises in pattern of fingers

Belt marks

Cigarette burns

with no splash marks, a result of the child's body being held in scalding water (Fig. 15.30).

Other observable injuries include teeth marks, with bruising caused by human bites, and raised areas or welts caused by spankings with sticks, paddles, or belts on the buttocks or legs. A fracture, usually greenstick in nature, of a long bone may be noted.

Often the child is withdrawn, avoids eye contact, and does not respond appropriately to painful stimuli. When asked how the injury happened, the child denies any abuse and protects the abuser out of fear. In other cases, the child exhibits unusually aggressive behavior and has a neglected appearance.

Neglect often is also considered a form of child abuse. When children are not provided with food or shelter, the caregiver is considered to be neglectful. Leaving young children unattended, thus endangering their well-being, is also a form of neglect. Child abuse or neglect is a reportable crime in all states, and the health care giver caring for the child victim can be found liable if the case is not reported to the appropriate agency.

Patient Screening

Any reports of child abuse require immediate investigation. An appointment is an urgent matter and should be scheduled as soon as possible, and if none is immediately available, a referral to an emergency facility should be made. Follow up promptly if treatment is necessary.

Etiology

Child abuse has many causes. These include emotional immaturity of the abuser; stress caused by economic, social, or employment difficulties; poor parenting skills; drug or alcohol abuse; the abuser having a history of child abuse himself or herself; unrealistic expectations of the child; and the limitations of a physically or mentally challenged child.

Diagnosis

The diagnosis is made on the basis of history and the clinical findings. Many times, health care providers are often the first professionals who are aware of child abuse or neglect; therefore careful documentation is critical if the case goes to court. If the medical assistant suspects that child abuse or neglect is involved, further evaluation by an appropriate health care provider is necessary. Child abuse is not easy to diagnose; nevertheless, health care providers, teachers, and day care providers are required, by law in most states in the United States, to report suspected child abuse to the local or state law enforcement agency or child protective agency.

Treatment

Any injuries must be treated in an appropriate manner. Documentation of the injuries is necessary, and the health care provider must remain alert for patterns of injuries. Radiographic studies of the long bones and the skulls of

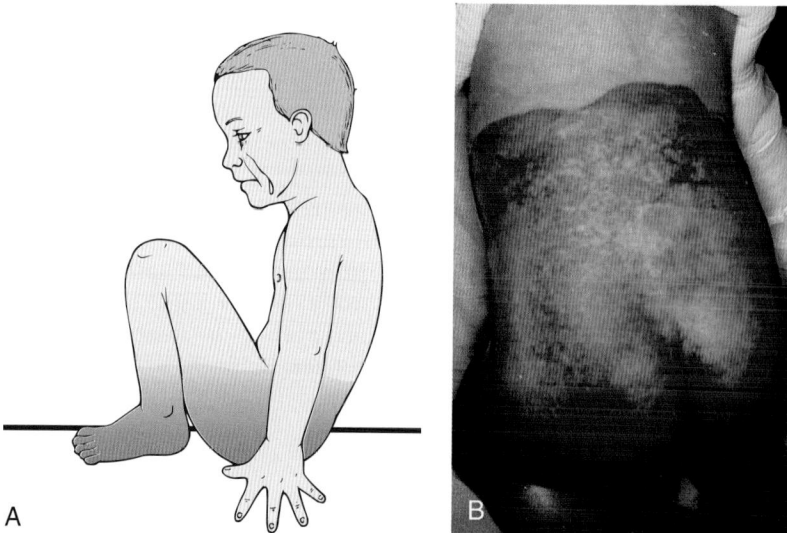

• **Fig. 15.30** (A) Typical pattern of scald dip burn. (B) Scalded child. (B, From slide set for Behrman RE, Kliegman RM, Arvin AM, editors: *Nelson textbook of pediatrics,* ed 15, Philadelphia, 1996, Saunders.)

infants and toddlers should be performed to investigate the extent of abuse. Emotional support for the child should be given unconditionally. The child abuse hotline, the hospital protection team or the local or state protection service, and the local police department should be contacted, as indicated. Abusive parents and other perpetrators could use help from the appropriate agencies.

Prognosis
The prognosis varies, depending on the duration and extent of the abuse and the identity of the perpetrator of the abuse, that is, whether the abuser has custody of or easy access to the child. Removal of the child from the abusive environment by appropriate social service agencies usually is helpful. The emotional attachment of the child to the abuser may play a role in the resolution of this action. This is a difficult and sensitive issue that requires multiprofessional interaction.

Prevention
Prevention is the best treatment. Parents need to be taught good parenting skills and made aware of resources for crisis intervention. They need parenting skill classes to learn about alternatives to striking a child and methods of controlling their abusive reactions to the child's behavior (e.g., counting to 10).

Patient Teaching
Provide written information about prevention of child abuse. Assist the family in locating and contacting community resources. Encourage family and community awareness of signs of child abuse and appropriate interventions.

Shaken infant (baby) syndrome
Description
Shaken infant syndrome (SIS), or *shaken baby syndrome (SBS),* refers to the injuries incurred by the infant or toddler

who has been shaken forcibly enough to cause intracerebral bleeding, resulting in a closed head injury.

ICD-10-CM Code	T74.4XXA *(Shaken infant syndrome, initial encounter)*

Once diagnosis of the injuries has been confirmed, referral to the current edition of the ICD-10-CM coding manual for appropriate codes is recommended.

Symptoms and Signs
The shaken baby may experience altered levels of consciousness to complete loss of consciousness. Irritability, changes in skin color to paleness or cyanosis, vomiting, lethargy, and convulsions are additional symptoms. Most of the time, there is no outward indication of physical trauma. Fractured or dislocated bones and neck or spinal injuries may be found. Examination of the eyes may reveal retinal hemorrhages (Fig. 15.31). Babies shaken into unconsciousness are often put to bed in the hope that the injury will resolve, and thus the opportunity for life-saving treatment is usually lost.

Patient Screening
SBS is a life-threatening emergency. These infants require prompt medical intervention. Contacting EMS for immediate transport to an emergency care facility is a prudent action. For a parent asking to speak with the physician after the diagnosis about treatment for their child, an appointment should be scheduled as soon as possible.

Etiology
The repeated rapid shaking of an infant results in the brain continually striking the inside of the cranial vault and then recoiling against the other side of the skull. As a result, tiny vessels rupture, causing minor or even major bleeds in and around the brain. The swelling and

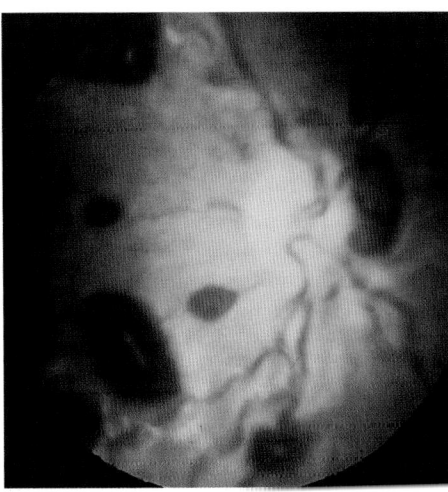

• **Fig. 15.31** Shaken baby syndrome (SBS): Retinal hemorrhages. (From Zitelli BJ, Davis HW: *Atlas of pediatric physical diagnosis,* ed 5, Philadelphia, 2008, Mosby. Courtesy Dr. Stephen Ludwig, Children's Hospital of Philadelphia.)

hemorrhage may lead to permanent severe cerebral (brain) damage or even death.

A form of child abuse, SIS usually occurs when the caregiver becomes irritated or upset and loses control, shaking the baby violently. Incidents of SIS resulting from tossing the baby into the air and catching him or her or even jostling the baby in a backpack as the caregiver jogs or runs, causing the baby to bounce up and down, have been documented. Young children have large heads and weak neck muscles and therefore are susceptible to intracerebral injury.

Diagnosis

The manifestation of three symptoms, subdural hematoma, cerebral edema, and retinal hemorrhage, leads to the diagnosis of SIS. CT should be performed to identify brain (bleeding) hemorrhages. However, it is not necessary for all three conditions to be present.

Treatment

Immediate and aggressive intervention, including life-sustaining measures, is necessary. Bleeding and cerebral edema must be controlled and intracranial pressure reduced. Nevertheless, damage may be permanent, even fatal. If the child survives, he or she may have visual deficits from retinal insults, including blindness, intellectual developmental disorder, or cerebral palsy. Trauma centers with traumatic brain injury programs are best prepared to handle these emergencies.

Prognosis

The prognosis varies, depending on the extent of the injury. Often the injuries to the brain are nonreversible or even fatal. Those children who do survive may be left with blindness, neurologic insults, and intellectual developmental disorder.

Prevention

SIS may be prevented by educating caregivers about the dangers of shaking a baby in anger and about methods of controlling their rage. Parents should be made aware of the importance of providing their children with competent caregivers. All caregivers, including parents, should develop a safe plan for dealing with and comforting a crying baby. When suspicions of nonaccidental injuries are raised, appropriate agencies must be notified.

Patient Teaching

Provide all parents with infants or young children written information about SBS. Encourage all parents to have competent child care for their children. Assist parents of shaken babies to locate and contact support groups in the community.

Elder abuse/neglect

Description

Elder abuse and neglect take on different forms: physical abuse, self-neglect, verbal abuse, psychological abuse, abandonment, violation of personal rights, and financial abuse. Withholding actions that result in harm or threatened harm to the health or welfare of older adults is considered abuse or neglect, depending on the extent of harm. The most commonly observed form is physical because the injuries are visually apparent. Psychological abuse may never be uncovered. Sexual abuse may be discovered incidentally with complaints of discomfort in the genital region or if reported by the older adult.

ICD-10-CM Code   T74.91XA *(Unspecified adult maltreatment, confirmed, initial encounter)*
                      T76.91XA *(Unspecified adult maltreatment, suspected, initial encounter)*

Once diagnosis of the injuries has been confirmed, referral to the current edition of the ICD-10-CM coding manual for appropriate codes is recommended. Additional codes are available for various forms of adult abuse.

Symptoms and Signs

It is rare for an older adult abuse victim to complain of abuse. Evidence of the abuse usually is discovered during examination for another purpose. Signs are similar to those of other forms of abuse, are varied, and often are hidden by clothing. Signs include bruising, fractures, malnutrition, skin breakdown (decubitus), poor hygiene, alopecia (hair loss) caused by repeated pulling or tugging of hair, and poor general health status. Other signs may include a series of missed appointments or frequently changing health care providers.

Similar to child abuse and domestic violence, victims often do not report or confirm the violence. One reason is that they love their abusers. Another is fear of losing a home and financial support. Additionally, they are afraid of more abuse from the abuser as a response to any complaint. Some older adults, as parents of the abuser, may feel that they have failed in raising their children.

Neglect often is also considered a form of elder abuse. When these individuals are not provided with food or shelter, the caregiver is considered to be neglectful. Leaving the disabled older adult unattended, especially for long periods, thus endangering their well-being, is also a form of neglect.

Patient Screening

Reports of signs of elder abuse require prompt attention. Schedule an appointment for the patient to be seen as soon as possible. Often the abuse is discovered during a routine examination, and follow-up appointments will then be scheduled.

Etiology

As with other forms of abuse, abuse of older adults is a complex situation. Often older adults may become more childlike or ill and dependent on their children for survival, including financial support and physical care. Society presumes that this group of people are protected by love, gentleness, and caring. Some of the older adults requiring care have diminished mental capacity and are confused. The care of these persons can be a source of stress to the caregiver, not only because of the physical care demands but also because of financial and emotional pressures. With the breakdown of the nuclear family structure and the stresses of being a single parent, the additional task of caring for an older person can become an overwhelming burden.

Additionally, current society puts emphasis on youth. Often, the "sandwich" generation no longer can cope, and abuse takes place. Other cases of elder abuse have a financial basis, either in the caregiver being unable to afford the necessities that the older person requires or in taking control of the older person's finances for the abuser's personal gain.

Diagnosis

The diagnosis is made on the basis of an evaluation of the situation and physical examination. Psychological abuse is difficult to diagnose. Many of the victims believe that revealing their child's abusive behavior toward them will suggest that they have failed as parents or that it will jeopardize the living arrangements.

Treatment

Treatment consists of treating any trauma with the appropriate care and determining the need for appropriate protective services. Counseling should be made available to all parties involved. If necessary, the victim should be removed from the abusive environment. Prevention is the best treatment; however, that is not always possible.

Prognosis

The prognosis varies, depending on the extent and duration of the abuse and the perpetrator of the abuse. Removal of the older individual from the abusive environment usually is helpful.

Prevention

The primary goal is to protect the patient from harm; however, prevention is not always possible. Close monitoring of situations in which an older person is dependent on others for care may be helpful. Suggestions of respite care may be helpful. Recognition of signs of extreme stress in the caregiver and suggestions of assistance for care provision may be helpful.

Patient Teaching

Assist family members in locating and contacting community resources that are available.

Psychological or verbal abuse

Description

Psychological or emotional abuse is the intentional and systematic diminishment of another's self-worth or self-esteem.

ICD-10-CM Code   T74.31XA *(Adult psychological abuse, confirmed, initial encounter)*
                      T76.31XA *(Adult psychological abuse, suspected, initial encounter)*
                      T74.32XA *(Child psychological abuse, confirmed, initial encounter)*
                      T76.32XA *(Child psychological abuse, suspected, initial encounter)*

Symptoms and Signs

Symptoms of psychological or verbal abuse, the systematic diminishment of another, take on many forms. Often the abused person makes no complaints. Although emotional battering occurs in all age groups, children are the most frequent victims. The guilt that is imposed on these victims often leads to self-destructive behavior, including anorexia, bulimia, obesity, alcoholism, self-mutilation, drug addiction, depression, and suicide. Others manifest their guilt feelings by emotional guarding and turn their anger and rage inward against themselves. These persons display lack of self-esteem and self-worth and often are unable to bond with others.

Patient Screening

Psychologically or emotionally abused individuals usually do not have enough mental strength to seek help. Many of these individuals are unaware of the abusive actions directed toward them and feel that they deserve any abusive psychological behavior directed at them. Many are often referred from emergency care facilities and require an immediate appointment. The situations often are discovered on a visit to the physician for another reason.

Etiology

The cause of this form of abuse is unknown. Often a parent, partner, or caregiver is the abuser, denying the victim (child or partner) love and protection. The abuse can be active, with the parent telling the child, "You're stupid," "I'm ashamed of you," or "You'll never amount to anything." It can be passive in the form of intentional neglect. Often it is a combination of the two. The abuse can take on the verbal form, or it may be shown by the abuser's actions. The response to the abuse often is buried so deep that it does not surface until later in life. Most verbal abuse is done in secret; usually only the victim hears it. Emotional abuse becomes more intense over time; the victim begins to adapt to it. Verbal and emotional abuse can take on many forms and disguises; verbal abuse consistently discounts the victim's perception of the abuse.

Diagnosis

Emotional abuse is difficult to diagnose because no physical contact occurs. The comments usually are made to the victim in private or in the home environment. The abusive behavior takes place over time, making it difficult to identify its occurrence at a given time. The victim believes that he or she is responsible for the behavior of the abuser and does not realize that it is a form of abuse. The victims often defend the abusive behavior, believing that they deserve it. Victims feel lost, not knowing where to turn. These relationships are filled with inequity, competition, manipulation, hostility, control, and negation and create feelings of inadequacy, frustration, rejection, disappointment, sadness, fear, and confusion.

Treatment

The best treatment is prevention. Education of the population as to what constitutes emotional abuse and ways to prevent the many forms is important. A building of self-esteem and self-worth is necessary to begin the healing process. Because of the varied forms of emotional abuse, each individual must believe in himself or herself and address the specific guilt felt, possibly with the help of a therapist.

Prognosis

The prognosis varies, depending on the duration of the abusive relationship. Psychological therapy may be helpful; however, many of these abused individuals are unable to accept the diagnosis of abuse and resist treatment.

Prevention

Prevention relies on the education of society as to what constitutes psychological or emotional abuse and how society can be helpful.

Patient Teaching

Help victims to build self-esteem and realize their self-worth. Assist them to locate and contact community resources.

Intimate partner violence

Description

IPV is the result of threatened or actual physical abuse, a pattern of behavior in which the victim is repeatedly physically assaulted by her or his partner. Other terms for IPV include domestic violence, spouse abuse, and battered spouse syndrome.

| ICD-10-CM Code | T74.11XA *(Adult physical abuse, confirmed, initial encounter)* |
| | T76.11XA *(Adult physical abuse, suspected, initial encounter)* |

Symptoms and Signs

Victims of IPV in heterosexual and homosexual relationships are most frequently women. The victim has evidence of bruising in various stages of healing, usually in an area of the body that is concealed by clothing, and has a tendency to avoid making eye contact with the examiner.

Patient Screening

An individual reporting physical assault by a spouse or partner requires prompt attention and should be reported to the police according to state guidelines.

Etiology

IPV is a complex issue; no one specific cause is known. Stress is suggested as an important factor, along with alcohol ingestion and possible intoxication. Cultural and societal values that made wives their husbands' "property" and the mindset that women are expected to be submissive to their mates have contributed to spouse abuse. Some women are victimized because they do not have the physical or emotional strength that their partners do. Many of these victims have low self-esteem, adding to their inability to escape the victimization. Women can be the abusers as well, and some women abuse their partners even to the point of dismemberment, setting the partner on fire, or murder. It is believed that in many of these cases, the actions are in retaliation for the battering that the woman received.

Diagnosis

The diagnosis is made on the basis of the information provided by the victim or by others. Physical examination indicates physical injuries. As with child abuse and sexual abuse, the injuries are varied and often occur on areas of the body that normally are covered by clothing. Assessment of the emotional state is difficult but necessary. Proper evaluation and direct, appropriate questions should be a part of the examination. For example, "You have a bruise on your face. Did someone hit you?" Often intervention results from law enforcement involvement; other times, the abusive trauma is discovered by the physician and other health care staff when the victim is seen for another reason in the office or health care facility. Information obtained and physical findings should be carefully documented; photographs of the injuries should be included in the documentation.

Treatment

Treatment involves the normal protocol for treating physical injuries. Discussing the situation in a nonjudgmental way is imperative. Referral to the appropriate agencies for counseling is indicated; nevertheless, the health care provider must recognize that the victim may not want or seek counseling and may elect to stay in the abusive situation. Listening is of the utmost importance; however, it is inappropriate to impose one's opinion of the situation on the victim.

Prognosis

The prognosis varies, depending on the duration and extent of the battering. Additionally, the circumstances of the relationship in which the battering has taken place will affect the long-term outcome of any intervention. Moreover, the willingness of the battered individual to leave the situation and to report the battering to law enforcement also will affect the outcome.

Prevention

Prevention is difficult because many abused partners feel that they deserve the battering and that it is accepted behavior in society as they know it. Raising awareness of the issue in the community and in the educational system and teaching that battering is not acceptable behavior may prevent battering and acceptance of battering occurring in future generations. In some states, the individual committing the violence also faces additional charges if a minor child witnesses the violent act. The state, not the victim, is the complainant, removing the responsibility of filing a charge from the victim. Additionally, intervention programs for

the batterer are becoming part of the sentencing protocols in domestic violence cases. The legal responsibilities of the health care provider in battered spouse syndrome vary by state, but all health care providers should be aware of them.

Patient Teaching

Reinforcing to the victim that no one deserves to be treated in such a manner may be helpful. Acceptance of the victim as an individual with inherent self-worth is a valuable tool in establishing rapport and in building trust between the caregiver and the individual. Provide the victim with local telephone contact numbers to be used in an emergency situation to obtain help. Additionally, assist them in locating and contacting community resources if they desire to do so. Local IPV organizations are well informed regarding the process of providing protection and can assist the victim with civil protective orders, shelters, and information regarding protective laws.

Sexual Abuse

Description

Any form of nonconsensual sexual contact or activity is considered sexual abuse. Sexual abuse may involve either gender and may be perpetrated by either gender. Another important factor is that the victim of sexual abuse may be of any age, from an infant to an older adult.

ICD-10-CM Code	T74.21XA *(Adult sexual abuse, confirmed, initial encounter)*
	T76.21XA *(Adult sexual abuse, suspected, initial encounter)*
	T74.22XA *(Child sexual abuse, confirmed, initial encounter)*
	T76.22XA *(Child sexual abuse, suspected, initial encounter)*

Symptoms and Signs

Sexual abuse takes on many forms; thus symptoms and signs can be numerous and different from one patient to the next. Any form of nonconsensual sexual activity can be considered sexual abuse. Some examples of sexual abuse are fondling of the genitals or breasts, penetration of the vagina or rectum with fingers or other objects, and forcing the victim to touch the perpetrator on or around the sex organs. Exposing a child to pornography is also considered abuse, as is taking pornographic photos of a child. The victim often does not report unwanted advances or activity and usually appears subdued. If the victim is a young woman, she may have itching or burning in the urethral and vaginal areas and exhibit symptoms of a urinary tract infection. Sexually abused children have an unusual obsession with the genital region and frequently touch themselves abnormally. They often exhibit aggressive behavior.

Patient Screening

Any individual reporting sexual abuse requires prompt attention. If no immediate appointments are available, refer the patient to a sexual abuse or emergency facility for immediate intervention. Some victims may be resistant to this option; if so, schedule an appointment as soon as possible.

Etiology

As with other forms of abuse, the cause of sexual abuse is a complicated matter. Domination, control, and power issues can be reasons for this unacceptable form of behavior. Many of the perpetrators were sexually abused as children, and they do not regard what they are doing as wrong. Some simply have a sociopathic approach to society and its norms. It is important to consider that victimization of both sexes occurs and that the abuser can be of either sex. There are reported cases of women sexually assaulting men of all ages.

Diagnosis

The diagnosis is made on the basis of the history given by the victim and is confirmed on physical examination. Often the sexual abuse is combined with physical abuse, and treatment of that abuse may lead to the victim confiding in the caregiver or healthcare provider regarding the unwanted sexual activity. Many times, the removal of the victim from a physically abusive environment allows the victim to feel safe enough to discuss the sexual abuse. Perpetrators of sexual abuse of children or infants have been babysitters, relatives, or even a parent. Sexual abuse can affect a person of any age.

Treatment

Immediately after the assault, strict legal guidelines must be followed when performing a physical examination if the assault occurred within 72 hours. Emergency treatment of a victim of sexual assault involves both medical and forensic examinations. Any trauma is treated according to the protocol of the facility. Law enforcement agencies should be notified, with the victim's consent, or according to local or state policy. Prophylactic sexually transmitted disease (STD) treatments and pregnancy prevention therapy may be offered. If possible, the victim is removed from the abusive situation. Emotional support is provided, and reinforcement is given to the victim that he or she is not responsible for the sexual abuse. If the victim is receptive to counseling, arrangements are made to assist the victim in dealing with the abuse. If the victim is a child, child protective services are usually involved, and when the situation warrants, the child is removed from the environment. The social services agencies involved usually determine when a child is to be removed from this type of environment.

Prognosis

The prognosis varies, depending on the form, duration, and extent of sexual abuse. The physical wounds may heal quickly, but the emotional wounds often leave permanent scars. When possible, direct the victim to follow-up counseling. A resulting pregnancy or STD will require additional intervention.

Prevention

Prevention is difficult. It is not often possible to predict who may be a sexual abuser; nor is it possible to predict where or when sexual abuse may take place.

Patient Teaching

Assist the victim in locating and contacting community resource agencies that can provide support and assistance. Reinforce that sexual abuse is not accepted behavior; however, it is important to maintain a nonjudgmental attitude toward the victim.

◆ ENRICHMENT

DNA Parentage Testing

Deoxyribonucleic acid (DNA) parentage testing is the most reliable and powerful method of providing proof of parentage for legal and medical reasons. It conclusively answers difficult questions, resolves disputes, and helps streamline court proceedings.

Testing is based on a highly accurate analysis of the genetic profiles of the mother, the child, and the alleged father. DNA, the unique genetic blueprint within each nucleated cell of a person's body, determines the genetic pattern and individual characteristics. A child inherits half of this DNA pattern from the mother and half from the father. If the mother's and child's patterns are known, the alleged father can be included or excluded as the biologin father of the child.

There are no age restrictions for DNA testing because the DNA makeup is set at conception. Testing can be performed before a child is born, and newborns can be tested safely at delivery by using umbilical cord blood. In fact, samples can be taken from persons of any age, even post mortem. A buccal swab is typically collected for paternity testing.

DNA technology is so powerful that the genetic profile of a deceased father can often be reconstructed from grandparents, siblings, or other children to determine paternity.

(From DNA Diagnostics Center, Fairfield, OH.)

Rape/Sexual assault

Description

Intercourse forced on a person against her or his will is termed *rape* or *sexual assault*.

ICD-10-CM Code	T74.21XA (*Adult sexual abuse, confirmed, initial encounter*)
	T76.21XA (*Adult sexual abuse, suspected, initial encounter*)
	T74.22XA (*Child sexual abuse, confirmed, initial encounter*)
	T76.22XA (*Child sexual abuse, suspected, initial encounter*)

Symptoms and Signs

The symptoms and signs of rape/sexual assault vary with the degree of violence incurred by the victim. Many come to an emergency care facility, physician's office, clinic, or a law enforcement agency stating, "I've been raped." Some report having pain in the pelvic and perineal regions or being choked or restrained in some manner. Others report threat of death. Bruising may be noted in any area of the body, not just the pelvic area. Signs of rape include torn clothing, dirt and debris ground into clothing or hair, disheveled appearance, withdrawal, anxiousness, avoidance of eye contact, and bruising, tears, or lacerations around or on the genitals, rectum, or mouth. Pelvic and rectal examination often reveals tenderness in those areas and evidence of trauma. If the victim has not bathed or douched, evidence of semen may be present on the inner aspects of the thighs, genital areas, mouth, nares, or pubic region. Any part of the body, including the breasts, may be traumatized. If the victim is male, bruising or lacerations in the anal region are indicative of sodomy. Bruises and lacerations also may be discovered in the anal region of the woman if she has been sodomized.

Patient Screening

Many rape victims will go to or be transported to an emergency facility for a sexual assault examination, which includes the gathering of any evidence. However, some victims resist reporting the attack to authorities and request an appointment to see the physician. Other victims may seek anonymity and seek a physician with whom they have had no previous contact. It is important to remember that men can also be victims of sexual assault and may be one of the most underreported of all groups. For any individual reporting rape or sexual assault, an appointment should be scheduled as soon as possible and the person treated using complete discretion.

Etiology

Rape is a crime of violence and domination, not a sexual act. It occurs when there is no mutual consent between both parties involved in the sexual act, and it is a forced act. Rape can happen to either women or men; most often, the victims are women. Rape can be in the form of date rape, acquaintance rape, rape by the victim's spouse or partner, or a violent act perpetrated by an unknown assailant.

Diagnosis

The diagnosis is made by evaluating the findings from the history, clinical examination, physical examination, including pelvic examination, and sex crime evidence gathering. Samples of debris, clothing, saliva, hair, pubic hair, fingernails, and scrapings from under the nails are collected. A specimen for urinalysis is obtained, along with specimens for blood tests for STDs, acquired immunodeficiency syndrome (AIDS), and possible pregnancy. Photographs may be taken for documentation of injuries. It is recommended that this type of complete examination take place in a facility with staff professionally educated in treating sexual assault victims. Many communities offer sexual assault response teams (SARTs) that are called in to perform sexual

assault medical and legal examinations. All personal belongings of the victim must be handled carefully, and all items must be marked as evidence. Rape examinations for most victims are performed at no cost.

Treatment

Any patient who has suffered trauma is treated in an appropriate manner. Sexual assault victims should receive an emergent priority and be placed in a safe and secure location. Counseling at a rape crisis center should be offered. Information concerning the risks of possible pregnancy, STDs, and AIDS is given, along with an explanation of the protocol for follow-up testing. If the patient has no religious objection, prophylaxis for pregnancy may be considered.

Reinforcement that the victim is a survivor of a violent crime and is not responsible for the incident is necessary. The victim needs to believe that she or he just happened to be in the wrong place at the wrong time. Everyone dealing with the victim and her or his family must be nonjudgmental and supportive. According to state laws, victims must be informed that law enforcement must be notified, when applicable. (Refer to the Enrichment box about Sexual Assault Response Teams and Evidence Maintenance.)

◆ ENRICHMENT

Sexual Assault Response Teams and Evidence Maintenance

Some states and communities have enacted legislation about providing mandatory services to sexual assault victims. A major factor is the requirement that a community-based sexual assault response team (SART) be involved in the investigation of the assault and be available as a support mechanism for the victim. For example, in Indiana, any evidence collected during the sexual assault examination must be maintained in a secure, refrigerated facility for a minimum of 7 years, in a manner that provides confidentiality for the victim. The cost of the sexual assault examination is reimbursed to the examining facility by the state. The statute also mandates that a victim should be required to submit to a polygraph or other truth-telling device examination. Another portion of the statute requires the hospital to give notice to victims about certain rights and to contact law enforcement. The prosecutor's office becomes involved after the initial investigation.

The sexual assault team includes a coordinated group of people who serve victims of sexual assault. They are educated to provide both emotional and physical assistance and also gather specimens that may be used as forensic evidence. Additionally, the sexual assault nurse examiner is also trained to be an understanding support person for the victim during the investigation. Other members of the SART include a law enforcement officer and a victim advocate. All are trained in assisting the sexual assault victim while gathering evidence.

Prognosis

The prognosis for victims of rape varies. Physical healing may take place without any complications. However, a resulting pregnancy or STDs will present a complication that needs to be addressed. Ongoing psychological counseling may be required for lengthy periods. Undoubtedly, the physical and psychological effects on the victims will be longstanding, if not lifelong.

Prevention

It is difficult to prevent rape because it is difficult to predict who might be a perpetrator or what place might be a potential location of a rape. On the one hand, social media have played a role in strangers meeting each other for various purposes, which can give perpetrators easy targets, because some individuals post a lot of information about their routines and personal lives. On the other hand, social media has also been used to help solve cases. Security cameras may deter some from committing crimes in those locations.

Patient Teaching

Have a nonjudgmental approach in providing care for rape victims. Assist them in seeking counseling and in contacting the local rape crisis center; and encourage them to follow through with the contact.

Suicide

Description

Suicide is taking one's own life or intentionally causing one's own death.

ICD-10-CM Code	T14.91XA (Suicide attempt, initial encounter)

Symptoms and Signs

Individuals contemplating suicide may appear depressed or may be making remarks about how they look forward to dying. They may give away certain items. They may state that they want to die and are thinking about committing suicide. Some may say, "You would be better off without me." They may withdraw from the family or the situation. They may say they are just tired, the body is tired, their mind is tired, and they are just exhausted. They may have tried cutting themselves or may be ingesting different drugs. To them, life is hopeless, and there is no relief. They feel that the only relief they will get will be by dying. Death is the final escape.

Patient Screening

When a patient or a family member calls about impending suicide, it is best to offer them the next available appointment. Additionally, the health care provider should be alerted and his or her instructions followed.

Etiology

Many factors may cause depression. Personal relationships may go bad. Difficult money situations may trigger the thought of escape. Loss of employment is a discouraging factor. Not being able to meet parental or partner expectations often is difficult.

Diagnosis

Some clients may be placed on a suicide watch if they have expressed a desire to end their life. Text messages, written messages, or letters indicating that the world or specific people would be "better off if I were dead" should be taken seriously. A psychologist or a psychiatrist is helpful in screening for this type of ideation.

Treatment

If the patient is seen in the office, treatment may include antidepressant medications. Once the person expresses suicidal intentions, 72-hour detention in a mental health facility is an available option. In the state of Indiana, an explanation of all symptoms is necessary for the judge to order the holding of the individual in a locked facility. Contacting the suicide hotline should be encouraged. The national suicide prevention hotline telephone number is 1-800-273-1825 and is answered 24 hours a day, 7 days a week. If the suicidal individual will not call the number, the individual attempting to help could call the number for advice on what to say and what to do.

Prognosis

When the individual has committed suicide, nothing more can be done. His or her family should receive counseling to help them deal with the circumstance. Grief counseling is recommended and arranged, if desired.

Prevention

Suicide may be stopped by recognizing sadness, depression, and intent to commit suicide. Talking with the person contemplating suicide and allowing him or her to know you care and want to help may stop or delay an impending suicide.

Patient Teaching

When an individual has attempted suicide or has expressed suicidal thoughts, express your recognition of the feeling. Recommend counseling, and discuss contacting the suicide hotline. Inform family members about the suicide hotline and its telephone number. Encourage the individual contemplating suicide to talk about his or her feelings. Suicide is a fatal action.

Review Challenge

Answer the following questions:
1. What are the major types of trauma?
2. What are some ways in which environmental factors can result in trauma?
3. What is the difference between an abrasion and an avulsion?
4. When is it appropriate to use tetanus toxoid in prophylactic treatment?
5. When is débridement of a wound necessary?
6. How are the depth and extent of burns assessed?
7. What are the possible effects of an electrical shock?

8. What are the types of lightning strikes? Which treatments may be required?
9. How are the signs and symptoms of heat stroke and heat exhaustion different?
10. What is the treatment for heat stroke? For heat exhaustion?
11. What are some precautions in the treatment of frostbite?
12. Which spider bites require emergency care?
13. What is Rocky Mountain spotted fever, and how is it transmitted?
14. Why is an animal quarantined after biting a human?
15. What are the signs and symptoms of a poisonous snakebite?
16. What is the relationship between repetitive activities and carpal tunnel syndrome?
17. Which physical patterns may be observed in child abuse?
18. How may elder abuse and neglect, child abuse and neglect, sexual abuse, or intimate partner violence (IPV) be noted during the history and physical examination?
19. What testing is available for the rape/sexual assault victim?
20. How can parentage be determined in the laboratory?

Real-Life Challenge: Heat Exhaustion

The mother of a 14-year-old girl called the office about her daughter, who had just come home from attending marching band practice for approximately 3 hours. The girl was complaining of nausea, weakness, and headache. On questioning, the mother revealed that her daughter's skin appeared pale, cool, and moist. The weather had been hot and humid, and the girl told her mother that she had been practicing the marching routines for about 2.5 hours before she felt ill. When the mother took the girl's temperature, it was 98.2°F, and the girl's pulse was faint and fast.

The mother was advised to have her daughter lie down in a cool environment, with feet slightly elevated; to loosen her clothing; and to place cool compresses on the girl's face, forehead, neck, chest, abdomen, arms, back, and legs. She also was instructed to give her daughter 4 ounces of cool water to drink every 15 minutes. The office advised that they would call back in 1 hour to get a progress report.

The diagnosis was heat exhaustion.

Questions

1. What is the significance of the cool, moist skin?
2. What measures could have been taken to prevent the onset of heat exhaustion?
3. Compare the moist, cool skin and sweating of heat exhaustion with the skin condition of heat stroke.
4. What could be the anticipated outcome of treatment which was suggested to the mother?
5. If the girl's condition did not improve in 1 hour, what would you expect the next step in treatment to be?
6. What is the significance of loosening clothing and applying cool compresses?
7. Why would the mother be instructed to use cool compresses and not ice?
8. Why would the patient with heat stroke require treatment in an emergency facility versus the heat exhaustion victim, who can be treated at home?

Real-Life Challenge: Intimate Partner Violence

A 36-year-old woman is in the office being treated for pain and reduced hearing in the left ear. She is very vague about any history, saying only that her left ear is painful; she has noted some blood coming out of the canal, and she has reduced hearing in her left ear. Bruising is noted around the ear on the left cheek, on the left side of the neck, and behind the left ear on the skull. These areas are tender to touch. The patient is very quiet, at times is tearful, and is wearing a long-sleeved turtleneck shirt and long pants. She is hesitant to remove her shirt for blood pressure measurement or for any other examination.

Examination reveals recent trauma to the left ear, blood is visualized in the canal, and otoscopic examination confirms a ruptured tympanic membrane. Audiometry confirms reduced hearing capability in the left ear. Bruises in various stages of healing are noted on the arms, neck, and chest. Further examination discloses similar bruising to the legs. The patient denies any abusive trauma and says she incurred the injuries in a fall. She avoids eye contact, tending to keep her eyes downward. Her demeanor is subdued, and her posture also appears subdued, with the shoulders slumped.

Gentle questioning eventually reveals that her husband, a man of large stature, recently lost his job as a result of drinking and aggressive or near-violent behavior. She also admits that in the past 2 weeks since the loss of his job, her husband has been "slapping her around" and that last night he struck her on the left side of her face and across the ear with his open hand. The patient does not want to file a police report and says she cannot leave the abusive situation.

She is referred to an ear, nose, and throat (ENT) specialist for treatment of the ruptured tympanic membrane. An appointment for follow-up is made for 2 days later, at which time additional support for the psychosocial situation will be supplied. She is instructed to call immediately in case of any recurrence of the abusive behavior. She also is advised to see whether she can get her husband to make an appointment for an examination.

Questions

1. What is typical behavior for a "battered" spouse or victim of intimate partner violence (IPV)?
2. What are the significance of the alcohol consumption and the loss of employment in the onset of abuse?
3. Why didn't the victim want the abuse reported?
4. What are the legal responsibilities of your office in this situation?
5. What might be the reasons that the victim feels she cannot leave the abusive situation?
6. Explain the mechanics of the impact of the slapping causing rupture of the tympanic membrane.
7. Discuss the implications of both the abusive husband and the battered wife being patients of the practice.

Internet Assignments

1. Research the support available to families of major trauma victims at the American Trauma Society. Check this same website for suggested preventive measures.
2. Research suggested measures available to the victim of domestic violence at the National Coalition Against Domestic Violence.
3. Research the Bair Hugger concept.
4. Research your state's guidelines for reportable incidents.
5. Research your state's required reporting for workers' compensation injuries.
6. Access the SART digital toolkit at https://www.nsvrc.org/sarts. What are some of the tools that can assist members of the SART team?

Critical Thinking

1. Working in a facility where you see many patients filling out worker's compensation forms, you recently have noted that several from the same facility have been experiencing the same type of injury. What do you feel your role is in making someone aware that there might be a problem at that facility? How do you make sure that reports concerning this condition exist?
2. What teaching techniques would you use to explain to parents the importance of training their children not to place any objects in their noses? How would you attempt to explain to children the reason that they should not put things in their ears or their noses? What happens to cereal when they put it in their nose?
3. Explain the "rule of nines" when it comes to assessing a burn patient and the percentage of burns on their bodies.
4. Why is it important to have an understanding about radiation effects and burns? Explain how you would protect yourself from radiation.
5. Explain the guidelines in your community about animal bites. Are the animals quarantined? What are the reportable guidelines for animal bites? Are animals held for a certain length of time before being put down?
6. Family violence is escalating. What is happening to the statistics in your community? Can you remain objective while dealing with all members of the family?
7. After and while working with victims of abuse, what explanation do you have for why older adults and children are reluctant to come forward about being abused? Discuss some of the reasons older adults are abused.
8. Research the Duluth Model Power and Control Wheel, and discuss why you think this has an effect on family violence, domestic violence, and even sexual abuse.

Common Laboratory and Diagnostic Tests

Values may vary, depending on laboratory reference values. These values are for reference only. Results of one test alone usually are not conclusive and should be considered with the results of other diagnostic procedures, the symptoms and signs, and the physical examination findings to arrive at a diagnosis.

Blood Analysis

Complete Blood Count

A complete blood count is the evaluation of cellular components of blood. It includes red blood cell (RBC) count, RBC indices, white blood cell (WBC) count, WBC differential, hemoglobin (Hgb), hematocrit (Hct), and platelet count. Sometimes it is referred to as *hemogram*. Often the differential must be ordered specifically as complete blood count (CBC) with differential.

Red Blood Cell Count

RBC count is the count of erythrocytes in a specimen of whole blood.

Normal Levels
Adult men: 4.5–6.1 million/μL
Adult women: 4.0–5.5 million/μL
Infants and children: 3.8–5.5 million/μL
Newborns: 4.1–6.1 million/μL

An elevated RBC count is indicative of many disorders, including, but not limited to, erythremia, polycythemia, erythrocytosis, dehydration, burns, hypoxia, diarrhea, cardiovascular disease, poisoning, pulmonary disease, and smoking. A reduced RBC count also is indicative of many disorders, including, but not limited to, anemias, bone marrow suppression, hemorrhage, lead poisoning, liver diseases, thyroid disorders, cardiovascular disease, malnutrition, vitamin deficiency, and adverse effects of certain drugs. When the RBC count is abnormal, cell morphology should be examined. As with most blood tests, results should be evaluated with those of other tests, along with symptoms and signs, to determine a diagnosis.

Hemoglobin Count

An Hgb count is the measurement of the oxygen (O_2)-carrying pigments of the RBCs.

Normal Levels
Adult men: 13.0–18.0
Adult women: 12.0–16.0
Infants and children: 9.5–15.5
Newborns: 14–24

An elevated Hgb count is indicative of many disorders, including, but not limited to, congestive heart failure (CHF), chronic obstructive pulmonary disease (COPD), dehydration, burns, diarrhea, erythrocytosis, polycythemia, high altitude sickness, and thrombotic thrombocytopenia. A reduced Hgb count also is indicative of many disorders, including, but not limited to, iron deficiency anemia, hemorrhage, hemolytic reaction to drugs or chemicals, liver diseases, and systemic lupus erythematosus (SLE) and indicative of pregnancy.

Hematocrit Count

Hct count is the measurement of the percentage of RBCs in a volume of whole blood.

Normal Levels
Adult men: 37%–52%
Adult women: 36%–48%
Infants and children: 28%–50%
Newborns: 45%–64%

An elevated Hct count is indicative of many disorders, including, but not limited to, dehydration, burns, diarrhea, eclampsia, pancreatitis, shock, and polycythemia. A reduced Hct count also is indicative of many disorders, including, but not limited to, anemia, bone marrow hyperplasia, CHF, fluid overload, burns, thyroid disorders, pancreatitis, pneumonia, malnutrition, and adverse effects of certain drugs and indicative of pregnancy.

White Blood Cell Count

The WBC count is the count of WBCs in a whole blood specimen.

Normal Levels
Adult men: 4500–11,000/µL
Adult women: 4500–11,000/µL
Infants and children: 6000–17,500/µL
Newborns: 9000–35,000/µL

An elevated WBC count is indicative of many disorders, including, but not limited to, acquired hemolytic anemia, anorexia, abscess, appendicitis, bacterial infections, bronchitis, burns, biliary disorders, respiratory disorders, disorders of the gastrointestinal (GI) tract, renal disorders, blood disorders, lactic acidosis, SLE, poisoning, rheumatoid arthritis, sepsis, shock, tonsillitis, trauma, uremia, and adverse effects of certain drugs, and indicative of pregnancy. Similar to an abnormal RBC count, a differential should be evaluated, and as with most blood tests, results should be evaluated with those of other tests—along with symptoms and signs—to determine a diagnosis. A decreased WBC is indicative of many disorders, including, but not limited to, acquired immunodeficiency syndrome (AIDS), anemias, chemical toxicity, Hodgkin disease, influenza, legionnaires disease, radiation therapy, rheumatoid arthritis, vitamin B12 deficiency, cirrhosis, hepatitis, hypothermia, leukopenia, tuberculosis (TB), and adverse effects of certain drugs.

Differential White Blood Cell (Leukocyte) Count

The differential WBC (leukocyte) count is an assessment by percentage of leukocyte distribution in a specimen of 100 WBCs.

Leukocyte Count

Normal Levels
Segmented neutrophils (SEGs; mature "fighter" cell), adults: 50%–62%
Band neutrophils (immature "fighter" cells), adults: 3%–6%
Eosinophil granulocytes (eosinophils), adults: 0%–3%
Basophil granulocytes (basophils), adults: 0%–1%
Monocytes, adults: 3%–7%
Lymphocytes, adults: 24%–44%

Increased neutrophils are indicative of many disorders, including, but not limited to, allergies, asthma, acute infections, appendicitis, burns, diabetic acidosis, cardiovascular disorders, disorders of the GI tract, leukemia, respiratory disorders, poisoning, pyelonephritis, septicemia, tonsillitis, and adverse effects of certain drugs. A decrease in neutrophils is indicative of many disorders, including, but not limited to, endocrine disorders, anaphylactic shock, carcinoma, chemotherapy, anemias, pneumonia, influenza, septicemia, radiation therapy, and adverse effects of certain drugs.

An increase in eosinophils is indicative of many disorders, including, but not limited to, allergies, asthma, cancer, dermatitis, diverticulitis, eczema, Hodgkin disease, leukemia, parasitic infection, pernicious anemia, radiation therapy, sickle cell anemia, TB, and adverse effects of certain drugs. A reduction in eosinophils also is indicative of many disorders, including, but not limited to, aplastic anemia, CHF, eclampsia, infections, stress, and adverse effects of certain drugs.

An increase in basophils is indicative of many disorders, including, but not limited to, allergic reactions, Hodgkin disease, hypothyroidism, radiation therapy, sinusitis, urticaria, and adverse effects of certain drugs. A decrease in basophils also is indicative of many disorders, including, but not limited to, acute infections, anaphylactic shock, endocrine disorders, cancer, radiation therapy, stress, and adverse effects of certain drugs and indicative of pregnancy.

An increase in lymphocytes is indicative of many disorders, including, but not limited to, endocarditis, infectious mononucleosis, leukocytosis, lymphocytic leukemia, syphilis, toxoplasmosis chronic bacterial infection, viral infections, and adverse effects of certain drugs. A decrease in lymphocytes also is indicative of many disorders, including, but not limited to, aplastic anemia, Hodgkin disease, immunoglobulin deficiencies, leukemia, renal failure, SLE, anemia, sepsis, and adverse effects of certain drugs.

An increase in monocytes is indicative of many disorders, including, but not limited to, Epstein-Barr virus, Hodgkin disease, leukemia, rheumatoid arthritis, syphilis, SLE, TB, chronic inflammatory disease, and adverse effects of certain drugs. A decrease in monocytes is primarily indicative of aplastic anemia and hairy-cell leukemia.

Platelet (Thrombocyte) Count

The platelet (thrombocyte) count is the count of platelets in a whole blood specimen. Platelets help the blood clot.

Normal Adult Levels
150,000–400,000/µL

An increase in the platelet count (thrombocytosis) is indicative of many disorders, including, but not limited to, anemias, carcinoma, fractures, liver disorders, heart disease, hemorrhage, acute infection, inflammation, leukemia, pancreatitis, rheumatoid arthritis, surgery, and adverse effects of certain drugs and indicative of pregnancy. A decrease in platelet count (thrombocytopenia) is indicative of many disorders, including, but not limited to, anemias, bone marrow disorders, autoimmune disorders, severe burns, carcinoma, liver disorders, disseminated intravascular coagulation (DIC), hemolytic disease of the newborn, infections, radiation therapy, leukemia, celiac disease, vitamin K deficiency, and adverse effects of certain drugs.

Blood Chemistries

Chemistries

A normal chemistry profile may contain blood serum levels for albumin, alkaline phosphatase, aspartate aminotransferase (AST), bilirubin, calcium, creatinine, lactate dehydrogenase (LDH), phosphorus, total protein, urea nitrogen, and uric acid. Blood chemistries are often ordered in a panel of tests, which gives a profile of a certain organ or a number of organs. Chem7 is a basic metabolic panel consisting of seven tests: blood urea nitrogen (BUN), carbon dioxide (CO_2), creatinine, glucose, serum potassium, and serum sodium levels. A comprehensive metabolic panel generally consists of albumin, alkaline phosphatase, alanine aminotransferase (ALT), AST, BUN, calcium, chloride, CO_2, creatinine, LDH, glucose, potassium, sodium, total bilirubin, and total protein. These tests provide the health care provider with information regarding how the patient's liver and kidneys are working, blood sugar and calcium levels, electrolyte levels (sodium, potassium, chloride), and protein levels.

Albumin

Serum albumin is the measurement of one of two major protein factions of blood.

Normal Adult Levels
3.5–5.0 g/dL

Increased levels of serum albumin are indicative of many disorders, including, but not limited to, dehydration, diarrhea, hepatitis, meningitis, carcinoma, myeloma, nephrosis, nephrotic syndrome, peptic ulcers, pneumonia, rheumatic fever, SLE, uremia, vomiting, and adverse effects of certain drugs. Below normal levels of serum albumin are indicative of many disorders, including, but not limited to, ascites, alcoholism, burns, CHF, Crohn disease, cystic fibrosis, diabetes mellitus, edema, hypertension, kidney disorders, malnutrition, GI disorders, trauma, stress, and adverse effects of certain drugs.

Alanine Transaminase

ALT is the measurement of the enzyme found in the liver.

Normal Adult Levels
4–36 units/L

ALT is released into blood when the liver is damaged. Elevated levels are indicative of cirrhosis of the liver, hepatitis, liver ischemia, mononucleosis, or inflammation of the pancreas.

Alkaline Phosphatase

Alkaline phosphatase level is the measurement of the enzyme found in bones, the liver, intestines, and the placenta.

Normal Adult Levels
25–100 units/L

Elevated alkaline phosphatase levels are indicative of many disorders, including, but not limited to, alcoholism, liver disorders, diabetes mellitus, fractures, GI disorders, endocrine disorders, hepatitis, Hodgkin disease, leukemia, neoplasms, myocardial infarction (MI), bone disorders, disorders of the pancreas, kidney disorders, and adverse effects of certain drugs. Below normal levels of alkaline phosphatase are indicative of many disorders, including, but not limited to, pernicious anemia, cretinism, hypothyroidism, malnutrition, nephritis, and adverse effects of certain drugs.

Aspartate Aminotransferase (Serum Glutamic Oxaloacetic Transaminase)

AST (serum glutamic oxaloacetic transaminase [SGOT]) is the measurement of enzyme found primarily in the heart, liver, and muscles.

Normal Adult Levels
Women: 10–36 units/L
Men: 14–20 units/L

Elevated AST levels are indicative of many disorders, including, but not limited to, acute MI, alcoholism, liver disorders, mononucleosis, insult and injury to tissue (including trauma), cerebral and pulmonary infarctions, and adverse effects of certain drugs. Reduced AST levels are indicative of many disorders, including, but not limited to, diabetic ketoacidosis, liver disease, uremia, vitamin B_6 deficiency, and adverse effects of certain drugs.

Bilirubin

Bilirubin is a by-product of Hgb breakdown. Bilirubin is produced in the liver, spleen, and bone marrow.

Normal Adult Levels
Total: < 1.5 mg/dL
Direct: 0.0–0.3 mg/dL
Indirect: 0.1–1.0 mg/dL

Total bilirubin is divided into direct bilirubin, primarily secreted by the intestinal tract, and indirect bilirubin, primarily circulating in the bloodstream. Obstructive or hepatic jaundice results in an increased amount of direct bilirubin entering the bloodstream rather than entering the GI tract and being filtered and eliminated by the kidneys. Conditions that cause an increase in direct bilirubin include, but are not limited to, biliary obstruction, pancreatic cancer (head of the pancreas), cirrhosis, hepatitis, and adverse effects of certain drugs. Hemolytic jaundice causes the indirect bilirubin to accumulate in blood because of the increased breakdown of Hgb. Conditions that cause an increase in direct bilirubin levels include, but are not limited to, pernicious and sickle cell anemias, autoimmune hemolysis, cirrhosis, hepatitis, intracavity and soft tissue hemorrhage, MI, septicemia, hemolytic transfusion reaction, and adverse effects of certain drugs.

Creatinine

Creatinine level is a measurement of an indicator of renal function.

Normal Adult Levels
Women: 0.5–1.1 mg/dL
Men: 0.6–1.2 mg/dL

Serum creatinine is excreted continually by the renal system, and elevated levels are indicative of slowing of glomerular filtration. Other conditions that may contribute to elevation of serum creatinine include, but are not limited to, CHF, diabetes mellitus, kidney disorders, hypovolemia, metal poisoning, endocrine disorders, subacute bacterial endocarditis, SLE, and adverse effects of certain drugs. Decreased serum creatinine levels are indicative of diabetic ketoacidosis and muscular dystrophy.

Lactate Dehydrogenase

LDH level is the measurement of body tissue intracellular enzyme released after tissue damage.

Normal Adult Levels
100–250 units/L

Elevated LDH levels are indicative of many disorders, including, but not limited to, alcoholism, anoxia, burns, cardiomyopathy, cerebrovascular accident (CVA), cirrhosis, CHF and MI, neoplasms, anemias, leukemia, renal disorders, pancreatitis, mononucleosis, muscle and bone pain, respiratory disorders, shock, trauma, and adverse effects of certain drugs. The levels of LDH decrease after radiation and after adverse effects of oxalates.

Total Protein

Total protein is the measurement of the total amounts of albumin and globulins in serum.

Normal Adult Levels
6.0–8.0 g/dL

Increased total protein is indicative of many disorders, including, but not limited to, Addison disease, dehydration, diarrhea, renal disease, vomiting, protozoal diseases, chronic inflammation or infection (including human immunodeficiency virus [HIV] infection and hepatitis B or C), and adverse effects of certain drugs. Decreased total protein is indicative of many disorders, including, but not limited to, autoimmune diseases, burns, cholecystitis, cirrhosis, CHF,

Crohn disease, diarrhea, hyperthyroidism, edema, leukemia, peptic ulcer, nephrosis, malnutrition, ulcerative colitis, and adverse effects of certain drugs.

Urea Nitrogen/Blood Urea Nitrogen

Urea nitrogen/BUN is the assessment of the urea content in blood and gives an indication of the functioning of the renal glomeruli.

Normal Adult Levels
5–20 mg/dL

An elevated urea nitrogen level can be indicative of many disorders, including, but not limited to, kidney disease, CHF, shock, dehydration, burns, urinary tract blockage, and a high-protein diet. Decreased urea nitrogen level can be indicative of many disorders, including, but not limited to, malnutrition, overhydration, and liver damage.

Uric Acid

Uric acid is an end product of the metabolism of purines.

Normal Adult Levels
Women: 2.4–6.0 mg/dL
Men: 3.4–7.0 mg/dL

Elevated uric acid levels are indicative of many disorders, including, but not limited to, gout, hyperuricemia, hemolytic and sickle cell anemias, hypothyroidism, acute infections, lead poisoning, leukemia, neoplasms, nephritis, kidney stones and polycystic kidney disease, renal failure, malnutrition, psoriasis, uremia, urinary obstruction, and adverse effects of certain drugs. Reduced uric acid levels are indicative of many disorders, including, but not limited to, acromegaly, carcinomas, Hodgkin disease, pernicious anemia, and adverse effects of certain drugs.

Thyroid Function Tests

An evaluation of the levels of all three thyroid hormones is important in diagnosing thyroid disorders.

Thyroxine

The hormone thyroxine (T_4) is produced in the thyroid gland from iodide and thyroglobulin in response to stimulation by thyroid-stimulating hormone (TSH) produced by the pituitary gland. T_4 stimulates triiodothyronine (T_3) to be produced. It also stimulates basal metabolism. In the process of negative feedback, circulating levels of T_4 influence the levels of TSH.

Normal Adult Levels
5.0–12.0 mcg/dL

Increased levels of T_4 usually indicate the presence of hyperfunctioning thyroid disorders, including Graves disease, hyperthyroidism, thyrotoxicosis, and adverse effects of certain drugs. Decreased levels of T_4 are indicative of hypothyroid disorders, including acromegaly, cretinism, and goiter, as well as hypothyroidism, liver disease, endocrine disorders, GI tract disorders, pituitary tumor, and adverse effects of certain drugs.

Triiodothyronine

T_3 stimulates the basal metabolic rate for metabolism of carbohydrates and lipids, protein synthesis, vitamin metabolism, and bone calcium release. T_3 is the most active thyroid hormone and affects all body processes, including gene expression.

Normal Adult Levels
80–230 ng/dL

An increase in T_3 levels is indicative of many disorders, including, but not limited to, Graves disease, hyperthyroidism, thyrotoxicosis, and adverse effects of certain drugs. Decreased levels of T_3 are indicative of many disorders, including, but not limited to, iodine and thyroid deficiency disorders, such as goiter and myxedema; renal failure; starvation; thyroidectomy; and adverse effects of certain drugs.

Thyroid-Stimulating Hormone

TSH, produced in the anterior lobe of the pituitary gland, stimulates the production and release of T_3 and T_4 by the thyroid gland.

Normal Adult Levels
0.4–4.2 units/L

An increase in TSH levels may be indicative of many disorders, including, but not limited to, Addison disease, goiter, hyperpituitarism, hypothyroidism, thyroiditis, and adverse effects of certain drugs. A decrease in TSH may be indicative of many disorders, including, but not limited to, Hashimoto thyroiditis, hyperthyroidism, and hypothyroidism.

Lipid Profile

A lipid profile consists of comparison of results of four serum lipids: total cholesterol, triglycerides, high-density lipoproteins (HDLs), and low-density lipoproteins (LDLs). One consideration is the ratio of HDL:LDL; the recommended ratio is 3.4:5.0.

Total Cholesterol

Total cholesterol measures a widely distributed sterol that facilitates the absorption and transport of fatty acids. Cholesterol helps build cells and produce hormones.

Normal Adult Levels
Desirable: < 200 mg/dL

Borderline: 200–240 mg/dL

High risk: > 240 mg/dL

Elevated serum cholesterol levels are indicative of many disorders, including, but not limited to, atherosclerosis, CHF, biliary disorders, kidney disorders, lipid disorders, and adverse effects of certain drugs. Decreased levels of serum cholesterol are indicative of many disorders, including, but not limited to, anemias, carcinoma, cirrhosis, liver disease, hepatitis, endocrine disorders, GI tract disorders, and adverse effects of certain drugs.

Triglycerides

Triglycerides, the principal lipids in blood, are simple fat compounds of three molecules of fatty acid: oleic, palmitic, or stearic. Triglycerides give energy to muscles and store energy.

Normal Adult Levels
Normal: Below 150 mg/dL

Borderline: 150–199 mg/dL

High: 200–499 mg/dL

Very high: Above 500 mg/dL

Elevated triglyceride levels are indicative of many disorders, including, but not limited to, arteriosclerosis, MI, aortic aneurysm, hypercholesterolemia, hyperlipoproteinemia, alcoholism, diabetes mellitus, gout, renal disease, and malnutrition. Decreased triglyceride levels are indicative of many disorders, including, but not limited to, cirrhosis, malabsorption, hyperalimentation, and adverse effects of certain drugs.

High-Density Lipoprotein Cholesterol

HDL transports cholesterol and other lipids to the liver for excretion. HDL is believed to reduce the risk of coronary artery disease. It is often referred to as the *good cholesterol.*

Normal Adult Levels
Desirable: 60 mg/dL or higher

Acceptable: 40–59 mg/dL

Undesirable: Less than 50 mg/dL

Increased levels of HDL are indicative of many disorders, including, but not limited to, alcoholism, hepatic disorders, cirrhosis, and adverse effects of certain drugs. Reduced levels of HDL are indicative of many disorders, including, but not limited to, arteriosclerosis, hypercholesterolemia, hyperlipoproteinemia, CHD, diabetes mellitus, liver disease, kidney disease, bacterial infections, and adverse effects of certain drugs.

Low-Density Lipoprotein Cholesterol

LDL has high cholesterol content, and it delivers lipids to body tissues. It is often referred to as the *bad cholesterol.*

Normal Adult Levels

Optimal: Less than 100 mg/dL

Near optimal: 100–129 mg/dL

Borderline: 130–159 mg/dL

High: 160–189 mg/dL

Very high: 190 and above

Elevated levels of LDL are indicative of many disorders, including, but not limited to, diabetes mellitus, anorexia nervosa, renal failure, hepatic disease, and adverse effects of certain drugs. Decreased levels of LDL are indicative of many disorders, including, but not limited to, hyperlipoproteinemia, arteriosclerosis, pulmonary disease, stress, and adverse effects of certain drugs.

Electrolytes

Electrolytes are examined in serum to test for chloride, potassium, sodium, carbon dioxide levels. Other electrolytes that may be included or can be tested individually are calcium, magnesium, and phosphorus.

Chloride

Chloride is an anion found predominately in extracellular spaces. It helps keep the balance of fluid inside and outside the cells.

Normal Adult Levels

97–106 mEq/L

Increased blood serum levels of chloride may be the result of several disorders, including, but not limited to, metabolic disorders, dehydration, diabetes insipidus, hyperventilation, hyperparathyroidism, acidosis, respiratory alkalosis, CHF, Cushing disease, nephritis, renal failure, and adverse effects of certain drugs. Reduced blood serum levels of chloride may be the result of several disorders, including, but not limited to, metabolic alkalosis, diabetes, severe vomiting, burns, overhydration, salt-losing diseases, some diuretic therapies, central nervous system (CNS) disorders, diaphoresis, fasting, fever, heat exhaustion, acute infections, gastric obstructions, uremia, and adverse effects of certain drugs.

Potassium

Potassium is the major positive ion found inside of cells. Potassium is important in nerve conduction, muscle function, osmotic pressure, acid-base balance, and myocardial activity.

Normal Adult Levels

3.5–5.3 mEq/L

Increased blood serum levels of potassium may be the result of several disorders, including, but not limited to, renal failure, dehydration, burns, trauma, chemotherapy, metabolic acidosis, Addison disease, uncontrolled diabetes, dialysis, hemolysis, intestinal obstruction, sepsis, shock, pneumonia, uremia, and adverse effects of certain drugs. Reduced blood serum levels of potassium may be the result of several disorders, including, but not limited to, alkalosis, anorexia, vomiting, diarrhea, malabsorption, starvation, diuresis, excessive sweating, draining wounds, severe burns, endocrine disorders, pancreatitis, cystic fibrosis, GI stress, and adverse effects of certain drugs. Abnormally elevated or decreased potassium can cause life-threatening cardiac arrhythmias.

Sodium

Sodium is the major positive ion found outside the cell and is the main base in blood. Its functions include chemical maintenance of osmotic pressure, acid-base balance, and nerve transmission.

Normal Adult Levels

135–145 mEq/L

Increased blood serum levels of sodium may be the result of several disorders, including, but not limited to, dehydration, excessive fluid loss caused by vomiting, diarrhea, sweating, Cushing disease, kidney disease, diabetic ketoacidosis, diabetes insipidus, hyperaldosteronism, hypertension, hypovolemia, edema, and adverse effects of certain drugs. Decreased blood serum levels of sodium may be the result of several disorders, including, but not limited to, CHF, cirrhosis, cystic fibrosis, hypothyroidism, poor nutrition, psychogenic polydipsia, syndrome of inappropriate antidiuretic hormone secretion (SIADH), severe burns, sweating, vomiting, diarrhea, and adverse effects of certain drugs.

Carbon Dioxide

CO_2 in normal blood plasma comes from bicarbonate. CO_2 levels in blood are affected by abnormal kidney and lung functions.

Normal Adult Levels

20–30 mEq/L

Increased blood serum levels of CO_2 may be the result of several disorders, including, but not limited to, emphysema, aldosteronism, severe vomiting, dehydration, COPD, Cushing disease, bradycardia, cardiac disorders, renal disorders, and adverse effects of certain drugs. Decreased blood serum levels of CO_2 may be the result of several disorders, including kidney failure, alcoholic ketosis, dehydration, high fever, head trauma, malabsorption syndrome, uremia, and adverse effects of certain drugs.

Calcium

Calcium studies include measurement of calcium levels in blood.

Normal Adult Levels

8.2–10.2 mg/dL

Ionized Calcium

Ionized calcium is the amount of calcium that is not attached to protein in blood. It is also called *free calcium*.

Normal Adult Levels

4.4–5.3 mg/dL

Calcium is the most abundant mineral found in the human body. Calcium acts in bone formation, impulse conduction, myocardial and skeletal muscle contractions, and the blood-clotting process. Elevated serum calcium levels are indicative of many disorders, including, but not limited to, endocrine disorders, hepatic disease, respiratory acidosis, leukemia, neoplasms, blood disorders, respiratory disorders, and adverse effects of certain drugs. Reduced serum calcium levels are indicative of many disorders, including, but not limited to, alkalosis, bacteremia, burns, chronic renal disease and other renal disorders, endocrine disorders, osteomalacia, rickets, vitamin D deficiency, and adverse effects of certain drugs.

Magnesium

Magnesium studies include measurement of magnesium levels in blood.

Normal Adult Levels

1.5–2.4 mg/dL

Magnesium is an important mineral found in bones and inside cells. It is needed for proper nerve function, muscle maintenance, and bone strength. Elevated levels of magnesium are indicative of many disorders, including, but not limited to, chronic renal failure, dehydration, Addison disease, and diabetic ketoacidosis. Decreased levels of magnesium are indicative of many disorders, including, but not limited to, pancreatitis, alcoholism, cirrhosis of liver, chronic diarrhea, preeclampsia, and malabsorption disorders.

Phosphorus

Phosphorus studies include measurement of phosphorus in blood.

Normal Adult Levels

2.4–4.1 mg/dL

Phosphorus is the second most abundant mineral found in the human body. It is needed in the building of bone and teeth, contraction of muscles, and nerve function. Elevated levels of phosphorus maybe indicative of many disorders, including, but not limited to, renal disease, diabetic ketoacidosis, liver disease, and hypoparathyroidism. Decreased levels of phosphorus maybe indicative of many disorders, including, but not limited to alcoholism, malnutrition, hypercalcemia, and hyperparathyroidism.

Clotting and Coagulation Studies

Activated Partial Thromboplastin Time

The activated partial thromboplastin time (aPTT) test is an evaluation of the time necessary to generate fibrin through the intrinsic pathway of coagulation. This test is a screening process used to detect coagulation factor deficiencies and to monitor the effectiveness of heparin therapy.

Normal values or standardized times used by the laboratory must be checked because various processes may be used.

Increased standardized times may be indicative of many disorders, including, but not limited to, hemophilia A or B, SLE, cardiac surgery, DIC, abruptio placentae, factor defects, hemodialysis, obstructive jaundice, vitamin K deficiency, presence of circulating anticoagulants, and adverse effects of certain drugs. Decreased standardized times are indicative of acute early hemorrhage and cancer spread.

Prothrombin Time

Prothrombin time (PT, also called *Pro Time*) is a measurement of the time taken for clot formation after the addition of reagent tissue thromboplastin and calcium to citrated plasma. In the clotting process, prothrombin converts to thrombin. Adequate vitamin K is necessary for adequate prothrombin production. This test helps in the evaluation of the extrinsic and common coagulation pathways and in monitoring oral anticoagulant therapy.

Normal Adult Levels

INR ≤ to 1.1

(INR 2.0–3.0 is an effective therapeutic range)

10.0–13.0 seconds may vary from laboratory to laboratory

PT test results are generally reported as an international normalized ratio (INR), which is a standardized result used with anticoagulation therapy. PT can also be reported in seconds.

Critical value: An INR of 4.9 or higher is considered a critical or panic value.

An increase in PT may be indicative of several disorders, including, but not limited to, vitamin K deficiency, liver disorders, adverse effects of anticoagulant therapy, prothrombin deficiency, salicylate intoxication, DIC, SLE, clotting disorders, biliary obstruction, CHF, pancreatitis, snakebite, vomiting, toxic shock syndrome, and adverse effects of certain drugs. A reduced PT may be indicative of certain disorders, including, but not limited to, deep vein thrombosis, MI, peripheral vascular disease, spinal cord injury, pulmonary embolism, and adverse effects of large amounts of foods rich in vitamin K or certain drugs.

Bleeding Time

Bleeding time is a screening test for coagulation disorders, a measurement of the time required for the platelet clot to form. It is often measured by using the Ivy method. The Ivy method involves placing a blood pressure cuff on the patient's arm, inflating the cuff to 40 mm Hg, and using a lancet or scalpel to make an incision on the underside of the forearm. The incision is to be shallow at 1 mm depth and about 10 mm long. Filter paper is used to "wick" blood from the cut every 30 seconds until bleeding ceases.

Normal time at most laboratories is between 1 and 9 minutes.

Increased bleeding times are indicative of several disorders, including, but not limited to, thrombocytopenia, DIC, aplastic anemia, platelet dysfunction, vascular disease, leukemias, liver disorders, aspirin ingestion, and adverse effects of certain drugs. Decreased bleeding time is clinically insignificant.

Erythrocyte Sedimentation Rate

Erythrocyte sedimentation rate (ESR) is the rate at which RBCs (erythrocytes) fall out of well-mixed whole blood to the bottom of the test tube. An alteration in blood proteins occurs during inflammatory and necrotic processes, causing an aggregation of RBCs, thereby making them heavier and thus causing them to fall rapidly when placed in a special vertical test tube. A higher ESR is the result of faster settling of RBCs. Although not diagnostic of any particular disease process, an elevated ESR gives an indication of an ongoing disease process.

Normal Values by Westergren Method (most labs use this method, which is more accurate)
Adult men: 0–15 mm/h

Adult women: 0–20 mm/h

Children: 0–10 mm/h

Normal Values by Wintrobe Method
Adult men: 0.41–0.51 mm/h

Adult women: 0.36–0.45 mm/h

Increased ESRs may be indicative of many disease processes, including, but not necessarily limited to, collagen diseases, infectious processes, inflammatory disorders, cancer, heavy metal poisoning, toxemia, pelvic inflammatory disease (PID), anemia, pain, pulmonary embolism, renal disorders, arthritis, subacute bacterial endocarditis, and adverse effects of certain drugs, and indicative of pregnancy. Decreased levels may be found in CHF, sickle cell anemia, polycythemia, and as adverse effects of certain drugs.

Glucose Monitoring

Glucose Tolerance Test

Glucose tolerance test (GTT) is a test that evaluates patients who have symptoms of diabetes mellitus or diabetic complications and screens for gestational diabetes. The test measures blood glucose levels at the following intervals: fasting, 30 minutes, 1 hour, 2 hours, and 3 hours after ingestion of a dose of glucose. Urine samples also are taken at these intervals.

Normal Adult Levels
Fasting: 70–110 mg/dL

30 min: 110–170 mg/dL

1 h: 120–170 mg/dL

2 h: 70–120 mg/dL

3 h: 70–120 mg/dL

All urine samples should test negative for glucose.

Increased glucose values or decreased glucose tolerance are indicative of certain disorders, including, but not limited to, diabetes mellitus, excessive glucose ingestion, certain endocrine disorders, hepatic damage, CNS lesions, pancreatitis, pheochromocytoma, and adverse effects of certain drugs. Decreased glucose values or increased glucose tolerance may be indicative of certain disorders, including, but not limited to, Addison disease, hypoglycemia, malabsorption, pancreatic disease, liver disease, hypoparathyroidism, hypopituitarism, and adverse effects of certain drugs.

Fasting Blood Glucose Levels

Fasting blood glucose (FBG) levels are measured by the amount of glucose found in blood after 8 hours of fasting.

Normal Adult Levels
Serum: 70–99 mg/dL

Increased levels of blood glucose are indicative of several disorders, including, but not limited to, diabetes mellitus, excessive glucose ingestion, certain endocrine disorders, hepatic damage, status post gastrectomy, CNS lesions, pancreatitis, pheochromocytoma, and adverse effects of certain drugs. Decreased glucose values may be indicative of certain disorders, including, but not limited to, Addison disease, hypoglycemia, malabsorption, pancreatic disease, liver disease, hypoparathyroidism, hypopituitarism, and adverse effects of certain drugs.

Two-Hour Postprandial

Two-hour postprandial levels indicate blood glucose levels after fasting for 10 to 12 hours and then again 2 hours after consuming a normal meal.

Normal Adult Levels
70–145 mg/dL

Increased postprandial levels of blood glucose are indicative of several disorders, including, but not limited to, diabetes mellitus, excessive glucose ingestion, certain endocrine disorders, hepatic damage, status post gastrectomy, CNS lesions, pancreatitis, pheochromocytoma, and adverse effects of certain drugs. Decreased postprandial glucose values may be indicative of certain disorders, including, but not limited to, Addison disease, hypoglycemia, malabsorption, pancreatic disease, liver disease, hypoparathyroidism, hypopituitarism, and adverse effects of certain drugs.

Glycosylated Hemoglobin/Glycohemoglobin

Glycohemoglobin (HgbA1c) is the measurement of the blood glucose bound to Hgb and gives an overall view of the past 3 months of glucose saturation.

Normal Adult Levels
Normal: < 5.7%
Prediabetic: 5.7%–6.4%
Diabetic: 6.5% and higher

Increased glycohemoglobin levels are indicative of several disorders, including, but not limited to, poorly controlled diabetes mellitus, iron deficiency anemia, splenectomy, alcohol or lead toxicity, and hyperglycemia. Decreased levels of glycohemoglobin may be indicative of certain diseases, including, but not limited to, hemolytic anemia, chronic blood loss, and chronic renal failure, and indicative of pregnancy.

Toxicology Studies and Drug Screens

Toxicology studies are conducted on blood, primarily serum, and on urine. Blood levels of various medications are checked by toxicology levels to determine whether a medication is at the therapeutic level or is approaching or at a toxic level. Blood alcohol levels are the preferred method of screening for blood alcohol content to provide the required qualitative information. Urine drug screens are used to detect the presence of various drugs or substances, primarily drugs of common abuse and/or of illegal origin and blood alcohol. Drugs detected by urine screening include depressants, hallucinogens, sedatives, and stimulants.

Blood Screening Tests

Drug Levels

Common blood serum testing for therapeutic drugs includes, but is not limited to, digoxin, digitoxin, theophylline, lidocaine, lithium, and various drugs for therapeutic or toxic levels.

Digoxin

Digoxin is a cardiac glycoside used to treat CHF and cardiac arrhythmias. Blood level studies produce information about therapeutic or toxic levels.

Normal Therapeutic Level
0.8–2 ng/mL

Levels above 2.5 ng/mL indicate toxicity of the drug. Medical intervention is necessary to return to therapeutic levels. Levels below 0.8 ng/mL indicate that more digoxin is necessary to achieve the expected therapeutic effect.

Theophylline

Theophylline, a bronchodilator, is used to treat asthma and obstructive respiratory disorders. Blood level studies give information about therapeutic or toxic levels.

Normal Therapeutic Level
10–20 mcg/mL

Levels above 20 mcg/mL indicate toxicity of the drug. Chronically poisoned patients may be asymptomatic but are at high risk for seizures and arrhythmias with levels 30 mcg/mL or greater. Medical intervention is necessary to return to therapeutic levels. Levels below 8 mcg/mL indicate that more theophylline is necessary to achieve the expected therapeutic effect.

Lidocaine

Lidocaine is used to treat acute ventricular arrhythmias resulting from MI or cardiac surgery. Blood level studies give information about therapeutic or toxic levels.

Normal Therapeutic Level
1.5–6 mcg/mL

Levels above 6 mcg/mL indicate potential toxicity of the drug, and levels greater than 9 mcg/mL are definitely toxic. Medical intervention is necessary to return to therapeutic levels. Levels below 1.5 mcg/mL indicate that more lidocaine is necessary to achieve the expected therapeutic effect. **Note:** The routine prophylactic use of lidocaine to prevent arrhythmia associated with fibrinolytic administration or to suppress isolated ventricular premature beats, couplets, runs of accelerated idioventricular rhythm, and nonsustained ventricular tachycardia (VT) is not recommended (American College of Cardiology Foundation [ACCF]/American Heart Association [AHA]; [O'Gara, 2013]). Therefore this drug is used only in acute cases and not routinely.

Lithium

Lithium is used to treat bipolar disorder.

Normal Therapeutic Level
0.6–1.2 mEq/L

Levels above 1.5 mEq/L indicate toxicity of the drug. Medical intervention is necessary to return to therapeutic levels. Levels below 0.6 mEq/L indicate that more lithium is necessary to achieve the expected therapeutic effect.

Prograf (Tacrolimus)/FK-506

Prograf (Tacrolimus)/FK-506 is an immunosuppressive medication used in patients who have received organ transplants. It is used prophylactically to prevent organ rejection.

Normal Therapeutic Level
5–20 mcg/L

Therapeutic levels vary, depending on other factors, such as organ of transplant, length of time with the transplant, patient's race, and other medication therapies.

Phenytoin (Dilantin)

Phenytoin (Dilantin) is an anticonvulsant medication used to control seizures.

Normal Therapeutic Level
10–20 mcg/mL

Levels above 20 mcg/mL indicate toxicity of the drug. Medical intervention is necessary to return to therapeutic levels. Levels below 10 mcg/mL indicate more phenytoin is needed to achieve expected therapeutic effect.

Alcohol Levels

Normal Level
0%

States have established blood levels or content of alcohol that are considered *legally drunk or intoxicated.* Refer to state guidelines for these levels.

Cardiac Enzymes/Cardiac Isoenzymes

Cardiac enzymes and isoenzymes are released by the myocardium as a result of an MI. Monitoring the levels of these enzymes helps evaluate the extent of the insult to the myocardium and the progress of the healing process.

Cross-Reactive Protein

The tissues of the body release cross-reactive (C-reactive) protein, a protein that can be detected and helps evaluate the general amount of inflammation in the body. In addition, a high-sensitivity C-reactive protein test measures the risk for coronary artery disease and thus potential heart problems. Baseline studies are recommended as a reference for future measurement of arterial condition.

Normal Adult Levels
Low risk: < 1.0 mg/dL
Average risk: 1.0–3.0 mg/dL
High risk: > 3.0 mg/dL

An elevation may be indicative of MI, rheumatic fever, rheumatoid arthritis, TB, cancer, pneumococcal pneumonia,

SLE, or use of oral contraceptives. This protein is normally elevated in the last half of pregnancy. An inflammation in the body's tissues also must be considered a source of the elevation.

Creatine Kinase

Creatine kinase (CK), an enzyme found in certain body tissues, becomes elevated with damage to cardiac and skeletal muscles.

Normal Adult Levels
Women: 26–140 units/L
Men: 30–174 units/L
Values may vary from laboratory to laboratory.

In MI, levels begin to rise in 4 to 6 hours, peak at 12 to 24 hours, and return to baseline 3 to 5 days after the onset of MI. The increased levels should be part of the total evaluation to confirm MI.

Creatine Kinase Isoenzymes (Creatine Phosphokinase Isoenzymes)

Isoenzymes increase during MI and are more specific in the diagnosis of MI.

Normal Values
MM-CK (muscle): 97%–100%
MB-CK (heart): 0%–1%
BB-CK (brain): 0%

MB-CK begins to rise within 2 to 6 hours after the myocardial insult; it usually peaks at 15 to 24 hours and then returns to normal within 72 hours.

Lactate Dehydrogenase

LDH, an enzyme found in the tissues of the kidneys, heart, skeleton, brain, liver, and lungs, is released from cells, increasing serum levels and indicating cellular necrosis.

Normal Values
100–250 units/L
Values may vary among laboratories.

LDH levels begin to rise at 12 hours after the insult, reach a peak at 24 hours, and return to normal later than CK levels.

Lactate Dehydrogenase Isoenzymes

LDH isoenzymes are found in many body tissues and are released when tissue necrosis occurs. There are five different LDH isoenzymes, and elevation of LDH1 and LDH2 usually point to cardiac involvement and subsequent necrosis of myocardial tissue.

Normal Values: Percentage of Total

LDH1: 17%–32%

LDH2: 25%–40%

LDH3: 19%–27%

LDH4: 5%–13%

LDH5: 4%–20%

LDH1 and LDH2 usually are increased in myocardial insult and necrosis. Normally LDH-2 is greater than LDH-1. When these values "flip," it is indicative of MI. The ratio will return to normal within 48 hours. When LDH-5 values are greater than those of LDH-4, liver damage or disease is indicated.

Aspartate Aminotransferase (Serum Glutamic Oxaloacetic Transaminase)

AST (SGOT) is a measurement of enzyme found primarily in the heart, liver, and muscles.

Normal Adult Levels

Women: 8–20 units/L

Men: 8–26 units/L

Elevated AST levels are indicative of many disorders, including, but not limited to, acute MI, alcoholism, liver disorders, insult and injury to tissue (including trauma and cerebral and pulmonary infarctions), and adverse effects of certain drugs. Low levels of AST in blood are considered normal.

Alanine Aminotransferase (Serum Glutamic Pyruvate Transaminase)

ALT (SGPT) evaluates liver insult and is a measurement of an enzyme product found primarily in the liver.

Normal Adult Levels

Women: 7–35 units/L

Men: 10–40 units/L

Elevated ALT levels are indicative of certain disorders, including, but not limited to, liver insult and liver disease, CHF, muscle injury, MI, pancreatitis, nonalcoholic fatty liver disease (NASH), mononucleosis, severe burns, trauma, shock, and adverse effects of certain drugs. Decreased levels of ALT are never found.

Urine Studies

Urinalysis/Clean Catch Urinalysis

Urinalysis/clean catch urinalysis is a physical, chemical, or microscopic analysis of a urine specimen. Clean catch is the method of collection used. Measurements include pH and specific gravity of urine and the presence of ketones, protein, sugars, bilirubin, and urobilinogen. Color and odor

are noted, as is the presence of abnormal blood cells, casts, bacteria, other cells, and crystals.

Routine Urinalysis

Normal Characteristics

Color and clarity: Pale to darker yellow and clear

Odor: Aromatic

Chemical nature: pH is generally slightly acidic, 6.5

Specific gravity: 1.003–1.030; reflects amount of waste, minerals, and solids in urine

Normal Constituent Compounds

Protein: None or small amount

Glucose: None

Ketone bodies: None

Urobilinogen and bilirubin: None

Casts: None or small amount of hyaline casts

Nitrogenous wastes: Ammonia, creatinine, nitrites, urea, and uric acid

Crystals: None to trace

Fat droplets: None

Refer to Table 11.1 for abnormal findings and related pathology.

Culture and Sensitivity of Urine

Culture

The urine specimen is placed in/on culture medium to see whether microbial growth occurs. If growth occurs, the pathogenic microbe is identified. Growth indicates pathogens residing in the urinary tract.

Normal Result

No growth

Sensitivity

Once the pathogen has been isolated, it is plated on the culture medium, and disks impregnated with specific antibiotics in specific concentrations are placed on top. Zones of inhibition of growth are measured around each disk to identify antimicrobials to which pathogens are sensitive.

Cardiology Tests

Electrocardiography (12-Lead)

Electrocardiography (ECG) is the recording of electrical activity of the myocardium used to diagnose ischemia, arrhythmias, conduction difficulties, and activity of cardiac medications.

Normal Result

No dysrhythmias/arrhythmias

The 12-lead ECG consists of three limb leads: I, II, III; three augmented limb leads: aV_R, aV_L, aV_F; and six precordial chest leads: V_1, V_2, V_3, V_4, V_5, and V_6. The conduction of an impulse through the myocardium is traced by three specific areas of the systolic and diastolic complex. The P wave represents atrial depolarization, the conduction of the stimulus from the sinoatrial (SA) node through the atrium to the atrioventricular (AV) node. The QRS complex represents ventricular depolarization, that is, the conduction of the stimulus from the upper portion of the ventricle and below the AV node through the AV bundle, through the right and left bundle branches, and through the Purkinje fibers, followed by its relay throughout the ventricular myocardium. The T wave represents the repolarization of the ventricular myocardium. The 12-lead ECG is used to detect conduction abnormalities, dysrhythmias, myocardial ischemia, and myocardial damage; to monitor recovery from an MI; and to assist in evaluation of the effectiveness of cardiac medications. Lead II normally is used to evaluate cardiac rhythm. Refer to Table 10.1 for an explanation of cardiac arrhythmias/dysrhythmias.

Echocardiography

Echocardiography is the ultrasound (acoustic imaging) examination of the cardiac structure to define the size, shape, thickness, position, and movements of cardiac structures, including valves, walls, and chambers.

Normal Result
Shows no abnormalities

This noninvasive procedure assists in diagnosing cardiac diseases and disorders, including structural abnormalities, congenital defects, myocardial damage, and blood flow through all structures of the heart.

Cardiac Stress Echocardiography

A cardiac stress echocardiography uses ultrasound imaging at rest and then during stress to evaluate the heart's walls, valves, and pumping action. The stress part of this examination can be accomplished in two different ways: (1) by walking on a treadmill or use of a stationary bike or (2) by using the chemically induced method. The chemical agent that can be used to simulate exercise in the body is dobutamine, which is given intravenously. This test is performed in a safe environment, and a physician or cardiologist is present, along with specially trained staff.

Normal Result
Negative
Low risk of cardiac disease
Normal appearance of heart chambers and valves
No significant changes on ECG

Holter Monitor

A Holter monitor is a miniature electrocardiograph that records the electrical activity of the heart for an extended period, usually 24 to 48 hours. The patient records all activities during the period to allow the examiner to correlate activity with cardiac abnormalities.

Cardiac Event Recorders

Cardiac event recorders are battery-powered, portable devices that record electrical activity of the heart while the patient goes about his or her everyday activities. The monitors record the heart's rate and rhythm. Some monitors are attached to the chest with electrodes, whereas some are placed on the wrist. There are two types of monitors: (1) the loop memory recorder and (2) the symptom event monitor. The *loop memory recorder* records the ECG reading for a short period. The person must push a button when symptoms (e.g., feeling faint, dizziness, or feeling of irregular heartbeat) occur, and the monitor records the readings for the period before and after the event. The *symptom event monitor* is similar to the loop memory recorder in that one must place or activate the recorder during a symptom or event. But unlike the loop recorder, it is unable to record an ECG reading prior to the event. Both recorders have the capability to have their records transmitted over the phone to the physician's office. They may be worn for several days to several weeks, depending on what the physician deems necessary.

Normal Result
No dysrhythmias
Refer to ECG

Multiple Gate Acquisition Scan

Multiple gate acquisition (MUGA) scanning is a nuclear medicine scanning method that assesses the function of the left ventricle, evaluates cardiac output, and identifies abnormalities of the myocardial walls.

Normal Result
50%–70% ejection fraction
Symmetric contraction of the left ventricle

A radioactive isotope "tracer" is injected, which attaches to RBCs to show all four chambers and the great vessels simultaneously. A series of images are taken during both systole and diastole, and then is shown as a movie (or superimposed) to relate ventricular function and to allow the ejection fraction to be calculated. This test may be performed with or without the stress factor.

Cardiac Stress Test (Cardiac Perfusion Scanning)

A cardiac stress test called *cardiac perfusion scanning* is used to detect and evaluate coronary artery disease. This test measures blood flow to the heart during stress and rest. The stress part of this examination can be accomplished two different ways— (1) by walking on a treadmill or (2) by using a chemically induced method. Chemical agents that can be used to simulate exercise in the body are dobutamine, dipyridamole (Persantine), adenosine, or regadenoson (Lexiscan). Myoview, Cardiolite, and thallium are all radioactive agents used, and this test may be referred to accordingly. This test is performed in a safe environment, and a physician or a cardiologist is present, along with a specially trained staff.

> **Normal Result**
> Good blood flow during both the resting and exercise portions of test
> No coronary blockage

Exercise Tolerance Test

The exercise tolerance test is an assessment of cardiac function during moderate exercise on a treadmill or stationary bicycle after a 12-lead ECG. No chemical agent is used to stress the heart during exercise.

> **Normal Result**
> Negative

The stress test measures the effects of exercise on myocardial output and O_2 consumption by the concurrent evaluation of the monitored ECG readings and O_2 consumption. This test is performed in a safe environment to identify individuals who are prone to myocardial ischemia during activity.

Hepatobiliary (Gallbladder) Scanning With Ejection Fraction

A hepatobiliary iminodiacetic acid (HIDA) or gallbladder scanning with ejection fraction is a nuclear imaging scanning method used to evaluate the gallbladder and the ducts leading into and out of the gallbladder. It is also known as *cholescintigraphy* and *hepatobiliary scintigraphy*.

> **Normal Results**
> Negative scan
> Ejection fraction: 30%–50%

Cardiac Catheterization

Cardiac catheterization is the fluoroscopic visualization of the right or left side of the heart by passing a catheter into the right or left chambers and injecting dye. In angiography, the catheter is passed into the coronary vessels, where the dye is injected and fluoroscopic images are recorded.

> **Normal Results**
> Varies with the area being assessed
> Indicates normal anatomy and physiology, normal chamber volumes and pressures, normal wall and valve motion, and normal patent coronary arteries

> **Normal Value for Cardiac Output**
> 5–8 L/min

Imaging Studies

Radiography

Radiography helps visualize internal organs and structures with electromagnetic radiation. Radiography of bone; the abdomen; the chest; paranasal sinuses; kidneys, ureters, and bladder (KUB); and mammography do not require contrast medium. Contrast medium is used to distinguish soft tissues and some organs (e.g., the gallbladder, esophagus, stomach, and small and large intestines). Normal results vary, depending on the area being studied with the imaging process. The images are interpreted by the radiologist, and a report is then dictated and transcribed for the ordering physician. The ordering physician often visually inspects the films or images to evaluate the area himself or herself.

Magnetic Resonance Imaging/Magnetic Resonance Angiography

Magnetic resonance imaging (MRI)/magnetic resonance angiography (MRA) uses a magnetic field, instead of radiation, to visualize internal tissues. It is possible to view tissues and organs in three dimensions with MRI. MRA is used to examine major blood vessels in the body and to study the condition of blood vessels to detect tumors, to differentiate healthy and diseased tissues, and to detect sites of infection. It helps determine blood flow to tissues and organs. The patient is not exposed to ionizing radiation during MRI. A contrast material (gadolinium) may be required for some examinations. Gadolinium does not contain iodine and is given intravenously. It is important to screen patients before the procedure to determine if they have any metal implants or pacemaker, if they work with metal shavings, or if they are claustrophobic.

Normal results vary, depending on the area being studied on MRI. The MRI scan is interpreted by the radiologist, and a report is then dictated and transcribed for the ordering physician. The ordering physician may ask to see the films so that he or she may evaluate the area of concern.

Computed Tomography

Computed tomography (CT) is a radiographic technique that uses a scanner system, which can provide images of the internal structure of tissue and organs both geographically and characteristically. Depending on the area to be scanned and the reason indicated for scanning, oral and/or intravenous (IV) contrast media may be required. Iodinated contrast media may result in nephrotoxicity and renal failure, and therefore it is important to screen patients before they receive IV contrast media. Any patient receiving IV contrast media should be screened for the following risks:

- History of kidney disease, including tumor, surgery to kidneys, or transplantation

- Myeloma
- Diabetes
- Potentially nephrotoxic medications (e.g., metformin, chemotherapy, and/or long-term use of nonsteroidal antiinflammatory drugs [NSAIDs])
- 70 years of age and older

If any of these risk factors are present, serum creatinine level needs to be measured to determine the glomerular filtration rate (GFR). If the GFR is below 45 mn/min/1.73 m², intervention to protect the kidneys may be required before administration of contrast.

Normal results vary, depending on the area being studied on CT. The scan is interpreted by the radiologist, and a report is then dictated and transcribed for the ordering physician. The ordering physician often visually inspects the films or images to evaluate the area.

Fluoroscopy

A real-time imaging process, fluoroscopy provides continuous visualization of the area being imaged. Films of the process are made for more extensive examination. Fluoroscopy is used in certain procedures and to study the functioning of tissues and organs.

Normal results vary, depending on the area being studied on fluoroscopy. The film is interpreted by the radiologist, and a report is then dictated and transcribed for the ordering physician. The ordering physician often requests for fluoroscopy, which can be a diagnostic tool and also a guide for the treatment procedure.

Sonography, Ultrasonography, and Echography

Sonography, ultrasonography, and echography all use an imaging system that projects a beam of sound waves into target tissues or organs and receives waves as they bounce back off the target structure. An outline of the structure is produced and recorded on film for examination. Tissues, organs, and systems that may be studied by using ultrasonography include, but are not limited to, the abdominal aorta, brain, breasts, gallbladder, pelvis for gynecologic and obstetric diagnostic examinations, heart, kidneys, liver, lymph nodes, pancreas, prostate, spleen, thyroid, urinary bladder, and upper GI tract.

Normal Result
Varies, depending on the area being examined

The ultrasound scan is interpreted by the radiologist, and a report is then dictated and transcribed for the ordering physician. The ordering physician may request to visually inspect the films or images to evaluate the area himself or herself.

Myelography

Myelography is an imaging examination of the spinal cord and spinal nerve roots. Contrast medium (dye) or air

is injected into the subarachnoid space and recorded on radiographic film. Fluoroscopy generally is used in this procedure.

Normal Result
No lesions or abnormalities

It is used to diagnose ruptured or bulging disks, spinal cord lesions and tumors, spinal cord and spinal nerve trauma and edema, and other conditions involving the spinal cord and spinal nerves.

Positron Emission Tomography

Positron emission tomography (PET), a molecular imaging study, indicates how organs and tissues are actually functioning. It measures blood flow, O_2 use, and sugar metabolism. It is used to diagnose a variety of diseases, including many types of cancers, heart disease, and certain brain abnormalities and other CNS disorders. It is also helpful in assessing the effectiveness of cancer therapy.

A radioactive material, called a *radiotracer*, is injected intravenously or sometimes is inhaled as a gas. The energy that the tracer gives off is then detected and recorded by the gamma camera and PET scanner, and with the aid of a computer, three-dimensional images are created.

Results are interpreted by a nuclear radiologist with specialized training in nuclear medicine and are available in 2 to 3 days. Standardized uptake value (SUV) is the amount of chemical activity in a certain spot and assists the radiologist in interpretation. Generally, cancer has an SUV greater than 2.5 and creates what is known as a "hot spot" on the scan. However, many other factors and variables are taken into consideration by the physician.

Stool Analysis

Hemoccult/Guaiac Test/Fecal Occult Blood Test

The hemoccult/guaiac test looks for hidden (occult) blood in a stool sample. It is a qualitative detection of RBCs in the stool.

Normal Result
Negative

Presence of blood in the stool specimen is indicative of trauma, lesion, or other insult to the GI mucosa, producing blood. Blood in the stool may also be a sign of colorectal cancer. Fecal occult blood testing is used as a screening test for early detection (and thus treatment) of colorectal cancer. There are also tests that patients can perform in the privacy of their homes to determine blood in the stool.

Cologuard

Cologuard is a screening test for colorectal cancer. It can be used in those who do not have any family history of colorectal cancer (those who do have family history should undergo colonoscopy). Cologuard detects certain altered deoxyribonucleic acid (DNA) in cancer cells. Abnormal cells or blood in the stool could indicate cancer, precancerous tumors, or polyps.

Normal Result
Negative

The Cologuard test is not definitive for cancer diagnosis. If the test shows a positive result, further testing (colonoscopy) must be performed.

Tests for Ova, Larvae, and Parasites

These tests are microscopic examinations of the stool to detect the presence of parasites at various stages of development.

Normal Result
None detected

A positive examination result indicates parasitic infection of the GI tract.

Endoscopy Tests

Endoscopy

Endoscopy is the visual inspection of internal organs or body cavities through the use of a fiberoptic instrument with the appropriate scope. In addition, pathology may be removed, and insult to the tissue may be repaired during the diagnostic procedure.

Esophagogastroduodenoscopy/Upper Endoscopy

Esophagogastroduodenoscopy (EGD)/upper endoscopy helps visualize the esophagus, stomach, and duodenum in a single procedure by using an endoscope. Biopsy and endoscopic therapies, such as esophageal dilation, may be performed.

Normal Result
Appearance of esophagus, stomach, and duodenum within normal limits

Abnormal findings may include, but are not limited to, hiatal hernia, Barrett esophagus, gastroesophageal reflux disease (GERD), esophagitis, and ulcers.

Esophagoscopy

Esophagoscopy is the visualization of the esophagus by using an esophagoscope.

Normal Result
Appearance of the esophagus mucosa normal

Foreign bodies may be visualized and removed. Inflammation may be noted, and biopsy specimens can be taken.

Gastroscopy

Gastroscopy is the visualization of the stomach by using a gastroscope.

Normal Result
Appearance of upper GI tract within normal limits

Hemorrhagic areas or erosion of a vessel may be revealed. Additional abnormal findings may include neoplasms, gastric ulcers, hiatal hernia, gastritis, and esophagitis.

Colonoscopy

Colonoscopy is the visualization of the colon by using a colonoscope.

Normal Result
Appearance of large intestinal mucosa normal

Inflammation, areas of ulceration, bleeding areas, strictures, polyps, colitis, diverticula, benign or malignant tumors, or foreign bodies may be observed in abnormal findings.

Sigmoidoscopy

Sigmoidoscopy is the visualization of the sigmoid portion of the colon and the rectum by using a sigmoidoscope.

Normal Result
Normal appearance of mucosa of sigmoid colon

Inflammatory bowel disease, polyps, benign and cancerous tumors, and foreign bodies may be some of the abnormal findings during a sigmoidoscopic examination.

Proctoscopy

Proctoscopy is the visualization of the rectum by using a proctoscope.

Normal Result
Normal appearance of rectal mucosa and anal canal

Rectal prolapse, hemorrhoids, rectal strictures, fissures, abscesses, and fistulas are some of the abnormal findings during a proctoscopic examination of the rectum.

Cystoscopy

Cystoscopy is the visualization of the structures of the urinary tract by using a cystoscope.

Urethra, urethral orifices, urinary bladder interior, and male prostatic urethra appear normal

Cancer of the bladder, benign prostatic hyperplasia (BPH), bladder calculi, prostatitis, ureteral strictures, urinary fistulas, vesicle neck stenosis, ureterocele, polyps, and abnormal bladder capacity are some of the abnormal findings during a cystoscopic examination of the urinary bladder.

Ureteroscopy

Ureteroscopy is the visualization of the ureters and pelvis of the kidney.

Normal Result
Normal appearance of the ureters and pelvis of the kidney and its structures

Renal or ureteral stones, inflammation or bleeding of the urethral mucosa, and lesions or abnormal structures of the renal pelvis are some of the abnormal findings in a ureteroscopic examination.

Bronchoscopy

Bronchoscopy is visualization of the trachea and bronchi by using a bronchoscope.

Normal Result
Nasopharynx, larynx, trachea, and bronchi are normal in appearance.

Abnormalities revealed in a bronchoscopic examination include, but are not limited to, bronchitis, carcinoma and other tumors, inflammatory processes, TB, abnormal structure and disorders of the larynx and trachea, foreign bodies, and various pulmonary infections.

Arthroscopy

Arthroscopy is the visualization or inspection of the inner aspect of a joint by using an endoscope called an *arthroscope*. Biopsy specimens may be obtained.

Normal Result
Normal appearance of the inner aspect of the joint

Abnormal findings in the knee may include tears of meniscus, bone or cartilage fragments, and damage to other structures within the joint. Surgical repair may be attempted. Refer to Chapter 7 for additional information on arthroscopy.

Arterial Blood Gases

Arterial Blood Gas Analysis

Arterial blood gas (ABG) analysis is the measurement of dissolved O_2 and CO_2 in arterial blood. It is also a measurement of pH and O_2 saturation of the arterial blood. ABGs are used to assess oxygenation and ventilation, along with acid-base balance. In addition, they produce information about the effectiveness of therapy and the status of critical patients and are used in conjunction with pulmonary function studies.

Normal values are listed; however, these studies are complex and require interpretation by a physician, along with the results of other diagnostic studies, and consideration of symptoms and signs to arrive at a diagnosis or an evaluation.

Normal Adult Values
Acidity (pH): 7.35–7.45
CO_2 tension ($Paco_2$): 35–45 mm Hg
Arterial O_2 tension (Pao_2): 75–100 mm Hg
Amount of bicarbonate (HCO_3) in the blood: 22–30 mEq/L
O_2 saturation: 95%–100%

Increased pH is indicative of several disorders, including, but not limited to, alkali ingestion, diarrhea, vomiting, hyperventilation, high-altitude sickness, metabolic acidosis, fever, and adverse effects of certain drugs. Decreased pH is indicative of several disorders, including, but not limited to, asthma, COPD, cardiac disease, MI, renal disorders, pulmonary disorders, respiratory acidosis, sepsis, shock, and malignant hyperthermia.

Increased $Paco_2$ is indicative of several disorders, including, but not limited to, late-stage asthma, brain death, CHF, respiratory disorders, hypoventilation, renal disorders, poisoning, pneumothorax, respiratory acidosis, near drowning, and adverse effects of certain drugs. Decreased $Paco_2$ is indicative of several disorders, including, but not limited to, early-stage asthma, hyperventilation, dysrhythmias, respiratory alkalosis, metabolic acidosis, and adverse effects of certain drugs.

Increased Pao_2 is indicative of several conditions, including, but not limited to, hyperventilation and hyperbaric O_2 exposure. Decreased Pao_2 is indicative of several disorders, including, but not limited to, acute respiratory distress syndrome (ARDS), asthma, cardiac disorders, head injury, anoxia, hypoventilation, respiratory disorders, pneumothorax, respiratory failure, shock, smoke inhalation, and CVA.

Increased O_2 saturation is indicative of hyperbaric oxygenation. Decreased O_2 saturation is indicative of several disorders, including, but not limited to, anoxia, cardiac anomalies and disorders, carbon monoxide poisoning, ARDS, CVA, hypoventilation, respiratory disorders, pneumothorax, shock, smoke inhalation, and near-drowning.

Pulmonary Function Studies

Pulmonary function studies are complex and include evaluation of results from several tests. Most tests are performed by respiratory therapists and can be done with or without the use of bronchodilators. Results usually are reported to a pulmonologist for evaluation and correlation with symptoms and signs. Normal values are reported; however, the significance of these values is incomplete without the review and opinion of the pulmonologist, which is often assisted by the respiratory therapist.

Pulse Oximeter

A pulse oximeter is an instrument (spectrophotometer) that produces a noninvasive measurement of the O_2 saturation of arterial blood.

Normal Result
Arterial blood O_2 saturation $\geq$ 95%

Peak Flow

Peak flow is a measurement of inspiratory effort.

Normal Results
Approximately 300 L/min

Based on gender, height, and age

Spirometry

Spirometry is a measurement of lung capacity, volume, and flow rates used in the evaluation of asthma, bronchitis, COPD, and emphysema.

Methacholine Challenge

Methacholine challenge (also known as *bronchoprovocation test*) is a measurement of lung volumes before and after inhalation of methacholine chloride, which is used for the diagnosis of asthma.

Normal Result
Negative

The challenge is considered positive if there is a 20% or **greater** reduction in breathing compared with **baseline values.** A positive test indicates **that the** airways are "reactive," and an asthma diagnosis should be considered.

Sputum Studies

Sputum studies are analyses and cultures of sputum (material expelled from the respiratory tract) to detect the presence of pathogens. Common studies on sputum that are ordered include cytology testing, Gram staining, and culture and sensitivity (C&S).

Normal Result
Negative

Positive results might include respiratory disorders, such as fungal infections, mycobacterial infections (e.g., TB), or carcinoma.

Pulmonary Function Test

Normal findings are reported in percentages of observed values and by expected values calculated to include allowances

for age, gender, weight, and height. Abnormal results are considered to be less than 80% of calculated values. A respiratory therapist or pulmonologist should be consulted for interpretation of values.

Normal Values
Tidal volume: 500 mL

Expiratory reserve volume: 1500 mL

Residual volume: 1500 mL

Inspiratory reserve volume: 2000 mL

Miscellaneous Tests

Culture and Sensitivity Studies

For wound, drainage, and blood C&S studies, specimens are obtained from various tissues and fluids of the body, placed on or in a medium to grow, and then studied for the presence of microbes. The specimens are placed on Mueller Hinton agar, and a variety of antibiotic disks are added on top of the specimen. Zones of growth inhibition determine which antibiotic will be effective in destroying or curbing the reproduction of the microbe.

Tissues and fluids that are sampled include blood, sputum, cerebrospinal fluid (CSF), urine, exudates from lesions, nasal secretions, stool, wound drainage, and any excised tissue.

Normal Result
No growth

The growth of any microbes requires microscopic identification. The antibiotic-impregnated disk requires inspection and identification of antibiotics showing effectiveness against the microbes.

Bone Marrow Studies

For bone marrow studies, aspiration of bone marrow is obtained with a needle from the sternum, the posterior superior iliac spine, or the anterior iliac crest for the diagnosis of neoplasms, metastases, and blood disorders. Bone marrow studies provide a basis for the evaluation of hematologic disorders and infectious diseases.

Immune and Immunoglobulin Studies

Immune and immunoglobulin studies examine the functioning and malfunctioning of the immune system.

Normal Adult Levels
Immunoglobulin A (IgA): 60–400 mg/dL

Immunoglobulin G (IgG): 700–1600 mg/dL

Immunoglobulin M (IgM): 40–230 mg/dL

Immunoglobulin D (IgD): 0.13–15.27 mg/dL

Immunoglobulin E (IgE): 3–42 units/mL

Increased levels of immunoglobulins are indicative of many disorders, and the results need to be evaluated by a physician.

Some disorders include arthritis, cancer, chronic infections, sinusitis, asthma, food and drug allergies, liver disease, SLE, and adverse effects of certain drugs. Decreased levels of immunoglobulins are indicative of many disorders, including, but not limited to, AIDS, bacterial infection, advanced cancer, hypogammaglobulinemia, and adverse effects of certain drugs.

Biopsy

Biopsy is the excision of tissue from the living body, followed by microscopic examination, for the purpose of arriving at an exact diagnosis.

Normal Result
No abnormal cells seen

Abnormal findings depend on cell structure discovered during microscopic examination.

Lumbar Puncture

Lumbar puncture is a surgical procedure to withdraw spinal fluid for analysis. It involves measurement and analysis of the chemical components of CSF and is used in the diagnosis of CNS diseases and disorders.

Normal Adult Results
Appearance: Clear, colorless
Specific gravity: 1.006–1.009
Pressure: 110–100 mm H_2O
AST: 05–35 units
Bicarbonate: 22.9 mEq/L
WBC count: 0.0–0.8 mm^3
RBC count: None
Glucose: 40–80 mg/dL
Total protein: 15–45 mg/dL
Lactic acid: 10–24 mg/dL
Venereal Disease Research Laboratory (VDRL): Negative titer for syphilis
Bacteria or viruses: None present

Pressure depends on height and whether patient is positioned in the sitting or horizontal position.

Abnormal findings are indicative of disorders or insults to the CNS.

Electroencephalography

Electroencephalography (EEG) is the recording of the electrical activity of the brain. A neurologist interprets the brain wave activity to determine the presence of a neurologic disorder or any other medical condition.

Normal Result
Symmetric patterns of electrical brain activity

Abnormal findings include information indicative of CNS or brain insults, hematomas, CVAs, epilepsy, brain tumors, and seizure activity. Lack of any activity is an indication of brain death.

Electromyography

Electromyography (EMG) is **the** electrodiagnostic assessment and recording of the electrical activity of skeletal muscle at rest and **in** contraction. It is a nerve conduction study used to differentiate between muscle weakness **caused by** nerve injury and weakness **caused by** muscle diseases. EMG tests and nerve conduction tests are often done in combination.

Normal Results
Nerve conduction normal
Muscle action potential normal

Abnormal findings help identify the site and cause of muscle disorders and neuronal lesions, particularly of involvement of the anterior horn of the spinal cord.

Gastric Analysis

Gastric analysis is used in the diagnosis of pernicious anemia and peptic ulcers. The contents of the stomach are analyzed for acidity, appearance, and volume.

Normal Adult Levels
Bile: 0 or minimal
Mucus: Evenly mixed
Blood: 0 or scant
Fasting acidity: 2.5 mEq/L
Quantity: 62 mL/h
pH: 1.5–3.5

Increased levels of gastric acid are indicative of certain disorders, including, but not limited to, status post small-intestinal resection, gastric or duodenal ulcer, hyperplasia, Zollinger-Ellison syndrome, and hyperfunction of gastric cells. Reduced gastric acid levels are indicative of several disorders, including, but not limited to, pernicious anemia, status post vagotomy, renal failure, rheumatoid arthritis, gastric cancer, and atrophic gastritis.

Human Chorionic Gonadotropin

Human chorionic gonadotropin (hCG) is measured for diagnosis of pregnancy, abortion, ectopic pregnancy, and uterine pathology.

Normal Result
Negative

A positive result is indicative of pregnancy, either intrauterine or ectopic. A positive result can also occur with testicular cancer in men, a trophoblastic tumor, hydatidiform moles, and ovarian cancer.

Screening

Tuberculosis Screening (Mantoux Test)

An intradermal injection of tuberculin is given, usually on the inner aspect of the lower arm. Results are read between 48 and 72 hours. A two-step TB test may be indicated for certain populations.

Normal Result

Negative

Positive Result

Red, raised, hardened area at injection site; induration measures ≥ 10 mm

Positive reaction requires further investigation, usually including chest radiography.

Cancer/Tumor Markers as Screening Tools

Certain substances, including enzymes, antigens, and hormones, are produced by some tumors or cancers. These substances may be present in blood in higher-than-normal levels, indicating the presence of a tumor. Cancer/tumor markers cannot be used alone to diagnose cancer or a tumor. Some benign tumors may stimulate the production of these markers. In addition, elevated cancer markers are not always present, especially in the early stages of the disease process. Some physicians use these markers track the progress of tumor growth, and to measure the effectiveness of treatment, and to detect possible recurrence of the tumor. There are several markers, and many are specific in nature. The most widely used screening tool of this nature is the prostate-specific antigen (PSA) test. Other markers include CA 125, carcinoembryonic antigen, alpha-fetoprotein (AFP), CA 19-9, CA 15-3, and Papanicolaou (Pap) smear.

Prostate-Specific Antigen

The PSA test is a blood test used to determine the level of PSA in serum. This is a screening test that should be followed by a digital rectal examination (DRE) of the prostate gland to identify any abnormalities. Additional diagnostic studies often are indicated.

PSA blood test results are reported in nanograms per milliliter (ng/mL).

PSA is considered a marker in the screening for prostatic cancer. Usually 0 to 4 ng/mL is considered to be in the normal range; 4 to 10 ng/mL is considered borderline; values greater than 10 ng/mL are considered high. Increasing age makes slightly higher values acceptable:

- 40 to 49 years: 0 to 2.5 ng/mL
- 50 to 59 years: 0 to 3.5 ng/mL
- 60 to 69 years: 0 to 4.5 ng/mL
- 70 to 79 years: 0 to 6.5 ng/mL

Any increase of 20% or greater in the PSA value in 1 year raises suspicion and requires further investigation.

Above-acceptable levels may be indicative of cancer. Additional investigations, including biopsy, are recommended.

PSA screening should be completed before DRE. A constant increase in the PSA level leads to suspicion of prostate cancer. Fluctuating PSA levels usually are not indicative of cancer but indicate an inflammatory process in the prostate or BPH. The PSA test is a screening tool and must be combined with DRE for more accurate screening. Men older than 50 years of age are encouraged to undergo prostate screening on an annual basis; men older than 70 years of age may or may not be required to undergo regular screening because of the high incidence of prostatic cancer in this group and the treatment protocol of watchful waiting without significant intervention.

CA 125 Test

The CA 125 test measures the production of the protein marker CA 125. Increases in levels of CA 125 may be indicative of cancer of the ovaries.

Normal Levels

<35 units/mL (conventional units)

An elevation above normal may be indicative of cancer of the ovaries, pelvic organs (including the uterus and the cervix), pancreas, liver, breasts, colon, lungs, and digestive tract.

CA 19-9 Test

The CA 19-9 test measures the production of the protein marker CA 19-9. CA 19-9 levels may increase in the presence of pancreatic or colorectal cancer.

Normal Levels

<37 units/mL (conventional units)

An elevation may be indicative of the presence of colorectal, pancreatic, stomach, or bile duct cancer.

CA 15-3 Test

The CA 15-3 test measures the production of the protein marker CA 15-3. CA 15-3 levels may increase in the presence of breast cancer.

Normal Levels

<35 units/mL (conventional units)

An elevation may be indicative of the presence of breast cancer, benign conditions of the breast, ovarian disease, PID, endometriosis, and hepatitis and indicative of pregnancy and lactation.

Carcinoembryonic Antigen

Carcinoembryonic antigen (CEA) is normally found in developing fetuses and decreases to very low levels after birth. CEA may be elevated in some individuals without any form of cancer. This test is not a screening test. It is used to monitor recurrence or metastasis of colorectal cancer and other cancers after the disease has already been diagnosed.

Reference values vary, depending on the health of the individual, smoking history, and the presence of existing intestinal or other disease processes. A baseline value should be established and monitored to determine effectiveness of treatment or exacerbation of the condition.

Alpha-Fetoprotein

Under normal circumstances, AFP is produced by the liver of developing fetus and passes through the placenta to the mother's blood. Maternal levels decrease after birth. Certain conditions may cause an abnormal elevation of this protein as pregnancy progresses, suggesting a possible neural tube defects or other anomaly in the developing fetus(es). This test is not to be confused with the AFP tumor marker test, which is used in conjunction with other tests to diagnose liver, ovarian, or testicular cancer or to monitor the effectiveness of treatment of these cancers.

To compare or confirm normal values for amniotic fluid levels and serum AFP levels, their normal levels should be checked with reference laboratory.

Elevations in maternal serum levels and amniotic fluid may be indicative of neural tube defects.

Papanicolaou Smear

Pap smear is the cytologic examination of cells that have been scraped or aspirated from the cervix and the cervical os. This screening test is recommended every 2 to 3 years, and yearly pelvic examinations are recommended.

The results of Pap smear are now reported to the physician in two different formats: (1) a system based on classes and (2) the Bethesda system, which uses descriptive diagnostic terms.

Class System

The *class system,* based on classes, is used to report Pap smear results to the physician is as follows:

- Class I: Negative with no abnormal or unusual cells seen.
- Class II: Negative smear—but with some reservation based on the presence of inflammatory cells or evidence of infection. Additional causes may be regeneration of cervical cells or changes related to trauma, infections, or childbirth. A repeat Pap smear and treatment of the underlying cause may be indicated.
- Class III: Presence of some abnormal cells that may be considered premalignant. Changes may vary from mild dysplasia to severe dysplasia. Further evaluation is indicated, possibly including colposcopy.
- Class IV: Indicative of a high degree of suspicion for malignancy. Prompt and complete evaluation is indicated.
- Class V: Indication of high probability of more extensive malignancy. Prompt and complete evaluation to determine the extent of disease is indicated.

Bethesda System

When using the *Bethesda system,* the physician may relate the results as normal or abnormal because surface cervical cells may appear abnormal but are not always malignant.

The descriptive diagnostic terms are as follows:

- *Dysplasia:* Although not cancer, dysplasia may develop into very early cancer of the cervix. The cells in dysplasia undergo a series of changes in their appearance, appear abnormal in microscopic examination, and have not invaded nearby healthy tissue. The cells are described as *mild, moderate,* or *severe* according to their appearance under the microscope.
- *Squamous intraepithelial lesion (SIL):* This term describes the appearance of abnormal changes on the surface of the cervix. SIL cells are classified further as low grade, having early changes in size, shape, and number, or high grade, containing a large number of precancerous cells with an appearance very different from normal cells.
- *Cervical intraepithelial neoplasia (CIN):* This is a description of a new abnormal growth of surface layers of cells. Additional information is provided by using CIN with the numbers 1, 2, and 3 to describe how much of the cervix contains abnormal cells.
- *Carcinoma in situ:* This refers to preinvasive cancer that has not invaded deeper tissues and contains only surface cells.
- *Atypical glandular cells of undetermined significance (AGC-US):* This term describes slightly abnormal glandular cells of the cervix.
- *Atypical squamous cells of undetermined significance (ASC-US):* This describes slightly abnormal squamous cells of the cervix, possibly caused by a vaginal infection or by human papillomavirus (HPV).
- *Inflammation:* Inflammation is present in the cervical cells, and WBCs also are seen.
- *Hyperkeratosis:* This term describes dried skin cells on the cervix, often resulting from cervical cap or diaphragm usage or a cervical infection.

Abnormal results range from insignificant to precancerous to invasive cancer of the cervix. A repeat Pap smear in 6 months is often all that is indicated for mild dysplasia and class II Pap smears. Colposcopy and further investigation may be indicated with other abnormal findings. The physician discusses the abnormal findings with the patient, and a course of treatment or follow-up is determined.

Mammography

Mammography is the radiographic examination of the soft tissues of the breast. This is a screening test performed on an annual or biennial basis in women older than 40 years of age to detect the presence of breast disease. This screening should be accompanied by manual examination of the breast tissue by a physician. Monthly breast self-examinations are recommended.

Normal Result
Negative for disease

Identification of abnormal conditions may indicate the need for further investigation. Various benign disorders, including fibrocystic disease of the breast, calcifications, and asymmetric densities, may be responsible for a positive result and require additional mammographic views with ultrasonography. It may also be recommended that in 6 months, repeat mammography and/or ultrasonography be done to follow up on any abnormality. Ultrasound-guided breast biopsy or stereotactic breast biopsy may be indicated to confirm the presence of a malignant neoplasm.

Breast Self-Examination

Breast self-examination is a screening test conducted monthly by the woman herself at home for early detection of changes in breast tissue. The best time to conduct the test is 3 to 5 days after the menstrual cycle begins.

Normal Result
No changes

If any changes are noted, the patient should follow up with a doctor immediately for further testing. Changes may indicate breast cancer; however, more diagnostic tests are necessary. It should be noted that, although rare, breast cancer can occur in men.

Testicular Self-Examination

Testicular self-examination is a screening test conducted monthly by the man himself at home for early detection of changes in testicular tissue.

Normal Result
No changes

If any changes are noted or a small hard lump is found, the physician should be contacted immediately. These findings could indicate testicular cancer, and further testing is required.

BRCA1 and *BRCA2* Gene Testing

BRCA1 and *BRCA2* are genes that suppress malignant tumors in humans. People with mutations in these genes are at higher risk of cancers.

Normal Result
Negative for mutation

Even if the test is negative for mutation, cancer development is still possible. A positive test indicates a higher risk for cervical, uterine, colon, pancreatic, biliary, testicular, prostate, or stomach cancer. The individual is also at higher risk for melanomas. **Note:** Only 5% of breast cancers and 10% to 15% of ovarian cancers are associated with *BRCA*1 and *BRCA*2 mutations.

Appendix II

Pharmacology

Pharmacology is defined as a branch of medicine concerned with the study of drug action. Drugs may be human-made, natural, or endogenous molecules and exert their effect on cells, tissues, organs, or organisms. Pharmacology is not only about how a drug works but, more importantly, why a drug works in the way it does.

Side effects are listed by various groups of medications and are not specific to any one drug in that group. Referral to the current edition of the *Physician's Desk Reference* (PDR) or other pharmacology reference is recommended to confirm side effects for a specific drug.

This table presents the major drug groups, organized by the actions of medications. The examples are just that—examples—to represent the multiple medications found in each group. The example drugs are commonly prescribed and may be familiar in some way. Once again, refer to the current edition of the PDR or other pharmacology reference to locate additional drugs in the group.

Body System/ Drug Purpose	Drug Category	Drug Action	Examples	Side Effects	Comments
Chapters 1 and 2					
Drugs for pain and fever	Analgesics and/or opioids (narcotics)	Relieve pain	codeine, meperidine morphine, oxycodone hydrocodone, oxymorphone, hydromorphone, fentanyl	May cause drowsiness; blurred vision, dizziness, sedation; constipation can occur	May lead to physical and mental dependence. Patients should not drive or operate machinery while taking the drug.
	Nonopioids	Relieve pain and fever	acetaminophen (Tylenol), acetylsalicylic acid (aspirin), ibuprofen, naproxen, indomethacin	Aspirin and NSAIDs may cause GI irritation, anticoagulant effects, antiprostaglandin effects	Acetaminophen overdose has been linked to hepatic injury. The dose of acetaminophen based products is limited to 4 g or less per day.
	Anesthetics[a]	Produce loss of sensation by interfering with nerve impulses			
	A. General		midazolam (Versed), propofol (Diprivan), etomidate (Amidate)	Versed: May cause amnesia, hypotension, headache	Versed is used for conscious sedation.
	B. Local		cocaine, tetracaine, prilocaine, lidocaine	May cause skin rashes and/or edema	Lidocaine may be topical form; also used systemically as a cardiac drug.
Drugs for infectious diseases	Antibiotics	Destroy or inhibit the growth of bacterial strains of microorganisms but have not been found to be effective for viral infections	penicillin, amoxicillin, amoxicillin/clavulanic acid (Augmentin), tetracycline, doxycycline, minocycline, ciprofloxacin (Cipro), azithromycin (Zithromax)	Nausea, GI upset, urticaria	Caution must be used when administering IM penicillin and all antibiotics with regard to observation after injection for potential of anaphylaxis.
	A. Penicillins		penicillin V amoxicillin/clavulanic acid amoxicillin, piperacillin/ tazobactam (Zosyn)	Stomach upset and diarrhea	Most contraindications involve hypersensitivity to the drug.
	B. Tetracyclines		minocycline, doxycycline, tetracycline	Stomach upset, diarrhea, vomiting	Should not be taken with dairy or antacids. Cause photosensitivity.
	C. Cephalosporins[b]		cefazolin (Ancef), cephalexin, cefaclor, cefdinir, cefepime	Nausea, vomiting, headache	Patients allergic to penicillin may also be allergic to cephalosporins.
	D. Quinolone antibiotics		ciprofloxacin (Cipro), levofloxacin, moxifloxacin	Nausea, vomiting, dizziness.	Cause photosensitivity. Are contraindicated during pregnancy.
	E. Macrolide antibiotics		erythromycin, clarithromycin, azithromycin (Zithromax)	Stomach upset, nausea, vomiting	Should be taken with food.

Class	Action	Examples	Side Effects	Notes
F. Miscellaneous antibiotics		vancomycin (Vancocin), clindamycin, metronidazole (Flagyl), sulfamethoxazole/trimethoprim (Bactrim)		Vancocin: Used primarily for methicillin-resistant Staphylococcus aureus (MRSA). Flagyl: Patients should avoid alcohol. Bactrim: Patients should drink 6–8 glasses of water daily to avoid renal crystallization of the drug.
Antifungals	Inhibit and kill fungal growth		Systemically administered antifungals may be nephrotoxic, and hepatotoxic	Some are available in oral form for systemic treatment; others are available in topical form.
A. Polyene antifungals		amphotericin B, caspofungin, natamycin, nystatin		
B. Imidazole antifungals		clotrimazole, econazole, ketoconazole, miconazole, tioconazole		
C. Triazole antifungals		fluconazole, itraconazole, terconazole, voriconazole		
D. Allylamine antifungals		butenafine, terbinafine		
E. Echinocandin antifungals		anidulafungin, caspofungin, micafungin		
Antivirals	Inhibit viral growth	acyclovir, valacyclovir, boceprevir, zidovudine, amantadine	GI disturbances, headache, malaise, insomnia, dizziness	Should be taken at first sign of onset of viral attack for best relief of symptoms.
Antiprotozoals	Inhibit protozoal infections	chloroquine hydrochloride (Aralen Hydrochloride), artemether/lumefantrine (Coartem)	Headache, pruritus, GI disturbances, tinnitus	Also known as antimalarials.
Antituberculars	Suppress mycobacterium causing tuberculosis	isoniazid (Nydrazid), ethambutol, (Myambutol), rifapentine (Priftin)	GI disturbances, hepatic disturbances	These drugs usually are given in combination.
Drugs used to treat cancer — Antineoplastics	Used as chemotherapy to inhibit the growth of neoplasms	cyclophosphamide (Cytoxan), methotrexate, fluorouracil (5-FU), ofatumumat (Arzerra), sipuleucel-T (Provenge)	Nausea; vomiting; hair loss; interference with blood cell production, resulting in anemia and suppression of the immune system	Historically used in combination to treat cancer. May be used in conjunction with radiation or surgery. Arzerra is a monoclonal antibody used for the treatment of chronic lymphocytic leukemia. Provenge is used for the treatment of advanced prostate cancer. Fluorouracil is used topically to treat actinic keratosis and basal cell carcinoma.
Kinase inhibitors	Treat renal cell carcinoma	sorafenib (Nexavar), lenvatinib (Lenvima)	Hypothyroidism, GI disturbances, fatigue	

continued

Body System/ Drug Purpose	Drug Category	Drug Action	Examples	Side Effects	Comments
	CDK 4/6 inhibitors	HR-positive HER2-negative breast cancer	palbociclib (Ibrance), abemaciclib (Verzenio), ribociclib (Kisqali)	Neutropenia, respiratory issues, GI disturbances, hair loss	
	Angiogenesis inhibitors	Treat colon, lung, kidney, cervical cancers	bevacizumab (Avastin), remucirumab (Cyramza)	Hemorrhage, blood clots, hypertension, GI issues	
	Checkpoint inhibitors	Treat melanoma, lung cancer, Hodgkin lymphoma	Pembrolizumab (Keytruda), nivolumab (Opdivo)	Rash, fever, cough, GI disturbances, respiratory issues, hormonal issues	
	Antimetabolites	Treat carcinomas and sarcomas	methotrexate mercaptopurine (Purinethol), pazopanib (Votrient)	Bone marrow depression, stomatitis, mouth ulcers, GI upset, loss of hair, fever, chills	
	Estrogen receptor blockers	Used to treat breast cancer	tamoxifen (Nolvadex), anastrozole (Arimidex)	Reduce platelet count; may cause hot flashes, night sweats, insomnia	Side effects are relatively mild. Blood counts and liver studies are recommended.
Drugs used as nutritional supplements and alternative medicine	Electrolytes	Replace electrolytes	potassium chloride (K-Tab), 0.9% sodium chloride (normal saline), sodium polystyrene sulfonate (Kayexalate)	Rapid heart rate when levels are abnormally high	Potassium replacement therapy in use of diuretics. Potassium levels should be monitored.
	Vitamin/mineral supplements	Supplement or replace essential vitamins and minerals	cyanocobalamin (vitamin B_{12}), multiple vitamins, vitamins with minerals, carbonyl iron (Feosol)	Oral iron supplements may cause constipation; excessive oral iron intake may cause GI bleeding; caution must be used to avoid excessive ingestion of fat-soluble vitamins and iron to prevent toxicity	Vitamin B_{12} for treatment of pernicious anemia is by injection. Folic acid supplements are encouraged for women of childbearing capability to reduce incidence of neural tube deficits in the developing fetus.
Chapter 3					
Drugs used to treat disorders of the immune system, immunizations	Immunizations	Provide artificially acquired active immunity to diseases; produce an antigen-antibody reaction	diphtheria, tetanus, and acellular pertussis (DTaP) vaccine, measles, mumps, rubella (MMR) vaccine, oral poliovirus vaccine (OPV; Sabin vaccine), inactivated poliovirus vaccine (IPV; Salk vaccine)	Redness may develop at injection site, generalized malaise, fever	Follow the American Academy of Pediatrics' schedule recommendation.
	Immune globulins and antitoxins	Provide artificially acquired passive immunity	Rho(D) immune globulin (RhoGAM), immune globulin (GamaSTAN), tetanus antitoxin	Local inflammation at the injection site, slight fever	RhoGAM is given prenatally and postnatally to Rh-negative mothers to prevent Rh incompatibility in the infant and in subsequent pregnancies.

	Action	Drugs	Side effects	Notes
Immunosuppressants	Reduce the body's autoimmune response to its own tissues	methotrexate, cyclosporine, azathioprine, mycophenolate, tacrolimus, adalimumab (Humira), abatacept (Orencia) etanercept (Enbrel), brilumab (Siliq)?, golimumab (Simponi) interferon beta-1a, fluoride (Arbagio)	Imuran: Lower white blood cell count, upper GI symptoms, fatigue, alopecia, diarrhea, joint pain	Used to prevent rejection in transplant recipients and to treat rheumatoid arthritis. Increases risk of cancer in long-term use.
Drug therapy for HIV infection	Prevent and reduce viral reproduction	efavirenz (Sustiva), emtricitabine (Emtriva), atazanavir (Reyataz), raltegravir (Isentress), darunavir (Prezista)	Various	Therapy is given per various protocols using combinations of antivirals.

Chapter 4
Drugs for the endocrine system

	Action	Drugs	Side effects	Notes
Hypoglycemics				
A. Insulin and insulin analogues — Rapid-acting: Onset of action varies from 10–30 min		insulin lispro (Humalog), insulin glulisine (Apidra), insulin regular (Humulin R, Novolin R)	Hypoglycemia, insulin shock	Glucophage reduces absorption of glucose from the intestine, helps prevent gluconeogenesis, and increases insulin use.
Intermediate-acting		insulin isophane (Humulin N, Novolin N)		
Long-acting		insulin glargine (Lantus), insulin detemir (Levemir)		Long-acting basal insulin. Once daily dosing.
Other analogues		exenatide (Bydureon, Byetta), liraglutide (Victoza), pramlintide (SymlinPen 120, SymlinPen 60)		
B. Oral hypoglycemics	Stimulate insulin release	glipizide, glimepiride (Amaryl), glyburide	Sulfonylureas also may cause hypoglycemia	
Biguanides	Enhance insulin sensitivity in muscle and fat	metformin (Glucophage)	Stomach upset, gas	Patients taking Glucophage should be warned about the danger of iodine medium-based contrast imaging studies and the importance of advising any imaging technicians that they are taking Glucophage.
Glitazones	Stimulate peroxisome proliferator-activated receptors (PPARs)	pioglitazone (Actos), rosiglitazone (Avandia)	Reports of acute pancreatitis. Have a boxed warning regarding potential cardiovascular issues.	Should not be used by patients with pancreatitis.
DPP-4 inhibitors	Inhibit degradation of incretins and increase insulin secretion	sitagliptin (Januvia), saxagliptin (Onglyza), alogliptin (Nesina), linagliptin (Tradjenta)	Headache, respiratory tract infection	
SGLT-2 inhibitors	Cause kidneys to remove sugar in the body through urine	canagliflozin (Invokana), dapagliflozin (Farxiga)	Dehydration, ketoacidosis, kidney problems	

continued

Body System/Drug Purpose	Drug Category	Drug Action	Examples	Side Effects	Comments
	Alpha-glucosidase inhibitors	Slow the breakdown of carbohydrates to glucose	acarbose (Precose), miglitol (Glyset)	Gas, bloating, diarrhea	
	Insulin antagonists or hyperglycemic agents	Elevate blood sugars	glucagon	Increase in blood glucose	Glucose tablets and gels are effective in emergency situations of low blood glucose levels.
	Corticosteroids	Regulate immune response and control of artificial immune response	hydrocortisone (Cortef), dexamethasone (Decadron), prednisone (Deltasone), methylprednisolone (Medrol)	Nervousness; sleepiness; hypertension; muscle weakness; dry, itching, burning skin; depression	Must be "weaned" off by reducing dosages. Long-term use may cause severe effects.
	Thyroid replacements	Treat hypothyroidism	thyroid extract, levothyroxine, liothyronine, liotrix	Increased or irregular heartbeat, shortness of breath, headache, nervousness, irritability, sleeplessness, tremors, heat intolerance, weight changes, vomiting, diarrhea	Should be taken 30 min before breakfast on empty stomach. Once diagnosed with hypothyroidism, patient must take replacement therapy for life.
	Antithyroid preparations	Inhibit the production of thyroid hormone	methimazole (Tapazole), propylthiouracil (PTU)	Blood dyscrasias	Medication should be taken around the clock. Used to treat Graves disease.
Chapter 5 Drugs for the sensory system					
A. Eyes	Mydriatics	Dilate the pupil of the eye	epinephrine (Epifrin, Glaucon), phenylephrine ophthalmic (Isopto Frin, Prefrin Liquifilm)	Systemically cause increased heart rate, increased BP	Adrenergic drugs
	Miotics	Constrict pupil of the eye	pilocarpine (Isopto Carpine, Ocusert Pilo), carbachol ophthalmic (Isopto Carbachol)	May slow heart rate and cause drop in BP	In the beta-blocker class
	Prostaglandin analogues	Decrease eye pressure from glaucoma	latanoprost ophthalmic (Xalatan), travoprost ophthalmic (Travatan), bimatoprost ophthalmic (Lumigan), unoprostone ophthalmic (Rescula)		
	Alpha-adrenergic receptor agonists	Decrease eye pressure from glaucoma	brimonidine ophthalmic (Alphagan P)		
	Ophthalmics	Treat allergic conjunctivitis, topical antibiotics	gatifloxacin (Zymaxid), alcaftadine (Lastacaft), bepotastine (Bepreve), besifloxacin (Besivance), neomycin/polymyxin B		Mast cell stabilizers

continued

B. Ears	Cerumenolytics	Soften and emulsify ear wax		carbamide peroxide (Debrox)	Should not be used if tympanic membrane is ruptured or there is a discharge from ear.
	Antiinfectives	Inhibit growth of bacteria, as in swimmer's ear	Rash	boric acid solution, hydrogen peroxide/ethyl alcohol, ciprofloxacin	Used routinely after swimming.
Chapter 6 Drugs for the integumentary system	Anesthetics	Produce lack of sensation to pain or abolish sensation to pain	Neurotoxicity, local reaction	Topical ethyl chloride or lidocaine (Nupercainal), Local lidocaine (Xylocaine), bupivacaine (Marcaine HCl)	May be mixed with epinephrine, causing vasoconstriction and extending duration of anesthesia.
	Antiparasitics	Rid body of parasites (e.g., lice)	Possibly carcinogenic	lindane (Kwell, Scabene, pyrethrins, piperonyl (RID), permethrin topical (Elimite), spinosad topical (Natroba)	May be a blood toxin; must be used with care; all directions should be followed completely.
	Antipruritics	Stop itching	Skin rash may rarely occur	calamine lotion, diphenhydramine cream, corticosteroid creams	Provide topical relief for dermatitis type of irritation.
	Antiseptics	Inhibit bacterial growth, usually used on living tissue	pHisoHex: Dermatitis, may be toxic when absorbed systemically Silvadene: Has a sulfa base; may cause reactions in those allergic to sulfa-based products Betadine: May cause skin rash when applied to those who have allergic reactions to topical iodine	hexachlorophene (pHisoHex), silver sulfadiazine topical (Silvadene), hydrogen peroxide, povidone-iodine (Betadine), isopropyl alcohol	Used as preoperative scrubs and cleansing. Silvadene is used on burn patients.
	Disinfectants	Kill or inhibit bacterial growth; usually used on inanimate objects	Not for use on humans; may cause skin rash	formaldehyde, glutaraldehyde, phenol	Effective as disinfectant on inanimate objects.
	Emollients/demulcents	Soothe and/or protect irritated tissue	None likely	A+D Cream, Eucerin, Lubriderm, many varients, vitamin E ointment, Desitin, Sween Cream	Frequently used to treat diaper rash or other localized skin irritation.
	Keratolytics	Control abnormal skin scaling or promote peeling of overgrowths/neoplasms of skin	Retin A: Erythema, crusting lesions on skin; itching, burning, dryness of skin	topical tar (coal tar, Tegrin Dandruff Shampoo, Neutrogena T/Gel), salicylic acid, benzoyl peroxide (Clearasil) fluorouracil topical (Efudex) tretinoin (Retin A)	Efudex is used to treat actinic keratosis and basal cell carcinoma.
Chapter 7 Drugs for the musculoskeletal system	Antigout agents	Treat chronic gout	Rash, headache, GI disorders, blood dyscrasias	colchicine (Colcrys), allopurinol (Zyloprim), probenecid (Benemid), febuxostat (Uloric)	Helpful in reducing excessive amounts of uric acid produced by the body.

Body System/Drug Purpose	Drug Category	Drug Action	Examples	Side Effects	Comments
	Antiinflammatories	Reduce inflammation in joints and muscles			
	A. Steroidal (see Drugs for the endocrine system, Corticosteroids)		prednisone, dexamethasone, methylprednisolone	GI upsets and bleeds, renal disturbances; steroids may mask infections	Patients usually are instructed to follow directions carefully and report any side effects as soon as possible.
	B. NSAIDs		ibuprofen (Motrin, Advil), naproxen (Aleve, Naprosyn), indomethacin (Indocin), celecoxib (Celebrex), meloxicam (Mobic)	GI symptoms, bleeding tendencies, changes in liver enzymes	Celebrex is a COX-2 inhibitor reported to have fewer gastric side effects.
	Bone replacement therapeutics	Treat and prevent osteoporosis	alendronate, ibandronate, risedronate, zoledronate, calcitonin-salmon (Miacalcin Nasal Spray)	Abdominal pain, muscle pain, constipation or diarrhea, nausea, flatulence	Instruct patients to take drug on an empty stomach with a glass of water and not to eat for at least 30 min.
	Muscle relaxants	Relax skeletal muscles	metocarbamol, cyclobenzaprine, baclofen, metaxalone, carisoprodol	GI upset, miosis, increased bronchial secretions, muscle cramps, tachycardia, elevated liver enzymes	May make patients drowsy; advise against driving or operating machinery.
Chapter 8					
Drugs used for the gastrointestinal system	Antacids	Neutralize stomach acid	calcium carbonate (Tums), magaldrate,	Heartburn, indigestion, stomach upset	Chronic use of antacids may cause acid rebound effect.
	Antidiarrheals	Control diarrhea	bismuth subsalicylate (Pepto-Bismol), loperamide (Imodium), diphenoxylate hydrochloride (HCl)/atropine (Lomotil)	Constipation, abdominal cramping, diarrhea	Prolonged uncontrolled diarrhea should be reported to a physician.
		Used as antiprotozoal/infant use Used as antiprotozoal for diarrhea caused by Cryptosporidium parvum or Giardia lamblia in pediatric patients	nitazoxanide (Alinia) aluminum hydroxide/magnesium hydroxide		
	Antidotes	Neutralize toxins and poisons	syrup of ipecac, activated charcoal	Charcoal causes stool to be black	Syrup of ipecac is never given if the ingested substance is corrosive (e.g., lye, Drano) or is petroleum based, or if patient is lethargic or unconscious.

Syrup of ipecac: Administration is followed by drinking a minimum of four to six glasses of water (adults). Vomiting should be expected and be prepared for. Activated charcoal is given after the vomiting has ceased; clothing should be protected; drug is given with a straw to get medication to back of mouth and prevent charcoal staining teeth.

Classification	Action	Examples	Side Effects	Comments
Antiemetics	Prevent and treat nausea and vomiting	prochlorperazine (Compazine), metoclopramide (Reglan), dimenhydrinate (Dramamine), ondansetron (Zofran)	Drowsiness, dizziness, blurred vision, anticholinergic effects, hypotension, skin reactions	Slow peristalsis, may cause abdominal cramping and related constipation. Zofran may be given to patients with cancer on chemotherapy to treat nausea and vomiting.
Antiflatulents	Provide symptomatic relief of gastric bloating and intestinal gas	simethicone (Mylicon, Phazyme)	None noted	Also used to treat colic in infants.
Anthelmintics	Eradicate helminths (worms)	mebendazole (Vermox), pyrantel pamoate (Antiminth)	Abdominal pain, diarrhea	Treatment of entire family is recommended.
Antispasmodics	Relieve smooth-muscle spasms of the stomach and intestines	hyoscyamine (Levsin), belladonna alkaloids/phenobarbital (Donnatal), dicyclomine (Bentyl)	Decreased peristalsis, dry mouth, headache, dizziness, palpitations, fatigue	Used to treat irritable bowel syndrome and similar intestinal disorders.
Antiulcer agents	Reduce gastric acid secretions by acting as histamine-2 (H2)-receptor antagonists	cimetidine (Tagamet), ranitidine (Zantac), nizatidine (Axid), famotidine (Pepcid)	Headache, fatigue, myalgia, alopecia, diarrhea, rash, dizziness	Helpful in treatment of GERD.
	Act as proton pump inhibitors	omeprazole (Prilosec), pantoprazole (Protonix), esomeprazole (Nexium), lansoprazole (Prevacid)		More effective than H2-receptor antagonists.
Digestants	Assist with digestion of food by replacing pancreatic enzymes	pancrelipase (Ultrase, Pancrease, pancreatin (Creon)	GI upset, rashes	Patient should be instructed not to chew or crush capsules.
Emetics	Induce vomiting	syrup of ipecac		Syrup of ipecac is never given if the ingested substance is corrosive (e.g., lye, Drano) or is petroleum based, or if patient is lethargic or unconscious. Syrup of ipecac administration is followed by drinking a minimum of four to six glasses of water (adults). One should be prepared for vomiting.

continued

Body System/ Drug Purpose	Drug Category	Drug Action	Examples	Side Effects	Comments
	Laxatives/ cathartics	Induce defecation and relieve constipation	bisacodyl (Dulcolax), sennoside alkaloids, mineral oil psyllium (Metamucil)	Cramping, diarrhea	Patients should be cautioned about excessive continued use, which may cause a reverse reaction.
	Stool softeners	Soften feces	docusate sodium (Colace), docusate calcium (Surfak), polyethylene glycol (MiraLAX)	Leakage of oil-like substances from rectum, increased peristalsis, cramping	Used to ease evacuation of bowel contents.
Chapter 9					
Drugs used for the respiratory system	Asthma prophylactics Leukotriene receptor antagonists	Prevent exercise-induced asthma	cromolyn sodium (Intal), montelukast (Singulair) roflumilast (Daliresp)	Bronchospasm, cough, wheezing, nasal congestion	Have best action when used before exposure.
	Antihistamines	Inhibit histamine to relieve allergy symptoms	diphenhydramine (Benadryl), clemastine (Tavist), chlorpheniramine (Chlor-Trimeton), fexofenadine (Allegra), cetirizine (Zyrtec), loratadine (Claritin) desloratadine (Clarinex), levocetirizine (Xyzal)	Drowsiness, dry eyes, dry mouth, hypotension constipation, anorexia, palpitations	May cause drowsiness. Patient should be advised not to drive or operate machinery while taking medication. Contraindicated in patients with glaucoma.
	Antitussives	Suppress cough	dextromethorphan, codeine, hydrocodone, benzonatate	CNS stimulation, blurred vision, palpitations, anxiety, weakness, insomnia	Patients should be instructed to follow directions. Hydrocodone and codeine may be habit forming.
	Bronchodilators	Relax smooth muscle of bronchial tree; relieve bronchospasm	albuterol sulfate (Proventil), levalbuterol (Xopenex), epinephrine (Primatene), theophylline (Theo-Dur), ipratropium (Atrovent), tiotropium (Spiriva)	Hyperactivity, excitement, tremor, nervousness, insomnia, tachycardia	Routine theophylline blood level studies are recommended.
	Decongestants	Shrink nasal mucous membranes	oxymetazoline (Afrin), pseudoephedrine HCl (Sudafed), phenylephrine (Neo-Synephrine)	Nasal sprays may cause irritation to nasal membrane Constrict vessels; cause hypertension	Prolonged use of sprays may cause rebound effects. Should not be used by pregnant women because of possible constriction of vessels.
	Expectorants	Increase respiratory secretions and reduce viscosity to allow for the expulsion of sputum	guaifenesin (Robitussin, Mucinex)	Excitability, constipation, nausea, vomiting, drowsiness	May cause drowsiness. Patient should be advised not to drive or operate machinery while taking medication.
	Mucolytics	Liquefy respiratory secretions	acetylcysteine (Mucomyst)	Runny nose, throat irritation, nausea	Used to treat asthma and cystic fibrosis. Also used as antidote in acetaminophen overdose.

Chapter 10

Drugs used for the cardiovascular system and for hematology

Category	Use	Examples	Side effects	Notes
Smoking cessation aids	Reduce nicotine levels while assisting with smoking-cessation programs	nicotine (Nicorette, ...Derm), bupropion (Zyban), varenicline (Chantix)	Tobacco withdrawal symptoms, local effects from patches or sprays, dry mouth, insomnia	Patient may require emotional support while using these products. Chantix may elicit vivid dreams.
Antianginals	Used for prophylactic treatment of angina; dilate coronary arteries	nitroglycerin (Nitro..., Transderm Nitro), isosorbide mononitrate, isosorbide dinitrate	Lightheadedness, headache	Nitrostat sublingual tablets should be placed under the tongue to treat angina. May be repeated every 5 min, three times, to relieve angina. If no relief, entry into the emergency medical system is advised.
Antiarrhythmics	Suppress cardiac arrhythmias	propranolol, verapamil, procainamide, dronedarone (Multaq), dofetilide (Tikosyn)	Hypotension, GI upset, headache, fatigue	Regular monitoring of arrhythmias is recommended.
Anticoagulants	Prevent formation of clots	warfarin (Coumadin), heparin sodium, ticagrelor (Brilinta), prasugrel (Effient), rivaroxaban (Xarelto)	Tissue or organ hemorrhage, rash, abdominal pain, headache	Blood coagulation studies are performed on a regular basis.
Antihypertensives	Treatment and management of hypertension			
A. Calcium channel blockers		amlodipine, diltiazem, verapamil	Constipation, dizziness	
B. Beta-blockers		atenolol, carvedilol, metoprolol, propranolol (Inderal)	Hypotension, lethargy, GI symptoms, slow heart rate, dizziness	
C. ACE inhibitors		enalapril, benazepril, lisinopril, fosinopril, ramipril, quinapril, trandolapril	Dizziness, hypotension, dry cough	
D. Angiotensin receptor blockers		azilsartan medoxomil, candesartan, irbesartan, losartan, valsartan		
E. Diuretics		hydrochlorothiazide (HCTZ), furosemide, bumetanide, spironolactone		
Antihyperlipidemics	Reduce serum cholesterol and low-density lipoproteins	gemfibrozil, fenofibrate, cholestyramine (Questran), niacin, fish oil, simvastatin (Zocor), atorvastatin (Lipitor), pravastatin (Pravachol), rosuvastatin (Crestor), ezetimibe (Zetia), pitavastatin	Myalgia, GI upset, headache, rash, dizziness, elevated liver enzymes. Zetia: Stomach pain, tiredness	Statin drugs are reported to reduce existing arterial plaque. Zetia is a cholesterol-lowering drug with less myalgia reported.

continued

Body System/ Drug Purpose	Drug Category	Drug Action	Examples	Side Effects	Comments
	Cardiotonics/ cardiac glycosides	Strengthen heartbeat	digoxin (Lanoxin), digitoxin (Crystodigin)	Irregular heartbeat, palpitations, loss of appetite, nausea, vomiting, diarrhea, visual changes	Patient should be instructed to take the drug in the morning, record daily weights, and take apical pulse before taking medication. If pulse rate is over than 60 bpm, dose should be withheld and pulse recounted in 1 h. If pulse rate is still less than 60 bpm, medication should be withheld and the physician contacted. Patient may be prone to digitalis toxicity.
	Coagulants/ hemostatics	Control or stop bleeding by promoting coagulation	phytonadione (AquaMEPHYTON), menadiol sodium (Synkayvite), vitamin K	Normal aspirin side effects. Persantine : Dizziness, headache, rash, GI upset	Administered to newborns to prevent hemorrhagic disease.
	Platelet inhibitors	Inhibit platelet clumping	aspirin, dipyridamole (Persantine), prasugrel (Effient), dabigatran (Pradaxa), clopidogrel (Plavix), rivaroxaban (Xarelto), ticagrelor (Brilinta)	Normal aspirin side effects Aspirin side effects may include GI distress, ulceration, increased bleeding time (international normalized ratio [INR],T). Persantine: Dizziness, headache, rash, GI upset	
	Thrombolytics	Dissolve blood clots	streptokinase (Streptase), alteplase (Activase)	GI bleeds, bleeding in other sites	Best if administration begins within 2–3 h after onset of chest pain in MI.
	Vasoconstrictors	Constrict blood vessels	metaraminol (Aramine), norepinephrine (Levophed), epinephrine (Adrenalin)	Nausea and vomiting, cardiac arrhythmias, decreased urine output	Used to treat shock.
	Vasodilators	Dilate blood vessels	nitroglycerin, isosorbide dinitrate (Isordil), isoxsuprine HCl (Vasodilan), isosorbide mononitrate (ISMO)	Lightheadedness headache	Nitrostat sublingual tablets should be placed under the tongue to treat angina. May be repeated every 5 min, three times, to relieve angina. If no relief, entry into the emergency medical system is advised.

continued

Chapter 11

Drugs used for the urinary system

Category	Use	Drugs	Side effects	Notes
Urinary analgesics	Lessen pain and burning of urinary tract infection	phenazopyridine HCl (Pyridium)	Produces orange- to red-colored urine that may stain clothing	Patients should be advised about possibility of stains to clothing from the orange- or red-colored urine.
Urinary antiseptics	Used as specific antibacterials to treat urinary tract infections	nitrofurantoin (Furadantin), nitrofurantoin monohydrate/macrocrystals (Macrobid), sulfamethoxazole-trimethoprim (Bactrim)	GI disturbances, orange-colored urine	Patients should be informed about possibility of orange-colored urine and sanitary napkin suggest for protection of underwear.
Urinary antispasmodics	Relieve urgency, frequency, and incontinence	oxybutynin HCl, fesoterodine darifenacin (Enablex), mirabegron (Myrbetriq) fesoterodine (Toviaz) solifenacin (Vesicare), trospium (Sanctura)	Dry mouth, constipation, somnolence, tachycardia	Relax bladder muscles and help to reduce incontinence.
Diuretics	Remove excessive fluid from body tissues; increase urinary output	furosemide (Lasix), hydrochlorothiazide, bumetanide (Bumex), torsemide, spironolactone, metolazone	Hypokalemia, excessive diuresis, GI upset, dizziness, vertigo	Characterized by site of action. Many require monitoring of potassium levels and require daily potassium replacement. Patients should be instructed to take medication in morning to ensure restful nights. Recording of daily weights should be encouraged.
Enuretic agents	Control enuresis	desmopressin (DDAVP)	Dry mouth, constipation, somnolence, tachycardia	Relax bladder muscles and help reduce incontinence.

Chapter 12

Drugs used for the reproductive system

Category	Use	Drugs	Side effects	Notes
Contraceptives	Prevent conception/pregnancy			
A. Low-dose monophasic birth control pills	Estrogen: ethinyl estradiol (EE) Progestins: Levonorgestrel, norethindrone, desogestrel, drospirenone, or ethynodiol diacetate.	ethinyl estradiol/levonorgestrel (Aviane, Lessina, Lutera, Nordette, Orsythia) levonorgestrel/ethinyl estradiol (Famine, ethinyl estradiol/norethindrone (Brevicon Fe 1/20, Junel Fe 1/20, Loestrin Fe 1/20, Microgestin 1/20 ethinyl estradiol/norgestrel (Cryselle, LoOvral), ethinyl estradiol/desogestrel (Apri)	Thromboembolism associated with MI and CVA. Elevated blood pressure and blood glucose levels, acne, hair loss, gallbladder disease, hirsutism	A missed pill may result in pregnancy. Antibiotic therapy may render contraceptive ineffective. Now available in an intradermal patch form.
B. High-dose monophasic birth control pills		ethinyl estradiol/norethindrone (Ovcon-50), ethinyl estradiol/norgestrel (Ogestrel 0.5/50), Zovia (ethinyl estradiol/ethynodiol diacetate)		

Body System/ Drug Purpose	Drug Action	Examples	Side Effects	Comments
C. Biphasic birth control pills		ethinyl estradiol/desogestrel (Kariva, Mircette), ethinyl estradiol/norethindrone (Necon 10/11)		
D. Triphasic birth control pills		ethinyl estradiol/norethindrone (Estrostep Fe), ethinyl estradiol/norgestimate (Ortho Tri-Cyclen, TriNessa, Tri-Previfem, Tri-Sprintec), ethinyl estradiol/desogestrel (Cyclessa, Velivet), ethinyl estradiol/levonorgestrel (Enpresse, Trivora)		
E. Four-phase birth control pills		dienogest/estradiol (Natazia)		
F. Extended-cycle birth control pills		ethinyl estradiol/norethindrone/ ferrous fumarate tablets (Lo Lcestrin Fe), ethinyl estradiol/ levonorgestrel (Amethia Lo, Amethia, Seasonique), drospirenone/ethinyl estradiol/ levomefolate (Beyaz), drospirenone/ethinyl estradiol (Gianvi, Loryna, Yaz)		
G. Progestin-only pills (mini-pill)		norethindrone (Camilla, Errin, Nor-QD, Ortho Micronor)		
Emergency contraception		ulipristal (Ella), levonorgestrel (Plan-B, Next Choice)		
Alternative methods		medroxyprogesterone acetate (Depo-Provera), levonorgestrel intrauterine system (Mirena), etonogestrel (Nexplanon), ethinyl estradiol/ etonogestrel (NuvaRing)		Depo-Provera requires an injection every 3 months. Nexplanon implantation must be performed by a physician every 3 years. NuvaRing is a vaginal ring insert that is inserted/removed by the patient. Mirena releases levonorgestrel. Included in grouping as a non-pill-related method. Occurrence of multiple pregnancies is possible.
Fertility enhancers	Induce ovulation	clomiphene citrate (Clomid)	GI symptoms, CNS symptoms, acne, ovarian enlargement, ectopic pregnancies	

	Action	Examples	Side Effects	Notes
Hormone replacements	Replace reproductive hormones			
A. Androgens	Stimulate the development of male sexual characteristics	testosterone cypionate (Depo-Testosterone), methyltestosterone (Testred)	Urinary urgency, breast tenderness, priapism	Supplement low levels of testosterone
B. Estrogens	Stimulate the development of female sexual characteristics	estradiol (Estrace, conjugated estrogen (Premarin, estropipate (Ogen)	Anorexia, nausea, headaches, edema of lower extremities, hypercalcemia, thrombophlebitis	Used to treat symptoms of menopause; increases risk of breast and cervical cancers. Caution must be used in women who smoke; may cause deep vein thrombosis.
C. Progestins	Treat amenorrhea and abnormal uterine bleeding	medroxyprogesterone (Provera), medroxyprogesterone acetate (Depo-Provera)	Weight gain, stomach disturbances, edema, headaches, break-through bleeding	May be used for contraception, used in combination with estrogen for postmenopausal hormone replacement therapy.
Drugs used to treat prostatic conditions	Treats BPH and urinary retention	tamsulosin (Flomax), terazosin (Hytrin), finasteride	Hypotension, fatigue, edema, dyspnea	Used to relieve urinary retention and nocturia caused by enlarged prostate.
Drugs used to treat erectile dysfunction		sildenafil citrate (Viagra), tadalafil (Cialis), vardenafil (Levitra)	Nasal congestion, blurred vision, hypertension, dizziness, rash	Patients who have cardiac disease should be cautioned not to take Viagra. Drug should be taken on an empty stomach an hour before eating.

Chapter 13

Drugs used for the neurologic system	Action	Examples	Side Effects	Notes
Adrenergic drugs	Mimic sympathetic nervous system	epinephrine (AceTate), dobutamine (Inregan)	Increased blood pressure, rapid heart rate	Initiate "fight or flight" system.
Adrenergic blockers	Block the action of sympathetic nervous system	propranolol (Inderal), methyldopa (Aldomet)	Hypotension, bradycardia, constricted bronchioles	Used to treat hypertension; Inderal also used for migraine headaches.
Analgesics	Relieve pain			
A. Opioids (narcotics)		codeine, meperidine, hydrocodone, hydromorphone, oxycodone, oxymorphone, fentanyl, morphine	May cause drowsiness; constipation can occur	May become addictive. Patients should not drive or operate machinery while taking the drug.
B. Nonopioids		acetaminophen (Tylenol), acetylsalicylic acid (aspirin), NSAIDs	Aspirin: May cause stomach upset and tinnitus	Aspirin also has anticoagulant, antiprostaglandin effects. All are antipyretic medications.
Anesthetics	Produce loss of sensation by blocking nerve impulses			

continued

Body System/ Drug Purpose	Drug Category	Drug Action	Examples	Side Effects	Comments
	A. General		thiopental sodium (Pentothal), midazolam (Versed)	Versed: May cause amnesia, hypotension, headache	Versed is used for conscious sedation.
	B. Local		lidocaine (Xylocaine), procaine (Novocain)		Xylocaine may be topical form; also is used systemically as a cardiac drug.
	Anticholinergics	Block parasympathetic nervous system	atropine, scopolamine	Dry mouth, increased heart rate, constipation, urinary retention, dilated pupils	May be used in treatment of Parkinson disease.
	Antiepileptics	Reduce the number and/or the severity of seizures caused by epilepsy	phenytoin (Dilantin), phenobarbital, clonazepam (Klonopin), gabapentin (Neurontin), vigabatrin (Sabril), ezogabine (Potiga)	Reduced coordination, involuntary eye movement, slurred speech	Encourage good mouth care because Dilantin may cause gingiva hyperplasia. Neurontin may be prescribed to treat posttherapy neuralgia. These medications should not be stopped abruptly.
	Antiparkinsonism medications	Relieve symptoms and increase mobility of patients with Parkinson disease	levodopa (L-dopa), amantadine (Symmetrel)	Dystonia, GI symptoms, dry mouth, increased hand tremors	Used to increase levels of dopamine in the brain.
	Cholinergics	Mimic parasympathetic nervous system by liberating acetylcholine	neostigmine (Prostigmin), pilocarpine (Isopto Carpine)	Increased peristalsis	
	Hypnotics/ Sedatives	Produce sedation or sleep			
	A. Barbiturates		amobarbital (Amytal), secobarbital (Seconal)	Increased excitability, hostility, confusion, hallucinations	May cause drowsiness; patient should not drive, operate machinery, and consume alcohol while using the drug.
	B. Nonbarbiturates		zolpidem (Ambien), eszopiclone (Lunesta)	May be habit forming.	May cause confusion, sleep walking.
	Stimulants	Increase the activity of brain/spinal cord	caffeine, methylphenidate (Ritalin), amphetamines, modafinil (Provigil), armodafinil (Nuvigil)	Anorexia, euphoria, sleeplessness, dry mouth, GI disturbances, insomnia, weight loss	May be addictive. Ritalin is used to treat hyperactivity in children.
Drugs used in the treatment of Alzheimer disease	Alzheimer disease medications	Enhance transmission of cholinergic neurons to improve thought processes	tacrine (Cognex), donepezil (Aricept), memantine (Namenda)	GI disturbances, insomnia, vomiting, anorexia	Help with memory and thinking processes; improve everyday activities; improve behavior.

Category	Drug type	Use	Examples	Side effects	Comments/Precautions
Drugs used in the treatment of multiple sclerosis	Multiple sclerosis drugs	Used for relapsing forms of multiple sclerosis	interferon beta-1b (Betaseron), interferon-beta 1a (Avonex, Rebif), glatiramer (Copaxone), natalizumab (Tysabri), fingolimod (Gilenya), teriflunomide (Aubagio), dimethyl fumarate (Tecfidera)		Gilenya, Aubagio, and Tecfidera are oral agents. The remaining agents are given by injection.
Chapter 14 Drugs used for mental disorders	Antianxiety/anxiolytics/minor tranquilizers	Used for short-term treatment of anxiety disorders, some psychosomatic disorders, and nausea and vomiting	diazepam (Valium), lorazepam (Tranxene), alprazolam (Xanax), vigabatrin (Sabril), asenapine (Saphris), milnacipran (Savella), iloperidone (Fanapt)	CNS symptoms, GI disturbances, skin rash, nasal congestion. May be habit forming.	May cause drowsiness; use caution when driving or operating machinery. Patient should not stop medication abruptly but be "weaned" off by reducing dosages.
	Antidepressants/mood elevators	Treat depression	amitriptyline (Elavil), phenelzine (Nardil)	CNS symptoms, GI disturbances, weight gain, somnolence. SSRIs have a lower incidence of side effects	May take 2–4 weeks for effects to be realized. Consumption of alcohol should be avoided.
			sertraline (Zoloft), fluoxetine (Prozac), venlafaxine (Effexor), paroxetine (Paxil), fluvoxamine (Luvox), milnacipran (Savella), vilazodone (Viibryd)		
	Antimanics	Treat manic disorders	lithium (Litobid)	Dry mouth, excessive thirst, weight gain, GI disturbances, tremors, cardiac arrhythmias, visual impairment, unsteady gait	Used to treat bipolar disorders. Blood level should be monitored on a regular basis.
	Antipsychotics	Relieve symptoms of psychosis and severe neurosis	haloperidol (Haldol), asenapine (Saphris), iloperidone (Fanapt)	Tachycardia or bradycardia, vertigo, postural hypotension, dry mouth, constipation, urinary retention, anorexia, blurred vision, fever, CNS system reactions	May cause drowsiness; caution should be exercised when driving or operating machinery.
	A. Atypical antipsychotics		aripiprazole (Abilify), clozapine (Clozaril), olanzapine (Zyprexa), paliperidone (Invega), quetiapine (Seroquel), risperidone (Risperdal), ziprasidone (Geodon)		May cause significant drowsiness. Various agents may cause significant weight gain. Some may be weight neutral or produce weight loss.
	B. Neuroleptics/major tranquilizers		fluphenazine HCl (Prolixin), chlorpromazine (Thorazine), prochlorperazine (Compro), quetiapine (Seroquel)		May cause drowsiness; caution should be exercised when driving or operating machinery.

continued

Body System/ Drug Purpose	Drug Category	Drug Action	Examples	Side Effects	Comments
Chapter 15					
Drugs used for first aid, emergency situations	Sulfonamides	Treat burns topically	silver sulfadiazine (Silvadene), mafenide acetate (Sulfamylon)	Rash, redness	Helpful in treating infections; broad-spectrum agents effective against both gram-positive and gram-negative organisms.
	Antivenoms	Counteract toxins, such as those from snake-bites, spider bites	Crotaline polyvalent immune Fab (FAB) (rattlesnake), black widow spider antivenom	Made from sheep serum; less likely to produce severe reaction than antivenom from horse serum Compartment syndrome may occur in affected limb	Often preceded by administration of antihistamine to lessen any allergic effects. Observation of individual for a minimum of 24 h is usual protocol.

aAnesthetics may be used alone or in combination to produce effects.

bDifferent generations of cephalosporins are effective against different strains of bacteria.

ACE, Angiotensin-converting enzyme; *BP,* blood pressure; *BPH,* benign prostatic hyperplasia; *bpm,* beats per minute; *CNS,* central nervous system; *COX-2,* cyclooxygenase-2; *CVA,* cerebrovascular accident; *DPP-4,* dipeptidyl peptidase-4; *GERD,* gastroesophageal reflux disease; *GI,* gastrointestinal; *HIV,* human immunodeficiency virus; *IM,* intramuscular; *MI,* myocardial infarction; *NSAID,* nonsteroidal antiinflammatory drug; *SSRI,* selective serotonin reuptake inhibitor.

Glossary

Note: The Glossary contains the chapter Key Terms (unless they are defined in the text) and other important terms in the text. *Sp.,* Spanish

A

abduct (Sp. abducción, separar) move an arm or leg away from the body

ablation (Sp. ablación) excision or removal

abruptio placentae (Sp. desprendimiento de la placenta) detachment of the placenta from the uterus before birth; often results in severe bleeding

abscess (Sp. absceso) a localized collection of pus surrounded by swollen tissue

acetabulum (Sp. acetábulo) the cup-shaped cavity in which the ball-shaped head of the femur articulates

achalasia (Sp. acalasia) failure of the esophagogastric sphincter to relax with swallowing

acholic (Sp. arcilla) pale or clay-colored. Acholic stool usually results from problems in the biliary system

acidemia (Sp. acidemia) a decreased pH of blood (increased hydrogen ion concentration)

acidosis (Sp. acidosis) a pathologic condition resulting from an abnormal increase in the level of hydrogen ions in the body (decrease in pH), resulting from the accumulation of acid or loss of the alkaline reserve

acute abdomen (Sp. abdomen agudo) an abdominal condition of sudden onset, accompanied by pain resulting from intraabdominal inflammation or infection

acyanotic (Sp. acianótico) absence of a bluish appearance of the skin and mucous membranes

adenocarcinoma (Sp. adenocarcinoma, carcinoma glandular) a cancerous tumor arising from glandular tissue

adenoma (Sp. adenoma) a benign neoplasm in which cells are derived from the glandular epithelium

adenosarcoma (Sp. adenosarcoma) a cancerous glandlike tumor, such as Wilms tumor

adenovirus (Sp. adenovirus) a virus pathogenic to humans that causes conjunctivitis, upper respiratory infection, cystitis, or gastrointestinal infection; may persist in lymphoid tissue in latent period of the infection

adnexal (Sp. de los anexos) pertaining to accessory organs or tissues; appendage(s)

adrenocorticotropic hormone (ACTH) (Sp. hormona adrenocorticotrópica [ACTH]) a hormone secreted by the anterior lobe of the pituitary; also known as *corticotropin*

aerodigestive (Sp. aerodigestivo) pertaining to the respiratory and digestive tract considered together

agglutination (Sp. aglutinación) the clumping of antigens with antibodies or of the red blood cells from one type of blood with the red blood cells of another type

aggregation (Sp. agregación) the coming together of entities, such as platelets, blood cells, or diseases

agranulocytosis (Sp. agranulocitosis) a condition of the blood marked by a sudden decrease in the number of granulocytes (a type of white blood cell); occurs in lesions of the throat or other mucous membranes or as a side effect of the administration of certain drugs or radiation

alkalosis (Sp. alcalosis) excessive alkalinity of body fluids

allergen (Sp. alérgeno) an antigenic substance capable of producing an allergic response in the body

allograft (Sp. injerto alogénico) a graft of tissue between genetically different individuals of the same species

amblyopia (Sp. ambioplía) reduced vision in an eye without a detectable organic lesion

amnesia (Sp. amnesia) a loss of memory; inability to recall past experiences

amniogram, amniography (Sp. amniografía) radiography (after injection of radiopaque contrast medium into the amniotic fluid) of the pregnant uterus to determine placement of the placenta, the amniotic cavity, and the fetus

amniotic fluid (Sp. líquido amniótico) a transparent albuminous liquid made by the amnion and the fetus membranes and protects the fetus during pregnancy

amylase (Sp. amilasa) an enzyme produced in the salivary glands and pancreas that helps in digestion of starches

amyloid (Sp. amiloide) a waxy, starch-like protein that tends to build up in tissues and organs in certain pathologic conditions

analgesia, analgesic (Sp. analgesia, analgésico) relief of pain

analogue (Sp. análogo) a drug that resembles another but has different effects

anaphylaxis (Sp. anafilaxia) a severe systemic allergic response characterized by redness, itching, swelling, and water buildup (angioedema); in severe cases, life-threatening respiratory distress occurs, and blood pressure drops rapidly (anaphylactic shock)

anaplastic (Sp. anaplástico) a change in the orientation and structure of cells; a loss of differentiation that is characteristic of malignancy

anastomosis (anastomoses) (Sp. anastomosis) the surgical or pathologic connection between two vessels or tubular structures

anesthesia, anesthetic (Sp. anestesia, anestésico) partial or complete loss of sensation caused by injury, diseases, or the administration of an anesthetic agent

angina pectoris (Sp. angina de pecho) paroxysmal chest pain, which often radiates to the arms and may be accompanied by a feeling of suffocation and impending death; the most common cause is a shortage of oxygen to the cardiac muscle linked with coronary artery disease

angioplasty (Sp. angioplastia) repair of a narrowed blood vessel through surgery or other angiographic procedures

angiotensin-converting enzyme (ACE) (Sp. enzima de conversión de la angiotensina [ECA]) an enzyme found on the surface of blood vessels in the lungs and other tissues with vasopressive action

angiotensin-converting enzyme (ACE) inhibitors (Sp. inhibidores de la enzima de conversión de la angiotensina) agents that inhibit angiotensin-converting enzyme (a potent vasoconstrictor) and promote relaxation of blood vessels

ankylosis (Sp. anquilosis) immobility of a joint

anorexia, anorectic (Sp. anorexia, anoréxico) loss of appetite for food

anosmia (Sp. anosmia) impairment or loss of smell

antibody (antibodies) (Sp. anticuerpo) an immunoglobulin that may combine with a specific antigen to destroy or control it

anticholinergic (Sp. anticolinérgico) a drug used to block the transmission of parasympathetic nerve impulses

anticholinesterase (Sp. anticolina esterasa) any enzyme that counteracts the action of the choline esters

anticoagulant (Sp. anticoagulante) any substance that delays or prevents blood clotting

antiemetic (Sp. antiemético) a medication that prevents or relieves nausea and vomiting

antigen (Sp. antígeno) any substance that stimulates the immune system to produce antibodies

antimicrobial (Sp. antimicrobiano) a substance that kills microorganisms or suppresses their growth

antipyretic (Sp. antipirético) a drug or treatment that reduces or relieves fever

antiseptic (Sp. antiséptico) a substance that inhibits the growth of microorganisms

antitrypsin (Sp. antitripsina) a substance that inhibits trypsin, an enzyme that hastens the hydrolysis of protein

anxiolytic (Sp. ansiolítico) a substance that diminishes anxiety

aphasia (Sp. afasia) a nerve defect that results in loss of speech

aphonia (Sp. afonía) inability to produce normal speech sounds or loss of voice

aphthous ulcers (Sp. úlceras aftosas) recurrent painful canker sores in the mouth

apicectomy (Sp. apicetomy) surgical removal of the apex of an infected or damaged tooth root

apnea, apneic (Sp. apnea, apneico) the temporary cessation of breathing

apoptosis (Sp. apoptosis) a pattern of cell death affecting single cells; refers to programmed cell death

arrhythmia (Sp. arritmia) variation or loss of normal rhythm of the heartbeat

arthrodesis (Sp. artrodesis) the immobilization of a joint accomplished surgically

arthroplasty (Sp. artroplastia) surgical reconstruction or replacement of a diseased joint

ascites (Sp. ascitis) abnormal intraperitoneal accumulation of serous fluid

aspiration (Sp. aspiración) drawing in or out by suction

assay (Sp. ensayar) the analysis of biologic substances, including laboratory and clinical evaluations

asymptomatic (Sp. asintomático) without symptoms

asystole (Sp. asístole) the absence of contractions of the heart; cardiac standstill

ataxia (Sp. ataxia) an uncoordinated gait associated with pathology of the central nervous system; an individual with this gait may be described as being *ataxic*

atrophy (Sp. atrofia) a wasting away; a degeneration of a cell, tissue, organ, or muscle because of disease or other influences

audiogram (Sp. audiograma) the record of a hearing test

aura (Sp. aura) a sensation or phenomenon that signals the onset of an epileptic seizure or a migraine

auscultation (Sp. auscultación) a diagnostic technique of listening for sounds within the body, particularly the lungs, heart, or abdominal viscera

autoantibody (Sp. autoanticuerpo) an antibody that attacks and destroys the body's own cells

autoimmunity, autoimmune (Sp. autoinmunidad, auto-inmune) an immune response resulting in the presence of self-antigens or autoantigens on the surface of certain body cells; may result in allergy or autoimmune disease

autoinoculation (Sp. autoinoculación) refers to spreading a microorganism by contact with a lesion on one's own body

autonomic (Sp. autónomo) refers to the autonomic nervous system, which has two divisions (i.e., sympathetic and parasympathetic)

autosome, autosomal (Sp. autosoma, autosómico) any of the 22 ordinary paired chromosomes in humans, distinguished from the sex (X and Y) chromosomes

avulsion (Sp. separación) separation of a body part by tearing

azoospermia (Sp. azoospermia) an absence of spermatozoa in semen

azotemia (Sp. azotemia) an excess of urea or other nitrogenous bodies in blood

B

barium (Sp. bario) a pale, soft, alkaline metallic element; a radiopaque barium (barium sulfate) compound commonly used in radiographic studies of the gastrointestinal tract

Battle sign (Sp. signo de Battle) bogginess of the temporal region of the head that may indicate fracture at the base of the skull

bicornuate uterus (Sp. útero bicorne) a uterus having two horns or horn-shaped branches

bifurcate (Sp. bifurcado) split into two branches

bilirubinemia (Sp. bilirrubinemia) the presence of bilirubin in blood

bilirubinuria (Sp. bilirrubinuria) the presence of bilirubin (a yellow- or orange-tinged pigment in the bile) in urine

biopsy (Sp. biopsia) the excision of tissue from the living body, followed by microscopic examination, for the purpose of exact diagnosis

blood gases (Sp. gases sanguíneos) the gases present in blood as a result of use of oxygen and production of carbon dioxide during metabolism; the blood is analyzed for evidence of deviations (acidosis or alkalosis) from normal levels

blood urea nitrogen (BUN) (Sp. nitrógeno ureico en sangre [NUS]) a measurement of urea nitrogen (a substance formed during protein breakdown) in the serum or plasma; an elevated BUN level may indicate impaired renal function

breech (Sp. nalgas) buttocks

bronchoscopy (Sp. broncoscopía) examination of the bronchial tree with a bronchoscope to obtain a biopsy specimen, remove an obstruction, or diagnose a disease

bruit (Sp. ruido) an abnormal sound heard in auscultation

C

cachexia (Sp. caquexia) a profound and marked wasting disorder, usually associated with malnutrition and diseases, such as cancer and tuberculosis

calculus (calculi) (Sp. cálculo) a stone usually composed of mineral salts (e.g., kidney stones and gallstones) or calcified deposits on teeth

carcinogen, carcinogenic (Sp. carcinógeno) a substance that produces cancer or that causes transformation of a normal cell to a cancerous one

cardiac sphincter (Sp. esfínter cardiaco) the circular muscle at the opening of the esophagus into the stomach

cardiomegaly (Sp. cardiomegalia) enlargement of the heart

cardiomyopathy (Sp. cardiomiopatía) a defect of the heart muscle

cast (Sp. impresión) a negative mold or copy formed in a hollow organ or part (e.g., kidney or bronchi); a urinary cast is a small structure formed within the urinary system from mineral or protein matter and extruded from the body in urine

cataract (Sp. cataratas) a progressive disease in which the lens of the eye becomes cloudy, impairing vision or causing blindness

catatonic posturing (Sp. estado catatónico) a state of not being able to move, with the assumption of a rigid, often bizarre posture

cautery (Sp. cauterio) an instrument or chemical that destroys tissue as a therapeutic measure

cellulitis (Sp. celulitis) an acute, diffuse, spreading infection of the skin and subcutaneous tissue

centromere (Sp. centrómero) the constricted area of a chromosome

cephalgia, cephalalgia (Sp. cefalea) pain in the head; headache

cephalic (Sp. cefálico) referring to the head; cranial

cerclage (Sp. cerclaje) encircling of the cervix with a metal ring or suture ring to treat cervical incompetence during pregnancy to help prevent spontaneous abortion

chancre (Sp. chancro) a type of skin lesion usually associated with primary syphilis

cheilectomy (Sp. queilotomía) surgical removal of abnormal bone around a joint; also refers to surgical removal of a lip

cholangiogram, cholangiography (Sp. colangiograma) a diagnostic radiographic study of the gallbladder and bile ducts

cholecystogram, cholecystography (Sp. colecistografía) a diagnostic radiographic study of the gallbladder

cholinergic (Sp. colinérgico) an agent that produces the effect of acetylcholine at the connections of muscles and nerves

chorea (Sp. corea) the ceaseless occurrence of involuntary muscular movements of the limbs or facial muscles

chromosome (Sp. cromosoma) structures in the nucleus of a cell that function in the transmission of genetic information

cicatricial (Sp. cicatriz) refers to a scar or the nature of a scar

circadian rhythm (Sp. ritmo circadiano) the biologic clock in humans; the rhythmic repetition of certain phenomena, such as hunger, fatigue, and changes in blood pressure, that tend to fluctuate within a 24-hour period

circumoral cyanosis (Sp. cianosis circumoral) a bluish discoloration around the mouth

clean-catch urine specimen (Sp. espécimen de orina limpia) a urine specimen obtained by cleaning the genitalia and then capturing a midstream urine sample for laboratory analysis

clonic (Sp. clónico) pertaining to increased reflex activity

closed reduction (Sp. reducción cerrada) the nonsurgical manipulative reduction of a dislocation or fracture

coagulation (Sp. coagulación) the process of clot formation

cognitive (Sp. cognitivo) pertaining to the mental processes of thinking, knowing, remembering, and perceiving

collateral (Sp. colateral) a small side branch of a blood vessel or nerve

colporrhaphy (Sp. colporrafia) suturing of the vagina

colposcopy (Sp. colcospia) examination of the vagina and cervix with an optical magnifying instrument frequently associated with biopsy of the cervix

comedo (comedones) (Sp. comedón) a blackhead, as seen in acne

commissurotomy (Sp. comisurotomía) surgical incision of component parts at the sites of junction between adjacent cusps of the heart valves to increase the size of the opening

comorbid (Sp. comórbido) two or more existing medical conditions

computed tomography (CT) (Sp. tomografía asistida por computadora [TAC]) a diagnostic technique using ionizing x-rays passed through a patient around specific sections of the body at multiple angles; useful in the detection of tumors

continuous positive airway pressure (CPAP) (Sp. presión positiva continua de las vías respiratorias [CPAP]) a form of respiratory therapy in which ventilation is assisted by a flow of oxygen delivered at a constant pressure throughout the respiratory cycle

contracture (Sp. contractura) immobility of muscles or a joint caused by shortening or wasting of tissue or muscle fibers

contrecoup a type of brain injury in which the tissue damage is on the opposite side of the trauma site

controlled drug (Sp. drogas controladas) a drug regulated by the Federal Controlled Substance Act

corneal ulcer (Sp. úlcera de la córnea) ulcerative keratitis

corticotropin (Sp. corticotropina u hormona adrenocorticotrópica) a hormone secreted by the anterior lobe of the pituitary; also known as *adrenocorticotropic hormone (ACTH)*

cortisol (Sp. coritsol) major natural glucocorticoid synthesized in the adrenal cortex

craniotomy (Sp. craneotomía) incision into the skull—usually to relieve pressure, to remove a lesion, or to control bleeding

creatinine (Sp. creatinina) an important nitrogen compound that is a normal constituent of urine and blood; increased levels may indicate renal damage

Credé method (maneuver) (Sp. maniobra/método de Credé) manual external compression of the bladder to aid in expulsion of urine

cryoablation (Sp. crioablación) the removal of tissue by destroying it with extreme cold

cryotherapy (Sp. crioterapia) the therapeutic use of cold

cryptorchidism (Sp. criptorquidismo) failure of one or both testicles to descend into the scrotum

cul-de-sac (Sp. fondo de saco) an area at the end of the abdominal cavity that is midway between the rectum and the uterus

curettage (Sp. curetaje/legrado) the removal of growths or other material from the wall of a cavity or other surface

cyanosis, cyanotic (Sp. cianosis, cianótico) bluish appearance of the skin and mucous membrane that usually indicates reduced hemoglobin levels in blood

cytology, cytologic (Sp. citología, citológico) the scientific study of cells

cytoreduction (Sp. citorreducción) a decrease in the number of cells (such as in a tumor)

D

débride (Sp. desbridar) remove foreign material or dead tissue in a wound

deficit (Sp. déficit) a deficiency from what is normal

delusion (Sp. falsa ilusión) a fixed false belief

demise (Sp. fallecimiento) destruction or death

demyelination (Sp. desmielinización) loss of the myelin sheath of a nerve

dermatome (Sp. dermatoma) a configured zone of skin innervated by a spinal cord segment

dialysate (Sp. dializado) the fluid that passes through an impermeable membrane during dialysis

dialysis (dialyses) (Sp. diálisis) a procedure that filters out unwanted substances from the blood, usually in cases of renal failure

diaphoresis, diaphoretic (Sp. diaforesis, diaforético) profuse perspiration

diplopia (Sp. diplopía) double vision

discoid (Sp. discoide) shaped like a disk

diuresis, diuretic (Sp. diuresis, diurético) increased formation and excretion of urine

Doppler (Sp. Doppler) ultrasonogram, Doppler ultrasonography ultrasonographic technique used to evaluate blood flow velocity

dorsiflexion (Sp. dorsiflexión) to bend a joint toward the posterior aspect of the body; for example, the hand is dorsiflexed when it is extended or bent backward at the wrist

drusen (Sp. drusen) small yellowish deposits that develop beneath the retina; commonly associated with age-related macular degeneration

dyscrasia (Sp. discrasia) a pathologic condition; an abnormal condition of blood

dyspareunia (Sp. dispareunia) pain or discomfort in the pelvis or the vagina during or after sexual intercourse

dysphagia (Sp. disfagia) difficulty swallowing

dysphasia (Sp. disfasia) difficulty speaking, usually caused by a lesion in the central nervous system

dysphonia (Sp. disfonía) hoarseness; difficulty speaking

dysplastic, dysplasia (Sp. displástico) marked by abnormal adult cells

dyspnea (Sp. dispnea) labored or difficult breathing

dysrhythmia (Sp. disritmia) an abnormal cardiac rhythm

dysuria (Sp. disuria) painful or difficult urination

E

ecchymosis (Sp. equimosis) discoloration of the skin associated with a contusion

echocardiogram, echocardiography, echocardiographic (Sp. ecocardiograma, ecocardiografía, ecocar-diográfico) an ultrasonographic study of the motion of the walls or structures of the heart

ectopic (Sp. ectópico) out of normal position

effacement (Sp. borramiento) the thinning or obliteration of the cervix during labor

electrocardiogram (ECG), electrocardiography, electrocardiographic (Sp. electrocardiograma, electrocardiografía, electrocardiográfico) a record of the electrical activity of the heart

electromyogram (EMG), electromyography, electromyographic (Sp. electromiograma, electromiografía, electromiográfico) an electrodiagnostic assessment of the activity of skeletal muscles

embolization (Sp. embolismo) a treatment that blocks the flow of blood (i.e., to "starve" a tumor)

embolus (emboli), embolism (Sp. émbolo) a mass (e.g., foreign body, blood clot, or a piece of tumor) that breaks off and causes occlusion of an artery

emergency medical service (EMS) (Sp. servicios médicos de urgencia [SMU]) trained services provided on the scene

empyema (Sp. empiema) accumulation of pus in a hollow organ; abscess

encephalitis (Sp. encefalitis) inflammation of the brain

endarterectomy (Sp. endarterectomía) the surgical excision of the innermost lining of an artery to remove blockage

endemic (Sp. endémico) condition in which a disease is prevalent in a particular geographic area or in a population

endometriosis (Sp. endometriosis) a growth of endometrial tissue at various sites outside the uterus

endometrium (Sp. endometrio) the lining of the uterus that changes with the menstrual cycle; if the ovum is fertilized, the endometrium serves as the place where implantation occurs

endorphins (Sp. endorfina) one of the body's own morphine-like pain killers

endoscopy (Sp. endoscopia) examination of any cavity of the body with an endoscope

enzyme-linked immunosorbent assay (ELISA) (Sp. prueba de inmunoabsorción enzimática [prueba ELISA]) a test used to detect antibodies to the virus (human immunodeficiency virus [HIV]) that causes acquired immunodeficiency syndrome (AIDS) in serum

epidural (Sp. epidural) an anesthetic injected into the epidural space around the spine, often used in labor and delivery

epigastric (Sp. epigástrico) refers to the upper middle region of the abdomen

epiphysis (epiphyses), epiphyseal (Sp. epifisis, epifiseal) the long end of a bone where bone growth occurs

epistaxis (Sp. epistaxis) bleeding from the nose

ergonomics (Sp. ergonomía) the science concerned with people and their work; it explores mechanical principles enhancing efficiency and well-being in the work environment

ergot (Sp. cornezuelo) a drug obtained from a fungus that grows on rye plants

erythema (Sp. eritema) redness or inflammation of the skin produced by capillary congestion

erythrocyte sedimentation rate (ESR) (Sp. tasa de sedimentación eritrocítica) a measurable reflection of the acute-phase reaction in inflammation and infection

esophagoscopy (Sp. esofagoscopia) examination of the esophagus with an esophagoscope

exacerbation (Sp. exacerbación) an increase in the severity of a disease or aggravation of its symptoms

exotoxin (Sp. exotoxina) bacterial toxins excreted outside of the bacterial cell

exsanguination (Sp. desangramiento) excessive loss of blood from a body part

exudate, exudative (Sp. exudado) fluid, cells, or cellular debris that has oozed into tissue because of injury or swelling

F

fascia (Sp. fascia) a fibrous membrane that covers, separates, and supports the muscles

fasciculation (Sp. fasciculación) involuntary contraction or twitching of muscles

fibrin (Sp. fibrina) a protein material produced by the action of thrombin on fibrinogen

fibrosis, fibrotic (Sp. fibrosis, fibrótico) the abnormal formation of fibrous tissue

fissure (Sp. fisura) a crack or groove on a surface

fistula (Sp. fístula) an abnormal tubelike passageway

fluorescein angiography (Sp. angiografía fluoresceínica) a procedure in which light-sensitive material is injected into a blood vessel

foramen (foramina) (Sp. foramen) an opening or hole in a bone, allowing the passage of nerves or blood vessels

foramen ovale (Sp. agujero ovale) an opening in the septum between the right and left atria of the fetal heart

Fowler position (Sp. posición de Fowler) a semisitting position, usually at 45 degrees, used to facilitate breathing and drainage

fulguration (Sp. fulguración) tissue destruction with high-frequency electrical sparks

fulminant (Sp. fulminante) occurring with great intensity; refers to severe pain with sudden onset

G

gamete (Sp. gameto) male or female sex cell

gangrene (Sp. gangrena) death of tissue caused by a decrease or absence of blood supply

gastrectomy (Sp. gastrectomía) surgical removal of the stomach

gastroscopy (Sp. gastroscopía) visual examination of the stomach using a gastroscope

genitourinary (Sp. genitourinario) referring to the genital and urinary systems of the body

Giemsa stain (Sp. tinción de Giemsa) a process of staining bacteria for identification

glenoid (Sp. glenoideo) having the semblance of a socket

glomerulosclerosis (Sp. glomeruloesclerosis) hardening of the renal glomerulus

glomerulus (glomeruli) (Sp. glomérulo) a tiny ball of microscopic blood vessels on the end of the renal tubules

glucosteroid (Sp. glucosteroid) steroid produced by the adrenal cortex

goitrogenic (Sp. bociógeno) pertaining to substances causing goiters

gonadotropin (Sp. gonadotropina) a hormone that stimulates the testes and the ovaries to function

Gram staining (Sp. coloración de Gram) a process of staining bacteria for identification

Guthrie test (Sp. prueba de Guthrie) a test to detect phenylketonuria

gynecomastia (Sp. ginecomastia) abnormal enlargement of breast tissue in men

H

H2-receptor antagonist (Sp. antagonista del receptor H2) chemical agent that blocks the interaction of histamine or acetylcholine with receptors in stomach cells; drugs that inhibit secretion of gastric acid

hallucination (Sp. alucinación) a false perception of reality; may be visual, auditory, or olfactory

hallux (Sp. hallux) the great toe

hematemesis (Sp. hematemesis) vomiting of blood

hematocrit (Sp. hematocrito) the percentage of the total blood volume consisting of erythrocytes

hematoma (Sp. hematoma) localized swelling filled with blood as a result of a broken blood vessel

hematopoiesis, hematopoietic (Sp. hematopoyesis, hematopoyético) pertaining to the production and the development of blood cells or a substance that stimulates their production

hematuria (Sp. hematuria) blood in urine

hemiparesis (Sp. hemiparesia) paralysis affecting one side of the body

hemoccult (Sp. hemoccult) trademark for a guaiac reagent strip test for occult blood

hemochromatosis (Sp. hemochromatosis) a rare inherited disease of iron metabolism characterized by excess iron deposits in the body; a bronze color of the skin may be noticed

hemodynamic (Sp. hemodinámica) refers to forces involved in the circulation of blood within the body

hemolysis, hemolytic (Sp. hemólisis, hemolítico) the destruction of red blood cells with the release of hemoglobin

hemoptysis (Sp. hemoptisis) spitting up of blood

hemostasis (Sp. hemostasis) the condition of controlled bleeding

hepatomegaly (Sp. hepatomegalia) enlargement of the liver

histoplasmosis (Sp. histoplasmosis) a systemic respiratory disease caused by a fungus

homeostasis (Sp. homeostasis) a state of equilibrium within the body

human chorionic gonadotropin (hCG) (Sp. gonadotropina coriónica humana [GCH]) hormones produced by the placenta and detected in the urine and blood of a pregnant woman

humoral (Sp. humoral) refers to body fluids or substances found in them

hyaline membrane (Sp. membrana hialina) a membrane that forms in the lung sacs of a developing fetus; a respiratory distress syndrome of the newborn

hydronephrosis (Sp. hidronefrosis) accumulation of urine in the renal pelvis caused by obstruction, forming a cyst

hymen (Sp. himen) the membrane partially covering the entrance to the vagina

hyperabduction (Sp. hyperabducción) abduction beyond normal limits

hyperalimentation (Sp. hiperalimentación) infusion of life-sustaining fluids, electrolytes, and elements of nutrition intravenously or via the gastrointestinal tract

hypercapnia (Sp. hipercapnia) increased carbon dioxide levels in blood

hypercoagulable (Sp. hipercoagulable) refers to the increased ability of any substance to coagulate, especially blood

hyperemic (Sp. hiperémico) refers to an excessive amount of blood in a body part or area

hyperesthesia (Sp. hiperestesia) increased sensitivity to pain

hyperglycemia (Sp. hiperglicemia) an increase in the normal blood glucose level

hyperkalemia (Sp. hipercalemia) a greater than normal amount of potassium in blood

hyperkeratosis (Sp. hyperqueratosis) results when an excess of proteins called *keratins* are produced, leading to thickening of the skin

hyperlipidemia (Sp. hiperlipemia) an increase of fat levels in blood

hyperparathyroidism (Sp. hiperparatiroidismo) a condition caused by overactive parathyroid glands

hyperplasia (Sp. hiperplasia) abnormal multiplication of the number of cells resulting from an increased rate of cellular division

hypertrophy, hypertrophic (Sp. hipertrofia, hipertrófico) enlargement of an organ or structure

hyperuricemia (Sp. hiperuricemia) excessive uric acid levels in blood

hypoalbuminemia (Sp. hipoalbuminemia) low albumin levels in blood

hypocalcemia (Sp. hipocalcemia) low calcium levels in blood

hypogammaglobulinemia (Sp. hypogammaglobulinemia) a below normal concentration of gamma globulin in blood associated with a decreased resistance to infection

hypogonadism (Sp. hipogonadismo) a condition resulting from a deficiency in the secretions of the ovary or the testis

hypokalemia (Sp. hipocalemia) low potassium levels in blood

hypoparathyroidism (Sp. hipoparatiroidismo) a condition caused by greatly reduced function of the parathyroid glands

hypothalamus (Sp. hipotálamo) a portion of the diencephalon of the brain

hypovolemic shock (Sp. choque hipovolémico) a condition that occurs when blood in the circulatory system is decreased (e.g., as a result of hemorrhage)

hypoxia (Sp. hipoxia) low oxygen levels in tissues

hysterosalpingography (Sp. histerosalpingografía) radiographic images of the uterus and the fallopian tubes

I

iatrogenic (Sp. iatrogénica) pathology inadvertently introduced by medical treatment or a diagnostic procedure

idiopathic (Sp. idiopático) refers to a disease without a known or recognizable cause

immunocompetent (Sp. inmunocompetente) the immune system has the ability to defend the body against disease

immunocompromised (Sp. con inmunidad comprometida) refers to an immune system incapable of fighting disease

immunodeficiency (Sp. inmunodeficiencia) the diminished ability of the immune system to react with appropriate cellular immunity response; often the result of loss of immunoglobulins or aberrance of B- or T-cell lymphocytes

immunoelectrophoresis (Sp. inmunoelectroforesis) a technique used to separate and allow identification of complex proteins

immunogen (Sp. inmunógeno) an antigen (i.e., a substance capable of stimulating an immune response)

immunoglobulin (Sp. inmunoglobulina) a protein that can act as an antibody

immunoincompetence (Sp. inmunoincompetencia) immunodeficiency

immunosenescence (Sp. Inmunosenescencia) the gradual advanced age-related deterioration of the immune system that increases the risk for, and severity of, infection in the older adults

immunosuppressive (Sp. inmunosupresor) having the property of suppressing the body's immune response to antigens

incompetent cervix (Sp. cervix incompetente) premature painless dilation of the cervical os during pregnancy

infarct, infarction (Sp. infarto, infartado) an area of dead tissue caused by lack of blood supply

inguinal (Sp. inguinal) pertaining to the groin

insidious (Sp. insidioso) refers to the onset of a disease without symptoms

intractable (Sp. incurable) incurable or resistant to treatment

intravenous pyelogram, intravenous pyelography (Sp. pielograma intravenoso, pielografía intravenosa) radiographic study of the renal pelvis and ureter using injected dye

intravenous urogram, intravenous urography (Sp. urograma intravenoso, urografía intravenosa) radiographic study of the urinary tract using injected dye

intrinsic (Sp. intrínseco) refers to the essential nature of a substance or structure

intrinsic factor (Sp. factor intrínseco) a substance normally found in gastric juices; essential for the absorption of vitamin B_{12}

iontophoresis (Sp. iontoforesis) the therapeutic introduction of ions into the body tissues by direct current

Ischemia, ischemic (Sp. isquemia, isquémico) holding back or obstructing the flow of blood

ischemic necrosis (Sp. necrosis isquémica) the death or sloughing off of small areas of tissue or bone, caused by insufficient circulation or lack of blood supply

J

jaundice (Sp. ictericia) yellowing of the skin

K

karyotype (Sp. cariotipo) a picture of chromosomes in the nucleus of a cell

Kegel exercises (Sp. ejercicios de Kegel) isometric pelvic exercises used by women to strengthen pelvic muscles and/or to improve retention of urine

keratin (Sp. queratina) a hard protein substance found in hair, nails, and skin

keratoconjunctivitis sicca (Sp. queratoconjuntivitis seca) dryness of the conjunctiva resulting from a decrease in lacrimal function

keratolytic (Sp. queratolítico) a substance that causes shedding of skin

keratosis (Sp. keratosis) a skin lesion where there is overgrowth and thickening of cornified epithelium

keratotomy (Sp. queratotomia) surgical incision of the cornea

kernicterus (Sp. kernicterus) a form of icterus (bile pigmentation of tissues and membranes) occurring in infants

ketone (Sp. cetona) acid chemical that builds up in blood when the body burns fats instead of glucose

L

laparoscopy (Sp. laparoscopia) a surgical procedure to examine the abdomen by using an endoscope called a *laparoscope*

laryngectomy (Sp. laringectomía) surgical removal of the organ of voice (larynx)

laryngoscopy (Sp. laringoscopia) visual examination of the larynx by using a laryngoscope

laser ablation (Sp. ablación por láser) separation, detachment, destruction, or removal of a part using laser surgery

laser photocoagulation (Sp. fotocoagulación por láser) coagulation of the blood vessels in the eye by using a laser

lavage (Sp. lavado) the cleaning out of a cavity by using liquid

leukocoria (Sp. leucocoria) the appearance of a whitish "reflection" or mass in the pupillary area behind the lens of the eye

leukocytosis (Sp. leucocitosis) a slight increase in the number of white blood cells

leukopenia (Sp. leucopenia) a decrease in the number of white blood cells

leukorrhea (Sp. leucorrea) a white or yellow mucous discharge from the vagina

lipase (Sp. lipasa) a fat-splitting enzyme produced by the pancreas

liposome (Sp. liposoma) a small, spherical particle in an aqueous solution, formed by a bilayer of phospholipid molecules

lithotripsy (Sp. litotripsia) crushing of stones (e.g., kidney stones and gallstones)

lumbar puncture (Sp. punción lumbar) a surgical procedure to withdraw spinal fluid for analysis or the injection of an anesthetic solution

lumpectomy (Sp. tumorectomía) removal of just the tumor from the breast

lymph (Sp. linfa) a mostly clear, colorless, transparent, alkaline fluid found within the lymphatic vessels; formed in tissues throughout the body

lymphadenitis (Sp. linfadenitis) inflammation of the lymph nodes

lymphadenopathy (Sp. linfadenopatía) disease of the lymph nodes

lymphocyte (Sp. linfocito) one of two types (B cells and T cells) of leukocytes (white blood cells) found in blood, lymph, and lymphoid tissue

lymphocytosis (Sp. linfocitosis) an excessive number of lymph cells

M

macrophage (Sp. macrófago) a monocyte blood cell

macula (Sp. mácula) a small spot or a colored area

maculopapular (Sp. maculopapular) pertaining to or consisting of macules and papules

magnetic resonance imaging (MRI) (Sp. formación de imágenes por resonancia magnética [RM]) a procedure similar to computed tomography and does not require radiation; a large magnetic field is applied and creates an image; useful in visualizing the cardiovascular system, brain, and soft tissues

malaise (Sp. malestar) a feeling of discomfort, illness, or uneasiness

malocclusion (Sp. maloclusión) improper positioning and faulty contact of teeth

mastectomy (Sp. mastectomía) surgical removal of breast tissue; can be partial or radical

McBurney point (Sp. punto de McBurney) the point of special tenderness in acute appendicitis; corresponds with the normal position of the base of the appendix

meconium (Sp. meconio) the first stool of a newborn, greenish black and with a tarry consistency

mediastinal shift (Sp. desplazamiento mediastinal) abnormal movement of the structures within the mediastinum to one side of the chest cavity

mediastinum (Sp. mediastino) the area in the chest between the lungs

megakaryocyte (Sp. megacariocito) a large bone marrow cell having large or many nuclei

megaloblastic (Sp. megaloblástico) pertaining to abnormally large red blood cells found in pernicious anemia

meibomian gland (Sp. glándula de chalazion) a sebaceous gland on the posterior margin of each eyelid

melanin (Sp. melanina) the black pigment found in the basal layer of the epidermis

melena (Sp. melena) the passage of very dark, tarry stools stained with digested blood

meningitis (Sp. meningitis) inflammation of the coverings around the brain and the spinal cord (meninges)

menorrhagia (Sp. menorragia) painful menstruation

metabolic acidosis (Sp. acidosis metabólica) excessive acid in body fluids, caused by dehydration, diarrhea, vomiting, renal disease, or hepatic impairment

metaplastic (Sp. metaplástico) characterized by metaplasia (a reversible change of cells usually caused by stress or injury); cancer formation can occur with chronic inducing stimulus by injury or irritation

metastasis (metastases), metastatic, metastasize (Sp. metástasis, metastásico, metastatizar) spreading of a malignant disease or pathogenic microorganisms from one organ or body part to another not directly connected with it

metatarsophalangeal (Sp. metatarsofalángico) pertaining to the metatarsus and phalanges of the toes

metrorrhagia (Sp. metrorragia) irregular menstruation

monoclonal antibodies (MAB) (Sp. anticuerpos monoclonales [MAB]) antibodies produced from a single clone of B lymphocytes

monocyte (Sp. monocito) a phagocytic white blood cell that engulfs and destroys cellular debris

multiparous (Sp. multiparos) having had multiple pregnancies

murine (Sp. roedor) pertaining to mice or rats

murmur (Sp. murmullo) a blowing sound heard when listening to the heart or vessels with a stethoscope

mutation (Sp. mutación) a variation or change in genetic structure

mutism (Sp. mutismo) the condition of being unable to speak

myalgia (Sp. mialgia) muscle pain

mycoplasma (Sp. micoplasma) microscopic organisms that lack a rigid cell wall; some species cause infections in humans

myelin (Sp. mielina) the protective fat and protein covering around the axons of many nerves

myelogram, myelography (Sp. mielograma, mielografía) radiographic study of the spinal cord after the injection of a dye

myringotomy (Sp. miringotomía) a surgical incision of the eardrum performed to release fluid or pus from the middle ear

N

necrosis, necrotic (Sp. necrosis, necrótico) death of tissue

neoadjuvant therapy (Sp. quimioterapia) a preliminary cancer treatment

neonate (Sp. neonato) a newborn baby

neoplasm, neoplasia, neoplastic (Sp. neoplasma, neoplasia, neoplástico) abnormal formation of new tissue; can be benign or malignant

neovascularization (Sp. neovascularización) the formation of new blood vessels

nephrectomy (Sp. nefrectomía) the surgical removal of a kidney

nephron (Sp. nefrona) the functioning unit of the kidney or renal tubule

nephropathy (Sp. nefropatía) any disease or damage of the kidney

nephrotoxic (Sp. nefrotóxico) a quality of being destructive to kidney tissue

neurotransmitter (Sp. neurotransmisor) a chemical released by the terminal end fibers of an axon

nociceptor (Sp. nociceptor) nerve that receives and transmits painful stimuli

normal flora (Sp. flora normal) the presence of normal bacteria and fungi adapted for living in, and characteristic of, the area considered (e.g., skin, intestine, or vagina)

nuchal rigidity (Sp. rigidez en la nuca) neck stiffness

nullipara (Sp. nulípara) a woman who has never produced viable offspring

O

odynophagia (Sp. odinofagia) painful swallowing; a severe burning, squeezing pain while swallowing caused by irritation or muscular disorder of the esophagus

oligospermia (Sp. oligospermia) insufficient number of spermatozoa in semen

oliguria (Sp. oliguria) scanty urination

oncogene (Sp. oncógeno) a gene in a virus that can prompt a cell to become malignant

onycholysis (Sp. onicolisis) a spontaneous separation of the nail plate or supporting structures

oophorectomy (Sp. ovariectomía) the surgical removal of one or both ovaries

opacity (Sp. opacidad) the state of being opaque or not transparent

open reduction (Sp. reducción abierta) exposure of a fractured or dislocated bone through a surgical incision to realign the bone ends

ophthalmoscopy, ophthalmoscopic (Sp. oftalmoscopia, oftalmoscópico) an examination of the interior of the eye

opportunistic infection (Sp. infección oportunista) infection resulting from a defective immune system

orchiectomy (Sp. orquiectomía) the surgical removal of one or both testes; also called *orchidectomy*

orchiopexy (Sp. orquidopexia) surgical procedure to mobilize an undescended testis and bring it into the scrotum

orchitis (Sp. orquitis) inflammation of the testes

orthodontics (Sp. ortodoncia) branch of dentistry concerned with correction of dentofacial structures (e.g., teeth)

orthopnea (Sp. ortopnea) a condition in which breathing becomes easier in the upright standing position or in the sitting position

orthoptic training (Sp. entrenamiento ortóptico) eye muscle exercises

Ortolani sign (Sp. prueba de Ortolani) an assessment maneuver designed to detect a hip dislocation

ossification (Sp. osificación) the development of bone

osteogenesis (Sp. osteogénesis) the formation of bone tissue

osteophyte (Sp. osteofito) a bony outgrowth, usually branch shaped

ostomy (Sp. ostomía) a surgical opening of the bowel to the outside of the body

otitis media (Sp. otitis media) middle ear infection

otoscopy (Sp. otoscopia) visual examination of the ear by using an otoscope

oxygen saturation (Sp. saturación de oxígeno) refers to the oxygen content in blood, divided by oxygen capacity, and expressed in volume percent

P

palliative (Sp. paliativo) alleviating symptoms without curing the underlying cause

panhypopituitarism (Sp. panhipopituitarismo) a condition in which the entire pituitary gland ceases to function and is not producing any pituitary hormones

papule (Sp. pápula) a circular area on the skin that is reddened and elevated

parasympathetic (Sp. parasimpático) the division of the autonomic nervous system mediated by the release of acetylcholine, which has many effects on body functions, such as slowing heart rate and stimulating peristalsis

paresis (Sp. paresia) partial paralysis

paresthesia (Sp. parestesia) abnormal, usually increased, sensations

parietal (cells) (Sp. células parietales) the cells on the wall of a cavity, such as the stomach; pertaining to or located near the parietal bone (of the parietal lobe) of the skull

paronychia (Sp. paroniquia) inflammation of soft tissue surrounding the nail

partial thromboplastin time (PTT) (Sp. tiempo parcial de tromboplastina [TPT]) a measure of the coagulation sequence of plasma and screen for platelet abnormalities

patch test (Sp. prueba del parche) a screening test in which a small piece of material containing the allergy-causing substance is placed on the skin; redness or edema indicates a positive reaction

patent (Sp. de patente, accisible) open and unblocked

pathogenesis (Sp. patogénesis) the development of disease; pathologic mechanisms

pathologist (Sp. patologista) one who specializes in the study of disease

peau d'orange (Sp. piel de naranja) condition in which the skin is dimpled, resembling the skin of an orange

pelvic inflammatory disease (PID) (Sp. enfermedad inflamatoria pélvica [EIP]) inflammation of the female pelvic organs, usually caused by bacteria

perfusion (Sp. perfusión) delivery of oxygen and other nutrients to the tissue by blood

pericoronitis (Sp. pericoronitis) inflammation of gum around the crown of a tooth

periosteum (Sp. periostio) the fibrous covering of long bones

peritonitis (Sp. peritonitis) inflammation of the membrane that lines the abdominal cavity and covers the viscera

pessary (Sp. pesario) an object placed in the vagina to support the uterus

petechia (petechiae) (Sp. petequia) a tiny spiderlike hemorrhage under the skin

phagocyte, phagocytic, phagocytosis (Sp. fagocito, fagocítico, fagocitosis) the process by which cells surround and digest certain particles (e.g., bacteria, protozoa, debris)

phenotype (Sp. fenotipo) the entire physical appearance and biochemical and psychological makeup of an individual as determined by the interaction of genetic makeup and environmental factors

phlebotomy (Sp. flebotomía) surgical puncture of a vein to withdraw blood

phonologic (Sp. fonológico) refers to oral communication or vocal sounds

photocoagulation (Sp. fotocoagulación) the coagulation (clotting) of tissue by controlled use of a laser to seal off bleeding blood vessels

photon (Sp. foton) the smallest quantity of electromagnetic energy; a particle with no mass and no charge; may occur in the form of x-rays, gamma rays, or quanta of light

photophobia (Sp. fotofobia) unusual sensitivity to light

phototherapy (Sp. fototerapia) treatment of disease by exposure to light

plaque (Sp. placa) a deposit of hardened material lining a blood vessel; or a gummy accumulation of microorganisms that clings to teeth and is considered the forerunner of caries and periodontal disease

plasmapheresis (Sp. plasmaféresis) the process of separating blood into its components by centrifuging

polydipsia (Sp. polidipsia) excessive thirst

polyphagia (Sp. polfagia) excessive eating

polyposis (Sp. poliposis) a condition of multiple polyps

polyuria (Sp. poliuria) excretion of abnormally large amounts of urine

positive end-expiratory pressure (PEEP) (Sp. presión positiva al final de la expiración [PEEP]) mechanical ventilation with pressure maintained, thereby increasing the volume of gas remaining in the lungs at the end of expiration

positron emission tomography (PET) (Sp. tomografía por emisión de positrones [PET]) a noninvasive radiographic study of the blood flow in specific organs and body tissues

postprandial (Sp. posprandial) after meals

primipara (Sp. primípara) a woman who has delivered one child of at least 20 weeks' gestational age

probiotic (Sp. problotico) a substance that stimulates the growth of microorganisms with beneficial properties (such as those of the intestinal flora)

proctoscopy (Sp. proctoscopia) visual examination of the rectum by using a proctoscope

prodromal (Sp. prodrómico) refers to the initial stage of a disease before the onset of actual symptoms

prophylaxis, prophylactic (Sp. profilaxis, profiláctico) the prevention of disease

prostate-specific antigen (PSA) (Sp. antígeno específico de la próstata [APE]) an enzyme that is measured in a blood test to detect cancer of the prostate

proteinuria (Sp. proteinuria) the presence of protein in urine

prothrombin time (PT) (Sp. tiempo de protrombina [TP]) a measure of the time taken for clot formation

proton pump inhibitor (Sp. inhibidor de la bomba de pro-tones) a drug that blocks gastric acid secretion; used to treat ulcers of the gastrointestinal tract and gastroesophageal reflux disease (GERD)

pruritus (Sp. prurito) itching

pseudomembranous (Sp. membrana pseudo) a false membrane

pseudoneurologic (Sp. pseudoneurológico) refers to a neurologic symptom that is without clinical basis

pseudopregnancy (Sp. pseudoembarazo) false pregnancy, also known as *pseudocyesis*

psychosexual (Sp. psicosexual) refers to the relationship between the psychological and emotional aspects of sex

psychosis, psychotic (Sp. psicosis, sicopático) a major mental disorder usually accompanied by perceptional distortion of reality, regressive behavior, and diminished impulse control

psychotropic drugs (Sp. erogas psicotrópicas) drugs that have an effect on the mind or that alter a person's state of mind

ptosis (Sp. ptosis) drooping of one or both eyelids

purpura (Sp. púrpura) a red-purple discoloration of the skin caused by multiple minute hemorrhages in the skin or mucous membrane

purulent (Sp. purulento) containing pus

pustule (Sp. pústula) a small elevation of the skin containing pus

putrefaction (Sp. putrefacción) decomposition of organic matter

pyelogram, pyelography (Sp. pielografía) radiography of the pelvis of the kidney and ureter by using a contrast solution

pyelonephritis (Sp. pielonefritis) a purulent infection of the kidney tissue and renal pelvis

pylorus (Sp. píloro) the narrow part of the stomach toward the duodenum

pyuria (Sp. piuria) pus in urine

R

raccoon eyes (Sp. ojos de mapache) dark discoloration (bruising) around the eyes; a sign of possible basilar skull fracture

radioimmunoassay (Sp. radioinmunoanálisis) radiology used to detect the concentration of an antigen or antibody or other protein in serum

rale (Sp. estertor) an abnormal crackling sound made by the lungs during inspiration; indicative of fluid in a bronchus

Raynaud phenomenon (Sp. fenómeno de Raynaud) a temporary constriction of arterioles in the skin causing short episodes of numbness and color changes in the fingers and toes; this condition is usually idiopathic

reflux (Sp. reflujo) a backward flow

regenerative medicine (Sp. medicina regenerador) a field where stem cells are induced to differentiate into a specific cell type that can be used to repair damaged tissue

renal calculi (Sp. cálculo renal) kidney stones

reticuloendothelial (Sp. reticuloendotelial) refers to the system responsible for phagocytosis of cellular debris, pathogens, and foreign substances and for removing them from the circulation

retinopathy (Sp. retinopatía) refers to noninflammatory eye disorders

retrovirus (Sp. retrovirus) a family of viruses that contains ribonucleic acid (RNA) and reverse transcriptase; some retroviruses are oncogenic and can cause tumors

rheumatoid factor (Sp. factor reumatoide) a macroglobulin type of antibody; increased levels are found in the blood of persons with rheumatoid arthritis

rhonchus (rhonchi) (Sp. ronquido) dry rattling in the throat or bronchus caused by partial obstruction

ribonucleic acid (RNA) (Sp. ácido ribonucleico [ARN]) controls protein synthesis in cells and takes the place of deoxyribonucleic acid (DNA) in some viruses

S

salpingo-oophorectomy (Sp. anexectomía) the surgical removal of a fallopian tube and an ovary

Schick test (Sp. prueba de Schick) an intradermal skin test to detect immunity to diphtheria; a positive result indicates lack of immunity or negative immunity

Schilling test (Sp. prueba de Schilling) a 24-hour urine test for gastrointestinal absorption of vitamin B_{12}

sclerosis, sclerosing (Sp. esclerosis) hardening of a body part

sclerotherapy (Sp. escleroterapia) use of sclerosing chemicals to treat esophageal varices or hemorrhoids

seborrhea (Sp. seborrea) the excessive secretion of sebum from sebaceous glands

sebum (Sp. sebo) oily secretion of sebaceous glands

semi-Fowler position (Sp. posición semi-Fowler) position of lying on the back with the head elevated 8 to 10 inches and the knees flexed

senile (Sp. senil) refers to growing old with decreased physical and mental capacity

senile plaque (Sp. placa senil) microscopic patch of fragmented nerve around amyloid deposits found in the cerebral cortex of normal older people; found in larger amounts in people with Alzheimer disease

sensorineural (Sp. sensorineural) pertaining to a sensory nerve

septicemia (Sp. septicemia) a disease in which pathogenic microorganisms or toxins are present in blood

sequestrum (Sp. secuestro) a segment of dead bone; the result of an abscess from a bacterial infection in a bone and bone marrow

serology, serologic (Sp. serología, serológico) a study of blood serum to measure antibody titers

sigmoidoscopy (Sp. sigmoidoscopia) examination of the sigmoid colon by using a sigmoidoscope

sinopulmonary (Sp. sinopulmonar) pertaining to the paranasal sinuses and lungs

sinusotomy (Sp. sinusotomia) incision into the sinus

skeletal traction (Sp. tracción ósea) a method of immobilization and reduction of a long-bone fracture, in which traction is applied by means of pins and wires

somatoform (Sp. forma somática) psychogenic symptoms without an underlying disease process

somatotropin (Sp. somatotropina) growth hormone (GH) secreted by the anterior pituitary gland

spermicidal (Sp. espermicidal) destructive to sperm

splenomegaly (Sp. esplenomegalia) enlarged spleen

squamous cell (Sp. células escamosas) flat and scaly epithelial cell

status asthmaticus (Sp. estado asmático) severe asthmatic episode that does not respond to normal treatment

steatorrhea (Sp. esteatorrea) the presence of malabsorbed fat in feces

stenosis, stenosed (Sp. estenosis, estenosado) narrowing of an opening

stent (Sp. stent) a device used to hold tissue in place or provide support

Steri-Strips (Sp. Steri-Strips) trademarked brand name for sterile adhesive strips used to approximate and hold together the edges of a wound

stomatitis (Sp. estomatitis) an inflammatory condition of the mouth

stress incontinence (Sp. incontinencia por presión) leakage of urine when stress is placed on the perineum

stridor (Sp. estridor) a high-pitched respiratory sound caused by obstruction of air passageway

subluxation (Sp. subluxación) partial dislocation

substernal retraction (Sp. retracción del esternón) condition in which the chest wall under the sternum sinks in with each respiration

sulfonylurea (Sp. sulfonilurea) oral hypoglycemic agent that stimulates the pancreas to produce insulin

supine (Sp. supino) lying on the back

surfactant (Sp. agente de superficie) an agent (normally present in the lungs as a phospholipid) that lowers surface tension; abnormal in the lungs of premature infants or in hyaline membrane disease

symptomatic (Sp. sintomático) concerning the nature of a symptom indicative of a disease

syncope (Sp. sincope) fainting, lightheadedness

syncytial virus (Sp. virus de sincytial) a type of minute parasitic microorganism

synovial (Sp. sinovial) pertaining to a lubrication fluid around a joint, bursa, and tendon sheath

synthesize (Sp. sintetizar) to produce a substance by combining two or more elements or chemicals

T

tachycardia, tachycardic (Sp. taquicardia, taquicár-dico) rapid heartbeat; greater than 100 beats per minute

tachypnea (Sp. taquipnea) rapid and shallow respirations

tamponade (Sp. tamponar) compression of a part by pressure or a collection of fluid

tendinitis (Sp. tendinitis) inflammation of a tendon

tenesmus (Sp. tenesmo) ineffectual spasms of the rectum accompanied by a desire to empty the bowel; sometimes mistaken as constipation

tetany (Sp. tetania) hyperexcitability of nerves and muscles resulting from low serum calcium levels; a syndrome characterized by intermittent tonic spasms of the extremities, cramps, and convulsions

tetralogy of Fallot (Sp. tetralogía de Fallot) a congenital cardiac condition

tetraplegia (Sp. tetraplejia) another term for quadriplegia; the inability of a person to move the upper and lower extremities; impaired mobility includes the upper and lower extremities; the head, neck, and shoulders may or may not be affected, depending on the level of injury to the spine

thallium scan (Sp. escáner con talio) a cardiac stress test using intravenous thallium injection to diagnose ischemia and coronary artery disease

thoracentesis (Sp. toracentesis) surgical puncture into the parietal cavity for aspiration of fluids

thoracostomy (Sp. toracotomía) an incision in the chest wall for the purpose of drainage; a chest tube may be inserted for drainage of air or fluid from the pleural space

thrill (Sp. estremecimiento) vibration felt on palpation, especially over the heart

thrombocytopenia (Sp. trombocitopenia) reduced number of thrombocytes (platelets)

thrombus (Sp. trombo) a blood clot attached to the interior wall of a blood vessel, often causing vascular obstruction

thyroidectomy (Sp. tiroidectomía) surgical removal of the thyroid gland

thyrotoxicosis (Sp. thyrotoxicosis) a toxic condition caused by hyperactivity of the thyroid gland

thyrotropin (Sp. tirotropina) thyroid-stimulating hormone (TSH)

tinnitus (Sp. tinnitus) ringing or buzzing in the ears

tonometry (Sp. tonometría) measurement of intraocular pressure

toxin, toxic (Sp. toxina, tóxico) poisonous substance

toxoplasmosis (Sp. toxoplasmosis) a disease caused by infection with protozoa found in many mammals and birds

transcutaneous electrical nerve stimulation (TENS) (Sp. estimulación nerviosa eléctrica transcutánea [ENET]) electrical stimulation of nerves for relief of pain

transferrin (Sp. transferrina) globulin in blood serum that transports iron

triiodothyronine (T₃) (Sp. triyodotironina) a hormone that helps regulate growth and development, metabolism, and body temperature

trisomy (Sp. anormalidad chromosomal) one or more than the normal number of chromosomes

Trousseau phenomenon (Sp. fenómeno de Trousseau) sign in which pressure applied to the upper arm produces muscular spasms, indicating latent tetany

truss (Sp. braguero) a device that holds a reduced hernia in place

tumor necrosis factor (Sp. factor de necrosis de tumor) a natural body protein with anticancer effects; also produced in response to bacterial toxins (can be produced synthetically)

turgor (Sp. turgor) normal tension in a cell that results in normal strength and tension of the skin

tympanic membrane (Sp. membrana del tímpano) eardrum

Tzanck test (Sp. análisis de Tzanck) diagnostic test that examines the tissue of a lesion to determine the type of cell present

U

ulcer, ulceration (Sp. úlcera, ulceración) a craterlike sore on the skin or mucous membrane

ultrasonogram, ultrasonography (Sp. ultrasonografía) imaging deep structures of the body using high-frequency sound waves

ultrasound diathermy (Sp. diatermia por ultrasonidos) medical diathermy (heating of body tissue) by using ultrasound

uremia (Sp. uremia) toxic condition of excessive waste products, protein, and nitrogen in blood caused by renal insufficiency

urethritis (Sp. uretritis) inflammation of the urethra

urodynamics (Sp. urodinámica) study of the mechanics of urinary bladder, filling and emptying liquid

urothelium (Sp. urotelio) transitional epithelium in the wall of the bladder

V

vaginismus (Sp. vaginismo) a spasm of the muscles surrounding the vagina, causing painful contractions of the vagina

Valsalva maneuver (Sp. maniobra de Valsalva) forced exhalation with the mouth and nose closed, causing increased intrathoracic pressure, slowing of heart rate, increased venous pressure, and a reduced amount of return blood flow to the heart

varicocele (Sp. varicocele) a condition in which the veins in the scrotum near the testicles are swollen and enlarged

vector (Sp. vector) carrier of infectious agent of disease from one person to another (usually insects)

venom (Sp. veneno) poison secreted by an animal

ventricular shift (Sp. desplazamiento ventricular) lateral movement of one of the ventricles of the brain to one side caused by pressure on the other side

vertex (Sp. vertex) top of the head

vertigo (Sp. vértigo) loss of equilibrium or sensation of instability; dizziness

vesicle (Sp. vesícula) a small blister-like elevation of the skin containing clear fluid

vitrectomy (Sp. vitrectomía) a surgical procedure that removes the contents of the vitreous chamber of the eye

W

Western blot test (Sp. prueba Western blot) a laboratory blood test to identify and analyze specific protein antigens; sometimes used to confirm the validity of the enzyme-linked immunosorbent assay (ELISA) test

wheal (Sp. ampolla) a smooth, round, elevated area of the skin with red edges and a white center, usually accompanied by itching; hives

white blood cell (WBC), WBC count (Sp. glóbulos blancos, conteo de glóbulos blancos) see Appendix I, Common Laboratory and Diagnostic Tests, under Blood Analysis

X

xerostomia (Sp. xerostomía) dry mouth; reduced amount of saliva

Z

zygote (Sp. zigoto) fertilized ovum

Index

A

ABCDEs of malignant melanoma, 230b
Abdominal bloating, in ascites, 316f
Abdominal hernia, 307–309, 308f
Abdominal locations, of undescended
    testes, 63, 63f
Abdominal pain, in peritonitis, 320
Abducens nerve (VI), 164t, 536–537b
Ablation, cardiac, 414b
Abnormal curvatures of spine, 248–252
Abnormal skin pigmentation
    abnormal suntan, 233–234
    albinism, 231, 231f
    description, 231
    hemangiomas, 232, 233f
    melasma (chloasma), 232, 232f
    nevi (moles), 232–233, 233f
    patient screening, 231
    pityriasis, 233
    vitiligo, 231, 232f
Abortion, spontaneous, 517–518
Abrasion, 621
    corneal, 175–176
    description, 621
    treatment and prognosis, 622
Abruptio placentae, 521–522
Abscesses
    brain, 568–569
    furuncles and carbuncles, 218–219
    in peritonitis, 320f
    pulmonary, 360, 360f
    tooth, 289–290
Absence seizures, 558
Absorption atelectasis, 356f
Abuse
    alcohol, 589–592
    child, 652–654
    drugs of abuse, 592
    elder, 655–656
    psychological or verbal, 656–657
    sexual, 658–659
    substance, 592b
Acarbose, 156
Acid-base balance, respiratory system
    role in, 343
Acidosis, 154
Acinar cells, pancreatic, 330f
Acne vulgaris
    description, 214–215
    diagnosis, 215
    etiology, 215
    patient screening, 215
    patient teaching, 215
    prevention, 215
    prognosis, 215
    symptoms and signs, 215
    treatment and prognosis, 215
Acoustic neuroma, 200f
Acquired hypogammaglobulinemia, 109

Acquired immunodeficiency syndrome.
    See AIDS (acquired immunodeficiency
    syndrome)
Acquired rubella, 78, 79f
Acrochordon (skin tag), 226–227, 227f
Acromegaly, 140f
    etiology and diagnosis, 140
    patient teaching, 141
    symptoms and signs, 140
Acrophobia, 605t
Acrosome reaction, 32–33f
ACTH (adrenocorticotropic hormone),
    138t, 139f
    deficiency of, 154f
Actinic keratosis
    diagnosis, 227
    etiology, 227
    patient teaching, 227
    prevention, 227
    prognosis, 227
    treatment, 227
Active immunity, 103–105
Actos. *See* Pioglitazone
Acupressure, 26
Acupuncture, 23, 26
Acute angle-closure glaucoma, 178–179,
    179f
Acute appendicitis, 305–306, 305f
Acute bronchitis, 365–366
Acute cystitis, 467f
Acute disease, 2
Acute epiglottitis, 82–83, 82f
Acute glomerulonephritis, 451–454
Acute inflammation, 3
    conjunctivitis as, 173–174
Acute lymphocytic leukemia (ALL), 433
Acute myelogenous leukemia (AML),
    434–435
Acute necrotizing ulcerative gingivitis, 292
Acute otitis media, 189, 190f, 197
Acute pain, 23
Acute pancreatitis, 330–331, 331f
    etiology and diagnosis, 330–331
    symptoms and signs, 330
    treatment and prognosis, 331
Acute promyelocytic leukemia (APL), 435
Acute renal failure, 459
Acute stress reaction, 606t
Acute tonsillitis, 83
Acyanotic cardiac defects
    atrial septal defect, 58
    coarctation of aorta, 56
    patent ductus arteriosus, 56
    patient screening, 56
    ventricular septal defect, 56
Addison disease
    etiology and diagnosis, 153
    symptoms and signs, 153
    treatment and prognosis, 153

Addisonian crisis, 153
Adenocarcinoma, 294
    of distal rectum, 315f
    of oral cavity, 294–295
Adenohypophysis, 139f
Adenoid hyperplasia, 83–84
Adenosarcoma, Wilms tumor, 64–65, 473f
ADHD (attention-deficit/hyperactivity
    disorder), 581–582
Adhesions
    as intestinal obstruction, 313f
    in peritonitis, 320f
Adhesive capsulitis, 272
Adipose tissue, of breast, 480f
Adrenal cortex
    chronic hypersecretion of, 152
    secretions and functions of, 138t
Adrenal gland diseases, 152–153
    Addison disease, 153
    Cushing syndrome, 152–153, 152f
Adrenal glands, 136f
Adrenal medulla, secretions and functions
    of, 138t
Adrenocorticotropic hormone (ACTH),
    138t, 139f
    deficiency of, 154f
Adult onset diabetes, 154
Adult respiratory distress syndrome (ARDS)
    diagnosis and treatment, 375
    etiology, 375
    patient screening, 374–375
    patient teaching, 375
    prevention, 375
    prognosis, 375
    symptoms and signs, 374
Adverse effects, abnormal suntan as,
    233–234
Aerosols, abuse of, 593–595t
Affect, in depression, 600t
Affect (feeling), schizophrenia, 596
Afferent arteriole, 451f
Afferent lymphatic vessels, 437f
Afferent neuron, 535f
Agammaglobulinemia, X-linked, 110–111
Aganglionic megacolon, congenital,
    66–67
Age, as predisposing factor for disease, 2
Age-related macular degeneration (AMD),
    179–180
Agglutination, 442
    of RBCs, 442f
Aggregation, 444
Aging
    changes in hearing caused by, 198t
    as risk factor for health problems,
    15–16
Agoraphobia, 605t
Agranulocytes, 428f
Agranulocytosis, 430–432

AIDS (acquired immunodeficiency
    syndrome)
  caused by HIV, 105
  diagnosis and treatment, 107–108
  etiology, 106–107
  opportunistic infections, 106b
  pathologic changes associated
      with, 107f
  patient screening, 106
  patient teaching, 108–109
  prognosis and prevention, 108
  symptoms and signs, 105–106
Air cells, mastoid, 196f
Air, in pleural cavity, 370f
Albinism, 231, 231f
Alcohol
  blood alcohol content and body
      weight, 591t
  blood alcohol levels, 590t, 591b
  comparison of amounts of, 591f
  effects of, 593–595t
  metabolized in liver, 591
Alcohol abuse
  description, 589
  etiology and diagnosis, 590
  symptoms and signs, 589–590
  treatment, 590–591
Alcoholics Anonymous (AA), 590–591
Aldosterone, 138t
Algophobia, 605t
Alkalis, strong, 647t
Allergic disease, 14
  contact dermatitis, 206–207f
Allergic reaction, 14f
Alopecia (baldness)
  description, 234, 235f
  diagnosis and treatment, 235
  etiology, 234–235
  patient screening, 234
  patient teaching, 236
  prevention, 235
  prognosis, 235
  symptoms and signs, 234
Alopecia areata, 235f
Alpha-fetoprotein (AFP), in liver cancer,
    326, 327
Altitude sickness, 643b
Alveolar glands, 480f
Alveolar sac, 344f
Alveoli, 344f
  fluid-filled, in ARDS, 375
Alzheimer disease, 560f
  diagnosis and treatment, 584–585
  patient teaching, 586
  symptoms and signs, 584
Amblyopia, 168
Amenorrhea, 498, 499
American Burn Association, 633
Amnesia, transient global, 562–563
Amniocentesis, 34, 515f
Amniotic cavity, 32–33f
Amphetamines, 593–595t
Amphiarthrodial joints, 245
Amputation, 270b
Amsler grid, 180f
Amyloid material, 585
Amyotrophic lateral sclerosis (ALS),
    561–562

Anal canal, 321f
Analgesics, narcotic, 586
Anaphylaxis, 14
Anastomosis, 311
  cardiac arteries, 388f
  ileoanal, 311
Androgen deprivation therapy, 496
Androgenetic alopecia, 235, 235f
Androphobia, 605t
Anemias
  autoimmune hemolytic, 115–116
  description, 428–429
  diagnosis and treatment, 430
  etiology, 429–430
  pernicious, 116–117
  symptoms and signs, 429
Anencephaly, 52–55
Aneurysm
  aortic, in Marfan syndrome, 260f
  cerebral, 543b
  description, 422
  symptoms and signs, 422
  treatment and prognosis, 422–423
Anger, in mourning, 602t
Angina pectoris, 389–390
  cardiac arteries, 388f
Angiography, of cardiac stent, 392f
Angioplasty, 387, 388f
Angle-closure glaucoma, acute, 178–179,
    178f
Animal bites
  animals capable of biting, 643–645
  diagnosis and treatment, 644–645
  patient teaching, 645
  symptoms and signs, 643–644
Ankle sprain, 270f
Ankylosing spondylitis
  etiology and diagnosis, 127
  symptoms and signs, 127
  treatment and prognosis, 127–128
Ankylosis, in RA, 124f
Annulus fibrosus, 553f
Anorexia nervosa, 337f
  description, 337
  etiology and diagnosis, 337
  prognosis and prevention, 338
  symptoms and signs, 337
  treatment, 338
Anosmia, 351
Antabuse. See Disulfiram
Anterior chamber, 164
Anterior pituitary, 138t
  hypopituitarism and, 141
Anthracosis, 369
Anthrax, 652b
Antibiotics, nephrotoxic, 458b
Antibodies, 102
  classes of, 104t
  RBCs destroyed by, 115
Anticoagulant, lupus, 444b
Antidepressants, tricyclic, 586
Antidiabetic agents, 156
Antidiuretic hormone (ADH),
    138t, 139f
  in diabetes insipidus, 142
Antiemetics, 303
Antifungal medications, for tinea infections,
    222

Anti-GBM antibody disease. See
    Goodpasture syndrome
Antigen-antibody complex, 103
Antigens
  in allergic disease, 14
  HLA-B27, 127
Antihistamines, 345–346
  contraindicated in Alzheimer patients,
    586
Antipsychotics, 586
  atypical, 597
Antipyretics, 643
Antisocial disorder, 616
Antisocial personality disorder, 616
Anus
  female, 479f
  male, 478f
Anxiety disorders
  description, 603–604
  generalized anxiety disorder and panic
      disorder, 604
  obsessive-compulsive disorder,
      604–606
  phobic disorder, 604
  posttraumatic stress disorder,
      606–608
  symptoms and signs, 604
Aorta, 382f, 383f
  coarctation of, 56, 57f, 58f
Aortic aneurysm
  in Marfan syndrome, 260f
  types of, 423f
Aortic stenosis, 408f
Aortic valve, chronic rheumatic endocarditis
    of, 407f
Apex of heart, 382f, 383f
Aphasia, 537
Aphthous ulcers, 290
Aplastic anemia, 430, 431t
Apnea, sleep, 614–615
Appendicitis, acute, 305–306
Apple, toxicity of, 647t
Apricot, toxicity of, 647t
Aqueous humor, 164, 177
Arachnoid membrane, 534–535f
Arachnoid villus, 53f
Arachnophobia, 605t
Arch of aorta, 382f, 383f
Arcuate artery, 450f, 451f
Arcuate vein, 451f
ARDS (adult respiratory distress syndrome),
    374–375
Areola, 480f
Arm, 534–535f
  anatomy, 649f
  hyperabduction of, 651
Aromatherapy, 25
Arrector pili muscle, 205f
Arrhythmias, 411–412t
  description, 410
  symptoms and signs, 410
  treatment and prognosis, 410
Arterial blood gases, 679
Arterial embolism, 421f
Arterioles, 418f
Arteriosclerosis, 386–387, 419
Arteriovenous malformation, 540–541f,
    542b

Arthritis
  gout, 257–259
  juvenile RA, 125–126
  Lyme, 254–255
  osteoarthritis, 252–254
  rheumatoid (RA), 123–125
Arthroscopy, 277b
Asbestosis, 369
Ascites, 316, 316f, 322f
Asperger syndrome, 581
Aspiration pneumonia, 358
Aspirin
  contraindications, 345b, 348b
  gastritis caused by, 303f
Asthma, 367
  etiology and diagnosis, 84
  patient teaching, 86
  symptoms and signs, 84
  treatment and prognosis, 84, 85
Astigmatism, 166
Astrophobia, 605t
Asymptomatic patient, 2
Asystole, 392
Ataxic cerebral palsy, 47
Atelectasis
  diagnosis and treatment, 355–356
  etiology, 355
  patient screening, 355
  patient teaching, 356–357
  prevention, 356
  prognosis, 356
  symptoms and signs, 355
Atheroma, 386f
Atherosclerosis, 419
  consequences of, 307f
  systemic, 367f
Athetoid cerebral palsy, 47
Athlete's foot (tinea pedis), 221
Athletic events, prevention of disease spread
    during, 74b
Atopic dermatitis
  description, 209–211
  etiology and diagnosis, 210
  patient screening, 210
  patient teaching, 211
  symptoms and signs, 210
  treatment and prognosis, 210
Atresia, tricuspid, 57f
Atrial fibrillation, 411–412t
Atrial septal defect (ASD), 57f, 58, 58f
Atrial tachycardia, 411–412t
Atria, posterior view, 382f, 383f
Atrioventricular node, 410f
Atrophy, testicular, 322f
Attention-deficit/hyperactivity disorder
    (ADHD)
  description, 581
  diagnosis, 582
  patient teaching, 582
  symptoms and signs, 581–582
  treatment, 582
Atypical antipsychotics, 597
Auditory area, 534–535f, 586f
Auer rod cells, 435f
Aura, 557
Auricle
  of ear, 185, 185f
  of left and right atria, 382f

Autism spectrum disorder, 579–581
  diagnosis, 580
  symptoms and signs, 580
  treatment, 580
Autoimmune diseases, 15, 102
  connective tissue diseases, 120–128
  hematopoietic disorders, 115–119
  neurologic disorders, 128–131
  renal disorders, 119–120
  vasculitis, 131–132
Autoimmune hemolytic anemia
  etiology and diagnosis, 115, 116
  patient teaching, 116
  symptoms and signs, 115
  treatment and prognosis, 116
Autoinoculation, 184
Automated external defibrillator (AED), 392f
Autonomic nervous system (ANS), 535,
    538–539f
Autosomal dominant disease, Robinow
    syndrome, 43b, 44f
Autosomal dominant inheritance, 7
Autosomal recessive disease, Robinow
    syndrome, 44f
Autosomal recessive inheritance, 7
Avandia. See Rosiglitazone maleate
Aviophobia, 605t
Avoidant personality disorder, 616
Avulsion, 245, 621
Avulsion injuries, 622–623
Axon, 531, 535f, 585f
Azalea, toxicity of, 647t

B
Baby blues. See Postpartum depression
Bacterial endocarditis, 404f
Bacterial infection
  cellulitis, 219–220
  of CNS, 368t
  Lyme disease, 254–255
  in pneumonia, 358–359
  reservoir, 5t
Bacterial meningitis, 566, 566f
Balance equilibrium coordination, 534–535f
Baldness, 234–236, 235f
Ball-and-socket joint, 246f
Bariatrics, 334b
Barium swallow, 296
Barrel chest, in emphysema, 367, 367f
Barrett esophagus, 300b, 300f
Basal cell carcinoma
  description, 227–228
  diagnosis and treatment, 229
  etiology, 228–229
  patient screening, 228
  symptoms and signs, 228
Basilar skull fracture, 548b
Bed sore (decubitus ulcer), 222
Behavioral changes, in mourning, 602t
Behavioral reorganization, in mourning,
    602t
Bell palsy, 565–566
Benign paroxysmal positional vertigo (BPPV)
  etiology and diagnosis, 194
  symptoms and signs, 193–194
  treatment and prognosis, 194
Benign prostatic hyperplasia (BPH),
    494–495

Benign tumors
  compared with malignant tumors, 8t
  laryngeal, 352
  oral, 287–288
  of skin, 225–227
Benzodiazepines, 586
Beta-blockers, in glaucoma, 178b
Biceps brachii muscle, 244f
Biceps femoris muscle, 244f
Bicornuate uterus, 37
Bigeminy arrhythmia, 411–412t
Bile acids, 328
Biliary colic, 327–328
Biliary tract diseases, 322–332
Bioidentical hormone replacement, 137
Biopsies, 19
  chorionic villus, 34
Bioterrorism, 652b
Bipolar disorder
  diagnosis and treatment, 598–599
  patient teaching, 599
  symptoms and signs, 598
  unspecified, 598t
Bites
  animal/human, 643–645
  insect, 639f, 641f, 644f
  mosquito, malaria, 642–643
  reportable diseases and conditions, 640
  snakebite, 645–647
  tick
    Lyme disease, 254–255
    Rocky Mountain spotted fever,
      641–642
Bladder
  cystoscopy, 464b
  female, 479t
    cystocele, 508
  male, 478f
  neurogenic, 469–470
  obstruction, 462f, 469–470
  overactive, 471–472b
  site of helminthic infestation, 87f
  tumors, 473–474
Blastomycosis, 362b
Bleeding
  of esophageal varices, 296–298
  from nose, 352
Blepharitis, 171f
  etiology and diagnosis, 171
  symptoms and signs, 171
  treatment and prognosis, 171
Blepharoptosis, 173f
  description, 172–173
  etiology and diagnosis, 173
  symptoms and signs, 173
Blind spot, of eye, 164
Blisters
  herpes simplex, 291
  of shingles, 217f
Blood
  hemoptysis, 354–355
  in pleural cavity, 370f
  shunting patterns, in fetal circulation, 55
Blood alcohol levels, 590t, 591b
Blood analysis
  blood values in anemia, 431t
  laboratory and diagnostic tests, 17
Blood cell formation, 428f

Blood chemistries, 666–670
  alanine transaminase, 666
  albumin, 666
  alkaline phosphatase, 666
  aspartate aminotransferase, 666
  bilirubin, 666–667
  blood urea nitrogen, 667
  calcium, 670
  carbon dioxide, 669
  chemistries, 666
  chloride, 669
  creatinine, 667
  electrolytes, 669
  high-density lipoprotein cholesterol, 668
  ionized calcium, 670
  lactate dehydrogenase, 667
  lipid profile, 668
  low-density lipoprotein cholesterol, 669
  magnesium, 670
  phosphorus, 670
  potassium, 669
  serum glutamic oxaloacetic transaminase,
    666
  sodium, 669
  thyroid function tests, 667
  thyroid stimulating hormone, 668
  thyroxine, 667–668
  total cholesterol, 668
  total protein, 667
  triglycerides, 668
  triiodothyronine, 668
  urea nitrogen, 667
  uric acid, 667
Blood disorders of childhood
  anemia, 90–91
  erythroblastosis fetalis, 92
  lead poisoning, 93–95
  leukemia, 91–92
Blood dyscrasias, 427–432
  agranulocytosis, 430–432
  anemias, 428–430
  polycythemia, 432
  thrombocytopenia, 423–424
Blood glucose control, in diabetes,
    155, 156
Blood pressure, decreased in shock, 415f
Blood screening tests
  alcohol levels, 673
  digoxin, 672
  dilantin, 673
  drug levels, 672
  lidocaine, 672
  lithium, 672
  phenytoin, 673
  prograf (tacrolimus)/FK-506, 673
  theophylline, 672
B lymphocytes
  coated with immunoglobulins, 103
  formation of, 103f
Body image, anorexia nervosa and, 337–338
Body louse, 223
Body systems
  in autoimmune diseases, 115t
  responses to radiation exposure, 634b
Body weight, blood alcohol content
    and, 591t
Boils, furuncles and carbuncles, 218–219
Bone conduction system, 186

Bone disorders
  osteomalacia and rickets, 265
  osteoporosis, 263–264
  Paget disease, 259–260
  periodontitis, 286–287
  tumors, 261–263
Bone marrow
  formation of lymphocytes, 103f
  hematopoiesis, 244
  laboratory and diagnostic studies, 19
Bone marrow transplantation
  for SCID, 111
  terms used in conjunction with, 437b
  for Wiskott-Aldrich syndrome, 114–115
Bone matrix, breakdown of, 150f
Bones
  infection, osteomyelitis, 256–257
  lead deposits in children, 93–95
Bone tumors
  description, 261
  diagnosis, 262
  etiology, 262
  patient screening, 261
  patient teaching, 262
  prevention, 262
  prognosis, 262
  symptoms and signs, 261
  treatment, 262
Borderline personality disorder, 616
Botulinum toxin, 234b
Botulism, 652b
Bouchard nodes, 252, 253f
Bowel blockage, 312–313
Bowman's capsule, 451f
Boys, precocious puberty in, 159–160
BPH (benign prostatic hyperplasia),
    494–495
Brachial plexus (C5-T1), 538–539f
Brachial plexus injury, 650–651
Brachiocephalic trunk, 382f, 383f
Bradycardia, 383, 411–412t
Brain, 163f, 534–535f
  abscess, 568–569
  in Alzheimer disease, 585f
  degenerative diseases of, 560f
  intracranial tumors, 570–571
Brain stem, 534–535f
  displacement of, 570f
Breast
  mammogram, 19, 526f
  normal female, 480f
Breast cancer
  diagnosis and treatment, 529
  etiology, 528–529
  patient teaching, 530
  screening, 526t
  symptoms and signs, 528
Breast diseases
  fibrocystic breast condition, 526–527
  mastitis, 527
  Paget disease, 530–531
Breathing, paradoxical, 372
Breech presentation, 523f
Briquet syndrome. See Somatization
    disorder
Broca's speech area, 534–535f, 586f
Broken heart syndrome, 393–394
Bromocriptine, 156

Bronchi
  obstruction, in atelectasis, 356f
  primary, 344f
  tumor attached to, 376f
Bronchial asthma, 84
Bronchiectasis, 366, 366f
  diagnosis and treatment, 366
  etiology, 366
  patient screening, 366
  patient teaching, 367
  prevention, 366
  prognosis, 366
  symptoms and signs, 366
Bronchioles, 344f
  in influenza, 363f
  obstructed, in asthma, 85f
Bronchiolitis, 86
Bronchitis, acute and chronic, 365–366
Bronchomalacia, 40b
Bronchopulmonary dysplasia, 40–41
Bronchospasm, 85f
Brow presentation, 523f
Bruit, 422
Buerger disease, 425–426
Bugs, in ear, 626–628
Bulging disk, 552–554
Bulimia
  etiology and diagnosis, 338
  symptoms and signs, 338
  treatment and prognosis, 338
Bulla, 206–207f
Bundle of His, 410f
Bunion, 265–266
Burns
  cigarette, in child abuse, 653f
  depths of, 631f
  diagnosis, 630–631
  electrical, 632f
  etiology, 630
  scald dip, 654f
  sunburn, 632f, 633b
  symptoms and signs, 630
  treatment, 631–633
Burrow, dermatologic, 206–207f
Bursae, 247
Bursitis
  description, 255
  diagnosis, 256
  etiology, 256
  patient screening, 255–256
  patient teaching, 256
  prevention, 256
  prognosis, 256
  symptoms and signs, 255
  treatment, 256
Buttercup, toxicity of, 647t
Butterfly rash, of SLE, 120f
Bypass, coronary artery, 389f, 392f

C
Cachexia, 13
Caffeine, 593–595t
Calcaneal spur, 274–275
Calcitonin, 138t, 150f
  for Paget disease, 260
Calcitonin gene-related peptide (CGRP)
    inhibitors, 557
Calcium, blood levels, regulation of, 150f

Calculi
    gallstones, 327–329
    renal, 463f, 465–466
Calluses
    description, 236
    etiology and diagnosis, 236
    patient screening, 236
    patient teaching, 236
    prevention, 236
    prognosis, 236
    symptoms and signs, 236
    treatment, 236
Calyx, 450f
Cancer. *See also* Neoplasms; Tumors; specific
        types of cancer
    benign and malignant tumors, 8t
    classification by tissue of origin, 8–9t
    deaths from (2013 estimates), 10f
    general types of, 7
    hospice care, 13b
    patient teaching and, 29
    risk reduction recommendations, 9
    staging systems, 10
    stereotactic radiosurgery, 13b
    treatment regimens, 12
    tumor grade, 11–12
    tumor markers, 10
    vaccines, 12b
Candida albicans, 113
Candidiasis
    chronic mucocutaneous (CMC), 113–114
    thrush, 292
Canine teeth, 282f
Canker sores, 290
Cannabis synthetic, 592–595
Capillaries, 410f, 419f
    peritubular, 451f, 452f
    pulmonary, 344f
Carbon dioxide, acid-base balance and, 343
Carbon monoxide, 647t
Carbon tetrachloride, 647t
Carbuncles
    description, 218
    diagnosis and treatment, 219
    etiology, 219
    patient screening, 219
    patient teaching, 219
    prevention, 219
    prognosis, 219
    symptoms and signs, 219
Carcinoembryonic antigen (CEA), 149, 316
Cardiac ablation, 414b
Cardiac arrest, 392–394
    broken heart syndrome, 393–394
Cardiac cycle, 382–383, 384f
Cardiac enzymes and isoenzymes
    alanine aminotransferase, 674
    aspartate aminotransferase, 674
    creatine kinase, 673
    creatine kinase isoenzymes, 673
    creatine phosphokinase isoenzymes, 673
    cross-reactive protein, 673
    lactate dehydrogenase, 673
    lactate dehydrogenase isoenzymes,
        673–674
    serum glutamic oxaloacetic transaminase,
        674
    serum glutamic pyruvate transaminase, 674

Cardiac ischemia, mistaken for hiatal hernia
        symptoms, 306b
Cardiac muscle, 244, 245f
Cardiac tamponade, 417
Cardiogenic shock, 415–417
Cardiology tests, 18
    cardiac catheterization, 676
    cardiac event recorders, 675
    cardiac perfusion scanning, 675–676
    cardiac stress echocardiography, 675
    cardiac stress test, 675–676
    echocardiography, 675
    electrocardiography, 674–675
    exercise tolerance test, 676
    gallbladder scanning, 676
    hepatobiliary scanning, 676
    holter monitor, 675
    multiple gate acquisition scan, 675
Cardiomegaly, 401
Cardiomyopathy, 397, 400–402
    diagnosis and treatment, 401, 402
    etiology, 400–401
    hypertrophic, 45
    symptoms and signs, 400
Cardiopulmonary resuscitation (CPR), 393b
Cardiovascular diseases, 383–385
Carpals, 246f
Carpal tunnel syndrome
    etiology and diagnosis, 648
    symptoms and signs, 648
    treatment and prognosis, 648
Cartilage, 245
    costal, 248f
    osteoarthritis and, 461–462
Cataract, 177f
    etiology and diagnosis, 177
    symptoms and signs, 176
    treatment and prognosis, 177
Catatonic schizophrenia, 592, 596t
Catecholamines, 138t
Catheterization, urinary, 470b
Cautery, 644
CD8 cells, 102
Cecum, 305f
Celiac disease
    diagnosis and treatment, 335
    symptoms and signs, 335
Cell body, 534–535f
Cell-mediated immunity, 103
Cellulitis, 439
    description, 219, 220f
    diagnosis and treatment, 220
    etiology, 220
    patient screening, 220
    patient teaching, 220
    prevention, 220
    prognosis, 220
    symptoms and signs, 219
Cementum, 282f
Central fovea, 165t
Central nervous system (CNS), 534–535,
        535f
    abscess, 568
    site of helminthic infestation, 87f
Central sulcus, 534–535f
Cephalalgia (headache), 556
Cerebellum, 534–535f, 538–539f
Cerebral aneurysm, 543b

Cerebral circulation, 540f
Cerebral concussion, 545–546
Cerebral contusion, 546–547
Cerebral cortex, functional areas of, 586f
Cerebral palsy, 47–48
Cerebral syndrome, 634b
Cerebrospinal fluid
    flow of, 53f
    in hydrocephalus, 51
    in myelomeningocele, 50f
Cerebrovascular accident (CVA), 537–543,
        540–541f
Cerebrum, 534–535f, 538–539f
Cerumen, impacted, 186–188, 187f
Cervical cancer
    and HPV vaccine, 485b
    prognosis and prevention, 510
    symptoms and signs, 509
Cervical nerves, 534–535f
Cervical plexus (C1-C4), 538–539f
Cervical vertebrae, 249f
Cervix, 479f
Chalazion, 170f
    patient teaching, 170
    symptoms and signs, 169
    treatment, 170
Chancre, 486
    of primary syphilis, 486f
Chancroid, 487
Chemical agents
    injurious, 15
Chemotherapy
    in cancer treatment, 12
    systemic side effects, 10?
Chenodeoxycholic acid, 330
Cherry hemangioma, 233f
Chest cavity
    barrel chest, in emphysema, 367, 367t
    flail chest, 371–372
    movements, in respiration, 345f
Chiari malformation, 563b
Chickenpox (varicella zoster), 72–74
Child abuse/neglect
    description, 652–653
    diagnosis and treatment, 653–654
    patient teaching, 654
    symptoms and signs, 653
Childhood disintegrative disorder, 581
Childhood disorders, 72–98
    blood disorders, 90–95
    diaper rash, 96–97
    fetal alcohol syndrome, 96, 96f
    gastrointestinal disorders, 86–90
    infectious diseases, 72–80
    neuroblastoma, 97–98
    respiratory disorders, 80–86
    Reye syndrome, 95
Children
    depths of burns, 631f
    and play therapy, 576b
    PTSD in, 607
Chiropractic medicine, 25
Chlamydia, 481
Chloasma, 232, 232f
Cholecystitis, 329, 329f
    description, 329
    symptoms and signs, 329
    treatment and prognosis, 329

Cholecystogram, oral, 328f
Cholelithiasis, 327–329, 328f
    etiology, 328
    symptoms and signs, 327
    treatment and prognosis, 328
Cholesteatoma, 196f
    etiology, 196–197
    symptoms and signs, 196
    treatment and diagnosis, 197
Cholesterol gallstones, 328f
Cholinergic agent, 307
Cholinergic fibers, pre- and postganglionic,
    538–539f
Chondrosarcoma, 262
Chorea, 560–561
Chorionic villus biopsy (CVB), 34
Choroid, 163–164, 163f, 165t
Choroid plexus, 53f
Chromosomes, 6
    sex, abnormalities of, 70f
Chronic bronchitis, 365–366
Chronic disease, 2
Chronic glomerulonephritis, 454–456
Chronic inflammation, 3
Chronic kidney disease, 460–461
Chronic lymphocytic leukemia (CLL),
    433–434
Chronic mucocutaneous candidiasis (CMC)
    etiology and diagnosis, 113–114
    patient screening, 113
    symptoms and signs, 113
    treatment and prognosis, 114
Chronic myelogenous leukemia (CML),
    435–437
Chronic obstructive pulmonary disease
    (COPD)
    acute and chronic bronchitis, 365–366
    asthma, 367
    bronchiectasis, 366–367, 366f
    pneumoconiosis, 368–369
    pulmonary emphysema, 367–368
Chronic open-angle glaucoma, 178, 178f
Chronic otitis media, 190, 190f, 197
Chronic pain, 23
Chronic pancreatitis, 330–331
    etiology and diagnosis, 330–331
    symptoms and signs, 330
    treatment and prognosis, 331
Chronic passive congestion, 401f
Cialis. See Tadalafil
Ciliary body, 163–164, 165t
Cingulate gyrus, herniation, 570f
Circle of Willis, 540f, 543b
Circulation
    cerebral, 540f
    collateral, of heart, 388f
    fetal, 55–56, 55f
    pulmonary, 343
    through body, 383f
    through heart, 384f
Circulatory system disorders. See also Heart
        disease
    arrhythmias, 410–414
    blood dyscrasias, 427–432
    cardiovascular diseases, 383–385
    clotting disorders, 443–445
    leukemias, 432–437
    lymphatic diseases, 436–442

Circulatory system disorders. See also Heart
        disease (Continued)
    pulmonary edema, 400
    rheumatic fever, 405–408
    shock, 414–417
        cardiogenic, 415–417
        transfusion incompatibility reaction,
            442–443
    vascular conditions, 417–427
Circulatory system, orderly function of,
        382–398, 383f, 384f, 386f, 388f, 393t,
        400–402, 404–443, 413b
Circumflex artery, 382f
Circumoral cyanosis, 367
Cirrhosis of liver, 322–323, 322f, 325f
    etiology, 322
    prognosis and prevention, 323
    symptoms and signs, 322
Cisterna magna, 53f
Classic hemophilia, 443–444
Claustrophobia, 605t
Clavicle, 246f
Cleft lip, 62–63
    unilateral, 60f
Cleft palate, 62–63
CLL (chronic lymphocytic leukemia), 433–434
Closed head injury, 547f
    direct and contrecoup, 544
Clostridium difficile, in pseudomembranous
        enterocolitis, 318
Clotting and coagulation
    activated partial thromboplastin time, 670
    bleeding time, 671
    erythrocyte sedimentation rate, 671
    prothrombin time, 670–671
Clotting disorders
    classic hemophilia, 443–444
    disseminated intravascular coagulation,
        443–445
Clubfoot, 60–62
Cluster A personality disorders
    paranoid personality disorder, 616
    schizoid personality disorder, 616
    schizotypal personality disorder, 616
Cluster B personality disorders
    antisocial personality disorder, 616
    borderline personality disorder, 616
    histrionic disorder, 616
    narcissistic disorder, 616
Cluster C personality disorders
    avoidant personality disorder, 616–617
    dependent personality disorder, 616
    obsessive compulsive personality disorder,
        616–617
CMC (chronic mucocutaneous candidiasis),
    113–114
Coarctation of aorta, 56, 57f, 58f
Cocaine, 593–595t
Coccygeal nerve, 534–535f
Coccyx, 246f, 249f
Cochlea, 185f, 186
Cochlear implants, 186b
Cochlear nerve, 194f
Cognitive processing, 578
Cold
    common cold, 344–346
        in childhood, 80
    extreme (hypothermia), 638–639

Cold sores, 291–292
Colic, infantile, 86–87
Colitis, ulcerative, 310–311
Collagen, 120, 247
Collapsed lung, 356f
Collar bone, fracture of, 269
Colles fracture, 269
Cologuard, 677–678
Colonoscopy, 310f, 316–317
Colorectal cancer, 315–317
Colostomy, 315f
Colporrhaphy, 508
Coma
    diabetic, 155t
    myxedema, 147–148
Comedo, 206–207f, 206t
Comminuted fracture, skull, 547f
Commissurotomy, mitral, 408
Common bile duct, 330f
    impacted, 328f
Common cold
    in childhood, 80
    diagnosis and treatment, 345
    etiology, 345
    patient screening, 344–345
    patient teaching, 346
    prevention, 346
    prognosis, 346
    symptoms and signs, 344
Common variable immunodeficiency
    (CVID), 109
Communication disorders, stuttering, 579
Compensations, in progress of shock, 415f
Complementary and alternative medicine
    (CAM), 23, 25
Complement cascade, 104f
Complement system, activation of, 103
Complete blood count, 664
Concussion, 544
Concussion, cerebral, 545–546
Condoms, latex, and STDs, 480
Conduction disorders
    impacted cerumen, 186–188, 187f
    infective otitis externa, 188–189, 188f
    otitis media, 189–191, 190f, 191f
    otosclerosis, 192, 192f
    swimmer's ear, 189
Conduction system of heart, 410f, 412f
Conductive deafness, 186
Condyle of mandible, 289
Condylomata acuminata, 484–486
Congenital aganglionic megacolon,
    66–67
Congenital anomalies, 32–33
Congenital cardiac defects
    acyanotic defects
        atrial septal defect, 58
        coarctation of aorta, 56
        patent ductus arteriosus, 56
        ventricular septal defect, 56
    cyanotic defects
        tetralogy of Fallot, 59–60
        transposition of great arteries,
            59–60
    fetal circulation, 55–56, 55f
Congenital pyloric stenosis, 65–66
Congenital rubella syndrome, 79b
Congestion, chronic passive, 401f

Congestive heart failure, 396–398
  course of, 397f
  effects of, 399f
  radiography depicting, 398f
Conjoined twins, 36b
Conjunctiva, 163f, 164
Conjunctivitis, 173f
  etiology, 173
  patient teaching, 174
  symptoms and signs, 173
Connective tissue diseases
  ankylosing spondylitis, 127–128
  autoimmune, 120
  juvenile RA, 125–126
  Marfan syndrome, 260–261
  polymyositis, 128
  rheumatoid arthritis (RA), 123–125
  scleroderma, 121–122
  Sjögren syndrome, 122–123
  SLE, 120–121
Constipation, 296b
Contact dermatitis
  description, 208–209
  etiology and diagnosis, 209
  patient screening, 209
  patient teaching, 209
  prognosis, 209
  symptoms and signs, 209
  treatment, 209
Contact lenses, keratitis and, 170
Contact strike by lightning, 636
Contagious diseases
  chickenpox, 74–74
  German measles, 78–79
  impetigo, 217–218
  measles, 77–78
  mumps, 75–76, 76f
  scabies and pediculosis, 223–225
  STDs, 480–487
Continual Glucose Monitoring System, 157
Continuous ambulatory peritoneal dialysis, 456
Continuous cycling peritoneal dialysis, 456
Continuous positive airway pressure (CPAP), 615f
Contractures, in muscular dystrophy, 48
Contrecoup injury, 544, 588f
Contusion, cerebral, 546–547, 588f
Contusions, 544
Conversion disorder
  diagnosis and treatment, 609
  symptoms and signs, 608–609
COPD (chronic obstructive pulmonary disease), 365–378
Coracoid process, 277f
Cornea, 163f, 165t, 175
  keratitis, 170–171
Corneal abrasion
  etiology and diagnosis, 175
  symptoms and signs, 175
  treatment and prognosis, 175
Corneal ulcer, 175–176
Corns
  description, 236
  etiology and diagnosis, 236
  patient screening, 236
  patient teaching, 236
  prevention, 236
  prognosis, 236

Corns (Continued)
  symptoms and signs, 236
  treatment, 236
Coronary arteries, 382f, 383f
  bypass, 389f
  bypass graft, 392f
  stent, 392f
Coronary artery disease
  angina pectoris, 389–390
  etiology and diagnosis, 386–387
  myocardial infarction, 390–392
  patient teaching, 389
  symptoms and signs, 385
  treatment and prognosis, 387
Coronary sinus, 383f
Coronary vessels, 385f
Cor pulmonale, 398–400
Corrosive esophagitis, 298f
Corticotropin, 138t, 141
Cortisol, in Cushing syndrome, 152
Cosmetic dermatology, 234b
Costal cartilage, 246f
Cough suppressants, 345–346
Counseling
  genetic, 7
  psychological, 575f
Coupling arrhythmia, 411–412t
Cowper's gland, 478f
CPR (cardiopulmonary resuscitation), 393b
Crab louse, 224f
Cradle cap, treatment of, 207, 208f
Cranial nerves, 530–539f
  ocular, 168t
  types of fibers and functions of, 536–537b
Cranial sutures, 246f
Craniofacial abnormalities, in Robinow syndrome, 43b
Craniopagus twins, 36
Craniotomy, 544–545
Cranium, 246f
Crepitation, 252
Crest syndrome, of scleroderma, 122t
Cretinism
  etiology and diagnosis, 147
  patient teaching, 147
  symptoms and signs, 147
Crib death (SIDS), 80
Cri-du-chat syndrome, 44b
Crohn disease, 309–310, 309f
Cross-eye, 168
Croup, 81–82
Crown of tooth, 282f
Crushing injuries, 623–624
Crust, 206t
  of impetigo, 217
  oozing, 206–207f
Cryotherapy, 182
Cryptorchidism, 63–64, 63f
Crystals, uric acid, 258f
Cultural diversity, 20
Culture and sensitivity tests, 18
Cumulative trauma
  carpal tunnel syndrome, 648–649
  tendinitis, 651
  tennis elbow, 649–650
  thoracic outlet syndrome, 650–651
  trigger finger, 650
Curettage, 287, 514

Curvatures, abnormal, of spine, 248–252
Cushing syndrome
  clinical manifestations, 152f
  diagnosis, 152–153
  etiology, 152
  symptoms and signs, 152
  treatment, 153
Cutaneous nerve, 205f
Cuticles, paronychia, 239
CVA (cerebrovascular accident), 537–543, 540–541f
CVID (common variable immunodeficiency)
  diagnosis and treatment, 109
  etiology, 109
  patient screening, 109
  prognosis and patient teaching, 109
  symptoms and signs, 109
Cyanosis, circumoral, 367
Cyanotic cardiac defects
  tetralogy of Fallot, 59–60
  transposition of great arteries, 59–60
CyberKnife, 13b
Cycloset. See Bromocriptine
Cystic fibrosis, 67–69
Cystitis, infectious, 466–467
Cystocele, 508
Cystoscopy, 464b
Cysts
  epidermal (sebaceous), 226, 226f
  fluid filled, 206–207f
  ovarian, 500–501
Cytotoxic T cells (killer T cells), 102

D

Da Nang lung, 374
Deafness, central, 186
Death
  from cancers (2013 estimates), 10f
  crib death (SIDS), 80
Débride, 624
Decongestants, 345
Decubitus ulcer
  description, 222
  diagnosis, 222
  etiology, 222
  patient screening, 222
  patient teaching, 223
  prognosis, 223
  symptoms and signs, 222
  treatment and prevention, 222, 223
Defense mechanisms in body, 3
Deficits, in adaptive behavior, 577
Deformity, of nails, 238
Degeneration
  of hearing structures, 198t
  macular, 179–180, 180f
  myelin, in MS, 129f
  of peripheral nerves, 563–564
Degenerative disk disease, 549–552
Degenerative joint disease (osteoarthritis), 252–254
Degrees of uterine prolapse, 507f
Deltoid muscle, 244f
Delusions, 575
Dementia
  Alzheimer disease, 560f, 584–586
  caused by head trauma, 588–589
  vascular, 586–588

Demyelination, 567
Dendrites, 534–535f
Dental caries, 283–285, 284f
Dental implant, 284f
Dentin, 282f
Deoxyribonucleic acid (DNA)
    EBV, 349
    parentage testing, 659b
Dependent personality disorder, 616
Depressed skull fracture, 547–548, 547f
Depression, 599f
    continuum of, 600t
    postpartum, 603b
Depths of burns, 631f
De Quervain disease, 649b
Dermal papilla, 205f
Dermatitis
    atopic, 209–211
    contact, 208–209
    seborrheic, 207–208
Dermatofibroma, 225, 226f
Dermatomes, 216, 216f
Dermatophytoses
    description, 220
    patient screening, 220
    symptoms and signs, 220
    tinea capitis, 220
    tinea corporis (ringworm), 220–221
    tinea cruris (jock itch), 221–222, 221f
    tinea pedis (athlete's foot), 221
    tinea unguium, 221
Dermis, 206–207f
Dermopathy, 145–146
Designer drugs, 593–595t
Developmental and congenital disorders
    congenital anomalies, 32–33
    congenital cardiac defects, 55–60
    developmental characteristics, 32
    digestive system diseases, 65–67
    endocrine syndromes, 69–72
    genetic disorders and syndromes, 33–34
    genetic syndromes and conditions,
        43–47
    genitourinary conditions, 63–65
    metabolic disorders, 67–69
    methods of prenatal diagnosis, 34–36
    musculoskeletal conditions, 60–63
    nervous system diseases, 47–55
    prematurity, 35–43
Developmental dysplasia of hip, 62
Deviated septum, 350
Dextromethorphan, 593–595t
Diabetes insipidus
    etiology, 142
    prognosis, 143
    symptoms and signs, 142
    treatment, 142–143
Diabetes mellitus
    diagnosis, 155
    etiology, 154–155
    patient screening, 154
    patient teaching, 157
    primary forms of, 154
    prognosis and prevention, 156–157
    symptoms and signs, 154
    treatment, 155–156
Diabetic coma, 155t
Diabetic nephropathy, 468

Diabetic retinopathy, 181f
    description, 180
    etiology and diagnosis, 181
    symptoms and signs, 180
    treatment and prognosis, 181
Diagnosis of disease, 16
Diagnostic and Statistical Manual of Mental
    Disorders-V (DSM-V), 575
Diagnostic tests. See Laboratory and
    diagnostic tests
Dialysis, 456, 456–457f
Diaphragm, movements, in respiration, 345f
Diarrhea
    in childhood, 88–89
    traveler, 311
Diarthrodial joints, 245
Diastole, 384f
Diet
    avoidance of goitrogenic foods, 144
    and nutrition therapy, 26
DiGeorge anomaly (thymic hypoplasia or
        aplasia)
    etiology and diagnosis, 112
    patient screening, 112
    patient teaching, 113
    symptoms and signs, 112
    treatment and prognosis, 112–113
Digestive distress signals, 296b
Digestive system
    disorderly function of, 281–339
    orderly function of, 281
Digestive system diseases
    congenital pyloric stenosis, 65–66, 66f
    Hirschsprung disease, 66–67, 67f
Digestive system, main and accessory organs
    of, 281f
Dilated cardiomyopathy, 400
Dilation and curettage (D&C), 514
Dimpling, in breast cancer, 528f
Diphtheria
    diagnosis and treatment, 75
    symptoms and signs, 75
Diphtheria, tetanus, and pertussis (DTaP),
        73f
Diplopia, 168, 537
Direct strike by lightning, 636
Disaster, mock disaster drills, 629b
Discoloration
    around mouth, in emphysema, 367f
    of nails, 238
    of teeth, 285, 285f
Disease
    acute and chronic, 2
    autoimmune. See Autoimmune diseases
    genetic, 6–7
    immunodeficiency. See Immunodeficiency
        disorders
    life-threatening, patient teaching
        and, 29
    mechanisms of, 2–27
    prevention of spread during athletic events,
        74b
    produced by pathogens, 5t
    signs and symptoms of, 2
Disease-modifying antirheumatic drugs
    (DMARDs), 125
Disorganized schizophrenia, 596t
Dissecting aneurysm, 423f

Disseminated intravascular coagulation
        (DIC), 443–445
    pathophysiology, 445f
Disulfiram, 590–591
Diverticular Disease, 313–314
Diverticulitis, 314–315
Diverticulosis, 313–314
DNA (deoxyribonucleic acid)
    EBV, 349
    parentage testing, 659b
Down syndrome, 45–47, 46f
DPP IV inhibitors, 156
Drugs
    of abuse, 592
    for Alzheimer disease treatment,
        686–702t
    antithyroid, 146
    to be avoided in Alzheimer patients, 586b
    for cancer treatment, 686–702t
    for cardiovascular system, 686–702t
    DMARDs, 125
    for endocrine system, 686–702t
    erectile dysfunction treatment,
        686–702t
    for first aid, emergency situations,
        686–702t
    for gastrointestinal system, 686–702t
    for hematology, 686–702t
    immune system, disorders of, 686–702t
    for immunizations, 686–702t
    for infectious diseases, 686–702t
    for integumentary system, 686–702t
    for mental disorders, 686–702t
    for multiple sclerosis treatment, 686–702t
    for musculoskeletal system, 686–702t
    for neurologic system, 686–702t
    NSAIDs, 125
    ototoxicity caused by, 187
    for reproductive health, 471–472t
    for pain and fever, 686–702t
    prostatic conditions, treatment, 686–702t
    recreational, 592
    for reproductive system, 686–702t
    for respiratory system, 686–702t
    for sensory system, 686–702t
    for urinary system, 686–702t
    used as nutritional supplements and
        alternative medicine, 686–702t
Dry eye syndrome, 174
Ductal carcinoma in situ (DCIS), 529
Ductus deferens, 478f
Duodenal ulcer, 301–303
Duodenum, 330f
Dura mater, 534–535f, 544, 545f
Dusts
    containing Histoplasma capsulatum, 362
    in occupational lung diseases, 368
Dwarfism, 141–142
Dyscrasias, 428
Dyscrasias, blood, 427–432
Dysmenorrhea, 498, 499–500
Dyspareunia, 481
Dysuria, 481

E
Ear
    manifestations of Robinow syndrome, 43b
    normal anatomy, 185f

Ear cancer
description, 199
diagnosis, 200f, 201
etiology, 200–201
symptoms and signs, 200
treatment and prognosis, 201
Ear disorders, 185–201
benign paroxysmal positional vertigo, 193–194
cholesteatoma, 196–197, 196f
of conduction, 186–192
labyrinthitis, 194–195, 194f
mastoiditis, 197–198
Meniere disease, 193
ruptured tympanic membrane/ruptured eardrum, 195–196, 195f, 196f
sensorineural hearing loss, 198–199
Eardrum. See Tympanic membrane
Ear wax. See Cerumen
Eating disorders
anorexia nervosa, 337–338
bulimia, 338–339
motion sickness, 339
EBV (Epstein-Barr virus)
DNA, 349
and infectious mononucleosis, 374
Ecchymosis, 443
Eclampsia, 521
Ecstasy, club drug, 593–595t
Ectopic pregnancy, 518–519
Ectopic sites
of endometriosis, 502f
of tubal pregnancy, 518f
Ectropion, 172, 172f
Eczema
description, 209–211
etiology and diagnosis, 210
patient screening, 210
patient teaching, 211
symptoms and signs, 210
treatment and prognosis, 210
Edema
bronchiolar, in influenza, 363f
in cirrhosis of liver, 322f
in congestive heart failure, 396f
pulmonary, 400
Effector, 535f
Efferent lymphatic vessels, 437f
Efferent neuron, 535f
Ejaculatory duct, 478f
Elbow, 246f
tennis elbow, 649–650
Elder abuse/neglect
description, 655–656
prognosis and prevention, 656
symptoms and signs, 656
E-learning teaching, 28
Electrical activity procedures, and pacemakers, 413b
Electrical burns, points of entry and exit, 632f
Electrical shock, 635–636
Electrocardiogram (ECG) tracing, 412f
Electroencephalography (EEG), 19
Electromyelogram (EMG), 19
Ellipsoidal joint, 246f
Embolism, 419
pulmonary, 357–358, 357f

Embolus
causing TIA, 543f
in coronary artery disease, 386f
diagnosis and treatment, 419
patient teaching, 419
septic, from endocarditis, 405f
symptoms and signs, 418
venous and arterial, 421f
Embryonic disk, 32–33f
Emergency medical service (EMS), 629b
Emphysema, pulmonary, 367–368
Enamel, 282f
discoloration of, 285
Encephalitis, 567
Endarterectomy, carotid, 587
Endocarditis, 404–405
Endocardium, 383f
Endocrine dysfunction of pancreas, 154–159
diabetes mellitus, 154–157
gestational diabetes, 157–158
hypoglycemia, 158–159
Endocrine glands
dysfunction of, 136
hormone secreting, 136
secretions and function of, 138t
Endocrine syndromes
Klinefelter syndrome, 70–71, 71f
resulting from chromosomal nondisjunction, 69
Turner syndrome, 71–72, 71f
Endocrine system, orderly function of, 136–160
Endolymph, 194f
Endometrial cancer, 513–514
Endometriosis, 501–503
Endorphins, 23
Endoscopic retrograde cholangiopancreatography (ERCP), 328
Endoscopy, 297
Endoscopy tests, 18, 678–679
upper GI, 302f
End-stage renal disease (ESRD), 456b
Enterocolitis
necrotizing, 42–43
pseudomembranous, 317–318
Enteropathy, gluten, 335
Entrapment of median nerve, 649f
Entropion, 171–172, 172f
Environment
as predisposing factor for disease, 3
related factors resulting in trauma, 621
Enzyme-linked immunosorbent assay (ELISA), in AIDS, 107–108
Ephedrine, 593–595t
Epidemic hepatitis, 323
Epidemic parotitis (mumps), 75–76, 76f
Epidermal (sebaceous) cyst, 226, 226f
Epidermis, 206–207f
Epididymis, 478f
Epididymitis, 491–492
Epidural hematoma, 544–545
Epiglottis, 150f
Epiglottitis, acute, 82–83, 82f
Epilepsy (seizure disorder), 558
Episcleritis, 176b
description, 175
etiology and diagnosis, 176
patient teaching, 176
symptoms and signs, 176

Epistaxis, 352
Epstein-Barr virus (EBV)
DNA, 349
and infectious mononucleosis, 374
Ergonomic, 648
Erosion, 206–207f
Erythroblastosis fetalis, 92, 93f
Erythrocytes, 428f
sickled, 430f
Erythrocyte sedimentation rate (ESR), 671
Esophageal cancer, 299–300
Esophageal varices, 296–298, 297f, 322f
Esophagitis, 298–299
Esophagus, 201f
Barrett, 300b
carcinoma of, 299f
Esotropia, 168
Essential hypertension, 394–395
Estrogens, 138t
Ethmoid sinus, 346f
Eustachian tube, 185, 185f, 346f
Evidence maintenance, sexual assault response teams and, 660b
Ewing sarcoma, 261
Exercise, guidelines for adults, 24b
Exhaustion, heat, 637
Exocrine glands, in cystic fibrosis, 68f
Exophthalmos, 183–184
Exotropia, 168
Expectorants, 345
External auditory canal, 185f
External ear, 185f
External hemorrhoid, 321f
External oblique muscle, 241f
External ocular muscles, 165t
External otitis, 188f
Extracapsular surgery, for cataract, 177
Extracorporeal shock wave lithotripsy (ESWL), 328, 466
Extrapyramidal side effects, 597
Extrapyramidal side effects (EPSs), 597
Extrinsic muscles of eye, 164t
Exudate, pleural fluid, 369f
Eye
albinism-associated problems, 231
anatomy of, 163f
blind spot of, 164
in Down syndrome, 46f
foreign bodies in, 626–628
irrigation of, 627f
manifestations of Robinow syndrome, 43b
muscles of, 164t
raccoon, 97, 97f
shingles affecting, 215–217
site of helminthic infestation, 87f
structure and function of major parts of, 165t
Eyeball, 163, 167f
Eye cancer
etiology and diagnosis, 184
symptoms and signs, 184
treatment and prognosis, 185
Eye disorders, 163–185
of globe of eye, 175–184
in gonorrhea ophthalmia, 482f

Eye disorders *(Continued)*
  in Marfan syndrome, 260
  nystagmus, 167–168
  refractive errors, 166–167
  signs and symptoms of, 165
  strabismus, 168–169, 168f
Eyelid, 165t
Eyelid disorders
  blepharitis, 171, 171f
  blepharoptosis, 172–173, 173f
  chalazion, 169–170, 170f
  conjunctivitis, 173–174, 173f
  ectropion, 172, 172f
  entropion, 171–172, 172f
  hordeolum, 169, 169f
  keratitis, 170–171
  keratoconjunctivitis sicca, 174

F
Face, 534–535f
Facial bones, 246f
Facial nerve (VII), 536–537b
Facies, myxedema, 147f
Factitious disorder, 610–611
Factor VIII, in clotting cascade, 444f
Fallopian tube, 479f
False aneurysm, 423f
Family violence, 655b
Farsightedness, 166
Fascia, 245–247
  plantar, 275, 275f
Fasciculation, 561
Fasting blood glucose (FBG), 671
FAST method for stroke response,
    540–541f
Fat-soluble vitamins, hypervitaminosis and,
    333b
Female reproduction system. *See also*
    Pregnancy
  breast, 326–331
  infertility, 489–490
  menopause, 506–507
Female reproductive diseases
  amenorrhea, 499
  cervical cancer, 509–510
  cystocele, 508
  dysmenorrhea, 499–500
  endometrial cancer, 513–514
  endometriosis, 501–503
  genital herpes, 483f
  labial or vulvar cancer, 511–512
  ovarian cancer, 512–513
  ovarian cysts, 500–501
  pelvic inflammatory disease, 503–504
  premenstrual syndrome, 498–499
  rectocele, 509
  toxic shock syndrome, 505–506
  uterine leiomyomas, 504–505
  uterine prolapse, 507–508
  vaginal cancer, 510–511
  vaginitis, 505
Femur, 246f
Fentanyl-based drugs, 593–595t
Fertilization cycle, 479
Fetal circulation, 55–56, 55f
Fetus
  monthly changes during prenatal
      development, 34t

Fetus *(Continued)*
  movement, 520b
  presentations of, 523f
  spontaneous abortion, 517–518
  28-week ultrasonography, 515f
Fever
  glandular, 373
  Pontiac, 360–361
  rheumatic, 405–408
Fibrillation
  atrial, 411–412t
  ventricular, 411–412t
Fibroadenoma of breast, 527–528
Fibrocystic breast condition, 526–527
Fibroglial capsule, 568f
Fibroids, uterine, 504–505
Fibromyalgia
  description, 247
  diagnosis, 247–248
  eighteen tender points used to diagnose,
      248f
  etiology, 247
  patient screening, 247
  patient teaching, 248
  prevention, 248
  prognosis, 248
  symptoms and signs, 247
  treatment, 248
Fibroplasia, retrolental, 41, 41f
Fibula, 246f
Fibular collateral ligament, 247f
Fingers
  folliculitis, 237f
  Heberden node, 252
  in Marfan syndrome, 260f
  Raynaud phenomenon, 426
  trigger finger, 650
Fire ant bites, 641f
First-degree heart block, 411–412t
Fissure, 206–207f, 206t
Fissure of Sylvius, 534–535f
Fistula, 299
  tracheoesophageal, 299
Flail chest, 371, 372f
  diagnosis and treatment, 372
  etiology, 372
  patient screening, 372
  patient teaching, 372
  prevention, 372
  prognosis, 372
  symptoms and signs, 372
Flat bones, 245
Flow charts, steps in diagnosis, 17f
Flunitrazepam, 593–595t
Folic acid deficiency anemia,
    429, 431t
Follicle-stimulating hormone (FSH),
    138t, 139f
Folliculitis
  description, 237–238, 237f
  diagnosis and treatment, 237
  etiology, 237
  patient screening, 237
  patient teaching, 238
  symptoms and signs, 237
Food poisoning, 335–337, 336t
Food sources, of oxalates, purines, and
    phosphorus, 466b

Foot, 534–535f
  clubfoot, 60–62, 60f
  CMC of, 113f
  contracture, in muscular dystrophy,
      48, 48f
  corns and calluses, 236
  diabetic ulcer, 154f
  tinea pedis of (athlete's foot), 221
Footling breech presentation, 523f
Foramen ovale, 55
Foreign bodies
  in ear, 626–628
  in eye, 628–629
  in nose, 629–630
Fractures, 268–270
  rib, in flail chest, 372
  skull. *See* Skull fracture
Free-floating anxiety, 604
Frontalis muscle, 244f
Frontal lobe, 534–535f, 586f
Frontal sinus, 346f
Frostbite, 639–640
  diagnosis and treatment, 639–640
  symptoms and signs, 639
  usual sites of, 639f
Frozen shoulder, 272
Full-thickness burn, 631f
Fulminant, 310–311
Functional areas of cerebral cortex, 586f
Functional neurologic disorders
  amyotrophic lateral sclerosis, 561–562
  epilepsy, 558
  headache, 556
  Huntington chorea, 560–561
  migraine, 556–557
  Parkinson disease, 558–560, 560f
  restless legs syndrome, 562
  transient global amnesia, 562–563
Fungal infection
  CMC, 113–114
  dermatophytosis (tinea), 220–222
  histoplasmosis, 362
  pityriasis, 233
  reservoir, 5t
  thrush, 292
Furuncles
  description, 218
  diagnosis and treatment, 219
  etiology, 219
  patient screening, 219
  patient teaching, 219
  prevention, 219
  prognosis, 219
  symptoms and signs, 219
Fusiform aneurysm, 423f

G
Gait, 560f
Gallbladder, 281f
  cholecystitis, 329
  gallstones, 327–329
Gallstones, 327–329
Gamma hydroxybutyric acid (GBH),
    593–595t
Ganglion, 275–276
  parasympathetic, 538–539f
Gastric analysis, 19
Gastric cancer, 304–305

Gastric ulcer, 301–303
Gastritis, 303–304
Gastrocnemius muscle, 244f
Gastroenteritis, 311–312
Gastroesophageal reflux disease (GERD), 295–296, 295f
    and Barrett esophagus, 300b
Gastrointestinal (GI) disorders of childhood
    diarrhea, 88–89
    helminth (worm) infestation, 87–88, 87f
    infantile colic, 86–87
    vomiting, 90
Gastrointestinal syndrome, 634b
Gastrointestinal tract diseases, 295–322
    abdominal hernia, 307–309
    acute appendicitis, 305–306
    colorectal cancer, 315–317
    Crohn disease, 309–310
    diverticulitis, 314–315
    diverticulosis, 313–314
    esophageal cancer, 299–300
    esophageal varices, 296–298
    gastric cancer, 304–305
    gastric, duodenal, and peptic ulcers, 301–303
    gastritis, 303–304
    gastroenteritis, 311–312
    GERD, 295–296
    hemorrhoids, 321–322
    hiatal hernia, 306–307
    intestinal obstruction, 312–313
    irritable bowel syndrome, 319–320
    peritonitis, 320–321
    pseudomembranous enterocolitis, 317–318
    short bowel syndrome, 318–319
    ulcerative colitis, 310–311
Gastroscopy, 303
Gender
    dysphonia, 611–612
    as predisposing factor for disease, 2
Generalized anxiety disorder, 604
Generalized seizures, 558
Gene therapy, 20
Genetic counseling, 7
Genetic diseases, 6–7
Genetic disorders and syndromes, 33–34
Genetic syndromes
    cri-du-chat syndrome, 44b
    Down syndrome, 45–47, 46f
    hypertrophic cardiomyopathy, 45
    Robinow syndrome, 43–44
Genetic testing, 18
Genital herpes, 483–484
Genital hypoplasia, in Robinow syndrome, 43b
Genital warts, 484–486
Genitourinary conditions, 481
    cryptorchidism, 63–64, 63f
    phimosis, 65, 65f
    Wilms tumor, 64–65, 64f
Genotype, 6
German measles, 78–79, 79f
Germ cell tumors, testicular, 497
Germ layer formation, 32–33f
Gestational diabetes mellitus (GDM)
    etiology and diagnosis, 158
    symptoms and signs, 157
    treatment and prognosis, 158

Gigantism
    diagnosis, 139–140
    etiology, 139
    symptoms and signs, 139
    treatment, 140
Gilchrist disease, 362b
Gilles de la Tourette syndrome, 583
Gingiva, 282f
Gingivectomy, 293
Gingivitis, 285–286, 286f
    acute necrotizing ulcerative. See Necrotizing periodontal disease
    description, 285
    symptoms and signs, 285–286
    treatment and prognosis, 286
Girls, precocious puberty in, 160
Glandular fever, 373
Glasgow coma scale, 536–537b
Glaucoma
    acute angle-closure glaucoma, 178–179, 178f
    chronic open-angle glaucoma, 178, 178f
    description, 177–178
    patient screening, 178
Globe of eye disorders
    cataract, 176–177, 177f
    corneal abrasion or ulcer, 175–176
    diabetic retinopathy, 180–181, 181f
    episcleritis/scleritis, 175–176
    exophthalmos, 183–184
    glaucoma, 177–179, 178f
    macular degeneration, 179–180, 180f
    retinal detachment, 181–182, 181f, 182f
    uveitis, 183
Glomerular basement membrane (GBM), 119
Glomerulonephritis
    acute, 451–454
    chronic, 454–456
    poststreptococcal, 452f
Glossopharyngeal nerve (IX), 536–537b
Glucagon, 138t
Glucocorticoids, 138t
Glucophage. See Metformin; Metformin hydrochloride
Glucose monitoring
    fasting blood glucose levels, 671
    glucose tolerance test, 671
    glycosylated hemoglobin/glycohemoglobin, 672
    two-hour postprandial, 671–672
Glucose tolerance test (GTT), 671
Gluten enteropathy, 335
Gluteus maximus muscle, 244f
Glycated hemoglobin testing, 155
Glycohemoglobin, 672
Glycosylated hemoglobin, 672
Glycosylated hemoglobin test (HbA1c), 157
Goiter, simple, 144–145, 144f
Golden Gate Bridge, 601b
Gonadal dysgenesis in females
    Turner syndrome, 71
Gonadocorticoids, 138t
Gonadotropins, 136, 138t
Goniolens, 179
Gonorrhea, 481–482
Gonorrhea ophthalmia, 482f

Goodpasture syndrome
    description, 119
    etiology and diagnosis, 119
    symptoms and signs, 119
    treatment and prognosis, 119–120
Gout
    description, 257
    diagnosis, 258
    etiology, 258
    patient screening, 258
    patient teaching, 259
    prevention, 259
    prognosis, 259
    symptoms and signs, 257–258
    treatment, 258–259
Grading of cancer, 11–12
Graft coronary bypass, 401f
Gram stain, 19
Granulocyte count, 665
Granulocytes, 428f
Granulomas, in lung, 375
Graves disease, 146f
    description, 145
    etiology and diagnosis, 146
    symptoms and signs, 145–146
    treatment and prognosis, 146
Great arteries, transposition of, 57f, 59–60, 59f
Great cardiac vein, 382f, 383f, 385f
Great vessels
    anterior view, 382f
    posterior view, 383f
Grief response, 601b
Ground current lightning strike, 636
Groups at risk
    for influenza-related complications, 364b
    for lung cancer, 378
Growth hormone (GH), 138t, 139f
    abnormalities, 139f
    deficiencies, in dwarfism, 141–142
    hypersecretion
        in acromegaly, 140
        in gigantism, 139
Growth hormone-releasing hormone (GH-RH), 142
Guillain-Barré syndrome, 567–568
Guilt, in mourning, 602t
Gums
    inflammation of, 285–286
    necrotizing periodontal disease, 292–293
    periodontitis, 286–287
Gynecomastia, 71f, 322f
Gyrus, 534–535f

H
Haemophilus influenza type b (HIb), 73f, 82
Hair
    alopecia, 234–236
    analysis for drugs, 592b, 596f
    lice in, 223f
Hair follicle, 205f
    folliculitis, 237–238
Hair shafts, 224
Hallucinations, 596
    verbal/visual, 575
Hallucinogens, 593–595t

Hallux rigidus
  description, 266
  diagnosis, 267
  etiology, 266
  patient screening, 266
  patient teaching, 267
  prevention, 267
  prognosis, 267
  symptoms and signs, 266
  treatment, 267
Hallux valgus
  description, 265
  diagnosis, 266
  etiology, 266
  patient screening, 266
  patient teaching, 266
  prevention, 266
  prognosis, 266
  symptoms and signs, 265–266
  treatment, 266
Hammer toe
  description, 267
  diagnosis, 268
  etiology, 267
  patient screening, 267
  patient teaching, 268
  prevention, 268
  prognosis, 268
  symptoms and signs, 267
  treatment, 268
Hand, 534–535f
Hash, abuse of, 593–595t
Hashimoto thyroiditis
  etiology and diagnosis, 145
  symptoms and signs, 145
HbA1c, 157
Head abnormalities, in Robinow syndrome,
    43b
Headache, 556
Head louse, 223, 223f
Head trauma
  basilar skull fracture, 547f, 548b
  blunt, 545
  cerebral concussion, 545–546
  cerebral contusion, 546–547
  dementia caused by, 588–589
  depressed skull fracture, 547f
  epidural and subdural hematomas,
    544–545
Healing, course of inflammation and, 4f
Health care, preventive, 24–25
Health care providers, needlesticks, 624b
Health hazards of common molds, 359b
Hearing
  aging-caused changes in, 198t
  functioning organs of, 185–187
Hearing loss, 186
  sensorineural, 186, 198–199
Heart
  anterior view, 382f
  with cardiomyopathy, 45f
  circulation through, 384f
  collateral circulation of, 388f
  conduction system in, 410f, 412f
  locations of myocardial infarction,
    391f
  posterior view, 383f
Heart block, 411–412t

Heart defects, congenital, 55–60
Heart disease
  arrhythmias, 410–414
  atherosclerotic consequences, 387f
  cardiac arrest, 392–394
  cardiac tamponade, 417
  cardiomyopathy, 400–402
  congestive heart failure, 396–398
  coronary artery disease, 385–392
    angina pectoris, 389–390
    myocardial infarction, 390–392
  cor pulmonale, 398–400
  development of atheroma, 386f
  hypertensive, 394–396
    essential hypertension, 394–395
    malignant hypertension, 395–396
  myocarditis, 403
  pericarditis, 402–403
  rheumatic, 406–408
  valvular
    mitral insufficiency, 409
    mitral stenosis, 408–409
    mitral valve prolapse, 409–410
Heart failure
  congestive, 396–398, 399f
  left heart, 401f
Heart wall
  layers of, 385f
  pericardial effusion and, 403f
Heat exhaustion, 637
Heat stroke, 637
Heavy metals, nephrotoxic, 458b
Heberden node, 252
Helicobacter pylori, 302f
Helminth infestation, in childhood, 87–88,
    87f
Helper T cells, 102
Hemangiomas, 232, 233f
Hematemesis, 296
Hematocrit count, 664–665
Hematogenous metastases, in lungs, 377f
Hematomas
  epidural and subdural, 544–545
  subdural, 588f
Hematophobia, 605t
Hematopoiesis, 244, 432
Hematopoietic disorders
  autoimmune hemolytic anemia,
    115–116
  idiopathic thrombocytopenic
    purpura, 118
  immune neutropenia, 118–119
  pernicious anemia, 116–117
Hematopoietic stem cell transplantation
    (HSCT), 433, 436, 437b
Hematopoietic system, 102–103
Hematuria, in bladder tumor, 473–474
Hemiparesis, 537
Hemiplegia, 547, 548f
Hemodialysis, 456, 456–457f
Hemoglobin breakdown, in erythroblastosis
    fetalis, 93f
Hemoglobin count, 664
Hemolytic, 428–429
Hemolytic anemia
  autoimmune, 115–116
  blood values, 431t
Hemolytic disease of newborn, 92

Hemophilia, classic, 443–444
Hemopoietic syndrome, 634b
Hemoptysis
  diagnosis and treatment, 355
  etiology, 354
  patient screening, 354
  patient teaching, 355
  prevention, 355
  prognosis, 355
  symptoms and signs, 354
Hemorrhage
  intracranial, 544t
  from nose, 352
  retinal, in shaken baby syndrome, 655f
  skin, 322f
  spontaneous subconjunctival,
    176b, 176f
Hemorrhagic anemia, 430, 431t
Hemorrhoids, 321–322, 321f
Hemothorax, 370f, 371
Hepatic screening, 19
Hepatitis A, 323–324
  immunization schedule, 73f
Hepatitis B, 324–325
  and hepatocellular carcinoma, 326–327
  immunization schedule, 73f
Hepatitis B surface antigen (HBsAg), 324
Hepatitis C, 325–326
Hepatitis, viral, 323
Hepatocellular carcinoma (HCC), 326–327,
    326f
Hepatomegaly, 316
Herbal ecstasy, 593–595t
Herbal medicines, 25–26
Heredity, as predisposing factor for
    disease, 3
Hernias
  abdominal, 307–309, 308f
  hiatal, 306–307, 307f
Herniated disk, 552–554
Herniation
  of cingulate gyrus, 570
  as intestinal obstruction, 313f
Heroin, 593–595t
Herpes simplex (cold sores), 291–292
Herpes simplex virus type 1 (HSV-1),
    291f
  genital herpes caused by, 483–484
Herpes simplex virus type 2 (HSV-2),
    genital herpes caused by, 483–484
Herpes zoster
  description, 215
  etiology and diagnosis, 216–217
  patient screening, 216
  patient teaching, 217
  prevention, 217
  prognosis, 217
  symptoms and signs, 216
  treatment, 217
Herpetic whitlow, 484
Hiatal hernia, 306–307, 307f
Highly active antiretroviral therapy
    (HAART), 106–107
Hinge joint, 246f
Hip dysplasia, congenital, 60f, 62
Hirschsprung disease, 66–67, 67f
Histoplasmosis, 362
Histrionic disorder, 616

HIV
  AIDS caused by, 105
  diagnosis and treatment, 107–108
  etiology, 106–107
  opportunistic infections, 106b
  patient screening, 106
  patient teaching, 108–109
  prognosis and prevention, 108
  symptoms and signs, 105–106
Hives, 211–212
HLA-B27 antigen, in ankylosing spondylitis, 127
H1N1 infection, 364b
Hoarseness, laryngeal cancer and, 252–253
Hobnail liver, 322, 322f
Hodgkin lymphoma, 439–441
Hodophobia, 605t
Holistic medicine, 19
Homeostasis, definition of, 2
Hordeolum
  symptoms and signs, 169
  treatment and prognosis, 169
Hormonal methods, 491
Hormone replacement therapy, in Addison disease, 153
Hormones, 136
  bioidentical, 137
  endocrine, 136, 138t
  pituitary, 139f
Hormone therapy
  calcitonin, for Paget disease, 260
  in cancer treatment, 12
  in menopause, 507
  for precocious puberty in boys, 159–160
Hospice care, 13b
HPV (human papillomavirus)
  cervical cancer and, 510
  vaccine, 485b
HPV 16 infection, 294
Human bites
  diagnosis and treatment, 643–645
  patient teaching, 645
  symptoms and signs, 643–644
Human immunodeficiency virus. See HIV
Human papillomavirus (HPV)
  cervical cancer and, 510
  immunization schedule, 73f
  vaccine, 485b
Humerus, 246f
Huntington chorea, 560–561
Huntington disease, 560f
Hydatidiform mole, 525–526
Hydrocephalus, 51–52, 52f
  shunting procedures for, 54f
Hydronephrosis, 463–464
Hydrophobia, 605t
Hyoid bone, 150f
Hyperabduction, 651
  of arm, 651
Hyperactive responses, 101
Hyperemesis gravidarum, 516–517
Hyperextension, of spine, 550f
Hyperfunction of thyroid, 143t
Hyperglycemia, in diabetes mellitus, 154
Hyperkalemia, 153
Hyperopia, 166, 166f

Hyperparathyroidism
  description, 149
  diagnosis and treatment, 151
  etiology, 150–151
  symptoms and signs, 150
Hyperplasia
  adenoid, 83–84
  benign prostatic, 494–495
Hypertension
  development of, 395f
  essential, 394–395
  malignant, 395–396
Hypertensive heart disease, 394–396
  essential hypertension, 394–395
  malignant hypertension, 395–396
Hyperthermia, 630
  diagnosis and treatment, 637
  symptoms and signs, 637
Hyperthyroidism, Graves disease, 145
Hypertrophic cardiomyopathy, 401
Hypertrophic scars, 226, 226f
Hypertrophy, left ventricular, 408f
Hypervitaminosis, 333b
Hypnosis, 27
Hypocalcemia, 151
  signs of, 151f
Hypochondriasis, 610
Hypofunction of thyroid, 143t
Hypogammaglobulinemia, acquired, 109
Hypoglossal nerve (XII), 536–537b
Hypoglycemia
  etiology and diagnosis, 159
  symptoms and signs, 159
  treatment and prognosis, 159
Hypokalemia, 338
Hypoparathyroidism
  diagnosis and treatment, 152
  etiology, 152
  symptoms and signs, 151
Hypopituitarism
  etiology and diagnosis, 141
  patient teaching, 141
  symptoms and signs, 141
Hypothalamus, 136, 136f, 534–535f
Hypothalamus-pituitary-thyroid gland feedback mechanism, 137f
Hypothermia, 630
  symptoms and signs, 638–639
  therapeutic, 393b
Hypothyroidism, 146
  cretinism, 147
  myxedema and myxedema coma, 147–148, 147f
Hypovolemia, 414
Hypovolemic shock, 416f
Hypoxia, 398, 577
Hysteria. See Conversion disorder; Conversion disorders
Hysterosalpingography, 490

I
Iatrogenic disorders, 24
Iatrophobia, 605t
Idiopathic diseases, eczema, 209–211
Idiopathic thrombocytopenic purpura (ITP)
  description, 118
  etiology and diagnosis, 118
  patient screening, 118

Idiopathic thrombocytopenic purpura (ITP) (Continued)
  patient teaching, 118
  symptoms and signs, 118
  treatment and prognosis, 118
IgA (immunoglobulin A), selective deficiency, 109–110
Ileus, 312–313
Ilium, 246f
Imaging studies, diagnostic, 18
Immune disorders, 14–15
Immune neutropenia
  etiology and diagnosis, 119
  symptoms and signs, 119
  treatment and prognosis, 119
Immune response, 101
Immune system, orderly function of, 101–105
Immunity
  cell-mediated, 103
  passive and active, 103–105
Immunization
  immunization schedule, 73f
  influenza, target groups for, 364b
Immunocompetent, 101
Immunodeficiency
  as predisposing factor for disease, 3
  severe combined (SCID), 111–112
Immunodeficiency disorders, 15, 101
  AIDS, 105–109
  chronic mucocutaneous candidiasis, 113–114
  CVID, 109
  DiGeorge anomaly, 112–113
  SCID, 111–112
  selective IgA deficiency, 109–110
  Wiskott-Aldrich syndrome, 114–115
  X-linked agammaglobulinemia, 110–111
Immunoelectrophoresis, 110
Immunogen, 102
Immunoglobulin A (IgA), selective deficiency, 109–110
Immunoglobulins, classes of, 104t
Immunometric assay (IMA), 137
Immunotherapy, in cancer treatment, 12
Impacted cerumen, 187f
  etiology and diagnosis, 187
  patient teaching, 188
  symptoms and signs, 186–187
Impacted common bile duct, 328f
Impacted third molars, 283
Impaled object, in skin, 624
Impetigo
  description, 217, 217f
  etiology and diagnosis, 218
  patient screening, 218
  patient teaching, 218
  prevention, 218
  symptoms and signs, 217
  treatment and prognosis, 218
Implantable cardioverter-defibrillators, 413b
Implants
  dental, 284f
  radioactive, in vagina, 514
Impotence/erectile dysfunction, 488–489
Inactivated poliovirus, 73f
Incision, 626, 626f
Incisors, 282f

Incompetent valve, 408f
Incontinence
    stress, 470–472
    urinary, 471b
Incretin
    hormones, 156
Incretin hormones, 156
Incretin mimetics, 156
Incus, 185, 185f, 192f
Infantile atopic dermatitis, 210f
Infantile colic, 86–87
Infant respiratory distress syndrome (IRDS),
    39–40
Infants, premature, 38f, 39f
Infarction
    lung, 357f
    myocardial, 390–392
Infarcts
    myocardial
        thrombus over, 420f
    systemic
        emboli and, 421f
        endocarditis and, 405f
Infection
    bacterial
        of CNS, 568f
        Lyme disease, 254–255
        in pneumonia, 358–359
        reservoir, 5t
    bone, osteomyelitis, 256–257
    causing endocarditis, 404f
    cellulitis, 219–220
    control, and universal precautions,
        108b
    EBV, 374
    fungal
        CMC, 113–114
        dermatophytosis (tinea), 220–222
        histoplasmosis, 362
        pityriasis, 233
        reservoir, 5t
        thrush, 292
    hospital-acquired (nosocomial), 24
    keratitis as, 170–171
    latent TB infection (LTBI), 373b
    prevention of spread of, 3–6
    produced by pathogens, 5t
    standard precautions for body fluids, 480
    ulcerative blepharitis due to, 171
    upper respiratory, 344–346
    in urinary tract, 462f, 467
    viral
        hepatitis, 323
        herpes simplex (cold sores), 291–292
        in pneumonia, 358–359
        reservoir, 5t
Infectious cystitis, 466–467
Infectious diseases of childhood
    chickenpox, 72–74, 74f
    common cold, 80
    diphtheria, 75
    German measles (rubella), 78–79, 79f
    influenza, 80
    measles (rubeola), 77–78, 77f
    mumps, 75–76, 76f
    pertussis, 76–77
    tetanus, 79–80
Infectious hepatitis, 323

Infectious mononucleosis, 373, 374f
    diagnosis and treatment, 374
    etiology, 374
    patient screening, 374
    patient teaching, 374
    prevention, 374
    prognosis, 374
    symptoms and signs, 373–374
Infectious neurologic disorders
    brain abscess, 568–569
    encephalitis, 567
    Guillain-Barré syndrome, 567–568
    meningitis, 566–567
    poliomyelitis and post-polio syndrome,
        569–570
Infectious urethritis, 466–467
Infective otitis externa, 188f
    etiology and diagnosis, 188
    patient teaching, 189
    prevention, 188
Inferior parathyroid glands, 150f
Inferior vena cava, 383f
Infertility, 489–490
    Klinefelter syndrome, 70
Infestations, helminthic, 87f
Inflammation
    of appendix, 305f
    of brain tissue, in encephalitis, 567
    of bronchioles, 86
    course of, 4f
    of epiglottis, 82–83
    of larynx, 82f
    and repair, 3
    of skin (dermatitis), 205
Inflammatory diseases
    gingivitis, 285–286
    RA, 123–125
Influenza, 362–363, 363f
    in childhood, 80
    diagnosis and treatment, 363
    etiology, 363
    patient screening, 364
    patient teaching, 361
    prevention, 364
    prognosis, 364
    schedule for immunization, 73f
    symptoms and signs, 363
Influenza A (H1N1), 364b
Ingrown toenail, 238
Inguinal canal, 307
Inguinal hernia, 308f
Inhalants, abuse of, 593–595t
Inheritance, for genetic diseases, 7
Injectable fillers, 234b
Injury
    avulsion, 622–623
    brachial plexus, 650–651
    closed head, 544, 547f
    crushing, 623–624
    head, 546f
    to ligaments, 245
    lightning, 636–637
    penetrating, 625b
    rehabilitation after, 640b
    spinal cord, 548–549
Inner ear, 185f
    labyrinthitis, 194–195, 194f
    Meniere disease, 193

Insect bites
    diagnosis and treatment, 641
    insects capable of inflicting bites, 644f
    mosquito, malaria, 642–643
    symptoms and signs, 640
    tick
        Lyme disease, 254–255
        Rocky Mountain spotted fever,
            641–642
Insomnia, 612–613
Insulin, 138t
Insulin-dependent diabetes mellitus (IDDM),
    154
Insulin pump therapy, 155b
Insulin reaction, 155t
Integumentary system
    abnormal pigmentation of skin,
        231–234
    alopecia, 234–236
    benign and premalignant tumors,
        225–227
    carcinomas of skin, 227–231
    corns and calluses, 236
    folliculitis, 237–238
    nail deformation or discoloration, 238
    orderly functioning of, 205–240
    paronychia, 238–239
    verrucae (warts), 236–237
Intellect personality, 534–535f
Intellectual testing, 577
Interlobar artery, 450f
Intermittent peritoneal dialysis, 456
Internal hemorrhoid, 321f
Interneuron, 535f
Intervertebral disk disorders
    degenerative disk disease, 549–552
    herniated and bulging disk, 552–554
    sciatic nerve injury, 554–555
Intervertebral joints, 246f
Intestinal obstruction, 312–313, 313f
Intimate partner violence
    diagnosis and treatment, 658
    prevention and patient teaching, 659
    symptoms and signs, 657
Intracranial hemorrhage, 544t
Intrauterine devices (IUDs), 490
Intrinsic smooth muscles of eye, 164t, 165
Intussusception, 312, 313f
Involuntary movement of eye, 167–168
Iodized salt, in simple goiter, 144–145
Iridotomy, 179
Iris, 163–164, 165t
Iron-deficiency anemia, 429, 431t
Irritable bowel syndrome, 319–320
Irritation, contact dermatitis
    developed via, 208, 209f
Ischemia, 3, 385, 587
    cardiac, 306b
    renal, 459, 460f
Ischium, 246f
Itching. See Pruritus
Itch mite, 223, 223f
ITP (idiopathic thrombocytopenic purpura),
    118

J

Jaws, temporomandibular joint
    disorder, 289

Joints
    affected by RA, 123f
    function of, 245
    gout, 257–259
    in JVA, 125
    Lyme disease, 254–255
    osteoarthritis, 252–254
    temporomandibular, 289
    types of, 245, 246f
Juvenile onset diabetes, 154
Juvenile rheumatoid arthritis (JVA)
    etiology and diagnosis, 126
    patient teaching, 126
    symptoms and signs, 125–126
    treatment, 126
Juxtaglomerular apparatus, 451t

K
K2 (incense), 593–595t
Kainophobia, 605t
Kakorrhaphiophobia, 605t
Karyotype, 6f
    in Down syndrome, 47f
Keloids, 206t, 226, 226f
Keratitis
    patient teaching, 170–171
    symptoms and signs, 170
    treatment, 170
Keratoacanthoma, 225, 226f
Keratoconjunctivitis sicca, 174
Keratosis
    actinic, 227, 227f
    seborrheic, 225, 225f
Ketamine hydrochloride, 593–595t
Ketone bodies, 154
Kidney disease
    polycystic, 468–469
    Wilms tumor, 64–65, 64f, 473f
Kidneys
    anatomy of, 450f
    functions of, 450–451
    metabolic function of, 343
    transplantation, 456
Kidney stones, 465–466
Killer T cells (cytotoxic T cells), 102
Klinefelter syndrome, 70–71, 71f
Knee joint, ligaments and tendons of, 247f
Koplik spots, on buccal mucosa, 77, 77f
Kyphosis
    associated with Scheuermann disease, 250f
    description, 250
    diagnosis, 250
    etiology, 250
    patient screening, 250
    patient teaching, 251
    prevention, 251
    prognosis, 251
    symptoms and signs, 250
    treatment, 250–251

L
Labial cancer, 511–512
Labia majora, 479f
Labia minora, 479f
Laboratory and diagnostic tests
    arterial blood gases, 679
    blood analysis, 17, 664–665
    blood chemistries, 666–670

Laboratory and diagnostic
    tests (Continued)
    blood screening tests, 672–673
    cardiac enzymes/cardiac isoenzymes, 673–674
    cardiology tests, 18, 674–676
    clotting and coagulation studies, 670–671
    endoscopy tests, 18, 678–679
    glucose monitoring, 671–672
    imaging studies, 18, 676–677
    miscellaneous tests, 18–19, 680–681
    pulmonary function studies, 18, 679–680
    renal, 453t
    screening, 19, 682–684
    sputum analysis, 18
    stool analysis, 18, 677–678
    toxicology studies and drug screens, 672
    urine studies, 17–18, 674
Labor, premature, 519–520
Labyrinth, 186
    Meniere disease, 193
Labyrinthitis, 194–195, 194f
Lacerations
    avulsed, 625–626
    symptoms and signs, 625
    treatment and prognosis, 626
Lacrimal glands, 165t
Lactic acidosis, 156
Lactiferous duct, 480f
Lalophobia, 605t
Laparoscopic cholecystectomy, 328
Laparoscopy, 490
    in endometriosis, 502, 502f
Large intestine, 281f
    site of helminthic infestation, 87f
Laryngeal cancer, 353–354
Laryngitis
    diagnosis and treatment, 349
    etiology, 349
    patient screening, 349
    patient teaching, 350
    prevention, 350
    prognosis, 349
    symptoms and signs, 349
Laryngomalacia, 40b
Laryngopharynx, 344f
Larynx, 150f, 344f
    acute inflammation of, 82f
    cancer of, 353–354
    tumors of, 352–353
Latent TB infection (LTBI), 373b
Lateral patellar ligament, 247f
Lateral sulcus, 534–535f
Latex condoms, and STDs, 480
Latissimus dorsi muscle, 244f
Lead poisoning, 93–95
Learning differences. See Learning
    disorders
Learning disabilities. See Learning
    disorders
Learning disorders
    diagnosis, 578
    symptoms and signs, 578
    treatment, 578
Left bundle branch, 410f
Left occiput anterior presentation, 523f

Left-sided congestive heart failure, 399f
Leg, 534–535f
Legionellosis
    diagnosis and treatment, 361
    etiology, 361
    patient screening, 361
    patient teaching, 361
    prevention, 361
    prognosis, 361
    symptoms and signs, 360
Legionnaires disease, 360–361
Legs
    restless legs syndrome, 562
    varicose veins, 424–425, 424f
Leiomyomas, 504
    uterine, 504, 504f
Lens, 165f
    in presbyopia, 167
    shape of, 164
Lesions
    distribution in MS, 130f
    of oral cancer, 294–295
    skin, 206–207f, 206t
    skip lesions, in Crohn disease, 309
Leukemias, 432–437
    acute lymphocytic, 433
    acute myelogenous, 434–435
    in childhood, 91–92
    chronic lymphocytic, 433–434
    chronic myelogenous, 435–437
Leukocyte (white blood cell count), 665
Leukoplakia, oral, 293–294, 293f
Levitra. See Vardenafil
Lice (pediculosis), 223–225
Lichenification, 206t
Lifestyle
    and prediabetes, 157
    as predisposing factor for disease, 2–3
Ligaments, 245
    carpal, 649f
    of knee joint, 247f
Ligamentum arteriosum, 382f
Lightning injuries
    description, 636
    diagnosis and treatment, 637
    patient teaching, 637
    symptoms and signs, 636
Light rays
    in refractive errors, 166–167
    and sight, 164–165
Linear skull fracture, 547f
Lip, cleft, 60f, 62–63
Lithotripsy, extracorporeal shock wave, 328, 466
Liver, 281f
    rate at which alcohol is metabolized in, 591b
    site of helminthic infestation, 87f
Liver disease, 322–332
    cancer, 326–327
    cirrhosis, 322–323, 325f
    hepatitis A, 323–324
    hepatitis B, 324–325
    hepatitis C, 325–326
    viral hepatitis, 323
Long bones, 245
Loop of Henle, 451f

Lordosis
    description, 248
    diagnosis, 249
    etiology, 249
    patient screening, 249
    patient teaching, 249–250
    prevention, 249
    prognosis, 249
    symptoms and signs, 248–249
    treatment, 249
Lou Gehrig disease, 561–562
Lower esophageal sphincter (LES), 295f, 306
Lower respiratory tract, 344f
Lumbar nerves, 534–535f
Lumbar plexus (L1-L4), 538–539f
Lumbar puncture, 19
Lumbar vertebrae, 249f
Lung cancer
    description, 376
    diagnosis, 377–378
    etiology, 376–377
    patient screening, 376
    prevention, 378
    prognosis, 378
    symptoms and signs, 376
    treatment, 378
Lungs
    atelectasis, 356f
    effects of smoking, 367f
    metabolic function of, 343
    site of helminthic infestation, 87f
    thrombus lodged in, 421f
Lupus anticoagulant, 444b
Luteinizing hormone (LH), 138t, 139f
Luteinizing hormone-releasing hormone
    (LHRH) antagonists, 12
Lyme disease
    description, 254
    diagnosis, 254–255
    etiology, 254
    patient screening, 254
    patient teaching, 255
    prevention, 255
    prognosis, 255
    symptoms and signs, 254
    treatment, 255
Lymphangitis, 439
Lymphatic diseases, 436–442
    Hodgkin lymphoma, 439–441
    lymphangitis, 439
    lymphedema, 436–438
    lymphoma, 439
    non-Hodgkin lymphoma, 441–442
Lymphedema, 436–438
Lymph nodes
    in melanoma staging system, 11t
    sites for Hodgkin disease, 440f
    structure of, 437f
Lymphoblasts, 428f
Lymphocytes, bone marrow formation of,
    103f
Lymphoma, 439
Lysergic acid diethylamide (LSD), 593–595t

M
Macrophages, 102
Macula, 163f, 164, 165t
Macula lutea, 179

Macular degeneration, 180f
    etiology and diagnosis, 179
    patient teaching, 180
    symptoms and signs, 179
    treatment, 179–180
Macules, 206–207f, 206t
Magnetic therapy, 27
Major depressive disorder
    diagnosis and treatment, 599–603
    symptoms and signs, 599
Major depressive disorder, single episode,
    unspecified, 599t
Malabsorption syndrome
    etiology, 334
    patient teaching, 335
    treatment and prognosis, 334
Malaria, 642–643
Male hypogonadism, Klinefelter syndrome,
    70
Male pattern baldness, 235f
Male reproduction system, 478f
    infertility, 489–490
Male reproductive diseases
    benign prostatic hyperplasia, 494–495
    commonly affecting prostate gland, 491
    epididymitis, 491–492
    genital herpes, 483f
    orchitis, 492
    prostate cancer, 495–497
    prostatitis, 494
    testicular cancer, 497–498
    torsion of testicle, 492–493
    varicocele, 493
Malformation, Chiari, 563b
Malignant hypertension, 395–396
Malignant melanoma
    description, 229
    etiology and diagnosis, 230
    patient screening, 230
    patient teaching, 230–231
    prevention, 230
    symptoms and signs, 229–230
    treatment and prognosis, 230
Malignant tumors
    compared with benign tumors, 8t
    laryngeal, 352
    oral, 287–288
Malingering, 611b
Malleus, 185, 185f, 192f
Malnutrition, 15
    etiology and diagnosis, 332–333
    patient teaching, 333–334
    symptoms and signs, 332
    treatment and prognosis, 333
Malocclusion, 288, 288f
Mamillary body, 538–539f
Mammogram, 19, 526f
Mandible, 246f, 289
Marfan syndrome
    description, 260
    diagnosis, 261
    etiology, 260–261
    patient screening, 260
    patient teaching, 261
    prevention, 261
    prognosis, 261
    symptoms and signs, 260
    treatment, 261

Massage, 25
Masseter muscle, 244f
Mastitis, 527
Mastoid air cells, 196f
Mastoidectomy, simple, 197
Mastoiditis
    etiology and diagnosis, 197
    patient teaching, 198
Maxillary sinus, 346f
Measles (rubeola), 77–78, 77f
Measles, German (rubella), 78–79, 79f
Measles, mumps, rubella (MMR)
    schedule for immunization, 73f
Mechanisms of disease
    aging, 15–16
    cancer, 7–14
    cultural diversity, 20
    diagnosis of disease, 16
    gene therapy, 20
    genetic counseling, 7
    genetic diseases, 6–7
    immune disorders, 14–15
    infection, 3–6
    inflammation and repair, 3
    malnutrition, 15
    mental disorders, 16
    nontraditional medicine, 25–27
    pain, 21–23
    physical trauma and chemical agents, 15
    predisposing factors, 2–3
    preventive health care, 24–25
    psychological factors, 16
    stem cell research, 20–21
Medial patellar ligament, 247f
Median nerve, 649f
Medical alert bracelet, 143, 143f
Medical assistants, delegation of tasks
    to, 27
Medicine
    complementary and alternative, 23
    holistic, 19
    nontraditional, 25–27
Medulla, 534–535f
Medulla oblongata, 534–535f, 538–539f
Megacolon, congenital aganglionic, 66–67,
    67f
Meibomian glands, occlusion of, 169
Melanocyte-stimulating hormone, 138t
Melanoma
    malignant, 229–231
    ocular, 184
    staging system, 11t
Melasma (chloasma), 232, 232f
Melatonin, 138t
Melena, 296
Memory, 534–535f
Memory T cells, 103
Meniere disease, 193
Meningitis, 566–567
Meningocele, 49–51, 50f
Meningococcal (MCV4), 73f
Meniscectomy, 277
Menopause, 506–507
Menorrhagia, 498
Menstruation, 479
    amenorrhea, 499
    dysmenorrhea, 499–500
    PMS, 498–499

Mental disorders, 16
 anxiety disorders, 603–606
 attention-deficit/hyperactivity disorder
  (ADHD), 581–582
 communication disorders, 579
 dementia, 584–589
 gender dysphonia, 611–612
 learning disorders, 578
 mental retardation, 577–578
 mood disorders, 598–603
 oppositional defiant disorder (ODD),
  582–583
 pediatric autoimmune neuropsychiatric
  disorders associated with streptococcal
  infections, 606–608
 personality disorders, 615–617
 pervasive development disorders,
  579–581
 schizophrenia, 592–597
 sleep disorders, 612–615
 somatoform disorders, 608–611
 therapeutic approaches to, 575
 tic disorders, 583–584
Mental illness, 575–617
Mental retardation
 description, 577
 diagnosis, 577
 etiology, 577
 patient screening, 577
 patient teaching, 578
 prevention, 578
 prognosis, 578
 symptoms and signs, 577
 treatment, 577–578
Mental wellness, 575–617
Mesothelioma, 376f
Metabolic disorders
 cystic fibrosis, 67–69, 68f
 phenylketonuria, 69
Metabolic syndrome, 158b
Metacarpals, 246f
Metastasis, 7–9
 hematogenous, in lungs, 377f
 in melanoma staging system, 11t
Metatarsals, 246f
Metatarsophalangeal (MTP) joint, 265
Metformin, 156
Metformin hydrochloride, 156
Methamphetamines, 593–595t
Methicillin-resistant Staphylococcus aureus
  (MRSA), 4–6
Methylphenidate, 593–595t
Metrorrhagia, 498
Microcephaly, in fetal alcohol syndrome, 96f
Middle cardiac vein, 383f
Middle ear, 185f
 cholesteatoma, 196–197, 196f
Migraine, 556–557
Mineralocorticoids, 138t
Miscarriage, 517–518
Miscellaneous tests
 biopsy, 681
 bone marrow studies, 680
 culture and sensitivity studies, 680
 electroencephalography, 681
 electromyography, 681
 gastric analysis, 681
 human chorionic gonadotropin, 681

Miscellaneous tests (Continued)
 immune and immunoglobulin studies,
  680–681
 lumbar puncture, 681
Mites, itch mites (scabies), 223–225
Mitral commissurotomy, 408
Mitral valve, 407f
 insufficiency, 409
 prolapse, 409–410
 stenosis, 408
Mittelschmerz, 501b
Mock disaster drills, 629b
Molars, 282f
 missing, 282f
 third, impacted, 283
Molds, health hazards of, 359b
Moles (nevi), 232–233, 233f
Monitoring techniques, for diabetes
  mellitus, 157
Monoclonal antibodies, 12
Mononucleosis, infectious, 373–374
Monophobia, 605t
Mood disorders, 598–603
 bipolar disorder, 598–599
 major depressive disorder, 599–603
 postpartum depression, 603b
 seasonal affective disorder, 603b
Morning sickness, 516
Mosquito bite, malaria, 642–643
Motion sickness, 359
Motor cortex, 534–535f
Motor tics, 583
Mourning, experiences during, 602t
Mouth, 281f
 Koplik spots on buccal mucosa, 77t
 trench mouth (necrotizing periodontal
  disease), 292–293
 tumors, 287–288
 ulcers, 290–291, 290f
Movements
 of diaphragm and chest cavity in
  respiration, 345f
 fetal, 520b
 involuntary, of eye, 167–168
MRSA (methicillin-resistant Staphylococcus
  aureus), 4–6
MS (multiple sclerosis), 128–130
Mucous plug, 85f
Mucus, in asthma, 85f
Multifocal arrhythmia, 411–412t
Multiple pregnancies, 524b
Multiple sclerosis (MS)
 etiology and diagnosis, 129
 patient teaching, 130
 symptoms and signs, 129
 treatment, 129–130
Mumps (epidemic parotitis), 75–76, 76f
Munchausen syndrome. See Factitious disorder
Muscle
 of eye, 164t
 insertion and origin of, 245f
 types, 244, 245f
Muscle fiber, 244
Muscle relaxants, 586
Muscle tumors
 description, 262
 diagnosis, 263
 etiology, 263

Muscle tumors (Continued)
 patient screening, 263
 patient teaching, 263
 prevention, 263
 prognosis, 263
 symptoms and signs, 263
 treatment, 263
Muscle weakness, in polymyositis, 128
Muscular dystrophy (MD), 48–49, 48f
Musculoskeletal disorders. See also Traumatic
  and sports injuries
 bursitis, 255–256
 cleft lip and palate, 60f, 62–63
 clubfoot, 60–62, 60f
 developmental dysplasia of hip, 62
 fibromyalgia, 247–248
 gout, 257–259
 hallux rigidus, 266–267
 hallux valgus, 265–266
 hammer toe, 267–268
 Lyme disease, 254–255
 Marfan syndrome, 260–261
 osteoarthritis, 252–254
 osteomalacia and rickets, 265
 osteomyelitis, 256–257
 osteoporosis, 263–264
 Paget disease, 259–260
 spinal, 248–252
 tumors, 261–263
Musculoskeletal system
 bone composition, 244
 bursae, 247
 cartilage, 247
 collagen, 247
 fascia, 245–247
 joints, 244, 246f
 ligaments, 245
 muscle types, 244, 245f
 normal muscular system, 244f
 normal skeletal system, 246f
 tendons, 245
Musculoskeletal tumors
 bone tumors, 261–262
 description, 261
 muscle tumors, 262–263
Mushrooms, abuse of, 593–595t
Music therapy, 27
Mutation, 6, 634b
Mutism, 609
Myasthenia gravis
 etiology and diagnosis, 131
 symptoms and signs, 130–131
 treatment and prognosis, 131
Myelin degeneration, in MS, 129f
Myelin sheath, 534–535f
Myeloblasts, 428f
Myelomeningocele, 50f, 51
Myocardial infarction, 390–392
Myocarditis, 403
Myocardium, 385f
Myopia, 166, 167f
Myringotomy, 190–191, 191f
Myxedema
 etiology and diagnosis, 148
 facies, 147f
 patient screening, 148
 symptoms and signs, 147–148
 treatment and prognosis, 148

N

Nails
  deformed or discolored, 238
  paronychia, 238–239
Naltrexone, 590–591
Narcissistic disorder, 616
Narcolepsy, 613–614
Narcotic analgesics, 586
Nasal cavity, 344f
Nasal polyps, 351f
  diagnosis and treatment, 351
  etiology, 350
  patient screening, 350
  patient teaching, 351
  prevention, 351
  prognosis, 351
  symptoms and signs, 350
Nasopharyngeal carcinoma
  diagnosis and treatment, 348–349
  etiology, 348
  patient screening, 348
  patient teaching, 349
  prevention, 349
  prognosis, 349
  symptoms and signs, 348
Nasopharynx, 344f
National Burn Repository, 633
Natural killer (NK) cells, 12, 102
Nausea, in morning sickness, 516
Nearsightedness, 166
Neck, hyperflexion of, 550f
Necrotizing enterocolitis (NEC), 42–43
Necrotizing periodontal disease, 292–293,
  293f
Necrotizing vasculitis, systemic, 132
Needlesticks, contaminated, 624b
Neglect
  child, 652–654
  elder, 655–656
Neonatal intensive care unit (NICU), 38f
Neoplasms
  classification by tissue of origin, 8–9t
  of eye, 184
  of kidney, Wilms tumor, 64–65,
    64f, 473f
  oral, 287–288
  pancreatic, 331
  staging of, 10
  of urinary tract, 473f
Neoplastic lung disease, 377f
Nephron, 450f, 451f
Nephropathy, diabetic, 468
Nephrosis, 458–459
Nephrotic syndrome, 458–459
Nephrotoxins, 458b, 459, 460f
Nervous system
  autonomic (ANS), 538–539f
  central (CNS), 534–535
  chronic alcoholism effects, 589f
  cranial nerves, 536–537b
  neurologic assessment, 536–537b
  orderly function of, 534–536
  peripheral (PNS), 538–539f
Nervous system diseases
  anencephaly, 52–55, 54f
  cerebral palsy, 47–48
  hydrocephalus, 51–52, 52f
  muscular dystrophy, 48–49, 48f

Nervous system diseases (Continued)
  spina bifida
    meningocele, 49–51, 50f
    myelomeningocele, 50f, 51
    spina bifida occulta, 49
Neuralgia
  postherpetic, 217
  trigeminal, 564–565
Neural tube defects, 49
Neuritis/neuropathy, peripheral,
    563–564
Neuroblastoma, in childhood, 97–98
Neurofibrillary tangles, 585f
Neurogenic bladder, 469–470
Neurogenic shock, 416f
Neurohypophysis, 139f
Neuroleptic malignant syndrome, 597b
Neurologic assessment, 536–537b
Neurologic disorders
  functional disorders, 556–563
  head trauma, 544–548
  Infectious disorders, 566–570
  intervertebral disk diso, 549–555
  intracranial tumors, 570–571
  multiple sclerosis, 128–130
  myasthenia gravis, 130–131
  peripheral nerve disorders, 563–566
  spinal cord injury, 548–549
  vascular disorders, 537–544
Neuroma, acoustic, 200f
Neurons, 534–535f
  functional classification of, 535f
Neuroses. See Anxiety disorders
Neurotransmitter, 560
Neutropenia, 430–432
  immune, 118–119
Nevi (moles), 232, 233, 233f
Nicotine, 593–595t
Nipple, 480f
  in breast cancer, 528f
Nodules
  chalazion, 169
  description, 206–207f, 206t
Noise exposure, 199, 199f
Nonalcoholic Fatty Liver Disease (NAFLD),
    327b
Non-Hodgkin lymphoma, 441–442
Non-insulin-dependent diabetes mellitus
    (NIDDM), 154
Nonmelanoma skin cancers, 227–229
Nonpoisonous snakes, bite pattern,
    646f
Non-rapid eye movement (NREM) sleep,
    612
Non-small cell lung cancer (NSCLC),
    376–377
Nonsteroidal antiinflammatory drugs
    (NSAIDs), 125
Nonstriated (smooth) muscle, 244, 245f
Nontraditional medicine, 25–27
Nose
  foreign bodies in, 629–630
  short, in fetal alcohol syndrome, 96f
Nosebleed, 352
NSAIDs (nonsteroidal antiinflammatory
    drugs), 125
Nucleus, 534–535f
Nucleus pulposus, 553f

Nutrient intake and absorption disorders,
    332–339
  anorexia nervosa, 337–338
  bulimia, 338–339
  celiac disease, 335
  food poisoning, 335–337, 336t
  hypervitaminosis, 333b
  malabsorption syndrome, 334–335
  malnutrition, 332–334
  obesity, 334b
Nystagmus
  etiology and diagnosis, 168
  symptoms and signs, 167

O

Oak tree, toxicity of, 647t
Obesity, 334b
  childhood, 89b
Obsessive-compulsive disorder
  etiology and diagnosis, 605
  symptoms and signs, 604–605
Obsessive compulsive personality disorder,
    616–617
Obstruction
  atherosclerotic, 387f
  bladder, 462f, 469–470
  intestinal, 312–313
Obstructive atelectasis, 356f
Occipital lobe, 163f, 534–535f, 586f
Occlusion, 288
  coronary, 389f
  of meibomian glands, 169
Occupational hearing loss, 198–199
Ochlophobia, 605t
Ocular melanoma, 184
Ocular rosacea, 213, 214f
Oculomotor nerve (III), 164t, 536–537b
Older population
  conditions associated with, 16
  elder abuse/neglect, 655–656
  risks for, 15–16
Olfactophobia, 605t
Olfactory nerve (I), 536–537b
Olfactory receptors, 26f
Oligomenorrhea, 498
Ombrophobia, 605t
Oncogenes, 13
Oocyte, sperm penetration of, 32–33f
Open-angle glaucoma, chronic, 178, 178f
Open head injury, 544
Open trauma
  abrasions, 621–622
  avulsion injuries, 622–623
  crushing injuries, 623–624
  lacerations, 625–626
  puncture wounds, 624–625
Ophidiophobia, 605t
Opioids, abuse of, 593–595t
Oppositional defiant disorder
  diagnosis and treatment, 583
  symptoms and signs, 582–583
Optic chiasma, 163f, 538–539f
Optic nerve (II), 163f, 164, 165t, 536–537b
Optic tract, 163f
Oral cavity disorders, 281–295
  dental caries, 283–285
  discolored teeth, 285
  gingivitis, 285–286

Oral cavity disorders *(Continued)*
  herpes simplex (cold sores), 291–292
  impacted third molars, 283
  leukoplakia, 293–294
  malocclusion, 288
  missing teeth, 282–283
  mouth ulcers, 290–291
  necrotizing periodontal disease, 292–293
  oral cancer, 294–295
  oral tumors, 287–288
  periodontitis, 286–287
  thrush, 292
  TMD, 289
  tooth abscesses, 289–290
Oral cholangiogram, 329t
Oral tumors, 287–288
Orchitis, 492
Organic disorders, 575
Oropharynx, 344f
Orthopnea, 400
Ossicles, 196f
Ossification, 245
Osteitis deformans
  description, 259
  diagnosis, 259–260
  etiology, 259
  patient screening, 259
  patient teaching, 260
  prevention, 260
  prognosis, 260
  symptoms and signs, 259
  treatment, 260
Osteoarthritis
  description, 252
  diagnosis, 253
  etiology, 252–253
  patient screening, 252
  patient teaching, 254
  prevention, 254
  prognosis, 253
  symptoms and signs, 252
  treatment, 253
Osteogenesis, 245
Osteomalacia
  description, 265
  diagnosis, 265
  etiology, 265
  patient screening, 265
  patient teaching, 265
  prevention, 265
  prognosis, 265
  symptoms and signs, 265
  treatment, 265
Osteomyelitis
  description, 256
  diagnosis, 257
  etiology, 257
  patient screening, 257
  patient teaching, 257
  prevention, 257
  prognosis, 257
  symptoms and signs, 256–257
  treatment, 257
Osteopathy, 25
Osteophytes, 253f
Osteoporosis
  collapse of vertebrae due to, 250
  description, 263

Osteoporosis *(Continued)*
  diagnosis, 264
  etiology, 264
  patient screening, 264
  patient teaching, 264
  prevention, 264
  prognosis, 264
  in RA, 124f
  symptoms and signs, 264
  treatment, 264
Osteosarcoma, 262
Otitis externa, infective, 188–189, 188f
Otitis media, 346f
  acute, 189, 190f, 197
  chronic, 190, 190f, 197
  description, 189
  etiology and diagnosis, 190
  patient teaching, 191
  serous, 189, 190
  suppurative, 189, 190–191,
    190f, 195
  symptoms and signs, 189
  treatment, 190–191
Otosclerosis, 192, 192f
Otoscopy, 190
Ototoxicity, 187b
Oval window, 185f, 192f
Ovarian cancer, 512–513
Ovarian cysts, 500–501
Ovarian fimbriae, 479f
Ovaries, 136f, 479f
  mittelschmerz, 501b
  secretions and function of, 138t
Overactive bladder, 471–472b
Overuse syndrome, 646–651
Oxalates, 466b
Oxycodone, 593–595t
Oxytocin, 138t, 139f

P
Pacemakers, 413b
Paget disease
  of breast, 530–531
  description, 259
  diagnosis, 259–260
  etiology, 259
  patient screening, 259
  patient teaching, 260
  prevention, 260
  prognosis, 260
  symptoms and signs, 259
  treatment, 260
Pain
  abdominal, in peritonitis, 320
  in angina pectoris, 389f
  of bone tumors, 261
  classification of, 23
  describing, 21
  fear of, 605t
  headache, 556
  migraine, 556–557
  of mittelschmerz, 501b
  from myocardial infarction, 391f
  physiology of, 21–23
  psychological, 21, 575
  rating scales and instruments, 22f
  referred, 23f
  relief of, 23

Pain *(Continued)*
  sciatic nerve, 553f
  TENS for, 551–552
Pain disorder, 609–610
Palate, cleft, 60f, 62–63
Palliative treatment, of pancreatic cancer, 332
Pancreas, 281f, 322–332
  acute and chronic pancreatitis, 330–331
  cancer, 331–332
  endocrine dysfunction of, 154–159
  location and structure of, 330f
  secretions and function of, 138t
Pancreatic acinar cells, 330f
Pancreatic cancer, 331f
Pancreatic islets, 136f
Panencephalitis, subacute sclerosing, 78b
Panhypopituitarism, 141
Panic disorder, 604
Panic disorder [episodic paroxysmal anxiety]
    without agoraphobia, 604t
Papanicolaou (Pap) smear, 19
Papilla of hair, 205f
Papules, 206–207f, 206t
Paradoxical breathing, 372
Paralysis
  due to CVA, 540–541f
  types of, 548f
Paranoid personality disorder, 616
Paranoid schizophrenia, 596t
Paraplegia, 534–535f, 548–549, 548t
Parasomnias, 613
Parasympathetic division, 538–539f
Parasympathetic nerves, 535
Parathyroid gland diseases, 149–152
  hyperparathyroidism, 149–151
  hypoparathyroidism, 151–152
Parathyroid glands, 136f
  secretions and function of, 138t
Parathyroid hormone (PTH), 138t
  overproduction in hyperparathyroidism,
    149
  reduced production in
    hypoparathyroidism, 151
Parentage DNA testing, 659b
Paresis, 549
Parietal lobe, 534–535f, 586f
Parietal pleura, 343, 356f, 369f
Parkinson disease, 558–560, 560f
Paronychia, 238–239
Parotitis, epidemic (mumps), 75–76, 76f
Partial-thickness burn, 631f
Passive immunity, 103–105
Patella, 246f, 247f
Patellar ligament, 247f
Patent ductus arteriosus (PDA), 56, 57f
Pathogenesis, definition of, 2
Pathogens, causing infection, 3, 5t
Pathology, 2
Pathophobia, 605t
Patient teaching
  goals of, 28
  pre- and postoperative care, 29
  principles of, 27–28
  reasons for, 28
  role of medical assistants, 27b
  special considerations, 29
  specifics of, 28–29
Pectoralis major muscle, 244f

Pediatric autoimmune neuropsychiatric disorders associated with streptococcal infections (PANDAS), 606–608
Pediculosis
  description, 223
  etiology and diagnosis, 224
  patient screening, 224
  patient teaching, 224
  prevention, 225
  symptoms and signs, 224
  treatment and prognosis, 224
Pelvic inflammatory disease (PID), 503–504
Penetrating injuries, 625b
Penis, 478f
  phimosis, 65, 65f
Peptic ulcers, 301–303, 301f
Perfusion, 397
Pericarditis, 402–403
Pericardium, 385f
Periodontal disease, 286
  necrotizing, 292–293
Periodontal tissue, 282f
Periodontitis, 285–287, 286f
Peripheral nerve disorders
  Bell palsy, 565–566
  peripheral neuritis/neuropathy, 563–564
  trigeminal neuralgia, 564–565
Peripheral nervous system (PNS), 538–539f
Peritoneal dialysis, 456, 456–457f
Peritonitis, 306, 320–321, 320f
Peritubular capillaries, 451f, 452f
Permanent teeth, 282f
Pernicious anemia, 303, 429
  blood values, 431t
  etiology and diagnosis, 116–117
  patient teaching, 117
  symptoms and signs, 116
  treatment and prevention, 117
Peroxisome proliferator-activated receptors (PPARs), 156
Personality disorders
  antisocial disorder, 616
  cluster A
    paranoid personality disorder, 616
    schizoid personality disorder, 616
    schizotypal personality disorder, 616
  cluster B
    antisocial personality disorder, 616
    borderline personality disorder, 616
    histrionic disorder, 616
    narcissistic disorder, 616
  cluster C
    avoidant personality disorder, 616
    dependent personality disorder, 616
    obsessive compulsive personality disorder, 616–617
  description, 615–616
  diagnosis and treatment, 617
  patient teaching, 617
Pertussis (whooping cough), 76–77
Pervasive development disorders
  Asperger syndrome, 581
  autism spectrum disorder, 579–581
  childhood disintegrative disorder, 581
  pervasive development disorder not otherwise specified, 581
  Rett syndrome, 581

Pessary, 508
Petechiae, 444
Pet therapy, 575–576
Phacoemulsification, 177
Phagocytosis
  complement cascade and, 103
  by WBCs, 3
Phalanges, 246f
Phantom limb, 270b
  pain, 270b
Pharmacology, defined, 685
Pharmacophobia, 605t
Pharyngitis
  diagnosis and treatment, 348
  etiology, 347–348
  patient screening, 347
  patient teaching, 348
  prevention, 348
  prognosis, 348
  symptoms and signs, 347
Pharynx, 281f, 344f
Phasmophobia, 605t
Phencyclidine (PCP), 593–595t
Phenylketonuria (PKU), 69
Philodendron, toxicity of, 647t
Phimosis, 65, 65f
Phlebitis, 423
Phlebotomy, 398–399
Phobias, 604f, 605t
  objects initiating, 604f
Phobic anxiety disorder, unspecified, 604t
Phobic disorder, 604
Phobophobia, 605t
Phosphorus, 466b
Photocoagulation, 181, 182
Photophobia, 557
Physical activity, guidelines for adults, 24b
Physical and psychological assault trauma
  child abuse/neglect, 652–654
  elder abuse/neglect, 655–656
  intimate partner violence, 657–658
  psychological or verbal abuse, 656–657
  rape/sexual assault, 659–661
  sexual abuse, 658–659
  shaken baby syndrome, 654–655, 655f
  suicide, 661
Physical behavior, in depression, 600t
Physical therapy, 555b
Physical trauma, 15
Physicians, rheumatologist, 124b
Pia mater, 53f, 534–535f
PID (pelvic inflammatory disease), 503–504
Pigmentation of skin, abnormal, 231–234
Pineal gland, 136f
  secretions and function of, 138t
Pinna, 185, 185f
Pioglitazone, 156
Pituitary gland, 136f, 534–535f, 538–539f
  hormones, effect on target tissues, 139f
  secretions and function of, 138t
Pituitary gland diseases, 137–143
  acromegaly, 140–141, 140f
  diabetes insipidus, 142–143
  dwarfism, 141–142
  excess pituitary hormones secretion, 137
  gigantism, 139–140
  hypopituitarism, 141
Pityriasis, 233

Placenta
  abruptio placentae, 521–522
  hydatidiform mole, 525–526
Placenta previa, 522–524
Plague, 652b
Plantar fasciitis, 274–275
Plantar warts, 236
Plants, poisonous, 647t
Plaque, 206–207f, 206t, 386
  acid, in dental caries, 284
  in Alzheimer disease, 585f
  atherosclerotic, 422f
  corns, 225
  in coronary arteries, 386
  in gingivitis, 286
  of psoriasis, 212
  senile, 585f
Plasmodium protozoa, 642
Platelet count, 665
Platelets, 428f
Play therapy, 575, 576b
Pleura, visceral and parietal, 343, 356f
Pleuritis (pleurisy), 369–370, 369f
Plum, toxicity of, 647t
PMS (premenstrual syndrome), 498–499
Pneumococcal immunization, schedule for, 73f
Pneumococcal pneumonia, 359
Pneumoconiosis, 365
  diagnosis and treatment, 369
  etiology, 369
  patient screening, 368
  patient teaching, 369
  prevention, 369
  prognosis, 369
  symptoms and signs, 368
Pneumonia
  appearance of, 358f
  diagnosis and treatment, 359
  etiology, 358–359
  patient screening, 358
  patient teaching, 359
  prevention, 359
  prognosis, 359
  RSV, 361–362
  symptoms and signs, 358
Pneumothorax, 370f
  description, 370
  diagnosis and treatment, 371
  etiology, 370–371
  patient screening, 370
  patient teaching, 371
  prevention, 371
  prognosis, 371
  symptoms and signs, 370
Poinsettia, toxicity of, 647t
Poisoning
  food, 335–337
  ingested or swallowed poisons, 647b
Poison ivy, 647t
Poison oak, 647t
Poisonous plants, 647t
Poisonous snakes, bite pattern, 646f
Poliomyelitis, 569–570
Poliovirus, inactivated, 73f
Polycystic kidney disease, 468–469
Polycythemia, 432
Polydipsia, in diabetes insipidus, 142

Polymorphonuclear neutrophils (PMNs), 102
Polymyositis
etiology and diagnosis, 128
symptoms and signs, 128
treatment and prognosis, 128
Polyphagia, 154
Polyps
nasal, 350–351, 351f
vocal cord, 353
Polysomnography (PSG), 19
Polyuria, in diabetes insipidus, 142
Ponophobia, 605t
Pons, 534–535f, 538–539f
Pontine fever, 360, 361
Popliteal vein, 392, 393f
Postcentral gyrus, 386f
Posterior interventricular sulcus, 383f
Posterior pituitary, 138t
Postherpetic neuralgia, 217
Postoperative care, 29
Postpartum depression, 603b
Post-polio syndrome, 569–570
Poststreptococcal glomerulonephritis, 452f, 454f
Posttraumatic stress disorder (PTSD)
chronic, 606t
description, 606
diagnosis and treatment, 607–608
sources of, 607
symptoms and signs, 606
unspecified, 606t
Pothos, toxicity of, 647t
Pramlintide, 156
Prayer, 22
Precocious puberty, 159–160
in boys, 159–160
in girls, 160
Precose. See Acarbose
Prediabetes, 157b
Predisposing factors
for disease, 2–3
for duodenal ulcer, 302
for gastric cancer, 304
Preeclampsia, 521
Pregnancy
abruptio placentae, 521–522
amniocentesis, 515f
ectopic, 518–519
fetal alcohol syndrome and, 96
fetal movement, 520b
fetal presentations, 523f
hydatidiform mole, 525–526
hyperemesis gravidarum, 516–517
morning sickness, 516
multiple pregnancies, 524b
placenta previa, 522–524
and postpartum depression, 603b
preeclampsia and eclampsia, 521
premature labor, 519–520
spontaneous abortion, 517–518
ultrasonography, 515b
Pregnancy tests, 19
Premalignant tumors, of skin, 225–227
Premature atrial contraction, 411–412t
Premature labor, 519–520
Premature ventricular contraction, 411–412t

Prematurity
bronchopulmonary dysplasia and, 40–41
infant respiratory distress syndrome and, 39–40
necrotizing enterocolitis and, 42–43
preterm birth, 35–39
retinopathy of, 41–42
Premenstrual syndrome (PMS), 498–499
Premolars, 282f
Premotor cortex, 534–535f
Prenatal development, 32–33f, 34t
Prenatal diagnosis, methods of, 34–36, 35f
Preoccupation, in mourning, 602t
Preoperative care, 29
Presbyopia, 166–167
Pressure ulcer (decubitus ulcer), 222
Preterm birth, 35–39
Preventive health care, 24–25
Proctocolectomy, 311
Proctoscopy, 321
Prodrome, 291
Progesterone, 138t
Prolactin (PRL), 138t, 139f
Prolapse, 507
mitral valve, 407f, 409–410
uterine, 507–508
Prophylaxis, 621
Prostate cancer, 12
diagnosis and treatment, 496
prognosis and prevention, 496
symptoms and signs, 495
Prostatectomy, 491
Prostate gland, 478f
BPH, 494–495
prostatitis, 494
reproductive diseases commonly affecting, 491
Prostate-specific antigen (PSA), 19
age-specific reference ranges, 496t
Protein-energy malnutrition, 333f
Proton pump inhibitors (PPI), 317
Protozoal infection
Plasmodium, 642
reservoir, 5t
Protruding upper teeth, 288f
Proximal convoluted tubule, 451f, 452f
Pruritus, 154
of eczema, 211
of urticaria, 211–212
PSA (prostate-specific antigen), 19
age-specific reference ranges, 496t
Pseudomembrane, 317
Pseudomembranous, 317
Pseudomembranous colitis, 317–318, 317f
Pseudomembranous enterocolitis, 317–318
Psilocybin, 593–595t
Psoriasis
description, 212
etiology and diagnosis, 212
prognosis and prevention, 213
symptoms and signs, 212
treatment, 212–213
Psychological abuse, 656–657
Psychological evaluation, 16
Psychological pain, 21, 575
Psychosexual, 487

Psychosis, 575
Psychotic disorders, 575
Ptosis, 172–173
PTSD (posttraumatic stress disorder), 606–608
Puberty, precocious, 159–160
Pubic louse, 223, 224, 224f
Pubis, 246f
Pubis symphysis, 246f
Pulmonary abscesses, 360, 360f
diagnosis and treatment, 360
etiology, 360
patient screening, 360
patient teaching, 360
prevention, 360
prognosis, 360
symptoms and signs, 360
Pulmonary circulation, 343
Pulmonary edema, 400
Pulmonary embolism, 357f
diagnosis, 357
etiology, 357
patient screening, 357
patient teaching, 358
prevention, 358
prognosis, 358
symptoms and signs, 357
treatment, 358
Pulmonary emphysema, 367f
diagnosis and treatment, 368
etiology, 368
patient screening, 368
patient teaching, 368
prevention, 368
prognosis, 368
symptoms and signs, 367
Pulmonary function studies, 18, 679–680
Pulmonary system, undeveloped, in prematurity, 38
Pulmonary trunk, 382f
Pulmonary tuberculosis, 373f
description, 372
diagnosis and treatment, 373
etiology, 372–373
patient screening, 372
patient teaching, 373
prevention, 373
prognosis, 373
symptoms and signs, 372
Pulmonary valve, 407f
Pulmonary veins
anterior view, 382f
posterior view, 383f
Pulp, 282f
Puncture wounds
diagnosis and treatment, 625
symptoms and signs, 624
Pupil, 163f
Purines, 466b
Purkinje fibers, 410f
Purpura, 432
Pustules, 206–207f, 206t
of folliculitis, 237
Pyelonephritis, 460f, 461–463
acute, 454f
Pyloric stenosis, congenital, 65–66, 66f
Pyrophobia, 605t

Q

Quadrigeminy arrhythmia, 411–412t
Quadriplegia, 534–535f, 548–549, 548f

R

RA (rheumatoid arthritis), 123–125
Radial nerve, 649f
Radiation exposure, 634b
Radiation sickness, 634b
Radioimmunoassay (RIA), 137
Radius, 246f
Rai staging system, for CLL, 434
Rape, 659–661
Rapid eye movement (REM) sleep, 612
Rash
    butterfly, of SLE, 120f
    in measles, 77f
    pubic lice, 224f
    Rocky Mountain spotted fever, 642f
    scabies, 223f
Rattlesnake warning sign, 646f
Raynaud disease, 426–427
Receding upper teeth, 288f
Receptor, 535f
Recreational drugs, 592
Rectocele, 509
Rectum, 478f, 479f
Rectus abdominis muscle, 244f
Rectus femoris muscle, 244f, 247f
Rectus femoris tendon, 247f
Red blood cell count, 664
Red blood cells (RBCs), 428f
    agglutination, 442f
    in autoimmune hemolytic anemia, 115
    in pernicious anemia, 116
Reed-Sternberg cell, 440f
Reflex arc, 535f
Reflexes, affected by spinal cord damage,
    551f
Reflexology, 25
Refraction, 164–165
Refractive errors
    astigmatism, 166
    hyperopia, 166, 166f
    myopia, 166, 167f
    presbyopia, 166–167
Refractory sprue, 335
Regional enteritis, 309–310
Regional thyroid cancer, 149
Rehabilitation, after injury, 640b
Reiki, 27
Relaxation therapy, 27
Relief of pain, 23
Renal artery, 450f
Renal calculi, 463f, 465–466
Renal capsule, 450f
Renal cell carcinoma, 472–473
Renal cortex, 450f
Renal disorders, Goodpasture syndrome,
    119–120
Renal failure
    acute, 459
    chronic, 460–461
Renal medulla, 450f
Renal pelvis, 450f
Renal vein, 450f
Repetitive motion trauma, 646–651
Reportable diseases and conditions, 640

Reproductive system
    abnormal functioning of, 479
    breasts, 479
    female, 478–479, 479f
    fertilization cycle, 479
    male, 478f
    menstruation, 479
    normally functioning, 478–480
    sexual dysfunction, 487–490
Reproductive system diseases
    of breast, 526–531
    female, 498–514
    male, 491–498
    STDs, 480–487
Residual schizophrenia, 596t
Resistant bacterial infections, 6
Respective periodontal surgery, 287
Respiration
    external and internal, 343
    mechanism of, 344f
Respiratory disorders in childhood
    acute tonsillitis, 83, 83f
    adenoid hyperplasia, 83–84
    asthma, 84–86, 85f
    bronchiolitis, 86
    croup, 81–82, 82f
    epiglottitis, 82–83, 82f
    SIDS, 80–81
Respiratory distress syndrome, infant, 39–40
Respiratory failure, 343
Respiratory syncytial viruses (RSVs),
    358–359
Respiratory syncytial virus (RSV) pneumonia
    diagnosis and treatment, 361, 362
    etiology, 361
    influenza, 362–364, 363t
    patient screening, 361
    patient teaching, 361
    prevention, 361
    prognosis, 361
    symptoms and signs, 361
Respiratory system
    diaphragm and chest movements, 345f
    mechanism of respiration, 344f
    orderly function of, 343–364
    structural plan of, 344f
Respiratory system disorders
    anosmia, 351
    ARDS, 374–375
    atelectasis, 355–357
    common cold/upper respiratory tract
        infection, 344–346
    COPD
        acute and chronic bronchitis, 365–366
        asthma, 367
        bronchiectasis, 366–367, 366f
        pneumoconiosis, 368–369
        pulmonary emphysema, 367–368
    deviated septum, 350
    epistaxis, 352
    flail chest, 371–372, 372f
    hemoptysis, 354–355
    hemothorax, 371
    infectious mononucleosis, 373–374
    laryngeal cancer, 353–354
    laryngeal tumors, 352–353
    laryngitis, 349–350
    legionellosis, 360–361

Respiratory system disorders (Continued)
    lung cancer, 376–378
    nasal polyps, 350–351
    nasopharyngeal carcinoma, 348–349
    pharyngitis, 347–348
    pleuritis, 369–370, 369f
    pneumonia, 358–362
    pneumothorax, 370–371
    pulmonary abscesses, 360, 360f
    pulmonary embolism, 357–358
    pulmonary tuberculosis, 372–373
    sarcoidosis, 375–376
    sinusitis, 346–347
Response, 535f
Restless legs syndrome, 562
Restrictive cardiomyopathy, 401
Retina, 163f
    in hyperopia, 166f
    in myopia, 167f
    rods and cones in, 164
Retinal detachment, 181f
    description, 181–182
    etiology and diagnosis, 182
    large retinal tear with, 182f
    symptoms and signs, 182
    treatment and prognosis, 182
Retinoblastoma, 184, 184f
Retinopathy
    diabetic, 180–181, 181f
    of prematurity, 41–42
Retrolental fibroplasia, 41, 41f
Rett syndrome, 581
Reye syndrome, 95
Rheumatic fever, 405–408
Rheumatic heart disease, 406–408
Rheumatoid arthritis (RA)
    etiology and diagnosis, 123
    patient screening, 124
    patient teaching, 125
    symptoms and signs, 123–124
    treatment and prognosis, 125
Rh incompatibility, 92, 94f
Rhinitis, acute, 346f
Rhubarb, toxicity of, 647t
Ribs, 246f
    multiple fractures, in flail chest, 372f
Rickets
    description, 265
    diagnosis, 265
    etiology, 265
    patient screening, 265
    patient teaching, 265
    prevention, 265
    prognosis, 265
    symptoms and signs, 265
    treatment, 265
Right bundle branch, 410f
Right-sided congestive heart failure, 399f
Right ventricular failure, 401f
Ringworm (tinea corporis), 220–221,
    221f
Risk factors for disease, 2–3
    breast cancer, 528–529
    laryngeal cancer, 353–354
    melanoma, 230
    STDs, 479
Ritalin. See Methylphenidate
Robinow syndrome, 43–44, 43b, 44f

Rocky Mountain spotted fever, 641–642
  diagnosis and treatment, 643
  symptoms and signs, 642
Rods and cones, 164
Rohypnol. *See* Flunitrazepam
Root of tooth, 282f
Root planing, 286
Rosacea
  description, 213
  diagnosis, 214
  etiology, 214
  patient teaching, 214
  symptoms and signs, 213
  treatment and prevention, 214
Rosiglitazone maleate, 156
Rotator cuff injury, 277–278
Rotavirus, immunization schedule, 73f
Round window, 185f
RSV (respiratory syncytial virus) pneumonia,
  361–362
Rubella (German measles), 78–79, 79f
Rubeola (measles), 77–78, 77f
Rule of nines, 631f
Ruptured disk, 552–553
Ruptured tympanic membrane
  etiology and diagnosis, 195, 195f
  with purulent discharge, 196f
  symptoms and signs, 195
  treatment and prognosis, 196

S
Saccular aneurysm, 423f
Sacral nerves, 534–535f
Sacral plexus (L5-S3), 538–539f
Sacrum, 246f, 249f
Salivary glands, 281f
  in Sjögren syndrome, 122f
Salpingo-oophorectomy, 503
Saphenous vein grafts, 392f
Sarcoidosis
  diagnosis and treatment, 375, 376
  etiology, 375
  patient screening, 375
  patient teaching, 376
  prevention, 376
  prognosis, 376
  symptoms and signs, 375
Sartorius muscle, 244f
Scabies
  description, 223
  etiology and diagnosis, 224
  patient screening, 224
  patient teaching, 224
  prevention, 225
  symptoms and signs, 224
  treatment and prognosis, 224
Scalded child, 654f
Scale
  in cradle cap, 208
  dermatologic, 206–207f
  of dermatophytoses, 221
  of psoriasis, 212
Scaling and root planing (SRP), 287
Scapula, 246f
Scars, hypertrophic, 226, 226f
Scheuermann disease, kyphosis associated
  with, 250f
Schirmer tear test, 123f

Schizoid personality disorder, 616
Schizophrenia
  etiology and diagnosis, 596, 597
  prognosis and prevention, 597
  symptoms and signs, 592–596
  treatment, 597
Schizotypal personality disorder, 616
School absenteeism, recording of causes of, 74b
Sciatic nerve injury, 554–555
SCID (severe combined immunodeficiency),
  111–112
Sclera, 163, 163f, 165t
  rosacea involving, 213–214
Scleritis
  description, 175
  etiology and diagnosis, 176
  patient teaching, 176
  symptoms and signs, 176
Scleroderma
  chronic, progressive disease, 121
  etiology and diagnosis, 122
  symptoms and signs, 121
  treatment and prognosis, 122
Scleroplasty, 176
Sclerotic stage, 259
Scoliosis
  description, 251, 251f
  diagnosis, 251
  etiology, 251
  patient screening, 251
  patient teaching, 252
  prevention, 252
  prognosis, 252
  symptoms and signs, 251
  treatment, 251–252
Screening
  breast cancer, 526t
  drug, 592
  types of, 19
Screening test
  alpha fetoprotein, 683
  breast self-examination, 684
  cancer/tumor markers, 682
  carcinoembryonic antigen, 682–683
  CA 15-3 Test, 682
  CA 19-9 Test, 682
  CA 125 test, 682
  mammography, 683–684
  mantoux test, 682
  papanicolaou smear, 683
  prostate-specific antigen, 682
  testicular self-examination, 684
  tuberculosis screening, 682
Scrotal sac, 478f
  and abdominal hernia, 308f
Sea salt, in simple goiter, 144–145
Seasonal affective disorder (SAD), 603b
Seasonal pattern specifier. *See* Seasonal
  affective disorder
Sebaceous cysts, 226, 226f
Sebaceous glands, 205
Seborrhea, 171
Seborrheic dermatitis
  description, 207
  etiology and diagnosis, 208
  patient teaching, 208
  prevention, 208
  prognosis, 208

Seborrheic dermatitis (*Continued*)
  symptoms and signs, 207
  treatment, 208
Seborrheic keratosis, 225, 225f
Secondary hypopituitarism, 142
Secondary syphilis, 486f
Second-degree heart block, 411–412t
Seizure disorder (epilepsy), 557–558
Seizures, first aid for, 559f
Selective IgA deficiency
  etiology and diagnosis, 110
  patient screening, 110
  patient teaching, 110
  symptoms and signs, 109
  treatment and prognosis, 110
Semicircular canals, 185f, 186, 194f
Sense of smell, loss of, 331
Sensitization, contact dermatitis developed
  via, 209
Sensorineural hearing loss, 186
  patient teaching, 199
  prevention, 198–199
  symptoms and signs, 198
Sensory cortex, 534–535f
Septicemia, 482
Septum, deviated, 350
Serologic testing, 19
Serous otitis media, 189, 190
Serum markers
  CA 125, 513
  in testicular cancer, 497
Service animals, 575–576
Sesamoid bones, 245
Severe combined immunodeficiency (SCID)
  diagnosis and treatment, 111–112
  etiology, 111
  patient screening, 111
  patient teaching, 112
  symptoms and signs, 111
Severed tendon, 272–273
Sex chromosome abnormalities, 70t
Sexual abuse
  diagnosis and treatment, 658
  symptoms and signs, 658
Sexual assault, 659–661
  response teams and evidence maintenance,
    660b
Sexual dysfunction
  contraception/birth control, 490–491
  erectile dysfunction/impotence, 488–489
  male and female infertility, 489–490
Sexually transmitted diseases (STDs)
  chancroid, 487
  chlamydia, 481
  genital herpes, 483–484
  genital warts, 484–486
  gonorrhea, 481–482
  hepatitis B, 324–325
  risk factors for, 479
  syphilis, 486–487
  transmission of, 480–487
  trichomoniasis, 482–483
SGLT2 (sodium-glucose linked transporter 2)
  inhibitors, 156
Shaken baby syndrome
  etiology and diagnosis, 654–655
  prognosis and prevention, 655
  symptoms and signs, 654

Shiatsu, 27
Shingles, 215–217
Shin splints, 273–274
Shock
    cardiogenic, 415–417
    causes of, 416f
    diagnosis and treatment, 414
    spinal, 551f
    symptoms and signs, 414
Shock lung, 374
Short bones, 245
Short bowel syndrome, 318–319
Shoulder, 246f
    bursae, 255f
    major nerves of, 538–539f
Shunting procedures, for hydrocephalus, 54f
Sickle cell anemia, 430, 431t
Side flash lightning strike, 636
SIDS (sudden infant death syndrome),
    80–81
Sigmoid colostomy, 315f
Sigmoid diverticular disease, 314f
Sigmoidoscopy, 319
Sildenafil citrate, precautions, 489
Silicosis, 369
Simian crease, in Down syndrome, 46f
Simple goiter, 144f
    etiology, 144
    symptoms and signs, 144
    treatment, 144–145
Simple mastoidectomy, 197
Sinoatrial node, 410f
Sinus bradycardia, 411–412t
Sinuses, 346f
Sinusitis, 346f
    diagnosis and treatment, 347
    etiology, 347
    patient screening, 346–347
    patient teaching, 347
    prevention, 347
    prognosis, 347
    symptoms and signs, 346
Sinus rhythm, normal, 411–412t
Sinus tachycardia, 411–412t
Sitophobia, 605t
Sjögren disease, 281–282
Sjögren syndrome
    description, 122
    etiology and diagnosis, 123
    patient teaching, 123
    symptoms and signs, 122–123
    treatment and prognosis, 123
Skeletal muscle (striated), 244, 245f
    site of helminthic infestation, 87f
Skeletal system, 246f
    manifestations of Robinow syndrome, 43b
Skin
    abrasion, 621
    avulsion injury, 623f
    electrical, 635–636
    hemorrhages, 322f
    laceration, 626f
    layers of, 205, 205f
    lesions, 206–207f, 206t
    normal anatomy, 205f
    puncture wound, 624f
    site of helminthic infestation, 87f
    tag, 226–227, 227f

Skin cancers
    malignant melanoma, 229–231
    nonmelanoma, 227–229
Skin disorders
    abnormal pigmentation, 231–234
    benign and premalignant tumors,
        225–227
    cellulitis, 219–220
    corns and calluses, 236
    decubitus ulcers, 222–223
    dermatitis, 205–211
    dermatophytoses, 220–222
    furuncles and carbuncles, 218–219
    herpes zoster, 215–217
    impetigo, 217–218
    paronychia, 238–239
    psoriasis, 212–213
    rosacea, 213–214
    scabies and pediculosis, 223–225
    urticaria, 211–212
    warts (verrucae), 236–237
Skin tag, 227, 227f
Skip lesions, 309
Skull, 534–535f
    rebound, in contrecoup injury, 544
Skull fracture
    basilar, 547f, 548b
    depressed, 544, 547–548
SLE (systemic lupus erythematosus),
    120–121
Sleep apnea, 614–615
Sleep arousal disorders. See Parasomnias
Sleep disorders
    insomnia, 612–613
    narcolepsy, 613–614
    parasomnias, 613
    sleep apnea, 614–615
Sleep laboratory, 615f
Slipped disk, 552
Small cell lung cancer (SCLC), 376–377
Small intestine, 281f
    and abdominal hernia, 308f
    ileus, 312–313
    site of helminthic infestation, 87f
Smallpox, 652b
Small vessel vasculitis
    etiology and diagnosis, 131–132
    prevention, 132
    symptoms and signs, 131
Smoking
    Buerger disease resulting from, 426
    effects of, 367f
Smooth muscle (nonstriated), 244,
    245f
Snakebites
    description, 645
    diagnosis and treatment, 645
    symptoms and signs, 645
Sodium-glucose linked transporter 2
    (SGLT2) inhibitors, 156
Sofobuvir, 325
Soleus muscle, 244f
Solvadi. See Sofobuvir
Solvents, nephrotoxic, 458b
Somatic distress, in mourning, 602t
Somatization disorder
    diagnosis and treatment, 608
    symptoms and signs, 608

Somatoform disorders
    conversion disorder, 608–609
    factitious disorder, 610–611
    hypochondriasis, 610
    pain disorder, 609–610
    somatization disorder, 608
Somesthetic association area, 586f
Spastic cerebral palsy, 47
Speech disorder, stuttering, 579
Spermatic cord, varicose veins in, 493f
Sperm, penetration of oocyte, 32–33f
Spider bites, brown recluse, 641f
Spina bifida
    meningocele, 49–51, 50f
    myelomeningocele, 50f, 51
    spina bifida occulta, 49
Spinal accessory nerve (XI), 536–537b
Spinal cord, 534–535f
    compression of, 550f
    pressure on, 553f
Spinal cord injuries, paraplegia and
    quadriplegia, 548–549
Spinal disorders
    kyphosis, 250–251
    lordosis, 248–250
    scoliosis, 251–252
Spinal nerves, 538–539f
Spinal stenosis, 554–555
Spine
    abnormal curvatures of, 248–252
    ankylosing spondylitis in, 127f
    hyperextension of, 550f
    malformations, in Robinow syndrome,
        43b
    normal, 249f
Splint, 289
Splints, for TMD, 289
Spontaneous abortion, 517–518
Spontaneous subconjunctival hemorrhage,
    176b, 176f
Sprains, 270–271
Sputum analysis, 18
Squamous cell carcinoma (SCC)
    description, 227–228
    diagnosis and treatment, 229
    of esophagus, 299–300
    etiology, 228–229
    oral, 294–295
    patient screening, 228
    symptoms and signs, 228
Staghorn calculi, 465f
Staging systems
    for CLL, 434
    for colorectal cancer, 316
    for lymphomas, 439
    for melanoma, 11t
    TNM system, 10
Stapedectomy, 192
Stapes, 185, 185f, 192f
Staphylococcal infection, in TSS, 505–506
Stapled hemorrhoidectomy, 321
Status epilepticus, 557
STDs (sexually transmitted diseases),
    480–487
Stem cell
    hematopoiesis, 244
    lymphoid and myeloid, 428f
    research, 20–21

Stenosis
aortic, 408f
mitral valve, 408
pyloric, congenital, 65–66, 66f
spinal, 554–555
Stent
angiographic images of, 392f
coronary artery, 392f
Stereotactic radiosurgery, 13b
Sternocleidomastoid muscle, 244f
Sternum, 246f
Steroids, abuse of, 593–595t
Stimulants
abuse of, 593–595t
in treating ADHD, 582
Stimulus, 535f
Stomach, 281f
cancer, 304–305
gastritis, 303–304
gastroenteritis, 311–312
herniated portion of, 307f
ulcers, 301–303
Stomach flu, 311
Stool analysis, 18
Stool test, 677–678
Strabismus
etiology and diagnosis, 168
patient teaching, 169
symptoms and signs, 168
Strain, 245, 270–271
Strangulated hernia, 308f
Strawberry hemangioma, 233f
Streptococcal infection, rheumatic fever and, 406f
Stress incontinence, 470–472
Striated (skeletal) muscle, 244, 245f
Stride potential lightning strike, 636
Stroke, 537–543, 540–541f
heat stroke, 637
Stuttering, 579
Stye, 169
Subacromial bursa, 255f
Subacute sclerosing panencephalitis, 78b
Subarachnoid hematoma, 544t
Subconjunctival hemorrhage, spontaneous, 176b, 176f
Subcutaneous layer, 205f
Subdeltoid bursa, 255f
Subdural hematoma, 544–545, 545f, 588f
Submaxillary mumps, 76f
Substance abuse, 592b
Substance-related disorders
alcohol abuse, 589–592
drugs of abuse, 592
Subtypes of ADHD, 581–582
Subtypes of schizophrenia, 596
Sudden infant death syndrome (SIDS)
etiology and diagnosis, 80–81
patient screening, 80
prognosis and prevention, 81
symptoms and signs, 80
treatment, 81
Suicide, 661
depression and, 600–601
Sulcus, 534–535f
Sunburn, 632f, 633b
Sun exposure, excessive, 231b
Suntan, abnormal, 233–234

Superficial burn, 631f
Superior parathyroid glands, 150f
Superior vena cava, 382f, 383f
Suppressor T cells, 103
Suppurative otitis media, 189, 190–191, 190f, 195
Surgery
cataract, 177
for laryngeal cancer, 354
refractive, 167
stereotactic radiosurgery, 13b
treatment of solid cancers, 12
Sutures, cranial, 246f
Sweat ducts, 205f
Sweat glands, 205f
Swimmer's ear, 190
Swine flu, 364b
Symlin. See Pramlintide
Sympathetic division, 538–539f
Synarthrodial (immovable) joints, 245
Syncope, 385
Syndrome, 2
Syndrome X (metabolic syndrome), 158b
Synovial joints, 245
Synovitis, in RA, 124f
Syphilis, 486–487
Systemic lupus erythematosus (SLE)
etiology and diagnosis, 121
patient teaching, 121
symptoms and signs, 120
treatment and prognosis, 121
Systemic necrotizing vasculitis
etiology and diagnosis, 132
patient teaching, 132
symptoms and signs, 132
treatment and prevention, 132
Systemic sclerosis, 121–122
Systole, 384f

T
Tachycardia, 383, 411–412t
Tachypnea, 357
Tadalafil, precautions, 489
Takotsubo cardiomyopathy, 393–394
Tamponade, 383–384
cardiac, 417
Tanning beds, 231b
Tapeworms, 87, 88f
Target groups, for influenza immunization, 364b
Tarsals, 246f
Teeth
abscess, 289–290
dental caries, 284
discolored, 285
impacted third molars, 283
malocclusion, 288
missing, 282–283
structure of, 282f
Temporalis muscle, 244f
Temporal lobe, 534–535f, 586f
Temporomandibular joint disorder (TMD), 282, 289
Temporomandibular joints, 289
Tender points, in diagnosis of fibromyalgia, 248f
Tendinitis, 648, 651

Tendons, 245
of knee joint, 247f
passing through carpal tunnel, 649f
Tennis elbow, 649–650
symptoms and signs, 650
treatment and prognosis, 650
TENS (transcutaneous electrical nerve stimulation), 551–552, 552b
Terminal end fibers, 534–535f
Testes, 136f, 478f
atrophy, 322f
orchitis, 492
secretions and functions of, 138t
undescended, 63–64, 63f
Testicle
cancer of, 497–498
torsion of, 492–493
varicocele, 493
Testosterone, 138t
Tetanus
diagnosis and treatment, 80
etiology, 79–80
patient screening, 79
prognosis and prevention, 80
prophylaxis, 621
symptoms and signs, 79
Tetralogy of Fallot, 57f, 59–60, 59f
Tetraplegia, 548–549
Thalamus, 534–535f
Thanatophobia, 605t
Therapeutic hypothermia, 393b
Therapeutic touch, 26–27
Thermal insults
burns, 630–634
electrical shock, 634–636
frostbite, 639–640
hyperthermia, 637–638
hypothermia, 638–639
lightning injuries, 636–637
Thinking, in depression, 600t
Third-degree heart block, 411–412t
Third molars, impacted, 283
Thoracic nerves, 534–535f
Thoracic outlet syndrome, 650–651
Thoracic vertebrae, 249f
Thoracopagus conjoined twins, 36
3-day measles (rubella), 78–79, 79f
Thromboangiitis obliterans, 425–426
Thrombocyte count, 665
Thrombocytopenic purpura, idiopathic (ITP), 118
Thrombophlebitis, 423–424
Thrombosis, venous, 421f
Thrombus, 390
formation in coronary artery, 386f
sites of formation of, 420f
Thrush, 292
Thymic hypoplasia (DiGeorge anomaly), 112–113
Thymosin, 138t
Thymus, 136f
secretions and functions of, 138t
Thyroid cancer
diagnosis, 149
etiology, 148
patient teaching, 149
symptoms and signs, 148
treatment and prognosis, 149

Thyroid gland, 136f
  hypo- and hyperfunction of, 143t
  secretions and functions of, 138t
Thyroid gland diseases, 143, 144
  cretinism, 147
  Hashimoto thyroiditis, 145
  hyperthyroidism, 145
  hypothyroidism, 146
  myxedema, 147–148, 147f
  simple goiter, 144–145, 144f
  thyroid cancer, 148 149
Thyroid hormone (TH), 138t
Thyroid-stimulating hormone (TSH), 137f,
  139f, 141
Thyrotoxicosis, 145–146
Thyrotropin, 141
Thyrotropin-releasing hormone (TRH), 137f,
  138t, 139f
Thyroxine (T₄), 137f, 138t, 141, 143
TIA (transient ischemic attack), 542–544
Tibia, 246f
Tibial collateral ligament, 247f
Tic disorders, Tourette disorder, 583–584
Tic douloureux, 564–565
Tick-borne disease
  Lyme disease, 254–255
  Rocky Mountain spotted fever,
    641–642
Tinea
  capitis, 220, 221f
  corporis (ringworm), 220–221, 221f
  cruris (jock itch), 221–222
  pedis (athlete's foot), 221
  unguium, 221
Tinel sign, 649f
Tinnitus, 186
T lymphocytes
  formation of, 103t
  types of, 102–103
TMD (temporomandibular joint disorder),
  289
TNM staging system, 10
Tobacco, abuse of, 593–595t
Toenails
  ingrown, 238
  tinea unguium of, 221
Toes
  Buerger disease, 426f
  frostbite, 639f
Tongue, in Down syndrome, 46f
Tonic-clonic seizures, 558
Tonsillitis, acute, 83, 83f
Tonsils, coated, in mononucleosis infection,
  374f
Torn meniscus, 276–277
Torsion of testicle, 492–493
Total body irradiation, responses to, 634f
Tourette disorder, 583–584
Toxicity
  of cancer treatments, 13
  of nephrotoxic agents, 458b
Toxic shock syndrome (TSS), 505–506
Toxins, chemical, 647t
Toxiphobia, 605t
Trachea, 150f, 344f
Tracheomalacia, 40b
Transcutaneous electrical nerve stimulation
  (TENS), 551–552, 552b

Transfusion incompatibility reaction,
  442–443
Transient global amnesia, 562–563
Transient ischemic attack (TIA), 542–544
Transitional cell carcinoma
  in bladder cancer, 474f
  of ureter, 473f
Transplantation
  bone marrow
    for SCID, 111
    terms used in conjunction with, 437b
    for Wiskott-Aldrich syndrome, 114–115
  hematopoietic stem cell (HSCT), 433,
    436, 437b
  kidney, 456
Transplant rejection, 102b
Transposition of great arteries, 57f, 59–60,
  59t
Transurethral resection of bladder tumor, 474
Transverse lie presentation, 523f
Trapezius muscle, 244f
Trauma
  bites, 640–643
  cumulative trauma (repetitive motion,
    overuse syndrome), 646–651
  environmental factors resulting in, 621
  foreign bodies, 626–630
  head, 544–548
  open trauma, 621–626
  physical, 15
  physical and psychological assault trauma,
    651–661
  thermal insults, 630–640
  triage, 621
Traumatic and sports injuries
  adhesive capsulitis, 272
  fractures, 268–270
  ganglion, 275–276
  plantar fasciitis, 274–275
  rotator cuff tears, 277–278
  severed tendon, 272–273
  shin splints, 273–274
  strains and sprains, 270–271
  torn meniscus, 276–277
Traumatic ulcers, of mouth, 290
Traumatophobia, 605t
Traveler's diarrhea, 311
Treatment of disease, 19–20
Trench mouth, 292–293
Triage, 621
Triceps brachii muscle, 244f
Trichomoniasis, 482–483
Tricuspid valve, 407f
  atresia, 57f
Tricyclic antidepressants, 586
Trigeminal nerve (V), 536–537b, 564f
Trigeminal neuralgia, 564–565
Trigeminy arrhythmia, 411–412t
Trigger finger, 650
  etiology and diagnosis, 650
  patient teaching, 650
Triiodothyronine (T₃), 137f, 138t, 143
Triskaidekaphobia, 605t
Trisomy 21, 46, 46f
Trochlear nerve (IV), 164t, 536–537b
Trophoblast, 32–33f
Tropic hormones, 136
True vocal cords (vocal folds), 353f

Trunk, 534–535f
Trus, 308
TSS (toxic shock syndrome), 505–506
Tubercle bacillus, Mycobacterium tuberculosis,
  372
Tuberculosis (TB), 373f
  pulmonary, 372–373
  screening, 19
Tubes, myringotomy, 191f
Tubules, collecting, 451f
Tulip, toxicity of, 647t
Tumors
  benign and malignant, 8t
  bladder, 473–474
  bone, 261–263
  grade of, 11–12
  intracranial, 570–571
  laryngeal, 352 353
  markers for, 10
  muscle, 262–263
  ocular, 184
  oral, 287–288
  pituitary, transsphenoidal removal of, 140f
  skin, benign and premalignant, 225–227
  Wilms, 473f
Tunica externa, 417, 419f
Tunica intima, 417, 419f
Tunica media, 417, 419f
Turner syndrome, 71–72, 71f
Tutoring, 579f
Twins, conjoined, 36b, 36f
Tympanic membrane, 185f, 192f
  normal, 190f
  ruptured, 195–196, 195f, 196f
Tympanoplasty, 196
Type 1 diabetes mellitus, 154
Type 2 diabetes mellitus, 154

U

Ulcer
  corneal, 175–176
  decubitus, 222–223
  dermatologic, 206–207f, 206t
  diabetic, 154f
  gastric, duodenal, and peptic, 301–303
  mouth, 290–291, 290f
Ulcerative colitis, 310–311, 310f
Ulcerative gastric carcinoma, 304f
Ulna, 246f
Ulnar nerve, 649f
Ultrasonography, 492
Ultrasonography, 28-week, 515f
Umbilical hernia, 308f
Undescended testes, 63–64, 63f
Universal precautions, 108b
Upper GI endoscopy, 302f
Upper respiratory tract, 344f
Upper respiratory tract infection
  diagnosis and treatment, 345
  etiology, 345
  patient screening, 344–345
  patient teaching, 346
  prevention, 346
  prognosis, 346
  symptoms and signs, 344
Ureter, 450f
  stones in, 463f
  transitional cell carcinoma of, 463f, 473f

Urethra
  carcinoma of, 473f
  female, 479f
  male, 478f
Urethritis, 481
  infectious, 466–467
Uric acid, overproduction in gout, 257
Urinalysis, 453t
Urinary incontinence, 471b
Urinary system
  catheterization, 470b
  functional relationships of, 450f
  orderly function of, 450–454
Urinary system disorders
  acute glomerulonephritis, 451–454
  acute renal failure, 459
  bladder tumors, 473–474
  chronic glomerulonephritis, 454–456
  chronic kidney disease, 460–461
  diabetic nephropathy, 468
  hydronephrosis, 463–464
  infectious cystitis and urethritis, 466–467
  nephrotic syndrome, 458–459
  neurogenic bladder, 469–470
  polycystic kidney disease, 468–469
  pyelonephritis, 461–463
  renal calculi, 465–466
  renal cell carcinoma, 472–473
  stress incontinence, 470–472
Urinary tract infections, 467t, 467
Urinary tract neoplasms, 473f
Urine
  dilute, in diabetes insipidus, 142
  excretion of, 450
  formation of, 452f
  reflux, 462f
  stress incontinence, 470–472
Urine studies, 17–18, 674
Ursodeoxycholic acid, 328
Urticaria
  description, 211
  etiology and diagnosis, 211
  patient screening, 211
  prevention, 212
  symptoms and signs, 211
  treatment and prognosis, 212
Uterus, 479f
  fibroids in, 504–505
  normal uterine pregnancy, 514f
  prolapse of, 507–508
Uveitis, 183

V
Vaccines, 74b
  for adults, 24–25
  cancer, 12b
  hepatitis B, 323b
  for herpes zoster, 217
  HPV, 485b
  pneumococcal, 359
Vagina, 479f
  cancer of, 510–511
  cystocele, 508f
  rectocele, 509
Vaginitis, 505
Vagus nerve (X), 536–537b

Valvular heart disease
  mitral insufficiency, 409
  mitral stenosis, 408–409
  mitral valve prolapse, 409–410
Vancomycin-resistant enterococcal (VRE), 4–6
Vapors, abuse of, 593–595t
Vardenafil, precautions, 489
Varicella vaccine, 73f
Varicella zoster (chickenpox), 72–74, 74f
Varicella-zoster virus (VZV), 72
Varices, esophageal, 296–298, 322f
Varicocele, 493
Varicose veins
  of legs, 424–425, 424f
  in spermatic cord, 493f
Vascular conditions (circulatory system) (417–42)
  aneurysms, 422–427
  arteriosclerosis, 419
  atherosclerosis, 419
  emboli, 418–419
  phlebitis, 423
  Raynaud disease, 426–427
  thromboangiitis obliterans, 425–426
  thrombophlebitis, 423–424
  varicose veins, 424–425, 424f
Vascular dementia
  description, 586–587
  diagnosis and treatment, 587
  patient teaching, 587–588
  symptoms and signs, 587
Vascular disorders (neurologic)
  cerebral concussion, 545–546
  cerebral contusion, 546–547
  cerebrovascular accident, 537–544, 540, 541f
  depressed skull fracture, 547–548
  epidural and subdural hematomas, 544–545
  transient ischemic attack, 542–544
Vascular stage, 259
Vascular system, 418f
Vasculitis
  small vessel, 131–132
  systemic necrotizing, 132
Vasopressin, 138t
  in diabetes insipidus, 142
Vector, 643
Vegetations
  in endocarditis, 405f
  in rheumatic fever, 406f
  valvular thrombi, 420f
Vegetative signs, in depression, 600t
Veins
  testicular, varicocele, 493
  varicose
    of legs, 424–425, 424f
    in spermatic cord, 493f
Venous embolism, 421f
Venous thrombosis, 421f
Venous valves, 418f
Ventricles
  cardiac
    anterior view, 382f
    posterior view, 383f
Ventricles of brain, 534–535f
Ventricular fibrillation, 411–412t

Ventricular septal defect (VSD), 56, 57f, 58f
Ventricular tachycardia, 411–412t
Venules, 418f
Verbal abuse, 656–657
Verrucae (warts)
  description, 236
  diagnosis and treatment, 237
  etiology, 237
  patient teaching, 237
  prognosis, 237
  symptoms and signs, 236
Vertebrae
  collapse, due to osteoporosis, 250
  compression of, 550f
Vertebral body, 553f
Vertebral column, 246f
Vertebroplasty, 250–251, 269
Vertigo, 186
  benign paroxysmal positional, 193–194
Vesicles, 206–207f, 206t
  of shingles, 215
Vesicoureteral reflux, 462f
Vessel wall
  in Buerger disease, 426f
  structure of, 417, 419f
Vestibulocochlear nerve (VIII), 185f, 194f, 536–537b
Viagra. See Sildenafil citrate
Vincent angina, 292–293
Violence, 651–652
  family, 655b
  intimate partner, 657–658
Viral hepatitis, 323, 323b
Viral infection
  cold sores, 291–292
  hepatitis, 323
  hepatitis A, 323–324
  hepatitis B, 324–325
  in pneumonia, 358–359
  reservoir, 5t
Visceral pleura, 343, 356f, 369f
Vision, functioning organs of, 163–165
Visual area, 534–535f, 586f
Visual association, 534–535f
Visual field, loss of, 163f
Visual pathway, 163f
Vital centers, 534–535f
Vitamin A
  drugs derived from, 212–213
  toxicity, 333b
Vitamin B_{12}, for pernicious anemia, 116–117
Vitamin C, hypervitaminosis and, 333b
Vitamin D
  toxicity, 333b
Vitamin E, hypervitaminosis and, 333b
Vitamin K, toxicity, 333b
Vitamin therapy, for macular degeneration, 180
Vitiligo, 231, 232f
Vitreous body, 163f
Vitreous humor, 164
  in diabetic retinopathy, 181
Vivitrol. See Naltrexone
Vocal cords, polyp, 353f
Vocal tics, 583
Volvulus, 313f

Vomiting
  in bulimia, 338–339
  in childhood, 90
  in morning sickness, 516
VRE (vancomycin-resistant enterococcal),
  4–6
Vulvar cancer, 511–512

W

Warts (verrucae), 236–237
  genital, 485f
Wasting, in ACTH deficiency, 154f
Water hemlock, toxicity of, 647t
Weakness, muscle, in polymyositis, 128
Wenckebach heart block, 411–412t
Wet macular degeneration, 179
Wheal, of urticaria, 211, 211f
White blood cells (WBC), 3, 428f
  elevated count in appendicitis, 306

White blood cells (WBC) count,
  665
  leukocyte, 665
Whooping cough (pertussis), 76–77
Wilms tumor, 64–65, 64f, 473f
Wisdom teeth, impacted, 283, 283f
Wiskott-Aldrich syndrome
  etiology and diagnosis, 114
  patient teaching, 114–115
  symptoms and signs, 114
  treatment and prognosis, 114
Wisteria, toxicity of, 647t
Wong/Baker Faces Rating Scale, 22f
Worm infestation, in childhood,
  87–88, 87f
Wounds, puncture
  diagnosis and treatment, 625
  symptoms and signs, 624
Wrist, 246f

X

Xenophobia, 605t
Xerostomia, 281–282
Xiphoid process, 246f
X-linked agammaglobulinemia
  etiology and diagnosis, 110
  patient screening, 110
  patient teaching, 111
  symptoms and signs, 110
  treatment and prognosis, 110–111
X-linked recessive inheritance, 7

Y

YAG capsulotomy, 177
Yew, toxicity of, 647t

Z

Zonules, 164
Zoophobia, 605t